A SYNOPSIS OF
ANÆSTHESIA

A SYNOPSIS
OF ANÆSTHESIA

BY

J. ALFRED LEE

M.R.C.S., L.R.C.P., M.M.S.A., F.F.A.R.C.S., D.A.

Senior Consultant Anæsthetist to the Southend-on-Sea Hospital, etc.

AND

R. S. ATKINSON

M.A., M.B., B.Chir., F.F.A.R.C.S.

Consultant Anæsthetist, Southend General Hospital and Rochford General Hospital, Essex. Formerly Fellow in Anesthesiology, Hospital of the University of Pennsylvania, Philadelphia, U.S.A.

SIXTH EDITION

BRISTOL: JOHN WRIGHT AND SONS LTD.

1968

Distribution by Sole Agents:
United States of America : The Williams & Wilkins Company, Baltimore
Canada : The Macmillan Company of Canada Ltd., Toronto

By J. Alfred Lee

First Edition, January, 1947
Second Edition, November, 1950
Third Edition, December, 1953
Reprinted with minor amendments, May, 1955
Reprinted, February, 1956
Reprinted, January, 1957
Fourth Edition, June, 1959
Reprinted, November, 1960
Italian Edition, 1963

By J. Alfred Lee and R. S. Atkinson

Fifth Edition, November, 1964
Spanish Edition, 1966
Sixth Edition, December, 1968

SBN 7236 0215 8

PRINTED IN GREAT BRITAIN
BY JOHN WRIGHT AND SONS LTD., AT THE STONEBRIDGE PRESS, BRISTOL

PREFACE TO THE SIXTH EDITION

DURING the four years that have elapsed since the fifth edition of this Synopsis was published, there have been many additions to our knowledge of the scientific basis of anæsthesia, and these have had an influence on the administration of anæsthetics. We have tried to incorporate many of them in the text of this sixth edition in order to keep it up to date.

The chapters have undergone some rearrangement and each has been carefully revised. New ones deal with dental anæsthesia, the administration of anæsthetics in abnormal environments, resuscitation, the intensive therapy unit, and intractable pain. We have gone to some trouble to increase the number of references, hoping thereby to bring again to the attention of anæsthetists articles which aroused interest when first published, but since lost sight of.

We hope that the book will continue to be helpful to young anæsthetists in training, with examinations ahead, as well as to more senior workers who require a relatively short text which may direct them to some of the growing points in the specialty. We have also tried to keep in mind the occasional anæsthetist and the workers in underdeveloped countries.

July, 1968.

J. A. L.
R. S. A.

FROM THE PREFACE TO THE FIRST EDITION

THIS book is not designed to take the place of the larger textbooks of anæsthesia and analgesia. It is a summary of current teaching and practice, and it is hoped that it will serve the student, the resident anæsthetist, the practitioner, and the candidate studying for the Diploma in Anæsthetics as a ready source of reference and a quick means of revision.

January, 1947.

J. A. L.

To N. L. and V. A.

CONTENTS

"Eternal vigilance is the price of safety."

―――――――

"Relief from pain is purchased always at a price. The price in both morbidity and mortality does not greatly differ whatever the agent or agents used."―R. M. WATERS.

―――――――

"The duty of the anæsthetist towards his patient is to take care."

―――――――

"While the anæsthetist's chief function is to prevent and alleviate pain, his primary responsibility is to maintain respiration."

―――――――

Primum non nocere―"First of all, do no harm."

―――――――

"The proper dose of any drug is enough."―
Dr. J. H. DRYSDALE

―――――――

"It is a great mistake to suppose that Nature always stands in need of the assistance of Art . . . nor do I think it below me to acknowledge that, when no manifest indication pointed out to me what was to be done, I have consulted the safety of my patient, and my own reputation effectually by doing nothing at all."―THOMAS SYDENHAM (1624-1689).

A SYNOPSIS OF ANÆSTHESIA

CHAPTER I

NOTES ON THE HISTORY OF ANÆSTHESIA

Joseph Black (1728–1799).—The discoverer of carbon dioxide or " fixed air ". Born at Bordeaux, France, of Irish-Scottish parentage and educated at Belfast and at the Universities of Edinburgh and Glasgow. Became Professor of Anatomy and Lecturer in Chemistry in the University of Glasgow, and later Lecturer in Chemistry in Edinburgh, where one of his pupils was Thomas Beddoes, later of the Pneumatic Institute in Bristol. Was all this time a practising physician. In 1754 described " fixed air ", as he called carbon dioxide, and described its method of identification by lime water. He proved that the gas produced in respiration, during the fermentation of wine (this had been described by von Helmont), during combustion of charcoal in air, and that liberated from chalk by heat and acids was one and the same. He showed it to be toxic to animals and that it can be absorbed by alkalis, facts made use of by anæsthetists to-day.*

Joseph Priestley (1733–1804).—The discoverer of oxygen in 1771 and of nitrous oxide in 1772. He was also the first to describe fluorine, sulphur dioxide, and methane.

Born at Birstall, near Leeds, Yorkshire, and became a Unitarian minister. After an interregnum as secretary to Lord Shelburne returned to take charge of a church in Birmingham. Here he became intimate with Erasmus Darwin, James Watt, and Wm. Murdock, the inventor of gas lighting, and was elected to the Fellowship of the Royal Society. Because of his advanced political views and his sympathies with the French Revolution, his house was broken up by the mob and he was forced to flee the country in 1791. In 1794 he emigrated to Pennsylvania, where, in addition to carrying on with his scientific studies, he became a farmer. He died at the age of 70.

Humphry Davy (1778–1829).—Born in Cornwall, the son of a wood carver. Became apprenticed to J. B. Borlase, surgeon, of Penzance, in 1795. At the age of 17 he experimented with nitrous oxide and the effects of its inhalation. In 1798 Davy became superintendent of Thomas Beddoes's Pneumatic Institute in Clifton, Bristol, and in the following year published his book *Researches, Chemical and Philosophical; Chiefly Concerning Nitrous Oxide.*† In this, Davy suggested that nitrous oxide inhalations might be used to relieve the pain of surgical operations and named it " laughing gas ". A nitrous oxide container was made by James Watt in 1799 to assist this research. In later life,

---

* *See also* Foregger, R., *Anesthesiology*, 1955, **16**, 257.
† Excerpts reprinted in *Survey of Anesthesiology*, 1968, **12**, 92.

Humphry Davy, *continued.*

> Davy became famous. He invented the miner's safety lamp, was created a baronet in 1818, and was elected President of the Royal Society in 1820.

Michael Faraday (1791–1867).—Said to be the first man to note the narcotic effects of ether vapour, but this is doubtful.* Born at Newington Butts, near London, of poor parents, he became a paper boy and later graduated to book-binding, during which occupation he made his first contact with chemical literature. Deciding to become a chemist, he obtained the post of laboratory assistant to Humphry Davy at the Royal Institution in 1813, and a little later accompanied him on an extensive tour in Europe. Became Director of Laboratory of Royal Institution in 1825. His great ability soon threatened to rival that of his master, who became jealous. Later Faraday, too, achieved world-wide fame. Fullerian Professor of Chemistry, 1833. Discovered benzene. His observations on ether were published in 1818 in *The Quarterly Journal of Science and Arts*, **4**, 158.

Henry Hill Hickman (1800–1830).—Medical education received in Edinburgh. He settled in practice in Ludlow. While doing a locum at Shifnal, in Shropshire, his interest in gas therapy was aroused, as the village was the birthplace of Thomas Beddoes. Familiarizing himself with the pioneer work of Davy, Priestley, and Faraday, Hickman returned to Ludlow and commenced experiments on animals. He was able to perform surgical operations painlessly on them, by causing them to inhale carbon dioxide. This was the first work on surgical anæsthesia induced by inhaling a gas. His results were published in a paper, "A Letter on Suspended Animation" (Ironbridge, 1824),† but attracted no attention from scientific men in England. Even Sir Humphry Davy, who was approached by Hickman's friend, T. A. Knight, F.R.S., showed no interest. Charles X of France was appealed to in 1828, and the French Academy of Medicine agreed to investigate Hickman's results, but nothing came of the matter. Baron Larrey, one of Napoleon's surgeons, however, gave Hickman some encouragement. Hickman died prematurely, aged 29, and was buried in Bromfield churchyard, Shropshire.

Crawford Williamson Long (1815–1878).—Born in Danielsville, Georgia, in the U.S., son of a successful lawyer and merchant. Educated at Franklin College and the University of Georgia from which he graduated as Master of Arts at the age of 19. He studied medicine as an apprentice of Dr. George R. Grant of Jefferson and also at the Transylvania University in Lexington, Kentucky. Later he enrolled at the University of Pennsylvania in Philadelphia, the first medical school founded in the American Colonies. After eighteen months' postgraduate study in the hospitals of New York, Long returned to his home state and set up in practice in Athens, Ga. He was well aware of "ether frolics" as a form of

---

* Davison, M. H. Armstrong, *Brit. J. Anæsth.*, 1957, **29**, 575.
† Reprinted in *Survey of Anesthesiology*, 1966, **10**, 92.

social entertainment, and realized that an individual under the influence of ether vapour might sustain bruises without experiencing pain. He performed his first operation under ether, the removal of a tumour from the neck of a young man, James M. Venable who was accustomed to the effects of the vapour. This occurred on March 20, 1842, and caused the patient no pain whatever. The account of this pioneering effort was not published until seven years later (Long, C. W., *Sth. med. J.*, 1849, N.S., **5**, 705),* while Morton's first use of ether vapour was reported in a letter from H. J. Bigelow to the *Boston Medical and Surgical Journal* of Nov. 11, 1846.

A statue to Long was erected in 1926 in the Statuary Hall of the U.S. Capitol, and ten years later the town where he was born also honoured his memory in a similar way.†

Horace Wells (1815–1848).—In 1844, on Dec. 10, Gardner Q. Colton, a travelling lecturer in chemistry, gave a demonstration of the effects of inhaling nitrous oxide at Hartford, Connecticut. Horace Wells, a local dentist, was present and noticed that a young shop assistant Samuel Cooley while under the influence of the gas, banged his shin and made it bleed, but stated that he experienced no pain. Wells persuaded Colton to try the gas during a dental extraction, and on the following day, Dec. 11, 1844, the experiment was carried out with Colton as anæsthetist, Riggs as dentist, and Wells as patient. It was a big success. "A new era in tooth pulling", according to Wells. Wells learnt from Colton the method of manufacture of nitrous oxide and used it in his dental practice in 15 patients. It was administered from an animal bladder through a wooden tube into the mouth, while the nostrils were compressed. Later he went to Boston to interest a larger audience in his discovery. He demonstrated the method to the students of Harvard Medical School, but the patient complained of pain: the affair was a fiasco and Wells was hissed out of the room as a fraud. Morton was present at this operation in January 1845. Wells returned to Hartford and continued to use the gas, but the introduction of ether gradually ousted the use of nitrous oxide. In 1847 Wells published his letter "A History of the Discovery of the Application of Nitrous Oxide Gas, Ether, and Other Vapours to Surgical Operations" (Hartford, Conn., 1847; also *Survey of Anesthesiology*, 1958, **2**, 1). Wells gave up dentistry, became a chloroform addict, travelled round the country with a troop of performing canaries, and was incarcerated in jail after bespattering a New York prostitute with sulphuric acid. He committed suicide by cutting his femoral artery.

Colton reintroduced the use of nitrous oxide in dentistry in 1863, at New Haven.

William Thomas Green Morton (1819–1868).—Morton deserves the chief credit for the introduction of ether as an anæsthetic agent, although W. E. Clark, of Rochester, New York, gave ether for a dental extraction in 1842, and Crawford Williamson Long (1815–1878) removed a tumour from the neck of J. M. Venable quite

---

* Reprinted in *Survey of Anesthesiology*, 1960, **4**, 120.
† *J. Amer. med. Ass.*, 1965, **194**, 1008; and Taylor, F. L., *Ann. med. Hist.*, 1925, **7**, 267.

William Thomas Green Morton, *continued.*

painlessly, in Jefferson County, Georgia, a few months after Clark's experiment. By the time (1849) that Long reported his work, Morton's fame was well established.

Morton, born at Charlton, Worcester County, Massachusetts, was a dentist who became a student, and later a partner of Wells, at Hartford. He separated from Wells and, becoming a medical student in Boston, was present when Wells failed to satisfy the audience as to the efficiency of nitrous oxide. Charles A. Jackson, one of Morton's lecturers at Harvard, suggested that ether could be used as a surface analgesic in dentistry. Morton, however, went further; he experimented on dogs to find out the effect of giving ether vapour by inhalation. Impressed with the results, he gave the vapour to Eben Frost for the removal of a tooth on Sept. 30, 1846. The operation was painless. After gaining further experience, and while still a medical student, Morton gave a demonstration at the Massachusetts General Hospital on Oct. 16, 1846, when Dr. J. C. Warren removed a tumour from the jaw of his patient, Gilbert Abbott, without producing any pain. This success gained him the support of Warren and also of Jacob Bigelow, Professor of Materia Medica. Much wrangling occurred between Morton and Jackson as to who should be given credit for the discovery. Morton three times petitioned the U.S. Congress, and even obtained an interview with the President, but he was never in his lifetime officially recognized as the pioneer of ether anæsthesia. Time later vindicated his claim. He spent his later years farming, and died of cerebral hæmorrhage, a disappointed man. The inscription on his tombstone in Mount Auburn Cemetery, Boston, composed by Henry J. Bigelow reads: " Inventor and Revealer of Inhalation Anesthesia: Before Whom, in All Time, Surgery was Agony; By Whom, Pain in Surgery was Averted and Annulled; Since Whom, Science has Control of Pain ". His agent, which he tried to patent under the name Letheon, became widely used. It was given in London and Paris in 1846. Robert Liston was the first surgeon to operate under ether in England; this was at University College Hospital on Dec. 21, 1846, using Squire's inhaler when he amputated the leg of Frederick Churchill.* It was, however, probably given on Dec. 19 in the Dumfries and Galloway Royal Infirmary by William Scott and William Fraser (Baillie, T. W., *From Boston to Dumfries,* Dumfries, 1966; and *Brit. J. Anæsth.,* 1965, **37**, 952). This followed a verbal report of Morton's successful use of the agent, carried by Fraser, who arrived in Liverpool from Boston on Dec. 16.

The name anæsthesia was suggested by Oliver Wendell Holmes, but had been used by Plato in 400 B.C. to denote absence of feelings in a philosophical sense and also by Dioscorides in the first century A.D. to denote absence of physical sensation (Armstrong Davison). It also appeared in Bailey's *English Dictionary* in 1721.†

Ether became known in England through a letter written by Henry Bigelow, Jacob's son, to his friend, Dr. Boott, who, with

---

* Dawkins, R. J. Massey, *Anæsthesia,* 1947, **2**, 51.
† *See* Miller, A. H., *Boston med. surg. J.,* 1927, **197**, 1218.

Mr. Robinson, gave the first ether anæsthetic, a dental case, two days before Liston's first use of it. Malgaigne was the first man to use ether in France, on Jan. 12, 1847.

John Snow (1813–1858).—Born in York, the son of a farmer. After Morton, the first whole-time anæsthetist. Starting his medical studies in Newcastle, at the age of 14, as apprentice to Mr. William Hardcastle, Snow worked at the Newcastle Infirmary and became interested in a cholera epidemic at Killingworth Colliery in 1831–32. In 1833 he left Newcastle and worked for a time at Pateley Bridge in Yorkshire and in 1836 he migrated to London, travelling on foot via Liverpool, North and South Wales, and Bath, and attended lectures at the Hunterian School of Anatomy in Great Windmill Street, and also at Westminster Hospital. He became a member of the Royal College of Surgeons of England in 1838 and also passed the examination of the Apothecaries Hall; became M.D., London, in 1844, and was appointed lecturer (1844–1849) in Forensic Medicine at the Aldersgate School of Medicine. Snow took an active part in the discussions of the Westminster Medical Society (which became the Medical Society of London in 1849–50), eventually becoming its President in 1855. In 1841 he read before it a paper on resuscitation of newborn children. He became interested in ether soon after its introduction and quickly perceived that the common method of administration was faulty. To overcome this he invented an ether inhaler. He was appointed anæsthetist to Out-patients at St. George's Hospital, where his first anæsthetics (for dental extraction) were given, and in 1847 was promoted to the In-patient appointment. He also worked with Robert Liston at University College Hospital and with Sir William Fergusson at King's College Hospital. His health was poor and he suffered from phthisis and from nephritis, being treated for the kidney disease by Richard Bright. For many years he was a vegetarian and temperance advocate. He experimented with many substances to see if they possessed anæsthetic properties, trying many of them on himself.

Snow rapidly became the leading anæsthetist in London and wrote a book in 1847, *On the Inhalation of Ether in Surgical Operations*. He did much useful work on the physiology of anæsthesia, and described five stages or degrees of anæsthesia. He later abandoned ether for chloroform, but was familiar with the dangers of the newer drug, believing it to cause primary cardiac failure consequent on the use of too strong a vapour. To overcome this danger he invented a percentage chloroform inhaler. He gave over 4000 chloroform anæsthetics without a death. In 1853 Snow originated the method of "chloroform à la reine", when he acted as anæsthetist at the birth of Queen Victoria's eighth child, Prince Leopold, at the request of Sir James Clark, and in 1857 at the birth of Princess Beatrice. These royal occasions made anæsthesia in midwifery morally respectable. He gave his royal patient 15-minim doses intermittently on a handkerchief, the administration lasting 53 minutes: it met with the Queen's warm approval— "Dr. Snow gave that blessed chloroform and the effect was soothing, quieting, and delightful beyond measure." The birth of Leopold George Duncan Albert (1853–1884), later Duke of Albany, finally

John Snow, *continued.*

canonized "that blessed chloroform". Even the names of the Queen's attendants seemed to share the aura of purity which her royal participation had given to the subject: Mrs. Lilly and Mrs. Innocent the midwives, and of course Dr. Snow.* Snow introduced amylene as an inhalation anæsthetic in 1856. His income never exceeded £1000 per annum although during the last 10 years of his life he gave an average of 450 anæsthetics a year. His last work, *On Chloroform and Other Anæsthetics,* was published posthumously in 1858, Snow having been seized with paralysis while at work on the manuscript and dying a few days later on June 17, 1858. In later years he proved that cholera is a water-borne disease, when he ordered the removal of the Broad Street pump handle in 1854 in London and so terminated a cholera epidemic (although this particular epidemic had commenced to wane before the actual removal of the handle!). The theory of the mode of transmission of cholera was set out in the second edition of his book (first edition 1849, following the epidemic of 1848), *On the Mode of Communication of Cholera,* 2nd ed., 1855 (London: Churchill). Near the site of the pump, in Broadwick Street, a public house has been named "The John Snow" (although Snow was a teetotaller!). Snow's grave in Brompton Cemetery was restored in 1938 by anæsthetists from Britain and the United States. Benjamin Ward Richardson's (1828–1896) epitaph reads: "In Brompton Cemetery there was laid to rest, at the age of forty-five, John Snow (1813–1858), exemplary citizen and useful physician. He demonstrated that cholera is communicated by contaminated water; and he made the art of anæsthesia a science." Three of his case books with a record of his chloroform administrations 1848–1858, are in the possession of the Library of the Royal College of Physicians of London.†

James Young Simpson (1811–1870).—Born at Bathgate, near Edinburgh. Qualified 1830 ; M.D., 1832. Elected to Chair of Midwifery at Edinburgh, 1840, spending £500 on canvassing, etc. Started university career in atmosphere of hostility from his colleagues, but his ability as a lecturer soon attracted large classes of students. Four years afterwards was earning £4000 per annum. A later discovery was that of hæmostasis by acupressure. Created baronet, 1866. A memorial bust was erected in Westminster Abbey. Introduced chloroform into surgical practice in 1847.‡ This drug was independently discovered by von Liebig, Soubeiran, and Guthrie in 1831. Dumas gave it its name and wrote the first full description of its physical and chemical properties. The old name was perchloride of formyl. Chloric ether, or Dutch oil, is a solution of chloroform in alcohol. Flourens, in 1847, showed that on inhalation its vapour had anæsthetic powers on animals.

Waldie, 1813–1889, a Liverpool chemist, suggested that Simpson should try the effects of the inhalation of chloroform vapour to relieve the pains of labour. Simpson experimented on himself and

* Longford, E., *Victoria, R.I.,* 1964, p. 234. London: Weidenfeld and Nicolson.
† Atkinson, R. S., *Proc. 4th World Cong. Anæsth.,* 1968, in press.
‡ Simpson, J. Y., *Lond. Med. Gaz.,* 1847, N.S., **5**, 934; and *Lancet,* 1847, **2**, 549 (reprinted in *Survey of Anesthesiology,* 1961, **5**, 93).

his assistants, Mathews Duncan and George Keith, on Nov. 4, and four days later it was first used clinically and a report was read to the Edinburgh Medical and Chirurgical Society on Nov. 10. Although Simpson was the first obstetrician to employ ether (January, 1847), he held that chloroform has the following advantages over ether : (1) Action more rapid, complete, and persistent. (2) Smaller quantity required. (3) Pleasanter. (4) Cheaper. Chloroform was first given in London at St. Bartholomew's Hospital on Nov. 20, 1847.

Joseph T. Clover (1825–1882).—After the death of Snow, Clover became the leading scientific anæsthetic investigator and practical anæsthetist in Britain. He was born in Aylesham, Norfolk, and was educated at the Gray Friar's Priory School in Norwich and at University College Hospital in London (1844). It is likely that Clover was present in the operating theatre at University College Hospital on Dec. 21, 1846, when Robert Liston amputated the leg of Frederick Churchill when ether was given by Peter Squire, the first major operation performed under ether anæsthesia in England. Joseph Lister was a fellow student. Became R.M.O. at University College Hospital and took F.R.C.S. in 1850. He was the pioneer of the art of completely and immediately removing from the urinary bladder the calculus fragments produced by lithotrity and invented a bladder aspirator. He also devised "Clover's Crutch", a simple but effective piece of apparatus for maintaining a patient in the lithotomy position. Worked as general practitioner in London, later specializing in anæsthetics. Was appointed to staff of University College and Westminster Hospitals, and also worked at the London Dental Hospital. In 1862 he invented a chloroform inhaler which enabled percentage mixtures of chloroform and air to be accurately measured and administered. It took the form of a large bag, slung over the back of the anæsthetist, and it contained $4\frac{1}{2}$ per cent of chloroform vapour in air. Realizing the dangers of chloroform, Clover set to work to make the administration of ether more simple and easy. This he did by inducing anæsthesia with nitrous oxide, later adding ether to gas.[*] Was co-opted on to Committee of Royal Medical and Chirurgical Society which advised the use of a mixture of chloroform and ether, because of the danger of chloroform alone (1864). In 1868 published a paper "On the Administration of Nitrous Oxide", *Brit. med. J.*, 1868, **2**, 491. In 1877 he described his portable regulating ether inhaler which did much to make ether more popular at the expense of chloroform (*Brit. med. J.*, 1877, **2**, 69). Another of Clover's achievements was his teaching that ether could be safely given over long periods with anæsthesia carried to adequate depth. He was Lecturer on Anæsthetics at University College Hospital and died at the age of 57.[†]

Sir Frederick Hewitt (1857–1916).—Educated at Merchant Taylors' School, Christ's College, Cambridge, and St. George's Hospital, London, where he was a distinguished student. Became an

[*] Clover, J. T., *Brit. med. J.*, 1876, **2**, 75 (reprinted in *Survey of Anesthesiology*, 1964, **8**, 87).
[†] Lee, J. Alfred, *Ann. R. Coll. Surg.*, 1960, **26**, 280.

Sir Frederick Hewitt, *continued.*

anæsthetist as defective eyesight prevented his becoming a consulting physician, and was appointed to Charing Cross Hospital in this capacity in 1884, the National Dental Hospital in 1885, and the London Hospital in 1886. In 1902 became physician anæsthetist to his old teaching hospital, St. George's. He emphasized that nitrous oxide anæsthesia is possible without asphyxia and that chloroform is specially dangerous during induction. Hewitt modified Junker's chloroform bottle and redesigned Clover's inhaler, enlarging the bore of the central tube (as suggested by Wilson Smith in 1901) and arranging for its rotation within the ether reservoir. He devised a dental prop and also an airway (*Lancet*, 1908, **1**, 490), and wrote a popular text-book (1893) on anæsthesia (*Anæsthetics and their Administration*), the fifth edition of which appeared in 1922. He strongly advocated better teaching of anæsthetics to medical students. Hewitt invented the first practical machine for giving nitrous oxide and oxygen in fixed proportions in 1887 and the years following. In 1911 he was knighted. Administered an anæsthetic to Edward VII for his appendix operation in 1902.* He died at Brighton of a gastric neoplasm.

Edmund W. Andrews (1824–1904).—Born in Putney, Vermont, and graduated in medicine at the University of Michigan in 1855. Settled in Chicago and became one of the founders of the Chicago Medical College which later became the Medical School of Northwestern University. Served on the side of the North in the Civil War and thereafter resumed surgical practice in Chicago and became surgeon to the Mercy Hospital. Was a man of many accomplishments—scholar, speaker, artist, naturalist, and philologist.

His great contribution to anæsthesia was the addition of 20 per cent of oxygen to nitrous oxide and his work was published under the title of " The Oxygen Mixture ; A New Anæsthetic Combination", *Chicago Medical Examiner*, 1868, **9**, 656.† He claimed that his mixture was safer and pleasanter than any anæsthetic then known. His judgement of the mixture, with certain modern supplements, still holds to-day, one hundred years later.‡

Karl Koller (1858–1944).—Born in Schnetteuhofen in Bohemia and graduated at the University of Vienna in 1882. He trained as an ophthalmic surgeon and soon became dissatisfied with the results of the general anæsthetics given to his patients during eye operations. He performed experiments with many drugs in order to find better methods of pain relief and so he very readily accepted the suggestion of Sigmund Freud, later to become world famous as the founder of Psycho-analysis, to try out the alkaloid cocaine then used as a nerve tonic. In experiments on himself Freud had discovered that cocaine made his tongue numb when taken by mouth.§ Koller soon realized that he was working with a most

---

* *See* Edwards, George, *Ann. R. Coll. Surg.*, 1951, **8**, 233.
† Reprinted in *Survey of Anesthesiology*, 1963, **7**, 74.
‡ *Survey of Anesthesiology*, 1963, **7**, 74.
§ *Psychoanal. Quart.*, 1963, **32**, 309.

useful agent and after trying it out on animals he used it in his patients with astounding success. His findings were reported to the German Ophthalmological Congress meeting in Heidelberg, in September, 1884.* Thus was local analgesia born, as topical analgesia in the conjunctival sac, and its use spread throughout the world in a few weeks. Koller did not develop his discovery, preferring to concentrate on his chosen specialty of eye surgery. He later emigrated from Vienna to the U.S.A. in 1889, where he joined the staff of the Mount Sinai Hospital, New York. Here he died, aged 86, after a distinguished career in ophthalmology, in 1944.

August Karl Gustav Bier (1861–1949).—Bier was born in Helsen in Waldeck in Germany in 1861 and graduated in 1889 at Kiel where he later became assistant to the Professor of Surgery, von Esmarch. While there he supervised the transition from antiseptic to aseptic techniques in the operating theatres, following the teachings of von Bergmann and Karl Schimmelbusch. In 1898 he gave the first deliberate spinal anæsthetic† and to prove his faith in the method allowed his assistant, Dr. Hildebrandt, to inject into his own theca 2 ml. of 1 per cent cocaine solution. Leaving Kiel, Bier became Professor of Surgery successively at Griefswald, Bonn, and as successor to Ernst von Bergmann at Berlin, and in the capital he was to spend the greater part of his professional life. In addition to his discovery of spinal analgesia, he invented the method of treating chronic inflammation by the method of passive hyperæmia with Esmarch's bandage (1907), and pioneered intravenous procaine analgesia (1908)‡ (*see* Chapter XV for a modern description of this technique). He was one of the great figures of German surgery, as teacher, lecturer, and operator. Introduced the "tin helmet" into the German army in World War I. In later life he came to hold unorthodox ideas and deviated from the views of his colleagues. He died, aged 88, at Sauer in the German Democratic Republic in 1949.

Heinrich Friedrich Wilhelm Braun (1862–1934).—Braun has been called "The father of local analgesia" and he coined the term "conduction anæsthesia". He was born in Rawitch in Germany in 1862, and although intending to become a musician, he graduated in medicine in 1887, and after a period as assistant to von Volkmann, became director of the Deaconess Hospital in Leipzig where his interest in local analgesia was developed, having been stimulated by Oberst. In 1902 he introduced the use of adrenaline in local analgesic solutions of cocaine,§ and in 1905 became the pioneer of the new drug procaine.|| In this year, too, appeared the first edition of his classic text-book, *Local Anæsthesia*; the eighth edition was published in 1933. Braun was appointed to direct the new hospital at Zwickau in 1906, and here he passed the remainder of his professional life. He described the anterior approach to the cœliac plexus (anterior splanchnic block) and was

* Koller, K., *Klin. Mbl. Augen.*, 1884, **22**, 60; and *Wien. med. Wschr.*, 1884, **34**, 1276 and 1309 (translated in *Survey of Anesthesiology*, 1965, **9**, 288).
† Bier, A., *Dtsch. Z. Chir.*, 1899, **51**, 361 (translated in *Survey of Anesthesiology*, 1962, **6**, 352).
‡ Bier, A., *Verh. dtsch. Ges. Chir.*, 1908, **37**, 204.
§ Braun, H., *Arch. klin. Chir.*, 1902, **69**, 541.
|| Braun, H., *Dtsch. med. Wschr.*, 1905, **31**, 1667.

Heinrich Friedrich Wilhelm Braun, *continued.*

the inventor of the Braun splint. He was also interested in general anæsthetics and devised an apparatus for the safe administration of chloroform and ether vapour. Was president of the German Surgical Society in 1924. He died in 1934, aged 72.

Arthur Läwen (1876–1958).—Läwen was born in 1876 in Waldheim in Saxony, and qualified at Leipzig in 1900. He became a pupil of Heinrich Braun and later of Friedrich Trendelenburg. He held senior posts at Leipzig and Marburg and was appointed Professor of Surgery at Königsberg in East Prussia where his chief work was done. In 1912 he employed curare to reduce the amount of ether needed for relaxation, in an attempt to reduce the incidence of post-operative pulmonary complications which were then thought to be due to ether vapour.* This work was interrupted by the First World War. Läwen was the first to describe paravertebral conduction anæsthesia, and in 1910 he was the first to show that extradural analgesia was a safe and practical form of pain relief in pelvic and abdominal surgery. For this he used large volumes of 1·5 or 2 per cent procaine solution with sodium bicarbonate, injected through the sacral hiatus. He did a great deal to popularize local analgesia. After 1945 he became a refugee from Eastern Germany, having lost his sons, his possessions, and his university chair during the War. He died in 1958, aged 82.

Arthur E. Guedel (1883–1956).—Born in Cambridge City, Indiana, and received his medical education at the Indiana School of Medicine, Indianapolis, qualifying in 1908. Lecturer on anæsthesia in the University of Indianapolis (1920–1928), during which time he was a practising anæsthetist in that city. Gave anæsthetics in France during the First World War. Later moved to Los Angeles, where he became Associate Clinical Professor of Anesthesiology at the University of Southern California School of Medicine.

He made many contributions to his chosen specialty, including an early description of the self-administration of nitrous oxide and air for obstetrics and minor surgery (*Indianap. med. J.*, October, 1911); a description of the anæsthetic properties of divinyl oxide; a systematization of the signs of inhalation anæsthesia (*Curr. Res. Anesth.*, May, 1920; and *Inhalation Anesthesia, A Fundamental Guide*, The Macmillan Co., New York, 1937); the introduction of controlled respiration using ether, with Treweek (*Anesthesia and Analgesia*, December, 1934); and a classic description of the clinical use of cyclopropane (*Anesthesiology*, 1940, **1**, 1). He received the Hickman Medal from the Royal Society of Medicine in 1941.

Henry Edmund Gaskin Boyle (1875–1941).—Born in Barbados and qualified at St. Bartholomew's Hospital, London, in 1901, where as a student he was president of the Abernethian Society. Became casualty officer in Bristol and then returned to Bart's as junior resident anæsthetist, rising in due course to become head of the department. About 1912, became interested in nitrous oxide and oxygen anæsthesia and in 1917 got Coxeter, the instrument maker,

---

* Läwen, A., *Beitr. klin. Chir.*, 1912, **37**, 708.

to copy Gwathmey's gas–oxygen machine which became the first 'Boyle' apparatus. He introduced gas–oxygen into France for use in anæsthetizing wounded soldiers in World War I, and for this received the decoration of O.B.E. After the war he visited the U.S. and brought back with him Davis's gag which he introduced to British throat surgeons. He was an early user of Magill's endotracheal techniques and was elected F.R.C.S. and D.A. in 1935; was one of the original pair of examiners for the latter diploma. A founder member of the Association of Anæsthetists of Great Britain and Ireland in 1932.

In 1907 wrote the first edition of his textbook *Practical Anæsthetics*, the third edition of which was prepared by his junior colleague C. Langton Hewer. Boyle was a 'character' and was universally known as 'Cockie'.

His anæsthetic machine, modified in every particular, is used in most British hospitals today.

IMPORTANT DATES IN THE HISTORY OF ANÆSTHESIA

1516. Curare, South American arrow poison, described by Peter Martyr Angherius.

1540. Valerius Cordus (1515–1544) synthesized sweet vitriol (ether), possibly aided by Paracelsus (1493–1541).

1628. Wm. Harvey (1578–1657), pupil of Galileo (1564–1642) of Padua and contemporary of Bacon and of Descartes, described the circulation of the blood.

1657. First intravenous injection of a drug (tincture of opium) into an animal (a dog) by Sir Christopher Wren and Robert Boyle using a bladder attached to a sharpened quill.

1662. Boyle enunciated his law of the relationship of the volume and pressure of a gas.

1665. Richard Lower (1631–1691) transfused blood from one animal to another.

1754. Carbon dioxide discovered by von Helmont and isolated by Black.

1761. Auenbrugger described percussion of the chest.

1771. Discovery of oxygen by Priestley and Scheele, independently.

1775. Priestley discovered nitrous oxide.

1787. Charles's law, showing relationship of volume to temperature of a gas.

1788. Chas. Kite of Gravesend first used endotracheal tube in resuscitation of the drowned.

1792. Frobenius, a German, named sweet vitriol 'ether'.

1797. Publication of the description of the Venturi tube by Giovanni Battista Venturi (1746–1822) at Modena, Italy.

1800. Discovery of analgesic properties of nitrous oxide by Davy who named it " laughing gas ".

1806. Isolation of morphine from opium by Friedrich Wilhelm Adam Sertürner (1783–1841), a Hanover pharmacist.

1807. Baron Larrey performed painless amputations, using ice, on the battlefield.

1816. René Laënnec (1781–1826) invented stethoscope.

Important Dates, *continued.*

1818. Faraday is said to have discovered narcotic action of ether vapour.

1822. Magendie proved that while anterior spinal roots are motor, posterior roots are sensory.

1824. Henry Hill Hickman (1800–1830) carried out operations on animals under carbon dioxide, with freedom from pain, thus establishing the principle of inhalation anæsthesia.

1825. Chas. Waterton (1782–1865) published his *Wanderings in South America,* which contained an account of the actions of curare.

1831. Chloroform discovered independently by von Liebig (1803–1873) in Germany, Guthrie (1782–1848) in New York, and Soubeiran (1793–1858) in France.

Atropine prepared from *Atropa belladonna,* by Mein and by Geiger and Hesse.

1832. Thomas Aitchison Latta used intravenous saline in the treatment of circulatory collapse in cholera (not in surgical shock).

1834. Jean-Baptiste Dumas (1800–1884) described chemical composition of, and gave name to, chloroform.

1842. Ether given by W. E. Clark of Rochester, New York, for dental extraction, and by Crawford W. Long (1815–1878) in Jefferson, Georgia (the patient, John Venable), in the U.S.

Marie Jean Pierre Flourens (1794–1867) first isolated respiratory centre in medulla.

1844. Horace Wells (1815–1848) introduced nitrous oxide inhalation to produce anæsthesia during dental extraction.

Francis Rynd of Dublin invented hypodermic trocar.

1846. Wm. T. G. Morton (1819–1868) successfully demonstrated the anæsthetic properties of ether, Oct. 16. The word "anæsthesia" was suggested by Oliver Wendell Holmes for Morton's "etherisation".

First surgical operation performed in England under ether anæsthesia by Robert Liston, Dec. 21, when Frederick Churchill underwent amputation through the thigh and Peter Squire gave the anæsthetic at University College Hospital.

1847. Flourens described anæsthetic properties of chloroform and ethyl chloride vapour in animals.

James Y. Simpson (1811–1870) in November introduced chloroform into clinical work, to ease pains of labour in Edinburgh.

John Snow (1813–1858) published his book, *On the Inhalation of Ether in Surgical Operations,* the first scientific description of its clinical uses, physical and pharmacological properties.

Deaths from ether reported from Grantham and Colchester.

1848. Hannah Greener, aged 15, died from chloroform administered by Dr. Meggison, Jan. 28—the first recorded case—at Winlayton, Co. Durham.

Heyfelder first used ethyl chloride in humans.

1850. Wm. Gairdner, of Glasgow, differentiated between postoperative pneumonia and pulmonary collapse, the latter due to bronchial obstruction.

1853. Pravaz of Lyons (1791–1853) invented syringe made of glass.
John Snow gave chloroform analgesia to Queen Victoria at birth of Prince Leopold, hence " chloroform *à la reine* ".
Invention of hypodermic syringe and needle by Alexander Wood (1817–1874) of Edinburgh.

1855. Gaedicke, of Germany, isolated cocaine from coca plant.
Indirect laryngoscopy described by Manuel Garcia, a singing teacher.

1857. Claude Bernard (1813–1878) showed that curare acts on the myoneural junction.

1858. Publication of John Snow's book, *On Chloroform and Other Anæsthetics.*

1860. Nieman purified the alkaloid which Gaedicke had isolated from coca leaves. He named it cocaine.

1862. Thos. Skinner, a Liverpool obstetrician, introduced his domette-covered, wire-framed mask, frequently imitated since (e.g., by Carl Schimmelbusch, of Berlin, in 1890).
Clover's chloroform inhaler.
George Harley introduced his A.C.E. mixture (alcohol, 1 part ; chloroform, 2 parts ; ether, 3 parts).

1863. Colton popularized the use of nitrous oxide in dentistry, neglected since Wells's discovery.
Louis Pasteur (1822–1895) showed that micro-organisms cause fermentation, which led Lister to his discovery of antisepsis.

1864. Report of Chloroform Committee of Royal Medical and Chirurgical Society, which confirmed chloroform's position as first favourite.

1865. Professor J. Lister treated by means of carbolic acid the compound fracture of James Greenlee's leg—the birth of antiseptic surgery (Aug. 12).

1867. Introduction by F. E. Junker, a German surgeon on the staff of the Samaritan Free Hospital, London, of his chloroform inhaler, originally designed for use with bichloride of methylene (CH_2Cl_2), a drug first used clinically in this same year by Sir Spencer Wells and Benjamin Ward Richardson.
Joseph Lister (1827–1912), Professor of Surgery in Glasgow, described his antiseptic method of wound treatment (published in the *Lancet*, 1867, **1**, 326; and *Ibid.*, **2**, 353).

1868. Edmund Andrews combined oxygen with nitrous oxide.
T. W. Evans, an American dentist working in Paris, who had learnt about N_2O administration from Colton in 1867, introduced it to London dentists. In the following year, N_2O was supplied in cylinders in compressed form commercially, four years before U.S. manufacturers put it on the market. Supplies of nitrous oxide may well have been obtainable in London in 1856 from the Medical Pneumatic Appliance Co. (Barth).
C. A. Wunderlich (1815–1877) published his work on medical thermometry. He found fever a disease and left it a symptom.

1869. Nasal N_2O inhaler used (independently) by Clover and Coleman.

1871. Trendelenburg 1844–1924) gave anæsthetics via a tracheotomy wound.

Important Dates, *continued.*

1871. Hyoscine isolated.
      Mason invented his gag.   Modified by Fergusson three years later.

1872. Antisalivary effects of atropine described by Heidenhain.
      In England, use of ether became much more frequent following the visit of B. Joy Jeffries, an ophthalmic surgeon of Boston, Mass., U.S.A.   He 'sold' the American method of ether administration to British surgeons and anæsthetists, a method involving forcing ether on to the patient who was, if necessary, held down during induction.   Previously in Britain, chloroform was used almost exclusively.
      Pierre-Cyprien Oré of Bordeaux produced general anæsthesia with intravenous chloral hydrate in animals and two years later applied the method in man.
      Clover introduced his nitrous-oxide–ether sequence at B.M.A. Annual Meeting at Norwich.

1876. Hyperventilation with air shown to have analgesic effects by Bonwill, W. G. A., *Philad. J. Dent. Science*, 1876, **3**, 37 (*see Survey of Anesthesiology*, 1964, **8**, 348).

1877. Clover introduced his portable regulating ether inhaler.
      Forné, a French naval surgeon, gave chloral hydrate to produce sleep before chloroform anæsthesia.

1880. Macewen introduced intratracheal intubation by mouth.

1881. Klikovich used nitrous oxide to ease labour pains (*Arch. Gynaek.*, **18**, 81).
      Frederick Trendelenburg, Professor of Surgery at Rostock (afterwards at Bonn and Leipzig), introduced the head-down tilt with pelvic elevation, for abdominal surgery.

1882. Synthesis of cyclopropane by von Freund.
      Cervello introduced paraldehyde into medicine.

1884. Koller demonstrated local analgesic properties of cocaine on the cornea, at the suggestion of Freud, at Ophthalmological Congress at Heidelberg.
      Wm. Stewart Halsted (1852–1922) and Hall, in New York, did the first nerve-block with cocaine : the nerve, the mandibular.

1885. J. L. Corning produced analgesia by the accidental subarachnoid injection of cocaine.

1886. von Bergmann introduced heat sterilization, the beginning of aseptic surgery.

1887. Sir Frederick Hewitt invented the first practical gas and oxygen machine.

1888. First Hyderabad Chloroform Commission.

1889. Second Hyderabad Chloroform Commission.   Reports stated that chloroform is never a primary cardiac depressant.   This is now known to be untrue.

1890. Redard of Geneva introduced the ethyl chloride spray for local analgesia.
      Wm. Stewart Halsted, Professor of Surgery at the Johns Hopkins Hospital, Baltimore, introduced rubber gloves.

1891. Lumbar puncture demonstrated to be a practical clinical procedure by Quincke in Germany and by Essex Wynter in England.

1891. Giesel isolated tropococaine, the first alternative to the toxic cocaine.

1892. Karl Ludwig Schleich (1859–1922) introduced infiltration analgesia.

1893. London Society of Anæsthetists founded by F. W. Silk. It became the Anæsthetic Section of the Royal Society of Medicine in 1908.

1894. E. A. Codman and Harvey Cushing advocated use of anæsthetic record charts. Later, 1901, blood-pressure readings, taken with a Riva-Rocci instrument, were added to these charts.

1895. X-rays discovered by Wilhelm Konrad von Roentgen of Wurzburg.

First direct-vision laryngoscope devised by Kirstein.

1898. August Bier (1861–1949) induced first successful clinical spinal analgesia.

Tuffier developed and popularized spinal analgesia.

Alfred Coleman described nasal administration of nitrous oxide.

1900. Schneiderlinn combined hyoscine and morphine in psychiatry.

Landsteiner of the Univ. of Vienna described ABO blood groups.

1901. Extradural caudal block introduced by Sicard and Cathelin, both of Paris, independently.

Hewitt described his modification of Clover's portable regulating ether inhaler, using wider-bore tubes.

1902. Braun added adrenaline to cocaine solution to prolong its effect and retard its absorption.

A. G. Vernon Harcourt, F.R.S., described his chloroform inhaler.

E. H. Embley, of Australia, described death due to vagal inhibition of the heart during chloroform anæsthesia.*

1903. Barbitone (veronal) synthesized by Emil Fischer and von Mehring. This was the first barbiturate.

1904. Fourneau synthesized stovaine.

Procaine synthesized by Alfred Einhorn (1856–1917).

1905. The first society of anæsthetists founded in the U.S. by G. A. F. Erdmann, The Long Island Society of Anesthetists, later (1911) combined with a group from Manhattan to form the New York Society of Anesthetists; in 1935 the organization became national and in 1936 was named the American Society of Anesthetists Inc. In 1945 the title was changed to the American Society of Anesthesiologists Inc., at the suggestion of Paul Wood, the name 'anesthesiology' having been coined by Seifert in 1902.

Procaine used by Heinrich Braun (1862–1934).

1907. Barker made use of the curves of the vertebral column in spinal analgesia and introduced hyperbaric solutions.

Chevalier Jackson described his work on laryngoscopy.

Bellamy Gardner introduced his wire frame for open ether.

1908. Hewitt introduced his pharyngeal airway.

Massive collapse of the lungs described by Wm. Pasteur.

Louis Ombrédanne (1871–1956), a Parisian surgeon, described his ether–air inhaler.

---

* Reprinted in *Survey of Anesthesiology*, 1965, **9**, 511 and 634 from *Brit. med. J.*, 1902, **1**, 817, 885, and 951.

Important Dates, *continued.*

1908. Bier described intravenous procaine local analgesia.

George Washington Crile described his theory of 'anoci-association' (*American Surg.*, 1908, **47**, 864).

1909. Meltzer and Auer used intratracheal insufflation anæsthesia in animals.

Burkhardt used intravenous ether.

1910. Elsberg applied Meltzer and Auer's technique to man.

E. I. McKesson introduced the first intermittent-flow gas and oxygen machine, with percentage calibration of the two gases (*Surg. Gynec. Obstet.*, 1911, **13**, 456).

Arthur Läwen (1876–1958) of Königsberg showed that extradural analgesia via the sacral route was a useful and practical method of analgesia.

1911. Goodman Levy proved that chloroform can cause death (from ventricular fibrillation) in light anæsthesia.

Phenobarbitone (luminal) synthesized.

A. E. Guedel reported on the technique of self-administration of nitrous oxide in obstetrics (*Indianap. med. J.*, 1911, 141).

1912. Boothby and Cotton introduced a sight feed gas and oxygen flow-meter.

Kelly was first to use insufflation intratracheal anæsthesia in England.

A. Läwen (1876–1958) used curare to produce relaxation.

1913. Danis was first to describe trans-sacral analgesia.

Gwathmey introduced rectal oil-ether.

Noel and Souttar used intravenous paraldehyde.

1914. Hustin, of Belgium, was first to use citrate in blood transfusion.

Gwathmey's *Anesthesia* published.

1915. Use of carbon dioxide absorption in animals by Dennis Jackson, of Cincinnati (*J. Lab. clin. Med.*, 1915, **1**, 1).

1916. F. E. Shipway introduced his warm ether apparatus (*Lancet*, **1**, 70).

1917. Edmund Boyle described his portable N_2O and O_2 apparatus ; the chloroform bottle was added in 1920.

Avertin described by Eicholtz.

1919. The American Association of Anesthetists founded by James Gwathmey and Frank McMechan.

1920. Guedel's first paper on signs of anæsthesia. These supplanted Snow's signs.

Magill and Rowbotham developed endotracheal anæsthesia.

1921. Extradural analgesia described by Pagés, of Spain.

Carbon dioxide became common in anæsthetic practice, following the work of Henderson and Haldane.

1922. *Current Researches in Anesthesia and Analgesia* appeared in August.

Goodman Levy's *Chloroform Anæsthesia* published.

Labat's *Regional Anesthesia* published.

First Meeting of Section of Anæsthesia at Annual Meeting of B.M.A.

1923. Ethylene introduced by Arno B. Luckhardt (1885–1957) of Chicago.

1923. Carbon dioxide absorption used in man, by Waters.
British Journal of Anæsthesia appeared.

1924. Howard Wilcox Haggard (1891–1959) published his classic papers on "The Absorption, Distribution and Elimination of Ether" (*J. biol. Chem.*, 1924, **59**, 737 et seq.).

1926. Concept of "balanced anæsthesia" put forward by J. S. Lundy (*Minn. Med.*, 1926, **9**, 399).
Butzengeiger used tribromethyl alcohol (avertin) (*Dtsch. med. Wschr.*, 1927, **53**, 712).

1927. Pitkin introduced spinocain and popularized spinal analgesia.
Ocherblad and Dillon used ephedrine in spinal analgesia to prevent hypotension.
Pernocton used in Germany by R. Bumm. The first barbiturate routinely used for induction of anæsthesia.

1928. Introduction of circle method of carbon dioxide absorption, by Brian Sword.
Lucas and Henderson, in Toronto, proved that cyclopropane had anæsthetic properties.
I. A. Magill introduced blind nasal intubation.

1929. Sodium amytal used by Zerfas, the first use of rapidly acting barbiturates in anæsthesia, given into a vein.

1930. Waters introduced cyclopropane into clinical practice.
Nembutal and percaine described.
Leake and Chen discovered anæsthetic properties of divinyl ether.

1931. Achille Mario D. Dogliotti (1897–1966) re-introduced extradural analgesia, in Italy.

1932. Weese, Scharpff, and Rheinoff were the first to use hexobarbitone (evipan) (*Dtsch. med. Wschr.*, 1932, **2**, 1205).
Langton Hewer's *Recent Advances in Anæsthesia* appeared.
Gelfan and Bell, of the University of Alberta, first used divinyl ether in anæsthesia, Gelfan acting as the patient.
Foundation of the Association of Anæsthetists of Great Britain and Ireland.

1933. R. J. Minnitt, of Liverpool, designed his machine for the self-administration of N_2O and air in labour.
Guedel described his airway.

1934. Waters and associates reported on the clinical use of cyclopropane.
Lundy introduced thiopentone.

1935. First examination for D.A. held.

1937. Guedel's *Inhalation Anæsthesia* published.

1938. Positive-pressure respirator used in surgery by Crafoord—the spiropulsator of Frenckner in Stockholm.

1939. Pethidine synthesized by Schaumann and Eisleb at Hoechst Farbwerke, Germany.

1940. *Anesthesiology* first published.

1941. Trichloroethylene advocated by Langton Hewer and Hadfield.

1942. Allen reported his work on refrigeration analgesia.
Griffith and Johnson, of Montreal, used curare in anæsthesia.
Hingson and Edwards advocated their technique of continuous caudal analgesia.

Important Dates, *continued.*

1943. Macintosh described his curved laryngoscope in Oxford.
1946. The journal *Anæsthesia* appeared.
1948. First use of hypotensive anæsthesia by Griffiths and Gillies in Edinburgh.

Faculty of Anæsthetists formed by the Council of the Royal College of Surgeons of England.

First clinical use of lignocaine (xylocaine) by Gordh.
1949. Penta- and hexamethonium described by Paton and Zaimis.

Short-acting muscle relaxants described by Bovet and used clinically two years later in Italy and Sweden.

Melrose described his rotating disk oxygenator at the Postgraduate Medical School, Hammersmith, London.
1950. Induced hypothermia in cardiac surgery described by W. G. Bigelow and his colleagues from Toronto.
1951. Suckling synthesized halothane.
1953. First examination for Fellowship in Faculty of Anæsthetists of the Royal College of Surgeons of England in London.
1956. Michael Johnstone used halothane clinically.

(*See also* Davison, M. H. Armstrong, *The Evolution of Anæsthesia,* 1965. Altrincham: J. Sherratt and Son.)

CHAPTER II

SOME ANATOMICAL AND PHYSIOLOGICAL NOTES

CENTRAL NERVOUS SYSTEM

The Action of Anæsthetic Agents on the Brain Cells.—Many theories have been put forward, but so far no truly satisfactory explanation of how anæsthetic agents act has been produced. The site of action is more likely to be on synaptic transmission than on the cell-body itself. Multi-synaptic systems, such as the ascending reticular formation, are particularly susceptible to the effects of drugs.

Some of the most important theories are :—

1. That anæsthetics interfere with intracellular oxidation, possibly by influencing enzyme action (Quastel,[*] 1932). During anæsthesia there is inhibition of a carrier of energy which operates as an intermediate between the pyruvate of the cell and the cytochrome system. Cells of the central nervous system of most recent phylogenetic development are the most sensitive to oxygen lack.

2. That anæsthetic agents are readily absorbed by lipids, hence brain cells are specially susceptible to their action (Meyer,[†] Overton[‡]). Partition of a drug between lipid and water phases

---

[*] Quastel, J. H., *Proc. R. Soc. Med.,* 1932, **112**, 60.
[†] Meyer, H. H., *Arch. exp. Path. Pharmak.,* 1899, **42**, 109.
[‡] Overton, E. L., *Studien über Narkose,* 1901. Jena.

reflects its biological potency as a narcotic. This is true for volatile anæsthetics, but not for chloral hydrate or barbiturates which are both more hydrophilic than lipophilic.

3. That anæsthetics cause changes in cell metabolism of a physico-chemical nature, e.g., precipitation of colloids (Claude Bernard,* 1875), changes in surface tension, changes in permeability of cell membranes, changes in viscosity, etc.

4. That anæsthetics act by changing electric polarity of cells of nervous system. Both ether and chloroform reduce the frequency and voltage of action potentials. The brain usually is electronegative to the rest of the organism, but under anæsthesia it becomes more positive.

5. The inert gas effect. Ferguson† (1939) postulated that the narcotic potency of inert gases and vapours was inversely proportional to their vapour pressure, provided that they are chemically unreactive. This is roughly true for the common anæsthetic agents, though it does not explain how the brain cells are affected.

6. The hydrate micro-crystal theory of anæsthesia by non-hydrogen-bonding agents.‡ This involves primarily the interaction of the molecules of the anæsthetic agent with water molecules in the brain, rather than with molecules of lipids.

None of these theories is wholly satisfactory.

(See also: Mogey, G. A., Brit. J. Anæsth., 1955, **27**, 49; Pittinger, C. B., and Keasling, H. H., Anesthesiology, 1959, **20**, 204.)

Consciousness, Unconsciousness, the Anæsthetic State.—Hughlings Jackson (1884) propounded his basic theories On Evolution and Dissolution of the Nervous System. He suggested that the evolution of the central nervous system involved the successive addition of masses of nerve-cells to the rostral end of the neuraxis, the most recent addition being the development of the cerebral cortex. The higher centres exerted a measure of control over the lower centres, which were concerned with unconscious and reflex mechanisms.

The effect of anæsthetic drugs has been explained as a progressive depression of the central nervous system, beginning with the higher centres (cerebral cortex) and ending with the vital centres in the medulla. The standard sequence of depression of the brain has been used to explain the clinical signs of anæsthesia.§ Advances in neurophysiology, however, indicate that the system is more complex.

CEREBRAL CORTEX.—Experimental work shows that the cerebral cortex does not become inactive, even during deep planes of surgical anæsthesia. Nor does its activity by itself determine levels of consciousness. Even in deep anæsthesia, afferent impulses continue to flow into the cerebral cortex along the primary pathways and to excite cells in the appropriate sensory areas. Of more importance, in consideration of the anæsthetic

---

* Bernard, C., Leçons sur les Anaesthésiques et sur l'Asphyxie, 1875. Paris: Baillière.
† Ferguson, J., Proc. R. Soc. B, 1939, **127**, 387.
‡ Pauling, L., Science, 1961, **134**, 15; and Curr. Res. Anesth., 1964, **43**, 1.
§ Harris, T. A. B., The Mode of Action of Anæsthetics, 1951. Edinburgh: E. & S. Livingstone.

Consciousness, Unconsciousness, the Anæsthetic State, *continued.*

state, is the integration of the cerebral cortex with the reticular system via the reticulo-cortical projection. The electro-encephalogram is not a reliable indicator of consciousness or unconsciousness during nitrous-oxide–oxygen anæsthesia with fully paralysing doses of muscle relaxant.

RETICULAR FORMATION.—Anatomically poorly defined. Consists of scattered cells and neurons in the medulla, pons, and midbrain. Probably functionally continuous in a caudal direction with spinal-cord cells grouped around the central canal, and in a rostral direction with cells of the intralaminar group of thalamic nuclei. It does not include the cranial nerve nuclei or the sensory and cerebellar relay nuclei. It consists essentially of two parts—*descending* and *ascending.*

DESCENDING RETICULAR FORMATION.—Made up on each side of medial and lateral reticular tracts, continuous below with the reticulospinal tract in the anterior column of the spinal cord. Affects reflex muscle tone; medial tract inhibitory, lateral tract facilitatory.

ASCENDING RETICULAR FORMATION.—Receives afferent connexions involving most kinds of sensation, including spino-reticular, trigeminal and auditory afferents. Ascending reticular fibres connect with intralaminar thalamic nuclei. From here the diffuse thalamo-cortical projection connects with the cortex.

DIFFUSE THALAMO-CORTICAL PROJECTION.—The intralaminar nuclei are able to activate the whole cortex and de-synchronize the E.E.G. But the exact location of the anatomical pathway of the thalamo-cortical projection is far from certain.

PHYSIOLOGY.—The reticular formation is particularly concerned with integrative functions. Transmission is multi-synaptic, so that a wide range of synaptic phenomena may be displayed. Such a multi-synaptic system is particularly vulnerable to interference, e.g., by drugs. The reticular formation also has a rich blood-supply.

AROUSAL REACTION.—Direct electrical stimulation of the reticular system sets up diffuse nervous activity accompanied by changes in electrocortical activity (E.E.G.) identical with the transition from the sleeping to the wakeful state. Destruction of the reticular formation in animals produces permanent coma. It is likely that the ascending reticular formation is indispensable for the maintenance of consciousness, and that sleep-producing drugs have a predominant effect on this organization.

SIGNIFICANCE OF STIMULI.—Conscious attention is dependent more on the character than on the strength of an afferent stimulus. Thus a novel or unusual sensory stimulus may cause the sleeping patient to awake. A repetitive stimulus may provoke drowsiness and sleep. Induction of hypnosis, for example, is dependent on the nature and significance of repeated auditory or other stimuli.

(For further information *see* : Feldberg, W., *Brit. med. J.*, 1959, **2**, 771; Grey Walter, in *Modern Trends in Anæsthesia* (Ed. Evans, T. F.,

and Gray, T. C.), 1958, Ch.3, London: Butterworths; Hopkin, D. A.
Buxton, and Brown, D., *Anæsthesia*, 1958, **13**, 306 ; Symposium on the
Central Nervous System Related to Anæsthesia, *Brit. J. Anæsth.*, 1961,
33, 174 et seq.)

Reflex Action.—

A reflex arc consists of at least two neurons, afferent and efferent.
The stretch reflex, concerned with muscle tone, is an example
of a two-neuron reflex arc. More commonly, however, several
connecting or internuncial neurons are involved.

Reflex action is important in clinical anæsthesia. A significant part
of the practice of anæsthesia is the modification or abolition of
the normal reflex response to a noxious stimulus.

CHARACTERISTICS OF REFLEX ACTIVITY.—

1. *Synaptic Delay.*—The time between the afferent stimulus and
the effector response is nearly all taken up by transmission
across the synapses. Synaptic transmission takes about 0·5–
1·0 m. sec. and measurement of the total reflex time gives an
idea of the number of synapses involved.

2. *Subliminal Fringe.*—Stimulation of the afferent side of the
reflex arc results in the building up of post-synaptic potential.
This is of threshold value over a central area so that the
motor neurons are excited. Over a peripheral area a sub-
threshold potential is built up, and the motor neurons do not
become excited. This area is known as the subliminal fringe.

3. *Occlusion.*—The effect of two afferent impulses acting together
may be less than the sum of the effect of the two impulses
acting separately. This occurs when the central areas of
threshold potential overlap.

4. *Summation.*—This may be *spatial* or *temporal*. Spatial summation occurs when the subliminal fringes of two afferent
impulses overlap, so that the effector response is greater than
the sum of the effect of the two afferent impulses acting
separately. Temporal summation occurs when repetitive
stimuli evoke a response, but individual stimuli of the same
strength are ineffective.

5. *Recruitment.*—With continued excitation of an afferent nerve
with a stimulus of unaltered intensity, an increasing number
of motor neurons become activated, due to summation.

6. *After-discharge.*—After discontinuation of such an afferent
stimulation, tension of the muscle groups may remain unaltered for several seconds. Relaxation occurs more gradually than after a tetanic stimulation of the motor nerve.

7. *Successive Induction.*—This term applies to the facilitation
which one reflex exerts upon another immediately following.
It may be positive or negative. For example, the scratch
reflex is augmented by successive stimulation at different
points, as when an insect crawls over the skin. The cough
reflex is augmented by successive stimulation of irritant
vapours and the presence of an artificial airway or endotracheal tube.

8. *Rebound.*—If stimulation of an afferent nerve induces inhibition, augmentation of an excitatory reflex may occur when

Reflex Action, *continued.*

the inhibitory stimulus is withdrawn. An example of this phenomenon is the clonus which may occur after stretching a tendon, when a series of inhibitions and rebounds occurs.

9. *Irradiation.*—As the strength of an afferent stimulus is gradually increased, a progressively greater number of motor neurons becomes involved. Additional muscle groups take part in the reflex response. For example, stimulation of cough reflexes during light anæsthesia may result in spread of the motor response to other muscle groups, so that trunk muscles and limb muscles contract as the whole body takes part in the effector response.

10. *Reciprocal Inhibition.*—Reflex excitation of a muscle group is almost always accompanied by reflex inhibition of tone of the antagonists. Reflex inhibition has the same general characteristics as reflex excitation.

11. *Fatigue.*—Repeated stimulation may fatigue a reflex arc. For example, an endotracheal tube may be tolerated after the passage of time, even though the depth of anæsthesia remains unaltered.

12. *Susceptibility to Anæsthetic Drugs.*—During light planes of anæsthesia some reflex mechanisms are more easily elicited. For example, Stage II of anæsthesia has been called " the stage of uninhibited response ".* Vomiting is more likely to occur. Masseter spasm and ankle clonus readily occur in light planes of anæsthesia.

With deepening planes of anæsthesia reflex mechanisms are modified or obtunded. In deep anæsthesia many reflexes are abolished. The order of disappearance of certain reflexes is a guide to the depth of anæsthesia.

Pain.—

VARIETIES OF NERVE-FIBRE.—There are three main types of nerve-fibre† :—

A Fibres : All medullated somatic nerve-fibres of various diameter (1–20 μ). Rate of conduction rapid. Skeletal motor fibres, touch, proprioceptor, and some pain and thermal fibres. A fibres may be subdivided into α, β, γ, and δ. α are largest and most rapidly conducting, δ fibres smallest and slowest conducting. The larger fibres develop more current at each node to stimulate the next node. The smallest fibres are most easily affected by drugs. Local analgesic agents block some of the larger fibres before all of the smaller fibres. But if the concentration of local analgesic is kept low enough, all the small fibres will be blocked without affecting the larger fibres. Local analgesics block fibres in the order : C fibres, δ fibres, γ fibres, β fibres, α fibres, and recovery occurs in the reverse order.‡

---

* Mushin, W. W., in *General Anæsthesia,* 1959 (Ed. Evans, T. F., and Gray, T. C.), Vol. I, Ch. 12. London : Butterworths.
† Erlanger, J., and Gasser, H. S., *Amer. J. Physiol.,* 1924, **70**, 624.
‡ Nathan, P. W., and Sears, T. A., *J. Physiol.,* 1961, **157**, 565, and **164**, 375 ; and *Anæsthesia,* 1963, **18**, 467.

B Fibres : Medullated autonomic fibres, i.e., pre-ganglionic fibres, e.g., white rami. Diameter 1–3 μ.

C Fibres : Non-medullated fibres, both somatic and autonomic. All post-ganglionic sympathetic motor fibres (grey rami) and some pre-ganglionic. Some afferents convey pain and heat sensation. Diameter less than 1 μ. Visceral afferents are C fibres. Compression blocks A fibres before C fibres, while local analgesics block C fibres before A fibres.

Pain is carried in C fibres and δ fibres. The former conduct at 2 m./sec., the latter at up to 40 m./sec.

Anoxia lowers threshold of pain fibres. Stimulation of C fibres may cause a fall in blood-pressure.

The smaller the fibre the slower the conduction rate, and the more easily will local analgesic drugs produce a block. Cold slows the rate of impulse conduction.

PATHWAYS OF PAIN.—

1. FROM SKIN AND SUPERFICIAL STRUCTURES.—There is a network of fibres among the epithelial cells but no specialized receptor organs. Recent work distinguishes two separate pathways:—

   a. *The Lemniscal System.*—The first neuron passes up the sensory nerve to relay in the dorsal horn of the spinal cord. The cell body lies in the posterior root ganglion. The second neuron crosses to the other side within two to four segments to ascend in the lateral spinothalamic tract which terminates in the lateral nucleus of the thalamus. The third neuron passes through the internal capsule to reach the post-central gyrus of the cortex.

   b. *The Extra-lemniscal System.*—Fibres leave the spinothalamic tract to relay in the reticular formation, and are finally distributed to the cerebral hemispheres by the diffuse thalamo-cortical projection.

   Both systems appear to be virtually independent of one another below the level of the cerebral cortex. Both systems are interrupted by anterolateral chordotomy which is effective in the surgical relief of pain.

2. FROM MUSCLES, TENDONS, BONE.—The nervous pathways are the same, though the segmental innervation of these structures does not necessarily correspond with that of the overlying skin.

3. VISCERAL PAIN.—Transmitted *with* the sympathetic nerves through the sympathetic chain and white rami communicantes to the posterior root ganglia. The visceral afferent distribution is as follows :* The heart and aorta, T.1–T.5 ; The gall-bladder, T.4–T.10 ; The liver, T.6–T.10 ; The pancreas, T.6–T.10 ; The small intestine, T.8–T.11 ; The cæcum and appendix, T.10–T.12 ; The colon to the splenic flexure, T.11–L.1 ; The splenic flexure to the rectum, L.1–L.2 ; The adrenals, T.10–L.2 ; The kidneys, T.11–L.2 ; The ureters, L.1–L.3 ; The urinary bladder, T.11–L.2 ; The uterus, T.11–L.2.

* Mitchell, G. A. C., *The Anatomy of the Abdominal Nervous System*, 1953, pp. 120–3. Edinburgh and London : E. & S. Livingstone.

Pain, *continued.*

4. There is evidence that afferent C fibres are carried in the sympathetic nerves, and that they may ascend in the paravertebral sympathetic chain to enter the cord at levels which do not correspond with the somatic segments. It has been suggested that this pathway would explain tourniquet pain, pain from direct stimulation of the sciatic nerve, and phantom limb pain which may arise during an otherwise successful subarachnoid block.*

A careful distinction should be drawn between conscious feeling of pain and motor reaction to a painful stimulus. The integrity of the cerebral cortex is necessary for the full appreciation of pain. Motor reactions to painful stimuli may occur in decorticate animals and in anæsthetized man. It is postulated that pain produced by a thermal stimulus to skin differs neurologically from that caused by tibial pressure.†

AUTONOMIC‡ NERVOUS SYSTEM

Thoracico-lumbar Outflow (Sympathetic§).—This consists of a series of connector cells in the intermediolateral horn of grey matter, together with their connector fibres which are B type fibres, white and medulated. As they travel to peripheral ganglia, they are called pre-ganglionic. They synapse at these peripheral ganglia with excitor cells, which in their turn give off fibres which are of course post-ganglionic and usually are non-medullated and grey in colour. These run to the viscera and are C type fibres. Both of these are efferent.

The afferent neurons of the viscera are not strictly autonomic, although their fibres travel with autonomic fibres. Each travels from end-organs in the viscera, has a cell station in a ganglion of the posterior root, and sends a central process into the grey matter.

Anatomically the sympathetic outflow extends from the first thoracic to the second or third lumbar segments of the cord. In each segment the connector cells in the intermediolateral horn send off fibres which leave with the anterior nerve-roots. The fibres travel across the subarachnoid and extradural spaces, form part of the mixed spinal nerve and the anterior primary ramus, and then as *white rami* join the corresponding paravertebral ganglion of the sympathetic chain. Here they may end, synapsing with an excitor cell and being continued as a post-ganglionic fibre, or may pass, uninterrupted, through the ganglion to synapse with an excitor cell in a collateral ganglion (abdomen) or other paravertebral ganglion (e.g., superior cervical ganglion). In the thoracic region each white ramus measures about 1 cm. in length ; this increases to 2–3 cm. in the lumbar region.

* de Jong, R. H., and Cullen, S. C., *Anesthesiology*, 1963, **24**, 628.
† Robson, J. G., and others, *Ibid.*, 1965, **26**, 31.
‡ Term first used by J. N. Langley in 1898.
§ Term first used by Danish anatomist, J. B. Winslow (1669–1760), in 1732.

Craniosacral Outflow (Parasympathetic*).—Fibres leave in the 3rd, 7th, 9th, and 10th cranial nerves. The last is important to the anæsthetist, as it is not blocked by spinal analgesia. Stimulation of the vagal nerve-endings, e.g., in the stomach during gastrectomy, results in discomfort to a conscious patient, an effect removed by the infiltration of a local analgesic into the paraœsophageal tissues near the cardia.

Sacral fibres leave the cord with the 2nd, 3rd, sometimes 4th, sacral nerves. They leave in the cauda equina, and after the anterior sacral rami have passed through the anterior sacral foramina the white rami are given off. As pelvic nerves or nervi erigentes, one on each side, they do not pass through the sacral sympathetic chain, but run direct to the hypogastric ganglia and thence to the walls of the pelvic viscera. Their post-ganglionic or excitor fibres are given off from cells in the walls of the genitalia, bladder, and rectum. They cause contraction of the hollow viscera, relaxation of sphincters, and vasodilatation. In addition, visceral afferents travel with these nerves.

Ganglia.—

LATERAL GANGLIA.—This is the sympathetic chain and is composed of three cervical, eleven thoracic, four lumbar, and four sacral ganglia. There are also intermediate ganglia near the paravertebral sympathetic chain, the rami communicantes, and the anterior roots. These are not removed in surgical sympathectomy and may account for some of the bad results of what is in effect an incomplete operation. The chain receives white rami from T.1 to L.2, while from it every one of the spinal nerves receives a grey ramus communicans, which is composed of excitor or post-ganglionic fibres. One sympathetic ganglion may give off several grey rami. The grey rami carry pilomotor and vasomotor impulses, and secretory impulses to the sweat-glands. They reach their destinations via spinal nerves (each nerve receives a grey ramus) and blood-vessels. The inferior cervical and 1st thoracic ganglia unite to form the stellate ganglion at the level of the 7th cervical vertebra, posterior to the subclavian artery. In the neck, the chain of ganglia lies anterior to the transverse processes on the deep fascia covering the longus colli and longus capitis muscles. The thoracic ganglia lie anterior to the heads of the ribs ; the lumbar ganglia, irregular in shape, number, and position, lie in front of the anterolateral aspect of the bodies of the lumbar vertebræ. Certain pre-ganglionic fibres (connector) do not relay in the sympathetic chain ganglia ; from the 5th thoracic to the 2nd or 3rd lumbar segment, they pass directly as splanchnic nerves to the cœliac plexus, where excitor cells are placed and from where post-ganglionic fibres are distributed to the abdominal viscera. The cœliac plexus receives, in addition to the sympathetic connector fibres, fibres from the right vagus and the phrenic. It is continued downwards in the retroperitoneal, pre-aortic region, where it becomes the hypogastric plexus. Each pre-ganglionic (connector) fibre synapses with over a score of excitor or post-ganglionic neurons.

---

* Term first used by British physiologist, J. N. Langley, in 1905.

Ganglia, *continued.*

COLLATERAL GANGLIA.—Example, the cœliac.

TERMINAL GANGLIA.—Auerbach's myenteric (1862) and Meissner's submucosal (1864) plexuses in the walls of the gut.

Distribution of Vasoconstrictor Fibres.—Sudomotor fibres travel with vasomotor fibres.

HEAD.—Pre-ganglionic fibres arise in the lateral horn cells of 1st and 2nd thoracic segments. They leave in corresponding white rami and ascend in sympathetic trunk to synapse in the stellate and superior cervical ganglia. Post-ganglionic fibres (grey rami) go : (1) From the stellate ganglion to the vertebral nerve, a plexus surrounding the vertebral and basilar arteries. (2) From the superior cervical ganglion to the internal carotid, external carotid, and middle meningeal arteries. (3) To cervical plexus. (4) To the last four cranial nerves.

PARASYMPATHETIC.—Vasodilator nerves leave the brain with the 7th nerve and, at geniculate ganglion, enter the greater superficial petrosal nerve from which fibres travel with the internal carotid artery and its branches.

ARM.—Pre-ganglionic fibres arise in lateral horn cells of 2nd to 7th thoracic segments (some authorities say T.3 to T.7 ; others, T.5 to T.9). They travel in the anterior roots, mixed spinal nerves, and corresponding white rami and ascend in the sympathetic trunk to the middle cervical, stellate, and 2nd and 3rd thoracic ganglia. Post-ganglionic fibres pass up the chain to the stellate ganglion and middle cervical ganglion, from which, as grey rami, some go to the axillary artery and some to the brachial plexus and thence to vessels of arm. There may be a small grey ramus, the nerve of Kuntz, coming from the 2nd thoracic sympathetic ganglion direct to the lowest trunk of the brachial plexus, via the 1st thoracic nerve, so by-passing the stellate ganglion. A similar nerve described by Kirgis and Kuntz connects the 2nd and 3rd thoracic nerves. Hence to block all vasoconstrictors of arm there must be block of the 2nd and 3rd thoracic ganglia. If the stellate ganglion alone is blocked, Kuntz's nerve is missed ; if brachial plexus alone is blocked, fibres going to the axillary artery escape.

THORACIC AND ABDOMINAL WALL.—Pre-ganglionic fibres arise in lateral horn of corresponding segment of cord, leave in white rami, synapse in ganglia of sympathetic chain, and post-ganglionic fibres are thence distributed to spinal nerves as grey rami.

LEG.—Pre-ganglionic fibres arise in lateral horn cells of T.10 to L.2, pass out with anterior roots and white rami to corresponding ganglia, and descend in sympathetic chain to synapse with cells in L.1–3 ganglia for upper part of limb, and with cells in L.4 and 5 ganglia for lower part of limb. From these lumbar ganglia post-ganglionic fibres pass as grey rami to the nerves of the lumbar and sacral plexuses. The third lumbar ganglion is of practical importance as it sends a grey ramus to the fourth lumbar nerve and hence to the inner side of the foot via the femoral and saphenous nerves.

Blocking of the 2nd and 3rd ganglia interrupts sympathetic impulses to whole of limb. Blocking of the 1st lumbar ganglion on each side will cause temporary sterility ; extirpation will produce permanent sterility in the male.

Work by Kinmonth (1952)* would tend to show that the proximal parts of neither the brachial nor the femoral arteries have much vasoconstrictor nerve-supply. If this is correct, interruption of vasoconstrictor impulses is unlikely to relieve spasm due to trauma, embolism, or thrombosis of this part of their courses. Instead the local application of 2·5 per cent papaverine or of a local analgesic solution is of greater use.

THORAX.—Pre-ganglionic fibres from T.1 to T.6, passing in sympathetic chain to upper five thoracic ganglia and lower, middle, and upper cervical ganglia, where they synapse. Post-ganglionic fibres are the three cardiac nerves from the cervical ganglia to the cardiac plexus, which also receives post-ganglionic fibres direct from the upper five or six thoracic sympathetic ganglia. The efferent fibres to the lungs come from T.2 to T.6 or T.7 and synapse in the stellate and upper thoracic ganglia from which fibres pass to the posterior pulmonary plexus. The œsophagus derives its nerve-supply from T.4 to T.6.

VISCERAL AFFERENT FIBRES carrying pain from the heart and aorta (T.1–T.5) accompany the cervical and thoracic cardiac nerves and enter the cord via the white rami of the upper five thoracic nerves, to have their cell stations in the corresponding posterior root ganglia.

The thoracic part of the sympathetic trunk usually consists of ten or eleven ganglia and their connecting fibres, which lie anterior to the heads of the ribs, behind the pleura in the upper part, but on the sides of the vertebral bodies in the lower part.

ABDOMEN.—Pre-ganglionic fibres from T.5 to L.2. These pass through the ganglia of the sympathetic chain to form the three splanchnic nerves. Synapse occurs in cœliac (solar) plexus, from which post-ganglionic fibres reach the viscera with the arteries.

The sympathetic system probably contains vasodilator fibres, e.g., to blood-vessels of muscle, but vasodilatation is mainly humoral.

VISCERAL AFFERENT FIBRES from the alimentary canal and its offshoots travel with the splanchnic nerves, entering the cord on their way to the posterior root ganglia, via the white rami, from the 5th thoracic to the 2nd lumbar nerves.

Motor fibres to the alimentary canal travel with the splanchnic nerves.

Branches of the phrenic join the cœliac plexus (Hovelaque, 1927), as also do twigs from the right vagus.

Afferent Side of the Autonomic System.—There are afferent autonomic pathways carrying painful impulses from the viscera and probably from the limbs,† with cell stations in the posterior

---

* Kinmonth, J. B., *Brit. med. J.*, 1952, **1**, 59.
† de Jong, R. H., and Cullen, S. C., *Anesthesiology*, 1963, **24**, 628.

Afferent Side of the Autonomic System, *continued*.

root ganglia of the spinal nerves. They are similar to somatic afferent fibres—are not divided into pre- and post-ganglionic neurons. The long peripheral fibres travel from plexuses in the viscera with sympathetic fibres through grey and white rami to posterior roots. While the majority of these afferent fibres are medullated and larger in size than the efferent fibres, some are non-medullated. All the fibres enter the cord between T.1 and L.3, except those from the bladder, rectum, prostate, cervix uteri, and lower colon, which pass to the cord via nervi erigentes.

Physiology of Autonomic System.—The thoracico-lumbar outflow, the sympathetic, produces widespread diffuse effects. It activates the body for defence and is catabolic.

The craniosacral outflow, the parasympathetic, produces localized effects and is anabolic. When an organ is innervated by both systems they are antagonistic in effect.

The cranial parasympathetic supplies the heart and the gut with its outgrowths ; thus it is motor and secretory to the alimentary canal and constrictor to the pupil (3rd cranial nerve via ciliary ganglion and short ciliary nerves). The sacral parasympathetic is a mechanism for emptying, i.e., motor for bladder, rectum, and erection of penis. The sacral sympathetic, on the other hand, causes contraction of the smooth muscle in the bladder neck, prostate, and seminal vesicles ; inhibition of peristalsis in the lower colon ; contraction of internal anal sphincter ; and vasoconstriction.

All the vasomotor fibres of the body leave the cord between T.1 and L.3, and all inhibitory nerves of gut arise from the same region ; thus paralysis of this part of the cord will result in total vasomotor paralysis with low blood-pressure and contraction of the alimentary canal. (Paralytic ileus may be due to sympathetic preponderance and may sometimes be cured by blocking of the anterior roots.)

FUNCTIONS OF SYMPATHETIC SYSTEM.—

1. Inhibitory fibres to smooth muscle of alimentary canal and constrictor fibres to the sphincters.
2. Vasoconstrictor fibres to vessels.
3. Some vasodilator fibres to vessels.
4. Accelerator and augmentor fibres to the heart.
5. Secretory fibres to sweat-glands.
6. Pilomotor fibres.
7. Dilator fibres to bronchial tree.
8. Dilator fibres to coronary vessels.
9. Constrictor fibres to the spleen.
10. Dilator fibres to the pupil.
11. Secretory fibres to the adrenal gland (medulla).
12. Inhibitory fibres to bladder wall and constrictor fibres to internal urinary sphincter ; fibres to other pelvic viscera.

Paravertebral block is an easy way of blocking the vasoconstrictors to the limbs, especially as in the upper limb, Horner's syndrome (first thoracic, stellate ganglion) gives objective evidence of success. In addition, vasoconstrictor impulses can be removed by : (a) ganglionic blocking agents, (b) reflex heating (if arm is heated, leg vessels dilate and vice versa), (c) general anæsthesia, especially halothane.

CHEMICAL TRANSMISSION OF NERVE IMPULSES.—In 1905 T. R. Elliot suggested that adrenaline might be one transmitter of the nervous impulses in the autonomic system.* Bacq proposed noradrenaline as the transmitter rather than adrenaline.† Loewi established the chemical transmission theory firmly in 1921,‡ showing, with Dale, that there are two chemical transmitters.

In the autonomic nervous system, excitation is transmitted from pre- to post-ganglionic nerves by acetylcholine, while the post-ganglionic terminations liberate acetylcholine (cholinergic fibres) or noradrenaline or adrenaline (adrenergic fibres). All parasympathetic post-ganglionic fibres are cholinergic and most sympathetic post-ganglionic fibres are adrenergic (exceptions, fibres to sweat-glands and to vasodilators).

1. ADRENERGIC.—Adrenaline and noradrenaline are liberated at nerve-endings of adrenergic nerves (Barger and Dale, 1910).§ Noradrenaline is formed from tyrosine, which is first converted to DOPA, then under the influence of decarboxylase to dopamine, and then by β-oxidase to noradrenaline. The major portion of noradrenaline is found in the storage granules in the adrenergic nerve terminals, bound in an inactive form, but in equilibrium with a readily available pool from which it is released by nerve impulses. Recent evidence‖ suggests that the nerve-fibre may first release acetylcholine which then releases noradrenaline. This action of acetylcholine is nicotine-like and not muscarine-like and so is not abolished by atropine. Bretylium and guanethidine may act by blocking this action of acetylcholine so that it cannot liberate noradrenaline. Adrenaline and noradrenaline are destroyed in the body, the first step in the process being due to the action of the enzyme o-methyl transferase. Post-ganglionic sympathetic fibres are adrenergic. Exceptions to this are those supplying sweat-glands and those carrying vasodilator fibres, which are cholinergic. The adrenal medulla and the terminations of the post-ganglionic fibres of the thoracico-lumbar (sympathetic) division of the autonomic system produce neurohormones simulating adrenaline and noradrenaline and also store them from the blood-stream. Reserpine and guanethidine (ismelin) reduce the amount of noradrenaline in the sympathetic post-ganglionic fibres.

Two kinds of receptors are described:¶ Alpha and beta. Alpha receptors (mostly excitatory): sites where vasoconstriction, uterine contraction, and contraction of nictitating

* Elliot, T. R., *J. Physiol.*, 1905, **32**, 401.
† Bacq, Z. M., *Ann. Physiol.*, 1934, **10**, 467.
‡ Loewi, O., *Pflüg. Arch. ges. Physiol.*, 1921, **189**, 239; translated in 'Classical File' ,*Survey of Anesthesiology*, 1967, **11**, 506.
§ Barger, G., and Dale, H. H., *J. Physiol.*, 1910, **41**, 19.
‖ Burn, J. H., *Brit. med. J.*, 1961, **1**, 1623.
¶ Ahlquist, R. P., *Amer. J. Physiol.*, 1948, **153**, 583.

Physiology of Autonomic System, *continued.*

membrane are produced. Stimulated by adrenaline and noradrenaline. Blocked by phenoxybenzamine. *Beta receptors* (mostly inhibitory): sites where vasodilatation, bronchial dilatation, uterine inhibition, and cardiac stimulation occur. Stimulated by adrenaline and isoprenaline. Blocked by propranolol.

2. CHOLINERGIC (acetylcholine).—These include all nerve-fibres which release acetylcholine at their terminals.

a. Pre-ganglionic parasympathetic fibres which end, like pre-ganglionic sympathetic fibres (*d*), in autonomic ganglia. (Nicotine-like action.)

b. Post-ganglionic parasympathetic fibres. (Muscarine-like action. Muscarine was isolated in 1869 by Schmiedeberg and Koffe from *Amanita muscaria.*)

c. Post-ganglionic sympathetic fibres to sweat-glands (anatomically sympathetic, but functionally cholinergic), and vasodilators (antidromic fibres in posterior nerve-roots supplying skeletal muscle).

d. Pre-ganglionic sympathetic fibres (the receptor organs being in the sympathetic ganglia), including the splanchnic fibres to the medulla of the adrenals. (Nicotine-like action.)

e. Motor fibres are also cholinergic, impulses being inhibited by curare.

f. Certain neurons within the central nervous system.

Effects of Drugs on Autonomic System.—

1. Sympathomimetic drugs, e.g., adrenaline, ephedrine, methyl amphetamine, noradrenaline, methoxamine, phenylephrine, and metaraminol.

2. Adrenergic blocking agents ; *alpha* receptors are blocked by agents such as ergotoxine, dibenamine, and phenoxybenzamine. *Beta* receptors are blocked by propranolol. Propranolol can be used in treatment of angina, cardiac arrhythmias,* and in pre-operative control of phæochromocytoma. Methyldopa interferes with biosynthesis of catecholamines. Guanethidine and reserpine cause depletion of stores of catecholamines. Other blocking agents are phentolamine (rogitine), benzodioxanes (piperoxan), and tolazoline (priscol) alpha blockers.

3. Parasympathomimetic drugs (Dale, 1914, was the first to use this name);† e.g., acetylcholine; the anticholinesterases, e.g., neostigmine, edrophonium, physostigmine.

Acetylcholine has a muscarinic action corresponding to parasympathetic stimulation consisting of : (*a*) Increased tone of gastro-intestinal tract ; (*b*) Increased tone of urinary tract ; (*c*) Increased tone of bronchi ; (*d*) Relaxation of sphincters ; (*e*) Increased glandular secretion (e.g., salivary and bronchial glands) ; (*f*) Vasodilatation ; (*g*) Bradycardia ; (*h*) Constriction of the pupil. Atropine paralyses these effects. After muscarinic action has been paralysed by atropine larger doses of

---

* Payne, J. P., and Senfield, R. M., *Brit. med. J.*, 1964, **1**, 603 ; and Johnstone, M., *Brit. J. Anæsth.*, 1964, **36**, 224.
† Dale, H. H., *J. Pharmacol.*, 1914, **6**, 147.

acetylcholine cause a nicotinic effect, (a) stimulation of auto-nomic ganglia, (b) stimulation of voluntary muscle fibres, (c) stimulation of adrenaline secretion by adrenal medulla, the classic nicotinic effect of pharmacology. The nicotinic action can be abolished by larger doses of nicotine and by quaternary ammonium compounds, e.g., curare.

4. The cholinergic blocking drugs—the antagonists of acetylcholine acting on :—
   a. The autonomic ganglia : drugs antagonizing its nicotinic action, e.g., nicotine in excess, tetraethyl ammonium halides, hexa-methonium, trimetaphan, and halothane.
   b. The striated myoneural junction, e.g., tubocurarine, suxa-methonium.
   c. The plain muscle, glands, and heart : drugs antagonizing the muscarinic effects of acetylcholine, e.g., atropine, hyoscine, and their synthetic congeners.

THE CARDIOVASCULAR SYSTEM

Cardiac Rhythm.—
SINO-ATRIAL NODE.—Situated at the junction of the superior vena cava and the free border of the right atrial appendage, extending down the sulcus terminalis for 2 cm. These fibres normally initiate the heart-beat and are called the *pacemaker.*

ATRIOVENTRICULAR NODE.—Situated at the posterior and right border of the interatrial septum near the mouth of the coronary sinus.

BUNDLE OF HIS.—Composed of Purkinje fibres. Runs upwards from the atrioventricular node to the posterior margin of the membranous part of the interventricular septum and then forwards below it. It divides into two branches to left and right ventricles.

The conducting system is supplied by parasympathetic and sympathetic nerves. The sino-atrial node receives its main supply from the right vagus, the atrioventricular node from the left vagus.

EFFECT OF ELECTROLYTES.—Calcium ions cause an increase in the force of contraction. Excess interferes with relaxation of the muscle and the heart finally stops in systole. Potassium ions cause increasing relaxation of the heart, which eventually stops in diastole.

Blood-pressure.—
MAINTENANCE OF BLOOD-PRESSURE.—The blood-pressure is the pressure of blood on the arterial walls, the systolic blood-pressure being the maximal pressure during propulsion of blood, the diastolic pressure the minimal pressure occurring at the end of diastole. The difference between them is the pulse pressure. Depends on : (1) Force of the heart ; (2) Peripheral resistance ; (3) Volume of blood ; (4) Viscosity of blood ; (5) Elasticity of arterial walls.

The basic causes of low blood-pressure are :—
   1. Fall in cardiac output due to diminished venous return.
   2. Fall in cardiac output due to diminished cardiac action.

Blood-pressure, *continued.*

3. Fall in peripheral vascular resistance due to vasodilatation.

After induction of general anæsthesia there is a rapid onset of vasodilatation, due to: (1) A direct depressive action of the agent on the vasomotor centre, and (2) Direct action on the vessels. Later on, vasoconstriction is seen, especially in prolonged operations, and is an attempt at circulatory readjustment to maintain blood-pressure.

CAROTID AND AORTIC REFLEXES AND CIRCULATION.—

Pressoreceptors, when stimulated by increase in pressure inside artery or from outside its walls, cause bradycardia, vasodilatation, and a lowered blood-pressure (reflex stimulation of vagal nucleus). When, instead, decrease of pressure occurs, tachycardia, vasoconstriction, and raised blood-pressure result (Hering, 1927). There is also an increase in adrenaline secretion. The carotid sinus syndrome is seen in subjects with an irritable carotid sinus reflex mechanism. It comprises bradycardia and hypotension, and is seen when the sinus is stimulated from without by pressure or electricity (e.g., during operations on the neck). It can be prevented by injection of procaine around the sinus.

Chemoreceptors, when stimulated by oxygen lack or carbon dioxide excess, produce vasoconstriction and rise in arterial blood-pressure. The chemoreceptors are also stimulated by lobeline, acetylcholine, cyanide, nikethamide, and nicotine. Acetylcholine is probably the chemical mediator within the carotid body.

Afferent arc of these reflexes is via sinus nerve, a branch of the glossopharyngeal nerve ascending between internal and external carotid arteries ; also the aortic nerve, via the vagus, which also has connexions with the superior cervical sympathetic ganglion.

Efferent arc is via vagus to heart and via sympathetic outflow to vasomotor mechanism.

VASOMOTOR MECHANISM.—The circular involuntary muscular walls of the vessels, first described by Kölliker in 1849, are supplied by two types of nerve-fibres, excitatory and inhibitory, constrictor and dilator. These vasomotor nerves, first described by Claude Bernard in 1852, arise from cells in the lateral column of the grey matter of the cord from the first thoracic to the second or third lumbar segments.

Vasomotor nerves arrive at the arteries of the limbs in two ways :—

  a. A proximal innervation to the brachial and femoral arteries carried in fibres around these vessels.

  b. A distal innervation carried to the periphery by somatic nerves such as the median and sciatic, which receive them via grey rami.

Acute hypoxia, cerebral anæmia, and increase of intracranial pressure all stimulate the vasomotor centre directly and raise the blood-pressure.

VENOUS PRESSURE.—Central venous pressure can now be readily measured (Chapter XXXIII). It is affected by a multiplicity of factors of which the most important are venous tone and the amount of blood in the venous system. Venous tone is increased during hyperventilation and I.P.P.V. and in heart failure. Catecholamines cause increased venous tone as does a raised Pco_2 (central effect). Venous tone is diminished by drugs such as thiopentone, ganglion-blocking agents, histamine, and nitrites and by a raised arterial Pco_2 (peripheral effect). Central venous pressure falls with hæmorrhage or hypovolæmia, and rises when there is overloading of the circulation.

Normal central venous pressure lies between 30 and 100 mm. H_2O (2–8 mm. Hg) and values over 200 mm. H_2O are usually indicative of heart failure. Normal right atrial pressure is zero.

BLOOD-VOLUME.—The normal blood-volume for an adult may be taken as 30 ml. per lb. in males and 27·5 ml. per lb. in females. These values should be reduced by 10 per cent in the short obese subject and in the elderly patient.[*] Otherwise it can be obtained from formulæ, depending on height and weight,[†] or from nomograms. A simple rule where body-weight and height are in reasonable proportions is to take blood-volume as 7·7 per cent of body-weight.[‡] About half the total blood-volume is contained by the systemic venous system.

Regulation of Heart's Action.—

THE CARDIAC OUTPUT.—Determined by :—

1. THE VENOUS RETURN, which depends on the following : (a) The venous tone, controlled by vasomotor nerves, and chemical factors such as blood oxygen and carbon dioxide tension, and amount of adrenaline and noradrenaline in the blood. (b) Negative pressure in the thorax during inspiration. (c) Contraction of the diaphragm causing descent and squeezing out of blood from the abdomen towards the heart. (d) Tone of the arterioles, capillaries, etc., which may contain much or little blood. (e) Gravity. (f) Muscular activity (muscle pump).

2. THE FORCE OF THE HEART-BEAT, which depends on : (a) The length of the myocardial fibres at the beginning of each systole. (b) The duration of diastole, more blood being pumped out, the longer the diastole. (c) The coronary blood-flow, depending on the aortic diastolic pressure and coronary tone (vagus is vasoconstrictor, sympathetic is vasodilator). Chemical influences are also important, e.g., circulating catechol amines, blood oxygen and carbon dioxide tensions.

3. THE CARDIAC RATE.

4. THE ARTERIAL BLOOD-PRESSURE and TOTAL PERIPHERAL RESISTANCE, which influence the output of the heart through effect on venous return and venous pressure.

RATE.—Bears a relationship to the basal metabolic rate.

Increased by :—
   Muscular exercise, because of venous (auricular) reflex of Bainbridge, rise of carbon dioxide tension, etc.

---

* Albert, S. N., *Blood Volume*, 1963. Springfield, Ill.: Thomas.
† Nadler, S. B., Hidalgo, J. V., and Bloch, T., *Surgery*, 1962, **51**, 224.
‡ Scholar, H., *Amer. Heart J.*, 1965, **69**, 701.

Regulation of Heart's Action, *continued.*

Emotional excitement.

Environmental temperature.

Hæmorrhage and surgical shock.

Fever, cardiac arrhythmias, and hypoxia.

Also increased during digestion.

Decreased during sleep.

Influenced by action of : (1) Nerves ; (2) Chemical agents.

1. NERVES.—

a. The *vagus* is inhibitory (Weber, 1845). Pre-ganglionic efferent fibres originate in dorsal nucleus of vagus in the grey matter of the lower medulla and end in the intrinsic cardiac ganglia. Post-ganglionic fibres travel along the coronary vessels. Its cardiac branches are given off in the neck just below the origin of the superior laryngeal nerve, but a few leave nerve in thorax, so vagal stimulation there can cause vagal cardiac effects. Vagal effect is abolished if high doses of atropine are given, e.g., 4 mg., after which rate rises to 150 per minute. Fibres from right vagus terminate near sino-atrial node, those from left vagus near atrioventricular node. Vagi exert their effect on auricular muscle, and not directly on the ventricle. Slowing or stopping of ventricles is indirect effect due to auricular slowing or to block of conduction along A-V bundle.

Increased vagal activity can lead to generalized cardiac depression, with decrease in rate of pacemaker, force and duration of systole reduced, and refractory period lessened. On conductive system, vagal stimulation causes successively : (1) Increase in P–R interval ; (2) Partial A-V block ; (3) Complete A-V block. Bundle-branch block has also been demonstrated.

By decreasing cardiac output, hypotension may be caused, but this in turn, through the aortic and carotid sinus mechanisms, will result in sympathetic stimulation and tachycardia—the so-called vagal escape phenomenon.

On the heart, vagal effect is more pronounced than sympathetic effect.

b. The *sympathetic* is accelerator and augmentor, an effect described by von Bezold in 1863. Fibres arise in the lateral horn cells of the cord in segments T.3–4 and as white rami enter the lateral sympathetic chain, from which post-ganglionic fibres pass to the heart directly via the thoracic cardiac nerves. The superior cervical cardiac nerve is efferent only. The superior, middle, and inferior cervical sympathetic cardiac nerves pass behind the carotid sheath and on each side are joined by the superior cervical cardiac branches of the vagus and pass to the superficial and deep cardiac plexuses. In addition to accelerator efferent fibres the thoracic cardiac nerves contain afferent pain fibres. Other cardiac pain fibres run in the inferior and middle cervical cardiac sympathetic nerves. Stimulation of sympathetic causes increase in the rate and force of both auricles and ventricles, unlike vagal stimulation which affects only the auricles and junctional tissues. Arrhythmias, even ventricular fibrillation, may follow sympathetic stimulation, especially during chloroform, cyclopropane, halothane, or trichloroethylene anæsthesia.

Sympathetic stimulation causes : (1) Dilatation of coronary vessels ; (2) Increase of heart-rate ; (3) Increase of force of contractions ; (4) Facilitation of conduction ; (5) Increased irritability.

Sensation is through afferents having their cell stations in the posterior root ganglia of the upper thoracic nerves —especially the second—and running in the cervical (especially the middle and inferior) and thoracic cardiac nerves, thence entering cord via white rami of the upper six thoracic nerves.

Reflex slowing can be caused by pressure on the lateral part of the eyeball (oculocardiac reflex) or by stimulation of nasal branches of the fifth nerve.

Stimulation of afferent fibres of the vagus in the lungs, as by a too strong chloroform vapour, can cause reflex inhibition of heart, while stimulation of the structures in the abdomen can cause extrasystoles or bradycardia independently of anæsthesia.

c. *The sinus and aortic nerves* : Increase of pressure in the carotid and aortic sinuses produces bradycardia. Decrease of pressure here produces tachycardia.

Marey's Law :* Heart-rate is inversely proportional to blood-pressure.

The Bainbridge Reflex (the auricular or venous reflex):† Heart-rate varies directly with venous return to auricle. Pressoreceptors are present in the walls of the right auricle and the venæ cavæ. Afferent pathways of this reflex are probably in the vagus.

The regulation of cardiac rate and output occurs mainly through reduction of vagal tone.

2. CHEMICAL AGENTS.—May be: (a) drugs, (b) inorganic constituents, (c) acid metabolites.

a. Atropine antagonizes acetylcholine liberated at postganglionic terminals and so depresses vagal action. Muscarine has opposite effect, imitating that of vagal stimulation. Pilocarpine, physostigmine, acetylcholine are similar in effect to muscarine, and their action is antagonized by atropine. Nicotine first stimulates, then depresses, the vagus ; it affects the ganglion cells.

b. Beta-adrenergic blocking agents (e.g., propranolol) block sympathetic cardiac accelerator fibres and allow unopposed vagal action. Complete denervation by drugs is

* Marey, E. J. *La Circulation du Sang*, 1876-8. Paris: Masson
† Bainbridge, F. A., *J. Physiol.*, 1915, **50**, 65.

Regulation of Heart's Action, *continued.*

obtained when big doses of atropine and propranolol are given. The heart then beats at its own intrinsic rate.

c. Calcium increases contractility and prolongs systole. Potassium reduces contractility and prolongs diastole. Sodium is necessary for both systole and diastole.

d. Carbon dioxide and lactic acid have effect on cardiac and vasomotor centres and heart muscle. Mild excess causes tachycardia ; gross excess, bradycardia.

Causes of Rapid Pulse-rate.—(1) A speeding up of the normal sinus rhythm. (2) Supraventricular paroxysmal tachycardia. (3) Ventricular paroxysmal tachycardia (not usually more than 180 per minute). (4) Auricular fibrillation. (5) Auricular flutter.

The Coronary Circulation.—(1) Nerves : The sympathetic causes dilatation, the vagus constriction, when stimulated. The coronary vessels fill during cardiac diastole ; during systole the blood is squeezed out of them. (2) Blood Gases : A reduced oxygen tension increases blood-flow ; a raised carbon dioxide tension increases it. (3) The Aortic Blood-pressure : A fall in this reduces coronary flow. (4) The Cardiac Output : If this increases, the coronary flow also increases. (5) In Exercise : Violent exercise causes a great increase in blood-flow. (6) Drugs : (*a*) Constrictors; pituitrin; (*b*) Dilators; adrenaline, xanthine derivatives, papaverine, atebrine, ephedrine, amyl nitrite, sodium nitrite, nitroglycerin.

RESPIRATORY SYSTEM
Anatomy

Nasal Cavities.—Immediately inside the nostril is the nasal vestibule, lined by skin giving rise to hairs for coarse filtration, and sebaceous glands. The limen nasi, a ridge, separates the vestibule from the nasal cavity proper which is lined by mucous membrane, and extends from before backwards. This anteroposterior direction must be remembered when passing nasopharyngeal and naso-tracheal tubes. The upper part of the nasal cavity is olfactory, the lower part respiratory, in function. On the lateral walls are the superior, middle, and inferior conchæ or turbinate bones, with a meatus beneath each.

OPENINGS INTO THE NOSE.—

a. The sphenoidal sinus opens into the spheno-ethmoidal recess, above the superior turbinate.

b. The posterior ethmoidal sinuses open into the anterior part of the superior meatus.

c. The anterior and middle ethmoidal sinuses open into the middle meatus.

d. The frontal sinus opens into the middle meatus via the fronto-nasal duct.

e. The maxillary sinus opens into the middle meatus.

f. The nasolacrimal duct opens into the inferior meatus.

g. The pharyngotympanic (Eustachian) tube opens from the naso-pharynx, just behind the inferior concha. Nasal tubes have been blamed for originating infection in the accessory nasal sinuses and the middle ear. If such infections are established, nasal intubation may be contra-indicated.

Mucosa covering the conchæ is capable of great vascular engorgement during infection and allergic reactions, and following paralysis of the sympathetic chain in the neck (Guttman's sign), with production of narrowing of the nasal cavities. Vascularity is decreased by the application of adrenaline, noradrenaline, cocaine, ephedrine, and benzedrine ; also by cold air.

The nasal septum is formed by the perpendicular plate of the ethmoid, by the vomer, and by the septal cartilage.

Narrowing of the nasal cavities may be : (a) Congenital. (b) Due to bony deformities, e.g., nasal spurs, deviated septum. (c) Due to engorgement of the mucosa. Obstruction may be caused by foreign bodies, blood-clot, mucus. The degree of patency can be assessed by : (a) Inspection with a headlamp and speculum ; (b) Getting the patient to breathe deeply through the nose while occluding one nostril at a time.

The nasal cavities open into the nasopharynx, which is continuous with the oropharynx. Food and air pass through the oropharynx. When food passes the superior laryngeal aperture, the latter is reflexly closed, while inspiration is inhibited.

Squamous epithelium lines the oropharynx ; ciliated epithelium lines the respiratory part of the nasal cavities and the nasopharynx.

The nerve-supply of the nasal cavity :—

    1. The anterior ethmoidal (from nasociliary nerve).
    2. The anterior superior dental nerve (from the maxillary nerve).
    3. The long and short sphenopalatine nerves.
    4. The nerve of the pterygoid canal.
    5. The greater palatine and nasal branches of the sphenopalatine ganglion.
    6. The olfactory nerve supplies the upper part of the nasal cavity.

    The septum is supplied by the long and short sphenopalatine nerves from the sphenopalatine ganglion (second division of Vth) and the anterior ethmoidal nerve (nasociliary branch of first division of Vth)

Larynx.—The organ of voice, connecting the pharynx with the trachea. It extends from the root of the tongue to the trachea. (*Fig.* 1.) It is opposite the 3rd, 4th, 5th, and 6th cervical vertebræ ; higher in children and in females. The average length is 44 mm. in males, 36 mm. in females. Its transverse diameter 43 mm. in males, 41 mm. in females ; its anteroposterior diameter averages 36 mm. in males and 26 mm. in females. It is covered by the depressor muscles of the hyoid bone, by the thyroid gland, and by the cricothyroid muscles. Composed of the following cartilages, joined together by ligaments : thyroid, cricoid, two arytenoid, two corniculate (Santorini), two cuneiform (Wrisberg), and the epiglottis.

The cavity of the larynx extends from the superior laryngeal aperture to the lower border of the cricoid cartilage, when it is continuous with the trachea. The *piriform fossa* is a recess, on each side,

Larynx, *continued.*

bounded by the aryepiglottic fold medially and the thyroid cartilage and thyrohyoid membrane laterally. Beneath its mucosa lie twigs of the internal laryngeal nerve, which are blocked when local analgesic solutions are applied to this area.

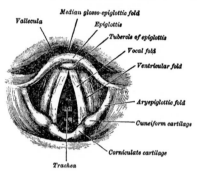

Fig. 1.—A laryngoscopic view of the interior of the larynx.
(From 'Gray's Anatomy', by kind permission of Professor T. B. Johnston.)

The depression between the dorsum of the tongue and the epiglottis is divided into two valleculæ by the glosso-epiglottic fold. The epiglottis is not essential for swallowing, breathing, or phonation.

The entrance to the larynx or superior laryngeal aperture is wider in front than behind, and slopes downwards and backwards. Bounded anteriorly by the epiglottis; laterally by the aryepiglottic folds containing the two small nodules on each side, cuneiform anteriorly and the corniculate posteriorly; posteriorly, by the arytenoids. This view is seen by laryngoscope. The vestibule of the larynx is the superior part of the cavity of the larynx and extends from the aryepiglottic folds to the vestibular folds. Each of the latter is a ridge formed by the vestibular ligament and extends from the angle of the thyroid cartilage anteriorly, backwards along the side cavity of the larynx to the cuneiform cartilage. The vestibular folds are the false cords, the space between them is the rima vestibuli, while a depression on the side-wall of the larynx between the vestibular fold and the vocal fold (false and true cords) is the saccule of the larynx.

The vocal cords (folds) stretch from the thyroid cartilage anteriorly, to the arytenoid cartilage of the corresponding side, posteriorly. The space between the cords is the glottis. It is bounded in front by the intermembranous part of the cords—the vocal folds; behind, by the intercartilaginous part. The glottis is the narrowest part of the larynx in adults and measures about one inch from front to back; less in females. In children, the narrowest part is found just below the cords at the cricoid ring.

The shape and width of the glottis vary with phonation and respiration and the tone of the muscles controlling it. When these are spastic, the glottis is obliterated.

Muscles.—The extrinsic muscles are the thyrohyoid and the sterno-thyroid and the inferior constrictor of the pharynx. The first elevates, the second depresses the larynx, while the third constricts the pharynx.

The intrinsic muscles: Those which open and close the glottis: (1) The posterior (open) and lateral cricoarytenoids (close) ; (2) The interarytenoid.

Those controlling the tension of the cords : (1) The cricothyroids lengthen cords ; (2) The posterior cricoarytenoids ; (3) The thyroarytenoids shorten cords ; (4) The vocales.

Those controlling the inlet of the larynx : (1) The aryepiglottics ; (2) The thyroepiglottics. In laryngeal spasm both the true and the false cords are adducted.

The lowest part of the pharynx extends from the vocal folds or cords to the cricoid cartilage. The mucosa of the upper part of the larynx is lined by squamous cells like the oropharynx ; the part above the cords, the ciliated epithelium ; the cords are covered by a thin layer of mucosa, closely adherent to them, white in colour. The lower larynx is lined by ciliated epithelium with mucous glands and goblet cells.

Intubation has been held responsible for the causation of small innocent tumours of the cords.* Traumatism in this area can result in dysphagia, dysphonia, and a husky voice. Duration is seldom more than a day or two.†

Nerve-supply of larynx is from the *vagus*. *The superior laryngeal branch* arises near the base of the skull and divides into the *internal laryngeal nerve*, the sensory nerve of the larynx, down to the level of the vocal cords and the *external laryngeal nerve* which supplies the cricothyroid muscle and the inferior constrictor of the pharynx, the division taking place slightly below and anterior to the greater cornu of the hyoid bone. The external laryngeal nerve may be injured during the ligation of the superior thyroid vessels, during thyroidectomy, such injury causing temporary huskiness of voice. Injury to the recurrent laryngeal nerve on one side from division or bruising causes huskiness, with fixation of one cord midway between abduction and adduction—the cadaveric position. With bilateral recurrent laryngeal nerve paralysis, there is respiratory difficulty as the cords lie together, and speech is difficult; the *recurrent laryngeal branch* supplies the remaining intrinsic muscles and the mucosa below the cords. It carries abductor and adductor fibres, but if it is injured abductor paralysis is greater than adductor paralysis. The superior aspect of the epiglottis is supplied by the *glossopharyngeal nerves*. Its stimulation, as by Macintosh's laryngoscope, does not, therefore, produce laryngo-spasm. The inferior surface of the epiglottis gets its nerve-supply

---

* Young, N., and Stewart, S., *Brit. J. Anæsth.*, 1953, **25**, 1.
† Jackson, Chevalier, *Anesthesiology*, 1953, **14**, 425.

Larynx, *continued.*

from the internal laryngeal. The sensory supply from the larynx ascends in the internal and recurrent laryngeal nerves to the nucleus solitarius in the medulla.

1. Incomplete paralysis of a recurrent laryngeal nerve causes paralysis of abductor before that of adductor muscles and results in respiratory distress from adduction of cords when bilateral.

2. Complete paralysis of recurrent nerve inactivates both abductor and adductor muscles. The tensing action of the cricothyroid muscles maintains cords in adduction.

3. Paralysis of both recurrent and superior laryngeal nerves together produces the cadaveric position. The cadaveric position, also seen when relaxants have had a full effect, is characterized by the cords being midway between abduction and adduction ; they are not under tension due to cricothyroid paralysis.

Topical analgesia of the larynx may, by paralysing twigs from the external laryngeal nerves going to the cricothyroids, cause both an alteration in the appearance of the cords and an alteration in the voice.

Movements of Larynx.—During inspiration, cords abduct. On expiration they return nearly to the midline. On phonation they actually touch.

Arteries are the laryngeal branches of the superior and inferior thyroid arteries. They accompany the nerves.

Trachea.—Length about 10–11 cm. It commences at the level of the 6th cervical vertebra and ends by dividing into the two bronchi at the carina, level of the 5th thoracic vertebra. Anteriorly, this corresponds with the junction of the body and manubrium sterni —the angle of Louis. In children, carina is on a level with 3rd costal cartilage. The diameter of the trachea is about $\frac{3}{4}$–1 in. (1·5–2 cm.) ; much smaller in the child, e.g., 3 mm. during first year of life, and thereafter the diameter in mm. corresponds to the age in years.

Abnormal narrowing of the trachea in its middle third, making it difficult to introduce a tube of adequate size, has been reported.[*] Abnormal dilatation of the trachea has also been described in a patient with chronic bronchial infection, treated by tracheostomy and insertion of a cuffed tube.[†]

Tracheostomy should be done below the first tracheal ring, to avoid stenosis.

Right Bronchus.—Shorter (1 in.—2·5 cm.) and more in line with the trachea than the left bronchus ; enters the right lung opposite the 5th thoracic vertebra ; greater in diameter than left bronchus —hence a long tube or a foreign body passes more easily into it than into the left bronchus. The main upper lobe bronchus, given off within $\frac{3}{4}$ in. of the commencement, arises above the

---

[*] Stewart, S., and Pinkerton, H. H., *Brit. J. Anæsth.*, 1955, **27**, 492.
[†] Robbie, D. S., and Feldman, S. A., *Ibid.*, 1963, **35**, 771.

right pulmonary artery and was accordingly called the eparterial bronchus. The opening is on a level with the carina. The right bronchus leaves the trachea at an angle of 25° from the vertical.

Left Bronchus.—Narrower, but longer, than the right. Length before dividing into upper and lower lobe bronchi, 2 in. (5 cm.). The aorta arches over it and it enters the left lung opposite the 6th thoracic vertebra. It leaves the trachea at an angle of about 45° from the vertical. In children under 3 years, the right and left main bronchi branch from the trachea at equal angles.*

Bronchial Tree.—This subdivides progressively, the terminal bronchioles being the last twigs. Air is carried by these twigs to the ' leaves ' of the tree, where active interchange of gases is carried on. The respiratory unit is composed of respiratory bronchioles, alveolar ducts and sacs, and pulmonary alveoli. These, together, form a primary lobule. Air in the alveoli is separated from blood in the capillaries by two thin layers of cells, the capillary and alveolar walls. Estimated area of respiratory epithelium—55 sq. metres, or over twenty-five times the skin area.

Elastic tissue is plentiful right down to the alveoli. Recoil of the lung during expiration is probably due to this tissue.

Muscular fibres surround the air-ducts, stopping at the end of the respiratory bronchioles. When strongly contracted they have a sphincter-like action: they also produce a peristaltic movement, to remove irritating foreign matter. This peristaltic action is depressed by morphine.

Bronchial arteries from the thoracic aorta (one for the right, two for the left lung) supply as far as the end of the respiratory bronchioles. Distal to this, blood-supply is from the pulmonary artery. There is a communication between the bronchial arteries and the pulmonary veins. The bronchial vessels are more under neural control than the pulmonary vessels.

Nerve-supply.—

Each vagus passes to the back of the hilum and is joined by branches of the sympathetic, from the second to the fourth or fifth thoracic sympathetic ganglia, and also from the inferior and middle cervical ganglia, forming the anterior and posterior pulmonary plexuses. From there, fibres go to the main bronchi and the pulmonary artery, and their branches.

Motor nerves are from the vagus (constriction) and the sympathetic (dilatation). Afferent impulses pass along the vagus.

Lining mucosa is of ciliated epithelium. The cilia have a wavelike motion resembling a cornfield in a breeze. The direction is upwards towards the mouth. The respiratory bronchioles are devoid of cilia, but above this level they are plentiful and act most efficiently. They are not under nervous control. Action depressed by general anæsthetics, sedatives, and cold air. Warm air stimulates ciliary action.

Dilatation of Bronchi.—Is seen : (1) On inspiration (together with lengthening) ; (2) On inhalation of cold air or gas ; (3) On

---

* Adriani, J., and Griggs, P., *Anesthesiology*, 1954, **15**, 466.

Bronchial Tree, *continued.*

inhalation of oxygen-rich atmospheres ; (4) Following hyper-capnia ; (5) Due to stimulation of the sympathetic or depression of the parasympathetic nerves ; (6) From depressant action of anæsthetic drugs on bronchial musculature, e.g., ether and halothane ; (7) After local analgesics sprayed into bronchi and trachea ; (8) After atropine and hyoscine; (9) After pethidine; (10) After aminophylline ; (11) After bromethol ; (12) After adrenaline and ephedrine ; (13) After procaine (intravenous) ; (14) After phenothiazine derivatives ; (15) After mid or high extradural or subarachnoid block causing hypotension which acts on baroceptors in the aortic and carotid sinuses, producing reflex bronchodilatation.

Constriction of Bronchi.—Is seen : (1) On expiration (together with shortening)—this narrowing causes a diminution of anatomical dead space ; (2) Following inhalation of hot gas or air (when a to-and-fro CO_2 absorber is used, the inhaled atmosphere can become quite hot) ; (3) Following stimulation of vagi and depression of sympathetic nerves (tone probably depends more on vagi than on sympathetic) ; (4) Following irritation of mucosa of tracheobronchial tree ; (5) Following morphine ; (6) Following paraldehyde (slight) ; (7) Following barbiturates and cyclopropane ; (8) Due to histamine (note possibility of histamine release when curare is used) ; (9) Following neostig-mine ; (10) After pituitary extract.

Inadequate suppression of reflex response because anæsthesia is too light is a potent cause of bronchospasm.

Cyclopropane constricts reflexly, but locally depresses bronchial muscle. Vinesthene and ethyl chloride first constrict, but later, by sympathetic stimulation, dilate bronchi. Strong ether and chloroform vapour given suddenly constrict, but if concentration is increased gradually, both cause dilatation because of sympathetic stimulation and muscular depression. The pulmonary arteries, like the arteries of the heart and the brain, are more under the influence of circulating metabolites than under neurogenic influence.

Foreign material, mucus, blood, etc., is removed from the bronchial tree by : (1) Cilia ; (2) Peristaltic bronchiolar contractions ; (3) Cough reflex.

Cough reflex is most active in the region of the carina. A short sharp inspiration is followed by an explosive expiration against a closed glottis which suddenly opens, allowing the built-up pressure to be released and with it carrying upwards the foreign material. Spasm of whole bronchial tree often accompanies spasm of larynx. Bronchi are very irritable in pulmonary tuberculosis, relatively insensitive in bronchiectasis.

Movements of Bronchial Tree during Respiration.—During inspiration, the bronchial tree elongates, while the smaller bronchi and bronchioles dilate during inspiration and contract during expiration. These movements are passive, unlike the peristaltic movement which helps to remove foreign bodies.

International Nomenclature accepted by the Thoracic Society.*—
THE RIGHT LUNG.—

    A. THE RIGHT UPPER LOBE.—(1) The apical bronchus and segment. (2) The posterior bronchus and segment. (3) The anterior bronchus and segment.

    B. THE MIDDLE LOBE.—(4) The lateral bronchus and segment. (5) The medial bronchus and segment.

    C. THE LOWER LOBE.—(6) The apical bronchus and segment. (7) The medial basal (cardiac) bronchus and segment. (8) The anterior basal bronchus and segment. (9) The lateral basal bronchus and segment. (10) The posterior basal bronchus and segment.

THE LEFT LUNG.—

    A. THE LEFT UPPER LOBE.—Upper division bronchus.—(1) The apical bronchus and segment. (2) The posterior bronchus and segment. (3) The anterior bronchus and segment. The lingula (lower division) bronchus. (4) The superior bronchus and segment. (5) The inferior bronchus and segment.

    B. THE LEFT LOWER LOBE.—(6) The apical bronchus and segment. (8) The anterior basal bronchus and segment. (9) The lateral basal bronchus and segment. (10) The posterior basal bronchus and segment.

    The absence of a medial basal (cardiac) segment involves omission of segment (7) in left lung.

Lungs.—Each lung is invaginated from the hilum into the closed sac of the pleura.

The pleura consists of a pulmonary part, a parietal part, and a diaphragmatic part. The two layers are in contact, gliding one over the other, the potential space being at a negative pressure of about 5 mm. Hg below atmospheric pressure. The elastic lungs collapse if air or liquid is admitted to the pleural cavity. If the thorax is laid open on both sides, a pressure of 7 mm. Hg in the trachea is necessary to keep the lungs from collapsing. The right lung has three lobes, the left lung two.

The lung roots are opposite the bodies of the 5th, 6th, and 7th thoracic vertebræ, and each contains the bronchus, pulmonary artery, two pulmonary veins, bronchial vessels, lymph-glands, etc.

When the pulmonary arteries are occluded, nutrition of lungs is partially carried out by bronchial arteries at normal systolic pressure (pulmonary B.P. being lower than general systemic B.P.). By extensive production of collateral bronchial arteries, respiratory function, too, can be partly taken over if pulmonary vessels become acutely or chronically occluded.

Expansion of the lungs at birth is due to descent of the diaphragm, which enlarges the thoracic cavity. The lung follows the thoracic walls while it becomes filled with air at atmospheric pressure. The lung is thus stretched out and remains so throughout life. The pressure on the pleural surface is less than the pressure on the alveolar surface.

Respiratory movements occur in utero, and are easily depressed by sedatives, anæsthetics, and carbon dioxide deficit.

---

* *Thorax*, 1950, **5**, 3, 222.

Lungs, *continued.*

If the free flow of air into and out of the lungs is obstructed, the intrapulmonary pressures will be increased beyond the normal range (from −40 mm. Hg to +40 mm. Hg) so that blood will be compressed from the auricles and great veins into the venous system, producing venous oozing—true engorgement with blue venous blood. Cyanosis unassociated with respiratory obstruction is not accompanied by increased venous engorgement.

Movements of Respiration.—The lungs are passive, air is moved as by a bellows, the walls of the thoracic cage causing the lungs to expand. During a normal inspiration, the chest capacity is increased by a combination of descent of the diaphragm and spreading of the ribs. The negative pressure in the intrapleural space is made greater and is responsible for expanding the underlying lungs.

During *inspiration* all thoracic movements are increased, although not equally. The diaphragm and the anterior parts of the ribs and sternum have the greatest movement, so the parts of the lungs in contact with these areas expand the most. During inspiration the lung roots move downwards, forwards, and laterally, while the trachea is stretched.

Anteroposterior diameter of the thorax is increased by the sternum and upper ribs moving upwards and forwards by the action of the external intercostals: the first and second ribs are immobilized by their attached scalene muscles and so become fixed points.

Transverse diameter is increased by the widening of the subcostal angle by the diaphragm and lower ribs.

Length of the thoracic cavity is increased by the diaphragmatic descent, which pushes down the abdominal viscera. In light anæsthesia this pushing down may cause inconvenience to the surgeon.

Expiration is chiefly passive, except when forced. The expanded thorax tends to resume its former position, the elastic lungs recoil, while the diaphragm is drawn up by the negative pressure in the thorax. The elastic recoil of lung tissue equals 5 mm. Hg on expiration, and 10 mm. Hg on inspiration. In forced expiration, the abdominal muscles contract and so help to push up the diaphragm, while the internal intercostal muscles help to depress the ribs.

Tracheal Tug.*—This is a sharp downward movement of the larynx and trachea on inspiration. Theories of causation include :—

1. Loss of tone of the sternocostal fibres of the diaphragm, the crural fibres contracting to produce a sharp pull on the central tendon transmitted to the mediastinal structures (Harris).

---

* Harris, T. A. B., *The Mode of Action of Anæsthetics*, 1951. Edinburgh and London : E. & S. Livingstone; Campbell, E. J. M., *The Respiratory Muscles and the Mechanics of Breathing*, 1958. London : Lloyd-Luke ; and Scurr, C. F., *Anæsthesia*, 1962, **17**, 111.

2. Loss of tone of the stabilizing muscles of the larynx (mylohyoid, stylohyoid, styloglossus, posterior belly of digastric). Unopposed action of diaphragm pulls larynx downwards (Campbell).

Tracheal tug may be associated with the following clinical states:—

1. Deep anæsthesia (Guedel Stage III, Plane 3 or 4).
2. Depression of the central nervous system by opiates, barbiturates, etc., and by moribundity.
3. Incomplete decurarization. This may be disputed if ventilation is adequate.
4. " Neostigmine-resistant curarization."*
5. Respiratory obstruction.
6. Post-operative pneumothorax.
7. Collapse and shock.
8. Respiratory acidosis.
9. Metabolic acidosis.

Muscles of Respiration.—

Inspiration: The diaphragm, the external intercostals, the scaleni (fixing ribs 1 and 2), the quadratus lumborum (fixing ribs 11 and 12).

Accessory muscles used in forced inspiration : trapezius, serratus anterior, latissimus dorsi, pectorales, sternomastoid—they all raise the upper part of the thoracic cage.

Expiration: In normal breathing this is passive. In forced breathing the muscles of the anterolateral abdominal wall, and the transversus thoracis.

THE DIAPHRAGM.—A dome-shaped partition between the thorax and the abdomen. The peripheral part is muscular, while the central tendinous part forms the muscles' insertion. The apex of the dome is at the level of the 5th rib in the mid-clavicular line, the right side a little higher than the left. Both are higher with the patient supine than standing. With the patient lying laterally the dome on the lower side falls slightly. The dome moves from 1·5 to 10 cm. depending on the depth of breathing. It is responsible for 60 per cent of the air breathed during deep inspiration.

Sternal part arises by two slips from the back of the xiphisternum ; the costal part from the inner surfaces of the lower six ribs and their cartilages, interdigitating with the transversus abdominis.

Vertebral part arises from the medial and lateral arcuate ligaments, and median arcuate ligament, connecting the crura.

Medial arcuate ligament (lumbocostal arch) covers the psoas major and extends from the body of the 1st or 2nd lumbar vertebra to the transverse process of the 1st lumbar vertebra.

Lateral arcuate ligament arches over the quadratus lumborum and extends from the tip of the transverse process of the 1st lumbar vertebra to the lower margin of the 12th rib.

The crura blend with the medial arcuate ligaments, the right arising from the anterior aspect of the bodies of the first

* Hunter, A. R., *Brit. med. J.*, 1956, **2**, 919.

Muscles of Respiration, *continued.*

three lumbar vertebræ, the left from the first two lumbar vertebræ. Fibres arching over the aorta from the crura form the median arcuate ligament.

The central tendon, trefoil in shape, receives the muscle-fibres from these various origins. It is adherent to the pericardium, above.

NERVE-SUPPLY.—The phrenic and the lower six intercostal nerves (which are sensory).

The phrenic nerve comes from C.4 with twigs from C.3 and C.5. It descends to the root of the neck, lying anterior to the scalenus anterior, which it crosses from lateral to medial.

The right nerve on leaving the medial side of the scalenus anterior passes between the cervical pleura behind and the innominate vein.

The left nerve leaves the scalenus anterior higher up, crosses the first part of the subclavian artery, and comes to lie between the pleura and the subclavian and the innominate vein.

The nerve then, on each side, descends in the thorax towards the diaphragm along the medial surface of the pleura in front of the root of the lung.

The phrenic nerve contains sensory and motor fibres in the proportion of 1 : 9, the former coming from the central parts of the diaphragm, the peripheral part getting its sensory supply from the lower intercostal nerves.

If both phrenic nerves are cut and lungs are functioning well, there is little respiratory difficulty.

Upper surface is related to the pericardium in the middle, and the right and left pleura on each side.

Under-surface is related to peritoneum, liver, right and left kidneys and adrenal glands, the stomach, and the spleen. The pancreas, kidneys, and adrenals lie on the crura.

OPENINGS.—There are three large and several smaller ones.

1. The aortic : opposite the 12th thoracic vertebra slightly to left of midline. Transmits the aorta, azygos vein, and thoracic duct.

2. The œsophageal : opposite the 10th thoracic vertebra. It is reinforced by a muscular slip from the right crus. Transmits the œsophagus and the vagi. Slightly to left of middle line. The left vagus is anterior, the right vagus posterior. The portal and systemic venous systems communicate at this point.

The cardiac sphincter is made up of* :—

   a. A muscular sphincter at the lower end of the œsophagus.
   b. Mucosal folds which plug the lumen.
   c. A valve-like arrangement due to the oblique angle at which the œsophagus joins the stomach.
   d. A muscular sling from the diaphragm which acts as a pinchcock on the lower end of the œsophagus (probably not important except where the other mechanisms are interfered with, e.g., hiatus hernia).

---

* *See also* article by Brown, H. G., *Brit. J. Anæsth.*, 1963, **35**, 136.

The lower 2 cm. of the œsophagus lie within the abdominal cavity and are subject to intra-abdominal pressures.*

3. The vena caval: opposite the 8th thoracic vertebra. Transmits the inferior vena cava and branches of the right phrenic nerve. Slightly to right of middle line.

The sympathetic trunk passes, on each side, behind the internal arcuate ligament.

The right crus transmits the greater, lesser, and lowest right splanchnic nerves.

The left crus transmits the greater, lesser, and lowest left splanchnic nerves and the hemiazygos vein.

The musculophrenic and the superior epigastric vessels pierce the diaphragm anteriorly.

MOVEMENTS OF DIAPHRAGM.—During inspiration, diaphragm descends and lower costal margin is raised and everted, so expanding the base of the thorax.

EXTERNAL INTERCOSTALS.—These are eleven in number on each side and extend from the tubercles of the ribs behind to a point near the costochondral junction in front; each is then continued as the anterior intercostal membrane. Fibres run downwards and forwards to the rib below and are attached to its upper border.

INTERNAL INTERCOSTALS.—These are smaller than the external muscles and are eleven in number on each side.

They extend from the sternum to the angles of the ribs and are then carried back to the vertebral column as the posterior intercostal membranes. Each passes in an upward and backward direction, from the inner surface of the rib above to the upper border of the rib below. The intercostales intimi are sometimes regarded as being parts of the internal intercostal muscles.

The two groups are supplied by the intercostal nerves and are believed to elevate the ribs and to prevent either indrawing or bulging during deep breathing. They aid inspiration but take no part in expiration.

The muscles of the anterior abdominal wall are muscles of expiration. They increase intra-abdominal pressure and draw the lower ribs inwards and downwards.

INTRAPULMONARY PRESSURE.—Pressure within the tracheobronchial tree varies between about 3 mm. Hg below atmospheric at the beginning of inspiration and about 3 mm. Hg above atmospheric at the beginning of expiration. During coughing or forced respiration, endotracheal pressures may range between −60 and +100 mm. Hg.

Respiration.—Defined as the gaseous interchange between an organism and its environment. Oxygen is absorbed and carbon dioxide excreted. External respiration takes place between the alveoli and the capillaries; internal respiration occurs in the tissue cells.

Pulmonary respiration has two phases: (1) A ventilatory phase or alternating movement of air between the atmosphere and the

Respiration, *continued.*

lung alveoli ; (2) An exchange phase, an interchange of oxygen and carbon dioxide between the alveolar air and the lung capillaries.

DIFFUSION RESPIRATION.*—The affinity of oxygen for hæmoglobin causes the amount of oxygen removed from the alveoli during apnœa to exceed the amount of carbon dioxide diffusing into the alveoli, thus reducing the alveolar pressure to less than atmospheric. If now a high concentration of oxygen occupies the lungs and dead space and if the circulation is adequate there will be a continuous inflow of oxygen—diffusion respiration. The terms *apnœic oxygenation*† and *aventilatory mass flow* have also been used.‡ Adequate oxygenation can be maintained by insufflation of a large volume of oxygen through a fine catheter (to allow for the blow-off of surplus oxygen), in the complete absence of respiratory movements. CO_2, however, accumulates at a rate of about 3·8 mm. Hg per minute, but does not reach an intolerable§ tension in the alveoli for 30–40 minutes.

Symbols used in Respiratory Physiology.‖—

1. GASES.—

PRIMARY SYMBOLS (Large capitals).—

V = gas volume.

P = gas pressure.

F = fractional concentration in a dry gas phase.

f = respiratory frequency (breaths per unit time).

D = diffusing capacity.

R = respiratory exchange ratio.

A dash above any symbol indicates a mean value:—

E.g., $\overline{P}$ = mean gas pressure.

A dot above any symbol indicates a time derivative:—

E.g., $\dot{V}$ = gas volume per unit time.

SECONDARY SYMBOLS (Small capital letters).—

I = inspired gas.

E = expired gas.

A = alveolar gas.

T = tidal gas.

D = dead space gas.

B = barometric.

STPD = 0° C., 760 mm. Hg.

BTPS = body temperature and pressure, saturated with water vapour.

ATPS = ambient temperature and pressure, saturated with water vapour.

* Draper, W. B., and Whitehead, R. W., *Anesthesiology*, 1944, **5**, 262; and *Ibid.*, 1947, **8**, 524.
† Nahas, G. G. *Fed. Proc.*, 1956, **15**, 134.
‡ Bartlett, R. G., and others, *J. appl. Physiol.*, 1959, **14**, 97.
§ Enghoff, H., Holmdahl, M., and others, *Nature*, 1951, **168**, 830; and Payne, J. P., *Acta anæsth. scand.*, 1962, **6**, 129.
‖ Comroe, J. H., Forster, R. E., Dubois, A. B., Briscoe, W. A., and Carlsen, E., *The Lung*, 2nd ed., 1962. Chicago: Year Book Publishers Inc.

2. BLOOD.—
    PRIMARY SYMBOLS (large capitals).—
        Q = volume of blood.
        C = concentration of gas in blood phase.
        S = percentage saturation of Hb with O_2 or CO.
    SECONDARY SYMBOLS (small letters).—
        a = arterial blood.
        v = venous blood.
        c = pulmonary capillary blood.

3. LUNG VOLUMES.—
        V.C. = vital capacity.
        I.C. = inspiratory capacity.
      I.R.V. = inspiratory reserve volume.
     E.R.V. = expiratory reserve volume.
    F.R.C. = functional residual capacity.
      R.V. = residual volume.
    T.L.C. = total lung capacity.

EXAMPLES OF USE OF SYMBOLS.—
    P_{AO_2} = alveolar O_2 pressure.
    D_{O_2} = diffusing capacity for oxygen.
    $\dot{Q}c$ = blood flow through pulmonary capillaries per min.
    $\dot{V}_{O_2}$ = O_2 consumption per min.
    F_{ICO_2} = fractional concentration of CO_2 in inspired gas.
    P_B = barometric pressure.
    Ca_{O_2} = ml. O_2 in 100 ml. arterial blood.

Lung Function.—Simple routine tests of lung function are :—
    a. Measurement of vital capacity (*see* (6) *below*).
    b. Measurement of forced expiratory volume (*see* (19) *below*).
    c. Measurement of peak expiratory flow rate (*see* (20) *below*).

1. TIDAL VOLUME (V_T).—The volume of gas inspired or expired during each respiratory cycle (400–500 ml.).

2. INSPIRATORY RESERVE VOLUME (I.R.V.).—The maximal amount of gas that can be inspired from the normal end-inspiratory position.

3. EXPIRATORY RESERVE VOLUME (E.R.V.).—Formerly reserve or supplemental air. The maximum amount of gas that can be expired from the end-expiratory position (average 1200 ml.).

4. RESIDUAL VOLUME (R.V.).—Formerly residual air or residual capacity. The volume of gas remaining in the lungs at the end of a maximal expiration (average 1200 ml.).

5. TOTAL LUNG CAPACITY (T.L.C.).—Formerly total lung volume. The amount of gas contained in the lung at the end of a maximal inspiration (average 6000 ml.). The sum of (1) to (4) above.

6. VITAL CAPACITY (V.C.).—The maximal volume of gas that can be expelled from the lungs by forceful effort following a maximal inspiration (average 4800 ml.). The sum of (1) to (3) above.

Lung Function, *continued.*

7. INSPIRATORY CAPACITY (I.C.).—Formerly complemental air. The maximal volume of gas that can be inspired from the resting expiratory level (average 3600 ml.). The sum of (1) and (2) above.

8. FUNCTIONAL RESIDUAL CAPACITY (F.R.C.).—Formerly functional residual air. The volume of gas remaining in the lungs at the resting expiratory level (average 2400 ml.). The sum of (3) and (4) above.

9. ALVEOLAR AIR.—The air in contact with the pulmonary capillaries, which therefore carries out gaseous interchange with the blood. Expired air is a mixture of alveolar air and dead space air. The air in the lower part of the trachea at the end of expiration is for all practical purposes identical with the alveolar air.

10. DEAD SPACE VOLUME (V_D).—

   a. ANATOMICAL DEAD SPACE.—Extends from the nostrils and mouth down to, but not including, the alveoli (about 1 ml. per lb. body-weight). Reduced by tracheostomy and by endotracheal intubation by about 75 ml.

   b. PHYSIOLOGICAL DEAD SPACE.—A dynamic volume, this denotes all air not available for respiratory exchange, as when alveoli have no capillary blood-flow or when alveoli become distended. It may therefore be greater than anatomical dead space. Physiological dead space cannot be measured directly, but a value can be derived using the Bohr equation:

$$\text{Physiological dead space} = V_T \left(\frac{P_{aCO_2} - P_{ECO_2}}{P_{aCO_2}} \right),$$

   where V_T = tidal volume, P_{aCO_2} = tension of CO_2 in arterial blood, and P_{ECO_2} = tension of CO_2 in expired air.

   c. Extra dead space produced by anæsthetic apparatus, face-masks, breathing tubes, etc.

Dead space takes no part in the actual respiratory exchange. Rapid shallow breathing is therefore less efficient than slower deeper respiration for the same minute volume. The nearer the tidal volume approaches the dead space volume, the less real respiratory exchange occurs. The *effective tidal volume* is the tidal air minus the dead space.

Factors affecting dead space include*:—

   i. Tidal volume and respiratory rate.
   ii. The pattern of respiration.
   iii. Lung volume.
   iv. Pulmonary blood-flow.
   v. Body position.
   vi. Alveolar P_{CO_2}.
   vii. Changes in bronchomotor tone.
   viii. Atropine.

---

* Editorial, *Anesthesiology*, 1964, **25**, 741.

ix. General anæsthesia.

x. Hypotension.*

11. MINUTE VOLUME.—The volume of air breathed each minute. Equals the tidal air multiplied by the number of respirations per minute. The normal pulmonary ventilation is 5 to 8 litres per minute. If the minute volume is reduced, care must be taken to prevent oxygen lack, and carbon dioxide accumulation, by assisting the minute volume by intermittent positive pressure. High extradural or spinal analgesia, halothane, cyclopropane, thiopentone, or deep ether may cause a reduced minute volume, and so may muscle relaxants if respiration is spontaneous and unassisted. A minute volume which is reduced may be adequate for the patient's oxygenation, but inadequate to remove his carbon dioxide.

12. ALVEOLAR VENTILATION ($\dot{V}_A$).—This is the effective tidal volume × rate of respiration. Average values are 2·0–2·5 l. per min. per sq. metre body surface area.

13. COMPLIANCE.—The volume change produced by each unit pressure increase, expressed as litre per cm. water pressure. It varies from person to person and in the same individual in different circumstances. Normal values for a healthy young man are pulmonary compliance 0·2 l. per cm. water, thoracic cage compliance 0·2 l. per cm. water, with a total compliance of 0·1 l. per cm. water.† With an open chest, compliance is due to the lungs alone.

Elastance is the reciprocal of compliance and measures the increase in airway pressure for a given increase in volume. Average elastance is 10 cm. of water per litre of air inhaled.

14. MEAN MECHANICAL RESISTANCE.—The amount of pressure necessary to obtain a certain flow rate. Expressed as cm. of water per litre per second. Normal value from 0·6 to 2·4 cm. water per litre per sec. In emphysema there is high resistance and low compliance. Airway resistance is increased in asthma and in a wide variety of disorders where there is airway obstruction.

15. DIFFUSION.—This can now be measured and in the lungs may be impaired as a secondary factor in disease, or it may occur specifically as ' alveolar capillary block ' which has been found present in some cases of Boeck's sarcoid of the lung, beryllium granulomatosis, asbestosis, pulmonary scleroderma, alveolar cell carcinoma, sulphur dioxide poisoning, certain metastatic lung lesions, and pulmonary œdema. The test requires the use of a gas which is considerably more soluble in blood than in the alveolar-capillary membranes. Apart from oxygen, only carbon monoxide fulfils this criterion because of its combination with hæmoglobin. The rate of carbon monoxide uptake is limited by diffusion, and the uptake is measured after adding 0·2 per cent CO to inspired air.

* Eckenhoff, J. E., Enderby, G. E. H., Larson, A., Edridge, A., and Judevine, D. E., *Brit. J. Anæsth.*, 1963, **35**, 750.

† Comroe, J. H., Forster, R. E., Dubois, A. B., Briscoe, W. A., and Carlsen, E., *The Lung*, 2nd ed., 1962. Chicago: Year Book Publishers Inc.

Lung Function, *continued.*

Pulmonary diffusing capacity for CO

$$= \frac{\text{ml. CO transferred from alveolar gas to blood per min.}}{\text{mean alveolar CO pressure} - \text{mean capillary CO pressure}}.$$

Normal values range from 17 to 25 ml. per min. per mm. Hg.[*]

16. VENTILATION–PERFUSION RELATIONSHIPS. — During normal spontaneous respiration in the healthy subject, there are some variations in the ventilation–perfusion ratio between different parts of the lung.[†] These variations account for the differences in oxygen tension between alveolar gas and arterial blood. The balance is upset to a greater degree in the diseased lung. In emphysema, for example, some distended alveoli may be underperfused (increased dead space effect) and some under-ventilated alveoli may receive normal perfusion (venous admix-ture effect).[‡] The result is a rise of Pco_2 and a fall of Po_2 of the arterial blood. Temporary changes in ventilation–perfusion relationships may occur during controlled respiration in anæs-thesia,[§] and also in the post-operative phase.[||]

17. MAXIMAL BREATHING CAPACITY (M.B.C.).—The maximum volume of air that can be breathed per minute. Usually measured for 15 sec. and expressed as flow per min. Average values 120 l. per min. May be only 25 l. per min. in emphysema. A disadvantage is that it is difficult for ill or post-operative patients to carry out the test. Equals $35 \times$ F.E.V.$_1$/ sec.

18. THE VITAL SPIROGRAM.—The patient expires and inspires maximally into a specially designed spirometer. The tracing obtained in the vital spirogram has characteristics from which lung function can be deduced.

19. FORCED EXPIRATORY VOLUME (F.E.V.).—There is a close correlation between the expiratory curve of the vital spirogram and the maximal breathing capacity. The volume exhaled in a given unit of time, usually 1 sec. from the start of expiration, is recorded, and this volume known as the F.E.V.$_{1.0}$ gives an indirect measure of the M.B.C. and is easier to obtain in ill patients. A normal individual can expire 83 per cent of his vital capacity in 1 sec. Where there is an obstruction to air flow (emphysema) the F.E.V.$_{1.0}$ is reduced to a much greater degree than the vital capacity. Where there is no resistance to air flow (restricted chest movement) the F.E.V.$_{1.0}$ shows a proportional reduction to that of the V.C. These measurements can now be made easily and rapidly using a dry spirometer, the Vitalograph.

This is a simpler test than the M.B.C. and is more applicable to the conditions of the pre- and post-operative periods.

* Comroe, J. H., Forster, R. E., Dubois, A. B., Briscoe, W. A., and Carlsen, E., *The Lung,* 2nd ed., 1962. Chicago: Year Book Publishers Inc.
† West, J. B., *Brit. med. Bull.,* 1963, **19**, 53.
‡ Hugh-Jones, P., *Brit. J. Anæsth.,* 1958, **30**, 107.
§ Nunn, J. F., *Ibid.,* 1957, **29**, 540.
|| Nunn, J. F., and Payne, J. P., *Lancet,* 1962, **2**, 631.

20. PEAK EXPIRATORY FLOW RATE.—This is the steepest part of the spirometer trace of a forced vital capacity estimation. It may be conveniently measured by using the Wright peak flow-meter.* The peak flow rate is usually 4 or 5 times the M.B.C. A small whistle, which can be carried in the pocket, has also been designed for the measurement of maximum expiratory flow rate.†

21. MATCH TEST.‡—Success or failure to blow out a lighted paper match held 6 in. from a patient's wide open mouth. It is essential that the lips are not allowed to come together. Patients who can perform this test should maintain adequate ventilation after thoracic or abdominal surgery. Patients who cannot extinguish the match require further investigation before operation.

Average Composition of Air.—(In parts per hundred.)

	Inspired Air	Expired Air	Alveolar Air
Oxygen	21	16·3	14·2
Carbon dioxide	0·04	4	5·5
Nitrogen	79	80	80

Atmospheric air contains less than 1 per cent of water vapour. The lungs contain over 6 per cent of water vapour at a tension of 47 mm. Hg.

Laws of Gases.—The kinetic theory of gases postulates that the molecules of a gas in an enclosed space are constantly moving and so are constantly bumping into each other and into the walls of the enclosing space. These bumpings give rise to the pressure or tension of the gas in the space. The greater the number of molecules the greater will be the tension. Temperature increases movement and so increases tension.

1. BOYLE'S LAW (1662; Robert Boyle, 1627–1691).—The volume of a gas varies inversely with the pressure it is subjected to, the temperature remaining constant.

2. CHARLES'S LAW (1787; Jaques Alexander César Charles, 1746–1823).—At constant pressure, the volume of a gas is proportionate to its absolute temperature.

3. DALTON'S LAW OF PARTIAL PRESSURE (John Dalton, 1766–1844).—The pressure of a gas in a physical mixture of gases equals the pressure which that quantity of gas would produce were it alone. Thus the total pressure of a mixture of gases equals the sum of the partial pressures of the individual gases. The partial pressure of a gas in a mixture is proportional to its percentage by volume in the mixture.

If a liquid is exposed to a gas at a given pressure, and equilibrium is established, the pressure of the gas in the liquid will equal the pressure of the gas in contact with it.

---

* Wright, B. M., and McKerrow, C. B., *Brit. med. J.*, 1959, **2**, 1041.
† de Bono, E. F., *Lancet*, 1963, **2**, 1146.
‡ Snider, T. H., and others, *J. Amer. med. Ass.*, 1959, **170**, 1631 ; Barry, C. T., *Lancet*, 1962, **2**, 964.

Laws of Gases, *continued.*

4. HENRY'S LAW OF SOLUTION OF GASES (1803; William Henry, 1774–1836).*—With temperature remaining constant, the volume of gas going into solution in a given liquid is proportional to the partial pressure of the gas.

5. GRAHAM'S LAW OF DIFFUSION OF GASES (1831; Thomas Graham, 1805–1869).—The rate of diffusion of a gas varies inversely as the square root of its density. Important in the theory of flow-meters (*see* p. 127).

6. AVOGADRO'S LAW (1811; Amadeo Avogadro, 1776–1856).—Equal volumes of a gas under standard conditions of temperature and pressure contain equal numbers of molecules. One gram molecule of a gas occupies 22·4 l. at N.T.P. This law is used in the calculation of the amount of a volatile liquid needed to make a known percentage of vapour in air. Provided the molecular weight is known and the density of the liquid, calculation is easy as in the following example:

Let the molecular weight $= x$ and the liquid density $= y$.

x grams will occupy 22·4 l. at N.T.P.

1 gram will occupy $\dfrac{22\cdot4}{x} \times 1000$ ml. at N.T.P.

1 ml. of liquid will occupy $\dfrac{22\cdot4 \times y}{x} \times 1000$ ml. at N.T.P.

For halothane, the molecular weight is 197 and the liquid density 1·86.

1 ml. liquid halothane will therefore $= \dfrac{22\cdot4 \times 1\cdot86}{197} \times 1000$ ml.

$\backsimeq 211$ ml. at N.T.P.

It is then a matter of simple proportion to make a known percentage of vapour in air, bearing in mind that a concentration greater than the saturated vapour pressure cannot exist.

7. OSTWALD'S SOLUBILITY COEFFICIENT (1894).—The volume of a gas which dissolves in unit volume of solvent, measured under the conditions of temperature and pressure at which solution takes place.

Critical Pressure.—Pressure required to liquefy a gas at its critical temperature.

Critical Temperature.—Temperature to which a gas must be cooled before it can be liquefied by pressure.

Vapour Pressure.—Pressure exerted by molecules of a gas escaping from a liquid. The saturated vapour pressure of a volatile anæsthetic agent is important in consideration of those systems which depend on dilution of a saturated vapour (e.g., copper kettle, Halox vaporizer). Saturated vapour

---

* Henry, W. *Phil. Trans. Roy. Soc.*, 1803, **93**, 29.

pressure varies with temperature. The boiling point of a liquid is that temperature at which the saturated vapour pressure equals atmospheric pressure.

SPECIFIC GRAVITY OF A GAS.—This is the ratio of the weight of a unit volume to a similar volume of air (regarded as 1), under the same conditions of temperature and pressure. Specific gravities of gases used by anæsthetists : Halothane vapour, 6·8 ; Trichloroethylene vapour, 4·5 ; Chloroform vapour, 4·12 ; Diethyl ether vapour, 2·6 ; Ethyl chloride, 2·28 ; Divinyl ether vapour, 2·2 ; Nitrous oxide, 1·53 ; Carbon dioxide, 1·5 ; Cyclopropane, 1·46 ; Oxygen, 1·1 ; Air, 1 ; Ethylene, 0·97 ; Nitrogen, 0·96 ; Water vapour, 0·6 ; Helium, 0·13.

SOLUBILITY OF GASES IN VOLUMES PER CENT AT 38° C. AND 760 MM. HG PRESSURE.—

	Water	Plasma	Blood
Oxygen	2·37	2·3	2·3
Nitrogen	1·2	1·2	1·1
Carbon dioxide	55·5	54·1	54·1

Air at atmospheric pressure or tension exerts a pressure of 760 mm. Hg. At higher altitudes or at lower barometric pressures, percentage composition of air does not alter, but partial pressure of each gas is reduced. Barometric pressure is reduced 20 mm. Hg for each 1000 ft. increase in altitude.

Exchange of Gases in Lungs.—Diffusion is aided by differences in pressure or tension. As inspired air is sucked into the alveoli, it mixes with air already there and so its oxygen becomes diluted, its carbon dioxide increased, and water vapour added. It is the partial pressure of the oxygen (104 mm. Hg) which drives it into the blood across the pulmonary epithelium and the walls of the pulmonary capillaries as the pressure of oxygen in these capillaries is about 40 mm. Hg. The result is that oxygen tension in the capillaries rises almost to the same level as it is in the alveolar air, so that the blood leaving the lungs in the pulmonary veins approximates that of the alveolar air in its oxygen tension. The small difference in oxygen tension between alveolar air and blood in the pulmonary veins is due to uneven distribution of blood-flow and ventilation in the normal lung. The ratio of ventilation to perfusion is greater at the apex of the lung and lowest at the base of the lung when the subject is in the upright position.[*] Transfer of oxygen from alveoli to blood depends on: (1) the pressure gradient, (2) the rate of pulmonary blood-flow, (3) the solubility coefficient. Equilibrium may not be reached if (1) is affected by high altitude or (2) is affected by heavy exercise. It is also affected by changes in ventilation–perfusion ratios and by incomplete diffusion of inspired air within the terminal airways.[†]

[*] West, J. B., *Brit. med. Bull.*, 1963, **19**, 53.
[†] *See also* West, J. B., in *A Symposium of Oxygen Measurements in Blood and Tissues and their Significance* (Ed. Payne, J. P., and Hill, D. W.), 1966. p. 13. London: Churchill.

Exchange of Gases in Lungs, *continued*.

Air in the alveoli is 98 per cent saturated with water vapour (tension of 47 mm. Hg).

The following table shows the partial pressures of gases in the lungs and blood :—

	INSPIRED AIR	EXPIRED AIR	ALVEOLAR AIR	ARTERIAL BLOOD	VENOUS BLOOD
Oxygen :					
Tension in mm. Hg	159·0	116·2	104·0	100·0	40·0
Volumes per cent	20·9	16·0	15·0	19·8	15·2
Carbon Dioxide :					
Tension in mm. Hg	0·3	28·5	40·0	40·0	46·0
Volumes per cent	0·04	4·5	5·6	50·0	55·0
Nitrogen :					
Tension in mm. Hg	601·0	576·0	570·0	570·0	570·0
Volumes per cent	79·0	79·0	79·0	0·83	0·83
Water Vapour :					
Tension in mm. Hg	5·0	47·0	47·0		
Volumes per cent	0·06	0·5	0·5		

Exchange of Gases in Blood.—Again, gas passes from a zone of high to a zone of low pressure, or, in other words, the pressure gradients enable oxygen to diffuse inwards from alveolar air to capillary blood ; and carbon dioxide to diffuse in the reverse direction. The diffusion coefficient of carbon dioxide (500) is greater than that of oxygen (25–45), i.e., it diffuses twenty times as readily, so this compensates for the lower pressure gradient of this gas as compared with that of oxygen.

This slower diffusion of carbon dioxide than oxygen explains why a tidal exchange sufficient to keep the arterial oxygen level up to normal may be too small to remove adequately the carbon dioxide. This is not inconsistent with the fact that carbon dioxide passes more rapidly across the alveolar membrane than oxygen, because of its greater solubility in water.

In whole blood 0·3 volume per cent of oxygen is carried in simple solution.

In whole blood 2·5 volumes per cent of carbon dioxide are carried in simple solution.

In arterial blood 19·8 volumes per cent of oxygen are carried, the greater part combined with hæmoglobin.

In arterial blood 40–55 volumes per cent of carbon dioxide are carried, the greater part as bicarbonate.

1 g. of hæmoglobin carries 1·34 ml. of oxygen when fully saturated.

15 g. of hæmoglobin (the normal amount in 100 ml. of blood) carry 20 ml. oxygen—actually about 19·5 ml. of oxygen, saturation not being maximal. The tissues require about 250 ml. of oxygen each minute—the basal oxygen.

Oxygen Carriage in Blood.—The oxygen dissociation curve of hæmoglobin (Barcroft and Poulton, 1913),* worked out for

---

* Barcroft, J., and Poulton, E. P., *J. Physiol.*, 1913, **46**, 4.

temperature of 37° C. and CO_2 tension of 40 mm. Hg, and plasma pH of 7.40 shows the relation between the partial pressure of oxygen (abscissæ) and the percentage saturation of the hæmoglobin (ordinates) (*Fig.* 2). It shows that at 104 mm. Hg partial pressure (i.e., partial pressure of O_2 in alveoli) hæmoglobin is 97 per cent

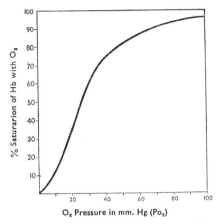

Fig. 2.—The oxygen dissociation curve of hæmoglobin.

saturated, whereas at 70 mm. Hg, hæmoglobin saturation is still 90 per cent. The dissociation curve may be altered by changes in the pH; it is shifted to the right in acidæmia and to the left in alkalæmia. Carbon dioxide increase causes a flattening of the curve to the right. An increase in temperature has a similar effect, while in hypothermia the curve is shifted to the left. Normally, oxygen in arterial blood is at a tension of 100 mm. Hg, at which hæmoglobin is 97 per cent saturated and the oxygen content is 19·8 volumes per cent, 0·3 ml. of this being dissolved in plasma. Venous blood has an oxygen tension of 40 mm. Hg and its oxygen content is 15 volumes per cent.

Results of Inhalation of Pure Oxygen.—If 100 per cent oxygen is inhaled the tension in arterial blood increases to 640 mm. Hg and hæmoglobin is fully saturated. Hæmoglobin is, however, fully saturated at an oxygen tension of a little over 300 mm. Hg. The arterial oxygen content increases from 19·8 volumes per cent to 22·0 volumes per cent, and of this increase 0·5 ml. is due to increased combination with hæmoglobin, the remainder to increased solution in plasma. As no more oxygen is used by the body, the venous blood also contains more oxygen. The saturation of hæmoglobin in mixed venous blood is 85 per cent and the partial pressure of oxygen is 55·3 mm. Hg, so after breathing pure oxygen

Results of Inhalation of Pure Oxygen, *continued.*

there is a significant increase in partial pressure of oxygen in venous blood over normal. (*See also* Chapter X.)

RESULTS OF INHALATION OF PURE OXYGEN*

	BREATHING AIR O_2 159 mm. Hg	BREATHING 100 PER CENT OXYGEN O_2 760 mm. Hg
ALVEOLAR AIR Oxygen tension	104 mm. Hg	673 mm. Hg
ARTERIAL BLOOD Oxygen tension Oxygen saturation Oxygen combined with hæmoglobin Oxygen in solution in plasma Total oxygen content	100 mm. Hg 97 per cent 19·5 ml. per cent 0·3 ml. per cent 19·8 ml. per cent	640 mm. Hg 100 per cent 20·1 ml. per cent 1·9 ml. per cent 22·0 ml. per cent
MIXED VENOUS BLOOD Oxygen tension Oxygen saturation Oxygen combined with hæmoglobin Oxygen in solution in plasma Total oxygen content	40 mm. Hg 75 per cent 15·07 ml. per cent 0·12 ml. per cent 15·19 ml. per cent	53·5 mm. Hg 85 per cent 17·19 ml. per cent 0·16 ml. per cent 17·35 ml. per cent

Arterial blood contains an additional 2·2 vol. per cent, a rise of more than 10 per cent, after inhalation of pure oxygen. This represents about 50 ml. O_2 transported to the tissues per minute, or about one-fifth of requirements.

Results of Breathing Oxygen at Increased Pressure.—The amount of oxygen carried in simple solution in the plasma increases significantly as the pressure is raised. This results in an increased rate of diffusion of oxygen into underperfused and hypoxic tissues (*see* Chapter X).

Oxygen Toxicity.—(*See* Chapter X.)

Stored Blood.—The oxygen and carbon dioxide dissociation curves in blood stored in an acid-citrate dextrose medium are shifted to the left. Such changes are progressive with storage and the effect lasts several hours after transfusion. As a result of these shifts the blood of an anæmic patient may for a few hours after transfusion be unable to release as much oxygen as it did before.†

Passage of Oxygen from Blood to Tissues.—Oxygen passes from alveolar air to blood by diffusion. The saturation of hæmoglobin depends on the oxygen tension of the blood or the amount of oxygen in solution in the plasma : this latter depends on the oxygen pressure in the alveoli.

Arterial blood containing a high oxygen content in solution, with oxyhæmoglobin in equilibrium with it, comes into contact through the capillary epithelium in the tissues with fluid poor

---

* Data obtained from Comroe, J. H., Forster, R. E., Dubois, A. B., Briscoe, W. A., and Carlsen, E., *The Lung,* 2nd ed., 1962. Chicago: Year Book Publishers Inc.
† Valtis, D. J., and Kennedy, A. C., *Lancet,* 1954, **1,** 119.

in oxygen. This results in oxygen flowing across the capillary membranes so that arterial plasma and oxyhæmoglobin cease to be in equilibrium : oxygen thus passes from the oxyhæmoglobin to the plasma. The difference in partial pressure of oxygen between red cell and tissue cell causes a steady flow of oxygen from the red cells to the tissue cells.

Carriage of Carbon Dioxide in Blood.—Total amount of carbon dioxide carried in blood is about 50–60 volumes per cent. Venous blood contains 5–10 per cent more carbon dioxide than arterial blood, its carbon dioxide combining power being greater.

The tension of carbon dioxide in arterial blood and alveolar air is 40 mm. Hg. In venous blood at rest it is 46 mm. Hg. Carbon dioxide output, about 200 ml. per minute.

Carbon dioxide is carried in blood in three forms :—

1. As dissolved carbon dioxide in plasma—from 3 per cent to 5 per cent. The amount of pre-dissolved carbon dioxide determines the partial pressure of the gas and it is this difference in partial pressure of carbon dioxide which accounts for carbon dioxide transport. The partial pressure of carbon dioxide in the body cell is greater than that in the capillary blood, so the gas passes into the blood. The partial pressure of carbon dioxide in mixed venous blood is 46 mm. Hg and is greater than that in the alveoli, which is 40 mm. Hg, so the gas passes from the blood to the alveoli and is exhaled.

2. As carbamino compounds formed by the combination of carbon dioxide with NH_2 groups from hæmoglobin in the red cells—called carbamino-hæmoglobin or carbhæmoglobin. Carbon dioxide also combines on a small scale with plasma proteins. Reduced hæmoglobin can take up more carbon dioxide in this way than oxyhæmoglobin. The formation and dissociation of carbamino compounds is a rapid process. About 2 per cent to 10 per cent of the total blood carbon dioxide is carried in this way, the amount depending on the degree of oxygenation of hæmoglobin.

3. As bicarbonate, chiefly of sodium and potassium. Mainly in plasma, but also in the corpuscles. Whenever carbon dioxide enters or leaves the blood-stream, an interchange of ions takes place across the membranes of the red cells, which have the property of admitting negatively charged anions such as bicarbonate and chloride ions, while holding back positively charged cations such as sodium and potassium ions. About 80–90 per cent carried in this way.

When in the tissue capillaries carbon dioxide enters the red cells, it rapidly combines with water with the help of carbonic anhydrase, an enzyme, to form carbonic acid H_2CO_3. (This enzyme likewise accelerates the splitting up again into water and carbon dioxide ; it is not present in plasma, only in the red cells.) H_2CO_3 being a stronger acid than reduced hæmoglobin, attracts base from the latter, in the form of potassium (hæmoglobin exists chiefly as potassium hæmoglobinate). Thus $KHCO_3$ is formed. Bicarbonate ions now leave the cells, while chlorine ions from the plasma take their place. Thus plasma chloride

Carriage of Carbon Dioxide in Blood, *continued.*

decreases while cell chloride and plasma bicarbonate increase. This is the so-called *chloride shift* or Hamburger phenomenon. The newly formed bicarbonate, arriving in the plasma from the cells, combines with the sodium there to form sodium bicarbonate. This sodium is set free when sodium chloride is split to enable the chloride ion to shift into the red cells, there to combine with the potassium ions. The purpose of the chloride shift is to allow some of the carbon dioxide entering the red cells to be converted into bicarbonate and in this form to be carried in the plasma.

Reverse changes occur in the lungs, the shift working the other way. Reduced hæmoglobin becomes oxyhæmoglobin and carbon dioxide is excreted into the plasma and so diffuses into the alveolar air. Reduced hæmoglobin, being a weaker acid, takes up carbon dioxide in the tissues more readily than oxyhæmoglobin. But oxyhæmoglobin when formed in the lungs liberates carbon dioxide more easily. In the lungs the relatively more alkaline reduced hæmoglobin unites with oxygen and so becomes relatively acid and thereby attracts the potassium ion from the potassium chloride, so liberating a chloride ion which diffuses out of the cells, while bicarbonate ions diffuse in. As this occurs, carbon dioxide is liberated and diffuses into the plasma and alveolar air.

In addition to transporting CO_2, sodium bicarbonate also acts as the alkali reserve, neutralizing strong acids which may enter the blood-stream. The pH of plasma depends on ratio of H_2CO_3 to bicarbonate. Breathing thus assists in the pH control of the blood.

Regulation of Respiration.—That rhythmical breathing is controlled by cells in the respiratory centre was for long the classic view of Legallois (1824) and Flourens (1842, 1858). Physiologists have tried to locate the anatomical centres in various ways—by observing the effect of section of parts of the brain, by observing the effect of electrical stimulation of small regions, and by recording the spontaneous activity of small regions using micro-electrodes. While there is now general agreement on some facts, their interpretation is open to dispute. There would, however, appear to be three main parts of the respiratory centre: (1) A medullary centre capable of initiating and maintaining sequences of respiration, though not of normal character; (2) An apneustic centre in the middle and lower pons, which if unopposed tends to produce inspiratory spasm or apneustic breathing;[*] (3) A pneumotaxic centre in the upper third of the pons that restrains the apneustic centre periodically. The chemoreceptor centre, whatever its site, has its own rhythm and is influenced by peripheral stimuli and humoral states, especially the tension of carbon dioxide. While essentially automatic, the centre may be influenced from many sources: (1) From changes in oxygen and carbon dioxide

---

[*] Wang, S. E., Ngai, S. H., and Frumin, M. J., *Amer. J. Physiol.*, 1957, **190**, 333.

tension in the blood. (2) By changes in body temperature. (3) By Hering-Breuer reflexes.* (4) By carotid-body reflexes, largely oxygen lack. (5) By proprioceptive impulses from intrathoracic structures and from muscles and joints throughout the body, the so-called ergoreceptors, so that respiration can fit in with exercise and movement, etc. (6) By reflexes which modify rhythm during talking, swallowing, etc. (7) Reflexes from the hypothalamus and cerebral cortex. (8) The will and emotional states. The respiratory centre is connected with the phrenic and intercostal nerves by fibres running in the anterior and lateral columns of the white matter of the cord and on the afferent side with the vagi, sinus, and aortic nerves.

Hering-Breuer reflexes have been known since 1868. Afferent impulses travel up the vagus and cause inspiration to be inhibited when alveoli are inflated : expiration is inhibited when the alveoli are deflated sufficiently. Stretch and deflator receptors are present in alveolar walls. Hypoxia exaggerates this reflex while hyperpnœa abolishes it. All volatile and gaseous anæsthetics increase excitability of the pulmonary receptors, which are stimulated by inflation. Deflation receptors are first stimulated, later depressed, by chloroform and ethyl ether. Trichloroethylene sensitizes deflation receptors without subsequent depression—hence tachypnœa seen with this agent. Thiopentone depresses the respiratory centre but exaggerates the Hering-Breuer reflex in direct proportion to depth of anæsthesia ; thus apnœa will result following reservoir-bag pressure, under this type of anæsthesia, sufficiently long for radiological investigations of the bile-ducts, for example.

Heat, cold, and pain stimulate breathing, while impulses arise in skeletal muscles during active exercise and have the same effect. Traction reflexes arising in the abdomen and chest stimulate respiration. Breathing is inhibited during swallowing (glossopharyngeal nerve). It is also inhibited by local irritation of the larynx by such vapours as strong ether, or by foreign bodies. Continuous stimulation of the inspiratory centre results in apneusis—maintenance of the inflated position.

EFFECTS OF CHEMICAL AGENTS ON RESPIRATORY CENTRE.—Carbon dioxide influences the chemoreceptors within the central nervous system, but their exact location is in dispute. A blood carbon dioxide tension increase of 5 mm. Hg will stimulate respiration, whereas the blood oxygen tension has to go down by about 60 mm. Hg (from the normal 100 mm. Hg to 40 mm. Hg) before hypoxia stimulates the centre. This corresponds to breathing 12 per cent oxygen instead of the normal 21 per cent, or breathing air at 13,000 ft. Thus we breathe primarily to get rid of carbon dioxide! Carbon dioxide is the normal respiratory stimulus, but changes in blood pH are also important. Ventilation which is adequate to get rid of carbon dioxide is more than adequate to replace oxygen in the alveolar air.

---

* Hering, E., and Breuer, J., *Sitz. Akad. Wiss. Wien.*, 1868, **57**, 672; and *Ibid.*, **58**, 909.

Regulation of Respiration, *continued.*

The oxygen tension is an important respiratory stimulant only when the patient is breathing hypoxic mixtures. Severe oxygen lack or gross hypercarbia depresses the respiratory centre.

If carbon dioxide is breathed, the carbon dioxide in the alveolar air does not diffuse out so readily, i.e., the gradient is not as steep. This results in a raised alveolar carbon dioxide tension with a similar change in the arterial blood ; the latter causes a stimulation of the respiratory centre.

If more than 6 per cent of carbon dioxide is inspired no amount of hyperventilation can keep the alveolar air below that figure, so the arterial carbon dioxide rises, producing an acidæmia or respiratory acidosis. If alveolar carbon dioxide is kept lower than normal by assisted or controlled breathing, apnœa results.

Noradrenaline and serotonin may be partially metabolized in lung tissue.*

Carotid and Aortic Reflexes and Respiration.—

Pressoreceptors are present in the carotid sinus, a slight enlargement of the common carotid artery just before its bifurcation and the internal carotid artery : they are also present in the aortic arch. Stimulation of the nerve-endings (stretch receptors) in the outer wall of the sinus and aorta inhibits respiration (Heymans, 1929). This occurs when pressure rises. Pressoreceptors are also present in the great veins, right auricle, and pulmonary artery, and increased pressure here may stimulate respiration. Such reflexes may be involved in the dyspnœa of heart failure and pulmonary embolism.

There is evidence that pressoreceptors, when stimulated by low blood-pressure, can produce reflex bronchial dilatation.

Chemoreceptors are present in the carotid body and the aortic bodies, small masses of polyhedral cells forming a rich network of capillaries. The carotid body is in relationship to the external carotid artery just after its commencement from the bifurcation of the common carotid artery. The aortic body lies between the descending aorta and the pulmonary artery. Other peripheral chemoreceptors sensitive to arterial Po_2 and Pco_2 are also present and may be situated in muscles, veins, and the pulmonary artery. Their main function is to prevent hypoxia by stimulating respiration when arterial Po_2 falls. The glomeric cells normally have a high oxygen usage. When the Po_2 falls, anaerobic metabolism causes the release of substances which diffuse out of the cells to stimulate pericellular chemosensory nerve-endings.† When stimulated by decreased oxygen tension or increased carbon dioxide tension, there is increase in rate and depth of breathing. Stimulation begins when oxygen tension falls to 70 mm. Hg, at which point the arterial blood is 92 per cent saturated with

---

* Webb, W. R., *Surg. Clin. N. Amer.*, 1965, **45**, 267.
† Joels, N., and Neil, E., *Brit. med. Bull.*, 1963, **19**, 21.

oxygen, i.e., about equal to that saturation resulting from inhalation of a mixture containing 18 per cent oxygen, or by ascending to a height of 4000 ft. Thus hypoxia directly depresses the respiratory centre, but secondarily stimulates it via this reflex. Stimulation only occurs if plasma oxygen tension is reduced, not blood-oxygen content (as in anæmia). Chemoreceptors are important when the respiratory centre is depressed, as by barbiturates, morphine, etc., when the resulting hypoxia stimulates respiration reflexly. If at such times oxygen in excess is given, the sole remaining stimulant to breathing is removed and hypopnœa may follow with its resulting hypercapnia. With ether, respiratory centre is not so greatly depressed.

Asphyxia.—The body is exposed to the twin insults of oxygen lack and carbon dioxide excess. First there is cardiac slowing secondary to rise in blood-pressure (Marey's law) consequent on stimulating effect on vasomotor centre. Later the blood-pressure falls due to depression of myocardium, the rate rises, and arrhythmias appear.

ACID-BASE BALANCE

Hydrogen Ion Concentration and pH.—pH expresses hydrogen ion concentration as its negative logarithm to the base 10. Normal range for arterial blood, pH 7·36–7·44. Normal hydrogen ion concentration can be taken as 36–44 micromilliequivalents per l. The range compatible with life is 20–160 micromilliequivalents per l. Hydrogen ions do not exist free in water, but as $(H_3O)^+$. Electrometric methods of determination measure ionic activity and not concentration.

pH units	Hydrogen Ions in micromilliequivalents/litre
7·0	100
7·2	63
7·4	40
7·6	25
7·8	16
8·0	10

Acidæmia and Alkalæmia.—In acidæmia, the hydrogen ion concentration is above, in alkalæmia below, the normal range.

Acidosis and Alkalosis.—Acidosis is a condition which would tend to cause acidæmia if uncorrected. Alkalosis tends to cause alkalæmia if uncorrected.

Respiratory Acidosis and Alkalosis.—Related to changes in carbon dioxide tension in arterial blood (P_{CO_2}). Normal range is 36–44 mm. Hg. Respiratory acidosis at higher tensions, and alkalosis at lower tensions.

Acidosis occurs as a result of underventilation, in central respiratory depression, in emphysema ; the body compensates by increased renal excretion of ammonium ions and plasma bicarbonate rises.

Respiratory Acidosis and Alkalosis, *continued.*

> *Alkalosis* occurs as a result of hyperventilation, whether active or passive; the body compensates by renal excretion of bicarbonate.

Metabolic or Non-respiratory Acidosis and Alkalosis.—This refers to acid-base disturbances due to any substance other than carbon dioxide. Acidosis means acid excess or base deficit (a deficiency of plasma bicarbonate). Alkalosis means base excess or acid deficit.

METABOLIC ACIDOSIS may occur :—

1. In diabetic ketosis, due to β-hydroxybutyric acid.
2. In renal failure.
3. In starvation.
4. In infantile diarrhœa.
5. In salicylate poisoning.
6. After severe muscular exercise.
7. During rewarming after hypothermia.
8. During cardiopulmonary by-pass causing tissue hypoxia.[*]
9. During ether anæsthesia if lactate metabolism is depressed (Cushing's disease, parenteral steroid therapy, cirrhosis of the liver, in infancy).[†]
10. In association with respiratory alkalosis.
11. Possibly in " neostigmine-resistant curarization ".[‡]
12. Shock. Inadequate tissue perfusion may result in anaerobic metabolism.
13. Prolonged intestinal obstruction.
14. Occlusion of large vessels.
15. Following cardiac arrest.

The body compensates by increased pulmonary ventilation to remove CO_2 and by increased renal excretion of hydrogen ions. Treatment may include infusion of sodium bicarbonate intravenously, as well as treatment of the primary condition causing acidosis. The use of agents, such as tris (hydroxymethyl) aminomethane (THAM), has not yet come in general use, though some workers believe it has advantages over bicarbonate infusion.[§]

> Sodium bicarbonate may be given : (*a*) as a 2·74 per cent solution.[‡] This has twice the osmolarity of plasma and contains 166 mEq. in 500 ml. Average dose 200 ml., which provides 1 mEq. per kg. in a 60-kg. man. (*b*) As an 8·4 per cent solution,[||] which contains 1 mEq. in each ml. Average dose about 50 ml.

METABOLIC ALKALOSIS may occur following ingestion of large amounts of bicarbonate or citrate, and in pyloric stenosis with loss of acid. The body compensates by underventilation and increased renal bicarbonate excretion.

Buffer Base.—Bicarbonate is the most important blood buffer in consideration of acid-base balance. It can be measured, but the

---

[*] Clowes, G. H. A., *Physiol. Rev.*, 1960, **40**, 826.
[†] Bunker, J. P., *Anesthesiology*, 1962, **23**, 107.
[‡] Brooks, D. K., and Feldman, S. A., *Anæsthesia*, 1962, **17**, 161.
[§] Tizard, J. P. M., *Proc. R. Soc. Med.*, 1967, **60**, 935.
[||] Stewart, J. S. S., *Lancet*, 1964, **1**, 106.

concentration is influenced by P_{CO_2}, so that this factor must be excluded in determination of metabolic acid-base state.

Base Excess is the surplus of fixed acid or base in mEq. per l. of blood. It is the amount of acid or base in mEq. per l. required for titration back to pH 7·40 at a P_{CO_2} of 40 mm. Hg at a temperature of 38° C. By convention an acid surplus (base deficit) is referred to as a negative base excess.

Equilibration Methods.—Blood is equilibrated *in vitro* with a gas mixture of P_{CO_2} = 40 mm. Hg and the bicarbonate determined.

Standard Bicarbonate is the concentration in plasma at a P_{CO_2} of 40 mm. Hg, with hæmoglobin fully saturated, at 38° C. No information is obtained about respiratory acid-base balance.

The Bicarbonate Buffer System.—Carbonic acid exists in a state of equilibrium with hydrogen ions and bicarbonate ions:

$$H^+ + HCO_3^- \rightleftharpoons H_2CO_3.$$

The Law of Mass Action states that, when such a reaction has reached equilibrium, the product of the concentrations of the reagents on one side of the equation is proportional to the product of the concentrations of reagents on the other side of the equation:—

$$[H^+] [HCO_3^-] = K \times [H_2CO_3],$$

where K is a constant, which may be rewritten:—

$$[H^+] = K \times \frac{[H_2CO_3]}{[HCO_3^-]}.$$

The carbonic acid in the equation can be replaced by P_{CO_2} if the solubility factor is known. If the units of measurements are defined, the value of K can be calculated.

The equation can then be written in a form which is more useful for clinical work:—

$$[H^+] = 24 \frac{P_{CO_2}}{[HCO_3^-]}.$$

The Henderson-Hasselbalch Equation.*—This classic equation links the same factors, expressed in logarithmic notation:—

$$\log [H^+] = \log K + \log \frac{[H_2CO_3]}{[HCO_3^-]},$$

$$- \log [H^+] = - \log K - \log \frac{[H_2CO_3]}{[HCO_3^-]}.$$

$- \log [H^+]$ can then be written as pH, $- \log K$ as pK, and $- \log \frac{[H_2CO_3]}{[HCO_3^-]}$ as $+ \log \frac{[HCO_3^-]}{[H_2CO_3]}$.

The equation then becomes the familiar one:—

$$pH = pK + \log \frac{[HCO_3^-]}{[H_2CO_3]}.$$

---

* Henderson, L. J., *Amer. J. Physiol.*, 1908, **21**, 173, and *Ibid.*, **21**, 427; and Hasselbalch, K. A., *Biochem. Zeitschr.*, 1916, **78**, 112 (*see also* 'Classical File', *Survey of Anesthesiology*, 1964, **8**, 486 and 607).

The Henderson–Hasselbalch Equation, *continued.*

As before, carbonic acid can be expressed in terms of P_{CO_2}:—

$$pH = pK + \log \frac{[HCO_3^-]}{0.03 P_{CO_2}}.$$

pK varies with temperature and pH. An average figure at 38° C. is 6.1. The solubility factor of carbon dioxide in plasma is taken as 0.03 mEq. per l. per mm. Hg. Total carbon dioxide content of plasma is expressed as $[HCO_3^-] + 0.03\, P_{CO_2}$.

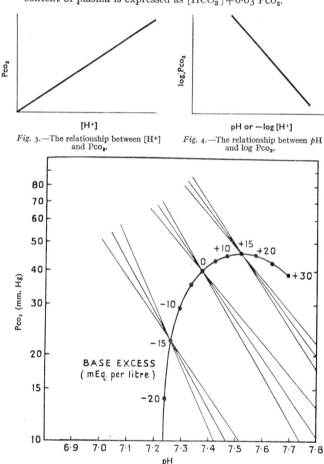

Fig. 3.—The relationship between [H+] and P_{CO_2}.

Fig. 4.—The relationship between pH and log P_{CO_2}.

Fig. 5.—The effect of addition of hæmoglobin and buffer base. (*By permission of Dr. Siggaard-Andersen and the Editor of the 'Lancet'.*)

Other Buffers.—Hæmoglobin is the most important buffer after the bicarbonate system. Reduced hæmoglobin is a stronger base than oxyhæmoglobin. Plasma proteins also act as buffers, but their capacity in mEq. per l. in the blood is only one-third of that of hæmoglobin.

The relationships can also be expressed graphically. When any two factors are used as co-ordinates, iso-lines can be constructed for the third.

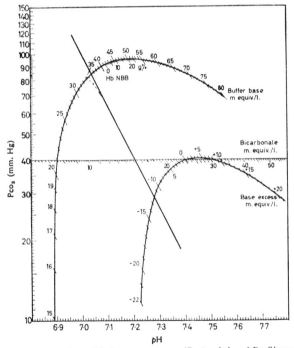

Fig. 6.—The Siggaard-Andersen nomogram. (*By permission of Dr. Siggaard-Andersen and Radiometer, Copenhagen.*)

The pH/log Pco_2 Diagram (Siggaard-Andersen).—If hydrogen ion concentration is plotted against Pco_2, a straight line is obtained (*Fig. 3*).

The graph may be plotted logarithmically, though, as pH is a negative logarithm, the slope of the line will be in the opposite direction in the pH/log Pco_2 graph (*Fig. 4*).

The ordinates can be so arranged that the slope is 45° when the bicarbonate/carbonic acid system above is considered. Whole

The $pH/\log P_{CO_2}$ Diagram (Siggaard-Andersen), *continued.*

blood contains other buffers, and the slope of the line will be increased when these buffers are present. Thus addition of hæmoglobin to plasma will change the slope of the line (*Fig. 5*).

The line can be drawn for various additions of hæmoglobin and when known amounts of base are added (bicarbonate). If the points of intersection of these lines are joined, a curved line is obtained, which is the base excess/base deficit line of the Siggaard-Andersen nomogram.*

The full diagram (*Fig. 6*) enables reading off of plasma bicarbonate levels and total buffer base in addition to base excess and P_{CO_2} (*see also* Chapter XXXIII).

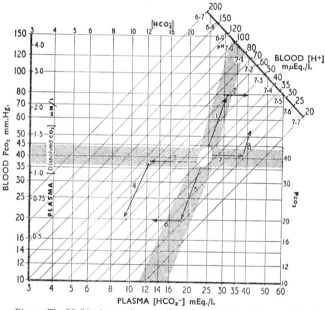

Fig. 7.—The CO_2/bicarbonate diagram. (*By permission of E. J. M. Campbell and Blackwell Scientific Publications, Ltd.*)

For details of the micro-Astrup technique of acid-base analysis *see* Chapter XXXIII.

The CO_2/Bicarbonate Diagram.†—This is a useful diagram for the understanding of acid-base changes in a patient. Straight iso-lines are drawn for pH (or $[H^+]$) (*Fig. 7*). The diagram is useful to follow

---

* *See* classic papers, Andersen, O. S., and Engel, K., *Scand. J. Lab. Invest.*, 1960, **12**, 177; and Astrup, P., Jorgensen, K., Andersen, O. S., and Engel, K., *Lancet*, 1960, **1**, 1035.

† *See* Campbell, E. J. M., Dickinson, C. J., and Slater, J. D. H., *Clinical Physiology*, 3rd ed., 1968. Oxford: Blackwell.

the progress of a patient by serial estimations. Arrow 1: Respiratory acidosis. Arrow 2: Compensatory metabolic alkalosis. Arrow 3: Metabolic acidosis. Arrow 4: Compensatory respiratory alkalosis. Arrow 5: Respiratory alkalosis. Arrow 6: Compensatory metabolic acidosis. Arrow 7: Metabolic alkalosis. Arrow 8: Compensatory respiratory acidosis.

(*See also* Nunn, J. F., in *Modern Trends in Anæsthesia*, No. 2 (Ed. Evans, T. F., and Gray, T. C.), Ch. 1, 1962. London: Butterworths.)

HYPERCAPNIA

(ὑπέρ (hyper), over + καπνόσ (kapnos), smoke)

Causes in Anæsthetic Practice.—

1. Gross impairment of ventilation due to respiratory obstruction, profound narcosis, or relaxants.
2. Severe bilateral lung disease, perhaps complicated by thoracotomy.
3. Accidental administration of carbon dioxide.
4. Faulty carbon dioxide absorption. Defective soda lime in faulty circuit.
5. The technique of apnœic insufflation oxygenation.

Hypercapnia has been classified by Nunn* as follows :—

1. MILD HYPERCAPNIA (arterial Pco_2 44–80 mm. Hg).—Tolerable in conscious subjects for a short time—common during clinical anæsthesia with spontaneous respiration. May not be recognized clinically. No cyanosis usually, even when breathing air. May cause arrhythmias during cyclopropane anæsthesia.
2. MODERATE HYPERCAPNIA (arterial Pco_2 80–200 mm. Hg). —Associated with progressive narcosis ; coma above 120 mm. Hg. Clinical picture variable. Cyanosis probable if the patient breathes air, may be absent with oxygen-rich mixtures.
3. SEVERE HYPERCAPNIA (arterial Pco_2 over 200 mm. Hg).— Profound narcosis and impending respiratory failure, often preceded by tracheal tug. May resemble curarization. A dangerous state of affairs.

Supercarbia, over 400 mm. Hg, is associated with a zone of acute tolerance in animals, when respiration is possible again.

Effects of Hypercapnia.—

1. CENTRAL NERVOUS SYSTEM.—
   a. Increased cerebral blood-flow.
   b. Inert gas effect (*see* p. 19).
   c. Rise of cerebrospinal fluid pressure.
   d. Progressive narcosis.

In patients with chronic hypercapnia, e.g., in emphysema, a relatively high Pco_2 may be compatible with mental alertness.

2. AUTONOMIC NERVOUS SYSTEM.—
   a. Sympathetic activation with a rise of circulating catecholamines ;

---

* Nunn, J. F., in *Modern Trends in Anæsthesia*, No. 2 (Ed. Evans, T. F., and Gray, T. C.), 1962. London : Butterworths.

Effects of Hypercapnia, *continued.*

but with reduced sensitivity of the end organs to these catecholamines. Sweating.

    b. Parasympathetic activation (though in general this is overshadowed by the sympathetic effect).

3. RESPIRATORY SYSTEM.—

    a. Carbon dioxide provides a most powerful stimulus to respiration. The precise site of action and the part played by carbon dioxide itself or by *p*H changes has been the subject of discussion. (*See* review by Lambutsen, C. J., *Anesthesiology*, 1960, **21**, 642.)

    b. Severe hypercapnia produces respiratory failure.

    c. Bohr effect. More oxygen is released from combination with hæmoglobin at the same oxygen tension in the presence of hypercapnia. Oxygen is more readily liberated in the tissues but less is taken up in the lungs. The dissociation curve is shifted to the right.

4. CARDIOVASCULAR SYSTEM.—

    a. Cardiac output. Force of contraction of the isolated heart is weakened, but effect variable in the intact animal.

    b. Tachycardia, due to catecholamine release.

    c. Arrhythmias. Arrhythmia CO_2 thresholds are described during cyclopropane and halothane anæsthesia.

    d. Peripheral resistance. A central vasomotor effect leads to vasoconstriction. A peripheral effect in the vessels themselves leads to dilatation except in the coronary arteries. The central effect is abolished by sympathetic block.

    e. Blood-pressure. Rises in the absence of anæsthesia. During anæsthesia there is no absolute rule, and hypertension, normotension, or hypotension may occur.

5. BIOCHEMICAL.—

    a. *p*H changes. Respiratory acidosis.

    b. Compensatory metabolic alkalosis. Secretion of acid urine with retention of bicarbonate and sodium.

    c. Metabolic acidosis sometimes occurs. This may, however, be difficult to assess after gross changes in Pco_2.

    d. Electrolytes. Rise of serum potassium. Of the order of 0·5 mEq. per l. at $Pco_2 = 150$ mm. Hg. A further rise may take place in sudden withdrawal, causing cardiovascular changes which may be serious.

    e. Rise of plasma 15-hydroxycorticosteroids.

6. EFFECTS ON ACTION OF DRUGS.—

    a. Changes of *p*H affect the ionization of many drugs thereby altering the concentration of the active fraction.

    b. Changes of *p*H affect the fraction of some drugs which is bound to protein (e.g., respiratory acidosis increases the dosage requirements of thiopentone).

    c. Tubocurarine is potentiated in hypercapnia. Other relaxants are antagonized.

Deliberate Hypercapnia.—Recently some anæsthetists of repute have advocated the deliberate addition of carbon dioxide to inspired mixtures, to produce vasodilatation during induced hypothermia,[*] carotid endarterectomy,[†] and in arteriosclerotic patients.[‡]

Carbon Dioxide Withdrawal.[§]—Sudden fall of Pco_2 following a period of hypercapnia may itself produce untoward effects:—

1. Hypotension. Sudden reversal of hypercapnia may produce the Brown and Miller effect of acute circulatory depression.[||] Not pronounced unless there has been moderate or severe hypercapnia for some time. More frequently seen after cyclopropane anæsthesia. Mechanism not established.
2. Arrhythmia. The reasons for this are not clear. It would appear that electrolyte (hyperkalæmia) and pH changes are insufficient to account for the clinical observations. Release of catechol amines may play a part—vagal inhibition of the heart is reduced and the resulting sympathetic preponderance may be important. Hyperkalæmia would potentiate such effects. Another contributory factor might be hypoxia—when marked hypercapnia is terminated by ventilation with air (diffusion anoxia).

Rapid lowering of the chronic hypercapnia in respiratory failure can lead to convulsions and death,[¶] unless the alkalæmia produced is corrected.

While every care should be taken to avoid hypercapnia, mild degrees of this condition may not be as serious as was once thought.

HYPERVENTILATION

Produces hypocapnia and rise of blood pH. There is a compensatory metabolic acidosis, but this is not of the same order as the respiratory alkalosis. I.P.P.V. under clinical conditions may reduce the Pco_2 from a normal of 40 to 25–20 mm. Hg.

Effects of Hyperventilation.—
1. CENTRAL NERVOUS SYSTEM.—
   a. Reduction in cerebral blood-flow,[**] and shrinkage of brain.[††]
   b. Reduction in cerebral oxygen tension.[‡‡]
   c. Clouding of consciousness and analgesia, due to depression of the reticular formation. The threshold to pain may be increased by up to three times, as evidenced by a study in volunteers in whom the pH rose from normal to 7·7.[§§]
2. CARDIOVASCULAR SYSTEM.—
   a. Protects against arrhythmias (caused by hypercapnia).

[*] Benazon, D. B., *Int. Anesth. Clin.*, 1964, **2/4**, 941; Sellick, B. A., *Proc. World Cong. Anæsth.*, 1964, **3**, 149; Broom, B., and Sellick, B. A., *Lancet*, 1965, **2**, 452; Sellick, B. A., in *Recent Advances in Anæsthesia and Analgesia* (Ed. Hewer, C. Langton), 1967. London: Churchill.
[†] Wells, B. A., Keats, A. S., and Cooley, D. A., *Surgery*, 1963, **54**, 216.
[‡] Horni, J., Smart, J. F., and Wasmuth, C. E., *Proc. 2nd Eur. Cong. Anæsth.*, 1966, **1**, 629.
[§] Price, H. L., *Anesthesiology*, 1960, **21**, 652.
[||] Brown, E. B., and Miller, F., *Amer. J. Physiol.*, 1952, **169**, 56.
[¶] Severinghaus, J. W., *Proc. 2nd Eur. Cong. Anæsth.*, 1966, Abstracts, p. 91.
[**] Kety, S. S., and Schmidt, C. F., *J. clin. Invest.*, 1946, **25**, 107.
[††] Whitwam, J. G., and others, *Brit. J. Anæsth.*, 1966, **38**, 846; and Allen, G. D., and Morris, L. E., *Ibid.*, 1962, **34**, 296.
[‡‡] Sugioka, K., and Davis, D. A., *Anesthesiology*, 1960, **21**, 135.
[§§] Robinson, J. S., and Gray, T. C., *Brit. J. Anæsth.*, 1961, **33**, 62.

Effects of Hyperventilation, *continued.*

  b. May protect the heart against the effect of atropine and neo-stigmine* though it is more important to prevent hypoxia than to produce hypocapnia.†

  c. Fall of blood-pressure if intermittent positive-pressure anæsthesia is not carried out with due regard to mean intrathoracic pressure (*see* Chapter VIII). Peripheral vasoconstriction. Little evidence that hypocapnia, *per se*, has any effect on blood-pressure.

 3. CHANGES IN THE BLOOD.—

  a. Increase of circulating red cells.

  b. Loss of plasma water from the circulation.

  c. Fall of plasma sodium.

  d. Small fall of plasma potassium.

  e. Fall in ionized calcium, but slight increase in total plasma calcium.

  f. Hinders the liberation of oxygen from oxyhæmoglobin.

 4. FŒTUS.—There is some evidence that hyperventilation during anæsthesia for Cæsarean section carries some risk to the fœtus. Recent work has shown that fœtal asphyxia is more likely if the Pco_2 falls below 17 mm. Hg,‡ and work on animals indicates that there is a fall in fœtal oxygen associated with maternal hyperventilation.§ The clinical importance of these observations are debatable,‖ but in the light of present knowledge it is probably best to avoid hyperventilation during anæsthesia in obstetrics.¶ There is some evidence that pH is the important factor rather than Pco_2 and that it causes intraplacental shunting in lambs.**

 5. TETANY.—Not commonly associated with clinical anæsthesia.

After hyperventilation, there may be a brief period of hypoxæmia followed by several hours of hypercapnia after operation.††

Active and Passive Hyperventilation.—Active respiratory effort increases the metabolism of the muscles resulting in increased carbon dioxide production. There is a minute volume of about 60 l. per min. where the increase in ventilation would be offset by the increased CO_2 production.‡‡

Advantages of Hyperventilation Techniques in Anæsthesia.—

  1. Full oxygenation is maintained, provided there is adequate oxygen concentration in the inspired gases.

  2. A mild respiratory alkalosis is generally held to be safer than a respiratory acidosis.

  3. The respiratory alkalosis itself contributes to the anæsthetic state. Smaller doses of anæsthetic drugs are required. (*a*) A reduction

* Riding, J. E., and Robinson, J. S., *Anæsthesia*, 1961, **16**, 346.
† Baraka, A., *Brit. J. Anæsth.*, 1968, **40**, 27.
‡ Moya, F., Morishima, H. O., and Shinder, S. M., *Amer. J. Obstet. Gynec.*, 1965, **91**, 76.
§ Motoyama, E. K., Acheson, F., Reward, G., and Cook, C. D., *Lancet*, 1966, **1**, 286.
‖ Coleman, A. J., *Ibid.*, 1967, **1**, 813.
¶ James, L. S., *Anesthesiology*, 1967, **28**, 804.
** Motoyama, E. K., Reward, G., Acheson, F., and Cook, C. D., *Ibid.*, 1967, **28**, 891.
†† Lees, M. M., Scott, D. B., and Taylor, S. H., *Brit. J. Anæsth.*, 1966, **38**, 179.
‡‡ Otis, A. B., *Physiol. Rev.*, 1954, **34**, 449.

in the dose of intravenous barbiturates. (b) A reduction in analgesic agents. (c) A reduction in non-depolarizing relaxants and an increase in their potency. These effects are probably due to the production of general analgesia and the depression of other cerebral functions, e.g., a decrease in the frequency of discharge from the reticular activating system. They are due not to a decrease in cerebral blood-flow and tissue hypoxia but to changes in the Pco_2 and pH values. Inhalation of pure oxygen and removal of vasoconstriction in the retinal vessels (and so presumably in the cerebral vessels) do not decrease analgesia.*

4. The biochemical effects of hyperventilatory hypocapnia are unlikely to be harmful.† Moderate hyperventilation causes no significant increase in metabolic acidosis or in tissue hypoxia.‡
5. Cardiac effects of neostigmine minimized.
6. Hypocapnia is important during the production of induced hypotension.§
7. Incidence of peripheral atelectasis reduced.
The analgesic effects of hyperventilatory hypocapnia is discussed by Geddes and Gray.‖

Disadvantages of Hyperventilation in Anæsthesia.—
1. In unskilled hands, undesirable sequelæ may follow due to faulty technique, e.g., hypotension.
2. Where cerebral perfusion is borderline (e.g., in cardiopulmonary by-pass) cerebral vasoconstriction may be undesirable.
3. In obstetrics (see p. 72).
If a relaxant is adequately reversed, respiration will start even in the presence of hypocapnia, always provided that the respiratory centre is not depressed (e.g., by narcotic analgesics) and that the peripheral receptors in the upper respiratory tract are not inactivated by local analgesic sprays or ointments.¶

HISTAMINE

Physiology of Histamine in Man.—Histamine causes : (1) Arteriolar dilatation. (2) Capillary paralysis. (3) Consequent hypotension. (4) Contraction of smooth muscle, e.g., in bronchi, intestine, spleen, and uterus. (5) Increased glandular secretion, e.g., of the stomach. (6) Locally in the skin a triple response, e.g., a red line, a flare, and a weal.

The following drugs used in anæsthesia may liberate histamine : tubocurarine, laudexium, benzoquinonium, morphine, codeine, dihydrocodeine bitartrate, papaverine, pethidine, atropine, trimetaphan, and dextran.

---

* Robinson, J. S., and Gray, T. C., *Brit. J. Anæsth.*, 1961, **33**, 61.
† Robinson, J. S., *Ibid.*, 1961, **33**, 69.
‡ Sykes, M. K., and Cooke, P. M., *Ibid.*, 1965, **37**, 372.
§ Prys-Roberts, C., *Proc. 2nd Eur. Cong. Anæsth.*, 1966, Abstracts, p. 91; and Eckenhoff, J. E., Enderby, G. E. H., and others, *J. appl. Physiol.*, 1963, **18**, 1130.
‖ Geddes, I. C., and Gray, T. C., *Lancet*, 1959, **2**, 4.
¶ Utting, J. E., and Gray, T. C., *Brit. J. Anæsth.*, 1962, **34**, 785.

CHAPTER III

PRE-ANÆSTHETIC CARE AND PREPARATION

The Anæsthetic Out-patient Clinic.—It is often convenient to see the patient in the out-patient clinic as soon as his name is placed on the waiting list for surgical operation. He should be referred to the clinic either routinely or : (1) when the operation is likely to be severe ; (2) when special techniques (e.g., controlled hypotension) are envisaged ; (3) in the presence of systemic disease which is likely to add to the risk of operation. In the clinic a full history and examination can be undertaken and special investigations ordered. Treatment can be instituted as an out-patient to render the patient as fit as possible by the time he is admitted to hospital. When necessary, the patient can be followed up by repeated attendances at the clinic.

Look for the following points in the history :—

1. Previous illnesses, operations, and anæsthetics. Complications may be avoided on this occasion.
2. Drug therapy,* e.g., corticosteroids, insulin, hypotensive drugs, tranquillizers, digitalis, mono-amine oxidase inhibitors. Drug allergies.
3. Symptoms referable to the respiratory system. Respiratory reserve, cough, sputum, bronchospasm. Smoking habits.
4. Cardiovascular system. Exercise tolerance. Anginal pain. Decompensation.
5. Tendency to vomiting. This may affect the choice of anæsthetic drugs and technique so as to reduce the likelihood of postoperative nausea and vomiting.

Give the patient a full clinical examination, bearing in mind :—

1. Signs of respiratory disease.
2. Signs of heart disease. Blood-pressure.
3. The airway. Teeth, jaws, neck. Intubation hazards.
4. The state of nutrition, malnutrition, or obesity.
5. Colour. Cyanosis or pallor.
6. Examination of the nervous system, particularly where spinal or extradural block is envisaged.
7. Examination of the urine for sugar and albumin.
8. Assess the psychological state of the patient. Calm, apprehensive, unstable, etc.

Simple tests which can be carried out in the clinic include:—

1. The breath-holding test of Sebrasez. The resting patient takes a full inspiration and holds his breath. A time of 25 sec. or longer may be taken as normal. A time of 15 sec. or less indicates a lack of cardiorespiratory reserve.
2. The forced expiratory volume and vital capacity can be readily measured using the vitalograph (p. 52).
3. The Wright Peak Flow-meter can be used to measure peak expiratory flow rate (p. 53).

---

* Grogono, A. W., and Jones, A. E. P., *Anæsthesia*, 1968, **23**, 215.

Special investigations may be ordered where indicated. They may include :—
1. Hæmoglobin and blood groups.
2. Blood-urea.
3. Chest radiograph.
4. Electrocardiogram.

In certain cases it may be desirable to refer the patient to other departments for advice (e.g., cardiology).

ASSESSMENT OF PHYSICAL STATUS (P.S.).—The American Society of Anesthesiologists classified patients into a number of grades according to their general condition and " risk ". There were originally seven grades, but the classification has been amended by the 1962 House of Delegates of the Society* as follows :—
1. A normal healthy patient.
2. A patient with a mild systemic disease.
3. A patient with a severe systemic disease that limits activity, but is not incapacitating.
4. A patient with an incapacitating systemic disease that is a constant threat to life.
5. A moribund patient not expected to survive 24 hours with or without an operation.

In the event of emergency operation, precede the number with an E.

An attempt may be made to put patients into their proper grade for purposes of comparison and assessment of risk.

TREATMENT.—Some forms of treatment may be instituted in the out-patient clinic.
1. DENTAL TREATMENT.—Refer the patient to the dental surgeon.
2. TREATMENT OF ANÆMIA.—Valuable time can be saved by treating anæmia before admission. Oral iron is effective in most cases, but occasionally when this is not tolerated or when time is short intramuscular iron may be indicated, e.g., Imferon 250 mg. twice a week.
3. RESPIRATORY DISEASE.—No patient should undergo a non-urgent operation while he is suffering from an acute infection of the upper respiratory tract. Chronic chest disease is more difficult to control, but much can be done.

   Smoking should be completely given up for the three weeks before operation. There is statistical proof that in abdominal operations post-operative chest complications are six times more frequent in smokers than in non-smokers.

   If the patient gives a history of chronic winter cough which improves during the warm weather, he should, if possible, have his operation postponed until he is at his best. Chemotherapy, penicillin, postural drainage, etc., may be suggested in suitable cases, e.g., the technique described by Palmer and Sellick,† in which postural drainage and physiotherapy are combined with inhalation of the bronchodilator isoprenaline sulphate, can be employed.

* *Anesthesiology*, 1963, **24**, 111.
† Palmer, K. N. V., and Sellick, B. A., *Lancet*, 1953, **1**, 164.

The Anæsthetic Out-patient Clinic, *continued.*

Post-nasal catarrh and sinus infection should be sought out and treated, while viscosity of sputum can often be reduced by the daily administration of potassium iodide 1–2 g. for a few days before operation.

Breathing exercises should be started in the clinic and should be conducted if possible by the same personnel who will later be met in the ward after operation, though they do not necessarily improve respiratory function.* Group therapy has a place here, and classes of patients can be put through a suitable drill with advantage both to their physique and their morale.

4. MALNUTRITION.—In appropriate cases high-protein diets, vitamins, etc., can be ordered.

5. OBESITY.—This is the enemy of both surgeon and anæsthetist. If treated properly by a 1000-calories diet excellent results may be obtained, even in the few weeks at the anæsthetist's disposal. It is important to give the patient a diet sheet he can readily understand, to explain to him the purpose of the diet, and for him to attend the out-patient clinic at regular (fortnightly) intervals for weight check and for interview so that the anæsthetist can give appropriate encouragement or scolding.

6. PSYCHOLOGICAL FACTORS.—Occasionally patients are terrified of anæsthesia, or they may fear a particular anæsthetic technique (face-mask, spinal anæsthesia). A little time spent in discussion with these patients is invaluable and may in fact bring some patients into hospital who would otherwise default. It should rarely be necessary to force an unwelcome technique on a patient.

One other advantage of the thorough pre-operative investigation of the patient is the assurance and confidence that the anæsthetist feels, should medico-legal proceedings be instituted by the patient after operation. " It is the fate of those who toil at the lower employments of life, to be exposed to censure without hope of praise ; to be disgraced by miscarriage or punished for neglect, where success would have been without applause, and diligence without reward." (Dr. Samuel Johnson.)† Among these unhappy mortals is the administrator of anæsthetics, and he must cover himself in every way possible.

Pre-operative Preparation.—The patient should be seen in the ward a day or two before his operation takes place. The anæsthetist then has an opportunity to check the notes made in the out-patient clinic and to look for any recent change in the patient's condition. If the patient has not been seen before, a more detailed history must be taken, and appropriate examination made. At this visit the anæsthetist should check laboratory findings and if necessary order cross-matching of blood. Sedation and pre-operative medication may then be prescribed.

---

* Saunders, K. B., and White, J. E., *Brit. med. J.*, 1965, **2**, 680.
† Preface to *The Dictionary of the English Language*, 1755.

Pre-operative preparation in special cases is discussed in Chapter XXVI.

THE DAY OF OPERATION.—Food and drink should be withheld during the six hours preceding operation. It is often wise to order nothing by mouth on the day of operation, but excessive starvation and dehydration are to be avoided.

Lipstick, nail varnish, and other cosmetics should be removed before the patient comes to theatre so that the anæsthetist can readily appreciate cyanosis, etc.

Dentures, artificial limbs, artificial eyes, etc., should be removed before the journey to the theatre.

The patient should not come to theatre with a full bladder.

The patient is dressed in a linen theatre gown. It is wise to tie an identification label around his wrist or neck. This should state the name and case record number. Where indicated the side or number of digit should be marked on the patient's skin with indelible ink.

Emergency cases should be delayed if possible to allow the stomach to empty. Remember that gastric emptying may be considerably delayed after accidents, in labour, and in the anxious patient. Resuscitative measures, such as intravenous infusion, may be required to improve the patient's condition.

THE EFFECTS OF DRUG THERAPY*

The majority of drug reactions can be explained as follows†:—

1. Potentiation, additive or synergistic effect, e.g., barbiturates and alcohol.
2. Enzymatic inhibition by one drug preventing normal metabolism of another, e.g., monoamine oxidase inhibitors and pethidine.
3. Stimulation of enzyme systems by one drug leading to an increased rate of metabolism of another. It is thought that phenobarbitone stimulates metabolism of anticoagulants so that dosage of the latter must be increased and a dangerous situation may arise if phenobarbitone is withdrawn.
4. Displacement of one drug from plasma or tissue protein by another. For example, phenylbutazone may displace a coumarin anticoagulant which has an enhanced effect with danger of bleeding.
5. Electrolyte imbalance. Loss of potassium induced by thiazide diuretics may cause abnormal reactions to digoxin and muscle relaxants.
6. Influence of drug on urinary pH may affect excretion of drugs.
7. Interference with other renal mechanisms affecting drug excretion.

Drugs affecting Sympathetic Responses.—Hypotensive agents produce their effects by a reduction in peripheral vascular tone. The hypotensive effect may be augmented by general anæsthesia, especially when this is combined with sudden change of position, head-up tilt, use of ganglion-blocking drugs, sudden hæmorrhage, etc. Care should be exercised in the use of spinal or extradural techniques.

---

* *See also* the table in the Appendix.
† McIver, A. K., *Pharm. J.*, 1965, **195**, 609.

Drugs affecting Sympathetic Responses, *continued.*

GANGLION-BLOCKING DRUGS.—These produce hypotension by ganglionic blockade.

GUANETHIDINE (ISMELIN).—Causes depletion of noradrenaline from the sites associated with adrenergic nerve function but also blocks transmission before significant depletion has occurred.

RAUWOLFIA COMPOUNDS.—Reserpine causes a depletion of the stores of catecholamines of the body, including the brain (adrenaline, noradrenaline, and 5-hydroxytryptamine). Effects last for two weeks after cessation of therapy. Side-effects include nasal congestion, increased salivation, weight gain, and mental depression.

METHYLDOPA.—An inhibitor of the enzyme decarboxylase which is necessary in the biosynthesis of adrenaline and noradrenaline. It also depletes the noradrenaline stores. Side-effects include nasal congestion, mental depression, abdominal colic, and diarrhœa.

ADRENERGIC α-RECEPTOR BLOCKERS.—Phenoxybenzamine and phentolamine are powerful blocking agents and too potent for use in the treatment of essential hypertension. There is no antagonist available and side-effects are common, so that these drugs are not used in antihypertensive therapy.

ADRENERGIC β-RECEPTOR BLOCKERS.—Pronethalol and propranolol prevent inotropic and chronotropic cardiac responses. Anæsthesia must be administered cautiously when these drugs have been administered.

DIURETICS.—Most diuretics potentiate the more effective hypotensive agents, though their action is not understood.

MONO-AMINE OXIDASE INHIBITORS.—Mono-amine oxidase is concerned in the breakdown of noradrenaline which escapes from the immediate vicinity of the storage granules in adrenergic nerve-endings. Mono-amine oxidase inhibitors cause an accumulation of certain amines in nerve terminals, so that nerve impulses release a mixture of catecholamines which has less pressor activity than noradrenaline itself. The result is that of a partial sympathetic blockade. Pargyline (eutonyl) is used in hypertension.

Significance of Antihypertensive Therapy.—

1. Threat to circulatory homeostasis. Sympathetic blockade is likely to interfere with the normal compensatory mechanisms of the cardiovascular system which are called into play during induction of anæsthesia. It may prevent the rise in circulating catecholamines which normally occurs during anæsthesia with ether and cyclopropane. Hypotensive episodes have been reported during anæsthesia and special care is necessary in the administration of thiopentone, intermittent positive-pressure ventilation, changes of posture, the treatment of hæmorrhage, etc.

2. The response to pressor amines may be altered. This will depend upon the nature of the sympathetic block and on the mechanism of the pressor itself (direct or via noradrenaline release). Drugs blocking the ganglia or the adrenergic nerve terminals deprive

the effector of tonic impulses and induce a supersensitivity to catecholamines. Drugs such as the α-receptor blockers induce a subsensitivity to catecholamines. Drugs which deplete noradrenaline in the nerve terminals diminish the activity of indirectly acting pressors, though methyldopa may be an exception. Mono-amine oxidase inhibitors preserve noradrenaline stores and may dangerously potentiate the indirect vasopressors, and care is necessary with adrenaline and noradrenaline. β-adrenergic blockers do not affect pressor action.

3. Effect on other drugs.—
   a. Though ganglion-blocking drugs potentiate non-depolarizing muscle relaxants, this is only important when they are used intravenously.
   b. There is some evidence that reserpine and iproniazid prolong anæsthesia.*
   c. The interaction between mono-amine oxidase inhibitors and pethidine is discussed below.
   d. Diuretics may cause hypokalæmia.

Tests for Sympathetic Reactivity.—Various tests have been suggested to attempt to identify the patient at risk:—
   1. Injection of a small dose of pressor drug with a minimal direct pressor activity. The action of the drug should be abolished in patients at risk. In practice these tests have proved disappointing owing to the mixed action of many pressors and the number of abnormal reactions encountered.
   2. Tilt tests to demonstrate postural hypotension.
   3. Response to the Valsalva manœuvre.† The patient blows against a mercury column to a pressure of 40 mm. Hg and sustains it for 15 sec. Evidence of sympathetic vasoconstriction is provided by the rise in systolic pressure which normally occurs on releasing the intrapulmonary pressure. This has the disadvantage that the transient overshoot is difficult to detect by indirect arterial pressure measurement, and the accompanying bradycardia is not always a reliable sign.

Cessation of Drug Treatment.—The activity of the drug ceases:—
   1. Within 24 hours. Ganglion-blocking agents, bethanidine (estabal), mecamylamide (inversine), bretylium, adrenergic α- and β-blockers.
   2. Prolonged action. Recommended period to allow for normal function: methyldopa, 7 days; guanethidine, 10 days; reserpine, 14 days; mono-amine oxidase inhibitors, 14–21 days.

Disadvantages of Withdrawal.—
   1. Possibility of renal damage if diastolic pressure rises.
   2. Possible precipitation of cardiac failure or cerebrovascular accident.
   3. Inconvenience to the patient and the hospital.
   4. The patient presents for anæsthesia in a state of hypertension, and there may be added systolic peaks as a result of intubation, hypoxia, etc.

---

* Wolfsohn, N. L., and Politzer, W. M., *Anæsthesia*, 1962, **17**, 64.
† Sharpey-Schafer, E. P., *Brit. med. J.*, 1955, **1**, 693.

The Patient maintained on Hypotensive Drugs.—Opinion now tends to favour keeping patients on antihypertensive medication. The safety factor is the knowledge that these drugs have been given and their pharmacology is known.* The first agent to be thought dangerous in this respect was reserpine, but there are now several workers who have concluded after careful investigation that there is no danger.† Whether this applies also to drugs such as guanethidine and methyldopa cannot be known for certain until further trials are undertaken.

There has been no conclusive demonstration that any particular anæsthetic technique is contra-indicated, apart from the reaction between mono-amine oxidase inhibitors and pethidine. Care should be taken during the induction and maintenance of anæsthesia, especially if halothane, ether, cyclopropane, or spinal techniques are used. Bradycardia, due to unopposed vagal action, should be treated with atropine or gallamine. Blood-loss requires careful replacement. Intravenous fluids are probably preferable to pressor drugs, and if the latter are used, careful selection is necessary. Carbon-dioxide accumulation should be prevented.

The pressor drug of choice in the patient treated with reserpine, guanethidine, or methyldopa is one of the group methoxamine, phenylephrine, metaraminol; and atropine should be given if associated with bradycardia. Extreme caution should be used if any pressor agent is given to a patient receiving mono-amine oxidase inhibitors, especially methylamphetamine.

(The reader is referred to the excellent review by Dingle, H. R., *Anæsthesia*, 1966, **21**, 151.)

Antibiotics.—There is convincing evidence that large parenteral doses of neomycin, streptomycin, and dihydrostreptomycin can cause a neuromuscular block, which is potentiated by ether or non-depolarizing muscle relaxants. Other antibiotics which may cause a similar effect include kanamycin, polymyxin B, biomycin, bacitracin, and colistin.‡ Clinical reports of prolonged apnœa have been associated with the administration of a large dose of antibiotic into the peritoneal or pleural cavity towards the end of an operation with ether or relaxant anæsthesia. The effect may not become apparent until the patient has returned to the ward. Use of depolarizing muscle relaxants does not obviate this danger since there has been a report of this syndrome when suxamethonium had been used as the relaxant,§ presumably due to the onset of dual block.

Phenothiazine Derivatives.—These cause peripheral vasodilatation and a fall in blood-pressure in some subjects, which may become severe during anæsthesia. Narcotics are potentiated. Other

---

* Vandam, L. D., Harrison, J. H., Murray, J. E., and Mewill, J. P., *Anesthesiology,* 1962, **23**, 783.
† Papper, E. M., *Canad. Anæsth. Soc. J.,* 1965, **12**, 245; Munson, W. M., and Jenicek, J. A., *Anesthesiology,* 1962, **23**, 741; and Katz, R. L., Weintraub, H. D., and Papper, E. M., *Ibid.,* 1964, **25**, 142.
‡ Parisi, A. F., and Kaplan, M. H., *J. Amer. med. Ass.,* 1965, **194**, 298.
§ Foldes, F. F., and others, *Ibid.,* 1963, **183**, 672.

side-effects include liver dysfunction, anti-analgesia, and pseudo-Parkinsonism.

Mono-amine Oxidase Inhibitors.—The action of this group of drugs is imperfectly understood. Their varied action cannot be explained solely in terms of mono-amine oxidase inhibition. They are used in psychiatry in the treatment of depressive states. Reactions to pethidine and morphine have been reported in patients taking these drugs, and deaths have occurred. They include severe depression, coma, muscle twitching, hypotension, ataxia, ocular palsies, cerebral excitement, and Cheyne-Stokes respiration and may be due to liver dysfunction, though relief has been obtained following administration of 25 mg. of prednisolone hemisuccinate and chlorpromazine. Only a small proportion of patients receiving treatment show adverse reactions. It has been suggested that a test dose of 5 mg. pethidine should be given intravenously and the effect on blood-pressure and pulse-rate observed.* This is followed by test doses of 10 mg. and 20 mg. If the patient has a stable blood-pressure and pulse, and is not comatose or cyanosed, the administration of pethidine is probably safe. Severe hypertensive effects and even death may occur when pressor drugs are given to patients on treatment with this group of drugs. Examples of mono-amine oxidase inhibitors are: tranylcypromine (parnate), which has some chemical resemblance to amphetamine; phenelzine (nardil), nialamide (niamid), isocarboxazid (marplan), pivhydrazine (tersavid), and mebanazine (actomol) are hydrazine derivatives. Other mono-amine oxidase inhibitors not now in general use include iproniazid (marsilid), etryptamine (monase), and pheniprazine (cavodil), pargyline (eutonyl), and phenoxypropazine (drazine). Parstelin contains tranylcypromine and trifluoperazine. The effects of these drugs may last for 14 days. For postoperative analgesia in patients receiving mono-amine oxidase inhibitors, a combination of chlorpromazine and codeine has been used without ill effect.†

Disulphiram (Antabuse).—Blocks the normal metabolism of alcohol causing an accumulation of acetaldehyde which is responsible for the 'disulphiram reaction'. Used in the treatment of alcoholics. There may be a synergistic depressant effect with thiopentone.

Steroid Therapy.—(*See* Chapter XXIII.)

Insulin.—(*See* Chapter XXIII.)

(*See also* Godwin, E., *Hosp. Med.*, 1968, **2**, 412, and Grogono, A. W., and Jones, A. E. P., *Anæsthesia*, 1968, **23**, 215.)

---

* Churchill-Davidson, H. C., *Brit. med. J.*, 1965, **1**, 520; and Evans-Prosser, C. D. G., *Brit. J. Anæsth.*, 1968, **40**, 279.
† Jacobson, J., *S.A. med. J.*, 1965, **39**, 10.

CHAPTER IV

THE PHARMACOLOGY OF DRUGS USED FOR PRE-OPERATIVE AND POST-OPERATIVE MEDICATION

Premedication.—This term was first used in the 1920's. Its purpose is the administration of drugs to facilitate the induction and maintenance of, and the recovery from anæsthesia. At the present time the intramuscular injection of doses of sedative and a drying agent, which has been customary for decades, is being questioned[*] as it is realized that: (1) Anxiety is not always relieved: drowsiness does not necessarily abolish apprehension; (2) Some patients have in fact little anxiety concerning the induction of anæsthesia; (3) Drying agents are not always required and may have undesirable side-effects.[†]

REASONS FOR ADMINISTRATION.—

1. Reduction of fear and anxiety before anæsthesia and operation.
2. Reduction of secretion of saliva.
3. Prevention of undesirable reflexes, e.g., cardiac arrhythmia due to: (*a*) drugs such as volatile agents and suxamethonium; or (*b*) afferent impulses from, e.g., the upper respiratory tract, the eye, abdominal and thoracic viscera.
4. As part of the anæsthetic technique, e.g., narcotic analgesics reduce the tachypnœa of trichloroethylene and the extra-pyramidal movements sometimes seen after the intravenous injection of methohexitone or thiopentone; they also provide analgesia; chlorpromazine aids the production of hypothermia.

DRUGS USED.—These may include:—

1. SEDATIVES.—E.g., barbiturates, chloral hydrate, paraldehyde, methylpentynol, phenothiazines, bromethol.
2. NARCOTIC ANALGESICS.—Opium and its derivatives, pethidine, methadone. Narcotic analgesics may be derived from opium, e.g., morphine and codeine; they may be semisynthetic and obtained by chemical alteration of the morphine molecule, e.g., diacetyl morphine (heroin); or they may be entirely synthetic, e.g., pethidine.
3. NEUROLEPTIC AGENTS such as dehydrobenzperidol (droperidol).
4. PARASYMPATHOLYTIC AGENTS.—Atropine and hyoscine. A dose of 1·5–3 mg. of atropine is probably necessary to block the cardiac vagus completely although half of this will inhibit salivary secretion.

---

[*] Editorial, *Anæsthesia*, 1963, **18**, 1; Inglis, J. M., and Barrow, M. E. H., *Proc. Roy. Soc. Med.*, 1965, **58**, 29; and Jolly, C., *Lancet*, 1965, **1**, 42.
[†] Tomlin, P. J., Conway, C. M., and Payne, J. P., *Ibid.*, 1964, **1**, 14.

Sedative action is helped by the administration of a suitable hypnotic the night before operation. Examples are pentobarbitone (nembutal), butobarbitone (soneryl), or quinalbarbitone (seconal) 100–200 mg. and promethazine (phenergan) 50 mg.

Post-operative Pain.—Pain relief is necessary for: (1) Humanitarian, and (2) Therapeutic reasons.

Severity of pain depends on: (1) The site of operation (in a recent report of a large series of operations, post-operative analgesia was required in 74 per cent of thoracic cases; 63 per cent of upper abdominal cases; 51 per cent of lower abdominal cases; and 23 per cent of body-wall operations),* (2) Age, (3) Sex, (4) Premedication employed, (5) Anæsthetic agents used, (6) Psychological factors.

Abdominal and thoracic wounds result in grunting, inefficient respiration with the production of hypoxia. Areas of spontaneous atelectasis may arise with regional underventilation, perfusion inequality, and shunting of venous blood. The normal periodic deep breaths are inhibited by pain so that its relief undoubtedly aids respiration.†

METHODS OF PAIN RELIEF.—

1. Narcotic-analgesic drugs.
2. Blockade of pain afferents by regional techniques, e.g., post-operative high extradural analgesia.‡
3. Inhalation of analgesic gases and vapours, e.g., nitrous oxide and oxygen or air; trichloroethylene and air.§

Morphine

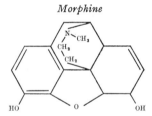

Morphine.—(From the Greek, Morpheus, god of dreams. Opium is derived from the Greek word for 'juice'.) Has been in use as opium for over 2000 years and is still the best available analgesic. ("Among the remedies which it has pleased Almighty God to give to man to relieve his sufferings, none is so universal and so efficacious as opium."—Thomas Sydenham, 1680, and still true in 1968.) Obtained from the seed capsules of the poppy plant.

Morphine isolated from opium by Sertürner in 1806.‖ Morphine salts are not destroyed by boiling.

---

* Loan, W. B., and Dundee, J. W., *Practitioner*, 1967, **198**, 759.
† Editorial, *Brit. J. Anæsth.*, 1967, **39**, 693.
‡ Bromage, P. R., *Ibid.*, 1967, **39**, 721.
§ Parbrook, G. D., *Ibid.*, 1967, **39**, 730.
‖ Sertürner, F. W. A., *J. pharm. Aeryte. Apoth. Chem.*, 1806, **14**, 47.

Morphine, *continued.*

First used as pre-anæsthetic drug by Lorenzo Bruno of Turin in 1850, by Claude Bernard in 1869,* in animals, and by Labbé and Guyon three years later.†

One of over 25 alkaloids contained in opium (*Papaver somniferum*), but only morphine, codeine, and papaverine have wide clinical use. Concentration of morphine in opium is 10 per cent.

PHARMACOLOGY.—Morphine is a direct metabolic depressant. Its chief effects are on the central nervous system, the respiratory system, and the bowel. Has been synthesized by Gates and Tschudi (1952).‡ Like codeine, it is related to phenanthrene and piperidine; this group of drugs being good analgesics and poor relaxers of smooth muscle. Papaverine is related to benzyl isoquinoline and like its congeners is a poor analgesic but a good relaxant of smooth muscle. Morphine may release histamine and 5-hydroxytryptamine from the tissues (sometimes seen in the skin weal following pre-operative injection of the drug).

CENTRAL NERVOUS SYSTEM.—It induces sleep and analgesia, the latter predominating. Mechanism of this action is unknown. More effective against dull, continuous, than against sharp, intermittent pain. Analgesia more efficient if given before onset of pain than if given to relieve existing pain. With high enough dosage analgesia adequate for the performance of surgical operations can be obtained but only at the expense of severe respiratory depression. Has no local pain-relieving effect. Analgesia usually, but not always, accompanied by euphoria. Very rarely, restlessness and delirium follow its injection (as in the horse and cat) and dysphoria follows. Depresses respiratory centre. Spinal cord reflexes sometimes exaggerated. Parasympathetic tone may be increased due to the anticholinesterase effect of morphine. The cerebrospinal fluid pressure is increased because of the augmented cerebral blood-flow consequent on a raised Pco_2. Intravenous injection causes a more rapid but less prolonged effect than intramuscular injection. It is a poor anticonvulsant.

EFFECT ON THE EYE.—It constricts the pupil, sometimes to a pinpoint size, by a central not a peripheral action, stimulating the pupillary fibres in the Edinger-Westphal nucleus, the oculomotor nerve being the efferent pathway. Atropine can counteract this miosis. Intra-ocular tension reduced in both normal and glaucomatous eyes.

RESPIRATORY SYSTEM.—The sensitivity of the respiratory centre to CO_2 is diminished. Respiratory rate, rather than tidal volume, decreased. Arterial and alveolar Pco_2 raised. Breathing may become periodic (Cheyne-Stokes) or irregular (Biot). Atropine does not reverse the respiratory depressant effects of morphine. There may be bronchoconstriction either from the anticholinesterase effect or due to histamine release, and this is worse in

* Bernard, C., *Lancet*, 1870, **2**, 285.
† Labbé, L., and Guyon, E., *C. R. Acad. Sci. Paris*, 1872, **74**, 627.
‡ Gates, M., and Tschudi, G., *J. Amer. Chem. Soc.*, 1957, **74**, 1109.

asthmatic patients. Maximal respiratory depression comes on 30 min. after intramuscular injection.

Factors which increase the likelihood of respiratory depression after morphine administration include: (1) Sleep, (2) Old age, (3) Certain pathological conditions, (4) Administration of other drugs, e.g., barbiturates, general anæsthetics, alcohol, and phenothiazines.

Factors which antagonize the depression include: (1) Pain, (2) Emotional states, (3) Tolerance and addiction, (4) Certain drugs, e.g., the specific antagonists: nalorphine, levallorphan, and naloxone, and non-specific agents, e.g., amiphenazole.

GASTRO-INTESTINAL TRACT.—Morphine constricts the sphincters of the gut. The movements of the stomach are reduced, while the pylorus is contracted. The tone of the muscles of the small and large intestines is increased, but peristalsis is reduced, and so constipation results from a state of spastic immobility of the bowel. The effects of morphine on the alimentary canal after injection are local and not central. Atropine and propantheline bromide, 15–30 mg., antagonize this action, neostigmine increases it.

Nausea and vomiting are due to stimulation of the medullary chemoreceptor trigger zone of Borison and Wang and not due to direct stimulation of the vomiting centres. This is seen most strongly with the allied drug, apomorphine. Vomiting after morphine depends partly on the movements of the body and the position of the patient: it sensitizes the vomiting centre to vestibular movements. Dimenhydrinate and histamine inhibitors have a protective effect and so has chlorpromazine. Perphenazine (fentazin) is one of the best antidotes to nausea and vomiting due to morphine; it can be given by mouth, per rectum, or by injection. Cyclimorph is a combination of morphine tartrate, 10–15 mg., with cyclizine tartrate, 50 mg. Ambulation after morphine will cause more nausea than quiet bed-rest.

Morphine produces a contraction of the muscle at the lower end of the common bile-duct (sphincter of Oddi), and so raises the bile-pressure in the bile-ducts by preventing emptying. Atropine does not fully antagonize this action, but nitroglycerin, nalorphine, levallorphan, adrenaline, aminophylline, and amyl nitrite do.

URINARY TRACT.—The tone and peristalsis of the ureters and other smooth muscle, e.g., of the hollow viscera, bladder sphincter, etc., is increased, an action antagonized by atropine. The tone of the Fallopian tubes is increased and spasm potentiated. The tone of the detrusor muscle and the vesical sphincter is increased and may hinder micturition. Urinary output decreased.

Little or no influence on uterus during labour. Crosses placental barrier and depresses fœtal respiration.

THE CARDIOVASCULAR SYSTEM.—Not greatly altered by clinical doses of morphine. There is sometimes a slight fall in pulse-rate and blood-pressure, especially if the drug is given intravenously. Vascular collapse may follow if a morphinized

Morphine—Pharmacology, *continued.*

patient suddenly sits up, or is moved. Sympathetic stimulants and leg bandaging will abolish this effect. There is vasodilatation of skin vessels, especially in the head and neck (the blush area). Skin weals may also be seen when morphine is applied to scarified skin, e.g., sometimes following an injection. Sweating may be stimulated.

Patients in shock should be given their morphine intravenously, so that it does not accumulate unabsorbed in the ischæmic tissues, only to produce a massive effect when absorption occurs with improvement in the circulation.

Morphine sometimes causes itching, especially of the nose. It may cause occasionally anaphylactoid and allergic reactions, ranging from slight syncope to anaphylactic shock with bronchial asthma due to histamine release.

Promotes glycogenolysis and so raises the blood-sugar.

THE ENDOCRINE SYSTEM.—Posterior pituitary and adrenal medulla stimulated, so antidiuretic hormone and blood catecholamine levels increased.

EXCRETION.—A small part detoxicated in the liver, a larger proportion being excreted by the kidneys, and by the gastro-intestinal tract after conjugation.

It appears in breast milk, saliva, and sweat.

The administration of opiates may be responsible for an increase in the serum glutamic oxalo-acetic transaminase activity in some individuals.*

ADVANTAGES AND DISADVANTAGES OF MORPHINE AS PREMEDICATION.—

ADVANTAGES.—

1. Relieves anxiety and produces tranquillity.
2. Reduces amount of anæsthetic needed.
3. Helps to prevent tachypnœa, e.g., after trichloroethylene.
4. Provides analgesia.

DISADVANTAGES.—

1. May produce post-operative constipation, vomiting, and ileus.
2. Causes respiratory depression and so may retard induction of inhalation anæsthesia or cause respiratory arrest when associated with halothane or cyclopropane. Morphine, in addition, depresses the cough reflex.
3. It interferes with pupil signs of depth of anæsthesia. When morphine is combined with atropine or hyoscine its miotic action usually proves stronger than their mydriatic effect.
4. It is habit forming. Tolerance follows repeated doses and addiction can occur. Abstinence symptoms are seen when addicts are suddenly deprived of their drug.
5. It may delay resumption of spontaneous respiration.

SPECIAL CARE IS NECESSARY.—

1. In infants under 6 months, the aged, feeble, and debilitated.
2. In patients with a raised Pco_2, Addison's disease, hypothyroidism, asthma, raised intracranial pressure (when codeine may be preferable).

---

* Foulk, W. T., and Fleisher, G. A., *Proc. Mayo Clin.*, 1957, **32**, 16, 405.

3. In some patients taking mono-amine oxidase inhibitors.
4. In patients who are to breathe spontaneously during cyclopropane or halothane anæsthesia because of the respiratory depression which may result.
5. In the period immediately following general anæsthesia.

Dose.—10–20 mg. The hydrochloride, sulphate, and tartrate are used, while the dose in adults is usually between 8 and 32 mg. ($\frac{1}{8}$–$\frac{1}{2}$ gr.). An adult weighing 10 stone will get maximum pain relief with minimal side-effects on a dose of 10 mg. ($\frac{1}{6}$ gr.). It can be given according to the formula, 1·5 mg. ($\frac{1}{40}$ gr.) per stone of body-weight, with 20 mg. ($\frac{1}{3}$ gr.) as a maximum dose. Should be given 90 minutes before anæsthesia, so that peak of respiratory depression is passed before induction commences. To make the ebbing life of a patient dying of carcinoma tolerable, the following "cocktail" may be given by mouth and repeated as required (Brompton Hospital): Morphine 16 mg. ($\frac{1}{4}$ gr.) and cocaine 10 mg. ($\frac{1}{6}$ gr.); Honey and gin, 5 ml. of each (or 5 ml. of syrup and 2·5 ml. of rectified spirit) ; Chloroform water to 15 ml.

[16 mg. = $\frac{1}{4}$ gr. ; 10 mg. = $\frac{1}{6}$ gr.]

Codeine Phosphate, B.P.—(Codeine is derived from the Greek name for 'poppy-head'.) This is methyl morphine and together with morphine and papaverine forms the chief alkaloidal derivative of opium. It was isolated in 1832 by Robiquet.
It depresses respiration less, causes less constipation, but is more depressing to cough reflex than morphine. Its analgesic effect is one-sixth that of morphine and it fails to produce progressive sedation with increasing doses. Useful as an analgesic after head injury. Less likely to cause addiction than morphine. Most of drug is excreted unchanged by kidneys. The usual dosage is 15–100 mg. ($\frac{1}{4}$–1$\frac{1}{2}$ gr.) of the phosphate. Increasing the total dose above 60 mg. does not increase analgesia.

Dihydrocodeine Bitartrate (D.F.118).*—This drug in 20–30-mg. doses is a very powerful analgesic, remarkably free from unpleasant side-effects such as nausea and respiratory depression. Duration of pain relief after hypodermic injection is about four hours. Put up in ampoules of 50 mg. in 1 ml. the solution has a pH of 3·2, so that it should be diluted before intravenous injection. Also in 30-mg. tablets. It releases histamine. Not a good substitute for pethidine as analgesic in light anæsthesia.† When 30 mg. are taken by mouth it tends to cause nausea and vertigo in women and constipation in men.‡

Diamorphine Hydrochloride, B.P.C. (heroin).—This is diacetyl morphine and is the most likely of the opium derivatives to become a drug of addiction, because of the euphoria it creates. Hence in the U.S. and in Australia its use is proscribed. It depresses the respiratory centre and the cough reflex more than morphine and is

* Gravenstein, J. S., and others, *New Engl. J. Med.*, 1956, **254**, 877 ; and Brittain, G. J. C. *Lancet*, 1959, **2**, 544.
† Swerdlow, M., and Foldes, F. F., *Brit. J. Anæsth.*, 1958, **30**, 515.
‡ Palmer, R. N., and others, *Lancet*, 1966, **2**, 670.

Diamorphine Hydrochloride, *continued.*

twice as efficient as an analgesic. Vomiting less common than after morphine, but constipation more common. An excellent post-operative analgesic although its effect does not last as long as that of morphine. In coronary occlusion, 5 mg. i.v. cause little cardio-vascular depression or vomiting.

Excretion is chiefly by the kidneys.

The usual dose is 2·5–10 mg. ($\frac{1}{24}$–$\frac{1}{6}$ gr.) of the hydrochloride.

Papaveretum, B.P.C. (omnopon, pantopon, alopon, opoidine).— Introduced in 1909 by Sahli.[*] These are mixtures of purified opium alkaloids in the proportion found in Nature. They contain 50 per cent of morphine, with codeine, thebaine, narcotine, and papaverine. Clinically 20 mg. papaveretum equals 13·3 mg. morphine sulphate, and its properties are not entirely due to its morphine content. The papaverine content is pharmacologically inert.[†] There is no evidence that papaveretum causes fewer unpleasant side-effects than morphine.

Dosage, 10–20 mg. ($\frac{1}{6}$–$\frac{1}{3}$ gr.).

PREMEDICATION IN CHILDREN WITH PAPAVERETUM-HYOSCINE.—A suitable dosage, worked out after careful clinical trial,[‡] is 2 mg. per stone of papaveretum with 0·04 mg. per stone of hyoscine—the normal adult dose reduced pro-portional to weight.

Papaverine, B.P.—Isolated by Merck in 1848 from opium. Related to isoquinoline and is different in constitution and action from morphine. Possesses an anti-spasmodic action but does not suppress intestinal peristalsis. Has an anti-fibrillating effect on the ventricles, but can cause cardiac arrhythmia and death if injected intra-venously quickly. Relieves spasm in arteries. Has almost no effect on the central nervous system, on respiration, or on mood, and causes no euphoria. Dose up to 30 mg. intravenously, very slowly; orally, 120–250 mg.

Apomorphine Hydrochloride, B.P.§—Prepared by treating morphine by strong mineral acids. Not used for premedication, but is derived from morphine. Used to treat delirium, e.g., that following cyclo-propane or hyoscine, in subemetic doses. Apomorphine 1–2 mg. in 10 ml. of saline injected 1 ml. at a time intravenously, provided that oxygen lack is not the cause of the delirium, will often quieten a grossly restless patient. Can be used to empty stomach, in emergency, by stimulating the vomiting centre before induction of anæsthesia. Dose 1·5 mg. intravenously with additional 1 mg. increments, if necessary. The addition of atropine 1·3 mg. will prevent possible vagal effects.

Pethidine Hydrochloride, B.P. (demerol, meperidine hydrochloride, isonipecaine, dolantin, dolantal, dolosal, pantalgin).—The

* Sahli, H., *Ther. Mh. (Halbruch.)*, 1909, **23**, 1.
† Loan, W. B., Dundee, J. W., and Clarke, R. J. S., *Brit. J. Anæsth.*, 1966, **38**, 891.
‡ Davies, D. A., and Doughty, A., *Ibid.*, 1967, **39**, 638.
§ Borison, H. L., and Wang, S. C., *Pharmacol. Rev.*, 1953, **5**, 193.

hydrochloride of the ethyl ester of 1-methyl-4-phenyl-piperidine-4-carboxylic acid.

First synthesized in 1939 by Schaumann and Eisleb at the Hoechst Farbwerke in Germany.* Intravenous dose 5–25 mg. repeated as necessary. First used in premedication by Schlungbaum in 1939† and by Rovenstine and Batterman in 1943.‡

PHARMACOLOGY.—

a. Has a morphine-like action on pain, about one-tenth as powerful as morphine, 100 mg. being the equivalent of about 10 mg. (⅙ gr.) of the latter drug. Duration of analgesia shorter than that of morphine. Relieves most types of pain, especially those associated with plain muscle spasm—except biliary colic. Produces sleepiness, but little euphoria or amnesia, and so is not the ideal drug for pre-operative sedation.§ Somewhat uncertain in its action. Depresses respiratory centre. Is a local analgesic. Raises the C.S.F. pressure. Can cause addiction.

b. Has a direct papaverine-like effect on the smooth muscle of the bronchioles, intestine, ureters, and arteries. In dilute solution is a vasodilator after intravenous injection. May cause hypotension. Will often relieve bronchial spasm. It causes spasm of the sphincter of Oddi, an effect counteracted by amyl nitrite, nitroglycerin, adrenaline, and aminophylline (not by atropine or papaverine). Reduces tone and amplitude of contraction of ureters. Does not lead to constipation.

c. Has an atropine-like effect on cholinergic nerve-endings, causing a dry mouth, dilated pupils, and depression of cholinergic nerve-supply to smooth muscle.

d. May release histamine from tissues, producing a typical triple response, causing urticarial weals over veins into which it is injected, and major or minor circulatory collapse. Weal reaction is lessened if solution is 1 per cent or less in strength and is abolished if made up to 1 per cent in 0·25 per cent procaine solution. Also has antihistamine properties.

e. Has a quinidine-like effect on myocardium and has been used to reduce the incidence of arrhythmia associated with cyclopropane anæsthesia.

f. Side-effects may include hypotension, nausea and vomiting, vertigo, and limb tingling. Post-operative nausea is similar to

* Schaumann, O., and Eisleb, O., *Dtsch. med. Wschr.*, 1939, **65**, 967.
† Schlungbaum, H., *Med. Klin.*, 1939, **35**, 1259.
‡ Rovenstine, E. A., and Batterman, R. I., *Anesthesiology*, 1943, **4**, 126.
§ Campbell, D., and others, *Brit. J. Anæsth.*, 1965, **37**, 199.

Pethidine Hydrochloride—Pharmacology, *continued.*

that following morphine, but comes on earlier.* These are worse after intravenous than after intramuscular injection. Like morphine, pethidine may cause hypotension if the head of the patient is raised or with sudden movement. May increase the incidence of post-operative nausea and vomiting, an effect reduced by its combination with atropine or hyoscine.† Because of its circulatory depressant effects it is probably not the ideal drug for the relief of pain in myocardial infarction.‡

ADMINISTRATION.—Can be given intramuscularly or intravenously. Effect comes on in 15 minutes, at maximum in 90 minutes, and lasts up to 2 hours after intramuscular administration. May be used as an analgesic to reinforce gas–oxygen and thiopentone anæsthesia, when it is given intravenously in repeated doses of 10 to 20 mg.§ Forms a precipitate with thiopentone solution.

EXCRETION.—Destroyed in body to extent of 80 per cent, probably by hydrolysis in liver, disease of which may retard its destruction. About 5–10 per cent is excreted unchanged by the kidneys. Renal excretion can be increased by forcing fluids and by making the urine more acid by the intravenous injection of sodium acid phosphate.‖

PETHIDINE IN LABOUR.—*See* Chapter XXV.

Congeners of pethidine include bemidone (hydroxypethidine), keto-bemidone, anileridine, and nisentil (alphaprodine), fentanyl and phenoperidine.

DANGER.—The administration of pethidine to patients under the influence of phenelzine (nardil) and some other mono-amine oxidase inhibitors may cause alarming reactions and even death.¶ There may be restlessness, hypertension, convulsions, and coma with absent tendon-jerks and an extensor plantar response; hypotension may also be seen. The reaction is said to be due to interference with the microsomes in liver cells which detoxicate pethidine. When the reaction does occur treatment with 25 mg. prednisolone** or chlorpromazine†† is worth trying. (*see also* table in Appendix), but not all patients are at risk.‡‡

There are with pethidine, as with other powerful drugs, two types of sensitivity. In the first the patient shows signs of overdosage following average amounts given, e.g., vasodilatation and hypotension. In the second the patient shows an abnormal reaction to the administration of the drug.

Phenoperidine and Fentanyl are related to pethidine, but are much more potent. (*See* Chapter XIV.)

* Dundee, J. W., and others, *Lancet*, 1965, **2**, 1262.
† Dundee, J. W., and others, *Brit. J. Anæsth.*, 1964, **36**, 703.
‡ Rees, H. A., and others, *Ibid.*, 1967, **2**, 863.
§ Neff, W., and others, *California med. J.*, 1947, **66**, 67.
‖ London, D. R., and Milne, M. D., *Brit. med. J.*, 1962, **2**, 1752.
¶ Palmer, H., *Ibid.*, 1960, **2**, 507.
** Shee, J. C., *Ibid.*, 1960, **2**, 507.
†† Papp, C., and Benain, S., *Ibid.*, 1958, **2**, 1070.
‡‡ Evans-Prosser, C. D. G., *Brit. J. Anæsth.*, 1968, **40**, 279.

Alphaprodine (nisentil, prisilidene hydrochloride).*—This is 1,3, dimethyl-4-phenyl-4 propionoxypiperidine and was synthesized by Lee in 1947.

It is structurally similar to pethidine. It does not produce tolerance on repeated injection, while it causes fewer side-effects than does pethidine. It leads to hyperglycæmia and is probably detoxicated by the liver. The effects of an intravenous dose last about 45 minutes. The recommended dose is 20–30 mg. intravenously and double this by mouth. In anæsthesia it is used instead of pethidine to supplement gas, oxygen, and thiopentone, and appears to be a better analgesic than pethidine and to cause, in proper analgesic doses, less respiratory depression. It raises the pressure of cerebrospinal fluid, an effect prevented by levallorphan. Its rapid onset and rather short effect make it useful in labour for pain relief. Dose: 20–30 mg. i.v.; 20–60 mg. i.m.

Anileridine (alidine).†—A new analgesic synthesized in 1956 by Weijlard and his colleagues. Chemically related to pethidine and similarly metabolized but between three and four times more potent; one-third the potency of morphine. Analgesic potency is as follows: morphine 10 mg. = pethidine 100 mg. = anileridine 30 mg. Does not cause much nausea and vomiting and euphoria uncommon. Non-constipating and non-spasmogenic. Active by mouth. A satisfactory supplement to thiopentone–gas–oxygen anæsthesia. Can cause addiction. Dose: 25–50 mg.

Dipipanone Hydrochloride, B.P. (pipadone).—An analgesic first described by Ofner, Thorpe, and Walton in 1949, chemically allied to methadone. Put up in ampoules each containing 25 mg. in 1 ml. Has similar action to pethidine but with less tendency to cause low blood-pressure. A poor hypnotic. Antagonized by nalorphine. Metabolized in liver. Analgesic effects last 4 or 5 hours. Nausea and vomiting are rare side-effects. In analgesic potency, 25 mg. is the equivalent of morphine or methadone 10 mg.

Can be used in obstetrics for pain relief (25 mg. intramuscularly), and to supplement nitrous-oxide–oxygen anæsthesia (2·5–5 mg. intravenously). Has been used like alphaprodine and pethidine to produce narcotic-induced controlled apnœa in patients in whom it is desirable to avoid the use of relaxants (e.g., in thoracic surgery‡). *Diconal* is dipipanone 10 mg. with cyclizine 30 mg. It is useful for the oral treatment of severe pain.

Pentazocine (fortral, talwin).—A benzomorphan derivative, first described in 1959. A non-addictive analgesic, 30–60 mg. of which give analgesia comparable to that following morphine 10 mg.§ No psychotic side-effects and is exempted from D.D.A. regulations in Britain. Sedation seen in only 30 per cent of patients so it is not a good drug for premedication. Causes little nausea and no marked

* Siker, E. S., Foldes, F. F., Pahk, N. M., and Swerdlow, M., *Brit. J. Anæsth.*, 1954, **26**, 405
† Swerdlow, M., and others, *Anæsthesia*, 1960, **15**, 280.
‡ Coleman, D. J., Levin, J., and Jones, P. O., *Brit. med. J.*, 1957, **1**, 1092.
§ Conaghan, J. P., and others, *Brit. J. Anæsth.*, 1966, **38**, 345; Finestone, S. C., and Katz, J., *Curr. Res. Anesth.*, 1966, **45**, 312; and Swerdlow, M., and Dalal, A., *Der Anæsthesist*, 1966, **15**, 43.

Pentazocine, *continued.*

effect on either C.S.F. or intra-ocular pressure. Increases tone of sphincter of Oddi. It is a narcotic antagonist akin to nalorphine. Its effects are antagonized by methylphenidate (ritalin).

Oxymorphone (numorphan).—Chemically closely related to morphine. A narcotic analgesic with morphine-like activity. A poor depressant of the cough reflex and produces little euphoria. Gastro-intestinal side-effects less marked than those caused by morphine. Reversed by nalorphine. Can cause addiction. Does not cause much respiratory depression. Used instead of pethidine to supplement gas and oxygen anæsthesia. It has been reported that pethidine 100 mg. is equal to oxymorphone 1·34 mg.* Analgesic potency of morphine : levorphan : oxymorphone is 1 : 5 : 10. Doses up to 5 mg. have little effect on the circulatory system. The *n*-allyl derivative is naloxone, a narcotic antagonist.

Dextromoramide Acid Tartrate (palfium).—A morphine-like analgesic but twice as potent. Dose 5-mg. tablet or 5–10 mg. by intramuscular injection.

Methadone Hydrochloride, B.P. (physeptone, amidone, dolophine, miadone, adanon, butalgin).—This is *d-l*-6-dimethylamino-4 : 4-diphenyl-heptan-3-1 hydrochloride. A white crystalline powder, soluble in water and alcohol. An analgesic with a similar effect to that of morphine. Can be given by mouth or by injection. In common with morphine, its analgesic effect is diminished if given together with hyoscine. Not a good sedative and so is not very useful as a drug for premedication, unless pain is severe. Its effect, in common with that of pethidine and morphine, is enhanced if neostigmine, 0·5 mg., is given at the same time. Most useful in treatment of post-operative pain, dysmenorrhœa, pain of spasm of bladder-neck, cough, renal colic, etc. Tolerance to its use is produced, while it has proved to be a drug of addiction. Side-effects are dryness of mouth, headache, nausea and vomiting, drowsiness, and euphoria; they are less troublesome than after either morphine or pethidine. Causes bradycardia, peripheral vasodilatation, and some hypotension. Has a similar effect in releasing muscle spasm to pethidine. Useful to relieve the pain associated with paralytic ileus, as it does not produce the spastic inactivity of the bowel seen with morphine. Does not increase tone of sphincter of Oddi and so is useful for pre- and post-operative sedation in biliary tract disease. As with morphine and pethidine, its side-effects are worse in ambulant patients than in those confined to bed. Causes less miosis than morphine; does not constipate. Is a mild local analgesic and antihistamine. Partly excreted in urine and partly in fæces. Powerful depressant of fœtal respiration. Dosage similar to morphine—5–10 mg. For the relief of cough, 2·5 mg. in a linctus is useful.

Phenazocine Hydrobromide, B.P.C. (narphen; prinadol hydrobromide; xenagol).—This is 2′-hydroxy-5,9-dimethyl-2-phenethyl-6,7-benzomorphan hydrochloride. An analgesic synthesized in

---

* Swerdlow, M., and Brown, P. R., *Brit. J. Anæsth.*, 1961, **33**, 126.

1957.* Effects of 3 mg. resemble those of morphine, 10 mg.† Has minimal sedative and narcotic properties, and the classic side-effects of morphine (nausea, constipation, etc.) not marked. May be used for minor surgery instead of general anæsthesia and to supplement thiopentone–relaxant–gas–oxygen anæsthesia—the dose being 0·5–2 mg. i.v. Respiratory depression can be reversed by nalorphine.

Levorphanol Tartrate, B.P. (dromoran, lævo-morphinan tartrate, levorphan, methorphan).—Was synthesized by Schnider and Grisner in 1949. Chemically is 3-hydroxy-n-methyl morphinan hydrogen tartrate dihydrate. The lævo-isomer is twice as active as the racemic drug. An analgesic, effective parenterally or by mouth, more potent and of longer duration than morphine. Has been used to supplement thiopentone–gas–oxygen anæsthesia.‡ A poor hypnotic. Nausea and vomiting rarely caused. Does not depress the cough reflex nor cause the drowsiness sometimes seen after morphine. May cause intestinal spasm and so is not the best agent to relieve the pains of colic. Dosage by mouth, 1·5–2 mg.; in severe pain 4 mg. By injection 1–5 mg.

Forms a precipitate with thiopentone, but not with gallamine or tubocurarine.

Dextromethorphan is a useful cough suppressant (romilar).

Amitriptyline.—This is a dibenzo-cyclo-heptadiene derivative and is an antidepressant and tranquillizer with antihistamine, anticonvulsive, and mild anticholinergic properties. It causes sedation without prolonging recovery. Does not result in hypotension. Dose: 0·33 mg. per kg. body-weight i.v.§

Methylpentynol, B.P.C. (oblivon, somnesin, dormison, atempol).—This is 3-methyl-1-pentyn-3-ol. An orally active depressant of the central nervous system with calming, sedative, and hypnotic actions.

$$\text{HC} \equiv \text{C}-\overset{\displaystyle \text{CH}_3}{\underset{\displaystyle \text{OH}}{\text{C}}}-\text{CH}_2-\text{CH}_3$$

Rapidly absorbed and its effects last about 1 hour. Crosses blood–brain barrier and enters placenta, its distribution in body being similar to that of ethyl alcohol. Even in large doses does not depress respiratory or cardiovascular systems. May act by its depressant effects on reticular-activating system and the thalamo-cortical circuits. Sedative action reversed by caffeine.

Introduced as an agent to banish apprehension and anxiety without causing sleep, but it has hypnotic activity—about 40 per cent of that of phenobarbitone or pentobarbitone. Has a reputation as a pre-anæsthetic drug in children undergoing tonsillectomy,

* Eddy, N. B., Murphy, J. L., and May, E. L., *J. Organ. Chem.*, 1957, **22**, 1370.
† Swerdlow, M., and others, *Brit. J. Anæsth.*, 1964, **36**, 782.
‡ Brown. A. K., *Brit. med. J.*, 1952, **2**, 1331.
§ Levesque, P. R., and others, *Canad. Anæsth. Soc., J.* 1965, **12**, 129.

Methylpentynol, *continued.*

when it interferes neither with the induction nor the recovery from anæsthesia. Dose 500–750 mg. for children under 8 years, 750–1000 mg. for those over 8 years, $1\frac{1}{2}$–2 hours before operation.

In obstetrics, 1000 mg. are given early in labour followed by additional doses of 500 mg. to a total of 3000 mg. Can be given per rectum, three or four 250-mg. capsules. Supplied in capsules of 250 mg., and as an elixir, each teaspoonful containing 250 mg.

See: *Brit. med. J.*, 1961, **2**, 170 ; Gusterson, F. R., *Ibid.*, 1958, **2**, 1229 (who gave one teaspoonful of the elixir per stone with hyoscine, 0·4 mg., dissolved in it for children under 3 and atropine, 0·6 mg., for older children. Intravenous thiopentone induction follows) ; Galley, A. H., and Trotter, P., *Lancet*, 1958, **1**, 343 ; Bartholomew, A. A., and others, *Ibid.*, 1958, **1**, 346.

Methylpentynol carbamate (oblivon-C) is three or four times as potent as the parent substance, while its effects last longer.

Methaqualone Hydrochloride (melsedin).—A sedative hypnotic. A dose of 150–300 mg. gives sedation for up to 5 hours, comparable to that of an opiate. Changes in heart-rate and blood-pressure minimal and nausea and vomiting not troublesome. Mandrax is a combination of methaqualone, 250 mg., and diphenhydramine, 25 mg.[*]

The potentiation of analgesic drugs by cholinergic agents such as neostigmine and pyridostigmine has been reported[†] and may be due to inhibition of destruction of the analgesic in the liver. Morphine, pethidine, levorphanol, and methadone may all act for a longer time after 1 mg. of pyridostigmine or 0·5 mg. of neostigmine.

Specific Narcotic Antagonists.—These are usually the *n*-allyl derivatives of narcotic analgesics. The more potent the narcotic, the smaller the dose of its allyl derivative necessary to antagonize narcotic-induced respiratory depression. Main difference between narcotics and their antagonists is that the latter do not: (1) cause euphoria, (2) lead to addiction, and (3) cause signs of withdrawal in narcotic addicts. Probable mode of action is competition at receptor sites on cell surfaces.

Specific antagonism to narcotics was first described in 1915 by Pohl.

Nalorphine Hydrobromide, B.P. (*n*-allyl normorphine hydrobromide, nalorphine, nalline, lethidrone).—This was first described by McCawley, Hart, and Marsh in 1940[‡] and synthesized by Weijlard and Erickson in 1942.[§] It was used as an antagonist to morphine by Eckenhoff in 1951.[||] It is closely related chemically to morphine, in which there is a nitrogen atom with a methyl group attached; in the new drug this methyl group is exchanged for an allyl group (C_3H_5). It combines with the receptors on which

[*] Norris, W., and Nisbet, H. I. A., *Brit. J. Anæsth.*, 1966, **38**, 886.
[†] Oehlandt, G., *Med. Klin.*, 1955, **50**, 2202.
[‡] McCawley, E. L., Hart, E. H., and Marsh, D. F., *J. Amer. chem. Soc.*, 1941, **63**, 314.
[§] Weijlard, J., and Erickson, E. A., *Ibid.*, 1942, **64**, 869.
[||] Eckenhoff, J. E., and others, *Amer. J. med. Sci.*, 1951, **222**, 112.

morphine acts (*see also* Annotation in *Brit. med. J.*, 1953, **1**, 35; Bodman, R., *Proc. R. Soc. Med.*, 1953, **46**, 11, 923; also Landmesser, C. M., Cobb, S., and Converse, J. G., *Anesthesiology*, 1963, **14**, 535).

It is effective in counteracting respiratory depression and narcosis produced by opiates, pethidine, methadone, methorphan, and metapon, but not that due to ether, cyclopropane, thiopentone, or other barbiturates. Intravenous dose 3–10 mg. Stimulation of respiration only lasts 10–15 minutes and may then increase drowsiness and lead to nausea, sweating, etc. Not suitable for use in ambulant patients. It restores the E.E.G. pattern of morphinized patients to normal.

It can be used :—

1. In the treatment of opium poisoning, e.g., in neonates ; in the ill or shocked or emphysematous patient suffering from right heart failure.

2. In the treatment of morphine addiction.

3. To aid diagnosis in patients whose symptoms are masked by morphine.

4. In midwifery, to reverse morphine- or pethidine-induced fœtal respiratory depression (Bodman).

Repeated doses may cause hypertension and should not be given unless respiratory depression is severe. It abolishes the increased intestinal tone due to morphine. When given to non-morphinized patients it causes nausea, miosis, sweating, slight sedation, and hallucinations. It is a tricky drug to use. Too little will not reverse morphine effects ; too much will potentiate them. In anæsthesia, respiratory depression due to morphine or pethidine is its chief indication. Useful in the treatment of asphyxia neonatorum due to fœtal respiratory depression from opiates or pethidine.[*] The dose in the baby is 0·25–0·5 mg. given into the umbilical vein, and repeated if necessary.

The ordinary solution contains 10 mg. per ml. The neonatal solution, 1 ml. equals 1 mg.

Levallorphan Tartrate (Lorfan, R-1-7700).—Levallorphan was synthesized in 1950 by Schneider and Hellerbach and used as an antidote to respiratory depression by Fromherz and Pellmond two years later.[†] Its effects last longer than those of nalorphine and than those of morphine and pethidine. It reverses the rise in cerebrospinal fluid pressure caused by pethidine. It is the *n*-allyl derivative of lævo-morphinan (lævo-dromoran) to which it bears a similar relationship as does nalorphine to morphine. It is 3-hydroxy-*n*-allyl morphinan tartrate and is an effective antagonist to the respiratory depression produced by morphine, pethidine, dromoran, etc., without reversing the sensory depressant effects. It potentiates the depressant effects of pentobarbitone. In anæsthesia it is used to reverse severe respiratory depression which may accompany nitrous-oxide–oxygen anæsthesia, supplemented with pethidine, alphaprodine, etc. Suggested dosage to reverse the respiratory depressant effects of the sedative is one-hundredth

---

[*] Eckenhoff, J. E., Hoffman, G. L., and Dripps, R. D., *Anesthesiology*, 1952, **13**, 242.
[†] Fromherz, K., and Pellmond, B., *Experientia*, 1952, **8**, 394.

Levallorphan Tartrate, *continued.*

the pethidine dosage, one-twentieth the morphine or alphaprodine dosage, and one-tenth the levorphan dosage, e.g., 0·5–1 mg. intravenously, repeated at 3–5-min. intervals. Put up in 0·1 per cent solution, 1 ml. equals 1 mg. *Pethilorfan* contains pethidine and levallorphan 100 to 1·25 (80 : 1). Recent reports have shown that the addition of levallorphan to pethidine reduces the analgesia and increases unwanted side-effects of pethidine, while respiratory depression may even be made worse.*

See also good review " Narcotic–Narcotic Antagonist Mixtures " by Telford, J., and Keats, A. S., *Anesthesiology*, 1961, **22**, 465.

Naloxone.—This is *n*-allyl noroxymorphone and is derived from the potent oxymorphone which is ten times as strong as morphine. It is a more effective antagonist of narcotic-induced respiratory depression than either nalorphine or levallorphan. These three antagonists show no specificity for any one narcotic, while each is no more effective against its parent compound than it is against the other narcotics. The antagonists counteract the analgesia produced by morphine, levorphan, pethidine, and oxymorphone although less so with morphine.†

Narcotic-induced Controlled Apnœa.—A technique introduced by Francis Foldes‡ in which a narcotic analgesic, such as pethidine, alphaprodine, oxymorphone, dipipanone, is given intravenously in incremental doses sufficient to cause, along with hyperventilation, apnœa. Anæsthesia can be induced by thiopentone and a tube inserted using suxamethonium. Movement of the patient or attempts at breathing are indications for more analgesic. Muscular relaxation can be obtained by small doses of suxamethonium or of a non-depolarizing drug. Levallorphan, 1–2 mg., will reverse the apnœa.

Barbiturates.—The parent molecule from which the barbiturates are derived is barbituric acid or malonyl urea.

$$\begin{array}{c} \text{HN---CO} \qquad \text{H} \\ \diagup \qquad\qquad \diagup \\ \text{OC} \qquad\qquad \text{C} \\ \diagdown \qquad\qquad \diagdown \\ \text{HN---CO} \qquad \text{H} \end{array}$$

This was described in 1882 by Conrad and Guthzeit, and introduced into medicine by Emil Fischer and von Mehring in 1903§ as barbitone (diethyl barbituric acid); pheno- and allobarbitone followed in 1912. Three groups are described:—

1. The ultra-short acting, e.g., thiopentone, hexobarbitone, methohexitone, thialbarbitone, and thiamylal, mainly detoxicated in the liver.

---

* Macris, S. G., and others, *Curr. Res. Anesth.*, 1963, **42**, 440; and Vasiloff, N., and others, *Canad. Anæsth. Soc. J.*, 1965, **12**, 306.
† Foldes, F. F., and others, *Anesthesiology*, 1965, **26**, 320.
‡ Foldes, F. F., *Amer. J. med. Sci.*, 1957, **233**, 1.
§ Fischer, E., and von Mehring, J., *Ther. d. Gegenw.*, 1904, **45**, 145.

2. The medium acting, e.g., sodium amytal, pentobarbitone, **quinal-barbitone**, butobarbitone, dial, ipral, neonal, phanodorm, partly eliminated unchanged, partly detoxicated in the liver.

3. The long acting, e.g., barbitone, phenobarbitone, eliminated unchanged by the kidneys.

The medium-acting barbiturates form useful pre-anæsthetic sedatives. They induce sleep, allay anxiety, depress the central nervous system without producing the same degree of respiratory depression as does morphine. They are anticonvulsant. They probably depress the cortex, reticular-activating system, spinal cord, and the medulla in that order. Large doses cause capillary dilatation and myocardial depression. As they are not analgesic and may even be anti-analgesic, they give rise to restlessness and loss of self-control in the presence of unrelieved pain. They reduce the B.M.R. and the blood-pressure and they depress the renal and hepatic function. Their effect on the E.E.G. is similar to that of natural sleep. They traverse the placental barrier. They reduce the tone of the gut. They are partly destroyed in the liver and partly excreted by the kidneys.

As pre-anæsthetic sedatives, barbiturates are administered by mouth or by the rectum. Three to five times the hypnotic dose usually produces coma. Suitable drugs of this type are:—

1. PENTOBARBITONE SODIUM, B.P. (nembutal).—First described in the U.S.A. Magill was the first to report its use in Great Britain.* It is sodium ethyl-methyl-butyl-barbiturate. Pentobarbitone can be administered parenterally dissolved in propylene glycol, each ml. containing 60 mg. of the drug. The usual dose is 60–90 mg. given deeply intramuscularly.† The ordinary intravenous solution of the sodium salt in water (7·5 per cent) can also be given intramuscularly.‡ Can be given per rectum to children 0·6 gr. (30–40 mg.) per stone of body-weight. Pentobarbitone is rapidly and completely eliminated and does not produce cumulative effects.

Pentobarbitone, 200 mg., slightly increases the pulse-rate and lowers the blood-pressure. Tidal exchange and minute volume are slightly decreased. It causes less respiratory depression than morphine, 16 mg.

It is supplied in yellow capsules containing 30–50 and 100 mg. (½, ¾, or 1½ gr.) and also in tablets. The adult dose is 100–200 mg. given two hours before operation by mouth. The elixir contains 2 gr. to the ounce.

2. QUINALBARBITONE SODIUM, B.P. (sodium seconal).—Was described in 1935. This is sodium propyl-methyl-carbinyl-allyl-barbiturate. Action is shorter, more intense, and more rapid in onset than that of pentobarbitone. Has been used intravenously dissolved in water and polyethylene glycol. Used similarly to intravenous pentobarbitone, i.e., before intubation, when it is less likely to cause laryngeal spasm than is thiopentone : used during regional analgesia to produce sleep. Usually given by

---

* Magill, I. W., *Lancet*, 1931, **1**, 74.
† Jarvis, J. R., *Ohio St. med. J.*, 1953, **49**, 308.
‡ Beecher, H. K., *Anesthesiology*, 1951, **12**, 863.

Barbiturates—Quinalbarbitone Sodium, *continued.*

mouth. Thioquinalbarbitone is known as thiamyl, surital, thioseconal.

Supplied in scarlet capsules each containing 50–100 mg. (¾ gr., 1½ gr.) and in 50–100 mg. tablets. Usual dose 100–200 mg.

3. BUTOBARBITONE, B.P. (sodium soneryl ; neonal). Sodium butylethyl-barbiturate. Supplied in white capsules containing 100 mg. of the drug.

Dosage is by body-weight and varies between two and five capsules.

Following 100-mg. doses of pentobarbitone, quinalbarbitone, and butobarbitone, the results are much the same. Following 200 mg. the hang-over is least with butobarbitone.

4. AMYLOBARBITONE, B.P. (sodium amytal).—Is sodium ethyl-isoamyl-barbiturate. Supplied in capsules of 60 mg. (1 gr.) and 200 mg. (3 gr.). The bed-time dose is 200 mg. Sodium amytal and sodium seconal, in 4 per cent solution, are also local analgesics.

Barbiturates antagonize the convulsant effects of local analgesic drugs, and so are suitable in the premedication of patients to be operated upon under local analgesia.

THE SIGNS OF ACUTE BARBITURATE OVERDOSAGE.— Depression of the central nervous system ; depression of respiration ; depression of reflex activity ; depression of the cardio-vascular system is a late result.

Mortality in special centres of admitted cases is less than 1 per cent.* Treatment consists of adequate respiratory care,† tracheal toilet, and perhaps I.P.P.V. if the minute volume is less than 4 l. per min. and blood gas estimations (which are useful for assessing changes in the patient's condition) call for it. Hypotension is managed by the i.v. injection of metar-aminol, plasma volume expanders, or hydrocortisone. Peritoneal dialysis, forced diuresis with 30 per cent urea or 10–20 per cent mannitol, and hæmodialysis may be required.

Estimation of serum barbiturate levels may be employed to monitor progress. The longer acting drugs being less protein-bound are more rapidly removed by hæmodialysis than shorter-acting agents. (*See* Annotation, *Lancet*, 1967, **1**, 200.)

Paraldehyde, B.P.—Introduced into medicine in 1882 by Cervello. A useful hypnotic in doses of one to two drachms (4–8 ml.). Effect comes on 30 min. after oral administration. Can be given in iced fruit juice or per rectum in twice the dosage with double its volume of olive oil. Its stench is its chief disadvantage. It does not depress the heart. Mostly destroyed in liver; a small amount excreted by lungs and kidneys. Can be given intramuscularly (10 ml.) when it is a useful sedative and anti-convulsant. Can be sterilized by heating to 130° C. for 30 min. without appreciable decomposition. Ampoules should be stored in a cool, dark place and used within 3 months of preparation. Intravenous injection of 2 ml. will often cause an explosive cough.

---

* Mathew, H., and Lawson, A. A. H., *Q. Jl. Med.*, 1966, **35**, 539.
† Nilsson, E., *Acta med. scand.*, 1951, suppl. 253.

Chloral Hydrate, B.P. ($CCl_3 \cdot CH(OH)_2$.—A needlessly neglected hypnotic introduced in 1869 by Liebreich (1839–1908),* a Berlin physician, and hence (apart from alcohol) the oldest. Hypnotic dose is 15–30 gr. (0·6–2 g.) suitably diluted. Effect comes on in less than an hour and lasts about eight hours. It leaves no hangover and is safe. Rather irritating to alimentary canal. It crosses the placental barrier. A portion is converted to trichloracetic acid and a part is excreted by kidneys after conversion to trichlorethanol (the substance responsible for its effects on the central nervous system), by conjugation in liver with glycuronic acid to form urochloralic acid. Supplied in tablet form as dichloral phenazonum (welldorm), which causes less gastric disturbance than the solutions of chloral hydrate. Dose: 1–2 g. Also as trichloroethyl phosphate, the phosphoric ester of trichlorethanol. Dose: 1–2 g. (triclofos, tricloryl).

Glutethimide (doriden).—This is alpha-ethyl-alpha-phenyl glutarimide. It is an analogue of bemegride, a central nervous system stimulant. A useful non-barbiturate hypnotic. Similar in effect to medium-acting barbiturates, e.g., pentobarbitone sodium. Dose 250–500 mg.

Methyprylone (noludar).—This is 3.3-diethyl-2 : 4-dioxo-5-methyl piperidine. A good hypnotic, similar in effect to amylobarbitone and butobarbitone. Dose 200–400 mg.

Droperidol.—This drug has been used in premedication, since it produces mental detachment and is anti-emetic. Large doses may cause extrapyramidal disturbances. It is often combined with phenoperidine or fentenyl. (*See* Chapter XIV.)

Phenothiazine Derivatives.—These have been given as sedatives before operation in various doses and in diverse combinations. They are also likely to reduce the incidence of vomiting. Chlorpromazine 25 mg. the night before operation, the morning of the operation, and continued for several doses post-operatively by mouth, is a popular prescription, while 300 mg. as a suppository per rectum is also successful.† Promethazine 50 mg. with or without pethidine has been used with considerable satisfaction; to this combination a drug to produce sleep can be added, e.g., an opiate, or pentobarbitone. *Trimeprazine tartrate* (vallergan) is another valuable member of this group of drugs. Dose: 25–50 mg. intramuscularly. (*See also* Chapter XIV.)

Ataraxic Drugs.—(From Greek *ataraxia* = peace of mind.) The tranquillizers have been used for pre-operative sedation ; one of these (pecazine, a phenothiazine derivative) has given good results. In addition to good pre-operative sedation, pecazine is said to decrease the amount of anæsthetic drugs necessary, does not alter the response to pressor drugs (unlike chlorpromazine), and reduces the incidence of vomiting. The dose suggested is 1 mg. per lb. body-weight in adults ; 1·5 mg. per lb. in children.

---

* Liebreich, M. E. O., *Das Chloralhydrat, ein Neves Hypnoticum und Anästheticum*, 1869. Berlin.
† Boulton, T. B., *Anæsthesia*, 1955, **10**, 233.

Ataraxic Drugs, *continued.*

Other ataraxic drugs include pipradol, atarax, ritalin, meprobamate, dioxolane, nostyn, promazine, compazine, reserpine, etc.*

Anti-analgesics.—Anti-analgesic effects may follow the administration of small doses of barbiturates.† These may be seen immediately after the injection of subnarcotic doses, or at a later stage as the effective concentration of the drug falls. A similar effect may be present with halothane in low concentration (0·5 per cent), with promethazine‡ and with hyoscine.

Parasympatholytic Agents

Atropine Sulphate, B.P. (from Atropos, the oldest of the Three Fates who severed the thread of life).—The alkaloid of the *Atropa belladonna* or deadly nightshade. Belladonna has been in use for many centuries: atropine isolated in 1831 by Mein. Bezold and Bloebaum demonstrated its blocking effect on the cardiac vagus in 1867 and Heidenhain discovered its antisalivary action in 1872, and, apart from hyoscine, it is still probably the best drug for this purpose.§ Not used in premedication before 1890. The atropine group of alkaloids are esters formed by the union of an aromatic derivative of benzyl alcohol, tropic acid, with organic bases—tropine (atropine) and scopine (hyoscine). The tropic acid is the active radical. Atropine is the racemic mixture of dextro- and lævo-hyoscyamine; hyoscine is lævo-rotatory. First synthesized by Willstaetter in 1896, and again by Robert Robinson in 1917.

ACTION ON AUTONOMIC NERVES.—It has a blocking action on effector organs of structures supplied by the post-ganglionic cholinergic nerves, i.e., smooth muscles, and secretory glands, acting on the effector cells, i.e., it interferes with the action of acetylcholine at these sites. It is a parasympathetic depressant, a parasympatholytic anticholinergic drug.

ACTION ON CENTRAL NERVOUS SYSTEM.—It stimulates the medulla and higher centres, and directly stimulates the respiratory centre sufficiently to counteract the depressing effect of morphine. Occasionally, restlessness and delirium are seen. With larger doses comes central depression. Atropine, like its allies the antihistamines, may cause slight drowsiness. The peak of its effect is one hour after hypodermic injection, wearing off rapidly.

EFFECTS ON EYE.—There is paralysis of the sphincter of the iris resulting in dilated pupils although a dose of 0·6 mg. does not greatly influence accommodation. (The sphincter muscle is innervated from the third cranial nerve via the ciliary ganglion and short ciliary nerves.) Used as drops, 1 per cent. Atropine does not appreciably raise the intra-ocular pressure in normal eyes, but in narrow-angle glaucoma this definitely occurs through interference of drainage of aqueous through the channels of

---

* Gold, M. L., and Stone, H. H., *Anesthesiology*, 1957, **18**, 357.
† Clutton-Brock, J., *Anæsthesia*, 1960, **15**, 71 ; and Dundee, J. W., *Brit. J. Anæsth.*, 1960, **32**, 407.
‡ Dundee, J. W., and Moore, J., *Anæsthesia*, 1960, **15**, 95.
§ Diamant, H., and Feinmesser, M., *Brit. J. Anæsth.*, 1959, **31**, 205.

Fontana and the canals of Schlemm. In angle-closure glaucoma, eserine drops may be desirable before operation as part of the premedication. Atropine is not contra-indicated in other types of glaucoma.*

It has recently been shown that atropine causes oxygen desaturation of the blood, possibly due to increased shunting of blood in lungs.† Other observers deny this.‡ Effect probably worse after subcutaneous than after intravenous or intramuscular injections.

Sweat, bronchial, and salivary glands are paralysed, while bronchial muscle is relaxed, causing a slight increase in the anatomical and physiological dead space. Must be used carefully in hyperthermic patients, especially in children.

Intramuscular injection 1 hour before anæsthesia suppresses salivation more efficiently than intravenous injection immediately before induction.

ACTION ON CIRCULATORY SYSTEM.—Rate of heart sometimes slowed at first, due to medullary (vagal) stimulation, but this effect is not seen after intravenous injection of clinical doses. It may occur after hypodermic injection or after intravenous injection of small amounts such as 0·05 mg.§ Later, rate is quickened by peripheral vagal paralysis and its effect on the S.A. pace-maker. This increase in heart-rate is not marked in infants and senile patients. Atropine 1·3 mg. subcutaneously will increase pulse-rate 20–30 per minute, effect lasting up to two hours. If 0·6 mg. is given intravenously, rate of heart will increase about 20 beats per minute. Reflexes involving vagal stimulation, and hence cardiac slowing and syncope, may be prevented by atropine. In cases of gross tachycardia, e.g., in thyrotoxicosis, hyperpyrexia, or heart disease, atropine is better avoided.

It has recently been shown:‖ (a) In patients not premedicated with atropine or hyoscine, doses less than 0·5 mg. i.v. cause a slow pulse; more than 0·5 mg. i.v. causes quickening, with or without preliminary slowing, depending on the rate of injection. (b) In patients premedicated with atropine or hyoscine, subsequent intravenous injection causes tachycardia, whatever the rate of injection. If premedication dose was given many hours previously its effects may wear off. Atropine premedication also tends to prevent the arrhythmias (A–V dissociation; A and V extrasystoles; multifocal ventricular tachycardia) sometimes seen after intravenous injection of atropine. Gallamine does not alter the basic effects of atropine on the heart-rate.

Atropine sometimes causes dilatation of the vessels of the face.

Blood-pressure not affected unless heart-rate is slowed by vagal overactivity, when atropine raises it.

* Mehra, K. S., and others, *Brit. J. Anæsth.*, 1965, **37**, 133; and Schwartz, H., and others, *J. Amer. med. Ass.*, 1957, **165**, 144.
† Tomlin, P. J., Conway, C. M., and Payne, J. P., *Lancet*, 1964, **1**, 14. *See also* Taylor, S. H., Scott, D. B., and Donald, K. W., *Proc. R. Soc. Med.*, 1964, **1**, 841.
‡ Gardiner, A. J. S., and Palmer, K. H. W., *Brit. med. J.*, 1964, **7**, 1433; Medrado, V., and Stephen, C. R., *Lancet*, 1966, **1**, 734; and Taylor, S. H., and others, *Ibid.*, 1964, **1**, 841.
§ Morton, H. J. V., and Kemp, S. W., *Anæsthesia*, 1962, **17**, 170.
‖ Thomas, E. T., *Ibid.*, 1965, **20**, 340.

Atropine Sulphate, *continued.*

ACTION ON ALIMENTARY CANAL.—The tone and peristalsis of the gut and urinary tract are decreased but it almost doubles the pressure that the cardia is able to withstand from the gastric aspect: it does not affect the resistance of the cardia to pressure from above. Thus it should always be given if regurgitation is at all possible.* Like hyoscine it is anti-emetic.

Has no effect on musculature of larynx. Inhibition of sweating may lead to increase in temperature.

Milk secretion is not affected, although the drug may be excreted into the milk. Passes placental barrier and may cause fœtal tachycardia preceded by bradycardia, or bradycardia alone.† Acts as a local anæsthetic, being half as potent as procaine.

It inhibits the muscarinic but not the nicotinic effects of acetylcholine. It raises the basal metabolic rate. It is active after inunction and after oral ingestion as reported by Sington‡ in 1926. Like morphine, may produce a skin weal after subcutaneous injection.

Effects of atropine on the eye, heart, and salivary glands less effective in Negroes than in white people.§

Excretion is partly by the kidneys, another part being destroyed in the body. Must be used carefully in thyrotoxicosis because of action on heart-rate and on B.M.R.

Given in adequate dosage 0·8–1·3 mg. intravenously, atropine blocks the muscarinic action of neostigmine on the heart, gut, and salivary glands. Its cardiac effects come on more rapidly than its antisalivary effects. Atropine has a wide therapeutic ratio and doses up to 200 mg. have been used in psychiatry.‖ To completely abolish vagal tone in fit adults, 3 mg. may be required.

If atropine is given in a dose of 0·8 mg. by mouth, 90 minutes before operation, it acts as well as 0·6 mg. hypodermically.¶

Usual dose, 0·4–0·8 mg. Even babies tolerate 0·3–0·4 mg.

Hyoscine Hydrobromide, B.P. (scopolamine).—The lævo-rotatory alkaloid is employed. Derived from *Hyoscyamus niger* (henbane). Isolated in 1871. Used, together with morphine, before anæsthesia in 1900 by Schneiderlinn.** It is a better drying agent than atropine.

Actions similar to atropine. Chief difference is that hyoscine is a depressant of the central nervous system, causing drowsiness, sleep, and amnesia in some patients. Occasionally it produces restlessness and excitement, especially in old patients and those with unrelieved pain. It decreases the intensity and duration of analgesia produced by opiates, pethidine, and methadone.†† It should not be the sole premedicant before methohexitone as it fails to prevent muscular movements.

---

* Clark, C. G., and Riddoch, M. E., *Brit. J. Anæsth.*, 1962, **34**, 875.
† John, A. H., *Ibid.*, 1965, **37**, 57.
‡ Sington, H., *Proc. R. Soc. Med.*, 1926, **19**, 1.
§ Kalow, W., *Anesthesiology*, **25**, 377.
‖ Miller, J. J., and others, *J. clin. exp. Psychiat.*, 1958, **19**, 312.
¶ Joseph, M. C., and Vale, R. J., *Lancet*, 1960, **2**, 1060.
** Schneiderlinn, J., *Aertz. Mitt. a. Baden*, 1900, **54**, 104.
†† Dundee, J. W., and Moore, J., *Anæsthesia*, 1961, **16**, 194.

It is a mild respiratory stimulant, while its action on the iris, the salivary, sweat, and bronchial glands is stronger than that of atropine. Has a beneficial effect on motion sickness. Tachycardia may occur, as after atropine.* After a dose of hyoscine sufficient to cause tachycardia, a secondary bradycardia may develop and last up to 3 hours.† Action on heart, intestine, and bronchioles is weaker than that of atropine. Is usually given with morphine in the proportion of 1 : 25.

Usual dose, 0·3–0·6 mg. ($\frac{1}{200}$–$\frac{1}{100}$ gr.).

Combination of hyoscine 0·4 mg. ($\frac{1}{150}$ gr.) with pethidine 100 mg. or papaveretum 20 mg. forms a useful sedative before operation.

L-Hyoscyamine (bellafoline).‡—The lævo-isomer of tropine tropate. (Atropine itself is racemic, an equal mixture of *d*- and *l*-tropine tropate, and is not found in the belladonna plant in Nature, but is formed during the process of isolation.) Hyoscyamine in doses of 0·2 mg. is said to be a better drying agent than atropine. It causes drowsiness and tachycardia and sometimes other undesirable side-effects.

Methantheline Bromide (banthine).—Has been recommended as a drying agent before anæsthesia§ (5 mg.) and so has **oxyphenonium bromide**‖ (antrenyl) 0·5 mg.

Note on Innervation of Salivary Glands.—

PARASYMPATHETIC.—To sublingual and submaxillary glands. Pre-ganglionic fibres from cells in the superior salivary nucleus through facial, lingual, and chorda tympani nerves, to glands directly. Post-ganglionic fibres lie along the chorda tympani, the submandibular ganglion. These are secretory and vaso-dilator fibres.

To parotid, pre-ganglionic fibres pass from cells in the inferior salivary nucleus, via the glossopharyngeal nerve, its tympanic branch (nerve of Jacobson), the lesser superficial petrosal nerve to the otic ganglion. Post-ganglionic fibres pass from the otic ganglion to the auriculotemporal branch of the fifth nerve. Secretory and vasodilator fibres.

SYMPATHETIC.—From cells in the intermediolateral horn of the first and second thoracic segments, via anterior roots of T.1–T.2 and corresponding white rami to the cervical sympathetic chain. Post-ganglionic fibres come from the superior cervical ganglion and go to the external carotid and internal maxillary arteries and so to glands. These are vasoconstrictor fibres.

Advantages and Disadvantages of Atropine and Hyoscine in Premedication.—

ADVANTAGES.—

1. Inhibits secretion which might interfere with airway or be aspirated into chest. This advantage is greater than the disadvantage of tenacious thick mucus formation.

* Gravenstein, J. S., and others, *Anesthesiology*, 1964, **25**, 123.
† List, W. E., and Gravenstein, J. S., *Ibid.*, 1965, **26**, 299.
‡ Galloon, S., *Brit. J. Anæsth.*, 1956, **28**, 113.
§ Burnstein. C. L., *Anesthesiology*, 1953, **14**, 484.
‖ Mushin, W. W., and Adams, A. S., *Brit. J. Anæsth.*, 1955, **27**, 519.

Advantages of Atropine and Hyoscine, *continued*.

2. Hyoscine produces sedation and amnesia.
3. Atropine depresses vagal nerve-endings in the heart and is useful when agents are employed which stimulate these, e.g.,
   halothane, trichloroethylene, and chloroform.
4. Atropine may help to prevent regurgitation.
5. May tend to prevent occurrence of bradycardia and arrhythmia
   following subsequent intravenous atropine doses, e.g., before
   neostigmine.*

DISADVANTAGES.—

1. Interferes with pupil reactions.
2. May cause thick tenacious mucus formation, which is removed
   from the bronchial tree only with difficulty.
3. May produce tachycardia.
4. May, owing to its anhidrotic effect, be liable to cause a rise in
   temperature.
5. Hyoscine may cause restlessness, especially in the aged.
6. Atropine may cause hypoxæmia.†

For a good comparison study of four techniques of premedication
see Feldman, S. A., *Anæsthesia*, 1963, **18**, 169.

RECTAL—BASAL NARCOSIS

Basal narcosis is deep premedication pushed to the stage of unconsciousness.

History—Pirogoff gave ether vapour into the rectum in 1847,‡
Wanscher of Copenhagen revived it in 1882, and Mollière of Lyons
used it again in 1884. Gwathmey introduced rectal oil-ether in
1913.§

Butzengeiger and Eicholtz (head of pharmacological section of Bayer
Products at Wuppertal-Elberfeld) used avertin in 1927.‖
Rowbotham used paraldehyde in oil in 1928.¶ Blomfield and
Shipway used avertin in England in 1928.** (*See also* Edwards, G.,
Proc. R. Soc. Med., 1945, **39**, 71.)

Anatomy of Rectum

The rectum is a hollow muscular tube, 5 in. long, extending from
the third sacral vertebra, where it is continuous with the sigmoid, and
ending below, where it bends sharply backwards into the anal canal.
It lies in the curve of the sacrum and coccyx and is S-shaped. Its
lower end is dilated to form the rectal ampulla. The average rectum
holds about 6 fl. oz.

When empty, the rectal mucosa is gathered into longitudinal folds.
There are also three transverse folds of circular muscle and mucosa,
the valves of Houston, which overlap when the viscus is empty, and

---

* Thomas, E. T., *Anæsthesia*, 1965, **20**, 340.
† Tomlin, P. J., Conway, C. M., and Payne, J. P., *Lancet*, 1964, **1**, 14.
‡ Pirogoff, N. I., *C. R. Acad. Sci. Paris*, 1847, **74**, 789.
§ Gwathmey, J. T., *Anæsthesia*, 1914. p. 433. Appleton: London and New York.
‖ Butzengeiger, O., and Eicholtz, F., *Dtsch. med. Wschr.*, 1927, **53**, 712.
¶ Rowbotham, E. S., *Proc. R. Soc. Med.*, 1928, **22**, 653.
** Blomfield, J., and Shipway, F. E., *Lancet*, 1929, **2**, 546.

help to support the fæcal mass when it is full, two on the left and one on the right.

Relations.—

To the peritoneum.   It has no mesentery :—
  a. The upper third is covered by peritoneum in front and at the sides.
  b. The middle third is covered only anteriorly, and from it the peritoneum is reflected on to the seminal vesicles in the male, and the posterior vaginal wall in the female.
  c. The lower third has no peritoneal covering.

Posterior relations are :—
  a. The superior rectal vessels.
  b. The left piriformis muscle and left sacral plexus.
  c. The coccyx and sacrum.
  d. The levatores ani.

Anterior relations are :—
  a. The rectovesical fold in the male, and, below it, the seminal vesicles, bladder, and prostate.
  b. The pouch of Douglas in the female, and, below this, the posterior vaginal wall.   The pouch of Douglas may contain coils of intestine.

Supports.—The rectum is held in position by :—
  1. The fascia of Waldeyer posteriorly.   It attaches the rectal ampulla to the hollow of the sacrum and encloses the superior rectal artery, veins, and lymphatics.
  2. A fibrous cord, the lateral ligament, on each side of the rectum, running from the third sacral vertebra to the rectum, just above the levator.   Through this fibrous tissue run the nervi erigentes (S. 2–3) and the middle rectal arteries.
  3. The connective and fatty tissue of the pelvis.

The Anal Canal.—Runs from the apex of the prostate to the anus. Is about 1 in. long and runs sharply backwards and downwards from its junction with the rectum.   It is surrounded from above downwards by the internal sphincter, the levatores ani, and the external sphincter.   Posteriorly is the anococcygeal body ; anteriorly, the urethral bulb and membranous urethra in the male, the perineal body in the female.
  The upper part is lined by mucosa which is thrown into vertical folds, the rectal columns of Morgagni : these end in valve-like reflections, the anal valves.

Blood-supply.—The superior rectal artery, branch of the inferior mesenteric, supplies the rectum as far down as the mucocutaneous junction.
  The middle rectal artery from the internal iliac, the inferior rectal from the internal pudendal, and the median sacral artery.   The anal canal receives its supply from the superior, middle, and inferior rectal arteries.
  The veins drain the hæmorrhoidal plexus, which is one of the communications between the portal and systemic circulations.
  The hæmorrhoidal plexus consists of two parts, one internal to the muscular layer, the other external to it.   The internal part

Rectum—Blood-supply, *continued.*

drains into the superior rectal vein which goes to the portal system via the inferior mesenteric vein. The external part drains into the superior, middle, and inferior rectal veins, which follow the course of the corresponding arteries.

Nerve-supply.—

The intrinsic nerve-supply is :—

1. Auerbach's myenteric plexus in the muscular layer.
2. Meissner's plexus in the submucosa.

These plexuses can take over automatic control of evacuation if impulses from the cord are removed.

The extrinsic nerve-supply is derived from somatic, sympathetic, and parasympathetic fibres.

1. Motor. From the pelvic nerves or nervi erigentes (S. 2–3).
2. Inhibitory. From the second and third lumbar, via lumbar splanchnic to the inferior mesenteric ganglion and thence to bowel via the inferior mesenteric and presacral (hypogastric) nerve. Paralysis of these fibres in a spinal analgesia may cause defæcation.
3. Afferent impulses from rectum travel via the nervi erigentes (S. 2–3). Afferent impulses from the anus and anal canal travel via the pudendal nerve and enter the cord with the S. 2, 3, and 4 roots.
4. The internal sphincter receives motor fibres from the sympathetic via the inferior mesenteric and presacral nerves. The nervi erigentes are inhibitory.
5. The external sphincter is composed of striated muscle and is partly under voluntary control. It is supplied by the inferior hæmorrhoidal branch of the pudendal (S. 2, 3–4), which also supplies the skin round the anus.

Lymphatics.—Lymphatic vessels accompany the arteries, the superior and middle rectal and the median sacral.

1. From the anus, to the superficial inguinal lymph-nodes.
2. From the anal canal, to the hypogastric lymph-nodes (internal iliac nodes).
3. From the rectum, to the pararectal nodes, nodes in the sigmoid mesocolon, and thence to the nodes around the origin of the inferior mesenteric artery.

Bromethol, B.P.
(Avertin—Tribromethanol)

This is tribromethyl alcohol, CBr_3CH_2OH. It was synthesized by Willstaetter and Duisberg in 1923 and was first used by Butzengeiger and Eicholtz,[*] in 1927, as a complete anæsthetic. It is now used for basal narcosis and requires in addition the use of a supplementary anæsthetic. Its popularity is dwindling and rectal and intravenous thiobarbiturates are taking its place. Used in treatment of eclampsia.

Preparation.—Tribromacetaldehyde is reduced with the aid of aluminium ethoxide in absolute ethyl alcohol in a nitrogen atmosphere ; the reaction product is then treated with aqueous

---

[*] Butzengeiger, O., and Eicholtz, F., *Dtsch. med. Wschr.*, 1927, **53**, 712.

sulphuric acid and the drug separated (Adriani). It is a white
crystalline powder which melts at 80° C., sold dissolved in amylene
hydrate so that 1 ml. of the solution contains 1 g. of bromethol.
The solution may decompose if exposed to light and heat above
70° C. or if left to stand when dissolved in water. Amylene
hydrate, $(CH_3)_2C(OH)C_2H_5$, is itself an anæsthetic and was reported
on by John Snow in 1856. In the solution used for basal narcosis
it does not greatly influence the anæsthetic potency nor does it
interfere with the pH indicator used. It is volatile and may
evaporate if kept exposed to air. Supplied in 100-ml. containers,
together with 10 ml. of Congo red solution. Should not be exposed
to light.

Dosage and Administration.—The dosage is 80–120 mg. per kg.
body-weight (0·6 g. per st.), depending on the metabolic rate of
the patient. Elderly, feeble, and obese subjects require a small
dose. Feverish patients and those in pain require a higher dose.
Children tolerate it well and need full doses. Morphine, if given
in addition, must be prescribed in small quantities to prevent
respiratory depression.

It is given in 2·5 per cent solution in distilled water, which must be
at 40° C. and not allowed to cool. Can be safely given in a
3 per cent solution which is less bulky. Vigorous shaking is
necessary to dissolve all the droplets. A higher temperature
may cause decomposition, a lower one may fail to allow complete
solution. Decomposition products are dibromacetic aldehyde
and hydrobromic acid, the former being irritating to the rectal
mucosa. To prevent this irritation 2 drops of Congo red (1–
1000 solution) are added to 5 ml. of the prepared solution just
before instillation ; the colour should be a clear bright red ; a
blue colour shows acid formation and the solution must be
discarded. A test for decomposition is essential, each time the
drug is used. The warmed solution can be stored for 12 hours
in a thermos flask, but must be tested just before use.

Bromethol in 1 per cent solution in saline can be given intravenously
as a continuous drip.*

The evening before administration, an enema is given. The solution
is run into the rectum from a funnel, through a catheter, the
patient being on his left side, with the foot of the bed raised.
It is run in slowly to prevent too rapid absorption. It is a
depressant of the central nervous system. It is rapidly absorbed
from the colon, 50 per cent of it disappearing from the bowel
during the first 10 minutes after injection.

The patient falls asleep in 10–15 minutes without any stage of excitement. The maximum effect is shown in 30 minutes and at the
end of an hour its effects begin to wear off as it is detoxicated.
The patient will usually be awake 3 hours after administration but may go to sleep again. It gives good amnesia. Large
doses give full surgical anæsthesia, accompanied by profound
respiratory depression. Normal narcosis with bromethol occurs
when blood concentration is 6–9 mg. per 100 ml. Constant

* Thornton, H. L., and Rowbotham, S., *Anesthesiology*, 1945, **6**, 580.

Bromethol—Dosage and Administration, *continued*.

supervision by a skilled person is required to prevent respiratory obstruction consequent on the muscular atony.

Pharmacology.—

CIRCULATION.—The blood-pressure falls during the first half-hour, but gradually picks up again. The fall is most severe in hypertensive subjects. It is capable of being controlled by pressor amines and is due to depression of the vasomotor centre in the medulla and relaxation of the muscular walls of the smaller blood-vessels. Large doses depress the myocardium. In addition, the cerebrospinal fluid pressure is increased.*

RESPIRATION.—Breathing depressed ; in overdosage central respiratory paralysis results ; this is the great danger of the drug. Relaxation of the jaw may result in respiratory obstruction, so that careful nursing attention is necessary to see that hypoxia is not present.

METABOLISM.—Body temperature is reduced ; the blood-sugar is slightly raised ; the basal metabolic rate is lowered.

The drug is toxic to the diseased liver and in the normal liver in excessive dosage it inhibits the secretion of bile acids. Ketosis may follow administration. Rarely, liver damage has been reported even in patients with no apparent liver disease. In the liver bromethol unites with glycuronic acid, which is excreted by the kidneys. Kidney disease retards excretion. The amylene hydrate is excreted by the lungs and kidneys in an unchanged condition.

It causes muscular atony.

Treatment of Overdosage.—

1. Assist respiration and prevent hypoxia. Endotracheal intubation if required.
2. Support the circulation :—
    a. Pressor amines.
    b. Intravenous saline or plasma.
    c. Tilt patient head down.
3. Rectal lavage with warm hypertonic sodium thiosulphate solution.

Advantages.—

1. Removes anxiety of induction of anæsthesia.
2. Produces post-operative sedation and amnesia.
3. Unlike paraldehyde, has no unpleasant odour.
4. Helps to produce muscular relaxation.

Disadvantages.—

1. Expert nursing required, before and after operation.
2. Danger of liver and kidney damage.
3. Excretion cannot be hurried as it is non-volatile.
4. Post-operative pulmonary morbidity increased, especially in abdominal cases.

Indications.—

1. Thyrotoxic cases. Modern pre-operative preparation of these patients has made it less useful than was formerly the case.

---

* Stephen, C. R., Woodhall, B., Golden, J. B., Martin, R., and Nowill, W. K., *Anesthesiology*, 1954, **15**, 365.

2. Frightened, anxious patients with an abnormal dread of anæsthesia.
3. Short intracranial operations ; bleeding is reduced.
4. Ophthalmic operations, because intra-ocular tension is decreased and the vessels of the conjunctiva are contracted and so bleed minimally.
5. Where induction of anæsthesia by inhalation is contra-indicated in the conscious patient and the veins are bad.
6. For cardiac catheterization in children.*

THERAPEUTIC USES OF BROMETHOL.—

   a. To control the contractions of tetanus, strychnine poisoning, eclampsia, and status epilepticus.
   b. To relax the muscles of the bronchioles in status asthmaticus.
   c. To quell delirium in acute alcoholism and toxic states, etc.

Contra-indications.—
1. Low basal metabolic rate because of delay in excretion.
2. Liver and kidney disease.
3. When a quick return of reflexes is required after operation, e.g., upper abdominal cases ; throat and nose operations.
4. Some anal and rectal diseases.
5. When adrenaline is to be used, lest the combination produce ventricular fibrillation.
6. In cases with respiratory obstruction.

In obstetrics, bromethol must be used in small dosage, lest it should depress the respiration of the child. It may produce restlessness if pain is left uncontrolled.

Paraldehyde

Paraldehyde was discovered by Wiedenbusch in 1829. It was introduced as a sedative into medicine by the Italian physician Cervello (1854–1918) in 1882.†

Rowbotham was the first, in 1928, to use paraldehyde in oil per rectum to produce basal narcosis.‡ Harold Sington used it for children in the following year, while in 1932 Rosenfield and Davidoff gave it per rectum to obstetrical patients.

The formula is $(CH_3CHO)_3$ and it is prepared by the action of concentrated sulphuric acid on acetaldehyde which causes the polymerization of three molecules of acetaldehyde into one of paraldehyde.

Paraldehyde is a clear, volatile, inflammable liquid, having a characteristic odour. It should be stored away from heat, light, and air. A relatively fresh preparation should be used as old paraldehyde may decompose with the formation of acetic acid, which may cause rectal sloughing.

It is administered like bromethol and is dissolved in either saline or olive oil, usually 4 ml. of paraldehyde to 50 ml. of solvent. The average dose is 4–5 ml. for each stone of body-weight (0·6 mg. per kg.), 40 ml. being the maximum. It should be given three-quarters of an hour before operation.

---

* Blundell, A. E., and others, *Curr. Res. Anesth.*, 1960, **39**, 499.
† Cervello, V., *Arch. per le sc. med.*, 1882, **6**, 177.
‡ Rowbotham, E. S., *Proc. R. Soc. Med.*, 1928, **22**, 653.

Paraldehyde, *continued.*

It has a low vapour pressure at room temperature, and so cannot be used as an inhalation anæsthetic. For the same reason, although it burns, it will not explode.

It acts more slowly and for a longer time than bromethol and is only slightly depressing to respiration. It has a constricting effect on the bronchi. Muscle tone is not lost and reflexes are not abolished. It is partly excreted unchanged by the lungs, partly metabolized by the liver, and a small amount is excreted in the urine.

It is a very useful and safe basal narcotic for children, its disadvantages being its smell, the long period of post-operative sedation, and the large volume of fluid to be instilled into the rectum. Has been used during labour.

It can be given in doses of 5–10 ml. either intravenously (diluted 1–10 in saline) or intramuscularly together with a little hyaluronidase to speed up its action, if necessary, and is a good anticonvulsant and remedy for restlessness.

Thiopentone (Pentothal)

Rectal use first described by Weinstein and Adams in 1939.*

Most useful in basal narcosis, with rapid onset of sleep and absence of prolonged post-operative sedation. Rectal thiopentone can be used to produce either pre-anæsthetic hypnosis in doses of 13·3 mg. per lb. or 1 g. per 75 lb., or basal anæsthesia in doses of 20 mg. per lb. or 1 g. per 50 lb. of body-weight. With the first, the patient is sleeping but is rousable ; with the second he cannot easily be roused, but will react to painful stimuli. Skilful nursing supervision is necessary after the drug is given. Can be given in suppository form† in doses of 125, 250, 500, and 750 mg. and also as a ready-made suspension. For children requiring additional anæsthesia 250 mg. for those weighing 6–12 kg. For those weighing 12–25 kg., 500 mg.

Dosage.—Dissolve 1 g. in 50 (or 75) ml. of tap water and give 1 ml. for each 1 lb. of child. More concentrated solutions may be used. It should be instilled into the rectum 15–30 min. before operation. The small bulk is an advantage in children, the strength of solution being anything between 1·5 per cent and 10 per cent. In children, maximum rectal dose should be 1·5 g. ; in adults 3–4 g. It should be preceded by atropine, and given on an empty stomach, no preliminary enema being necessary. It causes less restlessness than pentobarbitone after operation because it is excreted quicker, but following its use induction of anæsthesia, e.g., intravenous injection, may give rise to strong, although unremembered, resistance. Maximum blood levels are found after 20–30 min. After 24 hours the plasma concentration may be up to 15 per cent of the maximum.‡ Judgement is required in assessment of dosage, the strong, active, muscular hyperthyroid person requiring more than the obese, feeble, or anæmic patient. Contra-indicated in severe cardiac disease, severe respiratory embarrassment, and grave anæmia.

SPECIAL INDICATIONS.—

   1. For cardiac catheterization in young children.

* Weinstein, M. L., *Curr. Res. Anesth.*, 1939, **18**, 221.
† Aladjemoff, L., Kaplan, I., and Gestesh, T., *Anæsthesia*, 1958, **13**, 152.
  Buchmann, G., *Proc. 2nd Eur. Cong. Anæsth.*, 1966, **2**, 23.

2. Before eye examinations in young children as the sole sedative.
3. To produce quietness in young children during radiographic examination.
4. For cystoscopies.
5. For encephalography.
6. Before dissection of tonsils in children (provided the post-operative nursing is good).

Methohexitone has been given into the rectum with good results (10 mg. per lb.).*

Ether-oil

Rectal instillation of ether vapour was advocated by Pirogoff of St. Petersburg in 1847,† and of ether and water by Dupuy of Paris in the same year. It was revived by Gwathmey in 1913.‡

Ether 65 per cent is mixed well with olive oil 35 per cent, and 20 ml. of the mixture per stone of body-weight is the average dose; less should be given to obese and feeble patients. Anæsthesia, which may be complete, lasts for 2½–3 hours. A 50 : 50 mixture with olive oil can also be used.

The skin of the buttocks should be smeared with soft paraffin and the mixture run in from a funnel and catheter. As the solution enters the rectum cramp may be experienced.

It has been used in obstetrics, in status asthmaticus. and to induce anæsthesia in patients with cardiac decompensation.

CHAPTER V

INHALATION ANÆSTHESIA

THE UPTAKE OF ANÆSTHETIC GASES AND VAPOURS§

The general laws governing diffusion, solubility, and the relations of volume, pressure, and temperature apply to the anæsthetic gases and vapours. Uptake by the body can be divided into two phases :—

1. *The Pulmonary Phase.*—Inhalation of gas or vapour to build up a significant alveolar concentration and diffusion across the pulmonary membrane to reach pulmonary and hence arterial blood.

2. *The Circulatory Phase.*—Transfer to the brain and other organs by the circulation. The brain concentration must ultimately be proportional to the partial pressure of vapour in the alveolar air.

---

* Stetson, J. B., *Brit. J. Anæsth.*, 1963, **35**, 811; and Budd, D. C., Dornette, W. H. L., and Wright, S. P., *Curr. Res. Anesth.*, 1965, **44**, 222.
† Pirogoff, N. I., *Recherches pratiques et physiologique sur l'éthérisation*, 1847. St. Petersbourg: F. Bellezard et Cie.
‡ Gwathmey, J. T., *Lancet*, 1913, **2**, 1756; and *Anesthesiology*, 1942, **3**, 171.
§ *See also* Kety, S. S., *Anesthesiology*, 1950, **11**, 517; Bourne, J. G., *Nitrous Oxide in Dentistry*, 1960, London: Lloyd-Luke, p. 69 et seq.; Dripps, R. D., Eckenhoff, J. E., and Vandam, L. D., *Introduction to Anesthesia*, 1967, Ch. 9, Philadelphia and London: Saunders; and Bourne, J. G., *Anæsthesia*, 1964, **19**, 12 ; and Symposium on *Pharmacokinetics of Inhalation Anæsthetic Agents*, *Brit. J. Anæsth.*, 1964, **36**, 123 et seq.

The Uptake of Anæsthetic Gases, *continued.*

We can therefore speak of the *minimal alveolar concentration* of an anæsthetic agent which will produce general anæsthesia*(*see* p. 115).

The Pulmonary Phase.—Diffusion across the pulmonary membrane is rarely a limiting factor when the lungs are healthy. In general, arterial tension will equate with alveolar tension. We may consider some of the factors which regulate alveolar tension :—

1. INHALED CONCENTRATION.—The inspired concentration of the anæsthetic agent eventually determines the alveolar tension, the tension in arterial blood, and the degree of body saturation, but not until a state of equilibrium has been attained. Increasing the inspired concentration will speed up the rate of induction, provided that breath-holding, laryngospasm, or coughing are not caused.

2. ALVEOLAR VENTILATION.—The anæsthetic agent in inspired gases is immediately diluted by the functional residual air. It takes many breaths in and out before the concentration in alveolar air comes to approximate to inspired concentration. In a non-rebreathing circuit equilibration takes about 3 minutes in a healthy subject. Equilibration is hastened by increasing alveolar ventilation. Induction is therefore speeded by taking deeper breaths and slowed when there is rebreathing, respiratory depression, or respiratory obstruction.

3. BLOOD/GAS PARTITION COEFFICIENT.—The partition coefficient of a substance is the ratio, at equilibrium, of its concentration on the two sides of a diffusing membrane or interface. Alveolar concentration of anæsthetic agent does not in fact reach the inspired concentration because of the constant diffusion of molecules from the alveoli to the pulmonary blood. The solubility of the agent in blood is important. Approximate figures for the coefficient are :—

	Blood/Gas
Cyclopropane	0·46
Nitrous oxide	0·47
Ethyl chloride	2·0
Divinyl ether	2·8
Halothane	3·6
Chloroform	7·3
Trichloroethylene	9·0
Methoxyflurane	13·0
Diethyl ether	15·0

When blood solubility is high, alveolar concentration does not equilibrate with inhaled concentration. Induction is slow because alveolar tension, and hence arterial tension, remains low. It may be speeded by increasing alveolar ventilation (e.g., by adding carbon dioxide to the inhaled gases).

When blood solubility is low, alveolar concentration soon equilibrates with inhaled concentration. Induction is rapid and

---

* Merkel, G., and Eger, E. I., *Anesthesiology*, 1963, **24**, 346; and Eger, E. I., and others, *Ibid.*, 1965, **26**, 271.

is not materially affected by taking deeper breaths once the initial equilibration has occurred.

In other words, in the presence of a low blood/gas partition coefficient, a change in inhaled concentration is soon reflected as a change in arterial tension. When the coefficient is high the mechanism is ' buffered ' so that changes in inhaled concentration are not rapidly reflected in the arterial blood. The coefficient is an important physical characteristic in determination of the clinical potency of a drug.

4. PARTIAL PRESSURE OF ANÆSTHETIC AGENT IN BLOOD RETURNING TO THE LUNGS.—The tension in mixed venous blood, and hence in pulmonary arterial blood, depends on the redistribution of the agent in the circulatory phase. A high tension in pulmonary arterial blood will raise alveolar concentration. This occurs when redistribution to other tissues is slowed (e.g., in shock) and as total body saturation occurs.

5. PULMONARY BLOOD-FLOW.—Pulmonary blood-flow carries away the anæsthetic agent from the lungs. It is equivalent to cardiac output, except in some cases of congenital heart disease, pulmonary hæmangioma, etc.

6. THE ALVEOLAR MEMBRANE.—In health this is not a limiting factor. Disease, such as pulmonary œdema or pulmonary fibrosis, may interfere with diffusion across the membrane.

7. VENTILATION-PERFUSION RELATIONSHIPS.—Gross disturbances may delay the uptake of anæsthetic agents.

The Circulatory Phase.—

1. CARDIAC OUTPUT.—Under basal conditions about 70 per cent of the cardiac output goes to the brain, heart, liver, and kidney, which comprise about 7 per cent of the total body-weight. About 14 per cent of the cardiac output goes to the brain which comprises about 2·2 per cent of the total body-weight. During induction, therefore, a relatively high proportion of cardiac output goes to the brain.

With muscular activity, stress, fear, or thyrotoxicosis, conditions are not basal. The brain receives a smaller proportion of the cardiac output and onset of anæsthesia is delayed. In shock, dehydration, etc., circulation to the periphery is diminished. The brain receives a higher proportion of cardiac output and induction occurs rapidly.

2. CEREBRAL BLOOD-FLOW.—Depends on :—

   a. CEREBROVASCULAR RESISTANCE, which is influenced by blood viscosity (reduced in anæmia), the intracranial pressure, atheroma, and tone of blood-vessel walls. *Vascular tone* is influenced: (i) by carbon dioxide tension in the blood, e.g., inhalation of 5 per cent carbon dioxide increases cerebral blood-flow by 75 per cent ; low Pco_2, as in moderate hyperventilation, reduces blood-flow by 35 per cent ; (ii) by oxygen tension in the blood ; inhalation of 100 per cent oxygen decreases cerebral blood-flow by 12 per cent ; inhalation of only 10 per cent oxygen increases flow by 75 per cent; (iii) sympathetic nerves are no longer believed to affect cerebral vessels.

5

The Circulatory Phase, *continued.*

    b. ARTERIAL BLOOD-PRESSURE.—In essential hypertension cerebral blood-flow is not increased. But there is an arterial pressure below which cerebral circulation will not be adequately maintained, though it is hard to quote a figure. Gravity is important here, since 'fainting' may occur with low blood-pressure and head-up position ; head-down position protects the brain from this.

3. SECONDARY SATURATION OF BODY TISSUES.—The brain receives initially a high proportion of anæsthetic agent. But as time goes on there is a redistribution of the agent as it comes into equilibrium with the body tissues as a whole. Relatively large amounts of anæsthetic agent must be given during induction because of the recirculation of the agent to tissues other than the brain. As these depots become saturated, smaller amounts of anæsthetic are required to maintain anæsthesia (law of diminishing resistance of Gill). The rate of saturation of the non-nervous tissues depends on :—

    a. The tissue blood-flow. Fat has a poor blood-flow so that redistribution to the fat depots is slow and takes place later than redistribution to muscles and to the total body water compartment. Tissue blood-flow is increased in anxiety and thyrotoxicosis ; reduced in shock, dehydration, and old age.

    b. The tissue/blood partition coefficient for the anæsthetic agent :—

	Brain	*Fat*
Cyclopropane	—	20·0
Nitrous oxide	1·0	3·0
Halothane	2·6	60·0
Chloroform	1·0	68·5
Trichloroethylene	—	106·7
Diethyl ether	1·14	3·3
Methoxyflurane	2·34	38·5

RECOVERY FROM ANÆSTHESIA

Emergence from inhalation anæsthesia involves all the factors mentioned concerning the uptake of the anæsthetic agent. It is in fact a re-equilibration of the body with atmospheric air.

Recovery is more rapid when secondary saturation of the body tissues has not had time to occur. Tension of the agent in the arterial blood and brain falls rapidly because equilibration is occurring both with alveolar air and body tissues. For example, a child given ether in the anæsthetic room will rapidly lighten if allowed to breathe room air during transfer to the operating theatre (primary saturation) but recovery is slow after more prolonged anæsthesia.

Small amounts of trichloroethylene, cyclopropane, and ether are metabolized in the body, but this is not significant in the recovery from anæsthesia.* Halothane may also be broken down.

---

* Van Dyke, R. A., and Chenoweth, M. B., *Anesthesiology*, 1965, **26**, 348.

POTENCY

The potency of an anæsthetic drug is related to the concentration in the blood necessary to produce anæsthesia, and also to those physical and pharmacological characteristics which assist or prevent the achievement of this concentration during inhalation anæsthesia. It may also be considered that certain drugs have a selective action and reduce the reflex response to surgical stimuli without having a comparative effect on the brain as a whole.

1. **Minimal Alveolar Concentration.***—The minimal alveolar concentration of an anæsthetic agent to produce lack of reflex response to skin incision in 50 per cent of subjects tested has been studied in dogs. Equipotent concentrations (vols. per cent) of some agents were found to be as follows:† methoxyflurane, 0·230; halothane, 0·87; diethyl ether, 3·04; fluroxene, 6·0; cyclopropane, 17·5; xenon, 119; and nitrous oxide, 188. These values correlate with the oil/gas partition coefficient better than with other physical constants. Studies in man to determine the minimum anæsthetic concentration required to prevent muscular response to a skin incision give the following results (vols. per cent):‡ methoxyflurane, 0·16; halothane, 0·765; diethyl ether, 1·92; fluroxene, 3·4; cyclopropane, 9·2; nitrous oxide, 101.

2. **Physical Factors.**—
   a. THE SATURATED VAPOUR PRESSURE.—When this is low, it is not possible to make a high concentration available for inhalation. Thus, although methoxyflurane is the most potent agent in terms of minimal alveolar concentration necessary to produce anæsthesia, its low saturated vapour pressure means that induction is slow.
   b. BLOOD/GAS PARTITION COEFFICIENT.—When this is low, changes in inhaled concentration are quickly reflected as changes in alveolar and hence blood concentration. Anæsthesia can be deepened quickly and the agent is clinically potent.

3. **Pharmacology.**—Alveolar equilibration is delayed when an irritant agent produces breath-holding or laryngospasm, or when it produces marked respiratory depression.

4. **Chemical Structure.**—Potency can often be changed by substitution of one atom for another in the molecule, as can other pharmacological characteristics. For example, in the methanes potency increases progressively as chlorine replaces fluorine ($CHF_3 \rightarrow CHF_2Cl \rightarrow CHFCl_2 \rightarrow CHCl_3$), and when chlorine and bromine replace fluorine in an ethane series ($CF_2H-CH_3 \rightarrow CF_3-CH_3 \rightarrow CF_3-CHF_2 \rightarrow CF_3-CHFCl \rightarrow CF_3-CHFBr \rightarrow CF_3-CHClBr$).

The theoretical considerations which govern the ideal compound for inhalation anæsthesia are discussed by Artusio, J. F., in *Clinical Anesthesia—Halogenated Anesthetics* (Ed. Artusio, J. F.), 1/1963, Ch. I. Oxford: Blackwell.

---

* Merkel, G., and Eger, E. I., *Anesthesiology*, 1963, **24**, 346.
† Eger, E. I., Brandstater, B., Saidman, L. J., Regan, M. J., Severinghaus, J. W., and Munson, E. S., *Ibid.*, 1965, **26**, 771.
‡ Saidman, L. J., Eger, E. I., Munson, E. S., Bakad, E. A., and Muallem, M., *Ibid.*, 1967, **28**, 994.

CLINICAL APPLICATIONS

Factors which increase the Speed of Induction of Inhalation Anæsthesia.—
1. INHALED CONCENTRATION OF GAS OR VAPOUR.
2. CARBON DIOXIDE.—
    a. By increasing ventilation during early phase of equilibration, true for all anæsthetic agents.
    b. By increasing ventilation with those agents where equilibration with alveolar concentration is delayed due to high solubility in the blood (ether).
    c. By increasing cerebral blood-flow, all agents.
3. HYPERVENTILATION, VOLUNTARY OR CONTROLLED.—
    a. By increasing ventilation as in 2(*a*) and 2(*b*) above.
    b. By altering *p*H of blood so that the bound fraction of thiopentone is mobilized.
4. PRESENCE OF POOR CIRCULATION TO THE NON-VITAL ORGANS.—Shock, dehydration, old age, wasting of body tissues.
5. HIGH GAS FLOW SYSTEMS aid in speed of equilibration of alveolar gases with the anæsthetic mixture. Thus non-rebreathing methods allow for faster induction than closed systems.
6. UPTAKE AND ELIMINATION OF ANÆSTHETIC AGENTS is more rapid in infants than in adults, because of the relatively larger cardiac output and alveolar ventilation, and smaller functional residual capacity per unit of body-weight.

Factors which slow the Speed of Induction.—
1. RESPIRATORY OBSTRUCTION, LARYNGOSPASM, BRONCHIAL SECRETIONS
2. REDUCTION OF EFFECTIVE VENTILATION, BREATH-HOLDING, COUGHING.
3. RESPIRATORY DEPRESSION.—
    a. Due to premedication.
    b. Due to use of intravenous barbiturates for induction of anæsthesia.
    c. Due to the inhalation agent itself.
    This causes decreased effective ventilation directly and also decreases the response to carbon dioxide.
4. INCREASED CIRCULATION TO NON-VITAL ORGANS.—In anxiety, thyrotoxicosis, in children and young persons. Where the muscle mass is large, in robust subjects.
    (*See also* 'A Symposium on Pharmacokinetics of Inhalation Anaesthetic Agents', *Brit. J. Anæsthesia*, 1964, **36**, 123 et seq.)

METHODS OF ADMINISTRATION

Open Drop Administration.—
1. OPEN METHOD.—Introduced by Sir J. Y. Simpson for use with chloroform in 1847. He used a folded handkerchief. To-day, the Schimmelbusch mask is employed, which is a modification of Skinner's wire frame of 1862.* Plenty of air can be inhaled

---

* Skinner, T., *Retrosp. pract. Med.*, 1862, **46**, 185.

through the gap between the mask and the face. Useful to-day for giving chloroform, ethyl chloride, divinyl ether, and diethyl ether. Used by Lawson Tait, of Birmingham, from 1873 onwards, it was popularized by Prince, of Chicago, for use with ether, in 1895. Davis, of the Mayo Clinic, further popularized the method in the early 1900's.

2. SEMI-OPEN OR PERHALATION METHOD.—The mask is designed to fit the contour of the patient's face accurately. Examples are Ogston's mask and Bellamy Gardner's mask. A layer of gamgee between the mask and face further prevents air entry—other than through the gauze covering the mask. With this method some carbon dioxide build-up occurs.

These methods do not deserve the disdain they usually receive. *Advantages* are : (*a*) Immediate safety ; (*b*) Cheapness ; (*c*) Portability ; (*d*) Ease of administration ; (*e*) Minimal dead space. *Disadvantages* are : (*a*) Uneven anæsthesia due to variations in concentration of vapour ; (*b*) Risk of fire, except with chloroform and halothane ; (*c*) Wastefulness ; (*d*) Atmosphere of theatre becomes laden with vapour ; (*e*) Risk of damage to eyes or skin of patient from anæsthetic liquid. (*f*) Fall in oxygen concentration under the mask, easily remedied by trickling oxygen under the mask via small catheter.

Insufflation Techniques.—Endotracheal insufflation via a small catheter used by Elsberg in 1910 and popularized by C. Langton Hewer,[*] and recently shown to be reasonably efficient in avoiding hypercapnia.[†] The development of inhalation endotracheal anæsthesia with wide-bore (Magill) tubes supplanted this technique.

Endopharyngeal insufflation of an anæsthetic mixture can be carried out using the Boyle-Davis gag, the mouth hook, the side tube of a pharyngeal airway, or a catheter inserted down a pharyngeal airway. It is a useful method in children (e.g., in tonsillectomy or minor operations near the mouth) if endotracheal intubation is not desired.

Endotracheal insufflation with a high flow rate of oxygen is used to maintain oxygenation in the apnœic patient. Oxygen reaches the alveoli by diffusion, but hypercapnia occurs (*see* ANÆSTHESIA FOR BRONCHOSCOPY, Chapter XXI).

Semi-closed Methods.—These methods allow some degree of re-breathing, and may or may not be used in conjunction with carbon dioxide absorption. If the Magill attachment is used, effective carbon dioxide elimination requires spontaneous respiration, an expiratory valve of minimal resistance, and a total gas flow greater than the minute volume of the patient. Mapleson has made a theoretical study of various variations of the Magill attachment.[‡] He classifies them as shown in *Fig.* 8.

System A is the most satisfactory with spontaneous respiration. In assisted or controlled respiration the expiratory valve must be tightened. It opens only during the inspiratory phase, and all

* Hewer, C. Langton, *Brit. J. Anæsth.*, 1923–24, **1**, 113.
† Boulton, T. B., Cole, P. V., and Hewer, C. Langton, *Anæsthesia*, 1965, **20**, 442.
‡ Mapleson, W. W., *Brit. J. Anæsth.*, 1954, **26**, 323.

Semi-closed Methods, *continued.*

the expired gases are returned to the circuit. Very large flow rates are then required to flush carbon dioxide from the system. Studies* indicate that systems B and D, and possibly system C, can be used for controlled respiration, but it is better to use a non-rebreathing valve for soda-lime absorption of carbon

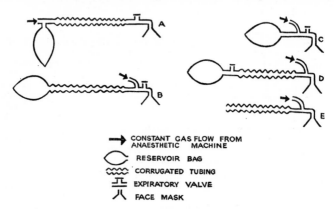

➡ CONSTANT GAS FLOW FROM ANAESTHETIC MACHINE

◗ RESERVOIR BAG

〰 CORRUGATED TUBING

⊥ EXPIRATORY VALVE

人 FACE MASK

Fig. 8.—The five semi-closed anæsthetic systems. (*By courtesy of William W. Mapleson and the 'British Journal of Anæsthesia'*).

dioxide. Recent measurements of end-tidal carbon dioxide and minute volume support the view that the Magill system is efficient with regard to carbon dioxide disposal.†

The closed-circuit apparatus can be used for the semi-closed technique, if excess gases are allowed to escape through an expiratory valve. High gas flows are not then necessary, since carbon dioxide is removed in the soda-lime canister provided that the patient's minute volume is adequate. With controlled ventilation, however, the method may not be economical unless unidirectional valves are placed one in each limb of the Y connexion to the patient, and the blow-off positioned immediately downstream from the valve in the expiratory limbs.‡ Without these precautions fresh gases are likely to be blown off before reaching the patient. Care must, however, be taken that the valves are in phase with those of the circle absorber.§

Non-rebreathing Valves.—Advantages are :—

1. No possibility of carbon dioxide build-up, provided the dead space of the valve itself is small.
2. Can be used for spontaneous or controlled respiration.

* Waters, D. J., and Mapleson, W. W., *Brit. J. Anæsth.*, 1961, **33**, 374.
† Kain, M. L., and Nunn, J. F., *Proc. R. Soc. Med.*, 1967, **60**, 749; Norman, J., Adams, A. P., and Sykes, M. K., *Anæsthesia*, 1968, **23**, 75; and Marshall, M., and Henderson, G. A., *Brit. J. Anæsth.*, 1968, **40**, 265.
‡ Eger, E. I., and Ethans, C. T., *Anesthesiology*, 1968, **29**, 93.
§ Rendell-Baker, L., *Ibid.*, 1968, **29**, 5.

3. Can be used to measure minute volume, if the flow-meters are accurate.

Disadvantages are :—

1. Wasteful of expensive agents (e.g., halothane).
2. Variations of minute volume during spontaneous respiration require frequent adjustment of the flow-meters to prevent collapse or distension of the reservoir bag.
3. Valves may stick.
4. Some valves are noisy.

Some examples of non-rebreathing valves :—

1. The Leigh valve, subsequently modified by Stephen and Slater.*
2. The Fink valve.†
3. The Ruben valve.‡ Dead space 9 ml. Low resistance. (*Fig.* 9.)
4. The circle absorber can be modified so that the valve on the inspiratory limb acts as a non-rebreathing valve.§

A recent investigation of these valves has shown that variable degrees of forward leak (escape from exhalation port during inflation) and rebreathing (sustained pressure preventing reseating of the valve) can occur with so-called non-rebreathing values during I.P.P.V.‖ The ideal valve should have no forward leak, no back leak, low resistance, minimal dead space, minimal opening pressure without sticking, light weight, transparency, easy cleaning and sterilizing, reliability and durability, and a single expiratory port for collecting and measuring exhaled air. The Fink valve and the Beaver valve do not allow back leak.

The T-piece Technique¶ (*Fig.* 10).—Advocated primarily for endotracheal anæsthesia in infants and young children. In order to prevent dilution of inspired gases with air on the one hand, or rebreathing with carbon dioxide accumulation on the other hand, it is recommended that the total fresh gas flow should be about twice the minute volume of the patient, and the volume of the reservoir tube equal to about a third of the tidal volume.

The following table may be a useful guide :—

Age	Total Gas Flow (l. per min.)	Volume of Reservoir Tube (ml.)
0–3 mth.	3–4	6–12
3–6 mth.	4–5	12–18
6–12 mth.	5–6	18–24
1–2 yr.	6–7	24–42
2–4 yr.	7–8	42–60
4–8 yr.	8–9	60–72

For adults, the technique has been recommended in anæsthesia for neurosurgery. A fresh gas inflow of 12–15 litres per min. with a reservoir tube of 150 ml. will usually suffice.

* Stephen, C. R., and Slater, H. M., *Anesthesiology*, 1948, **9**, 550.
† Fink, B. R., *Ibid.*, 1954, **15**, 471.
‡ Ruben, H., *Ibid.*, 1955, **16**, 643.
§ Bullough, J., *Brit. J. Anæsth.*, 1955, **27**, 181.
‖ Loehning, R. W , Gilbert-Davis, R. I. T., and Safar, P., *Anesthesiology*, 1964, **25**, 854.
¶ Ayre, T. P., *Lancet*, 1937, **1**, 561; *Curr. Res. Anesth.*, 1937, **16**, 330; *Brit. J. Anæsth.*, 1956, **28**, 520; and *Anæsthesia*, 1967, **22**, 359.

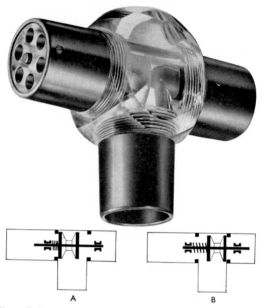

Fig. 9.—Ruben valve (British Oxygen Co. Ltd.). Diagrammatic. **A**, Inspiratory position. **B**, Expiratory position. (*By courtesy of C. Langton Hewer and the Publishers of 'Recent Advances in Anæsthesia'.*)

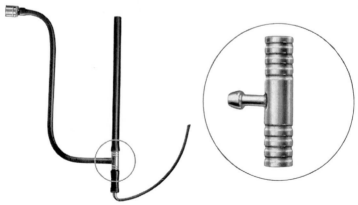

Fig. 10.—Ayre's **T**-piece. (British Oxygen Gases Ltd.)

Variations of the T-piece technique include the use of a Y-piece, the provision of a hole in the adaptor of the endotracheal tube, lifting up the diaphragm of the expiratory valve with a safety-pin, and the use of a reservoir bag on the open end for I.P.P.V.*

The main advantage of the T-piece technique is the absence of resistance to respiration, a factor of crucial importance in small children and in certain special operations (e.g., craniotomy).

Draw-over Methods.—Air, enriched if necessary by oxygen, is drawn over the surface of a volatile liquid or liquids. Inspiration of the patient is the motive force. Vaporization may be helped by the use of a gauze wick. Marrett's apparatus† is an example and so is the E.M.O. Inhaler, and the inhalers designed for the self-administration of trichloroethylene and air. Draw-over inhalers can be used for I.P.P.V. if a suitable bellows is incorporated (*see* Chapter XXX).

THE CLOSED CIRCUIT WITH CARBON DIOXIDE ABSORPTION

Introduced by John Snow in 1850; revived by Dennis Jackson of Cincinnati in 1915 for work on animals;‡ used by Waters, of Madison, in 1920 in clinical anæsthesia, and the first reports appeared in 1924.§ The circle or two-phase system was devised by Brian Sword‖ in 1926. W. B. Primrose, of Glasgow, used caustic soda solution as an absorber in 1931,¶ while Dräger patented an apparatus with a closed circuit in 1926.

Founded on principle that if sufficient oxygen is added to supply body's basal needs and carbon dioxide is absorbed, the same mixture of gases can be used repeatedly as it is exhaled unchanged. Basal oxygen varies between 200 and 400 ml. per minute, so that closed-circuit anæsthesia can only be used with a machine capable of delivering accurately measured small volumes of gases. The circuit may be completely closed as when cyclopropane is being used, or it may have a leak, which provides economy in gases and vapour, together with adequate removal of carbon dioxide from the circuit.

The vaporizer may be outside the breathing circuit (V.O.C.) in the fresh gas supply line and the circuit may be to-and-fro or circle.

The vaporizer may be inside the breathing circuit (V.I.C.) ; the patient's inspirations or expirations go through the vaporizer.**

Soda-lime.—Used to absorb the carbon dioxide. A mixture of 90 per cent calcium hydroxide with 5 per cent sodium hydroxide, with silicates to prevent powdering. It is essential for effective absorption that moisture (14–19 per cent) be incorporated within

---

* Rees, G. J., *Brit. J. Anæsth.*, 1960, **32**, 132.
† Marrett, R., *Brit. med. J.*, 1942, **1**, 643.
‡ Jackson, D. E., *J. Lab. clin. Med.*, 1915, **1**, 1 (reproduced in 'Classical File', *Survey of Anesthesiology*, 1965, **9**, 98).
§ Waters, R. M., *Curr. Res. Anesth.*, 1924, **3**, 20.
‖ Sword, B. C., *Ibid.*, 1930, **9**, 198.
¶ Primrose, W. B., *Brit. med. J.*, 1934, **1**, 478, and **2**, 339.
** Mapleson, W. W., *Brit. J. Anæsth.*, 1960, **32**, 298.

Soda-lime, *continued.*

the granule.* Moisture present in exhaled or humidified gases is not sufficient. The hydroxides combine with carbon dioxide in the presence of water to form carbonates. Wilson soda-lime, the type used in anæsthesia, is specially prepared; its granules are size 4–8 mesh to minimize resistance to breathing and to allow plenty of surface for absorption (4 mesh is 4 quarter-inch openings per inch; 8 mesh 8 eighth-inch openings per inch). Air space in the charged canister should equal the patient's tidal volume. Nearly half the volume in a properly packed canister consists of inter-granular space. The chemical change involved in absorption results in heat production, the heat of neutralization. The end-products of the reaction are water and the carbonate of the respective hydroxide. There is a gain in weight of the granule. Some regeneration of activity occurs if exhausted soda-lime is rested for two hours. Storing soda-lime in its container does not interfere with its efficiency.

Durasorb is an improved soda-lime with a prolonged effective life which does not overheat. Its pink colour turns to white when it becomes inactive.

Baralyme is 80 per cent calcium hydroxide with 20 per cent barium hydroxide. It is said to be less caustic, and to produce less heat than soda-lime. No silica is necessary to produce hardness.†

Amounts of carbon dioxide up to 2 per cent may be present in the respirable atmosphere without being detectable by clinical observation on the patient's tidal volume, respiratory rate, pulse, or blood-pressure changes, and may cause an unsuspected respiratory acidosis. It has, however, been stated‡ that 0·2 per cent is the highest permissible concentration of carbon dioxide in an anæsthetic circuit. It is therefore most important to see that the soda-lime is fresh and that tidal exchange is adequate for efficient ventilation. There is a tendency for gases to flow so that more absorption takes place in the soda-lime in contact with the walls of the canister than in that in the middle.§

SIGNS OF EXHAUSTION OF SODA-LIME.—

1. Rise in B.P. followed eventually by a fall.
2. Rise in pulse-rate.
3. Deepening of respiration and rise in P_{CO_2}.
4. Increased oozing from wound and perhaps sweating.
5. Increase in volume of gases in breathing bag, a late sign which should never occur. About 200 ml. of CO_2 per minute are excreted.

Some brands change colour when exhausted, but this is not a reliable sign. The one-pound canister will last about six hours intermittently, two hours continuously. In practice it is unwise to wait until the so-called signs of exhaustion of the soda-lime appear. Fresh absorbent should always be used if there is any doubt as to its efficiency.

* Wilson, R. C., *J. industr. Engng Chem.*, 1920, **12**, 1000.
† Kilborn, M. G., *Anesthesiology*, 1941, **2**, 621.
‡ Woolmer, R., and Lind, B., *Brit. J. Anæsth.*, 1954, **26**, 316.
§ Adriani, J., and Rovenstine, E. A., *Anesthesiology*, 1941, **2**, 1.

TEMPERATURE DURING ABSORPTION.*—*Sources of Heat.* Nearly all from the heat of the chemical reaction of neutralization which is exothermic. Small amounts from heat of solution in water formed, from heat liberated when moisture condenses in the apparatus, and from exhaled air.

The temperature within the canister may reach 60° C. in that part of the canister where active absorption is occurring. There are temperature gradients within the canister. Palpation of the canister jacket may yield little information about the temperature of the interior. Temperatures within the canister are likely to be about 5° C. less in the case of circle absorbers since there is a greater opportunity for heat loss.

Advantages.—
1. Economy in use of gases.
2. Less risk of explosion as no gas escapes into the surrounding atmosphere, providing the whole circuit is leakproof.
3. Conservation of heat and moisture.

Disadvantages.—
1. Tight fit of mask, tube, etc., to patient may cause trauma.
2. Alkaline dust may pass to patient.
3. Heat from chemically active soda-lime may cause sweating.
4. Resistance to breathing and dead space are high. The continued increase of inspiratory resistance may give rise to an increase of the negative intrapulmonary pressure and acute pulmonary œdema, while continued expiratory resistance may cause a positive intrapulmonary pressure increase, with increased peripheral venous pressure and decreased cardiac output. These factors, while relatively unimportant in the fit, may be harmful in the ill, the old, or the very young patient.
5. Increased carbon dioxide content of respired gases, as absorption is far from perfect.
6. Dilution of gases in reservoir bag by nitrogen which in the early part of the administration may be removed from the circuit by emptying the bag on several occasions.

Cross-infection from one patient to another is possible, and some machines incorporate a water bacterial trap. (*See also* Chapter XXXVIII.)

The present awareness of carbon dioxide accumulation in anæsthetic circuits has led many observers to question the efficiency of the closed-circuit system as a sufficiently reliable method of carbon dioxide absorption.† Monoethanolamine has been suggested as a substitute for soda-lime in closed circuits.‡

Apparatus.—
1. The Waters 'to-and-fro' single-phase system (*Fig.* 11).§ This consists of a mask separated from the breathing bag by a canister of soda-lime. Gases pass through the canister during both inspiration and expiration. Fresh gases are led to the patient close to

---

* Adriani, J., *The Chemistry and Physics of Anesthesia*, 1962. Springfield, Ill. : Thomas.
† Lund, I., Andersen, K. L., and Erikson, H., *Brit. J. Anæsth.*, 1956, **28**, 13.
‡ Derrick, W. S., and Smart, R. C., *Anesthesiology*, 1957, **18**, 551.
§ Waters, R. M., *Curr. Res. Anesth.*, 1926, **5**, 160 ; *Ann. Surg.*, 1936, **38**, 103 ; and *Proc. R. Soc. Med.*, 1936, **30**, 11.

Apparatus, *continued.*

the mask. Waters's canister was designed after much experimenting as to shape and size ; it measures 12 cm. long by 8 cm. in diameter, and holds 1 lb. of soda-lime. The air space between granules averages 400 ml. To obtain maximal efficiency, the tidal exchange should approximate the air space of the charged canister. If the tidal volume is greater than the air space the

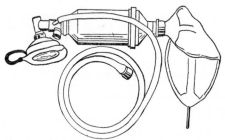

Fig. 11.—The Waters 'to-and-fro' carbon dioxide absorber.
(British Oxygen Gases Ltd.)

gases may pass through too rapidly for efficient absorption. If it is less than the air space, as when a large canister is used on a child, or when breathing is depressed, absorptive efficiency is sacrificed, because the soda-lime in the front of the canister becomes exhausted as the gases come into intimate contact with this part only and the result is an increase in dead space. In such circumstances a smaller canister should be used. It is heavy and rather awkward to use, but is cheap and can easily be sterilized. A rubber canister has been described[*] which weighs 8 ounces less than the metal one, is just as efficient, and gets no hotter. Resistance to gases 2–3 cm. water. In the to-and-fro system the pressure in the face-piece varies from +0·75 cm. of water to −0·75 cm. of water.

2. The circle or two-phase system (Brian Sword).[†] An inspiratory and an expiratory tube are used, with flap valves to ensure a one-way flow of gases ; breathing is thus divided into two phases and dead space is minimized. Efficiency is lost if the tidal volume is greater than the air space between granules. The soda-lime can be by-passed and the canister can be easily removed for recharging. The gases can be passed through or over ether or other volatile anæsthetic agent. The reservoir bag is either the bladder or concertina type. In this system, the canister does not drag on the mask, and there is less heating of inspired gases. Resistance to gases 2–3 cm. water. In the circle absorber face-piece the pressure varies from +2 cm. of water to −1·75 cm. of water.

[*] Kilpatrick, L. G., *Anæsthesia*, 1951, **6**, 236.
[†] Sword, B. C., *Curr. Res. Anesth.*, 1930, **9**, 198.

Circuits on the Coxeter-Mushin (1941), Boyle Absorber, Mark 2 or 3, McKesson, M.I.E., and Airmed machines are of this type. Circle and to-and-fro absorbers are equally efficient if properly designed, although resistance to respiration is nearly twice as great in the circle as in the Waters system because of the corrugated tubing and valves.

Dead Space.—Mechanical dead space is the addition to dead space which is produced by the anæsthetic apparatus.

Mechanical dead space in Waters's absorber is space between the face and the wire gauze of the canister. With a large mask, this may be 200 ml. Dead space may increase during use as the granules nearest to the patient become exhausted. The use of a simple nylon pot-scourer has been recommended.* This should be inserted after the canister has been filled and shaken down as tightly as possible. Its presence ensures that the canister is packed tight, so that gases cannot pass over instead of through the soda-lime when the canister is in a horizontal position.

Mechanical dead space in circle absorber is space between face and beginning of double corrugated tubing. A small mask reduces it, and so does an endotracheal tube connected directly to the anæsthetic breathing tubes.

Cope's modification of Waters absorber is designed to minimize dead space when anæsthetizing children. In the Coxeter-Mushin circuit, gases pass through soda-lime during both inspiration and expiration.

CARBON DIOXIDE ACCUMULATION.—Respiration normally keeps the alveolar carbon dioxide concentration at 5·6 per cent which gives a blood carbon-dioxide tension of 40 mm. Hg. If the tidal exchange is reduced by one-third, the alveolar concentration of the gas doubles, whereas a tidal exchange of more than 75 per cent above normal is required to halve the carbon dioxide concentration.† No matter how efficient the soda-lime, carbon dioxide will not be absorbed unless the tidal exchange is normal or above normal. During controlled breathing, too energetic artificial ventilation will result in a poorer absorption.‡

Circulatory collapse may occur after operation when carbon dioxide has been allowed to accumulate from stale soda-lime or from hypoventilation when the patient again breathes air. This may be seen after the patient has left the care of the anæsthetist.

NOTES ON APPARATUS

Apparatus for Administration of Inhalation Anæsthesia.—
Dates of introduction of some machines : Hewitt, 1898 ; Teter, 1902 ; McKesson, 1910 ; Water sight flow-meter of Boothby and Cotton, 1910 ; Connell, 1911 ; Foregger (water depression), 1914 ; Boyle, 1917.

---

* Robson, J. G., and Pask, E. A., *Brit. J. Anæsth.*, 1954, **26**, 333.
† Orton, R. H., *Anæsthesia*, 1952, **7**, 4.
‡ Lund, I., Lund, O., and Erikson, H., *Brit. J. Anæsth.*, 1957, **29**, 17.

Apparatus for Administration of Inhalation Anæsthesia, *continued.*

Machines are : (1) Continuous-flow ; (2) Intermittent-flow, the gas
flow being shut off during expiration.

CONTINUOUS-FLOW MACHINES.—

THE BOYLE MACHINE* (*Fig.* 12).—Gases are delivered from the
cylinders, via a reducing valve which reduces the pressure to

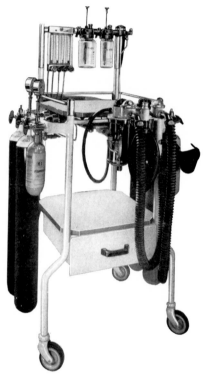

Fig. 12.—Boyle's machine with rotameters, Model H.   (British Oxygen Gases Ltd.)

5–7 lb. per sq. in. or 60 lb. per sq. in., to the flow-meters
where flow is controlled by a needle valve. Two vaporizing
bottles are usually provided and increasing amounts of the
gases can be diverted through them by means of a rotating
tap. If further concentration of vapour is required, a plunger,

---

* Boyle, H. E. G., *Brit. med. J.*, 1917, **2**, 653; Hewer, C. Langton, *Anæsthesia*, 1967, **22**, 357;
and Watt, O. M., *Ibid.*, 1968, **23**, 103.

progressively depressed, will give this by directing the gases so that they bubble through the liquid. Gases then pass into a Magill rebreathing attachment, a rubber bag (which can be cut out of the circuit), a length of wide-bore corrugated tubing, an expiratory valve, and a face-piece.

Modifications of the original Boyle machine of 1917, which was a two-gas water sight-feed, were :—

1920. Addition of vaporizing bottle to flow-meters.

1926. Addition of second vaporizing bottle and by-pass controls.

1927. Addition of third water sight-feed tube for carbon dioxide.

1930. Addition of plunger device.

1933. Dry-bobbin type of flow-meter displaced water sight-feed.

1937. Rotameters displaced dry bobbin flow-meters.

Cylinders.—The pressure inside a full nitrous oxide cylinder is 750 lb. per sq. in. (51 atmospheres), and the gas is liquefied. Full oxygen cylinders contain the compressed gas at 1950 lb. per sq. in. (120 atmospheres). Cylinders are made of molybdenum steel.* They are checked at intervals by the manufacturer for defects by subjecting them to tests: (1) *Tensile test.* This is carried out on at least 1 out of every 100 cylinders manufactured. Strips are cut and stretched—the 'yield point' should not be less than 15 tons per sq. in. (2) *Flattening, impact,* and *bend tests,* also carried out on at least 1 out of every 100 cylinders made. (3) *Hydraulic* or *pressure test.* Usually a water-jacket test. The filling ratio of a cylinder is the ratio of weight of gas in the cylinder to weight of water the cylinder could hold. Nitrous oxide cylinders are filled to a filling ratio of 0·69. Great care is taken that the gas is free from water vapour, otherwise when the cylinder is opened, temperature falls and water vapour would freeze and block the exit valve. Some reducing valves have fins to increase heat exchange and prevent freezing. Modern methods, however, provide gas free of water vapour so that fins are unnecessary. Cylinder outlet valves are now so arranged that it is impossible to connect cylinders to the wrong yokes or flow-meters.*

Reducing Valves.—These allow delicate control of gas flows. Without them constant adjustments are necessary to maintain constant flows, due to temperature and pressure falls within the cylinder. One of the commonest forms of reducing valve is the Adams valve (*Fig.* 13). A toggle mechanism occludes the orifice when pressure rises. In the Endurance valve a diaphragm moves a metal rod to occlude an orifice.

Flow-meters.—

THEORY.—Flow rate through a *tube* is proportional to the square root of the pressure difference. With a given pressure difference across an *orifice*, flow rate of gas is proportional to the square of

---

* *See also* Galley, A. H., in *General Anæsthesia* (Ed. Evans, F. T., and Gray, T. C.), 2nd ed., 1965, Ch. 15. London: Butterworths.

Flow-meters, *continued.*

the diameter of the orifice. Flow rate along a tube depends on the viscosity of a gas. Flow rate through an orifice depends on density, and varies as the reciprocal of the square root of the density.

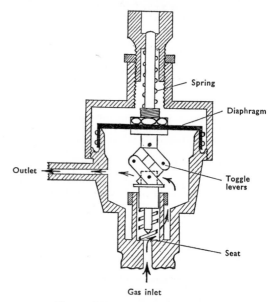

Fig. 13.—Diagram of the Adams valve.

TYPES OF FLOW-METER.—These may be divided into *Variable Orifice* and *Fixed Orifice* types:—

VARIABLE-ORIFICE METERS (or fixed-pressure difference).—

1. *The Water-sight-feed.*—Inaccurate and out-dated.
2. *Coxeter's Dry Bobbin Flow-meter.*—A bobbin floats in a vertical glass tube of uniform bore. Gas enters from below. As flow increases the bobbin rises and allows gases to pass through a series of orifices at the back of the tube. Now replaced by the more accurate Rotameter.
3. *The Rotameter.*—The type used to-day in most modern machines. This is an accurate meter with an error of ±2 per cent. As a gas-measuring device it was patented in Germany in 1908 by Karl Küppers, of Aachen, and used in anæsthesia by Maximilian Neu in 1910. Magill suggested its use independently in 1932 and used it a few years later. R. Salt

developed it further in 1937. Gas is led to the base of a finely wrought glass tube, slightly smaller on cross-section at bottom than at top. The tubes, usually three or four in number, are enclosed in a glass cylinder. A light metal float rides the gas jet and notches in its edge cause it to rotate. Height of top of float gives rate of flow, the gas escaping between the rim of the metal float and the walls of the glass tube. The glass tubes must be vertical. The calibrating of the glass tubes must take into effect both the density and the viscosity of the gases passing through them. Viscosity is important at low flows as gas flow round the float approximates to tubular flow (diameter of orifice less than length), but density is important at high flows (diameter of orifice greater than length). Consequently a rotameter calibrated for carbon dioxide will not read true for cyclopropane, because although their densities are similar (44 : 42) their viscosities are different (1 : 0·6). The design of the Rotameter unit itself is at present the subject of discussion and inquiry.*

4. *The Heidbrink Meter.*—A black, inverted, tapered float is free to rise within a metal tube. The upper end projects into a glass tube which is calibrated for gas flow.

5. *Connell Meter.*—A pair of stainless-steel balls move within a tapered glass tube on an inclined plane. They roll up the tube in the gas stream until the pressure difference above and below the balls counterbalances their weight component in the direction of the tube. Two balls are used, because a single ball tends to oscillate. Flow rate is read from the junction of the balls. The glass tube does not increase uniformly, but is compounded to allow measurement of high and low flows using a small length of tube. In the lower part of the tube work is so fine that internal diameter increases by only one-thousandth of an inch per inch length. The upper part opens rapidly to accommodate high flows.

FIXED-ORIFICE METERS (or variable-pressure difference).—Pressure differentials across an orifice vary with changes in flow. Pressure varies as the square of flow rate.

1. *Pressure Gauge Meter.*—The pressure build-up proximal to the constriction is measured utilizing a Bourdon pressure gauge which is then calibrated for flow.

2. *Water Depression Meter.*—Pressure on two sides of the fixed orifice is measured by means of a water manometer. Used on Foregger anæsthetic machines.

EFFECT OF BAROMETRIC PRESSURE.—Flow-meters are calibrated for use at atmospheric pressure (760 mm. Hg). They become inaccurate at high altitudes or in hyperbaric chambers.

Flow-meters also become inaccurate when a restriction at the outlet causes a pressure build-up. This may occur when some humidifiers, nebulizers, etc., are in use. Flow is then greater than indicated with variable-orifice-type flow-meters. In the fixed-orifice type a large flow may be indicated even when there

---

* Binning, R., and Hodge, E. A., *Anæsthesia*, 1967, **22**, 643.

Flow-meters, *continued.*

is complete occlusion of the outlet. These inaccuracies can be corrected by placing the control valve distal to the orifice. In the pressure-compensated flow-meter pressure in the flow-meter itself is the same as that in the supply line. The flow-meter is calibrated in terms of litres the gas will occupy after discharge to atmospheric pressure.

Vaporizers.—The Boyle and similar machines are supplied with two vaporizing chambers for volatile anæsthetics. Where a common flow of gases passes through vaporizers in series, the liquid having the lower boiling-point should be vaporized first. In this way vapour of the liquid from the first vaporizer is less likely to condense in the second vaporizer. Thus the ether vaporizer should be next to the flow-meters and the trichloroethylene or halothane vaporizer second in the serial gas train. If this is not done liquid trichloroethylene (boiling-point 87° C.), for example, can be recovered from the ether vaporizer (boiling-point 35° C.). In the older types of Boyle machine the J tubes and plungers of the vaporizing bottles should be interchanged.*

A wide variety of vaporizers is now available. In general they are designed for use with a particular agent (*see* Chapter VII) or in a particular situation (*see* Chapter XXX).

In modern practice it is often thought desirable to administer known concentrations of vapour of volatile agents. In the simple vaporizers mentioned above the concentration at any tap setting will vary according to ambient temperature, rate of evaporation, and the degree of insulation to prevent heat-loss. Efforts can be made to overcome these factors:—

1. To maintain the liquid at constant temperature. The use of water-baths helps to prevent heat-loss, but soon fall occurs unless special provision is made as in the original Oxford vaporizer for ether, where calcium chloride was used to maintain a constant temperature of 29° C.

2. Automatic variation of the inlet port with temperature. The use of bimetallic bars or a thermo-sensitive capsule.

3. The use of an apparatus such as the 'copper kettle' to provide a saturated vapour which can be diluted to obtain the desired concentration.

4. The Venturi principle has been utilized. A gas stream passes through a Venturi and sucks up liquid anæsthetic agents.

Warning Devices.—The ideal warning device should: (1) not depend on the pressure of any gas other than the oxygen itself, (2) an alarm system should not utilize battery or mains power, (3) the signal should be audible and of sufficient length, volume, and character.

The 'Bosun' Visual Audible Warning Device emits a reed-type whistle and switches on a red light supplied by a dry battery, when oxygen pressure falls. The audible signal, however, fails unless the nitrous oxide pressure is present, and regular maintenance of battery and bulb are necessary. The apparatus is useful but not infallible.

---

* Mushin, W. W., and Mapleson, W. W., *Brit. J. Anæsth.*, 1954, **26**, 3.

Attention has been drawn to a danger when certain artificial ventilators (e.g., Manley) are used with the 'Bosun' device. To overcome this the whistle must be set to blow at 3 lb. per sq. in. instead of the usual $1\frac{1}{2}$ lb. per sq. in.

More recently, devices have been made which are nearer to the ideal requirements. An apparatus is available* which is solely dependent on oxygen pressure, but it is designed for apparatus with a normal working pressure of 60 lb. per sq. in., and so cannot be used on many machines unless the reducing valves are changed. There is another device which is not confined to machines with a high second-stage pressure.† There is a pressure-sensitive switch and a separate low-voltage electrical unit. The electrical unit incorporates a warning buzzer, batteries, and a control knob.

Expiratory Valves.—These are one-way, spring-loaded valves. They should have minimal resistance to expiration and during spontaneous breathing should always be fully opened, as their setting determines the mean pressure in the anæsthetic circuit and in the patient's respiratory tract. Their opening pressure must, however, be greater than the collapsing pressure of the reservoir bag or the bag will not act as a reservoir. The amount of carbon dioxide rebreathed depends more on the provision of a plentiful flow of gases to the patient than on the tension of the expiratory valve.‡ Some workers remove the spring to reduce expiratory resistance to a minimum.

An expiratory valve may be combined with a suitable flap, making it into a non-return valve.

There are several types:—

1. The Magill, spring loaded.
2. The Coxeter-Heidbrink, spring loaded.
3. The McKesson: this can be set to blow off at definite pressures.
4. The Salt valve. Consists of a thin fibre disk on a knife-edge seating. Not spring loaded, so opens without appreciable resistance. Can be instantly closed by pressure on a spring plunger, so is very useful for assisted breathing when a semiclosed circuit is used.

Face-masks.—These should be of simple construction, easy to clean and sterilize, hard wearing, antistatic, and cheap. They should provide a good fit with the patient's face and add minimal dead space. Tests show that the increased dead space of a face-mask may be considerable (78–198 ml.) and this may equal or exceed the anatomical dead space of an average adult.§ In children and infants it is possible for the mask and attachments to double or treble the dead space. The face-piece connectors also add to the dead space (Ruben valve: 9 ml.; angle connexion and expiratory valve: 28–30 ml.).‖

---

* Adler, L., and Burn, N., *Anæsthesia*, 1967, **22**, 156.
† Cooke, M., and Waine, T. E., *Ibid.*, 1967, **22**, 487.
‡ Foster, A., and Todd, U. M., *Brit. J. Anæsth.*, 1956, **28**, 507; and Hunter, A. R., *Anæsthesia*, 1960, **15**, 61.
§ Harrison, G. G., Ozinsky, J., and Jones, C. S., *Brit. J. Anæsth.*, 1959, **31**, 269.
‖ Clarke, A. D., *Ibid.*, 1958, **30**, 176.

THE AIRMED APPARATUS is available in both hospital and portable forms. The makers stress its robust construction; minimal resistance to breathing; safety, in that trichloroethylene cannot contaminate soda-lime; compactness and simplicity. It is a compound machine which can be used with a straight-forward semi-open circuit, or with a closed circuit.

The MEDREX is a simplified form of this apparatus, designed for dental anæsthesia in the chair with nitrous oxide, oxygen, and halothane.*

INTERMITTENT-FLOW MACHINES.—

THE WALTON MACHINE.—Has been made in five models. The first appeared in 1925. Adams reducing valves lower pressure of issuing gases to 5–7 lb. to the square inch. Nitrous oxide and oxygen are led into separate bags which empty with the patient's inspiration, automatically fill again, and remain full until emptied. A lever, moving against graduations, controls the percentage of oxygen to be inhaled with the nitrous oxide. Another controls the pressure of the set percentage mixture. A rebreathing bag and vaporizing bottle can be used and a direct oxygen pressure supply is provided. These machines are used in dentistry and can also be employed to produce analgesia in obstetrics.

THE McKESSON MACHINE.—Designed and first manufactured in 1910 by Dr. E. I. McKesson (1881–1935), a pioneer anaesthetist of Toledo, Ohio, U.S.A.† He classified the signs of anæsthesia with nitrous oxide and oxygen, and introduced the method of secondary saturation. His description of fractional rebreathing appeared in 1915.‡

Reducing or regulating valves, set at 60 lb. to the square inch, admit gas and oxygen to two bags enclosed in metal drums, at equal pressures. From these bags, which empty only on inspiration, gases pass to a percentage mixing chamber, the proportion being controlled by a dial. Pressure of issuing gas from the mixing chamber varies between 0 and 40 mm. Hg. With pressures above 0, gases are released independently of the patient's inspiration and the machine becomes like a continuous-flow apparatus. Other features are a direct oxygen pressure supply, which can be used to inflate the chest ; a circle type carbon dioxide absorbing circuit ; flow-meters for carbon dioxide, basal oxygen, and cyclopropane ; and, independent of the closed circuit, a rebreathing bag which may be of the concertina type, with control of its volume and pressure. Expiratory valves are placed on the machine and near the mask. There is a vaporizing bottle for trichloroethylene or halothane.

To use the machine for ordinary induction, turn on the cylinders and see that both nitrous oxide and oxygen register 60 lb. to the square inch on the dials on the head of the machine.

---

* Marrett, H. R., *Anæsthesia*, 1963, **18**, 290.
† McKesson, E. I., *Surg. Gynec. Obstet.*, 1911, **13**, 456.
‡ McKesson, E. I., *Amer. J. Surg.* (Anes. Suppl.), 1915, **29**, 51.

Turn percentage mixture to o per cent oxygen, pressure to 3–5 mm. Hg, and open the expiratory valve near the mask. Gently lower mask to the patient's face until an airtight fit is secured.   He breathes in 100 per cent nitrous oxide, and oxygen can be added when it is indicated at any desired percentage.

A recent report* on intermittent-flow machines showed that unless frequently serviced, the accuracy of the gas mixtures delivered is not beyond reproach, particularly in apparatus which has been in use for several years.   There is an increasing tendency to use continuous-flow machines in out-patient departments and the dental surgery.

CLINICAL SIGNS OF ANÆSTHESIA

Since the early days of anæsthesia, it has been apparent that the anæsthetist must rely on a series of physical signs to indicate the onset of anæsthesia and to determine its depth.   This was appreciated by

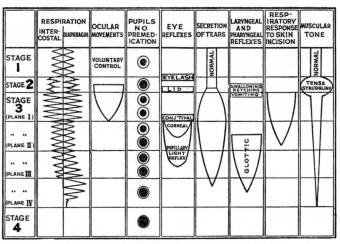

Fig. 14.—The levels of disappearance of reflexes (*after Guedel*).

the early anæsthetists, including John Snow (who described " five stages of narcotism "),† but it was not until Guedel‡ developed his classic table of the signs of anæsthesia, with division into stages and planes, using open ether, that a really detailed system became generally accepted.

---

* Nainby-Luxmoore, R. C., *Anæsthesia*, 1967, **22**, 545.
† Snow, J., *On Chloroform and Other Anæsthetics*, 1858. London : Churchill.
‡ Guedel, A. E., *Inhalation Anæsthesia*, 1937. London : Macmillan.

The Stages of Anæsthesia (using volatile agents, especially ether) (*Fig.* 14).—

FIRST STAGE—ANALGESIA.—From beginning of induction to loss of consciousness. Also known as " the stage of disorientation ". Artusio* has subdivided this stage into three planes in the deepest of which true analgesia is said to coexist with consciousness and co-operation from the patient. These planes are apparent during recovery from deeper stages of anæsthesia.

SECOND STAGE—EXCITEMENT OR UNINHIBITED RESPONSE.†—From loss of consciousness to onset of automatic breathing. These may be struggling, breath-holding, vomiting, coughing, swallowing, etc. Can be minimized by adequate premedication, psychological preparation of the patient, quiet surroundings, and rapid smooth induction. Emergence delirium may occur during recovery from anæsthesia, especially with cyclopropane.

THIRD STAGE—SURGICAL ANÆSTHESIA.—From onset of automatic respiration to respiratory paralysis. Guedel divided it into four planes :—

PLANE 1.—From onset of automatic respiration to cessation of eyeball movement.

PLANE 2.—From cessation of eyeball movement to commencement of intercostal paralysis.

PLANE 3.—From commencement to completion of intercostal paralysis.

PLANE 4.—From complete intercostal paralysis to diaphragmatic paralysis.

More recently there has been a tendency to divide the stage of surgical anæsthesia into only three planes :—

LIGHT ANÆSTHESIA.—Until the eyeballs become fixed.

MEDIUM ANÆSTHESIA.—Increasing intercostal paralysis.

DEEP ANÆSTHESIA.—Diaphragmatic respiration.

FOURTH STAGE—OVERDOSAGE.—From onset of diaphragmatic paralysis to apnœa and death. All reflex activity lost and pupils widely dilated.

The clinical signs of anæsthesia are the signs of: (i) a progressive increase of muscular paralysis (eyeball muscles, intercostals, diaphragm), (ii) a progressive abolition of reflex response.

Respiration.—Inspiration is active depending on muscular contraction ; expiration is normally passive, the accessory muscles only being used to overcome obstruction or in hyperpnœa.

FIRST STAGE.—Respiratory volume gradually becomes increased due to stimulation of respiration by the anæsthetic (especially ether). Too strong a vapour, or emotion, may interfere with breathing.

SECOND STAGE.—Breathing may show many abnormalities, but they are of no significance.

---

* Artusio, J. F., *J. Pharmacol.*, 1954, **111**, 343; and *J. Amer. med. Ass.*, 1955, **157**, 33.
† Mushin, W. W., in *General Anæsthesia* (Ed. Evans, T. C., and Gray, T. F.), 1959, Vol. I. London: Butterworths.

THIRD STAGE.—

PLANE 1.—Onset of regular, automatic breathing. Depth of breathing depends on the relationship between the respiratory threshold to stimulation and the amount of stimulant—carbon dioxide—in the blood. When ether is used there is usually some hyperpnœa which gets less after 15–20 minutes. Premedication depresses, while surgical trauma stimulates respiration in this and the two succeeding planes.

PLANE 2.—Breathing remains regular and deep, not very different from Plane 1.

With increasing muscular weakness both the diaphragm and the intercostals are depressed simultaneously, but because the intercostals work at a mechanical disadvantage, they are retracted and so appear to be paralysed.* Thus intercostal retraction is seen : (1) In muscular paralysis from : (a) Relaxant drugs ; (b) Peripheral action of general anæsthetics ; (c) Pathological conditions, e.g., myasthenia and poliomyelitis. (2) In respiratory obstruction. (3) In injury to the chest wall. This view has displaced the orthodox explanation of Planes 3 and 4 which were formerly described as follows :—

PLANE 3.—The plane of progressive intercostal paralysis, first described by John Snow ; later by Paul Bert, and again in 1899 by J. Hughlings Jackson and James Collier. Recognized as a sign of anæsthesia in 1924 by Albert Miller† and placed in its correct position in Guedel's table by Ralph Waters. Above Plane 3 intercostal and diaphragmatic breathing are synchronous, the chest and the abdomen rising together. With increasing intercostal paralysis, the chest lags behind the abdomen, a change often felt before it is seen. Depth of respiration is reduced, while the interval between inspiration and expiration increases at the expense of inspiration, which becomes relatively shorter in duration. Decreased depth of respiration may be made up for by increased rate. Passive expiration does not change as much as active inspiration. Increased diaphragmatic movement compensates for inactivity of the intercostals and may prove annoying to the abdominal surgeon, especially as it is sometimes jerky. Lightening of the level of anæsthesia will improve this. Diaphragmatic paralysis, preceding intercostal paralysis, has been reported.

PLANE 4.—The thorax becomes stationary, with complete intercostal paralysis. There may be retraction of intercostal spaces during inspiration. Tidal exchange may be inefficient so that oxygen lack and carbon dioxide excess may result. Breathing is slow, shallow, and irregular. When the thorax and abdomen move in opposite directions with complete intercostal paralysis, respiration is termed external paradoxical respiration ; a similar appearance may accompany

---

* Gray, T. C., *Ann. R. Coll. Surg., Engl.*, 1954, **15**, 402; and *Irish J. Med. Sci.*, 1960, **419**, 499.
† Miller, A. H., *J. Amer. med. Ass.*, 1925, **84**, 201.

Respiration, *continued.*

respiratory obstruction.   The term is not to be confused with internal paradoxical respiration in open pneumothorax.

With emphysema, increasing age, and rigidity of the thoracic cage, thoracic movements become less easy to assess.

Morton pointed out that the force of expiration is reduced with increasing depth of anæsthesia with volatile agents.

Rapid breathing may persist well into Plane 3.   It must be distinguished from tachypnœa due to oxygen lack.   Slow breathing is usually due to overdose of sedative premedication, or of pethidine, but this is not always so, even if ether is the agent.

FOURTH STAGE.—Marked by onset of apnœa.

During recovery, the same changes take place in the opposite order.

Eye Signs.—

1. EXTRINSIC MUSCLES.—Activity of the muscles of the eyeball is well marked in Stage I.   It is due to impulses coming from the superior colliculus to the pons and thence to the muscles by the third, fourth, and sixth nerves.   In Stage III, Plane 1, it is progressively reduced until it is abolished at the bottom of this plane.   The activity may consist of oscillation, squint, or the eyes may be pulled up or down.   When Plane 2 is entered the eyeballs usually rest in the normal centre position.   In extreme hypoxia the eyeballs may be strongly pulled either upwards or downwards, while the pupil is dilated.

2. PUPILS.—Opiates as premedication tend to produce miosis ; atropine and hyoscine in large doses, mydriasis.   If both are given the opiate effect usually predominates..   In the first stage the pupils may be dilated, reflexly, due to emotion and psycho-sensory impulses; in the second stage dilatation is due to sympathetic stimulation of the dilator muscle of the iris.   In Stage III, Plane 1, the pupils return to normal and then progressively dilate until the maximum is reached in Plane 4.   This is due to release of adrenaline from the adrenals and so is seen chiefly during ether and cyclopropane anæsthesia and not with intravenous barbiturates or halothane.   This maximum is not total dilatation, however, which is only seen as the result of anoxia and the paralysis of the sphincter it causes.   Dilatation of the pupil occurs also after the administration of ganglion-blocking drugs (e.g., hexamethonium, trimetaphan).

Horner's syndrome (small pupil, enophthalmos, and ptosis) may cause confusion.   It may follow cervical sympathetic paralysis associated with : (1) Birth injury ; (2) Retropharyngeal abscess ; (3) Tuberculosis of the apex of a lung ; (4) Intra-cranial lesions ; (5) Cervical rib, etc.

NOTE ON ANATOMY OF NERVE-SUPPLY OF IRIS.—

a. *Parasympathetic.*—The connector cells lie in the oculomotor nucleus in the floor of the aqueduct of Sylvius, from which fibres pass with the oculomotor nerve to the ciliary ganglion. From this, post-ganglionic (excitor) fibres pass in the short ciliary nerves to the constrictor muscle of the pupil and the ciliary muscle.   Function: contraction of pupil and accommodation.

   b. *Sympathetic.*—The connector cells lie in the lateral horn of
      the first and second thoracic segments, pass out in the
      anterior root of T.1, in the white ramus of T.1 to the inferior
      cervical ganglion, and ascend the sympathetic trunk to the
      superior cervical ganglion where excitor cells are located.
      Post-ganglionic fibres pass with the internal carotid artery
      into the skull and join the cavernous plexus in the cavernous
      sinus.   Further course : (1) In sympathetic root of ciliary
      ganglion and short ciliary nerves ; (2) To Gasserian ganglia,
      nasociliary nerves (1st division of 5th nerve), and long
      ciliary nerves to the eye.

3. OTHER EYE REFLEXES.—
   a. EYELASH.—Gently touching eyelashes causes contraction of the
      lids.   Reflex disappears on entering second stage.
   b. EYELID.—Gently raising the upper lid causes contraction of
      the lids.   Reflex disappears on entering third stage.
   c. CONJUNCTIVAL.—Gently touching palpebral conjunctiva causes
      blinking, a reflex which disappears at bottom of Stage III,
      Plane 1.
   d. CORNEAL.—Gently touching cornea produces contraction of lids.
      Reflex disappears in middle of Plane 2.   The afferent pathway
      is the fifth nerve; the efferent, the seventh.
   e. LIGHT.—Exposure to strong light causes the pupil to contract.
      Reflex abolished in upper Plane 3.
   f. LACRIMATION.—This is greater than normal in Planes 1 and 2,
      and is a useful sign of light anæsthesia.   Thereafter it rapidly
      decreases until the dull, glazed eye of deep anæsthesia results.

Other Reflexes.—
   1. SWALLOWING.—Occurs at upper border of Plane 1, i.e., in the
      lightest 3rd stage anæsthesia.   Rapid deepening of anæsthesia
      at this point may avoid vomiting.
   2. VOMITING.—Occurs at lower border of second stage, i.e., in
      the deepest 2nd stage anæsthesia.   These signs are also of im-
      portance in ascent from deeper anæsthesia, when swallowing
      may be a warning of impending vomiting.   Swallowing and
      vomiting mark the transition from the 3rd to the 2nd stage.
      Vomiting may indicate oxygen lack when nitrous oxide is the
      agent.
   3. SKIN.—Movement of limbs and deep breathing are the reflex
      responses to skin stimulation.   Abolished in Plane 2.
   4. POSTERIOR PHARYNGEAL.—Stimulation of the mucosa of
      the throat by airways, mucus, or vomitus produces gagging or
      coughing.   Abolished at bottom of Plane 1.   Afferent and
      efferent pathways, the ninth and tenth nerves.
   5. LARYNGEAL.—Coughing and adduction of the cords are pro-
      duced by stimulation of the nerve-endings in the larynx and
      epiglottis.   Reflex abolished in upper Plane 2.   Laryngeal
      spasm due to stimuli arising in the abdomen, anus, or cervix
      uteri, etc. (Brewer-Luckhardt reflex), may not be abolished until
      Plane 4.   Inflammation of upper respiratory tract increases
      its reflex irritability, so that coughing may persist well into
      Plane 2 or even Plane 3.   Thiopentone makes some patients
      cough, an effect sometimes very difficult to quell.

6*

Other Reflexes, continued.

6. TRACHEAL TUG.—This jerky depression of the thyroid cartilage, synchronous with inspiration, is often seen when the intercostal muscles are paralysed, either by deep anæsthesia or by a
relaxant (see also p. 44).

7. CARINAL.—Stimulation of the carina as by a long endotracheal
tube or bronchoscope may cause coughing anywhere above
Stage 4.

8. ANAL SPHINCTER.—If this is rapidly stretched, laryngospasm
or hyperpnœa may occur if the patient is above Stage 4. In the
days before I.P.P.V. was as frequently employed as it is now,
this reflex was used to stimulate breathing during periods of
apnœa.

9. TRACTION REFLEXES.—Pulling on peritoneum, mesentery,
liver, etc., may cause hyperpnœa, reflex contraction of the
muscles of the anterior abdominal wall, and laryngospasm.
Or it may cause temporary apnœa. Abolished in Plane 4.

Level of Anæsthesia for Various Operations

No hard-and-fast rules can be made. Operations on the limbs, body
wall, neck, and head can be performed in relatively light planes of
anæsthesia. Abdominal surgery demands adequate muscular relaxation, usually Planes 2–3, without muscle relaxant drugs. A light plane
of anæsthesia only is required for all operations, if undesirable reflex
manifestations can be inhibited, e.g., by muscle relaxants.

The Signs with Different Anæsthetic Agents

Ether.—The stimulus of strong ether vapour on the larynx is intense
and probably greater than that of skin incision. This means that
a patient breathing ether vapour without coughing, breath-holding,
or laryngospasm will almost certainly not react when the skin is
cut. This is not true of anæsthetic agents which are non-irritant
to inhale. The irritant stimulus of ether vapour also has an effect
on respiration, as do other painful stimuli. The constant stimulus
from the inhalation of ether vapour results in increased respiration
during light planes of anæsthesia.

Cyclopropane and Halothane.—These agents are relatively non-
irritant to inhale. Moreover they are powerful respiratory depressants. The patient may breathe quietly during light anæsthesia
and still react to skin incision. The respiratory centre is depressed,
hypercapnia is likely in the absence of intermittent positive-
pressure ventilation, and apnœa may occur even in light planes
of anæsthesia if the respiratory centre is already depressed by
other drugs. Tracheal tug is seldom seen in fit patients.

Trichloroethylene.—The stage of analgesia is well marked. Deep
planes of anæsthesia cannot be achieved safely. The early incidence of tachypnœa alters the respiratory signs.

Nitrous Oxide.—Deep planes cannot be obtained without hypoxia.
The signs of ' deep ' nitrous oxide anæsthesia are those of hypoxia.

BALANCED ANÆSTHESIA

Balanced anæsthesia really started in 1911 when George Washington Crile of Cleveland, Ohio, taught that psychic stimuli must be obliterated by light general anæsthesia, while the noxious impulses due to surgery must be blocked by local analgesia—the so-called theory of anociassociation.* In 1926 John S. Lundy of the Mayo Clinic introduced the term 'balanced anæsthesia' for a combination of agents such as premedication, regional analgesia, and general anæsthesia with one or more agents, so that pain relief was obtained by a nice balance of agents and techniques.†

The Triad of Anæsthesia

Rees and Gray‡ divided anæsthesia into three basic components : (i) Narcosis ; (ii) Analgesia ; (iii) Relaxation. The term 'analgesia' is not very satisfactory since it is without meaning in the unconscious patient. Gray§ has renamed the triad : (i) Narcosis ; (ii) Reflex suppression ; (iii) Relaxation. With selective drugs, it is possible to vary one component of the triad without affecting the others. In this context it should never be necessary to subject the patient to deep levels of central brain depression. The patient need not be 'deeper' than just unconscious.

Anæsthesia (or analgesia) is a process of modification of the normal physiological reflex response to the stimuli provided by surgery (and anæsthesia). The triad of anæsthesia may be considered as : (i) Inhibition of the afferent part of the reflex system ; (ii) Depression of the central synaptic mechanisms of co-ordination ; (iii) Block of the efferent part of the reflex arc.

We may consider various reflex systems which are of importance in anæsthesia. They may be hyperexcitable in light planes of anæsthesia, but progressively depressed in deeper planes.

1. Response to skin incision : (a) Gross limb flexion which interrupts the surgical operation ; (b) Minor limb movements which do not interfere with surgery ; (c) Subtle movements of facial muscles or digits, usually only noticed by the anæsthetist ; (d) No movement, but an increase in the depth of respiration ; (e) No response.

2. Cough reflex : (a) Muscles of trunk, neck, and limbs participate in the response ; (b) Confined to the respiratory muscles ; (c) Cough is present but ineffective ; (d) No cough, but expiration is forceful ; (e) No response.

3. Spasm : (a) Spasm of larynx, bronchi, and chest wall muscles, usually associated with cyanosis and difficulty in inflation of the lungs ; (b) Straining respiration ; (c) Laryngeal stridor or crowing ; (d) Quiet respiration.

Reflexes may be blocked centrally (general anæsthesia), or peripherally (local analgesia, muscle relaxants).

---

* Crile, G. W., *Lancet*, 1913, **2**, 7; *Surg. Gynec. Obstet.*, 1911, **13**, 170; *Ann. Surg.*, 1908, **47**, 866; and *Boston Med. Surg. J.*, 1910, **163**, 893 (reprinted in 'Classical File', *Survey of Anesthesiology*, 1966, **10**, 291).
† Lundy, J. S., *Minnesota Med.*, 1926, **9**, 399.
‡ Rees, G. J., and Gray, T. C., *Brit. J. Anæsth.*, 1950, **22**, 83.
§ Gray, T. C., *Irish J. med. Sci.*, 1960, **419**, 499.

The Triad of Anæsthesia, *continued.*

For further information on modern views of the clinical signs of anæsthesia *see*: Mushin, W. W., *Anæsthesia*, 1948, **3**, 154; Laycock, J. D., *Ibid.*, 1953, **8**, 15; Woodbridge, P. D., *Anesthesiology*, 1957, **18**, 536; Mushin, W. W., in *General Anæsthesia* (Ed. Evans, T. F., and Gray, T. C.), 1959, London: Butterworths; Symposium in *Irish J. med. Sci.*, 1960, **419**, 499, Nov.

ADMINISTRATION OF INHALATION ANÆSTHETICS

The patient's identity and diagnosis must be established and written permission for operation must be seen. False teeth must be removed; dose and time of premedication must be checked; presence or absence of stomach contents must be inquired about.

Induction of anæsthesia is now frequently carried out by the intravenous route, thiopentone being the most popular agent. The introduction of halothane, which is not unpleasant to inhale, does make inhalation induction more acceptable. If propanidid is used for induction, advantage should be taken of the period of hyperventilation to speed alveolar gas equilibration.

Difficulties.—

Delirium of the second stage must not be allowed to interfere with induction: the patient must be physically controlled by a nurse or porter, if necessary.

Swallowing, gagging, breath-holding, coughing, and laryngeal spasm may be due to emotion or to the use of too strong a vapour. In the latter case, vapour concentration must be decreased and later increased. Addition of a little carbon dioxide will also help.

RESPIRATORY OBSTRUCTION.—The signs are: (1) Inadequate tidal exchange, suggested by the small excursion of the reservoir bag, or the weakness of the sounds of breathing. (2) Retraction of the chest wall and of the supraclavicular, infraclavicular, and suprasternal spaces; (3) Excessive abdominal movement due to an overworking diaphragm; (4) Use of accessory muscles of respiration; (5) Noisy breathing (unless obstruction is absolute and complete); (6) Cyanosis; (7) The natural heave of the chest and abdomen becomes replaced by an indrawing of the upper chest and an outpushing of the abdomen because of strong diaphragmatic action: the lower thoracic region is almost at rest. This is the see-saw movement of complete respiratory obstruction and is one type of external paradoxical respiration. In partial cases it is not so marked. Respiratory obstruction is the cause of many deaths occurring in the operating theatre as well as in patients suffering from strokes, drug depression, coma, and head injury. It is evil in three ways:—

    a. It interferes with gaseous exchange.

    b. It calls for increased effort on the part of the patient. The increased negative pressure during inspiration may result in pulmonary œdema.

    c. It interferes with adequate anæsthesia and retards induction.

It must be remedied in all cases, after its cause has been diagnosed. It may be due to :—

1. OBSTRUCTION AT THE LIPS.—Especially in edentulous patients. A small mouth prop (e.g., Baker's airway ; London Hospital prop) is the cure.

2. OBSTRUCTION BY THE TONGUE.—Due to approximation of the tongue to the posterior pharyngeal wall (" swallowing the tongue "). It may be especially dangerous between the time that the patient leaves the hands of the anæsthetist and the return of his reflexes and muscle tone. It is very much less likely to occur if the patient is lifted into the semi-prone or ' tonsil ' position. May be accompanied by :—

   a. *Spasm of Jaw Muscles.*—Remedy is to push lower jaw forward by pressure behind the angles of the mandible. Occasionally elevation of the point of the jaw is sufficient. If obstruction is not thus relieved, a well-lubricated nasopharyngeal airway should be inserted into a nostril and manipulated so that its distal end lies just above the glottis. A safety-pin prevents it going too far down. The distance between nares and epiglottis equals that between naris and tragus of ear. With the tube in place and obstruction relieved, anæsthesia is deepened until the jaw can be easily opened for the insertion of a pharyngeal airway. A nasopharyngeal airway is tolerated at a lighter plane of anæsthesia than is a pharyngeal airway.

   To overcome jaw spasm it is sometimes necessary to prise the jaw open with a gag, draw the tongue forward, and insert a pharyngeal airway. The gag with Ackland's jaws is well adapted for this manœuvre. Care must be taken of the teeth. The use of short-acting muscle relaxants now enables the tightly clenched jaw to be opened atraumatically.

   b. *Flaccidity of the Jaw Muscles.*—Remedy is to manipulate the jaw and to insert a pharyngeal airway (e.g., Phillips, Guedel, or Waters), the chief function of which is to keep the tongue away from the pharyngeal wall.

3. OBSTRUCTION ABOVE THE GLOTTIS.—This may be due to a swab, a tooth, a foreign body, saliva, vomitus, blood, or œdema. The obstructing material must be removed by the fingers, gravity, swabbing, or suction. Very rarely, dislocation of the epiglottis or cysts or tumours of the epiglottis are encountered. Dislocation may be corrected digitally, so relieving obstruction. To relieve these cases, lower the head of the table, open the jaw, withdraw the tongue, apply suction, and administer oxygen. If unsuccessful, first feel the epiglottic region and then look at it through a laryngoscope : intubation may be necessary. The last remedy is tracheostomy, and it is extremely rarely necessary.

4. OBSTRUCTION AT THE GLOTTIS.—This is due to : (*a*) Impaction of the epiglottis into the larynx due to its abnormal overhanging shape, gravity, and muscular relaxation. The force of the inspiratory stream tends to maintain impaction while positive-pressure inflation will not overcome the obstruction. The

Difficulties, *continued.*

remedy is visual disimpaction via a laryngoscope after ensuring proper relaxation. (*b*) Sphincter-like closure of the ary-epiglottic folds allowing expiration but impeding inspiration. (*c*) Approximation of the ventricular ligaments or false cords. (*d*) Spastic closure of the rima glottidis by the vocal cords; their dome-shaped inferior surfaces allow escape of air, but their level superior surfaces prevent its entry. It may result from stimulation of the mucosa of the larynx or from stimuli arising at the site of operation (Brewer-Luckhardt reflexes) or from a combination of these factors with too light a plane of anæsthesia. It is usually worse on inspiration than expiration and causes a high-pitched 'tenor' sound. It is not influenced by altering the hold on the jaw, unlike the lower-pitched noise of pharyngeal obstruction. (*e*) Occasionally in patients who have had a large dose of relaxant which is incompletely reversed and have been intubated, respiratory obstruction develops after extubation because the relaxed cords, instead of becoming abducted during inspiration, become sucked in by the air-stream.

Local stimulation may be due to a vapour too concentrated, blood, or mucus, or to irritation from an airway: temporarily reduce vapour strength and partially withdraw airway: suck out blood or mucus.

Occasionally in operations on the neck, trauma to the recurrent laryngeal nerve causes spasm. Division of a nerve causes fixation of the cord midway between abduction and adduction. Difficulty only occurs during hyperpnœa in the non-intubated patient.

Peripheral stimulation causing partial or complete spasm suggests the need for deeper anæsthesia. Such stimuli occur when the cervix uteri or anal sphincter is stretched, when the cœliac plexus or its branches are stretched, when periosteum is separated from rib, etc. Addition of carbon dioxide and pressure on the breathing bag during inspiration will increase speed of induction and help separation of the cords. Temporary cessation of surgical stimuli may occasionally be necessary. The parasympathetic stimulants, thiopentone and, to a less extent, cyclopropane, favour the activity of this reflex especially if an artificial airway is inserted when the plane of anæsthesia is light.

If a volatile anæsthetic is being given, the vapour strength should be reduced and a little carbon dioxide given to increase the urge to breathe, after which the vapour strength is progressively increased. If the patient is under the influence of an intravenous thiobarbiturate, it may be necessary to ask the surgeon to interrupt his stimulating manœuvres for a few moments: the condition can cause considerable difficulty and may call for more active treatment. If this is considered necessary, one of the following can be given: (*a*) A short-acting relaxant; (*b*) A small dose of non-depolarizing relaxant is often sufficient to abolish partial laryngeal spasm, and may even result in increased tidal exchange.

The passage of an endotracheal tube between the cords completely abolishes the condition and is made easier after a relaxant has been injected. If laryngeal spasm does not pass off, and progressive hypoxia is in evidence, artificial respiration must be started at once if an endotracheal tube cannot be inserted :—

a. Apply pressure to reservoir bag filled with oxygen, after closing the expiratory valve and holding mask to face, or—

b. Blow into face-mask, or—

c. Compress the lower chest and then draw the costal margins upwards and outwards.

In any of these methods, an oropharyngeal or nasopharyngeal airway may be required.

If patient is *in extremis*, a large needle can be inserted into the larynx through the cricothyroid membrane and air can be injected from a 20-ml. syringe repeatedly, or half a litre of oxygen per minute can be insufflated. Cocaine can also be squirted on to the under-surface of the cords from a needle inserted through the cricothyroid membrane. Tracheostomy is needed only on the rarest occasions.

5. LOWER RESPIRATORY OBSTRUCTION.—This takes place in the bronchioles and is of great importance. " It is upon the patency of the bronchiolar lumen and the quiescence of the bronchial reflexes that smooth anæsthesia largely depends " (Nosworthy).* Bronchial and bronchiolar responses result from inadequate suppression of reflexes, either by afferent or efferent depression, and this may be associated with the stimulation of sputum, artificial airways, anæsthetic vapour, movement of the patient, and also from stimuli arising in the area of operation. The response is great or small, depending on the reflex irritability of the patient, his threshold of irritability. This is raised in the old and ill, and lowered in nervous and young patients and those in severe pain. The sensitivity of the respiratory tract increases from above downwards, being greatest at the carina. Acute infection increases sensitivity as also does tuberculosis : bronchiectasis does not increase sensitivity to the same degree. A tendency to asthma strongly predisposes to bronchial spasm and wheezing.

Anæsthesia is incomplete unless the threshold of irritability has been raised sufficiently to prevent the stimulus of the moment from breaking through.

6. Obstruction to respiration may be due to some fault in the anæsthetic apparatus, such as :—

1. Kinking of the endotracheal tube or breathing tube.

2. Obstruction of the endotracheal tube or breathing tube.

---

* Nosworthy, M. D., *Anæsthesia*, 1948, **3**, 86.

Difficulties, *continued.*

       3. Absence of gas flow to patient due to empty cylinders, faulty flow-meters, or reducing valve gauges.

OTHER RESPIRATORY ABNORMALITIES.—

    1. CESSATION OF BREATHING.—May be associated with : (*a*) Respiratory obstruction ; abortive attempts at breathing can usually be seen. (*b*) Depression of the respiratory centre by sedatives, general anæsthetics, etc. Easily caused by thiopentone and cyclopropane. (*c*) Hypocapnia following hyperventilation. (*d*) Depression of the Hering-Breuer reflexes during intermittent positive-pressure ventilation. (*e*) Reflexes resulting from stimulation of the cœliac plexus and its offshoots, e.g., traction on the gall-bladder. (*f*) Blood-pressure-raising drugs, e.g., adrenaline (action on aortic and carotid baroceptors). (*g*) Depression of aortic and carotid body (chemoreceptor) reflexes by a high oxygen tension following a period of hypoxia. (*h*) Bronchoconstriction, due to irritation of the upper respiratory tract, parasympathetic stimulating drugs (e.g., thiopentone, cyclopropane), light anæsthesia, and surgical stimuli. (*i*) Raised intracranial pressure. (*j*) The use of muscle relaxants.

    2. RAPID BREATHING.—This may occur in feverish patients and may also be due to respiratory obstruction. May follow oxygen lack or carbon dioxide accumulation. Frequent when halothane or trichloroethylene is given. Low blood-pressure, by failing to stimulate aortic and carotid sinuses, may cause rapid breathing. An increased venous return, causing a rise in pressure in the right auricle, stimulates receptors there and causes tachypnœa (Harrison and Marsh reflex).

    3. SLOW BREATHING.—May be caused by sedatives given before operation and by pethidine or morphine given intravenously during operation. Bilateral cervical vagotomy also causes slow breathing.

    4. HYPERPNŒA.—May follow severe surgical stimuli, e.g., abdominal traction reflexes. Otherwise it is likely to be due to respiratory obstruction, hypoxia, or carbon dioxide excess.

    5. HYPOPNŒA.—Shallow breathing may be due to :—
      a. Deep, i.e., 3rd or 4th plane, anæsthesia.
      b. Cyclopropane.
      c. Intravenous barbiturates used for induction of anæsthesia.
      d. Morphine or pethidine overdosage.
      e. Myoneural block.

    6. IRREGULAR BREATHING.—In deep anæsthesia, shows overdosage and heralds respiratory arrest. In light anæsthesia may indicate ascent into second stage.

    7. BRONCHOSPASM.—In addition to spasm of the bronchial muscle, there is often an œdema, a type of urticaria, of the bronchial mucosa and sometimes an œdema due to engorgement of the bronchial vessels. It is characterized by lower respiratory tract obstruction, with : (*a*) small tidal exchange, (*b*) prolonged forceful expiration, sometimes producing ' bucking ' movements, (*c*) wheezing.

Caused by vagal stimulation either central, e.g., cyclopropane, thiopentone, or peripheral, e.g., by endotracheal tube or pharyngeal airway or the surgical stimulus. Should be treated by the addition of a little halothane, trichloroethylene or ether, or by intravenous injection of : (a) procaine, (b) pethidine, (c) aminophylline (250 mg. repeated if required), (d) suxamethonium intravenously, (e) isoprenaline spray. May occur in asthmatics. Bronchospasm may well be due to inadequate suppression of reflexes.

8. TRACHEAL TUG.—This jerky type of inspiration is seen when the intercostal muscles and the sternocostal parts of the diaphragm are paralysed, either by deep general anæsthesia or by muscle relaxants. It may be due to the unopposed action of the crura pulling on the dome of the diaphragm and thence on the pericardium, lung roots, and tracheobronchial tree, during each inspiration. The degree of tug depends on the depth of respiration and so it is more marked if ether is given than if cyclopropane is used. It disappears as soon as the intercostal muscles and the sternocostal parts of the diaphragm regain their tone and is a useful guide to the degree of muscular relaxation, especially at the end of an operation.

9. APNEUSTIC BREATHING.—As anæsthesia deepens, the jerky type of breathing with tracheal tug may give place to a series of slow deep inspirations, each one held for 30–90 seconds, after which the air is suddenly expelled by the elastic recoil of the lungs. This may finally give place to gasping breathing and apnœa.

10. HICCUP.—This may be seen, especially when thiopentone, gas and oxygen, and a relaxant are used. It may be associated with too light a plane of anæsthesia, nervousness of the patient (i.e., high reflex irritability), stimulation of vagal nerve-endings (e.g., during gastrectomy), by a raised blood carbon dioxide content. It can be suppressed by adequate doses of relaxants. In addition, the following have been recommended as remedies: (a) Inhalation of amyl nitrite introduced into the circuit. (b) A short blast of strong ether vapour (Gray). (c) Inhalation of ammonia. The success of these three methods suggests that a reflex mechanism is involved as hiccup stops too rapidly to be due to absorption of the drug. (d) Intravenous injection of methylamphetamine. (e) Intravenous injection of pethidine. (f) Procaine block of the vagi at the œsophageal hiatus. (g) Vigorous hyperventilation via the reservoir bag. (h) Pressure on the eyeballs. After successful treatment the condition may recur later during the operation. The cause of this troublesome complication is not fully understood.

11. CHEYNE-STOKES BREATHING.—This may be seen after overdosage with respiratory depressant drugs, e.g., after chlorpromazine. It also occurs in heart failure, head injury, and more rarely in kidney disease. When not due to drugs it has a bad prognostic significance. Can be temporarily abolished by the intravenous injection of 250 mg. of aminophylline, and sometimes by inhalation of oxygen with or without carbon

Difficulties, *continued.*

dioxide. Biot's breathing is irregular periods of apnœa and hyperpnœa originally described in patients with meningitis.*

Technique.—

A. OPEN ETHER.—Atropine or hyoscine should be the premedication, given intravenously just before the induction, if necessary. If ether alone is used—an uncomfortable method—twenty or thirty minutes may be required to get the patient fully anæsthetized, as a rapid increase in vapour strength may cause coughing and breath-holding.

The mask is covered with fifteen thicknesses of gauze and, as induction proceeds, a gamgee pad with hole for nose and mouth can be allowed to separate the mask from the face, cutting down air leaks (technically, semi-open or perhalation). Ether is dropped on to mask as quickly as patient will tolerate it and during the first quarter-hour of surgical anæsthesia rate will approximate a hundred drops a minute : in second quarter-hour this rate will be halved. If the patient objects to the vapour it is diluted with air by raising the mask. A gentle flow of carbon dioxide under the mask will hasten induction. When neck muscles relax, head is turned to one side, while the jaw is supported to procure a good airway. Full rotation of head, with slight extension of neck, is frequently all that is required to ensure a good airway. If necessary, a pharyngeal airway can be introduced. The maximum concentration of ether under an open mask is about 15 per cent. With open ether there is always a reduction in the oxygen tension under the mask, so 500–1000 ml. of oxygen per minute should be added in every case. Reduction of oxygen tension under the mask falls, on average, from 150 mm. Hg to 105 mm. Hg, and is due to displacement of atmospheric oxygen by carbon dioxide and by ether vapour, which averages during induction 37–55 mm. Hg partial pressure.

A slow progressive increase in concentration and a good airway are the secrets of a successful induction. As the anæsthetic state becomes established, a given plane is maintained with the addition of less and less anæsthetic—the so-called ' law of diminishing resistance ' of Gill. This is because the body tissues are becoming saturated, there is less redistribution of ether from the brain, and a rising ether concentration in blood returning to the lungs.

Induction with *ethyl chloride* is quicker than with ether alone, though care is necessary owing to its high potency, and the anæsthetist should be aware of every breath. It is gently sprayed on to a mask, the concentration being increased as quickly as is tolerated by the patient. Normal breathing first becomes irregular, then automatic, and finally stertorous. Shortly after this point the mask is removed and a second one, well soaked with ether, is applied to the face, so that the patient's deep inspirations draw in sufficient ether vapour to

---

* Biot, *Lyon. méd.*, 1876, **23**, 517 and 561.

maintain surgical anæsthesia without an intervening stage of coughing or laryngospasm. The method needs experience, especially when robust individuals are being anæsthetized and is surely very rarely employed to-day.

Divinyl ether can also be used to provide a speedier induction before maintenance with diethyl ether. It can be used alone or in combination with diethyl ether as vinesthene anæsthetic mixture (V.A.M.). It is probably safer than ethyl chloride when used in this way, and so is generally to be preferred.

Induction with *chloroform* or *chloroform–ether mixtures* is seldom justified, as it is during the induction period that chloroform is especially dangerous.

Perhalational or semi-open methods increase speed of induction.

Anæsthesia by open mask results in considerable heat loss to the patient.

B. SEMI-CLOSED ETHER.—

1. CONTINUOUS-FLOW MACHINES (e.g., Boyle).

Nitrous oxide is used to produce unconsciousness. After seeing that the cylinders are correctly coupled up, a flow of 8–10 litres per minute of the gas is turned on, and the face-piece held a couple of inches over the patient's face. When consciousness is lost (abolition of eyelash reflex and automatic respiration) the flow is reduced to 8 litres a minute, the mask is applied to the face, while the ether tap is turned to its minimal vaporizing position, which varies from machine to machine. Two litres a minute of oxygen are now added and the ether tap progressively turned until it is full on, and then the plunger is depressed as fast as the patient will tolerate the increase in vapour strength. Addition of a half litre a minute of carbon dioxide will speed up induction. It is advisable that the total flow of gases should not be less than the alveolar ventilation rate, and usually should exceed this,* i.e., 8 litres a minute, and the oxygen percentage 25 or more, if patient is to be sure of receiving in his lungs at least 20 per cent of oxygen. It may be necessary in resistant patients to use both bottles with ether; first, the smaller one, and then the larger. Maintenance of anæsthesia can often be smoothly carried along with the gases passing over the surface of ether in one bottle. If the tension of the spring of the expiratory valve is relatively high, the mean pressure in the anæsthetic circuit and in the patient's respiratory tract will be increased and so will the effort required to expire through the valve. The main factors governing rebreathing are not the setting of the expiratory valve, but the relationship between the respiratory minute volume of the patient and the flow of fresh gases into the circuit. The tension on the valve should, however, always be as light as possible.

It is often convenient to follow nitrous oxide with a little trichloroethylene or halothane and then to add ether.

---

* Norman, J., Adams, A. P., and Sykes, M. K., *Anæsthesia*, 1968, **23**, 82.

Administration Technique, *continued.*

They are less irritating to the respiratory mucosa than ether and enable a smoother induction to be carried out.

2. INTERMITTENT-FLOW MACHINES (e.g., McKesson).—Gas mixtures at predetermined pressures and of predetermined percentage are delivered to the patient only when he inspires. The gases can be diverted over a halothane, ether, or trichloroethylene vaporizing bottle. The expiratory valve is opened ; the absorber indicator set at ' change ' ; the nitrous oxide at 100 per cent ; and the pressure at 3 to 5 mm. Hg. The mask is put on the patient's face and he inhales 100 per cent nitrous oxide until consciousness is lost, when the ether pointer is turned to its minimal vaporizing position and 20 per cent oxygen set on the percentage dial. Halothane, ether, or trichloroethylene concentration is increased as rapidly as possible, and here, too, the addition of 300–500 ml. of carbon dioxide a minute will hurry the induction along.

C. THE E.M.O. INHALER (*Fig.* 15).*—This has replaced the time-honoured and very useful Oxford Vaporizer† and, like it, was developed in the Nuffield Department of Anæsthetics in the

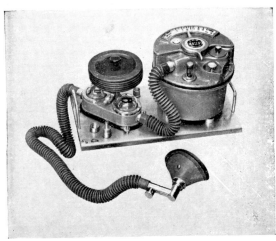

Fig. 15.—E.M.O. ether inhaler. (Longworth Scientific Instrument Co., Ltd., Abingdon.)

University of Oxford. It will deliver a predetermined concentration of ether vapour in air, irrespective of changes in the temperature of the liquid anæsthetic, and is controlled by an automatic thermocompensator mechanism. A water compartment acts

---

* Epstein, H. G., and Macintosh, R. R., *Anæsthesia*, 1956, **11**, 83.
† Epstein, H. G., Macintosh, R. R., and Mendelssohn, K., *Lancet*, 1941, **2**, 62.

as a heat buffer. It is usually employed as a ' draw-over ' apparatus, but if combined with an Oxford Inflating Bellows, can be used for intermittent positive-pressure respiration. Rebreathing is prevented by the use of unidirectional valves. The apparatus is useful in countries where nitrous oxide is not readily available or when portability is important. Ether and air can be used combined with a small dose of thiopentone or halothane for induction, and with a muscle relaxant and controlled respiration for major intra-abdominal or intrathoracic surgery. For light anæsthesia with spontaneous respiration the patient should breathe ether in concentrations gradually increasing to 15 per cent, after which it may be reduced to about 7 per cent for maintenance. For controlled respiration, induction with thiopentone and non-depolarizing muscle relaxant, intubation, and controlled respiration with 5 per cent ether in air reducing to 2–3 per cent is very satisfactory. Explosions have not been described during the administration of ether and air even when diathermy has been used. The use of a small halothane vaporizer during induction speeds the induction with ether.* *See also* Chapter XXX.

D. THE CLOSED CIRCUIT WITH CARBON DIOXIDE ABSORPTION. (*See also* p. 121.)—If ether is to be used, induction is often quicker when a semi-closed circuit is used to start with. When the required level of anæsthesia has been reached, the bag is filled with the mixture of gases being breathed, the gases are shut off, the expiratory valve is closed, and the mask strapped firmly to the patient's face. A basal oxygen flow of 250–400 ml. per minute is turned on and regulated so that the volume of gas in the bag remains constant. The soda-lime is brought into circuit. Increased depth is obtained by carrying the total gases over the ether vaporizer as in the McKesson and Coxeter-Mushin apparatus, or by bubbling the basal oxygen through both the bottles full of ether in the Boyle machine. In the last machine, alternatively, the circuit can be opened temporarily and a large volume of gas can be bubbled through ether to deepen the anæsthesia.

CHAPTER VI

THE ANÆSTHETIC GASES

NITROUS OXIDE [N₂O] ANÆSTHESIA

Gas first prepared by Priestley in 1772. Anæsthetic properties suggested by Sir Humphry Davy in 1799. Colton demonstrated its effects to Horace Wells in 1844, who used it in dentistry and had one of his own teeth painlessly extracted by John M. Riggs on Dec. 11. After an unsuccessful demonstration before John Collins Warren the surgeon and the students at the Massachusetts General Hospital, Wells continued to use it in his practice, but its use was temporarily

* Parkhouse, J., *Anæsthesia*, 1966, **21**, 498.

Nitrous Oxide Anæsthesia, *continued.*

forgotten and it was overshadowed by ether. Gardner Quincy Colton (1814–1898) revived its use in 1867–8 and this time the American dental profession showed considerable interest. In 1863 he established himself in practice in New York City and there founded the Colton Dental Association. He had been a pupil of Willard Parker (1800–1884), a distinguished surgeon who had written of the exhilarating properties of nitrous oxide and may have acquainted Colton with its effects. T. W. Evans, a U.S. dentist living in Paris, introduced it to his colleagues in London in 1868,* having learnt its use the previous year from Colton at the International Congress of Medicine in Paris. Later in the same year, the gas was supplied compressed into cylinders. Edmund Andrews, of Chicago, combined it with oxygen, to give longer anæsthesia, in 1868, while in 1878 Paul Bert, of France, administered it under pressure and proved it to be a true anæsthetic, not a means of causing asphyxia.† Sir F. Hewitt and E. I. McKesson have been pioneers in its use, and to-day it is widely used as an analgesic, along with a relaxant and an intravenous barbiturate. The book *Nitrous-Oxide–Oxygen Anesthesia* by F. W. Clement appeared in 1939. The book *Untoward Effects of Nitrous Oxide Anæsthesia* by C. B. Courville appeared in 1939, and in 1956 H. C. A. Lassen of Copenhagen reported that very prolonged nitrous-oxide–oxygen anæsthesia could cause bone-marrow aplasia.‡

Manufacture.—By heating ammonium nitrate in an iron retort to 240° C. The issuing gas is collected, purified, and compressed into metal cylinders at 51 atmospheres—750 lb. per sq. in.

$$NH_4NO_3 \rightarrow 2H_2O + N_2O$$

Nitric oxide (NO) and nitrogen dioxide (NO_2) are produced as impurities, particularly if overheating should occur. The gases evolved are washed with water, caustic soda, and alkali in turn, before being passed through activated alumina to remove water vapour. Gases are liquefied and fed into cylinders. At various stages, monitors are used to detect the presence of harmful impurities such as nitrogen dioxide. As a further check, regular random sampling of cylinders is carried out.§

The amount present in the cylinder can only be ascertained by weighing, as the gas is in liquid form and the gas pressure above the liquid level remains constant as long as any liquid remains. About three-quarters to four-fifths of the contents of a full cylinder is in the liquid state, so, in use, cylinders must have their valves elevated above the horizontal. Just before exhaustion of the cylinder, when all the liquid is vaporized, the pressure very quickly drops to zero. Cylinders are filled to a filling ratio of 0·69 (i.e., ratio of weight of nitrous oxide to weight of water the cylinder could hold). The cylinder weights, full and empty, are stamped on it. 100 gallons of nitrous oxide weigh

* Evans, T. W., *Brit. J. dent. Sci.*, 1868, **2**, 196.
† Bert, P., *C. R. Soc. Biol. (Paris)*, 1878.
‡ Lassen, H. C. A., *Lancet*, 1956, **1**, 525.
§ *See also Brit. J. Anæsth.*, 1967, **39**, 440 et seq.; and Austin, A. T., and Kain, M. L., *Proc. R. Soc. Med.*, 1967, **60**, 1175.

30 oz. (1 U.S. gallon = $\frac{5}{6}$ Imperial gallon; 1 cubic foot = 6$\frac{1}{4}$ Imperial gallons; 1 Imperial gallon = 4$\frac{1}{2}$ litres). Blue is the colour of the cylinder. A reducing or regulating valve (Adams, 1923) is usually attached to the cylinder. It steps down the pressure of issuing gas from 750 lb. to 7 lb. per sq. in. or 60 lb. per sq. in.

For a full description *see* Galley, A. H., in *General Anæsthesia* (Ed. Evans, F. T., and Gray, T. C.), 2nd ed., 1965, Ch. 15. London: Butterworths.

Impurities in Nitrous Oxide.—Two cases of poisoning occurred in September 1966 and were subsequently reported in detail by Clutton-Brock.[*] Investigation showed that a batch of nitrous oxide had become contaminated with nitric oxide (NO) and nitrogen dioxide (NO_2). Both these substances are toxic and cause severe constitutional disturbances. One of the 2 cases died.

The clinical features are:—

1. Cyanosis, commencing within a few minutes of administration, and becoming severe and unrelieved by oxygen. This is due to formation of methæmoglobin, which reduces the hæmoglobin available for oxygen transport and shifts the dissociation curve to the left.
2. Respiratory difficulty. This is due to nitrous and nitric acids which are formed in the lungs and cause a non-specific œdema and bronchopneumonia, and may produce a clinical picture resembling that of Mendelson's syndrome.
3. Circulatory failure, which is probably secondary to hypoxia.

The suggested treatment[†] would be:—

1. Oxygen therapy to compensate for hypoxia.
2. Methylene blue to reconvert methæmoglobin.
3. The prevention and treatment of chemical pneumonitis, with antibiotics, steroids, I.P.P.V.
4. Correction of acid-base disturbances.
5. Circulatory support, e.g., pressor drugs.
6. Dimercaprol has been suggested in view of the protective action of this type of agents against the higher oxides of nitrogen.

A crude test for contamination[‡] is to put a piece of moistened starch-iodide paper into a large syringe and then fill this with the suspected nitrous oxide mixed with 25 per cent oxygen and wait for 10 min. If the gas is contaminated by over 300 parts per million, the starch iodide will turn blue.

See also a series of papers on the subject, *Brit. J. Anæsth.*, 1967, **39**, 343 et seq., and Editorial, *Lancet*, 1967, **2**, 930.

Physical Properties.—Sweet smelling, non-irritating, colourless gas; the only inorganic gas in common use possessing anæsthetic properties. Boiling-point −89° C. Molecular weight 44. Critical pressure 71·7 atmospheres. Critical temperature 36·5° C. Specific gravity 1·5—that is, 1$\frac{1}{2}$ times heavier than air. Neither flammable

---

[*] Clutton-Brock, J., *Brit. J. Anæsth.*, 1967, **39**, 388.
[†] Prys-Roberts, C., *Ibid.*, 1967, **39**, 432.
[‡] Kain, M. L., Commins, B. T., Dixon-Lewis, G., and Nunn, J. F., *Ibid.*, 1967, **39**, 425; and 'Discussion on Impurities in Nitrous Oxide', *Proc. R. Soc. Med.*, 1967, **60**, 1175.

Nitrous Oxide—Physical Properties, *continued*.

nor explosive, but supports the combustion of other agents, even in the absence of oxygen, if a high temperature (above 450° C.) is supplied to initiate decomposition into nitrogen and oxygen. The oil/water solubility ratio is 3·2. Water will take up 100 vol. per cent, while blood-plasma dissolves 45 vol. per cent. Nitrous oxide is fifteen times more soluble in plasma than nitrogen and one hundred times more soluble than oxygen. The partition coefficient is 0·47 between blood and gas, 1·0 between brain and blood, and 3·0 between fat and blood.

It is eliminated unchanged from the body, mostly via the lungs, within 2 minutes. It is very stable and is unaffected by soda-lime.

Mode of Action.—Nitrous oxide does not combine with hæmoglobin, but is carried in solution in the plasma. Even with adequate oxygen it has been shown to cause some cardiac dilatation.* It does not enter into chemical combination with any body tissue, depression of the central nervous system being its chief pharmacological action, and this is probably due to oxygen displacement from the cerebral cells. If given under pressure this displacement is increased, and at 3 atmospheres' pressure animals may die even though an adequate proportion of oxygen is present. At a barometric pressure of 1520 mm. Hg (2 atmospheres) a 50 per cent nitrous-oxide–oxygen mixture will rapidly produce unconsciousness and surgical anæsthesia without significant alteration in oxygen saturation of arterial blood. Reduction of oxygen to 5 per cent is the equivalent of ascending to nearly 30,000 feet, whereas reduction to 3 per cent of oxygen is equivalent to ascent to 40,000 feet.

The gas has definite anæsthetic properties due to its great solubility. This is supported by the following facts, which suggest that it is more than an asphyxiating agent :—

 a. Anæsthesia is produced under certain conditions in the presence of 40 per cent or even 50 per cent oxygen and a 50 per cent nitrous-oxide–oxygen mixture produces very effective analgesia very quickly and is more efficient as an analgesic than is pethidine.†

 b. There is a great difference in effect following the inhalation of 20 per cent oxygen with 80 per cent nitrous oxide, and following 20 per cent oxygen–80 per cent nitrogen (air).

 c. Respiratory arrest is produced much quicker after inhalation of pure nitrous oxide than after inhalation of pure nitrogen.

Nevertheless, some of the clinical signs of well-administered nitrous-oxide–oxygen anæsthesia are due to the asphyxial element, this being necessary owing to weak anæsthetic properties of nitrous oxide.

100 ml. of blood will dissolve (in its plasma) 47 ml. of nitrous oxide. The amount of gases which can be carried, other factors being equal, by a given volume of blood in simple solution depends on the

---

* Fisher, C. W., Bennett, L. L., and Allahwala, A., *Anesthesiology*, 1951, **12**, 19.
† Dundee, J. W., and Moore, J., *Brit. J. Anæsth.*, 1960, **32**, 453.

proportions or tensions of these gases in contact with the blood. Therefore, the proportions inhaled determine the tensions of those gases held in solution. The amount of nitrous oxide absorbed from the lungs is dependent on its concentration or partial pressure. It follows that the tension in arterial blood governs the depth of anæsthesia.

Side-effects of Nitrous Oxide.—Nitrous oxide is usually regarded as a non-toxic anæsthetic agent, provided that it is administered with a sufficient concentration of oxygen. Undesirable effects may, however, sometimes occur:—

1. Nitrous oxide augments the respiratory depressant action of thiopentone, especially after opiate premedication. The response to hypercapnia is diminished.[*]
2. Post-operative hearing loss has been attributed to changes in middle-ear mechanics due to the differential solubility of nitrous oxide and nitrogen causing pressure changes.[†]
3. Prolonged anæsthesia may result in diffusion of the gas into cavities such as the bowel, pneumothorax cavity,[‡] and in air encephalography.[§]
4. In the treatment of tetanus and poliomyelitis, prolonged administration of nitrous oxide has resulted in bone-marrow aplasia and fatal agranulocytosis.[||]
5. Teratogenic effects have been observed in pregnant rats exposed to nitrous oxide for prolonged periods. The critical period is when the embryo is 8 days old, corresponding to the human fœtus of 6 weeks.[¶]

Diffusion Hypoxia.[**]—Immediately the mask is removed from a patient who has for a longish period been breathing nitrous oxide with adequate oxygen, a high percentage of the expired volume may consist of nitrous oxide so that the outward diffusion of the gas lowers the partial pressure of oxygen in the alveoli. This gives rise to a condition known as diffusion hypoxia and it may be harmful in ill or handicapped patients. The remedy is to add oxygen to the inspired air during the quarter of an hour following the anæsthesia.

Stages of Anæsthesia.—The Guedel classification does not apply to nitrous-oxide–oxygen anæsthesia with full oxygenation. With full oxygenation greater depth than a point corresponding to Plane 1, Stage III, is impossible in healthy patients. When the factor of hypoxia is added, greater depth is obtainable, but the signs are then partly those of asphyxia.

---

[*] Eckenhoff, J. E., and Helrich, M., *Anesthesiology*, 1958, **19**, 240.
[†] Waun, J. E., Sweitzer, R. S., and Hamilton, W K., *Ibid.*, 1967, **28**, 846; and Matz, G. J., Rattenborg, C. G., and Holaday, D. A., *Ibid.*, 1967, **28**, 948.
[‡] Egu, E. I., and Saidman, L. J., *Ibid.*, 1965, **26**, 61; and Vandam, L. D., *Canad. Anæsth. Soc. J.*, 1965, **12**, 107.
[§] Saidman, L. J., and Egu, E. I., *Anesthesiology*, 1965, **26**, 67.
[||] Lassen, H. C. A., Henrickson, E., Neukirch, F., and Kristenson, H. S., *Lancet*, 1956, **1**, 527.
[¶] Fink, B. R., *2nd Eur. Cong. Anæsth.*, 1966, oral communication; and Fink, B. R., Shepard, T. H., and Blandau, R. J., *Nature, Lond.*, 1967, **214**, 146.
[**] Fink, B. R., *Anesthesiology*, 1955, **16**, 511.

Stages of Anæsthesia, *continued.*

Thus in clinical nitrous-oxide–oxygen anæsthesia it is possible to recognize :—

Stage I—analgesia.
Stage II—delirium.
Stage III—surgical anæsthesia.
Stage IV—bulbar paralysis due to acute asphyxia.

It is important to know if the patient in surgical anæsthesia is :
(1) Too lightly ; (2) Adequately ; (3) Too deeply anæsthetized.

Opinions differ as to the degree of oxygen lack permissible. Moderate hypoxia in fit patients for short periods is probably not harmful. The present trend is towards the addition of small amounts of supplementary anæsthetics, e.g., methohexitone, thiopentone, vinesthene, trichloroethylene, halothane, etc., rather than pushing pure nitrous-oxide–oxygen.

Nitrous Oxide in Anæsthesia.—Nitrous oxide is a weak anæsthetic agent, and smooth anæsthesia is difficult to obtain consistently even for short operations, without some degree of hypoxia. Even in the out-patient department and dental surgery adjuvants are now frequently employed (*see* Chapter XXIV). For major surgery, nitrous-oxide–oxygen mixtures are usually administered after pre-medication, thiopentone induction, and with a volatile or intra-venous supplement. Muscle relaxants may be used not only to pro-vide full muscular relaxation, but also to obtund reflex activity. Under these circumstances it is possible to have very light planes of anæsthesia in a totally paralysed patient. The question arises whether we can be sure that the patient is unconscious. There is evidence that occasionally patients have been conscious during full-relaxant paralysis, though they have not usually complained of pain. Factors which may be considered are:—

1. Reports of awareness.* These would seem to be more common where sedative premedication has been omitted and other adjuvants used in minimal dosage (e.g., in Caesarean section).

2. Recollection of incidents occurring during operation when the patient is later subjected to hypnosis,† though this does not necessarily indicate awareness at the time.

3. The electro-encephalogram is not helpful in determining the existence of consciousness or unconsciousness.‡

4. The awake, paralysed, terrified patient may show sympathetic activity, e.g., dilatation of pupil, rapid bounding pulse.

It is now common practice to ensure against awareness by adding small amounts of trichloroethylene or halothane to the nitrous-oxide–oxygen mixture during controlled ventilation. Where it is justified, heavy premedication, the use of intravenous supplements, and hyperventilation may achieve the same result.

Factors causing awareness during operation.§

---

* Hutchinson, R., *Brit. J. Anæsth.*, 1961, **33**, 463.
† Cheek, D. B., *Amer. J. clin. Hypnosis*, 1959, **1**, 101; Cheek D. B., *Ibid.*, 1960, **3**, 101; and Levinson, B. W., *Brit. J. Anæsth.*, 1965, **37**, 544.
‡ Clutton-Brock, J., in *Thoracic Anæsthesia* (Ed. Mushin, W. W.), 1963, Ch. 19. Oxford: Blackwell.
§ Waters, D. J., *Brit. J. Anæsth.*, 1968, **40**, 259.

Premixed Nitrous Oxide and Oxygen.—Pressurized nitrous oxide and oxygen (80 : 20 per cent) at a maximum cylinder pressure of 700 lb. per sq. in. were used in the U.S. in 1945.* Certain mixtures of nitrous oxide and oxygen will remain in the gaseous phase at pressures and temperatures at which nitrous oxide by itself would normally be a liquid (Poynting effect). Mixtures of 50 : 50 and 60 : 40 per cent nitrous oxide and oxygen have been used, the pressure in the cylinder being 2000 lb. per sq. in. If such cylinders are exposed to cold, some of the nitrous oxide separates as a liquid and may lead to delivery of uneven mixtures, too much oxygen at the beginning and too much nitrous oxide at the end of the cylinder life. In 60 : 40 per cent mixture, the nitrous oxide condenses at a temperature of 0 to −1° C.; in 50 : 50 per cent mixtures, at −8° C.; only the 50 : 50 mixture is now available commercially. This can be avoided by immersing the cylinder in water at 52° C. and inverting it three times.† Doubts have been expressed as to the safety in use of such cylinders which have been exposed to low temperatures, as adequate remixing may not in all cases have occurred.‡ The Entonox apparatus has been designed for the administration of premixed gases on a demand system with equal volumes of oxygen and nitrous oxide.§

Nitrous Oxide and Analgesia.—Nitrous oxide is a good analgesic agent, a 25 per cent concentration in oxygen being compared favourably with morphine for relief of post-operative pain while having little general effect on consciousness.|| Nitrous oxide is a valuable aid to post-operative physiotherapy, when a 50 per cent concentration can be conveniently administered using a premixed gas cylinder and the Entonox apparatus. Long-term nitrous oxide has been used in the U.S.S.R. for up to 96 hours after thoracic surgery.¶ The use of nitrous oxide in obstetrics is discussed in Chapter XXV.

CYCLOPROPANE

Cyclopropane or trimethylene was first synthesized by von Freund who reduced trimethylene dibromide with sodium in an alkaline solution in 1882;** its anæsthetic properties were shown by Lucus and Henderson, of Toronto, in 1929†† while investigating the narcotic properties of propylene in an effort to find a more satisfactory agent than ethylene. First used on a human volunteer by W. Easson Brown, the patient being Professor Henderson, soon followed by Lucus and Banting (of insulin fame). As its use was not encouraged by the anæsthetic staff of the Toronto General Hospital it was developed by workers in the Anesthetics Department of the State of Wisconsin Hospital at Madison : clinical reports by Waters and his colleagues

* Barach, A. L., and Rovenstine, E. A., *Anesthesiology*, 1945, **6**, 449.
† Tunstall, M. E., *Brit. med. J.*, 1963, **2**, 240.
‡ Cole, P. V., *Anæsthesia*, 1964, **19**, 3.
§ *See* Hill, D. W., *Physics Applied to Anæsthesia*, 1967, p. 44. London: Butterworths.
|| Parbrook, G. D., and Kennedy, B. R., *Brit. med. J.*, 1964, **2**, 1303; and Parbrook, G. D., Rees, G. A. D., and Robertson, G. S., *Ibid.*, 1964, **2**, 480.
¶ Petrovsky, B. V., and Yefuni, S. N., *Brit. J. Anæsth.*, 1965, **37**, 42.
** von Freund, A., *Monats. f. Chemie*, 1882, **3**, 625.
†† Lucus, G. H. W., and Henderson, V. E., *Canad. med. Ass. J.*, 1929, **21**, 173.

Cyclopropane, *continued.*

followed in the years after 1930, when he started its use.* Its pharmacology was worked out by Seevers, Meek, Rovenstine, and Stiles in 1934. Harold Griffith began using the agent in Montreal about the same time.

A saturated hydrocarbon, isomeric with propylene. In the U.S. the method of manufacture is founded on von Freund's method: 1,3,dihalide of propane, when added to a solution containing elemental metal—zinc, magnesium, or sodium—will react to form cyclopropane. In Britain, prepared from trimethylene glycol. Trimethylene glycol reacts with hydrobromic acid to form trimethylene dibromide which is then reduced by zinc.

(1)
$$CH_2OH \qquad\qquad CH_2Br$$
$$\dot{C}H_2 \quad + 2HBr \rightarrow \dot{C}H_2 \qquad + 2H_2O$$
$$\dot{C}H_2OH \qquad\qquad \dot{C}H_2Br$$

(2)
$$CH_2Br \qquad\qquad CH_2$$
$$\dot{C}H_2 \quad + Zn \rightarrow \quad / \quad \backslash \qquad + ZnBr_2$$
$$\dot{C}H_2Br \qquad CH_2\text{——}CH_2$$

Cyclopropane can also be prepared from chlorinated propane which is cheaper to manufacture than brominated propane.

Is also prepared from natural gas, found in the U.S.

Physical Properties.—Colourless gas with sweet smell. Molecular weight 42·05. Boiling-point $-32\cdot9°$ C. One and a half times heavier than air. Liquefies at ordinary temperatures if pressure of 5 atmospheres is applied ; hence is stored in light-alloy cylinders as a liquid at a pressure of 75 lb. to the sq. in., no reducing valves being required. One ounce is equivalent to 3·5 gallons (4·29 gallons U.S.). Almost insoluble in water (1 volume dissolves in 2·7 volumes at 15° C.), but very soluble in lipoids ; partition coefficients, blood/gas 0·46, fat/blood 20·0, oil/water 34·4. Very explosive with oxygen (between 2·5 and 50 per cent) and nitrous oxide throughout the anæsthetic range ; explosive in air between 3 per cent and 10 per cent. Propylene is the chief impurity and is harmless in small volumes. It is not decomposed by soda-lime, but slowly diffuses through rubber. The gas is supplied in aluminium-alloy cylinders, orange in colour.

Pharmacology.—

ABSORPTION AND ELIMINATION.—Taken up via the lungs. Undergoes no chemical change in the body. Excreted into the alveoli (very small amount diffuses through the skin). Major part eliminated in 10 min., but complete desaturation takes much longer. Both induction of anæsthesia and recovery are relatively fast.

CENTRAL NERVOUS SYSTEM.—It is the most potent of the anæsthetic gases so that it is always possible to use more than

---

* Stiles, J. A., Neff, W. B., Rovenstine, E. A., and Waters, R., *Curr. Res. Anesth.*, 1934, **13**, 56; and Waters, R. M., and Schmidt, E. R., *J. Amer. med. Ass.*, 1934, **103**, 975.

20 per cent of oxygen with it. It is said that a concentration of 4 per cent will produce analgesia, 8 per cent light anæsthesia, 20–25 per cent moderate anæsthesia, and 40 per cent respiratory failure ; 3–5 per cent cyclopropane in oxygen has been used to obtain pain relief in labour.*

RESPIRATORY SYSTEM.—Non-irritating to mucous membranes in concentrations under 50 per cent, but may cause reflex laryngeal spasm in high concentration. Because the gas is non-irritant, coughing, laryngospasm, and bronchospasm are uncommon, even though it is vagomimetic. Cyclopropane is a powerful respiratory depressant. Breathing is quiet and progressively more shallow. Carbon dioxide retention is likely to occur in the absence of assisted or controlled respiration. Heavy premedication with opiates increases the depression of respiration, so that apnœa may occur in a light plane of anæsthesia. Control of respiration is facilitated.

BLOOD-PRESSURE.—Usually well maintained. Vascular resistance is increased in proportion to inhaled concentration, and this results in decreased forearm blood-flow.† Pressure often rises above pre-operative level, possibly due to carbon dioxide retention and/or a rise in circulating catecholamines. In dogs this has been shown to be a central effect ; hypertension and increased plasma catecholamines can be prevented by section through the medulla oblongata during cyclopropane anæsthesia.‡ Fall in blood-pressure is a danger sign which may be associated with severe bradycardia, or due to overdosage with cyclopropane.

CARDIAC OUTPUT.—This is usually increased if premedication has not been given. At inspired concentrations greater than 20–25 per cent cyclopropane cardiac output falls. After morphine premedication cardiac output falls when cyclopropane is administered.

CENTRAL VENOUS PRESSURE.—Increased. The large intrathoracic veins are less compressible and the hypotensive effects of I.P.P.V. are diminished. Raised venous pressure may be a cause of increased bleeding during cyclopropane anæsthesia.

CAPILLARY OOZING.—Cyclopropane anæsthesia is sometimes associated with increased oozing. This may be due to dilatation of cutaneous and muscle vessels in light anæsthesia, raised central venous pressure, or may be secondary to carbon dioxide retention.

ARRHYTHMIA.—Cyclopropane anæsthesia may be accompanied by the development of arrhythmias of all kinds. Most significant are :—

1. VAGOTONIC ARRHYTHMIAS.—Bradycardia (below 50 per min.). Nodal rhythm. Seldom of significance provided blood-pressure is maintained.

2. VENTRICULAR ECTOPIC BEATS.—These may occur singly, as coupled beats, or as runs of ventricular tachycardia. Ventricular fibrillation, with sudden death, can occur. Factors which predispose to ventricular arrhythmias :—

* Shnider, S. M., and others, *Anesthesiology*, 1963, **24**, 11.
† McArdle, L., and Black, G. W., *Brit. J. Anæsth.*, 1963, **35**, 352.
‡ Price, H. L., and others, *Anesthesiology*, 1963, **24**, 1.

Cyclopropane—Pharmacology, *continued.*

   i. *Overdosage with Cyclopropane.*—This has been disputed. Guedel* (1940) believed that there was a zone of arrhythmia, and that when anæsthesia was deepened, arrhythmias disappeared. Deep anæsthesia was achieved rapidly utilizing controlled respirations, and hence carbon dioxide was removed (*see below*). Waters† (1945), on the other hand, recommended lightening of the plane of anæsthesia if arrhythmia occurred. Propranolol may abolish ventricular arrhythmias.‡

  ii. *Carbon Dioxide Retention.*—It has been shown that any given patient has a carbon dioxide threshold for arrhythmias during cyclopropane anæsthesia.§ Carbon dioxide retention is likely to occur during spontaneous respiration, owing to the depression of respiration. This explains the views of both Guedel and Waters (*above*). Guedel deepened anæsthesia and controlled respiration. Waters lightened anæsthesia to produce an increase in tidal volume.

 iii. *Catecholamines.*—Cyclopropane, unlike halothane, anæsthesia is accompanied by an increase in circulating catechol amines.‖ Adrenaline sensitizes the heart to the presence of cyclopropane, and all concentrations of cyclopropane sensitize the heart to circulating adrenaline. Adrenaline infiltration during cyclopropane anæsthesia caused ventricular arrhythmias in 30 per cent of patients in a recent study, despite careful attention to ventilation and depth of anæsthesia.¶ It would appear that adrenaline injected subcutaneously is more dangerous during cyclopropane than during trichloroethylene or halothane administration. Methoxamine and phenylephrine do not share this effect.

  iv. *Hypoxia.*—Griffith (1951)** stresses the importance of keeping a clear airway and of assisting respirations if they become depressed.

   v. *Atropine.*—Intravenous injection of atropine may give rise to transient arrhythmias in conscious volunteers. These are more common during cyclopropane anæsthesia.†† If it is necessary to give intravenous atropine for any reason (e.g., severe bradycardia), it is wise to dilute the drug and give it slowly (0·1 mg. at a time).

The cardiovascular and respiratory effects of cyclopropane have been the subject of intensive study by Price and others in the University of Pennsylvania. *See* a series of papers : *Anesthesiology,* 1958, **19**, 457 ; 1958, **19**, 619 ; 1959, **20**, 563 ; 1960, **21**, 380 ; and 1963, **24**, 1.

* Guedel, A. E., *Anesthesiology,* 1940, **1**, 13.
† Waters, R. M., *Surgery,* 1945, **18**, 26.
‡ Payne, J. P., and Senfield, R. M., *Brit. med. J.,* 1964, **1**, 603 ; and Johnstone, M., *Brit. J. Anæsth.,* 1964, **36**, 224.
§ Price, H. L., Jones, R. E., Price, M. L., and Linde, H. W., *Anesthesiology,* 1958, **19**, 457.
‖ Price, H. L., and others, *Ibid.,* 1959, **20**, 563.
¶ Matteo, R. S., Katz, R. L., and Papper, E. M., *Ibid.,* 1963, **24**, 327.
** Griffith, H. R., *Ibid.,* 1951, **12**, 109.
†† Jones, R. E., Deutsch, S., and Turndorf, H., *Ibid.,* 1961, **22**, 67.

AUTONOMIC NERVOUS SYSTEM.—Cyclopropane is parasympatheticomimetic (bradycardia, tendency to laryngobronchospasm, contraction of the gut) and also sympatheticomimetic (liberation of circulating catechol amines).

MUSCULAR RELAXATION.—Good muscular relaxation can be obtained, though this may be associated with respiratory depression and carbon dioxide retention. It may be necessary (i) to assist or control respiration, (ii) to use ether in addition to cyclopropane in order to stimulate respiration, (iii) to use small doses of muscle relaxants and control respiration.

ALIMENTARY SYSTEM.—In light planes, gut is contracted (parasympathetic effect). Peristalsis and tone abolished by deep anæsthesia. Nausea and vomiting may occur. Cyclopropane reduces splanchnic,* hepatic, and renal blood-flow, a neurogenic effect.

BIOCHEMICAL CHANGE.—No interference with liver function. A suitable agent in the presence of liver disease, because a high oxygen tension can be obtained in arterial blood. Blood-sugar may rise.

HÆMOPOIETIC SYSTEM.—Spleen may increase in size. Leucocytosis (maximum after 8 hours).

UTERUS.—Contractions not inhibited in light planes, but abolished in deep planes. Blood concentration in fœtus equals that of mother after 15 min.

Clinical Use of Cyclopropane.—Owing to its explosive nature and the high cost of administration in an open system, cyclopropane is usually used in a closed circuit.

Techniques of Administration.—

INDUCTION WITH CYCLOPROPANE AND OXYGEN.—It is wise to avoid the use of those premedication drugs which are powerful respiratory depressants (morphine, pethidine). Cyclopropane is a potent agent and rapid induction can be achieved, a few breaths of 50 per cent cyclopropane in oxygen being enough to render a patient unconscious. It is probably wiser to begin with a lower percentage, however, and the following technique is recommended :—

Test the apparatus for leaks and make sure the soda-lime is not exhausted. Fill the reservoir bag with oxygen and start the patient breathing 100 per cent oxygen with a basal flow of about 500 ml. per min. of oxygen. When a good fit is obtained and the reservoir bag is moving well, add cyclopropane 500 ml. per min., explaining to the patient that he will now smell the rather sweet odour of the gas. Although 50 per cent cyclopropane is being added to the closed system, this is immediately diluted by oxygen and nitrogen in the circuit, so that a much lower percentage is inspired, though the inspired concentration will rise as time passes. Keep talking to the patient throughout induction. Suggestion may help to

---

* Price, H. L., Deutsch, S., Cooperman, L. H., Clement, A. J., and Epstein, R. M., *Anesthesiology*, 1965, **26**, 312.

Cyclopropane—Techniques of Administration, *continued.*

prevent the stage of excitement. If this occurs, keep the face-mask on and continue the administration until surgical anæsthesia is obtained.

In suitable cases induction can be obtained with a sleep dose of thiopentone, continuing as above. If intubation is required, it can be performed with thiopentone–suxamethonium proceeding to oxygen–cyclopropane as outlined. Small doses of thiopentone only are desirable so that undue respiratory depression does not occur (unless I.P.P.V. is planned).

When surgical anæsthesia is reached, the flow of cyclopropane gas into the system should be cut down or deep levels of anæsthesia will occur. It should be cut down gradually over several minutes to a maintenance level of about 100 ml. per min. Pay due attention to the various stimuli applied to the patient (skin cleaning, skin clips, skin incision, etc.) to gauge the depth of anæsthesia. A suitable maintenance flow for the particular patient, depending on the level of anæsthesia required and escape of cyclopropane from any leaks in the system, is usually readily found. Cyclopropane can be added to the system as a small basal flow throughout operation (50–150 ml. per min.) or as intermittent additions, with cyclopropane turned off in between. The former method may produce smoother anæsthesia.

During cyclopropane anæsthesia look for the signs of *too light* anæsthesia or *too deep* anæsthesia and make adjustments accordingly. Remember that deep anæsthesia in the absence of I.P.P.V. is associated with respiratory depression and carbon dioxide retention.

Signs of anæsthesia being *too light* :—

1. Obvious response to surgical stimulation. Movements, laryngospasm, etc.
2. Inadequate muscular relaxation.

Signs which may indicate that anæsthesia is *too deep*:—

1. Severe bradycardia (below 50 per min.).
2. Hypotension unrelated to surgery or hæmorrhage.
3. Ventricular ectopic beats.

Other factors which suggest that the level of cyclopropane anæsthesia should be reduced :—

1. Time.—In long operations, as the patient becomes fully saturated with cyclopropane, less additional cyclopropane need be given.
2. Shock.—In shock, patients need less total amounts of any anæsthetic. In long operations exhausting the patient, smaller amounts of cyclopropane are necessary. If the patient's general condition begins to deteriorate, he will usually need less anæsthetic.

When administering cyclopropane always bear these facts in mind :—

1. The gas is explosive. Beware of the build-up of static electricity. Do not allow towels to drape the breathing tubes themselves. Ban the use of diathermy or cautery.

2. The agent is potent and deaths have been reported from ventricular fibrillation. Keep a careful watch on the pulse and blood-pressure and ensure a clear airway.

3. The agent is a potent respiratory depressant, and carbon dioxide retention is a factor in the development of arrhythmias. Be, therefore, prepared to assist or control respiration, or to allow anæsthesia to lighten to the point where respiration is adequate. Some anæsthetists use a little ether added to the mixture to stimulate respiration.

A build-up of carbon dioxide during operation, with a fall to normal at the end of operation when the mask is removed, may be the cause of *cyclopropane shock*. The blood-pressure may be maintained during anæsthesia due to hypercapnia and may fall quickly as the excess CO_2 is blown off.

CYCLOPROPANE AND CONTROLLED RESPIRATION.—If respirations are assisted or controlled and a state of hypo- rather than hypercapnia is maintained by hyperventilation, then many of the serious complications of cyclopropane anæsthesia are considerably minimized. Controlled respiration is indeed facilitated by the respiratory depressant action of cyclopropane.

The disadvantage of controlled respiration is that one of the physical signs of anæsthesia is lost. It is harder to tell the depth of anæsthesia. Sometimes it is difficult to obtain controlled respiration without obtaining a deeper level of anæsthesia than is necessary for the operation.

Light cyclopropane anæsthesia can be used with muscle relaxants to maintain controlled respiration and good muscular relaxation. Small doses only of tubocurarine or gallamine are required. The use of a muscle relaxant further modifies the signs of anæsthesia. But with practice and experience the necessary skill can readily be acquired. The signs of light anæsthesia (*above*) are still apparent with the small doses of muscle relaxant. The signs of too deep anæsthesia are also apparent. Between the two there is a reasonably wide margin.

USES OF CYCLOPROPANE.—Enthusiasts believe that cyclopropane is a safe drug which can be used over a wide range of operations provided precautions against the explosive risk are taken. In other centres cyclopropane is little used, due in large part to the great use of diathermy by modern surgeons, and also due to the development of many excellent non-explosive anæsthetic methods.

We can only point to various circumstances where cyclopropane may be of special interest :—

1. Cyclopropane is excreted unchanged via the lungs. Recovery is rapid and there is little metabolic upset. We do not rely on the detoxication and excretory mechanisms of the body. Cyclopropane may therefore be of value in old and ill patients particularly where these mechanisms are deranged (liver disease, uræmia).

2. *Cyclopropane for Laparotomy.*—Cyclopropane can be used to provide good muscular relaxation when used as described

7

Cyclopropane—Uses, *continued.*

    above. It may be superior to nitrous oxide and muscle relaxants in certain circumstances, e.g., when it may be undesirable to use a near saturation dose of muscle relaxant (intestinal obstruction, uræmia).

3. *Cyclopropane and Thoracotomy.*—Controlled respiration is facilitated. It can be achieved in a light plane of anæsthesia if small doses of muscle relaxants are given. Can be successfully used for lung resection and for cardiac operations. Transient arrhythmias occur during mechanical manipulations of the heart with all forms of anæsthesia, and are not serious during light cyclopropane anæsthesia. Surprisingly small amounts of cyclopropane are needed (e.g., in mitral valvotomy). Blood-pressure is usually well maintained, which may be an important factor in coronary artery perfusion and myocardial nutrition.

4. *Induction of Anæsthesia.*—Cyclopropane produces rapid induction of anæsthesia without hypoxia or hypotension. It is valuable when intravenous thiopentone may be contra-indicated (e.g., in shock, obstetrics). After a few breaths of 50 per cent cyclopropane, rapid intubation can be achieved using a short-acting muscle relaxant.

5. *Out-patient Anæsthesia.*—Smooth anæsthesia without hypoxia, but with increased incidence of post-operative nausea and vomiting. The explosive risk can be obviated by diluting the cyclopropane–oxygen mixture with an inert gas, and special types of apparatus have been described. Bourne* recommends a mixture of cyclopropane 50 per cent, nitrogen 25 per cent, oxygen 25 per cent. Hingson† recommends cyclopropane 40 per cent, oxygen 30 per cent, helium 30 per cent. Stephens‡ has developed the CON apparatus (cyclopropane 40 per cent, oxygen 30 per cent, and nitrogen 30 per cent).

The anæsthetist who is familiar with halothane now favours that agent in many of the situations where he might formerly have used cyclopropane. If carefully administered, halothane can be used with success without introducing the explosive risk. The indications for cyclopropane are therefore less strong, although it may still be preferred to halothane in that blood-pressure is less likely to fall.

Sequelæ.—Owing to the slight upset of the body chemistry, patients are usually fitter after cyclopropane than after a comparable ether anæsthesia. Similarly they are less sick. Circulatory disturbances are more frequent after this agent than after ether, e.g., tachycardia or arrhythmia persisting into the post-operative period.

    Cyclopropane Shock.—A type of circulatory collapse after the return of the patient to the ward is sometimes seen after deep anæsthesia. It is accompanied by slow pulse, unlike surgical shock.

---

* Bourne, J. G., *Nitrous Oxide in Dentistry*, 1960. London : Lloyd-Luke.
† Hingson, R. A., *J. Amer. med. Ass.*, 1958, **167**, 1077.
‡ Stephens, K. F., and Bourne, J. G., 1960, *Lancet*, **2**, 481.

Dripps* postulated that one cause might be the sudden return to normal of a blood carbon dioxide tension which had been high for some time, the supposition being that during cyclopropane anæsthesia the shallow breathing is accompanied by a raised blood carbon dioxide level which maintains the blood-pressure somewhat above normal. It is treated by intravenous fluids. After long operations under cyclopropane anæsthesia, some workers inject a blood-pressure-raising drug, e.g., methoxamine 20 mg. intramuscularly, before the patient leaves the theatre. If this theory is correct, the condition should not occur if the patient is properly ventilated during the operation.† The reasons why hypotension may occur following a period of hypercapnia are still far from clear.‡

Emergence Delirium.—A condition of muscular activity and restlessness during emergence from anæsthesia is sometimes seen, particularly in thyrotoxicosis and in young, muscular, and nervous individuals who have had a relatively minor operation. A little ether given towards the end of the operation may prevent or lessen this. The first dose of post-operative medication can be injected intramuscularly about 15 min. before the end of operation in those patients who are thought likely to suffer emergence delirium. Subemetic amounts of apomorphine (0·3 mg. repeated, intravenously), or intramuscular paraldehyde, 5 ml., have given good effects.

Contra-indications.—

1. During operations involving use of diathermy or cautery, unless circuit is really leakproof. This is a difficult achievement when controlled breathing with its increased pressure is used.
2. Some patients do not settle down well with this agent. They may show pallor early on, may develop laryngospasm, and bronchospasm, or show cardiac arrhythmias at a light plane of anæsthesia. In such cases cyclopropane should be abandoned.
3. When adrenaline is to be used. Although thousands of operations have been successfully performed in which adrenaline has been injected into patients under cyclopropane, a recent study shows that the danger is much greater than when adrenaline is injected during trichloroethylene or halothane administration.§
4. For the unskilled anæsthetist, cyclopropane is contra-indicated.
5. In very young children unless specially designed apparatus is used. Otherwise the amount of dead space will lead to carbon dioxide accumulation, while resistance to breathing may exhaust the child and produce jerky respiration. It can be given in open circuit, high flow rates not being required in small children and babies.

Safety.—Its cardiac effects make it less safe than ether. Sudden deaths have occurred, presumably due to ventricular fibrillation, not all of them in deep anæsthesia.

* Dripps, R. D., *Anasthesiology*, 1947, **8**, 15.
† Buckley, J. J., and others, *Ibid.*, 1953, **14**, 3.
‡ Price, H. L., *Ibid.*, 1960, **21**, 652.
§ Matteo, R. S., Katz, R. L., and Papper, E. M., *Ibid.*, 1963, **24**, 327.

Note for Beginners.—First become familiar with the closed circuit, using ether. Then commence the use of cyclopropane on minor cases with only atropine as premedication. For abdominal cases always have the patient intubated so that when respiratory depression occurs, interchange of gases can be carried out without the worry of having to maintain a difficult airway. Beware of tachycardia over 140 per minute.

ETHYLENE [C_2H_4]

This is rarely used in the United Kingdom to-day, because its advantages over nitrous oxide are very slight, while its explosibility is great. Discovered by Johannes Ingenhousz in 1779, or by Becher in the seventeenth century. May have been given as early as 1849 by Nunnelly of Leeds.

Anæsthetic properties first noticed by Hermann in 1864. Crocker and Knight (1908), the botanists, proved that ethylene contained in illuminating gas would prevent carnation buds from opening. This work was taken up by A. B. Luckhardt and J. B. Carter of Chicago in 1923,* and by W. Easson Brown of Toronto in 1923,† and they introduced it into clinical medicine, along with Isabella Herb who independently employed it in the Presbyterian Hospital, Chicago, in March, 1923.‡

Manufacture.—
1. Dehydration of ethyl alcohol by sulphuric or phosphoric acid.
2. Cracking of natural gas by heat.
3. Passing ethyl alcohol and superheated steam over a catalyst such as aluminium oxide.

Physical Properties.—A colourless non-irritating gas of unpleasant odour. Specific gravity 0·97, so it is lighter than air. Molecular weight 28·03. Boiling-point −103° C. Liquefies at 10° C. under pressure of 60 atmospheres. Oil/water solubility ratio 14·4. Flammable and explosive with certain proportions of air, oxygen, and nitrous oxide. Explosive range 2 per cent to 28 per cent with air; 2 per cent to 80 per cent with oxygen.
Eliminated from the lungs unchanged, the greater part in two minutes. Not altered by soda-lime.
Analgesia requires from 20 per cent to 35 per cent. Anæsthesia, from 80 per cent to 90 per cent.

Pharmacology.—Ethylene has almost no effect on the body's metabolism, other than causing a slight rise in blood-sugar and an inhibition of bile-acid secretion.

Induction.—More rapid than with nitrous oxide : no stimulation of respiration. Mucous and salivary secretions not increased.

Maintenance.—Ethylene is more powerful than nitrous oxide, because of its higher oil/water solubility ratio. It is less powerful than

---

* Luckhardt, A. B., and Carter, J. B., *J. Amer. med. Ass.*, 1923, **80**, 1440.
† Brown, W. E., *Canad. med. Ass. J.*, 1923, **13**, 210.
‡ Herb, I., *Curr. Res. Anesth.*, 1923, **2**, 230.

cyclopropane and ether. Anæsthesia differs from that due to nitrous oxide in that :—

    a. Muscular relaxation is greater.

    b. More oxygen can be used, so that cyanosis does not play such a part.

    c. Breathing is quieter.

Anæsthesia can be carried to lower Plane 1. About 10 per cent of oxygen can be given during induction, and when patient is settled and well premedicated, up to 20 per cent oxygen will not lighten the anæsthesia.

Recovery is rapid, but post-operative nausea and vomiting are more frequent than after nitrous oxide.

It does not depress the fœtal respiratory centre, or interfere with uterine contractions.

Methods of Administration.—Can be used in the same way as nitrous oxide. If the smell is objected to, induction can be carried out with nitrous oxide, with maintenance by ethylene ; otherwise a few inspirations of ethylene are taken and then 5 per cent oxygen added and a larger percentage gradually worked up to. The closed-circuit technique, with carbon dioxide absorption, lessens the chances of explosion. As with nitrous oxide with this technique, nitrogen must be removed from the bag from time to time.

Ethylene can be supplemented with ether, cyclopropane, or thiopentone. Very rarely used in the U.K.

Advantages of Ethylene.—Ethylene offers the same advantages as nitrous oxide—non-toxicity, rapid induction, and recovery, with the additional ones of producing greater muscular relaxation with less risk of hypoxia.

Disadvantages.—Its explosiveness. It slightly increases capillary oozing when compared with nitrous oxide. Unpleasant odour, which may upset theatre staff.

RARE GASES

Xenon [Xe].—First used in anæsthesia by Cullen and Gross in 1951.[*] Has a potency roughly equivalent to that of ethylene. Causes no respiratory depression and no cardiac arrhythmia. Biochemical change is not marked. Different electro-encephalographic changes are seen with xenon than with other inhalation agents.[†] Deep anæsthesia results from the inhalation of xenon at elevated pressures, and hypoxia is not seen if the partial pressure of oxygen in the respired atmosphere is maintained at 200 mm. Hg. The amount of xenon in the arterial blood is directly proportional to the partial pressure of the gas in the inspired atmosphere. It should be given in a 20–80 per cent mixture and is non-flammable.[‡]

[*] Cullen, S. C., and Gross, E. G., *Science*, 1951, **113**, 580 ; and Pittinger, C. B., Movers, J., Cullen, S. C., Featherstone, R., and Gross, E. G., *Anesthesiology*, 1953, **14**, 10.
[†] Morris, L. E., and others, *Ibid.*, 1955, **16**, 312.
[‡] Fink, B. R., *Ibid.*, 1955, **16**, 29.

Xenon, *continued.*

Radioactive xenon has been used in studies of cerebral blood-flow during anæsthesia.* Xenon has been used at elevated pressures in animal studies of the general theory of anæsthesia.†

Other Gases.—Argon is reported to have mild anæsthetic properties, as also is sulphur hexafluoride.‡ Teflurane (1,1,1,2-tetrafluoro-2-bromoethane) is a non-flammable gas which has anæsthetic properties and has been used in the human subject.§ Cardiac arrhythmias are said to occur.

CHAPTER VII

VOLATILE ANÆSTHETIC AGENTS

ETHER [$CH_3.CH_2—O—CH_2—CH_3$]

Prepared originally in 1540 by Valerius Cordus, who called it sweet oil of vitriol. Used clinically for anæsthesia by W. E. Clarke of Rochester, N.Y., and Crawford Long (1815–1893) of Jefferson, Georgia, in 1842, but they did not publish their results. Introduced to the profession by W. T. G. Morton, of Boston (1819–1868), on Oct. 16, 1846. The first account of its pharmacological and clinical properties appeared in John Snow's book *On the Inhalation of Ether Vapour*, published in 1847. It did not attain its wide popularity in Britain until B. Joy Jeffries came from the U.S., with the American towel cone method of forcible induction, in 1872. Two years later Clover introduced his gas–ether sequence. Before this time, chloroform had been used almost as a routine. 'Open ether' was reintroduced by Prince in America in 1895,‖ and popularized in the U.K. by Robert Lawson Tait (1845–1899), the well-known Birmingham surgeon and gynæcologist, former assistant to J. Y. Simpson. It is still the safest all-purpose anæsthetic. "I hold it therefore to be almost impossible that a death from this agent [ether] can occur in the hands of a medical man who is applying it with ordinary intelligence and attention." (John Snow, *On Chloroform and Other Anæsthetics*, 1858.)

Manufacture.—By heating together concentrated sulphuric acid and ethyl alcohol (below 130° C.), which thereby becomes dehydrated, according to the formula :—

$$C_2H_5OH + H_2SO_4 \rightarrow C_2H_5HSO_4 + H_2O$$
$$C_2H_5HSO_4 + C_2H_5OH \rightarrow H_2SO_4 + C_2H_5OC_2H_5$$

The concentrated sulphuric acid is mixed with 95 per cent alcohol and heated to 130° C. in a still, and alcohol vapour passed continuously into the mixture. The ensuing vapour, a mixture of ether, alcohol, and water, is scrubbed with sodium hydroxide

* Slack, W. K., and Walther, W. N., *Lancet*, 1963, **1**, 1082.
† Domino, E. F., and others, *Anesthesiology*, 1964, **25**, 43.
‡ Virtue, R. W., and Weaver, R. H., *Ibid.*, 1952, **13**, 605.
§ Artusio, J. F., and Van Poznak, A., *Fed. Proc.*, 1961, **20**, 312.
‖ Prince, L. H., *Chicago Med. Rec.*, 1897, **17**, 232.

Anaesthetic	Molecular Weight	Boiling-point (°C.)	Vapour Pressure at 20° C.	Liquid Density	Oil/Water Solubility	Limits of Flammability (Per Cent) a = in air; b = in O_2	Vapour Concentration for Anaesthesia (vol./per cent)	Minimal Alveolar Concentration for Anaesthesia (vol./per cent)	Blood Concentration for Anaesthesia (mg./per cent)
Diethyl Ether $\begin{matrix} C_2H_5 \\ C_2H_5 \end{matrix}\Big\}O$	74	35	442	0·7	3·2	a. 1·85–36·5 b. 2–82	3–20	3·04	50–150
Divinyl Ether $\begin{matrix} C_2H_3 \\ C_2H_3 \end{matrix}\Big\}O$	70	28·3	553	0·7	41·3	a. 1·7–27 b. 1·8–85	4	—	30–40
Cyclopropane C_3H_6	42	−34	—	—	39	a. 2·4–10·3 b. 2·4	7–23	17·5	2·5–17
Trichloroethylene C_2HCl_3	131	87·5	60	1·47	400	a. non-flammable b. 10–64	0·2–2	—	6–12
Chloroform $CHCl_3$	119	61	160	1·49	100	Non-flammable	0·5–2	—	25–70
Ethyl Chloride C_2H_5Cl	64·5	12·2	—	0·9	—	a. 4–14; b. 4–67	3–4·5	—	20–30
Ethyl-Vinyl Ether $\begin{matrix} C_2H_5 \\ C_2H_3 \end{matrix}\Big\}O$	72	35·8	428	0·76	45	a. 2·1 (lower limit)	4	—	20–30
Nitrous Oxide N_2O	44	−89	—	1·2	2·2	Non-flammable	50–80	188	23–30 (vol./per cent)
Halothane $CF_3CHClBr$	197	50	243	1·86	330	Non-flammable	0·5–2	0·87	4–35
Fluroxene $CF_3CH_2{-}O{-}CH{=}CH_2$	126	42	—	1·13	94	a. 4·2; b. 4	3–8	6·0	17–38
Methoxyflurane $CHCl_2{\cdot}CF_2{\cdot}OCH_3$	165	104·8	23	1·42	400	Non-flammable	Up to 4	0·230	—

Ether—Manufacture, *continued.*

to remove the sulphur dioxide and passed through a fractionating column from the top of which ether and alcohol come off as vapour.   This is treated with alkaline permanganate, dried over calcium chloride, and distilled.

Physical Properties.—Colourless volatile liquid of molecular weight 74, and specific gravity of 0·719. Boiling-point 35° C.; saturated vapour pressure at 20° C. is 442 mm. Hg; specific gravity of vapour 2·6 (i.e., it is two-and-a-half times heavier than air). Oil/water solubility ratio 3·2. Minimal alveolar concentration for anæsthesia 3·04. Ether vapour is inflammable in air between 1·83 per cent and 36·5 per cent. Explosive in oxygen between 2 per cent and 82 per cent.

Chemical Properties.—Relatively inert.   May contain acetaldehyde and ether peroxide as impurities, due to decomposition, which is favoured by air, light, and heat and retarded by copper, iron, mercury, diphenylamine, and hydroquinone.   Thus ether should be stored in dark cool places.   Peroxides are probably the first impurities to develop in ether.   They form within 6 months and persist for a year or more.   Old ether contains less peroxides because aldehydes are then being formed.   The greater the peroxide content, the less potent is the ether as an anæsthetic. Peroxides shown to be present if a yellow colour develops on addition of potassium iodide. (Shake 10 ml. ether with 10 per cent neutral potassium iodide ; allow mixture to remain in corked container in dark for 30 min. ; yellow colour in ether layer indicates liberation of iodine by peroxides.) Aldehydes in ether will cause Nessler's solution to turn turbid or yellow. (20 ml. of ether shaken with 3 ml. of reagent ; two layers allowed to form ; yellow colour in aqueous layer indicates presence of aldehydes.)
It is unaltered in the body, 85 per cent to 90 per cent being eliminated by the lungs.   The rate of elimination depends on the tidal exchange and blood-flow and can be expedited by hyperventilation.

Pharmacology.—

CIRCULATORY SYSTEM.—Heart-rate is increased at first due to : (1) Adrenaline liberated ; (2) Sympathetic stimulation ; and (3) Vagal depression.   Later, the heart-rate is relatively unchanged.   A light plane of anæsthesia causes vasoconstriction and a deep one vasodilatation, both effects on the vasomotor centre.   Return of consciousness causes an increase of tone to a level greater than the original tone—hence the pallor.

BLOOD-PRESSURE.—If level of anæsthesia is below Plane 2, a fall takes place after the first half-hour and is progressive, due to depression of smooth muscle in vessel walls ; depression of skeletal muscle and consequent lack of support to circulation, reduced cardiac output, and depression of the vasomotor centre.   There is peripheral vasodilatation, especially of face and head : the effect of this on the meningeal and cerebral vessels is to raise the cerebrospinal fluid pressure.   In deeper planes the vasomotor centre is paralysed so that peripheral vasodilatation is another cause of reduced blood-pressure.

A functioning sympathetic nervous system is essential for the maintenance of blood-pressure at normal levels during ether anæsthesia.* Ether normally produces an increase in sympatho-adrenal activity.† This may be abolished by high spinal or extradural block or by ganglionic blockade.

The cardiac output is increased at light planes, decreased at deep planes of anæsthesia. To produce cardiac standstill the ether concentration must be thrice that required to produce paralysis of the respiratory centre. This is in marked contrast to chloroform, which is twenty-five times more toxic to the heart than ether.

Other work‡ would tend, conversely, to show that cardiac dilatation is obtained even with subanæsthetic levels of blood-ether, increasing progressively as the level of blood-ether rises. Clinically, however, experience would tend to regard these changes as relatively harmless.

Arrhythmias are rare. Adrenaline is relatively safe with ether.

The blood shows a reduction in plasma volume and an increase in viscosity due to contraction of the spleen (sympathetic effect) causing an increase in circulating red cells and hæmoglobin. The white-cell count is also increased, the polymorphs by as much as 200–300 per cent, the increase lasting several days.

RESPIRATORY SYSTEM.—Respiratory movements first increase due to mildly stimulating effects of ether vapour on the tracheobronchial mucosa and stimulation of the respiratory centre. This effect may be masked when a barbiturate or opiate has been given. They later decrease as anæsthesia deepens, but do not become inadequate until Stage III, Plane 4. Respiratory rate increases, while amplitude decreases, as anæsthesia deepens, and the respiratory rate may be greater than thirty a minute during maintenance. In light surgical anæsthesia with ether, the respiratory centre continues to respond to carbon dioxide and the blood tension of this gas remains within fairly normal limits. This is not so in deep planes. Salivary, but not bronchial, secretions are increased, while bronchial muscles are relaxed. Bronchial and upper respiratory cilia not inhibited by ether vapour. Vapour is irritating, producing cough and laryngeal spasm and, perhaps, reflex apnœa, if introduced too rapidly. Hence induction of anæsthesia should be gradual, starting with a low ether tension. The Hering-Breuer reflex is depressed in Stage III, Plane 2, but in Plane 1 the reflex inhibition of inspiration on increasing intrabronchial pressure lasts five to ten seconds. Useful in patients with tendency to bronchospasm and emphysema. Possible explanations§ of the stimulating effect of ether on respiration include: (1) Direct stimulation of respiratory centre, (2) stimulation of receptors in the lower respiratory tract, (3) stimulation of pulmonary

* McAlister, F. F., and Root, W. S., *Amer. J. Physiol.*, 1941, **133**, 70.
† McArdle, L., Black, G. W., and Unni, V. K. N., *Anæsthesia*, 1968, **23**, 203.
‡ Fisher, C. W., Bennett, L. L., and Allahwala, A., *Anesthesiology*, 1951, **12**, 1.
§ Dripps, R. D., and Severinghaus, J. W., *Physiol. Rev.*, 1955, **35**, 741.

Ether—Pharmacology, *continued.*

stretch receptors (similar to effect of trichloroethylene), (4) stimulation of extrapulmonary receptors (muscles and joints), (5) mobilization of adrenaline, (6) development of metabolic acidosis.

CENTRAL NERVOUS SYSTEM.—Induces analgesia, followed by excitement and then anæsthesia. Medullary depression is late and precedes serious cardiac depression. Meningeal and cerebral vessels dilate—an undesirable state in neurosurgery. Pressure of cerebrospinal fluid rises.

THE SYMPATHETIC NERVOUS SYSTEM.—Central stimulation, resulting in increase of blood catecholamines which causes : (1) Increase of heart-rate. (2) Increased production of glycogen and a raised blood-sugar level. (3) Contraction of spleen. (4) Dilatation of the gut and inhibition of its movements. (5) Bronchial dilatation. (6) Dilatation of coronary arteries. (7) Dilatation of pupils.

THE PARASYMPATHETIC SYSTEM.—Central depression.

ALIMENTARY SYSTEM.—Nausea and vomiting occur in more than 50 per cent of patients after ether anæsthesia. However, after use in minimal concentrations (2–3 per cent) in air with muscle relaxants for major surgery, no significant difference was found in the incidence of post-operative vomiting compared with other methods.* Salivary glands are stimulated during induction and depressed later.

Gastro-intestinal atony is produced in deep anæsthesia and post-operatively is more marked in the small than in the large bowel. This is due to stimulation of sympathetic nerves and atony of plain muscle. Liver function decreased, but restored to normal within twenty-four hours. Ether depresses the secretion of bile and bile-salts.

THE URINARY SYSTEM.—Urinary flow is diminished because of reduction in plasma volume and renal vascular constriction, a neurogenic effect, which soon passes off when anæsthesia is stopped.

In normal kidneys there is slight reduction of renal function, and this is greatly increased in cases of nephritis, and is not mediated through the posterior part of the pituitary. Both ether and cyclopropane cause renal vascular constriction.

THE PREGNANT UTERUS.—Movements inhibited, so that in deep anæsthesia relaxation is good. Ether passes the placental barrier and soon reaches the same concentration in fœtal blood as in maternal. The oxygen-carrying capacity of the fœtal blood is not altered.

METABOLISM.—Reduction in plasma bicarbonate and pH of blood and increase in blood carbon dioxide in deep planes. The explanation is probably that in deep ether anæsthesia there is overall depression of the respiratory centre which allows increase in alveolar and hence blood carbon dioxide, and this further depresses the respiratory centre. The importance of adequate ventilation follows, manually assisted if necessary. Alterations in acid-base equilibrium are usually due to alterations in

* Holmes, C. McK., *Anæsthesia*, 1965, **20**, 199.

ventilation. Ketone bodies may appear and may be excreted in the urine. Metabolic acidosis is likely to occur in infants, or when disease causes depressed lactic acid metabolism (cirrhosis of the liver, Cushing's disease).* Hyperglycæmia is common and blood-sugar levels may be increased two- or threefold. One hour of surgical ether anæsthesia lowers the liver glycogen 50 per cent. It is due to stimulation, arising from the midbrain, via sympathetic nerves to adrenal glands, causing mobilization of glycogen through extra secretion of adrenaline. If nerves to adrenals are paralysed no hyperglycæmia is produced by ether. Barbiturate (pentobarbitone) premedication inhibits this hyperglycæmia ; morphine does not.

After long periods of ether anæsthesia, there is no microscopic change in the liver.

OTHER EFFECTS.—Body temperature is reduced owing to depression of heat-regulating centre and decreased metabolism. The intra-ocular tension is increased. Plasma noradrenaline and adrenaline raised.

The spleen is decreased in size up to 50 per cent—another effect of sympathetic stimulation : this action is opposed by barbiturates.

A tremor, chiefly affecting the legs, is sometimes seen in light ether anæsthesia (ether clonus). Passive stretching of the quadriceps extensors, together with deeper anæsthesia, will usually abolish these movements.

Advantages of Ether.—
1. It is relatively non-toxic and would appear to upset the patient clinically less than biochemical investigation would suggest.
2. It will produce excellent relaxation without undue respiratory depression.
3. Respiratory depression is not accompanied by serious cardiac damage—in the absence of hypoxia. Artificial respiration will usually overcome the effects of temporary overdosage.
4. Thus ether is a very safe anæsthetic. For the unskilled anæsthetist dealing with the unfit patient it has a lot to commend it.

Light Ether Analgesia.—The advantages of light ether narcosis have been pointed out by Artusio,† who separated the first stage into three planes, in the deepest of which he claims to produce true analgesia with a fully conscious and co-operative patient. The technique is recommended by its originator for cardiac surgery.

Disadvantages of Ether.—
1. Its tendency to cause mucus secretion from the upper airway.
2. Its tendency to upset the body chemistry.
3. Its tendency to cause albuminuria.
4. Its tendency to explode when in contact with sparks, flames, and hot surfaces in the presence of oxygen or nitrous oxide.

The concentration of ether in the blood ranges from 100 to 170 mg. per cent, from light anæsthesia to respiratory failure.

---

* Bunker, J. P., *Anesthesiology*, 1962, **23**, 107.
† Artusio, J. F., *J. Pharmacol.*, 1954, **111**, 343; and *J. Amer. med. Ass.*, 1955, **157**, 33.

Disadvantages of Ether, *continued.*

The acoustic gas analyser (Ridley and others, *Anesthesiology*, 1951, **12**, 276) shows that the inspiratory ether concentration necessary for laparotomy ranges from 6·1 to 13·7 vols. per cent.

Light anæsthesia can be maintained by 3 to 6 per cent (25–50 mm. Hg partial pressure) in inspired mixture.

Ether Convulsions.—These have been reported since 1926. The classic case is the feverish child with a perforated appendix, on a hot day, who receives atropine premedication and ether anæsthesia, with the surgeon continually requesting more relaxation. They are not due exclusively to ether and may occur during any inhalation anæsthetic. Cause not understood, many factors having been held responsible. Examples : overdosage of ether ; impurities in ether ; excessive temperature of the patient due either to his own illness or to the warmth and humidity of the operating theatre ; carbon dioxide excess ; carbon dioxide lack ; sepsis ; calcium deficiency ; cerebral congestion ; atropine excess ; a specific streptococcus producing a neurotoxin, situated in the nasopharynx. Many of the convulsions occur in children and young adults. Death may follow from anoxia.

It has recently been shown by electro-encephalography that patients who get convulsions are of the convulsion-prone type. Some non-specific factor associated with the anæsthesia or operation acts as a trigger, setting off the convulsions. The triad of depth of ether anæsthesia, hyperthermia, and hypercapnia would seem to be the chief causes, operating on a convulsion-prone nervous system. Experimentally, deep ether anæsthesia together with hyperthermia has been used to produce convulsions.*

Convulsions during anæsthesia may commence as occasional twitching of the muscles of the head and neck or limbs. These may give place to general epileptiform, clonic spasms, which soon result in deficient tidal exchange from inadequacy of the respiratory muscles. Permanent cerebral damage has been reported in cases recovering from convulsions.

Convulsions give rise to :—

　1. Hypoxia due to spasm of laryngeal and chest wall muscles.
　2. Exhaustion due to the muscular effort involved.
　3. Hyperpyrexia due to the muscular work done. Hyperpyrexia may be itself an aetiological factor of convulsions so that a vicious circle may be set up.

TREATMENT.—

　1. Relieve hypoxia. Stop administration of ether and give oxygen.
　2. Abolish convulsive movements :—
　　a. By use of a muscle relaxant, e.g., suxamethonium. This paralyses the muscles and prevents convulsions, though it does not affect the cortical discharge directly. Ventilation must then be controlled, if necessary with endotracheal intubation. If veins are inaccessible, suxamethonium may be given intramuscularly, with or without hyaluronidase.

---

* Owen, G., and others, *Anesthesiology*, 1957, **18**, 583.

    b. By intravenous injection of thiopentone, 50–100 mg. ; may need to be repeated. Disadvantage is that it causes depression of the central nervous system in a patient who is already deeply anæsthetized.

3. Prevent or treat hyperpyrexia. Remove unnecessary coverings. Use cold sponging and a fan, and measure the rectal temperature frequently.

4. Raise the head if venous congestion of the brain is suspected. Treatment should be prepared for on the first appearance of muscular twitching.

PREVENTION.—The possibility of convulsions must be borne in mind when ether is being given to patients who are hot. Feverish children should receive little or no atropine or hyoscine and are often better anæsthetized with an intravenous barbiturate, a relaxant, and gas and oxygen. The child should be kept as cool as possible during operation, with minimal covering. Macintosh sheets should not be used. The operating room should also be kept cool and air conditioning is recommended for new theatre suites.*

DIVINYL ETHER [$(C_2H_3)_2O$]

Known also as divinyl oxide. Proprietary names : vinesthene in Britain, vinethene in the U.S.A. Originally prepared by Semmler in 1887 ; anæsthetic properties discovered by Leake and Chen, in 1930,[†] in an effort to combine the advantages of diethyl ether and ethylene. Used clinically by Gelfen and Bell of the University of Alberta in 1932.[‡]

Manufacture.—Fusion of β β′-dichlor-ether with molten potassium hydroxide using ammonia as a catalyst.

Physical Properties.—A clear fluid with non-irritating odour. Molecular weight 70. Specific gravity of liquid 0·77. Boiling-point 28·3° C. Saturated vapour pressure at 20° C. is 553 mm. Hg. Specific gravity of vapour 2·2. Extremely volatile. Oil/water solubility ratio 41·3. Explosive with air between 1·7 per cent and 27 per cent, with oxygen between 1·85 per cent and 85 per cent, and with nitrous oxide between 1·4 per cent and 24·8 per cent.

Chemical Properties.—Very unstable. Decomposed by air, light, and heat, with formation of formaldehyde, acetaldehyde, formic acid, acetic acid, and complex peroxides. Stored in tightly stoppered, coloured bottles containing 4 per cent ethyl alcohol to decrease volatility and 0·01 per cent phenyl-alpha-naphthylamine to inhibit oxidation. Put up in bottles of 25 ml. and ampoules of 5 ml. and 3 ml. Unaffected by soda-lime.

Pharmacology.—

Elimination, unchanged mostly through the lungs, rapidly. Light anæsthesia produced by 4 per cent vapour ; respiratory arrest if 10 per cent to 12 per cent is inhaled for any length of time

---

* Gray, T. C. (Ed.), *Operating Theatres and Ancillary Rooms* (Symposium, Royal College of Surgeons), 1964.

† Leake, C. D., and Chen, M. Y., *Curr. Res. Anesth.*, 1931, **10**, 1; and Leake, C. D., Knoefel, P. K., and Guedel, A. E., *J. Pharmacol.*, 1933, **47**, 5 (reprinted in *Survey of Anesthesiology*, 1965, **9**, 199).

‡ Gelfen, S., and Bell, I. R., *J. Pharmacol.*, 1933, **47**, 1.

Divinyl Ether—Pharmacology, *continued*.

after induction. Blood level of 28 mg. per cent corresponds with light anæsthesia and 70 mg. per cent produces respiratory arrest.

Rapid induction with rapid recovery. Unpleasant smell. Respiratory irritation not so marked as with ether. Nausea and vomiting after operation rare. Anæsthetic potency four times that of ether. Eyeball movements may be active in presence of good muscular relaxation. No cholinergic action : bronchodilatation the only adrenergic effect.

CIRCULATORY SYSTEM.—Slight cardiac dilatation is seen, less than that caused by ether, but more than that due to cyclopropane. The following changes have been seen : (1) Auriculoventricular nodal rhythm ; (2) Auricular flutter ; (3) Ventricular arrhythmia ; (4) Alteration in sinus rate. Supraventricular displacement of pacemaker has been reported as occurring in 60 per cent of cases. No harmful effect in anæsthetic doses.

RESPIRATORY SYSTEM.—In light anæsthesia, breathing more rapid and shallow than normal. Does not have same stimulant effect on breathing as does diethyl ether, nor does it produce the same degree of bronchodilatation. Respiratory centre paralysed before heart.

ALIMENTARY TRACT.—Motility unaltered in light, inhibited in deep anæsthesia. Salivary reaction strongly stimulated in light planes. Early relaxation of masseter muscles.

URINARY TRACT.—Kidneys not affected ; they excrete a small amount of the drug. Kidney function slightly decreased.

PREGNANT UTERUS.—Labour slowed down in deep, not in light, anæsthesia. Passes the placental barrier. During Cæsarean section, it does not produce a hard, tonically contracted uterus, and so enables suture to be easily accomplished if a classic operation is performed.

THE LIVER.*—In anæsthesia lasting more than an hour, central necrosis of liver lobules has been found. Experimentally, this is made worse by coexisting hypoxia. In patients who have died, a central lobular necrosis has been found. Divinyl ether should never be used for longer than 45 min. The body chemistry is not greatly upset.

NERVOUS SYSTEM.—Convulsions have been reported during and after its use, generally when a closed system is employed. In children, some minutes after the administration of a single dose, fits have occurred. Abnormal movements are often seen and depend on depth of anæsthesia, the greater the depth, the more frequent the incidence of abnormal movements. Oxygen usually stops them. The eye signs are not reliable in assessing the depth of anæsthesia.

Methods of Administration.—

1. THE OPEN DROP METHOD.—Useful for induction of anæsthesia, especially in children. A freshly opened bottle should be

---

* *See also* Orth, O. S., and others, *Anesthesiology*, 1940, **1**, 246; Ravdin, I. S., and others *J. Amer. med. Ass.*, 1937, **108**, 1163; Hawk, M. H., Orth, O. S., and Pohle, F. J., *Anesthesiology* 1941, **2**, 288; and Little, D. M., and Wetstone, H. J., *Ibid.*, 1964, **25**, 815.

used, and 60–80 drops a minute are sprinkled on to an open mask covered with gauze. Owing to its high volatility, an even plane of anæsthesia is difficult to maintain. Method is wasteful and costly, but useful for induction or for short operations. Can be given to children for dental extractions by sprinkling it on to gauze placed over the nose. (*Fig.* 16.)

2. GOLDMAN'S INHALER.*—Specially useful for tonsillectomies with a guillotine and dental extractions in children. For children below 5 years old a 3-ml. ampoule is used ; for those

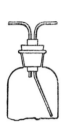

Fig. 16.—Bellamy Gardner's dropper.
(British Oxygen Gases Ltd.)

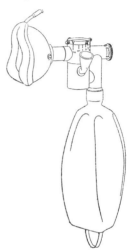

Fig. 17.—Oxford vinesthene inhaler.
(British Oxygen Gases Ltd.)

above 5, a 5-ml. ampoule. After shaking the contents of the ampoule into the inhaler, the mask is placed on the face and two exhalations are caught in the breathing bag. The mask is then firmly applied to the face and to-and-fro breathing takes place into the bag. Alternatively, oxygen or air is fed to the bag through a tap. The air breathed vaporizes the vinesthene and in about a minute regular breathing and the loss of the eyelid reflex indicate third-stage anæsthesia and the mask is removed. Anæsthesia lasts from 50 to 60 sec. If the mask is left too long, anæsthesia will lighten as the high concentration of anæsthetic in the brain diffuses into the other body tissues. Most patients can leave the theatre under their own power.

3. THE OXFORD INHALER† (*Fig.* 17).—A modification of Goldman's Inhaler. The vapour concentration can be gradually

---

* Goldman, V., *Brit. med. J.*, 1936, **2**, 122.
† Boston, F. K., and Salt, R., *Lancet*, 1940, **2**, 623.

Divinyl Ether—Methods of Administration, *continued.*

increased so that the patient does not get the full blast in his first few breaths. Should the bag empty, there is an inspiratory valve which allows air to be inhaled and exhaled into the bag.

4. SEMI-CLOSED AND CLOSED METHODS.—If vinesthene is put into the chloroform bottle of a Boyle machine it soon vaporizes away. It does less quickly if put in a Rowbotham's bottle. A drip-feed overcomes this difficulty and can be incorporated in the circuit of any standard gas machine.* An average of two drops for each inspiration is required. The drug then forms a useful supplement to nitrous oxide and oxygen, while it is useful to aid the change-over from nitrous oxide and oxygen to ether.

5. AS VINESTHENE ANÆSTHETIC MIXTURE.—This was advocated and introduced by Wesley Bourne† and consists of 25 per cent vinesthene with 75 per cent ether which approaches azeotropic proportions. The two liquids vaporize at a similar rate and the mixture combines the quick, easy induction of vinesthene with the good relaxation and absence of liver damage of ether. Useful for inducing anæsthesia in children either on an open mask or using a machine.

Advantages of Vinesthene.—
1. Quick induction and recovery.
2. Infrequency of post-operative nausea and vomiting.
3. Absence of pulmonary irritation.
4. Requires no heavy apparatus.

Disadvantages.—
1. Cannot safely be used for long operations.
2. Causes excessive salivation.
3. It is explosive.
4. Owing to its volatility it is wasteful and hard to hold.

Special Indications.—
1. For induction of anæsthesia.
2. For dental extraction and guillotine tonsillectomy in children.
3. For supplementing nitrous oxide and oxygen anæsthesia in resistant out-patients.
4. In obstetrics.

Contra-indications.—
1. Liver disease.
2. In presence of sparks or flames.
3. For long operations.

OTHER ETHERS

There are several ether compounds which have anæsthetic properties and which have been used in clinical anæsthesia. None of them has gained widespread popularity or threatened to replace diethyl ether or divinyl ether (methoxyflurane excepted).

---

* Goldman, V., *Brit. med. J.*, 1936, **2**, 122.
† Bourne, W., *Canad. med. Ass. J.*, 1935, **33**, 629.

Ethyl Vinyl Ether (vinamar).—Used by Krantz* in animals in 1947. Boiling-point 35·8° C. Explosive. Clinically resembles divinyl ether more than diethyl ether.

Methyl-n-Propyl Ether (neothyl, metopryl).—First described by Chancel in 1949. First used by Krantz† (1946). Neothyl is coloured green for identification. Explosive. Unpleasant smell. Oil/water coefficient 10. Boiling-point 39° C. Bradycardia, arrhythmias, and hypotension have been reported.‡

Fluroxene.—*See* p. 205.

Methoxyflurane.—*See* p. 206.

(*See also* Hewer, C. Langton, *Recent Advances in Anæsthesia and Analgesia*, 7th ed., 1953, Ch. VI. London : Churchill.)

ETHYL CHLORIDE [C_2H_5Cl]

Prepared by Valentine in the seventeenth century and again by Flourens in 1847, who described its anæsthetic properties, which led to investigation by Ernst von Bibra and Emil Harless. First used clinically by Heyfelder (1798–1869)§, of Erlangen, Germany, in 1848, but was used thereafter for many years only as a local analgesic. Carlson of Gothenburg, Sweden, in 1894, used it as a local spray to ease the pain of dental extraction and succeeded unexpectedly in producing general anæsthesia as the vapour was inhaled. Popularized by McCardie of Birmingham in 1901,‖ by Lotheissen, the well-known Austrian surgeon of Innsbruck, in 1896,¶ and in the United States by Ware in 1902.

Manufacture.—By action of hydrochloric acid on ethyl alcohol or ethylene.

$$HCl + C_2H_5OH \rightarrow C_2H_5Cl + H_2O \text{ or } C_2H_4 + HCl \rightarrow C_2H_5Cl$$

Physical Properties.—Clear fluid with ethereal odour. Boiling-point is below room temperature 12·5° C. Saturated vapour pressure at 20° C. is 1·3 atmospheres. Molecular weight 64; specific gravity of vapour 2·2. Five volumes of vapour dissolve in one volume of blood. Between 4 per cent and 14 per cent in air or 4 to 67 per cent in oxygen will burn with formation of irritating hydrochloric acid fumes. Oil/water solubility ratio high.

Supplied in a pure form for general anæsthesia and in a less pure form, with a smaller nozzle, for local analgesia. Eau-de-Cologne is added to some brands to disguise the odour. The pressure of ethyl chloride in its glass container is 30–40 mm. Hg above atmospheric pressure. It can be used as a gas and fed through the rotameter for cyclopropane on the anæsthetic machine, when it has little smell and only slight toxic action on the heart. It may, like trichloroethylene, cause tachypnœa.**

* Krantz, J. C., Carr, C. J., Musser, R. D., and Sauerwald, M. J., *J. Pharmacol.*, 1947, **90**, 88.
† Krantz, J. C., Evans, W. E., Carr, C. J., and Kebler, D., *Ibid.*, 1946, **86**, 138; and White, M. L. T., Shane, S. M., and Krantz, J. C., *Anesthesiology*, 1949, **7**, 663.
‡ Rees, G. J., and Gray, T. C., *Brit. J. Anæsth.*, 1950, **22**, 83.
§ Heyfelder, J. F. M., 1848. Erlangen: Heyder.
‖ McCardie, W. J., *Lancet*, 1901, **1**, 698.
¶ Lotheissen, G., *Arch. klin. Chir.*, 1898, **57**, 865.
** Cole, W. H. J., *Anæsthesia*, 1956, **11**, 156.

Ethyl Chloride—Physical Properties, *continued.*

Cannot be used in closed circuits, as it is hydrolysed by the soda-lime. Eliminated unchanged from lungs, mostly in five minutes.

Pharmacology.—Action on the central nervous system similar to that of the other volatile anæsthetics. Anæsthetic concentration is 3 to 4·5 vols. per cent in inhaled gases. Blood concentration during anæsthesia ranges from 20 to 30 mg. per cent. The safety margin is small owing to its volatility and relatively low blood/gas partition coefficient (2·0).

CARDIOVASCULAR SYSTEM.—Heart-rate first decreased, a vagus effect; later increased. The initial vagal stimulation necessitates that atropine should always be used as premedication. The heart muscle is directly depressed and ventricular fibrillation has been reported : this is extremely rare though. Adrenaline may increase myocardial irritability. No electrocardiographic changes were found in 106 patients who received an ethyl chloride induction to ether anæsthesia.*

The blood-pressure is decreased due to depression of vasomotor centre.

RESPIRATORY SYSTEM.—The respiratory centre is first stimulated, later depressed. The stage of hyperpnœa is sometimes taken advantage of to pass a blind nasal tube. It fails before the heart is seriously damaged. Only slightly irritating to mucous membranes, but laryngeal spasm not uncommon if drug is administered clumsily. Laryngeal spasm does not occur, however, during attempts at blind intubation.

MUSCULAR SYSTEM.—Masseters are liable to go into spasm, an effect which can be overcome by use of the nasopharyngeal airway. Other muscles may show twitching. Convulsions are often seen if the administration is prolonged.

ALIMENTARY SYSTEM.—Nausea and vomiting are frequent after anæsthesia.

Signs of Anæsthesia.—Induction may be stormy, but gives way in a matter of seconds to the regular breathing and muscular relaxation of surgical anæsthesia. Breathing is deeper than normal and becomes stertorous before overdosage causes it to become progressively shallower. If mask is removed after a few stertorous respirations when amplitude of breathing is maximal, about one minute of anæsthesia will result, followed by a shorter period of analgesia ; or blind nasal intubation can usually be performed, especially in children : should the attempt be unsuccessful, more ethyl chloride can be given and the manœuvre repeated. Occasionally, as after heavy premedication, this respiratory stimulation is not seen. After removal of the mask the patient will become a little deeper owing to diffusion into the blood of the vapour still in the air passages and lungs, and respiratory arrest has been known to occur even 60–90 seconds after removal of mask. A clear airway is most important, and every breath should be heard, seen, or felt by the anæsthetist. Apnœa from overdosage must

---

be overcome by artificial respiration. Peripheral vasodilatation usually produces flushing of the face. If this is replaced by pallor, anæsthesia may need to be lightened : it is a sign demanding extra caution. If in doubt as to depth of anæsthesia, regard the patient as deep until the contrary is proved.

Methods of Administration.—A prop or mouth gag should always be placed between teeth to facilitate the management of masseter spasm should it arise. The patient should inhale ethyl chloride through the mouth and not through the nose. In this way its unpleasant smell is not noticed, nor are its mildly irritating effects on the nose.

1. OPEN DROP METHOD.—The drug is sprayed on to a gauze-covered mask gradually, but as quickly as it is tolerated. With children, the mask can be held some distance from the face by the child itself. As vapour concentration increases, the mask is progressively moved nearer the face until unconsciousness is produced. The amounts used vary between 3 ml. and 20 ml., and vapour strength under mask should be 3·5 per cent to 5 per cent.

2. CLOSED METHOD.—The Goldman or Oxford vinesthene inhalers can be used. The amount of ethyl chloride sprayed into the apparatus varies between 2 ml. and 6 ml. and depends on the type of patient and length of anæsthesia required. If mask is kept on face after period of maximum respiratory amplitude is reached, the level of anæsthesia may become either too deep or too light. The open or closed method is often used to induce anæsthesia which is to be maintained with ether, the art being to carry the patient from deep ethyl chloride anæsthesia to ether anæsthesia without an intervening period of struggling and interruption of breathing. When the open method is employed, one mask should be used for ethyl chloride and a fresh one if ether is to follow.

3. AS SUPPLEMENT TO GAS–OXYGEN ANÆSTHESIA.—A few ml. can be introduced into the corrugated tubing of a continuous-flow or intermittent-flow gas machine, to augment the effects of nitrous oxide and oxygen. One plan is to place the ethyl chloride bottle in the breathing bag, manipulating its trigger through the rubber from outside.

In resistant or nervous patients having dental extractions under nasal gas–oxygen anæsthesia, mouth breathing can be used to get ethyl chloride into the lungs by spraying it on to a towel held over the mouth, or on to the mouth pad inside the mouth. With deepening anæsthesia nasal inhalation of the gas and oxygen proceeds, but hypoxia must be avoided.

4. FOR ANALGESIA.—Ethyl chloride has some use in the production of general analgesia in dental surgery. A special apparatus has been designed for its use.

As a local analgesic, ethyl chloride leaves a lot to be desired, but is useful before the extraction of loose deciduous teeth in children, if sprayed on to the gum.

Treatment of Collapse.—If this occurs in a young child suspend child by its feet and withdraw tongue while an assistant manually

Ethyl Chloride—Treatment of Collapse, continued.

compresses the chest. Sharp slapping of the precordium with a moist towel may stimulate the heart and respiration. If this does not rapidly improve the picture, the child should have an airway inserted (if necessary) and the anæsthetist should inflate the lungs, either from the reservoir bag of a gas machine, or from his own lungs, via a face-mask. Time should not be wasted over endo-tracheal intubation. True cardiac arrest must be treated by cardiac compression.

Advantages of Ethyl Chloride.—
1. Portability.
2. Rapid induction and recovery.
3. Economy.
4. Will not explode, though it burns.

Disadvantages.—
1. Post-operative nausea and vomiting.
2. Extreme potency and hence potential danger.

Indications.—
1. For induction before the use of ether. Not frequently employed to-day.
2. For short operations.
3. To supplement gas–oxygen anæsthesia in sturdy adults or nervous children, e.g., in the dental chair.
4. In domiciliary work, the (minimal) intravenous thiopentone → open ethyl chloride → blind nasal intubation → open ether sequence can be very useful.
5. To facilitate blind nasotracheal intubation in children. Absence of laryngeal spasm, deep breathing, and speed make this a most useful method.

CHLOROFORM [CHCl₃]

Prepared in 1831 by Justus von Leibig in Germany, by Samuel Guthrie in the U.S., and by Soubeiran in France. Jean-Baptiste Dumas described its physical and chemical properties in 1834 and gave it the name, chloroform, because of its relationship to chlorine and formic acid.* Anæsthetic properties discovered by Flourens (1794–1867) in 1847.† Used (in the form of chloric ether) at St. Bartholomew's Hospital by Holmes Coote (at the suggestion of Furnell) in the spring of 1847. Introduced to clinical practice and popularized by Simpson and his assistants, Mathews Duncan and George Keith, in Edinburgh in November, 1847, at the suggestion of David Waldie, a Liverpool chemist. Within a few months chloroform superseded ether as the most popular anæsthetic agent. John Snow gave over 4000 chloroform anæsthetics without a death. It was the favourite anæsthetic agent during the Franco-Prussian War. Following 1890, reports of liver damage appeared in the literature (Guthrie, 1894).‡ In 1911, Goodman

---

* Dumas, J.-B., *Ann. Chim. (Phys.)*, 1834, **56**, 115.
† Flourens, M. J. P., *C. R. Acad. Sci. Paris*, 1847, **24**, 340.
‡ Guthrie, L., *Lancet*, 1894, **1**, 193 and 257; and *Ibid.*, 1903, **2**, 10.

Levy showed that death due to ventricular fibrillation might occur in light anæsthesia, irrespective of a high concentration of vapour or overdosage.

See also Sykes, W. S., *Essays on the First Hundred Years of Anæsthesia*, Vols. I and II (Livingstone, 1960 and 1961); *Chloroform, A Study after One Hundred Years* (Ed. Waters, R.), 1951. Madison: University of Wisconsin Press; and Little, D. A., *Survey of Anesthesiology*, 1965, **9**, 508.

Manufacture.—By action of acetone or ethyl alcohol on bleaching powder. Commercially can be prepared by allowing hydrogen and carbon tectrachloride to react in the presence of iron :

$$CCl_4 + 2H \xrightarrow{Fe} CHCl_3 + HCl$$

Chloroform is stored in tinted bottles to prevent decomposition by light. One per cent ethyl alcohol is added to increase stability and to convert any trace of phosgene to diethyl carbonate.

Physical Properties.—Clear, sweet-smelling, heavy liquid. Molecular weight 119. Saturated vapour pressure at 20° C. is 160. Specific gravity of liquid 1·47 and of vapour 4·1. (Air = 1.) Non-flammable, but when heated with air in the presence of a cautery or open flame, phosgene ($COCl_2$) is formed. The liquid—though not the vapour—is irritating to skin and mucous membranes. Oil/water solubility ratio is 100. Boiling-point 61° C.

Chemical Properties.—Although it can be decomposed by alkalis, chloroform can be used with soda-lime. It is prepared with 1 per cent ethyl alcohol to convert any phosgene formed to diethyl carbonate.

Pharmacology.—Prolonged inhalation of 2 per cent vapour may produce respiratory arrest, but induction will require about 4 per cent. 25–40 mg. per 100 ml. blood = light anæsthesia ; 40–70 mg. per 100 ml. blood = respiratory arrest ; 20–30 mg. per 100 ml. blood may cause cardiac failure. Thus the safety margin is very slight. It is not altered in the body and is excreted mainly through the lungs. Complete desaturation takes many hours. Its use is largely given up because of tissue toxicity and action on heart. Its anæsthetic potency is ten times that of ether.

CARDIOVASCULAR SYSTEM.—Blood-pressure gradually falls and decreases with the depth of anæsthesia. The fall is due to: (*a*) Depressant effect on vasomotor centre. (*b*) Depressant effect on muscles of vessel walls. (*c*) Depressant effect on myocardium involving a reduction of its tone, a relaxation of the cardiac walls, and an impairment of its functional efficiency (MacWilliam, 1890). This may be enhanced by anoxia from respiratory depression if the vapour is given in air.

The effect on cardiac rhythm. Arrhythmia much more common than is the case with ether. Heart-block and nodal rhythm may occur. Arrhythmia is worst during induction and light anæsthesia. A light plane of anæsthesia causes vasoconstriction and a deeper one vasodilatation owing to action on the vasomotor centre, and this is reversible by lightening the plane of anæsthesia. The return of consciousness following anæsthesia is accompanied by increase in vascular tone in excess of tone prior to anæsthesia and hence pallor.

Chloroform—Pharmacology, *continued.*

Sudden cardiac standstill, occurring during light anæsthesia, may be due to either: (1) Vagal inhibition; (2) Ventricular fibrillation; or (3) Direct depression of the myocardium. Of these three, the first is the least important.

1. VAGAL INHIBITION.*—A sudden inhalation of a strong chloroform vapour may stimulate the vagus and so cause syncope, the so-called trigemino-cardiac reflex. In animals, large doses of atropine prevent this. An increase in the sensitivity of the aorticocarotid baroceptors may be the explanation of vagal inhibition in the induction stage of anæsthesia.†

2. VENTRICULAR FIBRILLATION.‡—Over half the deaths due to chloroform occur in the first few minutes of induction and are due to this cause. Waters and his colleagues think that this is rare. Deep anæsthesia protects against it. Causes are :—

   a. Irritation of the upper respiratory passages by too strong a vapour may irritate a reflex arc via the fifth nerve, brain-stem, stellate ganglion, and cardiac sympathetic nerves. Ventricular tachycardia and extrasystoles may precede the ventricular fibrillation.

   b. Adrenaline acts on the chloroform-sensitized myocardium to produce arrhythmia which may end as ventricular fibrilla-tion. Adrenaline may be autogenous—as from fear, or pain due to incision before anæsthesia is complete; or it may be exogenous, e.g., in nasal packs or along with local analgesic solutions. *Thus, adrenaline is contra-indicated during chloroform anæsthesia.*

   c. Direct effect of chloroform on heart muscle increases irrita-bility of ventricles and reduces the refractory phase of the myocardium. Depression increases with depth of anæs-thesia.

   d. An increase in the blood carbon dioxide level predisposes to ventricular fibrillation. This may easily occur in Stage II anæsthesia following apnœa and a stormy induction.

      Ventricular extrasystoles associated with chloroform anæs-thesia and raised arterial Pco_2 can be abolished by the intravenous injection of the adrenergic β-receptor antagonist, propranolol. The dosage is 0·5–1·0 mg. which can be repeated.§

Red and white blood-cells are increased in number.

Chloroform prevents the combination of hæmoglobin with oxy-gen as 65 per cent of the drug carried in the blood-stream is carried in the red cells because of their high lipoid content and chloroform's affinity for lipoids. Oxygen-carrying power of blood is reduced.

CENTRAL NERVOUS SYSTEM.—A complete and potent anæs-thetic which stimulates the sympathetic nervous system as does

---

* Embley, E. H., *Brit. med. J.*, 1902, **1**, 817, 885, 951 (reprinted in *Survey of Anesthesiology*, 1965, **9**, 511 and 634).
† Robertson, J. D., and Swan, A. A. B., *Anæsthesia*, 1957, **12**, 182.
‡ Levy, A. Goodman, *Heart*, 1913, **4**, 319; and *J. Physiol.*, 1911, **3**, 42.
§ Payne, J. P., and Senfield, R. M., *Brit. med. J.*, 1964, **1**, 603.

ether. Sub-anæsthetic concentrations have a good analgesic effect.*

RESPIRATORY SYSTEM.—The vapour does not irritate the bronchopulmonary mucosa during induction carried out with reasonable skill, while the bronchial musculature is relaxed. Salivation is not provoked. The respiratory centre is depressed and by the time that respiratory arrest occurs the circulation is so inadequate that efficient artificial respiration may fail to revive it. It is thus often difficult to know which fails first, the heart or the breathing. Muscles of respiration progressively depressed with increasing depth of anæsthesia.

ALIMENTARY SYSTEM.—Nausea and vomiting may occur after operation in 40 to 50 per cent of cases, a similar percentage to that caused by ether. The tone and movement of the bowel are inhibited during and for some time after anæsthesia.

URINARY SYSTEM.—Waters and his co-workers found that renal function, as tested by urine analysis and blood investigations such as non-protein nitrogen estimation, urea-clearance, phenol-sulphonphthalein tests, blood-sugar, and alkali-reserve estimations, is no more depressed after chloroform than after administration of other anæsthetics, provided always that hypoxia is avoided. Similarly they found that liver function was not significantly more depressed than in a comparable control series, using other anæsthetics.

PREGNANT UTERUS.—In light planes, contractions are not greatly affected, but are completely inhibited in deep anæsthesia. Chloroform easily passes through the placental barrier. It is very useful in the production of obstetrical analgesia and has a place in domiciliary obstetrics as an anæsthetic.

METABOLIC EFFECTS.—The serum bicarbonate and the pH of the blood are reduced, while acetone bodies may appear in the urine. Blood-sugar may be increased 200–300 per cent, owing to mobilization of glycogen from the liver, inhibition of insulin secretion, or direct effect on liver cells. The blood-sugar returns to normal in twenty-four hours. Non-protein nitrogen increased.

LIVER.—The function is decreased, with depletion of glycogen and diminished bile formation. Effects can still be found one week after chloroform anæsthesia. While careful work in America by Waters and his colleagues† absolves chloroform from blame in the production of liver dysfunction, a paper by Sheehan‡ tells rather a different tale. He regards the condition of the liver before anæsthesia as the important factor, and concludes : (1) If the patient is in a normal metabolic state, no liver effects are seen after a short—30-minute—chloroform anæsthetic. (2) If the patient is in normal nutritional state, a long anæsthesia or several short ones can produce definite pathological liver conditions observable histologically, but seldom causing clinical symptoms, other than slight vomiting

* Pittinger, C. B., Keasling, H. H., and Westerlund, R. L., *Anesthesiology*, 1960, **21**, 112.
† *Chloroform: A Study after One Hundred Years* (Ed. Waters, R.), 1951. Madison: University of Wisconsin Press.
‡ Sheehan, H. L., *Brit. J. Anæsth.*, 1950, **22**, 204.

Chloroform—Pharmacology, *continued.*

and perhaps jaundice. (3) If the patient has had prolonged vomiting, as after severe vomiting of pregnancy, chloroform will always cause necrosis of the central zones of the liver lobules. Clinically some of these patients will die without regaining consciousness, others recover consciousness, vomit, become jaundiced about the third day, and die a few days later. Prolonged labour and starvation may, with chloroform anæsthesia, result in this type of liver damage.

DELAYED CHLOROFORM POISONING.—First described by Caspar* in 1850. Guthrie† reported series of cases in 1894 and 1903, as did Beesly‡ in 1906. May occur from the first to the third day after anæsthesia.

The symptoms are increasing nausea and vomiting, with jaundice, prostration, and coma, and perhaps death. When recovery takes place there is no resulting permanent liver damage.

The condition is a toxic hepatitis like that produced by phosphorus poisoning. (Halothane, on the other hand, causes histo-pathological changes resembling those caused by infective hepatitis.) There is necrosis of tissue around the veins in the centre of the lobules. Death may occur on the fourth or fifth post-operative day, but if the fifth day is survived recovery is usual. In severe cases renal failure may accompany hepatic failure.

Protection is afforded by a high-carbohydrate, high-protein, and low-fat diet, prior to administration. As hypoxia makes the condition worse, it must be rigorously guarded against, and additional oxygen given. Sulphonamides may offer some protection.

Treatment consists in pushing fluids intravenously, together with plenty of carbohydrate and protein. If necessary, these are given intravenously as glucose and amino-acids respectively. Methionine may have a place in the treatment.

After one hour of chloroform anæsthesia, prothrombin formation by the liver is inhibited and oozing increases.

Methods of Administration.—Strength of vapour required for induction 2–4 per cent, for maintenance 0·2 to 1·5 per cent—average 0·6 per cent (Waters). The patient should be well stocked with carbohydrates and protein before anæsthesia. Morphine may depress respiration and mask signs of anæsthesia, so the tiro with chloroform should use it sparingly. A full dose of atropine may help to prevent vagal stimulation. Chloroform sleep must be distinguished from surgical anæsthesia. It is characterized by automatic respiration, but the eyelash reflex is present. Hypoxia must be carefully avoided, while administration of a little oxygen makes for safety during anæsthesia. Induction is helped by a trickle of carbon dioxide which keeps breathing regular and of equal volume.

---

* Caspar, J. L., *Wschr. ges. Heilk.*, 1850, **16**, 273.
† Guthrie, L., *Lancet*, 1894, **1**, 193 and 257 ; and *Ibid.*, 1903, **2**, 10.
‡ Beesly, L., *Brit. med. J.*, 1906, **1**, 1142.

Because of the fall of blood-pressure, chloroform should not be given to sitting patients. It should be administered regularly and not spasmodically, so that breath-holding followed by hyperpnœa is not produced, with its dangers of relative overdose of vapour. A relatively sudden, large increase in the concentration of vapour usually precedes cardiac depression, and inflation with oxygen will often retrieve the position. Before operation starts, depth of anæsthesia should be sufficient to prevent reflex hyperpnœa from surgical stimuli. If struggling or apnœa occurs, remove the anæsthetic temporarily so that the patient does not get a sudden lung-full of vapour when breathing is resumed.

As one of the chief dangers of chloroform is syncope during induction, a small dose of intravenous barbiturate can be used to produce unconsciousness, with chloroform used for maintenance.

1. OPEN DROP METHOD.—One drop of chloroform, weighing 20 mg., if vaporized in 500 l. of air forms a 1 per cent concentration of vapour in air. Chloroform burns of the eyes and skin must be avoided. One layer of lint on a Schimmelbusch mask

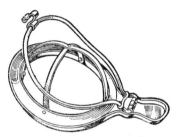

Fig. 18.—Schimmelbusch mask.

(*Fig.* 18) is satisfactory. It is held 2 in. (5 cm.) from the face and is gradually lowered. In the first half minute, one drop every three seconds is an average rate, speeding gradually to thirty drops each minute. With deep breathing or breath-holding, the mask is lifted away from the face. Pupils may be dilated and active to light in Stages I and II. Once Stage III is established, they are generally small. Subsequent dilatation with increasing depth is a sign of overdosage, together with pallor, weak pulse, and shallow breathing. Relaxation is easily produced. During anæsthesia with chloroform a close watch must always be kept on the patient's breathing, his colour, and his pulse.

2. PERCENTAGE INHALATION.—Chloroform vapour of known strength is inhaled by the patient. The method is a safe one, as sudden increases in vapour strength do not occur. Harcourt's 'draw over' inhaler (1903),* Rowling's bottle (1932),† and the E.S.O. (Epstein, Suffolk, Oxford) chloroform vaporizer and

* Harcourt, A. G. Vernon, *Brit. med. J.*, 1903, **2**, 142.
† Rowling, S. T., *Brit. J. Anæsth.*, 1932, **9**, 59.

Chlorofom—Methods of Administration, *continued*.

the Chlorotec (Cyprane Ltd.) are examples of apparatus used. (*See also* Davison, M. H. Armstrong, Essex, L., and Pask, E. A., *Anæsthesia*, 1963, **18**, 302.)

3. JUNKER'S INHALER (1867).*—A pump blows air (or oxygen) through a chloroform bubble bottle so that a small quantity of high concentration vapour is delivered to the patient, which is diluted with the air he breathes. Concentration depends on amount of chloroform in bottle and volume of air pumped. Useful in nose and throat operations. Important to see that liquid is not blown over to patient instead of air. Mennell's modification of Junker's inhaler is an improvement on the original. Now of historic interest only.

4. SEMI-CLOSED AND CLOSED METHODS.—Chloroform is placed in the vaporizing bottle. If nitrous oxide is used, hypoxia must be avoided. A very little chloroform vapour goes a long way and overdosage is easy. Rowbotham's bottle gives a fine control over concentration of vapour.

5. AS CHLOROFORM AND ETHER MIXTURE.—Harley's A.C.E. (1860) mixture was formerly much used. It consists of alcohol 1 part, chloroform 2 parts, ether 3 parts. It should be regarded as weak chloroform solution and used accordingly. As the ether stimulates respiration, it can be used for induction of anæsthesia. A mixture of C_2E_3 has had considerable vogue.

6. LINT AND MILL'S BOTTLE (St. Bartholomew's Hospital method).—Lint is folded and cut to shape. It is held away from the face while 'shakes' of chloroform are delivered from the Mill's chloroform bottle. One shake every 30 seconds is built up to 3–4 shakes every 30 seconds. (*See Modern Practice in Anæsthesia*, ed. Frankis Evans, 1949, p. 100, London: Butterworths, for fuller description.)

7. The anæsthetist who uses chloroform today is advised to avoid opiate premedication, to use an intravenous induction, to give the chloroform with pure oxygen, and to consider endotracheal intubation to ensure an adequate airway and adequate ventilation.

The conclusions of Waters and his colleagues, taken from their useful book,† are that while they do not recommend the widespread reintroduction of chloroform, they think that it still has a limited place in modern anæsthesia. They stress the following aspects of chloroform : (1) It is a most potent anæsthetic and really demands an apparatus capable of delivering increments of 0·1 per cent of vapour. Induction must be smooth, slow, and gradual, and extra oxygen should be administered throughout. (2) Its speed of action lies between ether and cyclopropane. (3) A light plane of anæsthesia is often sufficient for operation, once saturation has been established. (4) Too

---

* Junker, F. E., *Med. Times*, London, 1867, **2**, 590; and *Ibid.*, 1868, **1**, 171.
† *Chloroform: A Study after One Hundred Years* (Ed. Waters, R.), 1951. Madison: University of Wisconsin Press.

strong a vapour must not be given in the effort to speed induction. (5) Circulatory depression with increasing dosage occurs in two ways : (*a*) A sudden strong concentration of vapour may act on the heart and cause rapid hypotension with cardiac arrest ; (*b*) A gradual reduction in vasomotor tone. This may be used purposely to lower blood-pressure during operations and the effect can be reversed by lightening the anæsthesia. (6) Chloroform must only be given by anæsthetists who know what they are about. A finger must constantly be kept on the pulse, oxygen tension must not be allowed to fall, and vapour strength must not be allowed to increase unnecessarily or suddenly. The facilities for desaturation by artificial respiration must be available.

Waters and his colleagues had, it should be emphasized, 4 cases of cardiac arrest during their tests, 1 requiring cardiac massage, the other 3 responding to removal of the chloroform vapour and inflation of the lungs with oxygen.

Advantages.—
1. It is not a respiratory irritant (neither is cyclopropane, halothane, nor trichloroethylene).
2. Its vapour does not explode (nor does trichloroethylene or halothane).
3. It minimizes oozing from wounds (due to circulatory depression) and is one method of producing hypotension and wound ischæmia in such operations as radical mastectomy, extensive neck dissections, etc., a property shared with halothane.
4. It is well tolerated in obstetrics, especially in the production of analgesia. For domiciliary work it is very convenient, though no safer in the labouring mother than in any other type of patient.
5. It produces a quiet induction, free from respiratory obstruction, in acute inflammatory conditions of the neck and throat with œdema (e.g., Ludwig's angina) as does halothane.
6. Its relative non-volatility makes it useful in the tropics.
7. It can be used during bronchoscopy, œsophagoscopy, and laryngoscopy, especially in children, in whom trichloroethylene may not produce a sufficient depth of anæsthesia.
8. It can be used when diathermy is employed in the upper air-passages as can trichloroethylene and halothane.
9. It produces excellent muscular relaxation.

Disadvantages.—
1. It occasionally produces sudden cardiac failure, usually during induction, when cardiac standstill may occur with unexpected suddenness. This cannot always be avoided, even in skilled hands.
2. It may upset the body chemistry, including the liver, and should not be used in patients with diabetes, ketosis, or thyrotoxicosis.
3. It is incompatible with adrenaline, especially that produced by the patient's emotional response, e.g., the frightened, healthy young adult.
4. A respiratory or circulatory defect may cause delay in desaturation, with grave results.

Chloroform—Disadvantages, *continued.*

Many experienced anæsthetists now find few real indications for the use of chloroform but it has its loyal friends.* If it is used, the potentially dangerous induction stage should be with an intravenous barbiturate while inflation of the lungs with pure oxygen should immediately follow the first sign of circulatory collapse.

TRICHLOROETHYLENE, B.P. [CCl₂CHCl]
(Trichlorethylene, Trilene, Trimar)

First described in 1864 by E. Fischer,† since when it has been used in industry both as a fat solvent and in the dry-cleaning trade. Its poisonous properties have been long recognized (Plessner, 1916),‡ especially its power to produce analgesia in distribution of fifth cranial nerve (Oppenheim, of Berlin, 1915). On this account it has been used to relieve the pain of trigeminal neuralgia, the vapour from 1-ml. capsules being inhaled. Relief afforded is probably not a local action but part of a general analgesia. General anæsthetic effects described by Lehmann of Würzburg in 1911§ and by Dennis Jackson‖ of Cincinnati in 1933.

Striker¶ used it to anæsthetize 300 patients in 1935, but its present popularity is due to Langton Hewer, who published case reports in 1941.**

Manufacture.—Prepared by treating acetylene with chlorine, which forms tetrachlorethane and reacts with calcium hydroxide in ' lime slurry ' to form trichloroethylene.

$$C_2H_2 + 2Cl_2 \rightarrow C_2H_2Cl_4$$
$$2C_2H_2Cl_4 + Ca(OH)_2 \rightarrow 2C_2HCl_3 + CaCl_2 + 2H_2O$$

Physical Properties.—Colourless liquid with odour resembling chloroform. Molecular weight 131·4. Specific gravity 1·47. Boiling-point high 87° C., and saturated vapour pressure at 20° C. is 60 mm. Hg so volatility is low. Very soluble in lipoids, sparingly so in water; partition coefficients: oil/water 400, blood/gas 9·0, fat/blood 106·7. Will not burn or explode under clinical conditions but will ignite in concentrations above 10 per cent in oxygen or oxygen-rich mixtures (well above the concentration used in clinical practice). May be decomposed into phosgene and hydrochloric acid at temperatures above 125° C. Vapour nearly five times heavier than air, vapour density 4·35 (air = 1).

Stored in amber glass or aluminium containers, as it is decomposed by sunlight. Also decomposed by soda-lime, with formation of toxic products such as dichloracetylene. Thus the agent must not be used in closed circuits.

* *See*, e.g., Davison, M. H. Armstrong, *Brit. J. Anæsth.*, 1959, **14**, 127.
† Fischer, E., *Jena. Z. Med. Naturw.*, 1864, **1**, 123.
‡ Plessner, W., *Berl. klin. Wschr.*, 1916, **53**, 25.
§ Lehmann, K. B., *Arch. Hyg. Berl.*, 1911, **74**, 1.
‖ Jackson, D. E., *Curr. Res. Anesth.*, 1934, **13**, 198.
¶ Striker, C., Goldblatt, S., Wann, I. S., and Jackson, D. E., *Ibid.*, 1935, **14**, 68.
** Hewer, C. Langton, and Hadfield, C. F., *Brit. med. J.*, 1941, **1**, 924; and Hewer, C. Langton, *Proc. R. Soc. Med.*, 1942, **35**, 463.

For anæsthesia the proprietary form of the drug known as ' trilene ' is used. It is coloured blue for identification purposes (1 : 200,000 waxoline blue) and contains 0·01 per cent of thymol, to retard decomposition. Trichloroethylene is stable and does not seriously deteriorate with age. Trimar is another proprietary brand. Trichloroethylene may irritate the skin if rubbed on to it, e.g., before intravenous injection.

Pharmacology.—

CENTRAL NERVOUS SYSTEM.—Trichloroethylene should not be used to produce deep anæsthesia, since untoward side-effects (*see below*) are likely to develop. The stage of analgesia is well marked, so that trichloroethylene is useful for the production of analgesia (e.g., in obstetrics) without loss of consciousness. Concentration in blood of 6–12 mg. per 100 ml. is required for anæsthesia. Inhalation of 0·5 per cent leads to a blood concentration of 6–7 mg. per cent, 1 per cent inhalation to a blood concentration of 12–17 mg. per cent.[*] Convulsions have been reported, but are rare. Sometimes there is a tendency for headache afterwards.

TRICHLOROETHYLENE AND SODA-LIME.—If trichloroethylene is used in a closed circuit with soda-lime, toxic products may be formed (Morton,[†] 1943, and McAuley,[‡] 1943), the most important being dichloracetylene :—

$$C_2HCl_3 + NaOH \rightarrow C_2Cl_2 \text{ (dichloracetylene)} + NaCl + H_2O$$

This is a potent nerve poison and may produce paralysis of cranial nerves or even death. The fifth and seventh nerves are most commonly involved, but interferences with the third, fourth, sixth, tenth, and twelfth nerves have been reported. These lesions may be temporary or permanent.

This danger is much less with the brands of soda-lime now being used, which do not get so hot. The reaction to form dichloracetylene is much accelerated about 60° C. whereas present day soda-lime does not get much above 40° C. Addition of silica to soda-lime retards the reaction.

CARDIOVASCULAR SYSTEM.—Blood-pressure is not greatly altered. The main effect is on the production of arrhythmias which may go on to ventricular fibrillation and the clinical picture of cardiac arrest.

Arrhythmias are of two types :—

1. Associated with an increase of vagal tone. Some slowing of the pulse. Shift of the pacemaker towards the A.V. node. Without serious significance and often transient.

2. Premature contractions from ectopic foci, often ventricular. Extrasystoles; pulsus bigeminus (a normal beat followed by a premature contraction and a pause) ; multifocal ventricular tachycardia Barnes and Ives[§] reporting on the electrocardiographic behaviour of forty healthy patients under

[*] Clayton, J. I., and Parkhouse, J., *Brit. J. Anæsth.*, 1962, **34**, 141.
[†] Morton, H. J. V., *Brit. med. J.*, 1943, **2**, 838.
[‡] McAuley, J., *Ibid.*, 1943, **2**, 713.
[§] Barnes, C. G., and Ives, J., *Proc. R. Soc. Med.*, 1944, **37**, 528.

Trichloroethylene—Pharmacology, *continued.*

trichloroethylene anæsthesia found arrhythmias frequent, and a multifocal ventricular tachycardia in 10 per cent. However, they used no thiopentone for induction and probably pushed trichloroethylene to obtain anæsthesia. Ballantine and Jackson* using minimal concentrations to supplement nitrous oxide and oxygen after thiopentone induction in neurosurgical cases have not seen this change.

Trichloroethylene sensitizes the heart to the effects of adrenaline† and many anæsthetists believe that the two drugs should not be used in the same patient. Others believe that it is safe to use adrenaline in concentrations 1–250,000 during careful trichloroethylene anæsthesia. (A concentration of 1–500,000 adrenaline is often very effective if time is allowed for it to produce vasoconstriction.) A recent study showed that adrenaline could be safely used in a local infiltration provided that the total dose did not exceed 0·5 mg., the inhaled concentration of trichloroethylene did not exceed 0·6 per cent,‡ and that hypoventilation was avoided at all times.

A raised blood carbon dioxide tension increases the incidence of arrhythmia. This is particularly likely to occur if there is any obstruction to free respiration, or if tachypnœa is allowed.

If arrhythmias occur, they should be treated by reducing the trichloroethylene concentration, or by switching off for a time. Pethidine is useful in controlling tachypnœa and in providing an alternative analgesic supplement if arrhythmias occur.

RESPIRATORY SYSTEM.—The vapour is much less irritant than ether so that a smooth induction can be readily accomplished in most cases. A small amount of trichloroethylene vapour will often settle a patient whose pharyngeal or laryngeal reflexes are active. This is probably caused by depression of the afferent side of the reflex arc.

Tachypnœa is likely to occur. This is thought to be due to a peripheral action in the lung.§ Trichloroethylene stimulates both deflation-reflex fibres and stretch-reflex fibres, so that both expiration and inspiration are curtailed. The result is rapid shallow breathing, which is less efficient in terms of gaseous exchange than slow deeper breathing, for the same minute volume. This is because dead space takes up a greater portion of tidal volume with shallow breathing. Thus a fall in arterial oxygen saturation of 25 per cent has been found with severe tachypnœa,‖ and there is a rise in blood carbon dioxide tension, which in turn may predispose to arrhythmias.

* Ballantine, R. I. W., and Jackson, I. M., *A Practice of General Anæsthesia for Neurosurgery,* 1960. London : Churchill.
† Morris, L. E., Nottensmeyer, M. H., and White, J. M., *Anesthesiology,* 1953, **14,** 153.
‡ Matteo, R. S., Katz, R. L., and Papper, E. M., *Ibid.,* 1962, **23,** 156.
§ Whitteridge, D., and Bulbing, E., *Brit. med. Bull.,* 1946, **4,** 85.
‖ Dundee, J. W., *Brit. J. Anæsth.,* 1953, **25,** 1.

Tachypnœa occurs :—

1. In deep planes of anæsthesia, due to overdosage with trichloroethylene. Remedy—reduce the concentration or switch off.

2. In light planes of anæsthesia, due to surgical stimulation. The remedy here is not to increase the trichloroethylene concentration, but to deepen the level of ' basal narcosis ' with thiopentone or pethidine. Thiopentone is usually better where there is a marked and obvious reaction to a surgical stimulus. Pethidine is more satisfactory where there is a steady rise of respiratory rate over a period of time.

ALIMENTARY SYSTEM.—Post-operative nausea and vomiting are less common than after ether and chloroform. Salivation is not marked.

MUSCULAR SYSTEM.—Relaxation is poor. It is unwise to push the administration in an effort to obtain this.

METABOLISM.—Blood chemistry is not greatly altered. The liver is little affected.

ABSORPTION AND EXCRETION.—Trichloroethylene is administered by inhalation. Induction is relatively slow and it takes a long time for the patient to become saturated. Most of the drug is excreted, unchanged, by the lungs. Once a patient has become relatively saturated, excretion is slow and recovery from anæsthesia may take a long time. The longer the exposure to trichloroethylene, the longer the recovery time, and the sooner the vaporizer should be switched off before the end of operation.

A small amount undergoes change in the body with the formation of trichloracetic acid, which is pharmacologically inert, and which is excreted by the kidneys over a period of several days. After chronic exposure to trichloroethylene vapour (in industry) a diagnosis of trichloroethylene intoxication can be made if more than 7·5 mg. of trichloracetic acid per 100 ml. of urine is present. Recent work from Czechoslovakia* on the problem of industrial toxicity has also identified two other metabolites, monochloracetic acid, a toxic agent found in small amounts, and trichloroethanol (similar to tribromethanol in its action) in larger amounts.

SAFETY.—Several deaths due to primary cardiac failure have been reported.† It is difficult to estimate the incidence of such mishaps, but figures provided by Hewer‡ and Scragg§ suggest that, when properly used, the drug is extremely safe.

Trichloroethylene addiction, leading to psychosis, has been reported.

Methods of Administration.—Trichloroethylene is used either as a supplement to nitrous-oxide–oxygen in the production of full surgical anæsthesia at a light plane, or as an agent in its own right for the production of a state of analgesia.

* Soucek, B., and Vlachova, D., *Brit. J. industr. Med.*, 1960, **17**, 60.
† Edwards, G., Morton, H. J. V., Pack, E. A., and Wylie, W. D., *Anæsthesia*, 1956, **11**, 207.
‡ Hewer, C. Langton, *Ibid.*, 1959, **14**, 311.
§ Scragg, R. D., *Canad. Anæsth. Soc. J.*, 1958, **5**, 419.

Trichloroethylene—Methods of Administration, *continued.*

1. TRICHLOROETHYLENE AND SURGICAL ANÆSTHESIA.—
Low volatility makes open drop administration unsuitable.
Galley* has described a single dose method for children, using
an Oxford inhaler.

In most surgical operations, trichloroethylene can be used to
provide analgesia (as part of the triad of Gray). The drug is
employed in an analgesic rather than an anæsthetic concentration. It can be used in the chloroform bottle of the Boyle
machine with the Magill attachment. Or it can be put in a
Rowbotham chloroform bottle.

The standard chloroform bottle of the Boyle machine is not
likely to deliver more than 1·5 per cent vapour, provided that
gases are not bubbled through the trichloroethylene. Much less
than this is needed in practice. It should rarely be necessary to
depress the plunger, and the maintenance concentration of
vapour should be of the order of 0·5 per cent,† that is, slightly
more than can just be appreciated by smell.

Premedication with an opiate is desirable to prevent tachypnœa. It is wise to give something more than a sleep dose
of thiopentone for induction, so that a reasonable level of
' basal narcosis ' will exist and trichloroethylene will not have
to be ' pushed '. Following thiopentone, trichloroethylene
should be added gradually to nitrous oxide and oxygen. It
may be necessary to turn the lever full on (with plunger up) for
a few minutes to settle the patient, but it should then be returned
to a minimal position.

Do not expect trichloroethylene to act as more than a weak
anæsthetic agent. If there is obvious response to surgical
stimulation, it is best to deepen the level of ' basal narcosis '
with thiopentone. If respiratory rate rises, pethidine can be
given in doses of 10 mg., and this dose can be repeated so as to
' titrate ' the respirations to a satisfactory rate (20–30 per min.).

As an alternative to the use of thiopentone and pethidine the
patient can be settled with ether or halothane, and a change
then made to trichloroethylene. This may be useful in children
or in frail patients who tolerate thiopentone badly.

If the patient does not settle well on minimal trichloroethylene, and the laryngeal and cough reflexes remain active, a
small dose of muscle relaxant (e.g., tubocurarine, 5 mg.) will
often smooth the course of anæsthesia, and may actually increase
tidal volume by relaxing spasm of the respiratory muscles.

INTUBATION.—In some edentulous patients, where laryngoscopy
is easy, it is possible to intubate under nitrous-oxide–trichloroethylene. Usually it is best to give a muscle relaxant
or a supplementary dose of thiopentone‡ before intubation.

This method of administration of trichloroethylene is useful
in a wide range of surgical operations where muscular

---

* Galley, A. H., *Lancet*, 1945, **2**, 10.
† Ballantine, R. I. W., and Jackson, I. M., *A Practice of General Anæsthesia for Neuro-surgery*, 1960, London : Churchill.
‡ Ballantine, R. I. W., and Jackson, I. M., *Anæsthesia*, 1954, **9**, 4.

relaxation is not required, e.g., neurosurgery, laryngectomy, tonsillectomy, surgery of the limbs, mastectomy, etc.

2. TRICHLOROETHYLENE IN OUT-PATIENT ANÆSTHESIA. —Trichloroethylene can be used to supplement nitrous-oxide–oxygen anæsthesia in the out-patient department, e.g., in dental extractions. Addition of trichloroethylene makes the patient quiet without the need for hypoxia, and, in short operations, recovery time is little delayed.

3. TRICHLOROETHYLENE AND ANALGESIA. OBSTETRICS. —Trichloroethylene produces excellent analgesia in labour,* 0·5 per cent w/v in air being a suitable concentration for intermittent inhalation lasting several hours. In some patients drowsiness comes on after three hours, requiring reduction of vapour strength to 0·35 per cent. Trichloroethylene readily passes the placental barrier. Several methods of vaporization have been devised, among them the addition of a Rowbotham's bottle to a Minnitt gas–air machine.

Woodfield Davies's modification of Freedman's inhaler† (1943) consists of an unspillable bottle which cannot be overfilled. The patient draws air via a face-mask and corrugated tube, over trichloroethylene in the bottle. An inspiratory and an expiratory valve prevent rebreathing. It is designed to deliver about 0·6 per cent trichloroethylene vapour in air, but this is upset by environmental temperature, movement of the bottle, etc., so that the apparatus has not been accepted as safe for use by midwives working on their own.

Cyprane Inhaler : Another simple apparatus for self-administration of trichloroethylene in air.

The Tecota Mark 6 Trichloroethylene Inhaler (*see Fig.* 49, p. 626) : —A temperature-compensated inhaler which weighs, in its case, about 7 lb. It delivers either 0·5 per cent or 0·35 per cent trichloroethylene vapour in air over a range of room temperature between 55° and 95° F. Movement does not alter the vapour concentration.

Epstein, Macintosh, Oxford Inhaler‡ (Emotril) : Also for use as an auto-analgesia machine in obstetrics. It incorporates a compensating device, which for any rise in temperature reduces the amount of vapour leaving the vaporizing chamber. When patient inspires, a non-return valve opens and air enters through a variable opening into the trichloroethylene chamber and emerges mixed with vapour : another current of room air is drawn through a permanently open by-pass of fixed size and dilutes the mixture issuing from the vaporizing chamber. The size of the variable opening can be altered in accordance with the position of a pointer of a thermometer. It is also made with automatic temperature compensator for use by midwives. Normally vapour strength is 0·5 per cent, but a small disk can be rotated to make the apparatus deliver a

---

* Elam, J., *Lancet*, 1942, **2**, 309.
† Freedman, A., *Ibid.*, 1943, **2**, 696.
‡ Epstein, H. G., and Macintosh, R. R., *Brit. med. J.*, 1949, **2**, 1092.

Trichloroethylene—Methods of Administration, *continued.*

percentage of 0·35. There is a low resistance to respiration, and leaks due to an ill-fitting face-mask are of less consequence in diluting the mixture reaching the patient than in gas–air machines, owing to the greater efficiency of trichloroethylene vapour as an analgesic. (*Fig.* 19.)

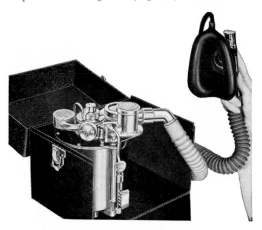

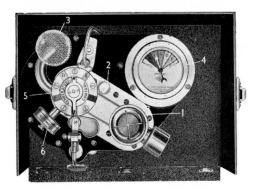

Fig. 19.—The Emotril apparatus. (Medical & Industrial Equipment Ltd.)

Machines to be used by midwives in Great Britain must fulfil strict conditions. They must deliver trichloroethylene vapour in air at 0·5 per cent and 0·35 per cent concentrations with an error of $\pm$ 20 per cent only, which must remain constant under all clinical conditions. Each machine must be individually certified and must be periodically checked. Examples of inhalers approved by the C.M.B. are the Tecota Mark 6 and the Emotril Automatic. Used under these conditions trichloroethylene vapour is as safe as gas and oxygen and more effective. Given with pethidine, labour may be prolonged, while depression of the infant's respiration may be seen.

Post-operative Analgesia.—Trichloroethylene analgesia has recently been advocated as an aid to physiotherapy.*

Advantages of Trichloroethylene.—
1. A good analgesic. Useful supplement of nitrous-oxide–oxygen.
2. Relative lack of irritation of upper respiratory tract. Smooth induction.
3. Non-flammable.
4. Does not depress cardiovascular system. Blood-pressure stable.
5. Does not depress respiration.
6. Safe, when used in minimal concentration.
7. Cheap.

Disadvantages.—
1. Tachypnœa may occur.
2. Arrhythmias may occur. Cardiac arrest has been reported, though it is extremely rare.
3. Does not provide muscular relaxation.
4. May cause post-operative nausea and vomiting.
5. Cannot be used with soda-lime.
6. Addiction has been reported.†

Uses of Trichloroethylene.—
1. To maintain light anæsthesia, as a supplement to nitrous-oxide–oxygen after thiopentone induction. For major and minor surgery, with or without an endotracheal tube, when muscular relaxation is not required.
2. To supplement nitrous-oxide–oxygen anæsthesia for short procedures in out-patients and dentistry.
3. To produce analgesia in obstetrics, to relieve post-operative pain during physiotherapy,* in various painful surgical procedures (e.g., wound dressings), and the first defæcation after hæmorrhoidectomy.
4. To avoid 'awareness' during maintenance of 'anæsthesia' with gas, oxygen, and a relaxant.

See also Ostlere, G., *Trichloroethylene Anæsthesia*, 1953, E. S. Livingstone: Edinburgh and London; review article, Atkinson, R. S., *Anesthesiology*, 1960, **21**, 67; and Dobkin, A. B., and Byles, P. H. in *Clinical Anesthesia—Halogenated Anesthetics* (Ed. Artusio, J. F.), 1963, Ch. 3. Oxford: Blackwell.

---

* Ellis, M. W., and Bryce-Smith, *Brit. med. J.*, 1965, **2**, 1412.
† *See* Leading Article, *Lancet*, 1949, **2**, 1205.

HALOTHANE
(*Fluothane*)

This is

$$F-C-C-Br$$

(2.bromo-2 chloro-1.1.1.trifluoroethane).

History.—Synthesized in the laboratories of Imperial Chemical Industries near Manchester by C. W. Suckling in 1951,[*] and studied pharmacologically by J. Raventós[†] in succeeding years. Used clinically by M. Johnstone[‡] of Manchester followed by Bryce-Smith and O'Brien[§] of Oxford. Because of its potency, its use calls for great care.

Physical Properties.—A colourless liquid volatile anæsthetic with molecular weight 197, specific gravity 1860 (ether is 713), boiling-point 50° C., saturated vapour pressure at 20° C. 241. Minimal alveolar concentration for anæsthesia 0·87 vol. per cent. Has a characteristic odour. Oil/water solubility coefficient 330. Blood/gas distribution coefficient 3·6; fat/blood 60·0; brain/blood 2·6. Decomposed by light (unless stabilized by 0·01 per cent thymol), but is stable when stored in amber-coloured bottles. Is not decomposed by soda-lime. In the presence of moisture it attacks tin and aluminium in vaporizers. Non-flammable and non-explosive when its vapour is mixed with oxygen in any concentration. May be decomposed by an open flame liberating bromine.[||]

Pharmacology.—As an anæsthetic it is four or five times as potent as diethyl ether and nearly twice as potent as chloroform. Vapour is pleasant to smell and is non-irritant. For induction of anæsthesia, 2–4 per cent vapour is necessary; for maintenance, 1–2 per cent. It is a very potent agent and has already caused several deaths from cardiac failure, probably because of relative overdosage.

CARDIOVASCULAR SYSTEM.—

BLOOD-PRESSURE falls, though not invariably. The fall is in proportion to the concentration of vapour inhaled. Hypotension is thought to be due to sympathetic blockade,[†] central vasomotor depression and direct depression of the myocardium,[¶] and depression of the smooth muscles of blood-vessels.[**] Sensitization of the baroreceptors may also result in hypotension.

Ganglionic blocking drugs must be given with extreme caution during halothane anæsthesia. Severe hypotension may follow administration of otherwise normal doses of hexamethonium, trimetaphan, tubocurarine, etc. The patient is

---

[*] Suckling, C. W., *Brit. J. Anæsth.*, 1957, **29**, 466.
[†] Raventós, J., *Brit. J. Pharmacol.*, 1956, **11**, 394.
[‡] Johnstone, M., *Brit. J. Anæsth.*, 1956, **28**, 392.
[§] Bryce-Smith, R., and O'Brien, H. D., *Brit. med. J.*, 1956, **2**, 969 ; and *Proc. R. Soc. Med.*, 1957, **50**, 193.
[||] Bullough, J., *Lancet*, 1964, **1**, 835.
[¶] Burn, J. H., and others, *Brit. med. J.*, 1957, **2**, 479.
[**] Burn, J. H., and Epstein, H. G., *Brit. J. Anæsth.*, 1959, **31**, 199.

also more subject to postural hypotension and hypotension following sudden blood-loss.

Shock.*—Halothane may protect the patient from the shock syndrome by producing vascular dilatation or ganglionic blockade. It allows a high concentration of oxygen to be given. Peripheral venous dilatation makes for easy rapid transfusion.

Hypotension during halothane anæsthesia responds to pressor drugs.

Arrhythmias.—(i) Increased myocardial excitability; ventricular extrasystoles, ventricular tachycardia, and even ventricular fibrillation. Less common than during cyclopropane anæsthesia, perhaps because halothane does not cause a rise in circulating catecholamines, and reduces the effectiveness of noradrenaline on vascular smooth muscle and on cardiac adrenergic receptors. Factors which increase the likelihood of ventricular arrhythmias include carbon dioxide retention† (though the threshold is higher than with cyclopropane‡), sensory stimulation in light anæsthesia, atropine injection,§ and the injection of adrenaline.‖ Cardiac arrest¶ (in asystole) has been reported following adrenaline infiltration during halothane anæsthesia. Other workers have used the combination without incident. Intravenous infusions of adrenaline or noradrenaline during halothane anæsthesia at rates of more than 10 μg. per min. have been found to provoke arrhythmias.** Katz and his colleagues†† recommend that adrenaline infiltration may be safely used in a dosage of 10 ml. of 1 in 100,000 concentration in a 10-min. period or 30 ml. per hour, provided ventilation is adequate. Ventricular extrasystoles can be abolished by the intravenous injection of adrenergic β-receptor antagonist, propranolol, dose 0·5–1·0 mg.‡‡ (ii) Bradycardia, which may be associated with hypotension. Atropine given intravenously may speed the pulse-rate and produce a rise in blood-pressure, but it should be given slowly as it may itself produce ventricular arrhythmias.

ALIMENTARY SYSTEM.—The secretion of saliva, mucus, and gastric juice is not stimulated, while post-operative nausea and vomiting are seldom severe. It has even been claimed that in subanæsthetic doses it has an anti-emetic effect.§§

CENTRAL NERVOUS SYSTEM.—It is a total anæsthetic like ether or chloroform, but not a good analgesic. Generalized convulsions following its use have been reported.‖‖ It increases cerebral

---

* Johnstone, M., *Brit. J. Anæsth.*, 1958, **30**, 435.
† Black, G. W., and others, *Ibid.*, 1959, **31**, 238.
‡ Price, H. L., *Ann. Surg.*, 1960, **152**, 1071.
§ Johnstone, M., and Nisbet, H., *Brit. J. Anæsth.*, 1961, **33**, 9.
‖ Millar, R. A., Gilbert, R. G. B., and Bundle, G. F., *Anæsthesia*, 1958, **13**, 164.
¶ Rosen, M., and Roe, R. B., *Brit. J. Anæsth.*, 1963, **35**, 51.
** Andersen, N., and Johansen, S. H., *Anesthesiology*, 1963, **24**, 51.
†† Katz, R. L., Matteo, R. S., and Papper, E. M., *Ibid.*, 1962, **23**, 597.
‡‡ Helliwell, J., and Potts, M. W., *Anæsthesia*, 1965, **20**, 269.
§§ Haumann, J. C. R., and Foster, P. A., *Brit. J. Anæsth.*, 1963, **35**, 114.
‖‖ Millar, T. W. P., *Anæsthesia*, 1958, **13**, 341.

Halothane—Pharmacology, *continued.*

circulation and raises the C.S.F. pressure.* It has been suggested that low concentrations of halothane might have an anti-analgesic effect,† though this has not been confirmed by other workers.‡

RESPIRATORY SYSTEM.—A respiratory depressant. Respiratory rate often increased and depth decreased, effects controllable with pethidine. Induction by halothane and air may result in arterial oxygen desaturation due to hypoventilation and assisted breathing may be necessary. The drug causes bronchodilatation and is very suitable for patients with bronchospasm, emphysema, and chronic bronchitis. Not a bronchial irritant; pharyngeal and laryngeal reflexes depressed early, and secretions not stimulated. Care must be taken that I.P.P.V. does not give rise to inadequate cardiac filling, otherwise severe hypotension may be caused. Control of respiration is facilitated by halothane.

MUSCULAR SYSTEM.—Moderate relaxation is produced by anæsthetic concentrations and the masseters are relaxed early, making laryngoscopy easy. Full abdominal relaxation is seen only with deep planes of anæsthesia.

THE LIVER.—Massive hepatic necrosis following halothane anæsthesia was reported in 1958,§ though widespread attention was not drawn to the problem until 1963.‖ Since then there have been large retrospective surveys,¶ including the National Halothane Study carried out by the American National Academy of Sciences.** The general conclusion is that the incidence of liver failure is no higher after halothane than after other anæsthetics, and there is no evidence that patients with biliary-tract disease are unduly susceptible. On general grounds it is recommended that unexplained fever and jaundice following halothane administration might be regarded as a contraindication to its subsequent use. Intensive study of a series of patients receiving halothane has likewise failed to incriminate halothane as more dangerous than other agents.††

After careful studies, no definite relationship has been found between halothane anæsthesia and post-operative liver damage. If halothane does have a toxic effect, it must be very rare. It remains a possibility that repeated halothane anæsthesia may cause a sensitivity type of hepatitis. The chance of the anæsthetist becoming sensitized may also be considered.‡‡

---

* Hunter, A. R., *Brit. med. J.,* 1963, **2**, 239; Wollman, H., and others, *Anesthesiology,* 1964, **25**, 180; Sondergard, W., *Danish med. Bull.,* 1961, **8**, 18; and Hunter, A. R., *Lancet,* 1964, **1**, 493.
† Dundee, J. W., Nicholl, R. M., and Black, G. W., *Brit. J. Anæsth.,* 1962, **34**, 158.
‡ Robson, J. G., Davenport, H. T., and Sugujama, R., *Anesthesiology,* 1965, **26**, 31.
§ Virtue, R. W., and Payne, K. W., *Ibid.,* 1958, **19**, 562.
‖ Bunker, J. P., and Blumfeld, C. M., *New Engl. J. Med.,* 1963, **268**, 531; and Brody, G. L., and Sweet, R. B., *Anesthesiology,* 1963, **24**, 29.
¶ Mushin, W. W., Rosen, M., Bowen, D. J., and Campbell, H., *Brit. med. J.,* 1964, **2**, 329; Green, K. G., and Mungarim, J. M., *Proc. R. Soc. Med.,* 1964, **57**, 311; and Pearce, C., and others, *Ned. Tijdschr. Geneest.,* 1966, **119**, 80.
** Bunker, J. P., *J. Amer. med. Ass.,* 1966, **197**, 775.
†† Dawson, B., and others, *Proc. Mayo Clin.,* 1966, **41**, 599.
‡‡ Belfren, S., Ahlgren, I., and Axelson, S., *Lancet,* 1966, **2**, 1416.

Impurities in halothane have also been implicated. Dichloro-hexafluorobutene (DCHFB) can rise to 0·03 per cent in the vaporizer, and is toxic to liver and kidneys.*

(*See also* Vickers, M. D., and Dinnick, O. P., *Anæsthesia*, 1964, **19**, 124.)

Professor Sheila Sherlock has reviewed this subject.† Damage to the liver due to drugs can be divided into three main groups:—

1. A direct toxic effect (carbon tetrachloride, phosphorus, chloro-form).
2. Hepatitis type. A sensitivity type of reaction which is not dose dependent (mono-amine oxidase inhibitors, halothane).
3. Cholestatic (obstructive) type. (Chlorpromazine and allied drugs, methyl testosterone.)

Halothane hepatitis, if it exists, produces a clinical, bio-chemical, and histological picture identical to that of infectious hepatitis.

When post-operative jaundice occurs, differentiation must be made from jaundice related to blood transfusion, shock, septic cholangitis, other drugs, and a coincidental virus hepatitis.‡

Blood-sugar is not affected, but sensitivity to insulin is in-creased. Care should be taken when halothane is administered to a diabetic patient receiving insulin lest hypoglycæmia should occur.

USE WITH MUSCLE RELAXANTS.—The myoneural effect of tubocurarine is moderately potentiated, while its somewhat weak ganglionic blocking effect is very markedly potentiated so that great care should be taken when the two are used together. The former of these effects is seen with gallamine, but as this agent has no ganglionic blocking effects, the combination of the two drugs is satisfactory and may, because of the specific effect of gallamine in paralysing the ability of the vagus to slow the heart, make it the relaxant of choice. Halothane somewhat antagonizes the effects of suxamethonium, but this is not important clinically.

TEMPERATURE.—Induction of anæsthesia with halothane is soon followed by a drop of up to 1° C. in œsophageal temperature, together with a rise of up to 4° C. in skin temperature.§ This is thought to be due to a redistribution of heat between core and peripheral tissues. Later, skin temperature may fall as peripheral vasodilatation aids heat loss. Halothane is used to aid heat loss by this mechanism during surface cooling to obtain hypothermia.

SHIVERING.—Shivering and tremor have frequently been reported during the immediate post-operative period following halothane anæsthesia. The evidence so far available indicates that post-operative shivering is not directly related to temperature falls during anæsthesia.§ It may be associated with a generalized increase in muscle tone, clonic or tonic.

* Cohen, E. N., Bellville, J. W., Budzikiewicz, H., and Williams, P. H., *Science*, 1963, **141**, 899; and Cohen, E. N., Brewer, H. W., Bellville, J. W., and Sher, R., *Anesthesiology*, 1965, **26**, 140.
† Sherlock, S., *Proc. R. Soc. Med.*, 1964, **57**, 305.
‡ Johnstone, M., *Brit. J. Anæsth.*, 1964, **36**, 718.
§ Cohen, M., *Proc. R. Soc. Med.*, 1967, **60**, 752.

Clinical Use.—

PREMEDICATION.—Atropine is usually recommended to obtain a degree of vagal block. Some anæsthetists prefer doses greater than 0·6 mg. ($\frac{1}{100}$ gr.), and prefer atropine to hyoscine as the better vagolytic agent. It is less necessary to give atropine before halothane than before other volatile agents to prevent salivary and bronchial secretions, as these are depressed by halothane. Arrhythmias may in fact be caused by atropine.[*]

Because halothane is a respiratory depressant, premedication with an opiate should be avoided unless it is intended to assist or control respiration.

HALOTHANE IN A HIGH GAS FLOW SYSTEM.—This method is wasteful of halothane, which is expensive. However, some anæsthetists think it is safer than closed or partially closed systems, since the concentration inspired by the patient is close to the concentration delivered from the machine.

Halothane can be used as a supplement to thiopentone-nitrous-oxide–oxygen. The analgesic properties are poor so that reflex activity (e.g., movement with skin incision) may occur in light planes. The potency of halothane, however, allows rapid increase of depth of anæsthesia so that the patient will tolerate surgical stimulation or an endotracheal tube and exhibit moderate degrees of muscular relaxation. Halothane has been used to speed the uptake of ether without breath-holding or coughing, and to settle the patient before changing to trichloroethylene.

Halothane is used to supplement nitrous oxide and oxygen in out-patient anæsthesia and in the dental chair.

HALOTHANE IN A LOW GAS FLOW SYSTEM WITH RE-BREATHING.—Halothane is an expensive drug. If it can be safely administered in a circuit with partial or total rebreathing, there is a significant reduction in cost. Halothane can be administered in conjunction with either a to-and-fro or a circle absorption system. The theory of administration differs according to whether the vaporizer is within the rebreathing circuit, or in the flow of fresh gases to that circuit.[†]

VAPORIZER IN CIRCUIT (V.I.C.) (e.g., the Marrett machine[‡] or the Goldman inhaler in a circle or to-and-fro system).—Halothane is vaporized by the patient's own respiratory effort. The deeper the breathing, the more halothane is vaporized. As anæsthesia deepens, respirations become depressed and less halothane is vaporized, a built-in safety mechanism. The vaporizer must be relatively inefficient (cf. V.O.C.) to prevent overdosage, and must offer little resistance to respiration. Controlled or assisted respiration must be used with the greatest care, since they result in the addition of a large amount of halothane vapour into the system. This is a technique for a

---

[*] Johnstone, M., and Nisbet, H., *Brit J. Anæsth.*, 1961, **33**, 9.
[†] Newman, H. C., *Ibid.*, 1958, **30**, 555; Mapleson, W. W., *Ibid.*, 1960, **32**, 294; Galloon, S., *Ibid.*, 1960, **32**, 310; and Mushin, W. W., and Galloon, S., *Ibid.*, 1960, **32**, 328.
[‡] Marrett, H. R., *Brit. med. J.*, 1957, **2**, 331 ; and *Anæsthesia*, 1959, **14**, 28.

completely closed circuit or total rebreathing, with basal oxygen flow only. It is then the most economical method for administration of halothane, because all the expired halothane is available for re-inhalation.

VAPORIZER OUTSIDE CIRCUIT (V.O.C.).—Halothane is vaporized by the flow of fresh gases to the circuit. If this flow is small, it follows that the vaporizer must be very efficient, and calibrated for low flows. Higher flows can be used if the expiratory valve is opened.

VAPORIZERS.—Because of the potency of halothane (twice that of chloroform and four times that of ether), accurate and fine control of vapour strength is required, and special vaporizers have been designed:—

1. Fluotec Vaporizer (Cyprane, Ltd.).* Remains accurate despite changes in temperature, passage of time, amount of liquid in the container, and gas flow (within limits). It utilizes the principle of a bimetallic strip as a temperature compensator. Different models give ranges of 1–3 per cent, 1–4 per cent, and 1–10 per cent (M.J. model). Suitable for a partially closed system (1–4 l. per min.) (V.O.C.), but not for total rebreathing, since the percentages are not accurate at very low flows. Calibration up to 10 per cent is useful in order to add sufficient vapour to the rebreathing system at low flow-rates. Johnstone† recommends induction with a 5-l. oxygen flow and up to 10 per cent halothane, and maintenance at 1 l. per min. oxygen flow and a setting at 3–4 per cent (30–40 ml. halothane vapour per min.) for light anæsthesia. This method is expensive for a short time during induction, but economical for maintenance (about 5 shillings per hour for halothane).

   Note that when intermittent positive-pressure is applied to the system, the vaporizer may deliver concentrations higher than those indicated on the dial.‡ This can be prevented by fitting a non-return valve between the Fluotec and the rebreathing system.

2. The Goldman Vaporizer.§ A simple apparatus without temperature control. The following table indicates the halothane percentage delivered (v/v) with 20 ml. in bowl at 20° C. after 1 min. for the Mark II vaporizer:—

POSITION	GAS FLOW		
	2 l./min.	8 l./min.	30 l./min.
1	0·1	0·1	0·1
2	0·5	1·0	1·0
3	1·5	2·5	1·5
ON	1·5	3·0	1·5

From Goldman, V., *Anæsthesia*, 1962, **17**, 537.

* Brennan, H. J. A., *Brit. J. Anæsth.*, 1957, **29**, 332.
† Johnstone, M., *Ibid.*, 1961, **33**, 29.
‡ Hill, D. W., and Lowe, H. J., *Anesthesiology*, 1962, **23**, 291.
§ Goldman, V., *Curr. Res. Anesth.*, 1959, **38**, 192.

Halothane—Clinical Use, *continued.*

3. The Copper Kettle.* This is a very efficient vaporizer described by Lucien Morris of Seattle in 1952. It employs the principle of metering the variable flow of oxygen as a carrier gas through liquid anæsthetic, and subsequently mixing it with known volumes of diluent gases to provide delicate control over the resultant vapour concentration as though the vapour itself were being metered. The vaporizer uses a sintered bronze disk in a copper container which rests on a copper table top and provides a highly efficient vaporizing surface as the disk disperses the oxygen into innumerable small bubbles so that the gas–liquid interface has a very large area. The heat required for vaporization is conducted from the copper vessel and the table top and makes use of the high specific heat and thermal conductivity of the metal.

   Oxygen passing through becomes maximally saturated with halothane vapour. The resultant oxygen–halothane mixture is led through a separate flow-meter, which can be calibrated at any given temperature so that a known amount of halothane vapour in ml. per min. is added to the system. Special flow-meters are necessary to measure the low flows required (0–100 ml. per min.). The mixture can be diluted as required by use of the regular oxygen flow-meter. The method is safe in that emergency oxygen does not pass through the vaporizer, but dangerous in that high concentrations of halothane (30 per cent) can be delivered. The vaporizer, which can be used for any volatile anæsthetic, is common in the U.S.A., but is not available in Britain. It is satisfactory for the very low flows required with total rebreathing.

4. The Halox Vaporizer.† This works on a similar principle to the Copper Kettle, but is made of glass. A thermometer is built in so that the temperature of the liquid halothane is known. A slide rule is used to read off the ml. of halothane vapour being added to the rebreathing system at any given flow rate and temperature. In a high gas flow system, the saturated vapour is diluted by measured flows of oxygen with or without nitrous oxide.

5. The Dräger Vaporizer. A temperature-compensated vaporizer which delivers constant and accurate concentrations of vapour over a range of gas flows between 0·3 and 12 l. per min. It is unaffected by pressure fluctuations produced by the action of a ventilator but offers a high resistance so cannot be used in the breathing circuit.

6. The Oxford Miniature Vaporizer,‡ with a range of up to 3·5 per cent, originally designed to pave the way for an ether maintenance, but can be used as a vaporizer in its own right.

---

* Morris, L. E., *Anesthesiology*, 1952, **13**, 587; Young, T. M., *Anæsthesia*, 1962, **17**, 328; Abajian, J., and others, *J. Amer. med. Ass.*, 1959, **171**, 535 ; and Feldman, S. A., and Morris, L., *Anesthesiology*, 1958, **19**, 650.
† Young, J. V. I., *Anæsthesia*, 1966, **21**, 551; and Collis, J. M., *Ibid.*, 1966, **21**, 558.
‡ Parkhouse, J., *Ibid.*, 1966, **21**, 498.

7. The Penlon Drawover Vaporizer, Mark 2. This is thermo-compensated, is efficient at flows from 4 to 14 l. per min., and provides a concentration up to 6 per cent.

8. The Blease Universal Vaporizer. This is a development of the Gardner vaporizer which can be used for vaporizing all volatile anæsthetic agents.*

The safety of closed circuit administration depends on the fact that saturation of the body tissues with halothane is not achieved for many hours.† This is because of the very high oil/water partition coefficient which is 330 (three times that of chloroform and one hundred times that of ether). Halothane is continually being removed from the blood as it passes to fat, and this is balanced by uptake of halothane from the alveoli. The concentration of halothane in expired gases is always less than that of the inspired gases. Hence the halothane concentration added to the system becomes diluted (V.O.C.). The inspired concentration is, therefore, always less than the concentration delivered from the vaporizer (V.O.C.), and if the vaporizers are switched off (V.O.C. or V.I.C.) the plane of anæsthesia lightens, even if there is apnœa. The Cardiff Calculator‡ has been devised to determine the inspired concentration of halothane at varying fresh gas flow, vaporizer concentration, and pulmonary ventilation.

OTHER METHODS.—Open drop administration or pharyngeal administration via a Boyle-Davis gag in children is extravagant because of the wastage of expensive agent which occurs, and there is little control over the inhaled concentration. Halothane in air may have some value in field or emergency conditions, but the respiratory depression which occurs means that there may be some arterial oxygen desaturation unless respiration is assisted or oxygen added to the mixture.

COST.—Halothane is an expensive agent and it is important to consider the relative cost of different methods of administration. Rough calculations indicate that halothane vapour costs about one penny per 30 ml. of vapour (in Britain).§ On this basis, 1 per cent halothane in a 6-l. flow will cost about 10s. per hour for halothane alone. 3 per cent halothane in a 1-l. flow to a rebreathing system will cost 5s. per hour. The cheapest method of administration is with vaporizer in the rebreathing system (V.I.C.). This is the only method which can be used as a completely closed circuit throughout; with V.O.C. the initial flow-rates must be high in order to obtain a rapid build-up of halothane in the rebreathing system.

Indications.—The indications for halothane in anæsthetic practice are by no means settled. Some anæsthetists believe that it is the agent of choice for practically all operations,‖ others have

* Dobkin, A. B., and others, N.Y. St. J. Med., 1963, **63**, 1815.
† Duncan, W. A. M., and Raventós, J., Brit. J. Anæsth., 1959, **31**, 302.
‡ Galloon, S., Anæsthesia, 1961, **16**, 96.
§ 1 ml. liquid halothane ≡ 211 ml. vapour at N.T.P.
‖ Johnstone, M., Brit. J. Anæsth., 1961, **33**, 29.

Halothane—Indications, *continued*.

pointed to the dangers of this potent agent, and deaths have been reported.

It may be of special value in certain circumstances :—

1. Where quiet respiration is required (e.g., neurosurgery ; it raises the C.S.F. pressure, however*).
2. Where the accompanying hypotension may be of value in reducing blood-loss at the operation site.
3. Where muscle relaxants are relatively or absolutely contra-indicated. Halothane is the only non-explosive inhalation agent besides chloroform which produces muscular relaxation. It may be of value in children, when intravenous techniques are difficult, or in poor-risk cases where large doses of muscle relaxants seem inadvisable.
4. In the bronchitic subject with bronchospasm and emphysema.
5. For external version.
6. It may have a special use in certain cases, e.g., dental surgery, prostatectomy, bronchoscopy, cystoscopy, etc.

Disadvantages.—

1. Potency. The drug is very potent and an overdose is easily given.
2. Poor analgesic properties. Full surgical anæsthesia must be achieved to prevent reaction to painful stimuli. There is also little or no post-operative analgesia.
3. High cost, unless used in closed circuit.
4. Hypotension, which may be undesirable.
5. Arrhythmias may occur, though they are seldom serious.
6. It may cause shivering or tremor, sometimes of a severe nature, in the immediate postoperative period.

Advantages.—

1. Rapid smooth induction.
2. Non-irritant to respiratory tract.
3. May produce bronchodilatation.
4. May protect against shock.
5. Rapid recovery.

Halothane may be used in clinical anæsthesia : (1) in minimal concentrations as a supplement to thiopentone–nitrous-oxide–oxygen, as part of a balanced technique ; (2) in greater concentration as the main anæsthetic agent. In the latter case addition of nitrous oxide to the anæsthetic mixture has little advantage.

The authors find halothane a most useful anæsthetic, though it can cause grave circulatory depression. This can be partially prevented by administering the agent with the patient tilted slightly head down and by vaporizing it with 100 per cent oxygen. Should circulatory depression occur, the reservoir bag should be emptied, the halothane vaporizer turned off, and the patient ventilated with pure oxygen. This will usually reverse the depression. Throughout the anæsthetic, the anæsthetist must be fully aware of what is happening to the patient's circulatory system.

---

* Hunter, A. R., *Brit. med. J.*, 1963, **2**, 239.

The authors employ halothane with considerable frequency and find it most useful in the following types of case : cystoscopy in emphysematous old men ; vaginal repairs ; operations on the middle and inner ear ; prostatectomy ; mastectomy ; external version and in ophthalmic surgery.

Comparison with Chloroform.—Halothane anæsthesia is said to resemble chloroform anæsthesia so closely that in a double blind study it is hard to differentiate between the two agents.* The advantage of chloroform lies in its cheapness. The advantages of halothane are the rareness of sudden cardiovascular collapse during induction (although this can occur) and the lower incidence of nausea and vomiting and other toxic effects. Chloroform is sympathomimetic and produces a rise in blood-sugar. Chloroform may cause toxic hepatitis, while the toxic effect of halothane on the liver has not been proven.

HALOTHANE–ETHER AZEOTROPE†

An azeotropic mixture of two (or more) volatile liquids is one which cannot be separated by fractional distillation, only by gas chromatography. Halothane and diethyl ether form such a mixture in the proportions halothane 68 to ether 32, by volume, with a boiling-point of 51·5° C. compared with 50·2° C. for halothane alone. The inflammability range is between 7·25 and 67 per cent in oxygen, so to keep it below 7 per cent it is better to induce anæsthesia with some other agent. Although circulatory depression has been reported to be minimal during anæsthesia with the azeotrope,‡ Black and Love§ found that arterial pressure in children was depressed to a greater extent than by either of its constituents used alone. The consensus of opinion is that the azeotrope has little or no superiority over halothane alone.

FLUROXENE
(Fluoromar)

This volatile agent, trifluoro-ethyl vinyl ether (CF_3—CH_2—O—CH=CH_2), was described by Lu and Krantz, and investigated by Krantz in 1953‖ and by Dornette in 1956.¶

Physical Properties.—It is a stable, clear fluid with boiling-point of 43·2° C. 0·01 per cent phenyl naphthylamine is added as a stabilizer. It is not altered by hot soda-lime. Its oil/water solubility is 94. Its lower limit of flammability in oxygen and in nitrous–oxide–oxygen (75 : 25) is 4 per cent and concentrations greater than 4 per cent are explosive.

Pharmacology and Clinical Uses.—It does not sensitize the heart to adrenaline, nor does it produce dangerous arrhythmias. Deepening

---

* Bamforth, B. J., Siebecker, K. L., Steinhaus, J. E., and Orth, O. S., Anesthesiology, 1960, **21**, 27.
† Hudon, F., Jacques, A., and Boivin, P. A., Laval. Med., 1958, **25**, 607; and Canad. Anæsth. Soc. J., 1958, **5**, 384.
‡ Dobkin, A. B., Drummond, K., and Purkin, N., Brit. J. Anæsth., 1959, **31**, 53.
§ Black, G. W., and Love, S. H. S., Anæsthesia, 1961, **16**, 324.
‖ Go Lu, Johnson, S. L., Lung, M. S., and Krantz, J. C., Anesthesiology, 1953, **14**, 466.
¶ Dornette, W. H. L., Cal. Med., 1956, **85**, 311.

Fluroxene—Pharmacology and Clinical Uses, *continued.*

the anæsthesia sometimes causes a fall in blood-pressure. While the induction period, when it is added to gas and oxygen, is relatively short, the recovery period is relatively rapid and there is a residual analgesic action. Jaw relaxation may be difficult to produce. It is less irritating than ether to the air passages but may, like cyclopropane, cause apnœa at light levels of anæsthesia, and like trichloroethylene it may give rise to tachypnœa which can be controlled by small doses of pethidine. The anæsthesia it produces cannot easily be fitted into the Guedel pattern and it may be most difficult to assess anæsthetic depth. The amount of abdominal relaxation it produces is variable, but so far no ill-effects have resulted from its combination with relaxants.

(*See also* Sadove, M. S., Balagot, R. C., and Linde, H. W., *Anesthesiology*, 1956, **17**, 591 ; and Dundee, J. W., Linde, H. W., and Dripps, R. D., *Ibid.*, 1957, **18**, 66 ; and Dornette, W. H. L., in *Clinical Anesthesia—Halogenated Anesthetics* (Ed. Artusio, J. F.), 1963, Ch. 4. Oxford: Blackwell.)

METHOXYFLURANE
(*Penthrane*)

Methoxyflurane is a halogen-substituted methyl ethyl ether :

$$
\begin{array}{ccc}
\text{Cl} & \text{F} & \text{H} \\
| & | & | \\
\text{H} - \text{C} - \text{C} - \text{O} - \text{C} - \text{H} \\
| & | & | \\
\text{Cl} & \text{F} & \text{H}
\end{array}
$$

The boiling-point is 104·6° C. and the saturated vapour pressure only 25 mm. Hg at room temperature. This means that concentrations higher than 4 per cent cannot be made available for inhalation. It is a chemically stable compound and does not react with soda-lime. It does not burn or explode at concentrations of less than 4 per cent.

It was first used in clinical anæsthesia by Artusio and Van Poznak (1960).* It can be used in most vaporizers and accurate control over the inhaled percentage is not necessary. Induction is slow (up to 10 min. for loss of consciousness by open-drop administration). The vapour is less irritating than that of diethyl ether, but coughing may occur if the strength is increased too rapidly. Analgesia develops early. Muscular relaxation is produced and non-depolarizing relaxants, if used, should be given in small doses. There is depression of respiration (especially if opiates have been given) and hypotension, which occurs slowly and is reversible by decreasing the inspired concentration. Ganglionic blocking drugs, such as trimetaphan, should be given with care. There may be an initial sharp rise in blood-sugar, which lasts for several hours.† Pallor has been reported post-operatively. It does not seem to be toxic to the liver or kidneys.

It is an extremely potent anæsthetic with a minimum alveolar concentration of 0·16 per cent. A high inspired concentration (difficult

---

* Artusio, J. F., Van Poznak, A., and others, *Anesthesiology*, 1960, **21**, 512.
† Roberts, R. B., and Cam, J. F., *Anæsthesia*, 1964, **19**, 126.

to attain) is required for induction and maintenance because of high blood and tissue solubility.*

Concentrations delivered from the Boyle's machine vary from 0·5 to 2·9 per cent, depending on the setting of the plunger. For use in closed circuit, the vaporizer should be within the rebreathing system (V.I.C.), since it is difficult to vaporize a sufficient quantity of methoxyflurane in a small basal flow (V.O.C.).

Because of the slow induction with methoxyflurane, induction of anæsthesia with some other agent is generally preferred, making use of the analgesic and relaxant properties of the drug during maintenance.

Ventricular extrasystoles are not a feature of methoxyflurane anæsthesia, nor do they appear when the Pco₂ rises.† Since hypercapnia is associated with a rise in circulating catecholamines, the inference is that exogenous adrenaline is relatively safe.‡ It is common practice in many centres to allow adrenaline infiltration during methoxyflurane anæsthesia but all workers do not agree with this.§

Methoxyflurane has been used to provide analgesia in obstetrics,‖ and as an adjunct to nitrous-oxide–oxygen in dental anæsthesia.¶

(*See also* Power, D. J., *Canad. anæsth. Soc. J.*, 1961, **8**, 488; Jarman, R., and Edgehill, H. B., *Anæsthesia*, 1963, **18**, 265; Torda, T. A. G., *Ibid.*, 1963, **18**, 287; Van Poznak, A., in *Clinical Anesthesia— Halogenated Anesthetics* (Ed. Artusio, J. F.), 1963, Ch. 6. Oxford: Blackwell; and Black, G. W., and Rea, J. L., *Brit. J. Anæsth.*, 1964, **36**, 26.)

CHAPTER VIII

ARTIFICIAL VENTILATION OF THE LUNGS

CONTROLLED RESPIRATION IN ANÆSTHESIA

History.—This was introduced by Guedel and Treweek in 1934,** using ether. Starting off in Stage III, Plane 2, they quickly increased the ether concentration and produced hyperventilation by bag pressure in a closed circuit with the soda-lime canister in operation. They thus caused a raised threshold of the respiratory centre together with a lowering of the stimulant to respiration— carbon dioxide, and apnœa followed in about 4 minutes—the so-called ether apnœa. Waters in 1936 first used the term ' controlled respiration ', but perhaps 'controlled apnœa' would be a better term. It is the temporary loss of respiratory drive due to either central or peripheral depression. Controlled apnœa, while

---

* Eger, E. I., and Larson, C. P., *Brit. J. Anæsth.*, 1964, **36**, 140.
† Black, G. W., and Rea, J. L., *Ibid.*, 1964, **36**, 26; and Black, G. W., *Acta anæsth. scand.*, 1967, **11**, 103.
‡ Jacques, A., and Hudon, F., *Canad. Anæsth. Soc. J.*, 1963, **10**, 53.
§ McIntyre, J. W. R., and Gain, E. A., *Ibid.*, 1962, **9**, 319.
‖ Romagnole, A., and Korman, D., *Ibid.*, 1962, **9**, 414; and Major, V., Rosen, M. and Mushin, W. W., *Brit. med. J.*, 1966, **2**, 1554.
¶ Unkles, R. D., and Murray Lawson, J. I., *Brit. J. Anæsth.*, 1965, **37**, 422.
** Guedel, A. F., and Treweek, D. M., *Curr. Res. Anesth.*, 1934, Dec.

History, *continued.*

formerly produced by cyclopropane, is now usually obtained by the use of muscle relaxants. Relative overdose of narcotic analgesics may also be employed. Crafoord reported on his spiropulsator in 1940, and in the following year Nosworthy's classic paper appeared.[*]
Apnœa can be produced during anæsthesia by:—

1. Raising the threshold of the respiratory centre, as by barbiturates, opiates, halothane, cyclopropane, phenoperidine or fentanyl, or a combination of these—a pharmacological method. The blood carbon dioxide no longer stimulates respiration. All volatile agents, if pushed, will cause apnœa in this way.
2. Depleting the physiological stimulus to respiration, carbon dioxide, by hyperventilation. When stimulus falls below the threshold there is respiratory depression. This is a physiological mechanism. In addition, a rich oxygen supply removes the respiratory drive originating in the aortic and carotid bodies.
3. Voluntary respiration is abolished by the use of curare or one of its substitutes, by paralysing the respiratory muscles, while anæsthesia is maintained by a combination of nitrous oxide, oxygen, and thiopentone.
4. A combination of the above methods.

A brief apnœic period, as is sometimes required in radiological procedures such as bronchography, pyelography, or cholangiography, can be produced by activation of the Hering-Breuer reflex brought about by continued pressure inflation of the lungs at the end of inspiration, if the anæsthetic in use has not inactivated this reflex response to inflation of the lung. Such agents as thiopentone, gas and oxygen, and light gas–oxygen–ether do not depress these reflexes. Deep ether, cyclopropane, and chloroform, on the other hand, inactivate these Hering-Breuer reflexes.

Apnœa may follow a sudden rise in blood-pressure, as by intravenous adrenaline, an effect mediated through the aortic and carotid sinuses.

Assisted Breathing.—Manually assisted inspiration implies some rhythmic activity of the respiratory centre and the respiratory muscles. Pressure on the reservoir bag should be synchronous with inspiration, while it is completely withdrawn to allow full passive expiration.

Intermittent Positive-pressure Ventilation (I.P.P.V.).—Includes both controlled and assisted respiration. If a mechanical ventilator is used there may or may not be a phase during expiration when the pressure is subatmospheric.

Physiological Changes associated with I.P.P.V.—In positive-pressure breathing, inspiratory, intrapulmonary, and intrapleural pressures are reversed from what they are during normal breathing —i.e., they become positive instead of negative. These effects are greater when the chest wall is intact than during thoracotomy.

---

[*] Nosworthy, M. D., *Proc. R. Soc. Med.*, 1941, **34**, 497.

Intrapulmonary pressure: During quiet spontaneous respiration, the difference is 2 cm. H_2O. During I.P.P.V. it averages 16–20 cm. H_2O.

Intrapleural pressure: During spontaneous respiration, the pressure is −5 cm. H_2O at end of expiration, and during inspiration it is −10 cm. H_2O. In I.P.P.V. pressure rises during inspiration from −5 cm. H_2O to +3 cm. H_2O and falls to −5 cm. H_2O during expiration.

Damage to lungs : Rupture is unlikely, as during coughing and straining pressure may rise to 100 cm. H_2O. It is difficult to increase pressure above 50 cm. H_2O by bag pressure.

Compliance: Artificial ventilation produces about a 50 per cent reduction in lung compliance.[*]

Dead space: There is an increase in the ratio of physiological dead space to tidal volume (V_D/V_T ratio).[†]

Respiratory alkalosis may be caused. This tends to increase the affinity of hæmoglobin for oxygen, to cause cerebral vasoconstriction, and to decrease cardiac output, but these changes are seldom clinically important. Over-ventilation raises the pain threshold possibly by depressing the ascending activating reticular formation.[‡]

Atelectasis: This can occur during prolonged I.P.P.V. Miliary areas of atelectasis may not be demonstrable radiologically, but are evidenced by a falling compliance and an increasing alveolar-arterial oxygen gradient. It has been suggested that periodic deep breaths or sighs are useful in the prevention of such atelectasis.[§]

Cardiovascular changes: (1) Abolition of thoracic pump. At the end of positive-pressure inspiration, right atrial pressure is raised and hence venous return and cardiac output are decreased. This is compensated for by a rise in the peripheral venous pressure which re-establishes venous return to its former level —due to venoconstriction. If the blood volume is reduced or venoconstriction is deficient (e.g., due to sympathetic blockade) or maximal (e.g., after hæmorrhage) harm may result. (2) Cardiac tamponade. Not clinically important. (3) Interference with pulmonary blood-flow. The pulmonary capillary pressure is 13 cm. H_2O, so even slight increases in pressure in lungs may strain right heart. This may be seen even with an open chest.

Oxygen consumption is reduced because of the easing of the patient's muscular effort.

It may be that the use of controlled apnœa reduces the necessary doses of relaxant and narcotic.[||]

Technique.—The circuit must be able to withstand the positive pressure applied to the breathing bag without leaking unduly.

---

[*] Howell, J. B. L., and Peckett, B. W., *J. Physiol.*, 1957, **136**, 1; and Opie, T. H., Spalding, J. M. K., and Stott, F. D., *Lancet*, 1959, **1**, 543.

[†] Watson, W. E., *Brit. J. Anæsth.*, 1962, **34**, 502.

[‡] Geddes, I. C., and Gray, T. C., *Lancet*, 1959, **2**, 4.

[§] Bendixen, H. H., Hedley-Whyte, J., and Laver, M. B., *New Engl. J. Med.*, 1963, **269**, 991; Bendixen, H. H., Smith, G. M., and Mead, J., *J. appl. Physiol.*, 1964, **19**, 195; and Pontoppidan, H., Hedley-Whyte, J., Bendixen, H. H., Laver, M. B., and Radford, E. P., *New Engl. J. Med.*, 1965, **273**, 401.

[||] Dundee, J. W., *Brit. med. J.*, 1952, **2**, 893.

Technique, *continued.*

Without an endotracheal tube the stomach may become distended with air but the exercise of care can often prevent this.   A Ryle's tube or an œsophageal tube will prevent and remedy it.   The former can be brought under the mask and aspirated occasionally, or a balloon can be fixed to it to distend the œsophagus as suggested by Macintosh.*   The junction between the machine and the patient also must be leak-proof and may be ensured by:—

    1. A well-fitting mask and harness.

    2, An endotracheal tube with inflated cuff or gauze pack.

    3. An endotracheal tube with the lower jaw bandaged backwards to occlude the pharynx (Pinson).

The pressure required to inflate the lungs varies with a number of factors, including: (*a*) The depth of anæsthesia. (*b*) Whether a relaxant has been used or not. (*c*) Whether the chest wall is open or closed. (*d*) The pathology of the lungs (pulmonary and chest wall compliance). (*e*) The patency of the airways.   Rupture of the lung and its sequelæ, pneumothorax, mediastinal emphysema, pulmonary interstitial emphysema, and subcutaneous emphysema, are unlikely if due care is taken.   Never should a pressure of 40 cm. H_2O be exceeded—even though during a severe bout of coughing an interbronchial pressure of 100 cm. H_2O has been recorded.

1. USING MUSCLE RELAXANTS.—Induction is by intravenous thiopentone and maintenance by nitrous oxide and at least 30 per cent of oxygen.   It may be preferred to induce anæsthesia with a volatile agent.   When the production of apnœa is desired the relaxant is injected intravenously in divided doses, and the patient is hyperventilated until apnœa is produced.   Further doses are given as may be necessary.   It is sometimes desirable to stop short of frank apnœa, in which case assisted breathing is required to ensure adequate gaseous interchange : the reservoir bag is gently compressed with each of the patient's shallow inspirations.   The necessity is again emphasized of seeing that breathing of normal depth has returned before the patient is sent from the theatre.   If necessary, neostigmine should be used to counteract a non-depolarizing block, preceded by atropine.

2. USING CYCLOPROPANE.—The respiratory centre is depressed by morphine premedication and a thiopentone induction, if thought desirable.   Depletion of carbon dioxide can be carried out by gently compressing the bag with each inspiration so that the expired carbon dioxide is absorbed in the soda-lime ; this hyperventilation soon produces a blood carbon dioxide level too low to stimulate the respiratory centre.   Tidal exchange is then maintained by compression of the breathing bag.   Bag pressure, whatever combination of drugs is being used, should be applied 15–35 times each minute at a pressure not exceeding 40 cm. H_2O, the duration of expiration being twice that of inspiration, so as to ensure complete elimination of carbon dioxide.   This also minimizes the circulatory effects of positive intrapulmonary pressure.   The more cyclopropane that is added the sooner will

---

* Macintosh, R. R., *Brit. med. J.*, 1951, **2**, 545.

apnœa appear. Thus breathing is directly controlled by the anæsthetist both as to rate and depth.

Small doses of muscle relaxant (e.g., tubocurarine 10–12 mg.) can be used in combination with light cyclopropane anæsthesia and hyperventilation. Toxic effects from cyclopropane are then very rare, and the small doses of muscle relaxant seldom require reversal by neostigmine. Cyclopropane anæsthesia may be deepened to provide for closure of the peritoneum towards the end of the operation, so saving muscle relaxant dosage.

Towards the end of the operation, the bag is emptied and refilled with 50 per cent nitrous-oxide–oxygen or air, and the absorber cut out of circuit. Tidal exchange is kept up as before, and the procedure repeated each minute. When active breathing recommences, the absorber is again employed and the patient finishes the operation breathing normally. If the early breaths are shallow they must be assisted by gentle bag pressure. If cyclopropane has been pushed, normal respiration may be delayed for 10–15 minutes after the end of the operation. The anæsthetist must not leave the patient until reasonably normal breathing has been re-established for a minute or two, lest apnœa should reappear and cause death from anoxia. Real danger from subsequent apnœa exists if a patient is suddenly removed from a circuit containing gases abnormally high in carbon dioxide content.

3. HALOTHANE.—The respiratory depressant action of halothane facilitates controlled respiration. Because the agent is potent and may produce hypotension, care must be taken that a sudden increase in depth of anæsthesia does not occur with onset of controlled respiration. Controlled respiration must be employed only with the greatest possible care when the halothane vaporizer is inside the rebreathing system. Gentle *assistance* of respiration is often useful with this agent.

4. INTRAVENOUS AGENTS.—The use of drugs which depress the respiratory centre—'narcotic-induced apnœa'. The new powerful agents, phenoperidine and fentanyl, can be used to produce apnœa. Narcotic antagonists may be given at the end of the operation to reverse their effect. Other narcotic analgesics can also be employed for this purpose, e.g., morphine, heroin, pethidine, alpha-prodine, dipipanone, etc.

Negative Pressure.—Use of negative pressure during the expiratory phase results in a lower mean intrathoracic pressure. An automatic ventilator with a negative phase can be used. It may decrease the circulatory upset produced by I.P.P.V., but should not exceed 5 cm. H_2O as it may lead to bronchial collapse, air trapping, and an increased physiological dead space. These harmful effects are particularly likely to occur in the emphysematous patient. Negative pressure is not of value during thoracotomy.

Assessment of Depth of Anæsthesia with Controlled Apnœa due to Central Depression.—(1) Anæsthesia is light if respiration

Depth of Anæsthesia with Controlled Apnœa, *continued.*

rapidly returns after a little carbon dioxide is allowed to accumulate. (2) The ease with which apnœa develops during hyperventilation through soda-lime is an index of depth and of respiratory centre depression, using any potent anæsthetic agent. (3) Resistance to inflation decreases with increased depth of anæsthesia, whether chest is open or closed. (4) Light anæsthesia is suggested if the chest, but not the abdomen, moves on squeezing the bag: good relaxation is only present when both chest and abdomen move on bag pressure. (5) Under thiopentone, the duration of apnœa, from activation of the Hering-Breuer reflexes by inflation of the lungs, is longer, the greater the depth of anæsthesia (this is before the onset of controlled apnœa). (6) The eye signs. (7) The presence or absence of swallowing. (8) Traction reflexes are more likely to break through apnœa due to overventilation than through that due to relaxants. (9) When cyclopropane is being used, the smell of the mixture should indicate its concentration. (10) Knowledge of the amounts of drugs used and length of time of anæsthesia. (11) Using gas–oxygen–ether and perhaps cyclopropane, but not gas–oxygen–thiopentone, when respiratory movements are present, if the reservoir bag is squeezed at the end of inspiration, so as to prevent expiration, a definite respiratory pause occurs in Planes 1–2, being longer the lighter the plane of anæsthesia and lasting for several respiratory cycles. This reflex disappears before intercostal activity ceases and its presence is a rough index of lightness.*

When employing the technique of controlled apnœa it is important for the anæsthetist to keep in mind : (*a*) The blood carbon dioxide tension. (*b*) The degree of depression of the respiratory centre. (*c*) The amount of muscular paralysis.

Advantages.—When muscle relaxants are used, controlled breathing is very often necessary in order to provide a proper interchange of gases. In thoracic surgery controlled or assisted respiration prevents paradoxical breathing, i.e., prevents inflation of the collapsed lung during expiration, and deflation during inspiration, with the inefficient interchange of gases so resulting. It also prevents mediastinal flap in those cases with a mobile mediastinum and makes breathing more efficient when the mediastinum is rigid. Controlled respiration is also frequently used nowadays in neuro-surgery. The quiescence of the diaphragm produced by controlled respiration aids the work of the surgeon when he is near this muscle, either in the upper abdomen or in the thorax. It may also reduce the amount of thiopentone and relaxant required during the operation, thus contributing to the speedy recovery of consciousness and muscle tone.† Assisted (or controlled) breathing is advisable at some time in almost all cases of inhalation anæsthesia requiring muscular relaxation (except when ether is the main agent) as it decreases the incidence of hypoxia and respiratory acidosis.

---

* Watrous, W. G., Davis, F. E., and Anderson, B. M., *Anesthesiology*, 1950, **11**, 558.
† Gray, T. C., and Jackson-Rees, G., *Brit. med. J.*, 1952, **2**, 891.

Disadvantages.—(1) The respiratory signs of anæsthesia are abolished. (2) Pressure changes in the chest may adversely influence the circulation and impede the venous return to the heart. (3) There is an increased resistance to pulmonary blood-flow.

Manually Operated Ventilators.—There are several simple contrivances which have been developed for ventilation of the lungs. They are portable and suitable for emergency or short-term use.

1. A bag and mask, provided there is a source of oxygen or compressed air.
2. The Ambu bag and Ruben valve.* Foam rubber is built into the walls of the Ambu so that its shape is automatically restored after compression and air is drawn in from the atmosphere.
3. The Oxford Inflating Bellows.† Air is drawn in through a non-return valve to a spring-loaded bellows which is compressed manually to push the air through a second non-return valve to the patient.
4. The Cardiff Inflating Bellows.‡ A compact apparatus working on similar principles.

Cuirass Ventilators.—A metal or canvas cuirass encloses the trunk. A rubber bag in contact with the chest and abdominal wall is distended and relaxed by a pump. This type of respirator has generally been intended for short-term use in anæsthesia with an oxygen-rich mixture, as during endoscopies.§ Respiratory exchange is achieved by forced expiration from the resting position and elastic recoil.

More effective ventilation can be obtained in some models where a rigid shell allows negative pressures to be obtained‖ so that the effect on the patient is similar to that of the tank respirator.

Automatic Ventilators.—For a full description of many of the machines available *see* Mushin, W. W., Rendell-Baker, L., and Thompson, P. W. (1959), *Automatic Ventilation of the Lungs*, Oxford : Blackwell. Some general principles only will be noted here.

DESIRABLE FEATURES OF AN IDEAL VENTILATOR.—

1. Must be capable of producing correct pulmonary ventilation.
2. A low mean intrathoracic pressure must be maintained.
3. Must be capable of output up to 80 l. per min.
4. Pressure must collapse immediately once the inspiratory phase is completed.
5. Negative pressure during expiration should be available.
6. Patient-triggering facilities should be provided.
7. It should be possible to use air or oxygen-enriched mixtures.
8. Humidification of the inspired air should be provided.
9. Must be reliable, and should have a warning system and provision for manual ventilation in an emergency.

* Ruben, H., and others, *Lancet*, 1958, **1**, 460.
† Macintosh, R. R., and Mushin, W. W., *Brit. med. J.*, 1955, **2**, 202.
‡ Hilliard, E. K., and Mushin, W. W., *Ibid.*, 1960, **2**, 729.
§ Pinkerton, H. H., *Brit. J. Anæsth.*, 1957, **29**, 421.
‖ Collier, C. R., and Affeldt, J. E., *J. appl. Physiol.* 1954, **6**, 531.

Automatic Ventilators, *continued.*

10. Gas loss in ventilator tubing should be minimized as far as possible. It is due to expansion of the corrugated tube leading to the patient and to the compression of the gas in these tubes. The tubes behave in a similar manner to the respiratory airways and may produce an increase in total dead space. The volume of gas losses may amount to 140 ml. per breath.* To obviate these factors non-expanding tubes should be used, or tidal volume measured at the catheter mount. A spirometer at the ventilator end of the expiratory limb may include gas losses in measured tidal volume.

CHARACTERISTICS OF VENTILATORS.—

1. Classification (Hunter)† into :—

   a. *Pressure preset*—build up to a preset pressure. Small leaks are automatically compensated for. Large leaks may cause the machine to stop if the preset pressure is not reached. Examples include Ble*ase, Aintree, Fazakerley, Radcliffe, Barnet, and Newcastle respirators.

   b. *Volume preset*—deliver a set volume of gas. Pressure will build up to overcome an obstruction. A safety blow-off is necessary, usually about 30 cm. H_2O. Example is the Beaver apparatus. Note that many machines can be used as either pressure or volume preset according to how the apparatus is employed (Bleal*e, Mortimer, Clutton-Brock, Manley respirators).

2. CYCLING.—This refers to the mechanism which brings about the change from the inspiratory to the expiratory phase. (The change from expiration to inspiration is usually controlled by a timing mechanism.) Machines may be *pressure cycled* (e.g., Newcastle respirator), *volume cycled* (e.g., Stephenson), or *time cycled*. In the strict sense, time cycled refers to machines with an auxiliary timing mechanism (e.g., the electronic time-cycled Barnet respirator), but in the wider sense it applies to any machine in which the duration of inspiration and expiration is set by the operator (e.g., Beaver, Mortimer, Radcliffe respirators).

3. WAVE FORM.—

   a. Pressure Generators.‡ A rapid inflationary stroke to produce a square wave form (e.g., Radcliffe, Barnet). Prolongation of inspiratory phase much above 1 sec. does not increase filling of lungs. May be advantageous in the presence of atelectatic or consolidated lung segments, in the severely crushed chest with flail segments and cause less over-riding of fractured ribs.§

   b. Flow Generators.‡ Triangular wave form. Inflation pressure increases steadily throughout inspirating phase (e.g., Aintree, Fazakerley, Bleal*e, Bird, Cyclator, Newcastle respirators).

---

* Bushman, J. A., and Collis, J. M., *Anæsthesia*, 1967, **22**, 664.
† Hunter, A. R., *Ibid.*, 1961, **16**, 231.
‡ Mapleson, W. W., *Ibid.*, 1962, **17**, 300.
§ Robinson, J. S., in *Modern Trends in Anæsthesia*, No. 3 (Ed. Evans, F. T., and Gray, T. C.), 1967, Ch. 8. London: Butterworths.

4. EFFECT ON INTRATHORACIC PRESSURE.—Positive-pressure respiration reverses the normal pressure gradient upon which venous return depends so that cardiac output falls. In most subjects compensatory mechanisms prevent a fall in blood-pressure. It is the mean intrathoracic pressure which determines the degree of circulatory upset in a susceptible patient. It is therefore desirable that the pressure in the lungs should fall as quickly as possible after the end of inspiration. Mean intrathoracic pressure can be reduced : (a) by shortening the duration of inspiration and allowing more time between inspirations, (b) by introducing a negative pressure in the expiratory phase of the respirator, although this increases the physiological dead space and may lead to bronchial collapse with respiratory trapping. Negative pressure should not exceed 5 cm. H_2O.

5. PATIENT-TRIGGERING.—It is desirable that a machine should be able to follow the patient's own respiratory rhythm. A triggered machine should be sensitive to 0·5 cm. H_2O pressure difference or 5–10 ml. volume displacement. Greater sensitivity than this may result in activation by the cardiac contraction. Delay in delivery of gas should not exceed 0·2 sec. There should be an automatic inflation of the lungs, should the patient fail to trigger the machine after a selected interval.

6. TYPE OF ACTIVATION.—

   a. Electrical—risk of explosion if flammable anæsthetic agents are in use.

   b. Compressed gas—no explosive risk if a cylinder is used, but cylinders are not satisfactory for long-term therapy although use of an entraining device reduces consumption to some extent. If a compressor is used the explosive risk may appear. A cheap substitute for a compressor is the blower unit of a domestic vacuum cleaner (Newcastle respirator).

Notes on Some Ventilators.—

Blease Pulmoflator. Various models available. Pressure preset and provided with negative phase and triggering device. Some models incorporate the anæsthetic flow-meters. Powered by electrically driven compressors. Cost is several hundred pounds.

Radcliffe.[*] Pressure preset and time cycled. An electric motor drives a four-speed bicycle hub through a gear-box. The concertina reservoir bag is raised by means of an arm fixed to the hub and then compressed by adjustable weights. Gases are delivered from an Oxford Inflating Bellows. The motor is powered by the mains or a 12V. battery. Provision is made for emergency hand control. The apparatus has been modified to provide negative pressure and to incorporate a soda-lime canister for use during anæsthesia.[†] The East-Radcliffe M2

* Russell, W. R., and Schuster, E., Lancet, 1953, **2**, 707 ; and Russell, W. R., and others, Ibid., 1956, **1**, 539.
† McDonald, I. R., Brit. J. Anæsth., 1957, **29**, 86.

Notes on Some Ventilators, *continued.*

ventilator is a version, which is a mechanically operated Oxford Inflating Bellows which delivers its stroke volume to the patient through an inflating valve. It can be used for anæsthesia in combination with a draw-over vaporizer and is then useful in the field.*

Barnet.† Pressure preset. Electronic time cycled, controlling the opening of solenoid valves. Transistorized. Patient triggering provided. Negative phase available. Powered by mains or battery. The electrical components have been sealed as a safety precaution when explosive agents are used. The noise of the solenoid valves has been reduced by the use of newer materials.

The Manley Ventilator. A simple apparatus which is operated by the gas flow delivered to it. The tidal volume is set, and the machine delivers the minute volume supplied to it at an appropriate rate. Not suitable for spontaneous or manual ventilation except for short periods as carbon dioxide accumulation then occurs.

The Loosco Amsterdam Infant Ventilator. A non-return system with minimal dead space. The inspiratory time is set by an electronically regulated valve using a modified Ayre's T-piece. The minute volume is set by flow-meter, and the tidal volume delivered depends on the electronic time setting. Easily operated by hand in the event of electrical failure. Suitable for premature babies, neonates, and babies up to age of 1–2 years.

Beaver.‡ Volume preset and time cycled. Electrically operated. Small and compact for transport.

Mortimer.§—Made from a suction-operated car windscreen wiper motor and the concertina bag from a Coxeter-Mushin absorber. It requires a negative pressure of 15–20 in. of mercury. Cost about £60 if a source of suction is available.

Newcastle.‖ A series of models have been devised, which are characterized by cheapness and simplicity of construction, so that they would be readily available for a poliomyelitis epidemic. They are operated by air at a pressure of about 35 cm. H_2O which may be delivered from a cylinder, a compressor, or a vacuum cleaner.

Clutton-Brock. *See* Clutton-Brock, J., *Brit. J. Anæsth.*, 1957, **29**, 517.

Aintree and Fazakerley. *See* Esplen, J. R., *Ibid.*, 1956, **28**, 176; and Hilliard, E. K., *Anæsthesia*, 1958, **13**, 347.

Cyclator. This is a pneumatically operated, pressure-cycled machine which is small and compact and can be fitted easily to the standard Boyle's machine. Patient triggering provided. The mechanism consists of a high efficiency injector which uses a stream of driving oxygen to entrain anæsthetic gases or air. It

---

* Collis, J. M., *Anæsthesia*, 1967, **22**, 598.
† Rochford, J., Welch, R. F., and Winks, D. W., *Brit. J. Anæsth.*, 1958, **30**, 23.
‡ Macrae, J., McKendrick, G. D. W., Claremont, J. M., Sefton, E. M., and Walley, R. V., *Lancet*, 1953, **2**, 971; and Macrae, J., and others, *Ibid.*, 1954, **2**, 21.
§ Mortimer, P. L. F., *Anæsthesia*, 1954, **9**, 312.
‖ *See* papers from Pask, E. A., and others, *Lancet*, 1957, **2**, 217; and *Ibid.*, 1957, **2**, 676; and *Brit. J. Anæsth.*, 1956, **28**, 169.

is designed to give a mean entrainment ratio of 3 to 1, at an input pressure of 60 lb. per sq. in. In other words, the driving oxygen forms 25 per cent of the mixture delivered to the patient. Cost about £100.

Cape-Waine Ventilator. A recent modification, the Cape Minor, is a portable version which can be used with a 'draw-over' vaporizer.*

Bird. Developed in the U.S.A. Automatic or patient triggered. Incorporates a nebulizer for inhalation therapy. Can be adapted for use in anæsthesia by interposing a 'bag in bottle'.

The MinEpac Emergency Ventilator.† Designed for the emergency treatment of patients with respiratory arrest. Portable and compact. Utilizes a non-return valve on the face-piece. Constant flow generator. Time cycled. Can be adapted for use in anæsthesia. Cost about £35.

The Minivent.‡ Small and simple. Fits on any continuous-flow machine, and the elasticity of the distended reservoir bag provides the driving force of inspiration. A bobbin is held against a magnet except when the pressure of gases serves to force it away. Cost about £26.

Vellore.§ A simple robust apparatus. Volume cycled. Powered by compressed gases.

East-Freeman 'Automatic Vent'. Small and simple. Fits any continuous-flow anæsthetic machine in place of the expiratory valve.

Other ventilators developed in the U.S.A. include the Bennett Assister, the Jefferson, and the Stephenson.

Care must be taken that air is not inadvertently admitted to the gas circuit.‖

(*See also* Robinson, J. S., in *Modern Trends in Anæsthesia*, No. 3 (Ed. Evans, F. T., and Gray, T. C.), 1967, Ch. 8. London: Butterworths.)

Humidification.—*See* Chapter XXXIV.

CHAPTER IX

ACCIDENTS OF INHALATION ANÆSTHESIA AND HOW TO TREAT THEM

1. Vomiting.—
   THE APPLIED ANATOMY OF VOMITING.¶—The expulsion through the mouth of material from the alimentary tract by muscular action. The act of vomiting is preceded by salivation, rapid breathing, pallor, sweating, and tachycardia.
   Like any other reflex arc, vomiting has its afferent and efferent pathways and its central connexion.

---

* Collis, J. M., *Anæsthesia*, 1967, **22**, 598.
† Burchell, G. B., *Ibid.*, 1967, **22**, 647.
‡ Cohen, A. D., *Ibid.*, 1966, **21**, 563.
§ Milledge, J. S., *Lancet*, 1967, **1**, 1090.
‖ Waters, D. J., *Brit. J. Anæsth.*, 1968, **40**, 259.
¶ Brown, H. G., *Ibid.*, 1963, **35**, 136.

Vomiting, *continued.*

AFFERENT PATHWAYS.—Impulses travel from many parts of the body and ascend in the visceral afferent fibres accompanying the vagus and, less importantly, the sympathetic.

Chemical changes occurring in the body do not stimulate the vomiting centre directly but reflexly by stimulating the chemoreceptor trigger zone of Borison and Wang; such chemicals being carried in the blood-stream or the cerebro-spinal fluid. Other chemical stimuli can arise from the alimentary tract (e.g., drugs, poisons, emetics, etc.) and impulses pass up the vagus and sympathetic.

THE VOMITING CENTRE.—This is closely related to other vital centres, e.g., the respiratory and vasomotor centres and the salivary and vestibular nuclei, in the dorsolateral border of lateral reticular formation. The chemoreceptor zone of Borison and Wang lies superficial to the true vomiting centre.

THE ACT OF VOMITING.—This commences with a deep inspiration followed by closure of the glottis and nasopharynx and is immediately followed by expiration together with contraction of the muscles of the abdominal wall and descent of the diaphragm. Now, while the body of the stomach relaxes, the antrum and also the pylorus and duodenum contract. This propels stomach contents into the œsophagus and mouth, and prevents escape from the stomach via the pylorus. A pressure of 40 cm. H_2O is needed to lift the contents of the stomach into the mouth in the upright position. The cardia is elevated during vomiting so that the abdominal part of the œsophagus rises into the chest.* While the glottis goes into spasm during the expulsive phase, it soon relaxes, so that aspiration of stomach contents into the bronchial tree is almost bound to happen in the unconscious patient. Predisposing factors during anæsthesia include: (a) Hypoxia; (b) Central stimulation during second stage general anæsthesia—either during induction or recovery; (c) Irritation of the base of the tongue or pharynx by airways, etc.

REGURGITATION, being a passive act, may be silent and un-heralded, and so even more potentially dangerous than vomiting. Predisposing factors include : (a) The head-down position if the cardia is inefficient ; (b) A stomach full of fluid.

THE CARDIAC SPHINCTER.—This is both a sphincter and a valve. It remains closed because of : (1) The angle at which the œsophagus meets the fundus of the stomach;† (2) Folds of thickened mucosa in the œsophagus;‡ (3) The presence of an anatomical muscular sphincter ; (4) The pinch-cock action of the crus of the diaphragm (in two-thirds of patients the right crus only).

NERVE-SUPPLY.—The vagus and sympathetic. Its activity is controlled reflexly. Its integrity is not affected by posture,

---

* Johnson, H. D., and Laws, J. W., *Lancet*, 1966, **2**, 1268.
† Marchand, P., *Brit. J. Surg.*, 1955, **42**, 504.
‡ Botha, G. S. M., *Ibid.*, 1958, **45**, 569.

anæsthetics, relaxants, autonomic blocking agents, or injecting the œsophageal mucosa with local analgesics.* Its integrity is affected and it is made incompetent by : (1) Anatomical abnormality, e.g., hiatus hernia;† (2) The presence of a stomach tube ; (3) Passage of anæsthetic gas from above during attempts at intermittent positive-pressure respiration ; (4) Attempts at active respiration in the presence of respiratory obstruction.

Thus, in normal patients under anæsthesia if the active vomiting reflex is suppressed, no material can regurgitate from the stomach into the œsophagus, no matter what position the patient is in, so long as the valve/sphincter mechanism is not interfered with.

THE CRICOPHARYNGEAL SPHINCTER.—This is at the upper end of the œsophagus at the level of C.6 and is composed of striated muscle. Its action is both voluntary and reflex. Its integrity is affected by both anæsthetics and relaxants. It acts as a sphincter normally but as a valve when paralysed. Normally it allows fluids to pass from the pharynx into the œsophagus, but not in the reverse direction. When paralysed by relaxants it tends to obstruct the passage of fluids from the pharynx to the œsophagus, but not in the reverse direction.

The lower part of the œsophagus contains plain muscle which is not affected by relaxants, but the upper part, the cricopharyngeal sphincter, behaves like striped muscle.‡

When considering this question, all anæsthetists should consult the first-class paper by Morton and Wylie§ dealing with vomiting during anæsthesia and its relationship to deaths on the table, in the causation of which it is one of the major factors.

CAUSES OF VOMITING.—

    a. Vomitable material in the stomach or œsophagus.—
1. Inadequate pre-operative preparation of the patient. Gastric emptying time varies between 4 and 8 hours: it is usually between 5 and 6 hours.‖
2. In pyloric obstruction.
3. When there is peritoneal irritation (e.g., perforated peptic ulcer, acute inflammatory lesions, etc.).
4. Blood in the stomach, following bleeding from ulcer, tonsil beds, œsophageal varices, or during gastric operations.
5. Gross abdominal distension.
6. Glucose solution mistakenly given to diabetic patients by mouth, instead of intravenously.
7. In cases of œsophageal disease, such as pouch or obstruction.

    b. Vomitable material returned into stomach from bowel, as in cases of intestinal obstruction.

    c. When stomach emptying time is delayed.—
1. In women in labour.
2. In cases of head injury.

* O'Mullane, E. J., *Lancet*, 1954, **1**, 1209.
† Dinnick, O. P., *Ibid.*, 1961, **1**, 470.
‡ Sinclair, R. N., *Brit. J. Anæsth.*, 1959, **31**, 15.
§ Morton, H. J. V., and Wylie, W. D., *Anæsthesia*, 1951, **6**, 190.
‖ Horton, R. E., *Brit. med. J.*, 1965, **2**, 1537.

Vomiting, continued.

3. When there is emotional strain associated with pain, accident, and the incident of hospitalization.
4. In seriously ill patients.
5. After drugs, e.g., opiates.

FACTORS PREDISPOSING TO PASSIVE REGURGITATION.*—
  a. Fluid in stomach.—
  1. In the emergency case.
  2. The patient prepared for elective surgery has a variable amount of resting gastric juice. In the nervous patient this is increased in both quantity and acidity.
  b. Incompetence of the cardia.—
  1. Hiatus hernia.
  2. Increased vagal tone.
  3. Presence of gastric tube.†
  c. Raised intra-abdominal pressure.—
  1. Posture, e.g., lithotomy position.
  2. Suxamethonium fasciculations.
  3. Pregnancy, especially where there is a high head or hydramnios.
  d. Lowered intrathoracic pressure.—This can occur with deep spontaneous respiration, and is exaggerated when there is respiratory obstruction as in a difficult induction of anæsthesia.
  e. Obesity.—There is both a raised intra-abdominal pressure,‡ and a greater likelihood of respiratory obstruction during induction of anæsthesia, particularly in unskilled hands.
  f. Pregnancy.—Incorporating several factors already mentioned.
  g. Relaxation of the cricopharyngeus by deep anæsthesia or muscle relaxants.

TIME OF ASPIRATION.—(1) Before anæsthesia. (2) During induction. (3) During anæsthesia—slow insidious regurgitation. (4) In immediate post-operative period. (5) During first few post-operative days in ill patients. Gastric contents can find their way into the lungs after death.

DANGERS OF VOMITING DURING ANÆSTHESIA.—These are :
  a. The inhalation of stomach contents into the lungs, with sequelæ such as pneumonitis, bronchopneumonia, atelectasis, and lung abscess. Food particles and liquid vomitus with a pH of less than 2·5 are particularly dangerous. Liquid vomitus with a pH greater than 2·5 (e.g., bile) is less harmful.§
  b. Hypoxia due to laryngeal spasm or obstruction of the air-passages by solid or liquid gastric contents.
  c. Cardiac inhibition from reflexes originating in the bronchi, due to acid contamination.
  d. Reflex chemical trauma to bronchial and alveolar mucosa—acute exudative pneumonitis or Mendelson's syndrome,‖ a syndrome following the aspiration of acid gastric contents.

---

* Dinnick, O. P., *Proc. R. Soc. Med.*, 1967, **60**, 623.
† Nagler, R., and Spiro, H. M., *New Engl. J. Med.*, 1963, **269**, 495.
‡ O'Mullane, E. J., *Lancet*, 1954, **1**, 1209.
§ Teabeaut, J. R., *Amer. J. Path.*, 1952, **28**, 51.
‖ Mendelson, C. L., *Amer. J. Obstet. Gynec.*, 1946, **52**, 191 (reprinted in *Survey of Anesthesiology*, 1966, **10**, 599).

While this is particularly likely to occur in obstetric patients, it is not confined to them. Following immediately, or after an interval of a few hours, the patient shows cyanosis, dyspnœa, bronchospasm, hypotension, and tachycardia. There are rhonchi and râles in the chest with a characteristic radiographic appearance, viz., irregular mottled densities. There are no signs of massive atelectasis or mediastinal shift. Severe cases may progress to acute pulmonary œdema with rapid death or the patient may succumb to pulmonary complications some days later.

PREVENTION.—This involves prevention of substances entering stomach, removal of substances from stomach, and prevention of substances leaving stomach in an uncontrolled manner. Except in the gravest emergency no general anæsthetic should be given to a patient whose stomach may contain vomitable material, i.e., a patient who has not been properly prepared for anæsthesia by preliminary avoidance of food and drink. This should be an infallible rule.

MANAGEMENT.—When an anæsthetic must be given for urgent reasons, a plastic Ryle's tube, e.g., size 6 gauge, should be passed from the nose into the stomach so that aspiration can take place and if necessary lavage. This should be done with the patient lying on his side to prevent soiling of lungs should he vomit. Information is thus obtained as to the amount and type of material still in the stomach. If the anæsthetist thinks that he can empty the viscus by the tube, well and good, but in all cases of doubt, an œsophageal tube such as size 12 E.G. should be inserted into the cocainized nostril and thence into the stomach, where it should remain until the patient gets his cough reflexes back at the end of the operation (although there is evidence that the presence of a tube interferes with the integrity of the sphincter mechanism, so that its withdrawal before induction is recommended by some authorities). This tube will allow fairly efficient drainage of liquid and semi-solid material, and so should prevent regurgitation even if actual vomiting is not prevented.

The insertion of a cuffed endotracheal tube into the larynx before the onset of vomiting or regurgitation is the only safe procedure when dealing with a patient who may have vomitable material in the stomach or œsophagus. A cuffed tube should always be used when in doubt about the contents of the stomach, and before induction commences, the availability of an efficient suction apparatus, source of oxygen, laryngoscope, endotracheal tubes, airways, etc., must be checked. It is wise to induce anæsthesia in these patients on the operating table, so that tilting can be employed easily. The inexperienced anæsthetist is perhaps well advised to tilt the patient's head downwards, and to induce anæsthesia with nitrous oxide, oxygen, trichloroethylene, and ether, helped with a little carbon dioxide to stimulate breathing and speed induction. By this technique the cough reflex is preserved until late so that this, together with suction and gravity, should prevent aspiration into the lungs.[*]

---

[*] Inkster, J. S., *Brit. J. Anæsth.*, 1963, **35**, 160.

Vomiting, *continued.*

In a patient lying horizontally, the long axis of the trachea is inclined at an angle of 30° downwards and backwards from the larynx so that a head-down slope of more than 30° is necessary if in fact gravity is to protect the trachea. Laryngoscopy may be difficult in this steeply inclined position.

INSERTION OF CUFFED TUBE INTO TRACHEA IN A PATIENT SUS-PECTED OF HAVING A FULL STOMACH.—Atropine should be given before all anæsthetics where regurgitation is at all possible. It almost doubles the pressure the cardia is able to withstand from the gastric aspect, but does not affect resistance to pressure from above.*

1. If the general condition of the patient will allow it, tilt the table 40° foot down.† If necessary the legs can be raised. Give pure oxygen for 2 min., followed by the intravenous injection of a rapidly acting thiobarbiturate, e.g., thiopentone 150–300 mg. and suxamethonium 25–100 mg. Then pass tube, immediately inflate its cuff, and level table.

2. Repeat the above method substituting gallamine 80–160 mg. for the suxamethonium.‡

3. If the condition of the patient makes the injection of thiopentone likely to be dangerous, substitute a mixture of equal parts of cyclopropane and oxygen in a 5-l. bag ; unconsciousness will supervene in a dozen breaths. Then give the relaxant as above.§

4. The lateral position with a head-down tilt, using a halothane-oxygen induction, followed by suxamethonium, has its advocates.‖

5. Topical analgesia of the upper airways will enable a tube to be inserted into the trachea in the conscious patient. Give an amethocaine lozenge, then : (*a*) spray throat, pharynx, and cords from above and inject 2 ml. of local analgesic solution by the transtracheal method (*see* Chapter XV); or (*b*) perform a bilateral superior laryngeal nerve-block (*see* Chapter XV) and then do the transtracheal injection.

An efficient, but not a particularly humane, method of reducing the risk of aspiration of stomach contents before induction of anæsthesia is to empty the patient's stomach by stimulating vomiting. Apomorphine 3 mg. is dissolved in 10 ml. of saline and 1 ml. is injected intravenously at short intervals until the patient vomits. Once the stomach is empty, nausea is abolished and relatively safe induction of anæsthesia should follow.¶

The prevention of regurgitation by occlusion of the œsophagus by backward pressure on the cricoid has been recommended

* Clark, C. G., and Riddoch, M. E., *Brit. J. Anæsth.*, 1962, **34**, 875.
† Edwards, G., Morton, H. J. V., Pask, E. A., and Wylie, W. D., *Anæsthesia*, 1956, **11**, 194.
‡ Snow, R. G., and Nunn, J. F., *Brit. J. Anæsth.*, 1959, **31**, 493.
§ Bourne, J. G., *Proc. R. Soc. Med.*, 1954, **47**, 416.
‖ Bourne, J. G., *Anæsthesia*, 1962, **17**, 379.
¶ Holmes, J. M., *J. Obstet. Gynæc. Brit. Emp.*, 1956, **63**, 239.

during induction of anæsthesia. This method must not be used during active vomiting as it may lead to œsophageal rupture.*

A further method, based on œsophageal occlusion by a balloon catheter, has been described many times,† most recently by Zohairy‡ who recommends a Foley catheter number 26 Fr., which has a strong balloon of 30–100-ml. capacity. This is passed with or without pharyngeal topical analgesia into either the lower œsophagus or into the stomach before induction of anæsthesia and its cuff inflated; upward passage of stomach contents is said to be prevented during the dangerous interval between loss of consciousness and the inflation of a cuffed endotracheal tube.

There is no fool-proof method of prevention of aspiration of gastric contents into the lungs.

Heavy sedation may result in aspiration of stomach contents in the ward before operation.

TREATMENT.—*If vomiting occurs.* The air-passages must if possible be spared contamination by tilting the head downwards or turning the patient on one side. Suction must be used, and oxygen carried to the alveoli in the most efficient way that is possible under the circumstances. Endotracheal intubation should only be attempted if relaxation is present and the manœuvre likely to be quick and easy, otherwise hypoxia may be made worse rather than better. Should the airways be contaminated, then suction and gravity should be employed to lessen the extent of the insult to the bronchi. Endotracheal suction may be sufficient in mild cases, whereas in others, suction through a bronchoscope will be required. The passage of a double-lumen tube (e.g., Bryce-Smith) will enable bronchial lavage to be performed down each bronchus separately, while ventilation is maintained down the other.§ It may be combined with lavage, 10 ml. of saline being injected and aspirated via the bronchoscope, and repeated until the washings are clear. This should not be done immediately but after the patient has recovered from the immediate effects of the catastrophe. Aminophylline and other bronchodilators may be helpful, while antibiotics and physiotherapy have a place too. Hydrocortisone can be given intramuscularly and instilled into the bronchial tree, where it is said to be of more benefit than either normal saline or sodium bicarbonate solution.||

To lessen the dangers of vomiting during recovery, the patient should, whenever possible, be returned to the ward with the head tilted downwards in the so-called tonsillar position, lying on his side with the bottom arm behind him to prevent his turning on to his back, and with pillows under the chest, to prevent his rolling into the prone position.

---

* Sellick, B. A., *Lancet*, 1961, **2**, 404.
† Kausch, W., *Berl. klin. Wschr.*, 1903, **40**. 753; Macintosh, R. R., *Brit. med. J.*, 1951, **2**, 545; Gilman, S., and Abrams, A. L., *New Engl. J. Med.*, 1956, **255**, 508; and Bizzari, D., and others, *Curr. Res. Anesth.*, 1965, **44**, 365.
‡ Zohairy, A. F. M., *Brit. med. J.*, 1967, **1**, 546.
§ Edwards, E. M., and Hatch, D. J., *Anæsthesia*, 1965, **20**, 461.
|| Lewinski, A., *Anesthesiology*, 1965, **26**, 37.

2. Coughing.—Occurs most commonly when ether is used and when patient has chemical (e.g., due to heavy smoking), or infective inflammation of the upper air-passages.

Concentration of gases and vapour must be increased slowly. A few breaths of trichloroethylene or halothane aid in the introduction of ether.

Coughing may also cause trouble during anæsthesia with thiopentone ; this is best controlled by nitrous-oxide–oxygen and minimal trichloroethylene or halothane. It may be due to irritation of the larynx from regurgitated gastric material, from the use of artificial airways, or from saliva.

3. Excessive Mucus.—This can often be avoided by adequate pre-medication, together with smooth induction.

It should be treated by clearing out the mucus with swabs or a sucker, and rotating head to one side.

Stimulation of the pharyngeal and laryngeal reflexes, as by artificial airways, may produce excessive mucus, especially in babies and children. If the table is lowered, head down, mucus tends to drain away from the hypopharynx. Patients who are ' moist ' should be thoroughly sucked out at the end of the operation.

4. Respiratory Arrest.—Due to obstruction of the airway or to peripheral or central respiratory depression.

TREATMENT.—After establishing the airway, using an endotracheal tube if necessary, oxygen must be carried to the alveoli :—

1. By blowing air into the lungs from a face-piece or by using a mouth-to-airway method (two Guedel airways glued together by their proximal ends).*

2. By forcing oxygen into lungs from a reservoir bag of a gas machine, with manual pressure, after closure of the expiratory valve.

3. By mechanical respirator. Small portable instruments are now available for emergency ventilation, e.g., MinEpac (p. 217).

4. By Silvester's method of artificial respiration (1858), whereby inspiration is produced by raising the arms above the patient's head with the production of expansion of the thorax, and expiration is aided by compressing the arms against the chest.

5. By Schaefer's method of artificial respiration (1903), with the patient prone on the floor and the anæsthetist applying pressure to lower ribs. This is seldom of use in anæsthesia, except in dental cases.

6. By Eve's rocking method (1932).

7. By Holger Nielsen's method of artificial respiration, which, although unsuitable for use on the operating table, should be known to anæsthetists. The patient lies prone with arms overhead, elbows flexed, one hand on the other, the cheek resting on the uppermost hand. The operator kneels on one knee at the patient's head facing his feet. The operator now grasps the patient's arms just above the elbows, lifts them and

---

* Cox, J. M., Woolmer, R., and Thomas, V., *Lancet*, 1960, **1**, 727.

rocks the thorax backwards ; this allows inspiration to take place. The arms are then dropped, the operator placing his hands just below the scapulæ ; air is expressed from the thorax. The cycle is repeated about twelve times each minute, allowing no pause between inspiratory and expiratory manœuvres. This arm-lift back-pressure technique produces a tidal exchange more than double that produced by Schaefer's method, and blood-oxygen levels should approach 90 per cent of saturation. It can, in addition, be carried out by persons of frail physique.

If it is impossible to establish an airway by a pharyngeal or endotracheal tube, tracheostomy or laryngostomy may be necessary. *See* Chapter XXXIV.

5. Atelectasis.—This may occur fairly suddenly during or immediately after the anæsthesia. Its signs are progressive hypoxia and absence of breath-sounds over part of the lung area. The diaphragm rises to occupy the space vacated by the lung. It may be caused by reflex bronchiolar spasm which by cutting off the return of blood by the veins could result in œdema of the mucosa and bronchial obstruction. Clinically it is shown by increasing difficulty in breathing or in inflation of the lungs. If the chest is open, the infiltration of the lung hilum with a local analgesic solution may do good. Spontaneous atelectasis of the left lung can occur if the right bronchus is accidentally intubated. Miliary areas of atelectasis can occur during I.P.P.V. (*see* p. 209).

Treatment consists in inflation of the lungs, and, if necessary, bronchoscopic examination and suction of the upper air-passages.

Closed pneumothorax has been reported and is presumably due to :
(1) The rupture of lung tissue—the result of excessive coughing or of intermittent positive pressure respiration carried out too vigorously. The treatment is to aspirate air from the pleural cavity. (2) Operations on the neck associated with respiratory obstruction, which causes an increase in the negative pressure in the mediastinum during inspiration and consequent trapping of air. This trapped air may rupture into the pleura or spread into the soft tissues of the neck, axilla, face, or thoracic wall, or along aorta and œsophagus into the abdomen. It may have to be evacuated by blunt dissection into the mediastinum from an incision just above the manubrium sterni.

6. Surgical Emphysema during Anæsthesia.—This was first reported in 1912 (Woolsey)* during insufflation endotracheal anæsthesia. Surgical emphysema commences as a pulmonary interstitial emphysema due to overdistension of the alveoli, i.e., at a pressure greater than 20 mm. Hg. The gas tracks along the sheaths of the vessels to the hilum—mediastinal emphysema, from which it may spread (*a*) to the neck, (*b*) to the abdomen, (*c*) behind the peritoneum, (*d*) into the pleura (tension pneumothorax). Once the mediastinal pleura is ruptured very little extra pressure will force gases into the pleural cavity. Tension pneumothorax

---

* Woolsey, W. C., *N.Y. St. J. Med.*, 1912, **12**, 171.

Surgical Emphysema during Anæsthesia, *continued.*

should always be looked for if surgical emphysema appears. Mediastinal emphysema often causes a crunching sound when the stethoscope is applied to the left border of the heart—Hamman's sign.* Radiologically there may be a small air space running parallel to the left or right border of the heart. Causes of mediastinal emphysema, other than anæsthetic, include pulmonary emphysema, asthma, pneumonia, childbirth, rupture of an air-passage or of the œsophagus, and penetrating wounds of the chest. Should circulatory or respiratory difficulty arise in the presence of mediastinal emphysema, an incision should be made at the root of the neck anteriorly and gas should be let out by blunt dissection.†

7. Convulsions.—Several types of abnormal muscular action may occur during anæsthesia :—

1. Deep ether convulsions (*see* p. 172).
2. Ether clonus—usually occurring in light anæsthesia and disappearing when anæsthesia is deepened. Commonly seen in the legs and may be stopped by raising thighs, leaving legs unsupported, or by injecting a small dose of muscle relaxant.
3. Epilepsy. Intubation may be required to ensure oxygenation.
4. Convulsions due to hypoxia, e.g., during nitrous oxide anæsthesia : the so-called jactitations.
5. Convulsions due to local analgesic drugs, e.g., lignocaine, procaine, amethocaine. Treat with intravenous thiopentone and oxygen inhalations and/or suxamethonium.
6. Tremor associated with the intravenous injection of thiopentone, usually a pronator spasm of the arm receiving the injection. Addition of more thiopentone together with nitrous oxide and oxygen will usually cure the condition which is commoner after 5 per cent solution than 2½ per cent solution.

8. Hyperpyrexia.—This is a condition which has recently been described.‡ The temperature rises rapidly and death may ensue. The mechanism of this rare reaction is not understood, but there is an inherited factor, since it has occurred in members of the same family. There may be increased muscle tone.

9. Damage to Eyes.—May follow accidental instillation into conjunctival sac of ether, blood, antiseptic lotion, etc., splashed from the operation site.

May be due to trauma from tightly applied face-mask or friction from gauze or fingers.

The eyes should be closed, oiled, and protected suitably, especially where there is exophthalmos.

Pressure on the eyeballs, e.g., from a mask, prolonged hypotension, and steep Trendelenburg position have all been blamed for causing occlusion of the central artery of the retina.

10. Status Lymphaticus.—Paltauf (1889) was first to describe the syndrome in recent times, but it has been discovered, forgotten,

---

* Hamman, L., *Trans. Ass. Amer. Phycns.*, 1937, **52**, 311.
† Spence, M., *Anæsthesia*, 1955, **10**, 50.
‡ Relton, J. E. S., Creighton, R. E., and Conn, A. W., *Anæsthesia*, 1968, **23**, 253; and Stephen, C. R., *J. Amer. med. Ass.*, 1967, **202**, 178.

rediscovered, and declared to be non-existent* from 1614 onwards. A condition occurring in children of fat lymphoid type. The condition may be suspected if there is a history of attacks of fainting, with shortness of breath; attacks of head retraction and stridor; X-ray evidence of an enlarged thymus gland.

Pathologically, there may be enlargement of the thymus ; hypertrophy of lymphoid tissue and fatty degeneration of the heart, and possibly suprarenal cortical deficiency.

Such children may be very sensitive to anæsthetic agents, requiring amounts much less than normal, and it is advised that children who "go under" without any signs of resistance, and who require only small amounts of anæsthetic, should be treated with extra special care, lest sudden death result from overdosage. Ether is probably the safest anæsthetic for such cases.

Many pathologists consider that no such condition exists as a definite entity (Report of Status Lymphaticus Commission, 1931), but it is sometimes stated that sudden death during anæsthesia in children is due to status lymphaticus, whereas it may well be due to error of technique or judgement on the part of the anæsthetist and be, in fact, an anæsthetic fiction.

11. Acute Hypoxia.—This may be associated with cardiac arrest or may by good fortune stop short of this calamity. It is most likely to be due to inattention on the part of the anæsthetist. Signs after anæsthesia may be coma, stertorous breathing, hyperpyrexia, restlessness, choreo-athetosis, and convulsions. For treatment *see* Chapter XXXIV.

12. Circulatory Collapse.—This, when it occurs during anæsthesia, may be due to : (*a*) Primary cardiac failure, or (*b*) Secondary or gradual cardiac failure. Shock, hæmorrhage, fat or air embolus may also cause circulatory failure, while pulmonary or cardiac infarction, and massive collapse of the lung, must be borne in mind. *See* Chapter XXXIV for treatment of cardiac arrest.

13. Hypertension.—This may be due to mild respiratory obstruction in its early stages, to hypercapnia, to over-vigorous transfusion, to abuse of pressor drugs, or to an unsuspected phæochromocytoma.

14. Post-operative Respiratory Distress.†—This may be due to reflex spasm of the smaller bronchi as a result of too light a level of sensory anæsthesia during operation. It should be prevented by deeper anæsthesia.

---

* Medical Research Council (Status Lymphaticus Commission), *Brit. med. J.*, 1931, **1**, 468.
†Gardiner, A. S., *Anæsthesia*, 1960, **15**, 246.

CHAPTER X

GASES USED IN ASSOCIATION WITH ANÆSTHESIA

OXYGEN [O_2]

Historical.—John Mayow* (1674) of Oxford showed that a component of air was used up by a burning candle or a live mouse. Priestley† (1772) discovered 'dephlogisticated air'. Lavoisier gave it the name 'oxygen' ('acid-producer'). Lavoisier and Laplace‡ were the first to show a quantitative relation between the heat production of animals and that resulting from combustion of carbon. They demonstrated a relationship between oxygen used and carbon dioxide produced. Liebig§ (1851) showed that carbohydrates and fats were important substrates and not carbon itself. Beddoes used oxygen in medical treatment in 1794 at Bristol.

Modern use of oxygen was popularized in 1917 by J. S. Haldane (1860–1936) during the First World War,‖ and by Yandell Henderson, the New Haven physiologist (1873–1944).

Preparation.—
1. The fractional distillation of liquid air (nitrogen comes off first), prepared by pressure and heat abstraction (Linde, 1895). Boiling point of oxygen −182·5° C.; of nitrogen −195° C.
2. The electrolysis of water.
3. The Le Brin process of heating barium oxide (BaO) to 500° C., so forming barium peroxide BaO_2, which is heated still more—to 800° C.—when it parts with oxygen, becoming barium oxide again.

Oxygen is supplied in cylinders, at a pressure of 132 atmospheres (1940 lb. per sq. in.). In the cylinder it is in the gaseous state. The gas is compressed to occupy 0·5 per cent of its volume at atmospheric pressure.

One volume of liquid oxygen is equivalent to 840 volumes of gas.

Cylinders are painted black with white shoulders.

Properties.—Molecular weight 32. Solubility in water at 37° C., 2·4 volumes per cent ; in water at 0° C., 4·9 volumes per cent. Specific gravity 1105 (air is 1000). Electric sparks convert it into ozone (O_3).

With oil or grease, oxygen under high pressure will cause an ignition. It encourages fires, although not itself flammable. Oxygen (and nitrous oxide) cylinders should be turned on outside

---

* Mayow, J., *Tractatus Quinque Medico-physici*, No. 2, 1674. Oxford.
† Priestley, J., *Phil. Trans.*, 1772, **52**, 147.
‡ Lavoisier, A., and Laplace, P. S., *Mém. prés. Acad. Sci.*, Paris, 1780, **103**, 566.
§ van Liebig, J., *Letters on Chemistry*, 3rd ed., 1851.
‖ Haldane, J. S., *Brit. med. J.*, 1917, **1**, 181.

the operating theatre, brought in faintly hissing, so that when reducing valve is connected, pressure is not built up in it suddenly, but gradually. At other times when the cylinders are turned on, the flow-meters should themselves be on. It is rapidly absorbed from the alveoli; this may be an argument for leaving an inert gas (nitrogen or helium) in the lungs after operation in order to prevent atelectasis after complete absorption of oxygen. Oxygen diffuses from an alveolus whose bronchus is blocked in 15 minutes. Nitrogen diffuses in 16 hours.

Some Relevant Physiological Data.—Oxygen content of air 20·93 per cent. Oxygen content of expired air 16·3 per cent. Oxygen content of alveolar air 14·2 per cent. Partial pressure of oxygen in air 160 mm. Hg. Partial pressure of oxygen in alveolar air 104 mm. Hg. Partial pressure of oxygen in venous blood 40 mm. Hg. Solubility of oxygen in arterial blood 0·3 ml. per 100 ml. Oxygen capacity of hæmoglobin 1·34 ml. per g. Hb. Oxygen capacity of arterial blood 19·8 vols. per cent. Oxygen saturation of arterial blood 97 per cent. Oxygen tension of arterial blood 100 mm. Hg.

Types of Oxygen Lack.—Oxygen lack not only stops the machine, but wrecks the machinery (J. S. Haldane). Hypoxia or anoxia is oxygen lack in tissues. Anoxæmia is oxygen lack in the blood.

Hypoxia	Oxygen Capacity	Arterial Oxygen		Venous Oxygen		Arteriovenous Difference
		Content	Tension	Content	Tension	
Hypoxic	Normal	Decreased	Decreased	Decreased	Decreased	Decreased
Anæmic	Decreased	Decreased	Normal	Decreased	Decreased	Decreased
Stagnant	Normal	Normal	Normal	Decreased	Decreased	Increased
Histotoxic	Normal	Normal	Normal	Increased	Increased	Decreased

Modified from Myer Saklad.*

Reduced utilization of oxygen by tissues may be of the following types: (1) Hypoxic (low arterial Po_2); (2) Anæmic (normal Po_2 but low hæmoglobin content); (3) Stagnant (normal Po_2 but slow blood-flow); (4) Histotoxic (normal Po_2 but poisoning of the cytochrome enzyme system of cellular oxidation). The first three were described by Joseph Barcroft† (1872–1947) (1920), the fourth by Peters and van Slyke‡ (1931).

1. HYPOXIC HYPOXIA.—Occurs when partial pressure of oxygen in blood is reduced. Saklad further subdivided this group into (a) atmospheric; (b) tidal; (c) alveolar. Seen in anæsthesia when oxygen tension of lung gases is deliberately cut down;

---

* Saklad, Myer, *Inhalation Therapy and Resuscitation*, 1953, p. 33. Springfield, Ill.: Thomas.
† Barcroft, J., *Lancet*, 1920, **2**, 485.
‡ Peters, J. P., and van Slyke, D. D., *Quantitative Clinical Chemistry*, 1932, Vol. 2, p. 579. Baltimore: Williams and Wilkins.

Types of Oxygen Lack, *continued.*

when airway is obstructed, respiratory muscles or respiratory centre are depressed; when there are changes in ventilation perfusion relationships in the lung, as after subcutaneous atropine, post-operatively, in emphysema and atelectasis; in the presence of pulmonary œdema, alveolar mucus, pneumothorax, hydrothorax, increased intra-abdominal pressure splinting the diaphragm, diffuse pulmonary hæmorrhages in blast injury. It is the type seen at high altitudes and in congenital heart disease with shunting of venous blood to the left side of heart, and conditions in which blood is circulating through unaerated alveoli. It is present during internal paradoxical respiration when there is an open pneumothorax.

The oxygen saturation of the arterial blood is reduced from its normal of 97 per cent while the oxygen content normally 19·8 vols. per cent is also reduced.

2. ANÆMIC HYPOXIA.—The oxygen content is reduced. Oxygen-carrying capacity of blood is reduced in proportion to degree of anæmia although the blood oxygen tension (Po_2) is normal. Also in carbon monoxide poisoning, when the affinity of hæmoglobin for carbon monoxide is several hundred times that for oxygen.

3. STAGNANT HYPOXIA.*—Occurs when circulation is slowed so that in spite of adequate oxygen saturation and oxygen tension of arterial blood, each red cell gives up a larger part of its oxygen owing to its longer stay in the capillaries. The oxygen content of venous blood is reduced. Typically seen in surgical shock and cardiac failure, in peripheral vascular disease, cerebral and coronary thrombosis, etc. Can occur in local areas such as finger-nails, owing to cold ; seen in obstruction to venous return of skin of face and forehead produced by anæsthetic harness.

4. HISTOTOXIC HYPOXIA.—Occurs when tissues are unable to utilize the normal supply of oxygen brought to them ; seen in cyanide poisoning and overdosage of narcotics and anæsthetics due to interference with dehydrogenase systems ; and when there is œdema of a tissue, œdema interfering with diffusion of oxygen from capillaries to tissue cells. The arterial oxygen content and tension are normal and the venous oxygen saturation is higher than normal.

Demand hypoxia is seen in hyperpyrexia and hyperthyroidism.

Diffusion hypoxia† may occur during recovery from nitrous oxide anæsthesia when the gas may diffuse into the alveoli in such volumes as to account for 12 per cent of the expired atmosphere ; this may so dilute the inspired air as to seriously reduce the oxygen saturation and so may prove dangerous to a handicapped patient, e.g., after pneumonectomy, in coronary disease, where there is residual respiratory depression. The remedy is to give oxygen in high concentration towards the end of the anæsthesia and for some time after its termination.

---

* Barcroft, J., *Nature*, 1920, **106**, 125.
† Fink, B. R., *Anesthesiology*, 1955, **16**, 511.

Diagnosis of Hypoxia.—The oxygen tension of the blood can be measured by polarography (oxygen electrode). Gas chromatography can also be used for blood-gas analysis.* Oximetry is used to measure oxygen saturation (*see* Chapter XXXIII).

Hypoxia can be suspected if the pulse-rate slows down ten or more beats within a few seconds of the administration of 100 per cent oxygen.

Central cyanosis occurs when oxygen saturation falls to about 75 per cent,† or when 3·3–5 g. reduced hæmoglobin are circulating in the blood. In anæmic states considerable falls in oxygen content can occur without cyanosis. In polycythæmic conditions cyanosis may be present without significant reduction in oxygen-carrying capacity. Cyanosis is therefore not always a reliable sign of hypoxia.

THE EFFECTS OF OXYGEN WANT.—There is considerable individual variation in this.

1. THE RESPIRATORY SYSTEM.—Hyperpnœa, which only appears if the oxygen percentage is below 16 per cent : it varies with individuals, and is due to reflex stimulation of respiratory centre by chemoreceptors in aortic and carotid bodies which react to the lowered oxygen tension, but not to a lowered oxygen content (as seen in anæmia and in carbon monoxide poisoning). The glomeric cells normally have a high oxygen uptake; when tension falls, anaerobic metabolism causes the release of substances which stimulate pericellular chemosensory nerve-endings.‡ The respiratory centre becomes less sensitive to carbon dioxide with increasing hypoxia. Dyspnœa and hyperpnœa are not necessarily indications for oxygen therapy, as both may be seen without hypoxia, just as hypoxia can occur without these symptoms.

2. THE CARDIOVASCULAR SYSTEM.—The coronary and cerebral vessels dilate, blood-pressure and pulse-rate are increased at first ; later they both decrease—the so-called hypoxic pressor and depressor phases. The E.C.G. T wave becomes inverted or decreased and there is slowing of conduction and a lengthening of the P–R interval. Capillaries lose their tone and their walls allow the leakage of fluid and cells into the tissues.

3. THE CENTRAL NERVOUS SYSTEM.—The nervous tissue is more susceptible to oxygen want than any tissue in the body. The blood-flow to the brain is increased, an effect also produced by the raised carbon dioxide tension which is often concurrent. Later œdema of the brain results from capillary damage. The C.S.F. pressure is increased. Vomiting may occur. Following acute or prolonged chronic hypoxia the following may be seen :§ (*a*) Acute psychoses ; (*b*) Increased psychomotor activity ; (*c*) Decerebrate states ; (*d*) Psychoneurotic states ; (*e*) Chronic psychotic states ; (*f*) Parkinsonism ; (*g*) Blindness or visual agnosia.

---

* Fothergill, W. T., *Proc. R. Soc. Med.*, 1968, **61**, 525.
† Meda, W. E., French, E. B., and Wylie, V. McA., *Thorax*, 1959, **14**, 247.
‡ Joels, N., and Neil, E., *Brit. med. Bull.*, 1963, **19**, 21.
§ Courville, C. B., *Med. Arts Sci.*, 1947, **1**, 1.

Diagnosis of Hypoxia, *continued.*

4. THE LIVER.—Inability to deaminate amino-acids ; damage to cells. Vasodepressor material (V.D.M.) formed in liver and muscles which interferes with capillary tone is destroyed in the presence of oxygen by vaso-excitor material (V.E.M.) formed in kidneys. V.D.M. accumulates during periods of hypoxia. The blood-sugar is raised.

5. THE KIDNEYS.—Hypoxia tolerated fairly well.

Causes of Hypoxia during Anæsthesia.—

1. Low oxygen percentage in inspired atmosphere.
2. Respiratory obstruction.
3. Deficient tidal exchange which causes dead space gases to be moved to and fro along gas tubes and air-passages.
4. Changes in ventilation perfusion relationships in the lung, which may arise after subcutaneous atropine due to atelectasis, or during the course of anæsthesia, and persist into the post-operative period.*
5. Delayed diffusion in lungs, because of abnormality of pulmonary epithelium or to mucus overlying it.
6. Shock and hæmorrhage.

Oxygen at 30–35 per cent may not be sufficient to maintain oxygenation during anæsthesia, particularly in elderly patients or those with pulmonary disease. Pulmonary hyperventilation may exacerbate this. The effects of diffusion hypoxia may be severe but can be largely avoided if 100 per cent oxygen is given for 5 min. at the end of the anæsthetic administration.†

Hypoxia depresses respiratory centre but may, if not great, stimulate the chemoreceptors of the carotid and aortic bodies with production of increase in rate and depth of breathing. This secondary stimulation disappears with the onset of gross hypoxia.

Post-mortem Changes caused by Hypoxia.—Brain : Punctate hæmorrhages in cortex and venous congestion in pia and basal ganglia. Microscopic changes in cells of cortex and basal ganglia : Necrosis of the third layer of the cerebral cortex, Purkinje cells, striate body, and globus pallidus ; necrosis of the thalamus. Hæmorrhages into epicardium and aorta ; systemic and pulmonary venous congestion ; congestion of submucosa of stomach and gut ; kidneys, liver.

OXYGEN THERAPY

The fundamental aim of oxygen therapy is to restore the tissue oxygen towards normal. A partial pressure of at least 10 mm. Hg is required at the cellular mitochondria.‡ An increase in the percentage of oxygen in the inhaled gases results in a rise in alveolar oxygen concentration and a rise in oxygen tension in the blood leaving the lungs. Oxygen therapy is most valuable when the blood oxygen tension is low (hypoxic hypoxia). In anæmic and stagnant hypoxia it does not greatly increase the amount of oxygen carried by hæmoglobin, though

* Tomlin, P. J., Conway, C. M., and Payne, J. P., *Lancet*, 1964, **1**, 14.
† Marshall, B. E., and Millar, R. A., *Anæsthesia*, 1965, **20**, 408.
‡ Flenley, D. C., *Lancet*, 1967, **1**, 270.

the rise in dissolved oxygen in the plasma is significant. It is doubtful whether histotoxic hypoxia is benefited by oxygen therapy.

Oxygen Tension and Hæmoglobin Saturation.—Examination of the dissociation curve (*Fig.* 2, p. 57) shows the relationship between oxygen tension and hæmoglobin saturation.* It will be seen that oxygen tension can fall considerably before there is an appreciable fall in saturation. Oxygen therapy can do little to increase hæmoglobin saturation unless the tension is already low.

The dissociation curve is shifted to the right in respiratory acidosis and to the left in hypothermia. Fœtal hæmoglobin has a dissociation curve shifted to the left, to aid the uptake of oxygen from the maternal blood.

Oxygen Availability.—The amount of oxygen available in the body can be calculated as follows: 100 ml. blood contains 19·8 ml. oxygen when fully oxygenated. If the cardiac output is 5 litres per min., then the oxygen available to the body is 19·8 × 50 = 990 ml. per min.

THE EFFECTS OF INHALATION OF 100 PER CENT OXYGEN.
Oxygen Carriage in the Blood (see p. 57).

Nitrogen is eliminated from the lungs in 2 min., from the blood in 5 min., from the brain in 20 min., and from the body in about 2 hours.

Carbon Dioxide.—As reduced hæmoglobin aids in the transport of carbon dioxide, inhalation of 100 per cent oxygen, by lessening the amount of reduced hæmoglobin, interferes with the transport of carbon dioxide, especially if the gas is given at a raised pressure.

Respiration.—This is often slightly depressed at first, owing to the removal of the stimulating effect through chemoreceptors. Later there may be some stimulation, because oxygen stimulates the mucosa of the lower respiratory tract, and by dilating pulmonary capillaries causes slight pulmonary congestion and hence respiratory stimulation.

Circulation.—There is decrease in the pulse-rate, from chemoreceptor effect. Cardiac output is lessened owing to effect both on rate and stroke volume. Slight increase in diastolic blood-pressure. Blood-vessels directly constricted; reflexly, via chemoreceptors, dilated—former effect predominating. Cerebral vessels constrict, coronary vessels also constrict, but pulmonary artery dilates, constricting in hypoxia. Very prolonged administration of oxygen may interfere with red-cell formation.

Physical Effects.—There may be rapid absorption of gas from the alveoli, leading to atelectasis; from the middle ear, leading to retraction of the drum if there is in addition obstruction of the Eustachian tube; from the nasal sinuses, causing headache.

ADVERSE EFFECTS OF HIGH OXYGEN CONCENTRATIONS.
CHRONIC BRONCHITIS AND EMPHYSEMA.—In patients who develop respiratory failure, oxygen is needed to correct hypoxia, but it

---

Oxygen Availability, *continued.*

must be given in a controlled manner otherwise a dangerous rise in arterial Pco_2 may occur. Chronic respiratory inadequacy results in elevation of arterial Pco_2, to which the patient acquires a tolerance. Respiratory activity becomes almost completely dependent on hypoxic drive. If the patient then develops an acute chest infection, acute respiratory failure may occur with hypoxia and further rise of Pco_2. Indiscriminate administration of oxygen may then remove the hypoxic drive so that respiration becomes depressed and Pco_2 rises still further. The danger is that a state of CO_2 narcosis may develop with loss of consciousness and ultimately death. The risk of this chain of events is said to be greater when arterial Pco_2 is already above 70 mm. Hg.

Controlled oxygen therapy is required. The aim is to give enough oxygen to relieve hypoxia, but not enough to remove the respiratory drive. The characteristics of the dissociation curve for hæmoglobin are such that a relatively small rise in oxygen tension will result in a relatively large increase in saturation in the middle part of the curve.

Campbell* recommends the administration of oxygen whenever there is a possibility of hypoxia in any patient with chronic lung disease. Arterial Pco_2 is estimated by the rebreathing method before commencing therapy. If the tension is over 50 mm. Hg, 25 per cent oxygen is given, and the concentration gradually increased if respiration is not depressed. Oxygen must be given continuously. Intermittent oxygen therapy is particularly dangerous since the increased alveolar CO_2 concentration which may then occur results in an even lower O_2 concentration when the patient breathes air.

Some workers† believe that it is necessary to undertake arterial blood-gas monitoring in these patients. The aim is to achieve an oxygen tension of at least 50 mm. Hg, without allowing the pH to fall below 7·25.

Should oxygen administration, however carefully regulated, fail to correct hypoxia without depressing respiration, then intermittent positive-pressure ventilation becomes necessary, usually after tracheostomy.

When a patient with chronic emphysema or similar complaint is to be anæsthetized, the immediate administration of high oxygen atmospheres, as with halothane or cyclopropane, is not always wise as apnœa may occur early.

FOLLOWING HYPOXIA.—The oxygen paradox was first described by Ruff and Strughold in 1939. Has subsequently been re-examined by Latham.‡ It is a temporary blackout due to the sudden administration of a high oxygen atmosphere, seen in airmen. If the gas is first inhaled at low tensions, and later gradually increased, ill effects are not seen.

* Campbell, E. J. M., *Lancet*, 1960, **2**, 10; and Campbell, E. J. M., *Brit. med. J.*, 1964, **2**, 630.
† Hutchinson, D. C. S., Flenley, D. C., and Donald, K. W., *Ibid.*, 1964, **2**, 1159.
‡ Latham, F., *Lancet*, 1951, **1**, 77.

RETROLENTAL FIBROPLASIA.*—The formation of a fibrovascular membrane, posterior to the lens, may occur in premature babies who have been exposed to high concentrations of oxygen causing an oxygen saturation of the blood greater than the normal 95 per cent. (There are other causes of this condition.) Premature babies should only receive oxygen if they are cyanosed, and then no more than 40 per cent concentration for as short a time as possible.

OXYGEN POISONING.†—*Acute* oxygen poisoning is manifest as convulsions.‡ These are similar in nature to idiopathic epilepsy, and do not occur except under hyperbaric conditions (3 atmospheres). The causes have not been fully elucidated, though the incidence appears to be related to an increased cerebral Pco_2.§ *Chronic* poisoning may occur when concentrations over 70 per cent are inhaled for prolonged periods at atmospheric pressure. Untoward effects reported include substernal distress, reduction in vital capacity, paræsthesia, joint pains, anorexia, nausea, contracted visual fields, vomiting, bronchitis, and atelectasis, and mental changes, first described in 1938.‖

While in a healthy person inspiration of 100 per cent oxygen may be harmful if continued for more than a few hours, 40 per cent can be inhaled indefinitely, with impunity.

INDICATIONS.—The relief of all forms of hypoxia other than histotoxic.

1. Cyanosis of recent origin. Acute heart failure, acute pulmonary œdema (should be given under positive pressure of 4 cm. of water), pneumonia, atelectasis, pulmonary embolism, etc. Venous to arterial shunts, intracardiac or intrapulmonary, are the only types of hypoxæmia not completely corrected by the inhalation of 100 per cent oxygen.

2. Following chest wounds, rib fractures, or major operations.

3. In shock and severe hæmorrhage and coronary occlusion. The central feature of shock is diminished cardiac output leading to reduction in cellular oxygenation. The stagnant hypoxia may be complicated by hypoxic hypoxia and anæmic hypoxia. In shock there is an increase in physiological dead space and a compensatory hyperventilation. Reduction of this hyperventilation by airway obstruction, chest injuries, drugs, etc., may be dangerous. Oxygen administration may prevent the vicious circles which end in death.¶

4. To decompress distended bowels, reduce surgical emphysema, pneumothorax, air embolism. The gas imprisoned in these cases is 70 per cent nitrogen. Prolonged inhalation of 100 per

* Campbell, K., *Med. J. Aust.*, 1951, **2**, 48; Forrester, R. M., and others, *Lancet*, 1954, **2**, 258; and Kinsey, V. E., *Arch. Ophthal.*, 1956, **56**, 481.
† Donald, K. W., *Brit. med. J.*, 1947, **1**, 667 and 712.
‡ Thompson, W. A. R., *Ibid.*, 1935, **2**, 208.
§ Bennett, P. B., in *A Symposium on Oxygen Measurements in Blood and Tissues and their Significance* (Ed. Payne, J. P., and Hill, D. W.), 1966, p. 41. London: Churchill.
‖ Barach, A. L., *Ann. intern. Med.*, 1938, **12**, 454.
¶ Brooks, D. K., Williams, W. G., Manley, R. W., and Whiteman, P., *Anæsthesia*, 1963, **18**, 363; and Freeman, J., in *A Symposium on Oxygen Measurements in Blood and Tissues and their Significance* (Ed. Payne, J. P., and Hill, D. W.), 1966, p. 221. London: Churchill.

Oxygen Availability, *continued.*

cent oxygen reduces the nitrogen tension in the blood, so that the molecules of gas in the tissues diffuse into the blood and are carried away.

5. When metabolic rate is raised, e.g., in post-operative thyrotoxicosis and hyperthermia, because in these conditions the demand for oxygen is increased.

6. In ill patients with liver damage, in the immediate post-operative period.

7. In carbon monoxide poisoning. Carbon monoxide is dangerous because : (*a*) Hæmoglobin has several hundred times greater affinity for it than for oxygen ; (*b*) Carboxyhæmoglobin alters the dissociation curve of the remaining oxyhæmoglobin, interfering with oxygen release to the tissues. Thus with a 50 per cent saturation of the blood with carboxyhæmoglobin the degree of hypoxia is greater than it would be in a simple anæmia with hæmoglobin reduced to 50 per cent of normal ; (*c*) Carbon monoxide may have a toxic effect of its own.

Treatment of Carbon Monoxide Poisoning.—This is designed to remove carbon monoxide from the body via the lungs. Oxygen given under pressure of 2 atmospheres increases the amount of oxygen dissolved in the plasma, circumvents the ill-effects of carboxyhæmoglobin on oxygen liberation, and hastens removal of carbon monoxide from combination with hæmoglobin.[*] More orthodox treatment consists in giving oxygen with 5–7 per cent carbon dioxide.[†] To maintain adequate ventilation, artificial respiration may be necessary.

If the patient has good respiratory exchange 30 min. after removal from the atmosphere containing carbon monoxide, there is little evidence that any form of active treatment will affect the ultimate prognosis, although he may remain unconscious for several days and require careful nursing supervision. In severe cases there may be residual neurological changes (confusional states).[‡]

8. As a routine following major operations to prevent fall in arterial oxygen saturation.[§]

9. In cases of severe headache due to retained intracranial air following encephalography. In migraine to produce vasoconstriction of cerebral vessels.

10. To assist denitrogenation before pure nitrous-oxide–oxygen anæsthesia.

Commercial oxygen is pure enough for inhalation and is much cheaper than medicinal oxygen. Oxygen therapy presents a definite fire hazard. In all cases it is important to see that a patent airway exists. At a height of 52,000 ft., oxygen pressure is one-tenth that at sea level. At 33,000 ft., one-quarter ; at

[*] Lawson, D. D., and others, *Lancet*, 1961, **1**, 800 ; and Smith, G., and Sharp, G. R., *Ibid.*, 1960, **2**, 905.
[†] Medical Research Council Report, *Brit. med. J.*, 1958, **2**, 1408 ; and Marriott, H. L., *Ibid.*, 1958, **2**, 1591.
[‡] Annotation, *Lancet*, 1962, **2**, 546.
[§] Conway, C. M., and Payne, J. P., *Brit. med. J.*, 1963, **1**, 844.

18,000 ft., one-half. Above 10,000 ft. symptoms of hypoxia appear.

A suggested new development is to utilize, at high altitudes, oxygen liberated by algæ under the influence of light.

MEASUREMENT.—This can be effected by :—

1. Dial flow-meters.
2. Any simple bobbin type flow-meter.
3. An anæsthetic machine.
4. The Cowan and Mitchell Injector (1942).* The air entrainment duct is covered by a rotating disk which has holes of varying size drilled in it, the size of the hole governing the volume of air mixed with oxygen. Between 40 per cent and 100 per cent of oxygen can be given and is led with air to a reservoir bag with non-return valves. No rebreathing takes place.

TECHNIQUE.—Modern oxygen therapy requires separate devices for administering oxygen in high and low concentration. A high dosage can be given to a patient whose breathing is not depressed by nasal catheter or by face-mask. Low doses are required in the treatment of hypoxia due to chronic lung disease, when there is a danger of further depression of respiration.

1. A NASAL CATHETER.—Size 9 (Jacques) is suitable, and its terminal 3–4 in. should be smeared with analgesic cream. The distal end lies in the nasopharynx. With it an oxygen flow of 3 litres a minute raises the alveolar oxygen from 14 per cent to 27 per cent. A flow of 5 litres per minute, which is uncomfortable for the conscious patient, raises the alveolar oxygen to 38 per cent. A humidifier should be used.†

2. Plastic nasal cannulæ are now available—the Addis‡ (Portex Ltd.).

3. Tudor Edwards's spectacle frame catheter carrier—now seldom used.

4. B.L.B. MASK.—The oronasal and the nasal types. Face-pieces may be of rubber or plastic. Two sizes in each type. The oxygen flow must be sufficient to prevent collapse of the bag at the end of inspiration. Useful for prolonged administration though has a large dead space and should not be used in those patients who are liable to carbon dioxide narcosis.

5. THE POLYTHENE DISPOSABLE MASK (Polymask) with its two communicating compartments, one to breathe into, the other to breathe out of. With a flow-rate of 8 litres a minute, an alveolar concentration of 50–60 per cent can be obtained but dead space is significant, and carbon dioxide is liable to rise. Suitable for delivery of high concentrations of oxygen (in the absence of hypercapnia).

6. EDINBURGH MASK§ (B.O.C.).—This is a semi-rigid mask designed to give controlled oxygen at low concentrations. With a flow-rate varying from 1 to 3 litres per minute, an alveolar concentration between 23 and 40 per cent can be obtained.

* Cowan, S. L., and Mitchell, J. V., *Brit. med. J.*, 1942, **1**, 118.
† Miller, W. F., *Anesthesiology*, 1962, **23**, 445.
‡ Addis, G. J., *Lancet*, 1963, **1**, 1084.
§ Flenley, D. C., Hutchison, D. C. S., and Donald, K. W., *Brit. med. J.*, 1963, **2**, 1081.

Oxygen Availability, *continued.*

The oxygen concentration varies according to flow-rate and pulmonary ventilation.

7. VENTIMASK (Oxygenaire).—Oxygen is entrained in air on the Venturi principle to provide a concentration of 27 per cent. The Venturi method is useful for providing controlled oxygen concentrations irrespective of flow-rate, such as is required in the treatment of chronic lung disease.*

8. THE PORTABLE OXYGEN APPARATUS.—This can be used in the patient's own home for use when climbing stairs, etc.† The weight is between 2 and 4 lb. and the capacity 100–120 litres; the flow-rate varies between 2 and 4 litres per minute and the cylinders can be refilled from standard oxygen cylinders. An example is the B.O.C. Portogen.

9. AN OXYGEN CHAMBER OR TENT.—This is best for babies and young children, and when prolonged administration is necessary.   It is the only means of giving oxygen to sleeping patients.   To enable real benefit to be obtained from a tent, it must be flushed with 10 litres per minute of oxygen and maintained with a flow of 8 litres per minute.   It gives lower levels of oxygen saturation than the various masks and spectacles.‡

A recent study of different methods of oxygen administration has been carried out.§ Patients find nasal cannulæ more comfortable than face-masks. The latter are likely to be hot and sweaty and patients cannot eat or spit. Oxygen tents held little advantage and the patient was less accessible and less easy to observe. With the Polymask or Pneumask at least 6 litres per minute were necessary to prevent the mask being sucked onto the face. This flow delivered an oxygen concentration of 60 per cent, too high for the patient with elevated Pco_2, but at 8 litres per minute flow they provided a concentration of 80 per cent suitable for treatment of cardiogenic shock. Nasal cannulæ were only comfortable when low flows (below 4 litres per minute) providing 40 per cent oxygen for inhalation. Cannulæ, the Edinburgh mask, and the Ventimask were without significant rebreathing. Oxygen given by cannula requires humidification. The patient with hypercapnia can be treated by nasal oxygen at 1 litre per minute or by Ventimask. If serious hypercapnia is present (over 70 mm. Hg) assisted ventilation is likely to be required. *See also* a study of dead space in various types of mask.‖

It has been suggested that hydrogen peroxide can be used for the oxygenation of bank blood.¶ Hydrogen peroxide is injected directly into the blood bottle through the rubber bung. One ml. of 30 per cent (100 vol.) solution contains enough oxygen to saturate more than 1·5 litres of venous blood.

* Campbell, E. J. M., and Gebbie, T., *Lancet,* 1966, **1**, 468.
† Cotes, J. E., and Gilson, J. C., *Ibid.,* 1956, **2**, 823.
‡ Ball, J. A. C., *Brit. J. Anæsth.,* 1963, **35**, 368 and 441.
§ Green, I. D., *Brit. med. J.,* 1967, **2**, 593.
‖ Bethune, D. W., and Collis, J. M., *Anæsthesia,* 1967, **22**, 43.
¶ White, D. C., and Teasdale, P. R., *Brit. J. Anæsth.,* 1966, **38**, 339.

Stored blood contains much less oxygen than venous blood and oxygen content falls during storage. There may be an application of hydrogen peroxide in systems such as the pump oxygenator.

OXYGEN AT HIGH PRESSURE.—

Solution of Oxygen in Plasma.—Breathing air, 100 ml. of plasma will dissolve 0·3 ml. of oxygen. For each 100 mm. Hg of oxygen tension 0·3 vol. per cent oxygen is dissolved in the plasma. Breathing 100 per cent oxygen, 100 ml. of plasma will thus dissolve 2·1 ml. of oxygen. Breathing 100 per cent oxygen at 2 atmospheres, 100 ml. of plasma will dissolve 4·2 ml. of oxygen. Breathing 100 per cent oxygen at 3 atmospheres, 100 ml. of plasma will dissolve 6·5 ml. of oxygen.

An efficient and rapid method of restoring cellular oxygenation is to give the gas under pressure. At 2 atmospheres' pressure, although the oxygen carried as oxyhæmoglobin will only increase by 1 vol. per cent, the gas carried in solution in the plasma rises from 0·3 to 4·2 vols. per cent. The pressure gradient is greatly increased between the arterial and the hypoxic tissue tension and this allows an increased rate of oxygen transport from blood to cells.

Vascular resistance is increased during hyperbaric oxygenation, especially in the brain and pulmonary circulation.

Oxygen at high pressure can be given from a pressure chamber into which patient and attendants enter. The patient then receives oxygen from an ordinary mask and cylinder. A pressure of 2 atmospheres is generally employed. Otherwise the hyperbaric oxygen bed can be used. This consists of a steel chamber with perspex dome in which the patient lies. Rate of compression and decompression is controlled from an adjacent console.

High-pressure Oxygen in Medical Conditions.—

1. In treatment of carbon-monoxide poisoning.[*]
2. In treatment of cerebral œdema associated with acute hypoxia, e.g., after cardiac arrest.
3. In the treatment of infections by anaerobic organisms, e.g., gas gangrene. The growth of aerobic organisms may also be inhibited.[†]
4. In the treatment of myocardial infarction,[‡] especially in the presence of acute pulmonary œdema.
5. In neonatal asphyxia, using a small hyperbaric oxygen chamber,[§] though work on experimental animals suggests that respiratory and metabolic acidosis are not corrected.[||]
6. In incipient gangrene and following intra-arterial injection of thiopentone.

[*] Smith, G., Ledingham, I. M., Sharp, G. R., Norman, J. N., and Bates, E. H., *Lancet*, 1962, **1**, 816.
[†] Sharp, G. R., Ledingham, I. M., and Norman, J. N., *Anæsthesia*, 1962, **17**, 136.
[‡] Moon, A. J., Williams, K. G., and Hopkinson, W. I., *Lancet*, 1964, **1**, 18.
[§] Hutchinson, J. H., Kerr, M. M., Williams, K. G., and Hopkinson, W. I., *Ibid.*, 1963, **2**, 1019.
[||] Barrie, H., and Miller, G., *Ibid.*, 1966, **2**, 1394; Denison, D. M., Ernshing, J., and Cresswell, A. W., *Ibid.*, 1966, **2**, 1404; and Cameron, A. J. V., and others, *Ibid.*, 1966, **2**, 833.

Oxygen Availability, *continued.*

7. In chronic osteomyelitis.*
Cases of respiratory failure in chronic chest disease are unsuitable for such treatment as it may result in respiratory acidosis leading to coma.

ELIMINATION OF CARBON DIOXIDE.†—During hyperbaric oxygenation, hæmoglobin remains fully saturated, even in the venous blood. The buffering capacity of the blood is not increased by the presence of desaturated hæmoglobin. Carbon dioxide is therefore transported in venous blood at a higher cost in terms of Pco_2. Arteriovenous difference in Pco_2, normally 6 mm. Hg, rises from 10 to 12 mm. Hg. The rise in venous and tissue Pco_2 occurs also at the respiratory centre to produce an increase in ventilation. The fall in arterial Pco_2 which results compensates in part for the raised tissue Pco_2 and is probably partly responsible for the cerebral vasoconstriction which occurs with hyperbaric oxygen.

The finding of a significant rise in Pco_2 of the blood during exercise in the hyperbaric chamber has little to do with the above. It is due rather to the increased density of the inhaled gas mixture, and occurs with both air and oxygen under pressure. The resistance to gas flow is such that there is an increase in the work of breathing. The body adapts by lowering alveolar ventilation and allowing a higher Pco_2.

SURGICAL OPERATIONS UNDER HIGH OXYGEN PRESSURE.‡— Professor Boerema, of Amsterdam, has given oxygen at 3 atmospheres' pressure using a cylindrical steel room, with air-locks for entrance and exit of patient, staff, and equipment. This method enables oxygen to be carried in solution in the plasma in sufficient quantity to supply the tissues, without utilizing hæmoglobin as an oxygen carrier. Circulation can be arrested for twice as long as is possible at normal atmospheric pressure with a moderate hypothermia of 29° C. The problems of anæsthesia under hyperbaric conditions are discussed in Chapter XXX.

HIGH PRESSURE OXYGEN DURING RADIOTHERAPY.§—There is evidence that the success of radiotherapy in the treatment of malignant disease is increased if during treatment the patient is breathing oxygen at a pressure greater than atmospheric, i.e., at 2 or 3 atmospheres. General anæsthesia may be desirable during treatment : (1) To keep the patient still ; (2) To avoid anxiety from claustrophobia ; (3) To reduce the incidence of oxygen convulsions. *See also* Chapter XXX.

DANGERS OF HYPERBARIC OXYGENATION.—These include:—
1. Risk of fires and explosions.‖

---

* Slack, W. K., and others, *Lancet*, **1**, 1093.
† Sluijter, M. E., Symposium on *Hyperbaric Oxygen, Proc. 2nd Eur. Cong. Anæsth.*, 1966, III, 67.
‡ Boerema, I., *Surgery*, 1961, **49**, 291; Vermeulen-Cranch, D. M. E., *Proc. R. Soc. Med.*, 1965, **58**, 319; and McDowall, D. G., *Ibid.*, 1965, **58**, 325.
§ Sanger, C., Churchill-Davidson, I., and Thompson, R. N., *Brit. J. Anæsth.*, 1955, **27**, 436.
‖ Denison, D. M., Ernshing, J., and Cresswell, A. W., *Lancet*, 1966, **2**, 1404.

2. 'Bends', unless nitrogen has been eliminated.
3. Acute oxygen toxicity and convulsions.
4. Avascular necrosis of bone.

(*See also Hyperbaric Oxygenation. Proc. 2nd Inter. Congr.*, Glasgow, 1964 (Ed. Ledingham, I. McA.), Edinburgh: Livingstone; and Slack, W. K., in *Recent Advances in Anæsthesia and Analgesia* (Ed. Hewer, C. Langton), 1967, 10th ed., Ch. 9. London: Churchill.)

CARBON DIOXIDE [CO₂]

Discovered by von Helmont and isolated by Joseph Black (1728–1799) in 1757. Became popular with anæsthetists soon after the work of Haggard and Yandell Henderson (1873–1944) in the U.S. (1921) who recommended 5 per cent of the gas in oxygen, and J. S. Haldane (1860–1936) in Britain (1926). The gas should always be provided on anæsthetic machines.

Properties.—Colourless gas with a pungent odour in high concentration. Molecular weight 44. Specific gravity 1500 (air is 1000). Dissolves in water 87·8 vols. per cent at room temperature.

It is non-flammable and is rapidly absorbed from the alveoli. It is stored in the liquid state in cylinders (painted grey) after compression to 50 atmospheres. Amount in atmosphere 0·04 per cent.

Preparation.—
1. Action of heat on calcium or magnesium carbonates during preparation of their oxides.
2. Action of acid on alkaline carbonate.
3. During fermentation of grain in preparation of alcohol.

Effects on Respiratory System.—Two hundred ml. of carbon dioxide are excreted each minute, i.e., about 300 litres per day. The gas diffuses twenty times as rapidly as oxygen, thus hypercapnia is never due to impairment of diffusion alone. It is carried in the blood: (1) In simple solution; (2) As bicarbonate in the plasma; (3) Combined with protein in red cells as carbamino compounds. The respiratory centre is stimulated, either specifically or owing to the acid properties of carbon dioxide in solution. Both rate and depth of breathing are increased. Respiration also reflexly stimulated by action of carbon dioxide on carotid and aortic bodies. If respiratory centre is depressed by morphine or anæsthetic agents, its power of responding to carbon dioxide is lessened. An increase of partial pressure in the blood of 3 mm. Hg increases the tidal exchange 100 per cent. A decrease of 4 mm. Hg may produce apnœa.

The usual clinical effects of hypercapnia include tachycardia, hypertension, sweating, and vasodilatation of arteries (except the coronaries).

Five per cent carbon dioxide is tolerated, but higher percentages cause distress, dyspnœa, headaches, etc. Above 10 per cent the narcotic effect becomes more marked, while at 30 per cent there is coma. At 40 per cent breathing is depressed. This so-called carbon dioxide reversal may occur at concentrations of even 5 per cent, if respiratory centre is deeply depressed by narcotics or hypoxia. Thus carbon dioxide should not be

Carbon Dioxide—Effects on Respiratory System, *continued.*

used for resuscitation in such cases. There is no relationship between the $Paco_2$ in anæsthetized patients and the bleeding or clotting times.[*]

Carbon dioxide at a partial pressure of 245 mm. Hg in the dog causes narcosis. Mechanism is closely related to the fall in pH of the cerebrospinal fluid, and this may be independent of arterial pH, Pco_2, and the Pco_2 of cerebrospinal fluids. Narcosis begins when the cerebrospinal fluid pH falls below 7·1 and reaches a maximum at pH 6·8. The narcosis resulting from carbon dioxide inhalation is thus likely to be due solely to the pH effect.[†] A concentration of CO_2 between 5 and 40 per cent causes no respiratory depression in anæsthetized cats.[‡]

In cats and dogs a state of *supercarbia* can exist, when there is spontaneous respiration with a Pco_2 in excess of 400 mm. Hg, and when the respiration is not apparently under the control of the arterial Pco_2.[§]

Carbon Dioxide in Anæsthesia.—Inspired air contains 0·04 per cent. Expired air contains 4 per cent. Alveolar air contains 5·6 per cent.

USE DURING INDUCTION.—

1. To stimulate breathing after heavy premedication, for a short time only, i.e., to increase the tidal volume in the presence of a normally active respiratory centre.

2. To expedite induction, when volatile agents are used. (*See* Chapter V.)

USE DURING MAINTENANCE.—

1. To increase depth of anæsthesia rapidly when volatile agents are in use. The addition of a little carbon dioxide at the first sign of returning reflex irritability—a sign of incomplete anæsthesia—may enable control to be re-established by increasing the patient's urge to breathe, and so to inspire more of the anæsthetic agent, e.g., during tonsillectomy under ether vapour. Its power to render the mucosa of the upper respiratory tract less sensitive to irritant vapours is here made use of.

2. To widen the glottis, either to overcome spasm or before blind intubation.

3. During induction of hypothermia, carbon dioxide has been used to increase peripheral vasodilatation and so lessen the degree of metabolic acidosis. ‖

4. Has been used during anæsthesia to increase cerebral blood-flow in arteriosclerotic patients undergoing surgery,¶ and to increase the tolerance to cerebral ischæmia during carotid endarterectomy.[**]

USE DURING RECOVERY.—

1. For short periods to promote pulmonary ventilation and avoid atelectasis.

---

[*] Robinson, J. E., *Anæsthesia*, 1966, **21**, 119.
[†] Eisele, J. H., Eger, E. I., and Muallem, M., *Anesthesiology*, 1967, **28**, 856.
[‡] Raymond, L. W., and Standaert, F. G., *Ibid.*, 1967, **28**, 974.
[§] Graham, G. R., Hill, D. W., and Nunn, J. F., *Der Anæsthesist*, 1960, **9**, 70.
‖ Broom, B., and Sellick, B. A., *Lancet*, 1965, **2**, 452.
¶ Homi, J., Smart, J. F., and Wasmuth, C. E., *Proc. 2nd Eur. Cong. Anæsth.*, 1966, **1**, 629.
[**] Wells, B. A., Keats, A. S., and Cooley, D. A., *Surgery*, 1963, **54**, 216.

2. To get rid of volatile anæsthetic agents from tissues via lungs. Beware of apnœa following deprivation of a high tension of carbon dioxide, especially if respiratory centre is depressed by morphine, cyclopropane, thiopentone, etc.
3. To stimulate the onset of respiration at the end of a period of controlled apnœa, especially in the emphysematous who are accustomed to a high PCO_2 in the blood.

USE FOR RESUSCITATION.—If normal people inhale $12\frac{1}{2}$ per cent carbon dioxide in oxygen, unconsciousness will result in a short time. This is because a narcotic and not a stimulant effect is produced when the concentration in the inhaled atmosphere is such (7 per cent) that increased ventilation can no longer prevent a significant rise in its concentration in the body. In an anæsthetized or narcotized patient with depression of the respiratory centre, even 5 per cent carbon dioxide in oxygen will cause increased narcosis.

The gas is, in fact, both a brain depressant and a respiratory stimulant in which the anæsthetic effect increases as the respiratory stimulating effect decreases. In the treatment of respiratory depression it is almost always contra-indicated.

USE IN CHRONIC LARYNGEAL OBSTRUCTION.—In this condition the retention of carbon dioxide accustoms the respiratory centre to a high tension of the gas. When obstruction is relieved, apnœa may follow unless carbon dioxide is added to the inspired gases, to be gradually reduced. Another method of avoiding apnœa is to relieve the obstruction gradually, as by partially occluding the tracheostomy tube temporarily.

USE IN RESPIRATORY OBSTRUCTION.—May be dangerous as the combination of the resulting hyperpnœa with respiratory obstruction may produce an increased negative intrathoracic pressure and onset of pulmonary œdema.

The role of carbon dioxide in carbon monoxide poisoning is as yet unsettled (*see* Marriott, H. L., *Brit. med. J.*, 1958, **2**, 1591, and Medical Research Council's Report, *Ibid.*, 1958, **2**, 1408).

NITROGEN [N_2]

First isolated by Rutherford in 1772.

Preparation.—
1. Fractional distillation of liquid air.
2. Heating ammonium nitrite.

Properties.—Molecular weight 28. Specific gravity 967 (air is 1000). Solubility in water and plasma at 37° C., 1·28 vol. per cent, liquefies at −140° C. at 75 atmospheres.

It is used to dry out medical gas cylinders and to displace air from the atmosphere surrounding chemical agents, e.g., thiopentone, during storage, thus retarding oxidation. It is chemically inert and will not support combustion or combine with water, but is dissolved in body tissues, from which it is displaced slowly. Solution in plasma is the sole method of transport of nitrogen in blood (unlike oxygen which combines with hæmoglobin, and carbon dioxide which forms carbamino compounds and,

Nitrogen—Properties, *continued.*

combined with base, is carried as bicarbonate). This accounts for the slow elimination of nitrogen. The elimination of nitrogen from the lungs, breathing pure oxygen from a semi-closed inhaler at a flow rate equal to or greater than the minute volume, and with no rebreathing, takes about $2\frac{1}{2}$ min. With a flow rate less than the minute volume, the time for elimination is proportionately increased. With all nitrogen eliminated, the refilling time equals the desaturation time if the patient breathes air. Once desaturation with nitrogen from the lungs has taken place, a patient breathing from a closed system with oxygen supplied at basal rates requires a considerable time to excrete nitrogen from the tissues.* This is important in closed circuit anæsthesia, when the breathing bag should be periodically emptied to get rid of the nitrogen accumulating there from the tissues. 1·28 ml. dissolve in 100 ml. of blood-plasma. The gas is five times as soluble in fat as in water.

Nitrogen diffuses from an isolated lung lobule, whose bronchus is tied, in 16 hours. Oxygen, under similar conditions, diffuses in 15 minutes.

HELIUM [He]

Isolated by Ramsey in 1895.

Preparation.—From natural gas in the U.S. Air contains 1 part in 85,000.

Properties.—Inert, colourless, odourless gas. Molecular and atomic weights 4. Specific gravity 178 (air is 1000).

When helium replaces the nitrogen of air the resulting mixture of helium and oxygen has a specific gravity of 341 (air is 1000). Because of its low density the gas will flow through an orifice three times as fast as air, so in patients with partial respiratory obstruction, 20 per cent of oxygen with 80 per cent of helium will enable more oxygen to get to the alveoli with the same effort, or the same ventilation will take place with less effort than when air is inhaled. There is a difference between viscosity and density when considering laminar and turbulent flow. Absorption rate from alveoli very slow, a property made use of at the end of an anæsthetic, when its introduction into the alveoli helps to prevent atelectasis. Helium has a low coefficient of solubility and high rate of diffusion, compared with nitrogen. It decreases the resistance to breathing and so is used with oxygen in treatment of respiratory obstruction in the larger air-passages. In asthma, a disease of the bronchioles, its use is doubtful.

If fed through a nitrous-oxide flow-meter the reading must be multiplied by 3·3 to get the approximate rate of flow in litres per minute. It diffuses through rubber.

---

* Miles, G. G., Martin, N. T., and Adriani, J., *Anesthesiology*, 1956, **17**, 213.

CHAPTER XI

ENDOTRACHEAL ANÆSTHESIA

History.—Endotracheal insufflation in animals described by Robert Hook in 1667.* C. Kite, of Gravesend, described oral and nasal intubation for resuscitation of the apparently drowned in 1788.† Intubation from the neck, through a tracheotomy wound, was performed in 1858 by John Snow, in anæsthetizing animals. Trendelenburg used the method in man in 1871, occluding the trachea by an inflatable cuff.‡

MacEwen, of Glasgow, in 1880 passed a tube from the mouth into the trachea, using his fingers as a guide.§ These early attempts were all made to prevent aspiration pneumonia in surgery of the upper air-passages. Karl Maydl of Prague employed O'Dwyer's tube, designed for the treatment of laryngeal diphtheria, in anæsthesia.‖

Fritz Kuhn of Cassel (1866–1929) in 1901 extended the technique by using a flexible metal tube introduced on a curved guide through the mouth: his preference was for inhalation anæsthesia, the patient breathing to and fro along the tube.¶

In 1907, Barthélemy and Dufour of Nancy, France, blew chloroform vapour and air from a Vernon Harcourt inhaler and a rubber catheter, guided into the trachea by touch, the first use of the insufflation endotracheal technique.**

Meltzer (1851–1920) and Auer (1875–1948), physiologists working in the United States, pioneered insufflation endotracheal anæsthesia in animals in 1909.†† This entailed blowing an anæsthetic vapour at a positive pressure through a narrow tube into the trachea near the carina, the gases returning either through a second tube or alongside the insufflation tube. Elsberg and others,‡‡ in the same year, applied the technique to man, while in 1912, Kelly, of Liverpool, brought the method to Britain.§§

Kirstein of Berlin and Killian of Freiberg—the original broncho-scopist—pioneered direct laryngoscopy in 1896 and Chevalier Jackson (1865–1958) published a book on the subject in 1907; this popularized direct laryngoscopy. Jackson did his first bronchoscopy in 1899.

As a result of their experiences during World War I, especially in plastic surgery, as anæsthetists to Sir Harold Gillies at the Queen's Hospital for Facial and Jaw Injuries, at Sidcup (1920), Rowbotham and Magill‖‖ used first insufflation through two

---

* Hook, R., *Phil. Trans. Roy. Soc.*, 1667, **2**, 539.
† Davison, M. H. Armstrong, *Brit. J. Anæsth.*, 1951, **23**, 238.
‡ Trendelenburg, F., *Arch. klin. Chir.*, 1871, **12**, 121.
§ MacEwen, W., *Brit. med. J.*, 1880, **2**, 122.
‖ Maydl, K., *Wien. med. Wschr.*, 1893, **43**, 102.
¶ Kuhn, F., *Zbl. Chir.*, 1901, **28**, 1281.
** Barthélemy and Dufour, *Pr. méd.*, 1907, **15**, 475.
†† Meltzer, S. J., and Auer, J., *J. exp. Med.*, 1909, **2**, 622.
‡‡ Elsberg, C. A., *N.Y. Med. Rec.*, 1910. **77**, 493; and *Ann. Surg.*, 1911, **54**, 749.
§§ Kelly, R. E., *Brit. med. J.*, 1912, **2**, 617 and 1121.
‖‖ Rowbotham, E. S., and Magill, I. W., *Proc. R. Soc. Med.*, 1921, **14**, 17.

History, *continued.*

narrow tubes—one for leading gases in from a Shipway apparatus (warm ether vapour), the other for carrying them away—and later inhalation endotracheal methods, the patient breathing in and out through a single wide-bore tube. Magill published his results of blind nasal intubation with a single wide-bore rubber tube during the years following 1928.* The first blind nasal intubation was performed by Stanley Rowbotham of London.

Inflatable cuffs have been used for many years, but were reintroduced by Waters and Guedel in 1928.

A pilot balloon was described in 1893 by Eisenmenger† and was reintroduced by Langton Hewer in 1939.

Before the days of muscle relaxants, blind nasal intubation was very popular as it was usually quicker than direct-vision oral intubation when inhalation agents were all that were available. Indirect laryngoscopy with a laryngeal mirror was pioneered by Manuel Garcia (1805–1906), a teacher of singing in London.‡

In recent years the attitude to intubation has altered radically because:—

1. The use of muscle relaxants,§ and especially the use of suxamethonium, has made intubation relatively easy, quick, and atraumatic.

2. The use of muscle relaxants has greatly increased the need for intermittent positive-pressure respiration, and this is usually more satisfactorily carried out if the patient is first intubated.

Apparatus.—

TUBES.—Those most commonly used are the wide-bore Magill tubes of mineralized rubber. They can be used for either nasal or oral intubation, the latter having thicker walls. The following are their sizes:—

BRITISH STANDARD ENDOTRACHEAL TUBE SIZES

MAGILL NUMBER	OLD INTERNAL DIMENSIONS IN MILLIMETRES	NEW INTERNAL DIMENSIONS IN MILLIMETRES	
		Cuffed and Oral	Nasal
None	None	2·5	—
oO	3·2	3·0	—
oA	3·6	3·5	—
o	4·4	4·0	—
1	4·8	4·5	—
2	5·2	5·0	5·5
3	5·6	5·5	6·0
4	6·0	6·0	6·5
5	6·8	6·5	7·0
6	7·1	7·0	7·5
7	7·5	7·5	8·0
8	7·9	8·0	8·5
9	8·8	9·0	9·0
10	9·5	9·5	10·0
11	10·3	10·0	11·0
12	11·1	11·0	—

* Magill, I. W., *Brit. med. J.*, 1930, **2**, 817.
† Eisenmenger, V., *Wien. med. Wschr.*, 1893, **43**, 199.
‡ Garcia, M., *Proc. R. Soc. London*, 1855, **7**, 399.
§ Bourne, J. G., *Brit. med. J.*, 1947, **2**, 654.

The custom now is for the number of the tube to correspond to the internal diameter in millimetres.

Other tubes are made of semi-rigid material, the Portex plastic tubes (polyvinyl chloride) being useful. Portex tubes if boiled and left to cool on a curved wire stylet will permanently take the curve of the wire. Another type of tube is made of a spiral coil of nylon embedded in latex to prevent kinking.* These reinforced latex tubes have been known to cause obstruction because of bubble formation in the rubber wall of the tube. The Oxford or inverted L-shaped tube† (*see Fig.* 21) has two limbs which are shaped to conform to the passage from the mouth to the trachea and so cannot kink, even when the head is fully flexed. Its internal diameter is the same throughout but the thickness of that part which lies in the mouth and pharynx is twice that of the distal part. The tube can be passed between the cords either as it is or else on a curved stylet. It comes in eight sizes with internal diameter rising by 1 mm. from 3 mm. to 10 mm. Inflatable cuffs can be incorporated with the rubber tubes, or loose ones can be slipped on, using french chalk as a lubricant. A new and relatively non-traumatic streamlined nasotracheal tube has been described: it is made with internal diameters of 7·5, 8, and 8·5 mm.‡

CLEANING.—Tubes should be cleaned with soapy water outside and inside with a test-tube brush. Repeated boiling softens the rubber and soon ruins the tubes, so sterilization should be by 1–1000 biniodide solution or by a solution containing 0·1 per cent chlorhexidine which should remain in contact with the tube for at least 1 hour. Heating to 75° C. for 10 min. (Pasteurization) will kill vegetative organisms which are potentially harmful (although the relatively harmless spores will not be killed).§ Rubber tubes can be autoclaved up to six times without much deterioration (134° C.—pure saturated steam at 30 lb. per sq. in. above atmospheric pressure, for 3 min.).‖ Magill tubes should be stored in a circular box, 7 in. in diameter, so that their curve is maintained. Rubber tubes can be softened if they are soaked for 1 to 12 hours in paraffin oil: this will also make the tube larger, a No. 3 equalling a No. 5 after soaking. A pen nib, dipped in 50 per cent solution of silver nitrate, can be used to write on tubes.

LARYNGOSCOPES.—The prototype is that of Chevalier Jackson, later modified by Magill,¶ Paluel J. Flagg, and Macintosh.** The blade and handle may be either parallel or set at an angle one to the other, the handle containing the 3-volt battery. Various types and sizes of blade are in use. While the usual laryngoscope blade is designed to lift the epiglottis forward, the Macintosh blade is shorter and its tip enters the vallecula, lifts the

* Hollinger, T. H., and Cassels, W. H., *Anesthesiology*, 1944, **5**, 583.
† Alsop, A. F., *Anæsthesia*, 1955, **10**, 401.
‡ Davies, J. A. H., *Ibid.*, 1967, **22**, 153.
§ Jenkins, J. R. E., and Edgar, W. M., *Ibid.*, 1964, **19**, 177.
‖ Stark, D. C. C., and Pask, E. A., *Ibid.*, 1962, **17**, 195.
¶ Magill, I. W., *Lancet*, 1926, **1**, 500.
** Macintosh, R. R., *Ibid.*, 1943, **1**, 205.

Apparatus, *continued.*

base of the tongue and, with it, the attached epiglottis, so that the cords can be visualized. The superior aspect of the epiglottis is supplied by the 9th nerve, the inferior (posterior) aspect by the internal laryngeal, and hence as the inferior aspect of the epiglottis is not touched and thereby stimulated, the Macintosh instrument can be used at a lighter plane of anæsthesia than the orthodox pattern, without producing laryngeal spasm. An additional advantage of the Macintosh instrument is that during intubation the tube does not hide the cords from view.

While the ordinary blade is designed to be inserted into the right side of the patient's mouth, moving the tongue over to the left, there is a blade available for the left side.*

Some of the many modifications which are available include:—

The Bowen-Jackson laryngoscope† is a modification of Macintosh's design. It has a rather long blade and the smallest possible 'step' consistent with adequate tongue deflexion. It occupies less room in the mouth than other instruments and is useful in difficult cases, while a 28-cm. Clerf bronchoscopic spray, with its distal end projecting beyond the tip of the endotracheal tube, can be used as an introducer.‡

The Larson blade§ is also a modification of the Macintosh design and is useful when introducing a latex-armoured tube between the cords. A bridge of metal projects into the lumen of the blade near the tip of its posterior part and this directs the soft and flexible tube into the larynx. It enables a curved stylet to be dispensed with.

A malleable illuminated introducer, 18 in. long, designed to project beyond the end of the tube, inside which it lies, has been developed for use in difficult cases.‖

INTUBATING FORCEPS.—Magill's instrument is commonly used and is made in two sizes. Lundy's modification is a small bulb attached to the tip of one of the blades, so that its illumination facilitates intubation.

ANGLE-PIECES.—These connect the endotracheal tube to the breathing tube of the gas machine. Several designs are in use and they are made in various sizes both of metal and plastic. The Rowbotham type makes a tight and secure joint. In other types there is an adjustable cap for insertion of a sucker tube where suction is required, e.g., Magill, Cobb. Gas flow is more turbulent and less laminar in right-angled than in curved connectors.

---

* Pope, E. S., *Anæsthesia*, 1960, **15**, 326.
† Bowen, R. A., and Jackson, I., *Ibid.*, 1952, **7**, 254.
‡ Bowen, R. A., *Ibid.*, 1967, **22**, 150.
§ Larson, A. G., *Ibid.*, 1966, **21**, 406.
‖ Macintosh, R. R., and Richards, H., *Ibid.*, 1957, **12**, 223.

Laryngoscopes, anæsthetic machines, and a great deal of other anæsthetic equipment were sold, over a long period of years, by A. Charles King (1889–1966), whose showrooms, opened in 1926 in Devonshire Street, London, became a meeting-place for anæsthetists. Charles King gave most valuable technical aid to the developing specialty of anæsthetics, and for his services was elected an honorary member of many Anæsthetic Societies in the U.K. and overseas.

INFLATABLE CUFFS (*Figs.* 20, 21).—Used to ensure airtight endo-tracheal anæsthesia, instead of pharyngeal gauze packing.* The Hewer pilot balloon shows the state of the cuff when it is hidden

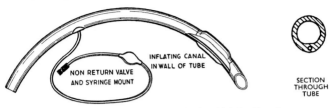

INFLATING CANAL IN WALL OF TUBE

NON RETURN VALVE AND SYRINGE MOUNT

SECTION THROUGH TUBE

Fig. 20.—' Streamline ' endotracheal tube with inflatable cuff.
(British Oxygen Gases Ltd.)

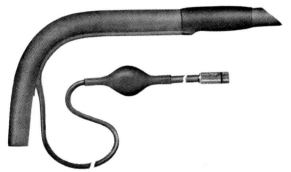

Fig. 21.—The Oxford non-kinking endotracheal tube.   (Medical & Industrial Equipment Ltd.)

in the trachea.† There is the danger, when using a cuff, of causing sloughing of the tracheal mucosa. The pressure in a cuff when comfortably inflated may be 120–180 mm. Hg, but this does not correspond to the pressure applied to the tracheal mucosa. Should sloughing occur, bronchoscopic removal of sloughs may be required. Cuffs should not be inflated to a pressure greater than that needed to prevent audible leakage of gas when the reservoir bag is compressed. The integrity of the inflatable cuff must always be tested before use.

Should gauze packing be used it must be well lubricated to prevent pharyngeal trauma. Failure to remove a gauze pack has resulted in many deaths.

Pinson pointed out that an airtight circuit results from firmly bandaging the lower jaw backwards so that the mouth is

---

* Guedel, A. E., and Waters, R. M., *Ann. Otol., etc.*, St. *Louis*, 1931, Dec.
† Hewer, C. Langton, *Recent Advances in Anæsthesia*, 3rd ed., 1939, p. 115. London: Churchill.

Apparatus, *continued.*

tied open. This places the base of the tongue in contact with the posterior pharyngeal wall. In edentulous patients a moistened 2-in. bandage inserted inside each cheek helps to get an airtight joint between mask and face.

As cuffs prevent leakage between the wall of the trachea and the outer wall of the tube, they are useful in intermittent positive-pressure anæsthesia. They also prevent blood, mucus, and vomitus from entering the lungs and so are essential in intestinal obstruction with regurgitant vomiting, and in operations on the upper air-passages.

LUBRICANTS.—To intubate atraumatically the tube and laryngo-scope should be smeared with either a greasy or a water-soluble lubricant, e.g., polyethylene glycol (555 M.*). Paraffin deteriorates rubber, and castor oil is preferable (Lunn, R. W.). A local analgesic can be incorporated, such as amethocaine 1 per cent, piperocaine 2–5 per cent, cinchocaine 1–10 per cent, lignocaine 2–4 per cent. Xylodase is useful for this purpose : it contains 5 per cent lignocaine and 0·015 per cent hyaluronidase in a water-miscible base. While petroleum jelly is the better lubricant for blind nasal intubation, its water-soluble substitutes will not cause pneumonitis if they reach the lungs. An analgesic-containing lubricant will reduce the incidence of extubation spasm.

Topical Analgesia.—The laryngeal reflex can be subdued if a suitable analgesic solution is sprayed on to the superior laryngeal aperture, the cords, and the mucosa of the larynx and trachea or by a combination of bilateral superior laryngeal block and transtracheal injection (q.v.). A German, Rosenberg, was the first to use a local analgesic (cocaine) to quieten the laryngeal reflexes (1895). Cocaine in 4–20 per cent solution is still a popular agent. It is said that the stronger solution is less rapidly absorbed because of the increased vasoconstriction that it causes, but the writers prefer the 4 per cent strength, each ml. of which contains 40 mg. of cocaine. Applied to the nares, it increases their patency by shrinking the mucosa covering the turbinates. Amethocaine 1 per cent, piperocaine 5 per cent, lignocaine or prilocaine 2–4 per cent, and cinchocaine 2 per cent solutions are also useful for the purpose of depressing the laryngeal reflexes. It is important not to poison the patient with these drugs (e.g., lignocaine 6 mg. per kg. or 10 ml. of 4 per cent solution for an 11-stone man should not be exceeded;[†] while other workers restrict the volume to 5 ml.; 10 ml. of 4 per cent prilocaine are probably safe).[‡]

SPRAYS.—An efficient atomizer such as that of Rogers, Macintosh[§] (*Fig.* 22), Magill, Rowbotham, Multicaine, Vale,[||] or de Vilbiss is essential, the patient inhaling the vapour into his larynx during

---

* Davies, Russell M., and Summers, F. H., *Brit. J. Anæsth.*, 1959, **31**, 325.
† Bromage, P. R., and Robson, J. G., *Anæsthesia*, 1961, **16**, 461.
‡ Thornton, J. A., *Proc. R. Soc. Med.*, 1965, **58**, 415.
§ Macintosh, R. R., *Lancet*, 1947, **2**, 54.
|| Vale, R., *Anæsthesia*, 1967, **22**, 314.

inspiration. Spraying is done either before or after induction of anæsthesia. More efficient analgesia is secured if, in addition, the piriform fossæ are treated with analgesic solution (*see* Chapter XV). The dental aerosol local analgesic spray with specially long nozzle has been used.*

The Macintosh laryngeal spray (*Fig.* 22) carries the local analgesic solution right down on to the cords, via a rubber tube inserted

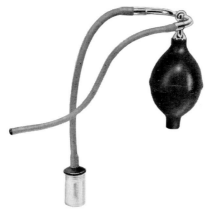

Fig. 22.—The Macintosh laryngeal spray. (British Oxygen Gases Ltd.)

through the nares. It is also convenient for applying an analgesic spray to the inside of the larynx, via a laryngoscope. Capacity 4 ml.†

Indications for Endotracheal Anæsthesia.—About this, experienced opinions vary. There are workers who intubate almost every patient and others who are much more conservative.

1. In operations—all but the shortest—in which a free airway cannot be otherwise maintained. Increasing skill lessens this indication.

2. In many abdominal operations, to ensure quiet breathing and absence of straining.

3. In cases of intestinal obstruction with regurgitant vomiting, performed under general anæsthesia, intubation and occlusion of the larynx prevent aspiration of infected material.

4. In intrathoracic operations, so that the airway is always patent, suction can be easily carried out, and control of intrapulmonary pressure and respiration made easy.

5. In cases operated on in positions making control of the airway difficult, e.g., operation in prone position.

* Binning, R., *Anæsthesia*, 1967, **22**, 529.
† Macintosh, R. R., *Lancet*, 1947, **2**, 54.

Indications for Endotracheal Anæsthesia, *continued.*

6. When intermittent positive-pressure ventilation is to be employed. To hold the jaw and support the airway, while rhythmically pressing on the breathing-bag for prolonged periods, is uncomfortable and may be dangerous. Without a cuffed tube inflation of the stomach may occur.
7. In operations on the head and neck.
    a. Intranasal operations : airway is secured and packing or an inflatable cuff prevents aspiration of blood.
    b. Tonsil dissection in adults. In children undergoing dissection, surgeons and anæsthetists vary in their prejudices.
    c. Œsophagoscopy and gastroscopy, when not performed under local analgesia.
    d. Major dental operations.
    e. All intracranial operations.
    f. Operation on the middle and inner ear ; the tube should avoid the nostril of the diseased side, if inserted through the nose.
    g. Certain eye operations, e.g., for squint, dacryocystitis, removal of the eyeball, cataract extraction, and insertion of anterior chamber implants, iridectomy, sclerectomy, etc.*
    h. Thyroid surgery. There are two schools of thought, the vast majority recommending intubation because of the good airway and position of the anæsthetist remote from the site of operation ; the minority avoiding intubation because of its tendency to cause post-operative tracheitis and dysphagia. Post-operative sore throat can, however, occur when no tube has been used. Pressure on the trachea by the tumour is an indication for intubation.
8. In patients likely to develop laryngeal spasm, e.g., some cases of cystoscopy, hæmorrhoidectomy, etc.
9. Where there is a tracheostomy.
10. In patients with fixation of the cords, e.g., in certain cases of rheumatoid arthritis and acromegaly.

In the authors' opinion endotracheal anæsthesia should not be abused and should not be employed without a real indication.

INTUBATION IN NON-SURGICAL CONDITIONS.—
1. In grave asphyxia neonatorum. The size 3 mm. (oo) Magill tube, with a knitting needle used as a stylet.
2. In resuscitating patients in whom respiration is obstructed, depressed, or absent, and who need frequent aspiration.
3. In grave laryngeal obstruction due to inflammatory exudates, tubes have been left in the trachea for four days and even longer, without serious results.
4. In patients with atelectasis and signs of exudate in lungs. A nasotracheal tube, passed blind after topical laryngeal analgesia, will serve as a channel down which a suction catheter can be passed. This will sometimes make unnecessary the more difficult bronchoscopic suction.
5. For bronchography in children for the instillation of radio-opaque oil—this is one of many techniques.

---

* *See* Discussion, *Proc. R. Soc. Med.*, 1967, **60**, 1273 et seq.

Where an artificial airway is likely to be required for longer than twenty-four to thirty-six hours, a tracheostomy is often preferable to prolonged intubation except in infants and young children.[*] More prolonged intubation in adults is being practised and studied.[†] Subglottic stenosis has, however, been reported.[‡]

Contra-indications.—These are relative.—

1. Aneurysm of aortic arch : trauma of tracheal walls may cause rupture.
2. Acute laryngitis : trauma may make condition worse or cause œdema. Intubation may, however, be life-saving.
3. In cases of open pulmonary tuberculosis : trauma may lead to tuberculous laryngitis.

Technique of Blind Nasal Intubation.—It is essential that extreme gentleness should characterize the whole procedure. It is a knack, only acquired by practice.

1. Examine nares for patency by listening to the patient's breathing with each naris alternately occluded.
2. Spray nares and upper respiratory tract with 4 per cent cocaine solution, realizing that it is toxic, or instil 1 per cent ephedrine in oil to shrink the nasal mucosa.
3. Select the largest size of tube that experience suggests will pass atraumatically through the larger naris : for a big man size 10, for a small woman size 5–7. See that the lumen of the tube is clean and patent. On the curve of the tube depends the position of the patient's head. The greater the curve, the more flexed should be the head during intubation. An average position of the head, advised by Magill, is that adopted when sniffing the morning air.
4. Induce anæsthesia and produce hyperpnœa by allowing carbon dioxide to be inhaled for a few breaths. A flow of 1 litre a minute is usually sufficient. Insert a drop of oil into the selected naris and remove mask. The Macintosh laryngeal spray can be used at this point if required.
5. Insert the tube into the naris so that its concavity is directed to the patient's feet. Thrust the tube directly backwards, not upwards. Movement of the bevel by rotation of the tube may be necessary to overcome resistance, either at this stage or when the tube enters the nasopharynx from the nose.
6. Slightly elevate the lower jaw to lift the epiglottis away from the posterior pharyngeal wall. Occlude the opposite nostril so that all breathing is taking place through the tube. If the right naris is used the head should be inclined slightly to the right, and vice versa.
7. As the tube is inserted the patient must be breathing actively. The ear is placed near the proximal end of the tube, which is so advanced that the audible tubular breathing is maximal. In

[*] Rees, G. J., and Owen-Thomas, J. B., *Brit. J. Anæsth.*, 1966, **38**, 901; and Harrison, J., and others, *Ibid.*, 1967, **39**, 645.
[†] Tonkin, J. P., and Harrison, G. A., *Med. J. Aust.*, 1966, **2**, 581; Annotation, *Brit. med. J.*, 1967, **1**, 321; and Markham, W. G., and others, *Canad. Anæsth. Soc. J.*, 1967, **14**, 11.
[‡] Taylor, T. H., Nightingale, D. A., and Simpson, R. B., *Brit. med. J.*, 1966, **2**, 451.

Technique of Blind Nasal Intubation, *continued.*

blind intubation, the anæsthetist should ' be led by the ear '. The anæsthetist's left hand may be able to move the larynx to meet the tube, by manœuvring the thyroid cartilage. The fingers often feel a slight snap as bevel passes between the cords, while there is usually some breath-holding or cough, except in deep anæsthesia. If the patient is at a light level of anæsthesia, laryngeal spasm may be produced. It is often worth waiting for the expulsive cough that may follow spasm of the cords, as the tube may slip between the cords which are widely abducted just before or after the cough.

8. Verify that the tube is in the trachea by the character of the breath-sounds issuing from the proximal end of the tube. With a tube of reasonable length, if breath-sounds are free, the distal end of the tube must lie in the trachea. If the tube can be inserted to its full extent and no breath-sounds can be heard, it is probably in the œsophagus. Free breathing through the tube, while the lower jaw is pushed backwards firmly, suggests successful intubation.

An experienced worker can usually intubate blindly, following the intravenous injection of thiopentone (0·2–0·3 g.) and suxamethonium chloride 25–40 mg., or a single injection of propanidid (250–750 mg.).

DIFFICULTIES.—If the tube does not enter the trachea it should be pulled out far enough for its tip to lie in the oropharynx before being thrust down again. A tube passed through the right naris comes to lie towards the left side of the glottis and vice versa. Should the tube not lie in the trachea it may be situated :—

a. In the œsophagus, i.e., posterior to its correct position, either because the tube is not sufficiently curved or because the head is too flexed.

b. On the anterior commissure of the larynx, i.e., anterior to its correct position, for reasons the opposite to those above.

c. In the vallecula, between the base of the tongue and the epiglottis. Rotation of the tube, so that it slips down the lateral wall of the pharynx, should overcome this obstruction.

d. In one or other pyriform fossa, lateral to its correct position. This is likely where the nose is asymmetric, and is overcome by rotating the tube, by moving the larynx laterally to meet the tube, or by rotating the patient's head.

e. Curled up in the pharynx. This will only occur with soft, worn-out tubes.

If unsuccessful, blind intubation should not be persisted in or postoperative local trauma may result. Tubes should always be handled daintily and not forcibly rammed down the patient's throat. If intubation through one naris is difficult, it may be found to be quite simple through the other.

Patients with *ankylosing spondylitis* and with ankylosis of the jaw may present special difficulties. Following the passage of the tube through the naris, the distal end can be guided into the trachea by:—

    a. The use of a wire hook in the oropharynx to guide the tube backwards or forwards.*

    b. Passage of a plastic catheter through the cricothyroid membrane via a Tuohy needle into the larynx and out through the nose; the catheter is then used as a guide for the nasal tube.

    c. The use of a fibre-optic endoscope (a modified choledochoscope).†

Technique of Direct-vision Nasal Intubation.—This is necessary if blind intubation fails and if a nasotracheal tube is desirable. It is the preferred method of nasotracheal intubation with intravenous barbiturate and relaxant.

The laryngoscope is inserted after anæsthesia is induced, as for direct orotracheal intubation. The tube tip, having been inserted as far as the hypopharynx, is guided between the cords, either by slight movement of the tube or with the aid of intubation forceps. If the tube is too curved it may impinge against the anterior commissure of the larynx and this can often be remedied by keeping the tube pressed against the anterior commissure, withdrawing the laryngoscope, flexing the head, and pushing the tube home 'blind'. Occasionally a tube cannot be guided successfully into the trachea from the nose ; it must then be withdrawn and inserted via the mouth.

Indications for Nasal Intubation.—

    1. When an oral tube is in the surgeon's way, e.g., in tonsillectomy, dental extractions, and operations on tongue.

    2. When the use of a laryngoscope is difficult owing to the anatomy of the patient.

    3. If direct vision intubation is unsuccessful.

    4. In lightly unconscious patients, for improvement of the airway.

Technique of Direct-vision Orotracheal Intubation.—The usual method consists of the injection of a sleep dose of barbiturate (e.g., thiopentone 100–500 mg.) followed by inhalation of pure oxygen: if this is maintained for 3 min. there will be no hypoxia following 4 min. of suxamethonium apnœa.‡ A little more barbiturate may be needed before the injection of suxamethonium 30–100 mg. Alternatively, the patient's lungs can be inflated with pure oxygen during the apnœa following the injection first of thiopentone, then of suxamethonium. Anæsthesia must be well established (in the second plane or below, with complete suppression of reflexes, if a volatile agent is being used), and relaxation must be profound. Less harm is done by getting the patient a little too deep than by using force in a patient with active reflexes and rigid neck muscles. Absence of reflexes and adequate muscular relaxation are necessary for laryngoscopy in all but expert hands. The angle formed by the mouth with the pharynx must be converted into a straight line by

* Bearman, A. J., *Anesthesiology*, 1962, **23**, 130; Munson, E. S., and Cullen, S. C., *Ibid.*, 1965, **26**, 365; and Singh, A., *Anæsthesia*, 1966, **21**, 400.

† Murphy, P., *Ibid.*, 1967, **22**, 429.

‡ Nolan, R. T., *Brit. J. Anæsth.*, 1967, **39**, 794.

Technique of Direct-vision Orotracheal Intubation, *continued.*

lifting up the base of the tongue and the tip of the epiglottis when using Magill's laryngoscope.

Before induction, the shape of the jaws and the condition of the teeth are carefully assessed. Loose or filled teeth, especially upper incisors, may be damaged by the blade of the laryngoscope and so should be protected by lead sheet, rubber, adhesive strapping, etc.

Difficulty may be expected in patients with :—

1. A short muscular neck and a full set of teeth.
2. A receding lower jaw. Increased distance between the mental symphysis and the lower alveolar margin, which requires wider depression of the lower jaw during intubation.
3. A long high-arched palate and a narrow deep mouth.
4. Protruding upper incisors—' rabbit teeth '.
5. Difficulty in opening the jaw, as in multiple arthritis involving the temporomandibular joints and spondylitis of the cervical spine causing rigidity of the neck so that the head cannot be satisfactorily positioned; scleroderma, neoplasms of the oropharynx, cicatricial contraction of the tissues of the mouth, face, and neck, achondroplasia,* trismus, etc.† Absence of upper incisors usually makes laryngoscopy relatively easy.
6. Contractures of the tissues in the front of the neck from burns, resulting in flexion of the neck.

The mouth and pharynx, usually at an angle, are brought nearest to a straight line if the head is elevated 5–6 in. on a pillow and extended at the atlanto-occipital joint. This is the best position for laryngoscopy, although Chevalier Jackson originally recommended that the head should be in full extension without a pillow. When the Macintosh laryngoscope is used, the head should be flexed moderately on the neck and the blade of the instrument should be inserted towards the right side of the patient's mouth to prevent his tongue from blocking the view of the larynx.

With the patient adequately anæsthetized and in the proper position, with a strip of adhesive protecting the upper incisor teeth and after artificial ventilation of the lungs with oxygen, the lubricated laryngoscope blade is gently inserted into the mouth and progressively advanced.

Landmarks are : (1) The base of the tongue ; (2) The uvula ; (3) The epiglottis.

When the epiglottis is seen it is elevated by the tip of the blade, care being taken not to scratch the posterior pharyngeal wall. The tongue and epiglottis are now lifted forwards, i.e., in the direction of the ceiling. The upper teeth must not be used as a fulcrum. As the curtain of the epiglottis is lifted forward the cords are exposed to view and are identified by their pallor. If the cords are obscured by spasm of the superior laryngeal aperture, the aryepiglottic and ventricular folds, the knobby

---

* Mather, J. S., *Anæsthesia*, 1966, **21**, 244.
† Cass, N. M., and others, *Brit. med. J.*, 1956, **1**, 488.

appearance of the arytenoids gives a clue to their position, these projections being behind the cords, and nearer the anæsthetist. Occasionally, only the posterior part of the glottis can be visualized, and then the tube must be inserted anterior to the arytenoids, using a fully curved tube encasing a fully curved wire introducer. Even the expert sometimes fails to get a good view of the cords. Should the reflexes or muscular tone return during laryngoscopy they must again be suppressed.

The blade can be either inserted in the middle line of the mouth, or along its right side, pushing the tongue to the left. With prominent teeth, the latter route may be preferable.

When using the Macintosh instrument, the blade is passed along the tongue to the vallecula and is tilted forwards so that the epiglottis is drawn away to reveal the cords. A tube with a curve is important, a straight one being difficult to insert.

When the cords are visualized and, if desired, sprayed with local analgesic solution the lubricated tube is passed either down the laryngoscope or at the side of it into the larynx and trachea. With the Magill laryngoscope a large tube obscures the view of the cords so that the tube may enter the œsophagus. As there may be apnœa, the anæsthetist may not be sure as to the lie of the tube. This can be determined by lightly blowing down the tube ; if it is in the trachea the chest will expand and the air will be heard issuing from the tube during the succeeding passive expiration. With the tube in the œsophagus chest expansion is not seen, and there is evidence of the insufflated air ' bubbling ' down the œsophagus. Another method of differentiation is to push sharply on the chest, when a short blast of air will be heard if the tube is in the trachea. Macintosh advises that if the mass of the tube hides the cords from view, the tube should be threaded over a long gum-elastic catheter, or curved, bulbous-ended wire which has previously been passed under direct vision, and after intubation can be withdrawn. This method is also useful if the patient's anatomy makes a good view of the cords difficult. Again the tube can be threaded over a Clerf bronchoscope spray.* The reflexes should of course be inactivated by topical analgesia and/or by muscle relaxants.

If, when visualized, the cords are in spasm, this must be allowed to relax before the tube is inserted. Forcing the cords is only justifiable in the presence of alarming hypoxia in patients whose condition under oxygen lack is particularly dangerous. If the cords are forced apart, a round-ended, semi-rigid tube, well lubricated, should be used. Once between the cords, it can be instantly blown down, with the rapid relief of the hypoxia.

With the tube in position, the laryngoscope is withdrawn and a pharyngeal airway, prop, or gag is placed between the teeth to prevent the tube from being bitten.

If a cuff is to be used its inflation should be delayed until the patient has settled down again and has become deeper, otherwise

---

* Bowen, R. A., *Anæsthesia*, 1967 ,**22**, 151.

Technique of Direct-vision Orotracheal Intubation, *continued.*

coughing and breath-holding may be produced and delay the onset of adequate anæsthesia.

Technique of Orotracheal Intubation without Laryngoscope.—This is very occasionally necessary when abnormal anatomy precludes the use of a laryngoscope.

1. The divided airway is an angled pharyngeal airway, split longitudinally into two parts held together by a pin. It is inserted into the mouth and through its lumen a rubber Magill tube is inserted blindly into the larynx. It can either be left in place or the pin can be removed so that the two parts will separate and can be withdrawn.

2. With the patient deeply anæsthetized and the anæsthetist standing to the left of the patient and facing him, and an assistant drawing the tongue forwards, the anæsthetist passes two fingers of his left hand over the dorsum of the tongue, so that the epiglottis is hooked forwards. The tube, which must be fully curved, is guided by the two fingers in the mouth into the glottis. Curved introducers have been used to aid this procedure, which was the one favoured by Fritz Kuhn in 1901.

3. The anæsthetist stands in his usual place at the head of the table and inserts his left thumb into the patient's mouth with his forearm pronated and his fingers on the patient's chin. The tip of the thumb makes contact with the base of the tongue as far back as possible. This gives good control of the lower jaw which with the tongue can be moved forward and backward, the patient being deeply anæsthetized. The tube is guided into the glottis with the right hand.*

4. Troup has suggested passing the tube 'blind' through a London Hospital prop held in the mouth, with the head of the anæsthetized patient in full extension. The tube must not be too fully curved.†

Extubation.—The normal response to extubation is a rise in blood-pressure and pulse-rate. After the operation the tube can be removed in the theatre, the air-passages sucked clear, and a pharyngeal airway inserted. Otherwise the patient returns to the ward with the tube still in position. In the latter case it is better that it should remain until the return of the cough reflex, when it can be removed by the post-operative observation ward sister.

Laryngeal spasm after extubation is sometimes seen, so it is important to fill the lungs with oxygen before extubation and to verify that breathing is free after the tube is removed. Extubation spasm can usually be prevented by the intravenous injection of 50–100 mg. of suxamethonium. Inflation of the apnœic patient with oxygen is then carried out until the return of normal breathing. This has the following advantages: (1) It prevents coughing and straining with increase of venous pressure, strain on suture lines, rise in intra-ocular pressure, rise in cerebrospinal

---

* Siddall, W. J. W., *Anæsthesia*, 1966, **21**, 221.
† Troup, G., *Curr. Res. Anesth.*, 1935, **14**, 249.

fluid pressure; (2) It enables a careful toilet of the upper air-passages to be carried out without disturbing the patient; (3) It minimizes post-operative sore throat. On the other hand, it is an unwise pharmacological venture to inject a depolarizing relaxant into a patient who has been for some time under the influence of a non-depolarizing agent.

Difficulty in extubation has been reported in patients in whom intubation was easy. Acute œdematous laryngitis has resulted from this complication.

Some Difficulties in connexion with Intubation.—

1. Kinking of the tube causing respiratory obstruction. Use as firm a tube for orotracheal intubation as possible. A reinforced latex tube kinks less easily than a rubber one. A pharyngeal pack may be used to support the tube. Kinking is rare with a naso-tracheal tube. Bourne's flexible metal guard helps to prevent kinking.*

2. Respiratory obstruction caused by use of too small a tube.

3. Separation of angle-piece from tube.

4. Blockage of tube by blood, mucus, etc. Tube may need to be sucked out.

5. Obstruction has resulted from a tube being pulled up so that its distal end becomes blocked by the inflated cuff. For this reason the cuff should not be too near the distal end of the tube.

6. Slipping out of tube owing to weight of attached breathing tubes, etc.

7. Obstruction by apposition of the bevel of the tube against the tracheal wall.

8. Epistaxis. This looks messy, but seldom interferes with the anæsthesia or causes post-operative discomfort.

9. Damage to teeth. If a tooth is knocked out it must be accounted for and prevented from disappearing into the trachea. If a radiograph shows it to be in a bronchus, it should be looked for with a bronchoscope as soon as possible.

10. Partial occlusion of tube by nasal spurs, deflected septa, etc., causing respiratory obstruction. The opposite naris or the oro-tracheal route may have to be substituted.

11. Grave laryngeal spasm. This will usually yield to a relaxant; if not, cricothyroid puncture with a wide-bore needle and subsequent oxygen insufflation may be life-saving.†

12. Intubation of the right bronchus. Due to use of too long a tube. Average distance between central incisors and carina is $10\frac{1}{2}$ in. in an adult male and 9 in. in a female. Distance from nares to carina is an additional $1\frac{1}{2}$ in. In a newborn baby, 2 in. separates the gums from the cords, and a similar distance separates the cords from the carina. Diagnosed by hypoxic appearance of patient, absence of air entry into left lung, unsatisfactory anæsthesia with jerky breathing.

Difficulties in Technique.—These may often be foreseen by experienced workers and may be due to:—

1. Receding lower jaw with obtuse angle of the mandible.

* Bourne, J. G., *Brit. med. J.*, 1947, **2**, 654.
† Boulton, T. B., *Anæsthesia*, 1966, **21**, 513.

Difficulties in Technique, *continued.*

2. A short muscular neck and a full set of teeth.
3. Prominent upper incisor teeth.
4. A long narrow mouth with high arched palate.
5. Carious or insecure upper teeth.
6. Abnormalities of the cervical spine including achondroplasia* because flexion of the skull on the neck at the atlanto-occipital joint is restricted.

   It may well be unwise to abolish spontaneous breathing in some of these patients before intubation.

Maintenance of Anæsthesia.—With the tube in position, the airway should take care of itself, while laryngeal spasm loses its importance. Anæsthesia can be maintained :—

1. By a continuous-flow gas machine, via an angle-piece and connecting tube ; or a face-mask.
2. By connexion to an automatic ventilating machine.
3. By the semi-open drop method on a mask placed over the tube.
4. By Flagg's can—a tin can with several openings in the top and containing ether. The endotracheal tube is connected to the can so that the patient breathes in air which is sucked over the surface of the ether.†
5. By Ayre's T-piece or one of its modifications (*see* pp. 119 and 264).

Anæsthetic Agents in relation to Endotracheal Intubation.—

1. SUXAMETHONIUM.—This short-acting muscle relaxant is probably the most popular drug used for making intubation quick, easy, and atraumatic when combined with an intravenous barbiturate. If the chloride is used, a suitable dose is 25–100 mg. ; if the bromide, then the dose should be 20–80 mg. active cations (i.e., 30–120 mg. of the salt). This is given after the patient is anæsthetized, it works in less than one minute, while its effects, including apnœa, seldom last more than a few minutes. For blind nasal intubation, a combination of thiopentone and suxamethonium shows great possibilities. Dosage suggested is 0·25 g. of the barbiturate, with suxamethonium chloride 25–40 mg. The relaxant removes the tone from the laryngeal and neck muscles. The muscle pain which may cause distress the day following operation can be lessened if gallamine 10–20 mg. is injected before the suxamethonium. An interval of 1 min. should separate the injections. There are, however, some pharmacological objections to this sequence.‡

   The drug can be given intramuscularly if veins are difficult, e.g., in infants.
2. THIOPENTONE–NON-DEPOLARIZING RELAXANTS.—This is an excellent method of direct-vision intubation. A test dose of 6 mg. of tubocurarine chloride is given (T. C. Gray) (or gallamine 20 mg.) and if uncontrollable ptosis and dyspnœa do not appear a further 9 mg. to 19 mg. are injected (or gallamine 40–140 mg.).

---

* Mather, J. S., *Anæsthesia*, 1966, **21**, 244.
† Flagg, Paluel J., *The Art of Anesthesia*, 7th ed., 1954, p. 148. Philadelphia: Lippincott.
‡ Churchill-Davidson, H. C., *Brit. med. Bull.*, 1958, **1**, 31.

This is followed by 2·5 per cent thiopentone solution injected through the same needle in amounts varying from 0·1 g. to 0·75 g. Oxygen should then be given for two or three minutes from a mask, using positive pressure on the reservoir bag when necessary. Laryngoscopy can then usually be performed with facility in the well-oxygenated patient. Occasionally additional doses of the drugs are necessary. This method is not for the beginner, who may be faced with an apnœic patient with cords which cannot be visualized.

3. ETHER.—This agent produces muscular relaxation without respiratory depression, so is very suitable for either method of intubation. It is the best and safest agent for the beginner but can be time-consuming.

4. CYCLOPROPANE.—Depresses respiration and makes blind intubation difficult, but the early relaxation of the jaw and neck muscles facilitates laryngoscopy. Anæsthesia lightens rapidly, so a speedy technique is often necessary. Suxamethonium aids intubation.

5. INTRAVENOUS BARBITURATES.—Intubation should seldom be attempted under thiopentone alone. Laryngeal irritability is increased, while muscular relaxation is poor with these agents given in reasonable dosage : respiration is depressed. The first makes blind intubation, the second makes laryngoscopy, difficult.

6. PROPANIDID (Epontol).—This can be used in place of the barbiturate. It can also be used as the sole agent for blind intubation (250–750 mg.) as it does not readily cause laryngeal spasm. Unconsciousness may be of short duration.

7. NITROUS-OXIDE–OXYGEN.—This agent, used alone, is not suitable for the passage of endotracheal tubes.
The addition of trichloroethylene to gas–oxygen makes blind intubation relatively easy, but does not produce relaxation suitable for laryngoscopy.

8. PHENOTHIAZINE DERIVATIVES.—Laryngoscopy and intubation is sometimes possible after intravenous injection of chlorpromazine, promethazine, and pethidine, without the addition of thiopentone or a relaxant.

9. HALOTHANE.—This agent fairly rapidly relaxes the pharyngeal and laryngeal muscles and can be used without relaxants for intubation in suitable patients who are reasonably deeply anæsthetized and with small doses of relaxants in others.

10. LOCAL ANALGESIA.—One or more of the following methods may be used: (a) Sucking an analgesic lozenge; (b) Spray of the mouth and pharynx and cords; (c) Bilateral superior laryngeal nerve-block (q.v.); (d) Transtracheal injection.
Voluntary hyperventilation, breathing pure oxygen, for a few minutes before intubation, minimizes blood-gas alteration associated with this manœuvre.

Advantages and Disadvantages of Intubation.—
ADVANTAGES.—
1. Avoidance of respiratory obstruction, and consequent absence of laboured respiration and capillary oozing.

Advantages and Disadvantages of Intubation, *continued.*

2. Absence of straining due to laryngeal spasm.

3. Artificial respiration and control of intrapulmonary pressure made easy.

4. Enables anæsthetist to keep away from the operative field.

5. Lessens the chance of inspiration of foreign matter and enables bronchial tree to be kept clear of blood or mucus by suction.

6. Dead space reduced to a minimum (when face-mask is not used).

7. Enables obstruction of tracheobronchial tree to be overcome as in obstructive goitre.

DISADVANTAGES.—

1. Trauma to lip, teeth, nose, throat, and larynx, resulting in hoarseness, dysphagia, pain, etc. Abrasion of the mucosa of the pharynx may result in extensive surgical emphysema. This can be partially relieved by aspirating air from beneath the deep fascia of the neck with a syringe and wide-bore needle. A subglottic slough may be caused by a cuffed tube if the cuff is too tightly inflated.

2. Safe use of laryngoscope may require a deeper plane of anæsthesia than the surgical operation or the use of a muscle relaxant which would otherwise not be employed.

3. Lack of contact of inspired gases with the mucosa covering the turbinates leads to cold dry gases reaching the alveoli : the use of a closed circuit prevents this.

There is no definite evidence that intubation increases the postoperative pulmonary morbidity.

Reflex Circulatory Responses to Laryngoscopy and Intubation.— During light general anæsthesia, and also under local analgesia, direct laryngoscopy and intubation, uncomplicated by hypoxia, hypercapnia, or cough, is capable of causing a rise in bloodpressure and an increase in heart-rate and arrhythmia because of stimulation of the nerve-endings of the vagus. These changes are not of great clinical significance, but are made much worse by changes in the blood-gases. For this reason pre-oxygenation by inhalation of pure oxygen for a few minutes or inflation with oxygen should be carried out following the injection of a relaxant and before intubation. Deep anæsthesia reduces the incidence of these reflexes, and may be used in certain cases of myocardial disease for this reason.* Arrythmias follow intubation, not laryngoscopy. Sudden death, presumably from ventricular fibrillation, has been reported to result reflexly from intubation and from endotracheal suction (for review *see* Gibbs†).

Electrocardiographic studies during intubation reveal that about 60 per cent of patients show some disturbance of a transitory nature. Most frequent are sinus tachycardia, premature ventricular contraction, nodal rhythm, and sinus bradycardia. Light planes of anæsthesia, clumsy technique, and hypoxia make the condition worse. Preliminary intravenous injection of 1 per cent procaine

* King, B. D., Harris, L. C., Greifenstein, F. E., Elder, J. D., and Dripps, R. D., *Anesthesiology,* 1951, **12**, 556.
* Gibbs, J, M., *N.Z. med. J.,* 1967, **66**, 465.

and atropine reduces their incidence, while cocainization makes them worse.* Procaine amide 300 mg. (in 10 per cent solution) injected intravenously one to five minutes before intubation reduces the incidence of arrhythmias but should seldom be necessary. Tubocurarine may be associated with a lower incidence of reflex cardiac disturbance than suxamethonium.† Extubation at light planes of anæsthesia causes no significant E.C.G. changes and so is safe.

Laryngeal Complications of Intubation.—

1. NON-SPECIFIC GRANULOMA OF THE LARYNX (GRANULOMA PYOGENICUM).—This is usually superimposed on a contact ulcer and takes some time to develop. The usual site is the tip of the vocal process of one or both arytenoids in the posterior one-third of the rima glottidis. The tips of the vocal processes are prominent and are covered with mucoperichondrium ; they are normally projected forcibly into the laryngeal lumen and slapped together. Contact ulcer is not necessarily due to trauma from the intubation but may be due to actual movements of the cords against the tube as it lies in the larynx. These movements are not necessarily abolished by anæsthesia.‡ The prognosis of a contact ulcer is good. Healing is usual but is hindered by phonation. If it is followed by granuloma formation, local removal will be necessary.

2. ACUTE ŒDEMATOUS STENOSIS.—This is very rare. More usual in children because of :—
   a. The amount of loose areolar tissue in the subglottic region.
   b. The small lumen which is easily occluded. Obstructive laryngeal œdema, from whatever cause, has the following signs:—
      i. Indrawing, during inspiration, at any of the following sites: (α) The suprasternal notch; (β) Around the clavicles; (γ) The epigastrium; (δ) The intercostal spaces.
      ii. Ashy grey pallor.
      iii. Choking and waking in terror every time the child falls asleep.
      iv. Restlessness.
   TREATMENT.—No sedatives. Further intubation contra-indicated. Low tracheostomy without delay.

3. BRUISING OF LARYNX.—This may result in dysphonia and dysphagia but usually clears up in a few days. It bears no constant relationship to the ease of intubation. In a series of 500 cases investigated, 15·9 per cent complained of some soreness of the throat after intubation.§ In another series of cases, 10 per cent of non-intubated patients receiving general anæsthesia and 40 per cent of intubated patients developed a sore throat after operation.‖

4. STRETCH INJURY OF RECURRENT NERVE.—This has been reported following intubation, and results in a paralysed cord. Suggested causes: (a) Stretching of nerve during acute

* Burstein, C. L., Lopinto, F. J., and Newman, W., *Anesthesiology*, 1950, **11**, 224, 229.
† Gibbs, J. M., *N.Z. med. J.*, 1967, **66**, 465.
‡ Jackson, Chevalier, *Anesthesiology*, 1953, **14**, 435.
§ Wolfson, B., *Brit. J. Anæsth.*, 1958, **30**, 326.
‖ Conway, C. M., Miller, J. S., and Sugden, F. L. H., *Ibid.*, 1960, **32**, 219.

Laryngeal Complications of Intubation, *continued*.

retroflexion during intubation; (*b*) Stretching during difficult extubation; (*c*) Rough handling of patient after operation.*
(*See also* Lewis, R. H., and Swerdlow, M., *Brit. J. Anæsth.*, 1964, **36**, 504.)

Endotracheal Intubation in Infants and Children.—Ayre's method (1937) does away with valves and rubber bags and allows the circuit to be open to the outside air. One end of the cross-piece of a metal T-tube 1 cm. in diameter is connected to an angle-piece of an endotracheal tube by about 1 in. of rubber. The upright of the T-piece is connected to a continuous-flow gas machine (*see Fig.* 10). Nitrous oxide, oxygen, and if necessary a volatile supplement are insufflated by a small inlet tube at right-angles to the main limb (the upright of the T). The other cross-piece has fixed to it rubber tubing—open to the air—which constitutes a small reservoir for the anæsthetic gases, most of which would otherwise escape into the outside air. The internal diameter of the reservoir tube should be 1 cm. so that each inch in length will have a capacity of about 2 ml.† (For adults a slightly larger tube with an internal diameter of 1·25 cm. and a capacity of 3 ml. per inch in length may be used.) These measurements should not be exceeded, otherwise increased 'dead space' will result. The fresh gas inflow should average twice the minute volume of the patient. Ayre gives the following table† as a guide to the gas inflow and tube (reservoir) capacity required for children of different ages.

Age	Gas Inflow in litres/min.	Reservoir Tube Capacity in ml.
0–3 months	3–4	6–12
3–6 ,,	4–5	12–18
6–12 ,,	5–6	18–24
1–2 years	6–7	24–42
2–4 ,,	7–8	42–60
4–8 ,,	8–9	60–72

After induction of anæsthesia the endotracheal tube is passed and connected up. Nitrous-oxide–oxygen in varying proportions—about 4 to 6 litres per minute—is allowed to pass over ether, or other volatile anæsthetic.

Ayre mentions the following advantages :—

1. No obstruction to respiration or hypoxia.
2. Amount of rebreathing adjustable by length of breathing tube.
3. Vascular congestion reduced.

The technique can be used in adults and is especially useful in intracranial surgery. The patient should be carried to Plane II, Stage 3, before being connected to the tube.

The T-piece principle can be modified by the addition of a small reservoir bag open at one end fitted on to the end of the reservoir tube. This enables intermittent positive-pressure ventilation with gas and oxygen to be employed, following the use of

---

* Bauer, H., *Der Anæsthesist*, 1958, **7**, 173.
† Ayre, P., *Brit. J. Anæsth.*, 1956, **28**, 520; and *Anæsthesia*, 1967, **22**, 359.

an intravenous barbiturate with a relaxant.* A further modification allows the fresh gas inflow tube and the expiratory tube to lie in the same plane.†

In children the laryngeal reflexes are very active, while the glottis is smaller relative to body size. A tube may pass readily into a naris, but be too big for the larynx, the narrowest part of which is at the level of the cricoid cartilage. The largest tube in a child's larynx, because of its rubber walls, reduces the capacity of the larynx very considerably.

The larynx is placed far forwards in infants and children.

Now that an endotracheal tube is numbered according to its internal diameter in millimetres, a rough guide is as follows : A child of 2 requires a 5-mm. tube ; a child of 4 requires a 5·5-mm. tube ; a child of 6 requires a 6-mm. tube ; a child of 8 requires a 6·5-mm. tube ; a child of 10 requires a 7-mm. tube ; a child of 12 requires a 7·5-mm. tube.

The smallest L-shaped tube has an internal diameter of 3 mm. Larger sizes increase by 1-mm. increments.

CHAPTER XII

CARE OF THE ANÆSTHETIZED PATIENT‡

Airway.—All mucus and blood, etc., must be aspirated from the air-passages before the patient leaves the table. Similarly, solid foreign matter, e.g., vomitus, should be removed via a broncho-scope without delay, if its presence is suspected.

If maintenance of the airway is difficult an oropharyngeal tube should be inserted before the patient leaves the table. An endotracheal tube can be removed either in the theatre and replaced by a pharyngeal airway, or later by the ward sister when the cough reflex has returned. In patients likely to be comatose for long periods, a tracheostomy is preferable to an endotracheal tube, which should probably be removed after 36 to 48 hours.

The anæsthetist must satisfy himself that the attendants taking the patient from the operating table back to his bed are capable of maintaining a good airway by manipulation of the lower jaw, or failing this, by the use of a gag and tongue traction. It is of course very important that the patient should not leave the anæsthetist's care until he is able to ventilate himself properly. Inhalations of carbon dioxide have no place in the treatment of post-operative respiratory depression, but can be given for short periods to cause hyperpnœa and so expedite the excretion of volatile anæsthetics.

An excellent position, recommended after all operations, is that usually adopted solely for patients returning to bed after operations on the upper respiratory tract, i.e., semi-prone with lower

---

* Rees, G. J., *Brit. med. J.*, 1950, **2**, 1419.
† Bethune, D. W., and Crichton, T. C., 1967, *Anæsthesia*, **22**, 160.
‡ Mushin, W. W., *Brit. med. J.*, 1955, **1**, 1116.

Airway, *continued*.

arm posteriorly and a pillow anteriorly ; upper leg flexed at knee-joint.

Trauma.—The minor sequelæ of anæsthesia* are often the cause of considerable discomfort to the patient. They include trauma to lips, gums, and teeth ; sore throat ; corneal abrasions ; superficial phlebothrombosis and simple ecchymosis following intravenous injections ; backache following lithotomy position ; nausea and vomiting. They occur in a disappointingly high proportion of patients and are only to be avoided by greater care in the handling of the unconscious.

Posture during Operation.—

TRENDELENBURG POSITION.†—Recent experimental work has shown that tilting into a steep Trendelenburg position in young patients under light anæsthesia had no effect on the gas tension of arterial blood, and none on the pH, minute volume, and respiratory rate.‡ In short stout patients, especially if there is an abdominal mass, pressure on the diaphragm from the bowel may produce cyanosis and dyspnœa and reduction of vital capacity by 15 per cent unless intermittent positive-pressure respiration is carried out. Cyanosis also occurs in the face and neck of plethoric patients in this position, as a result of stagnant hypoxia due to gravity even in the presence of adequate ventilation. If the arm is abducted, the elbow should be slightly flexed and pronated to prevent pull on the brachial plexus, but every care should be taken to avoid this position of arm abduction with the head-down tilt.

Position can be maintained by : (1) Shoulder supports (with risk of brachial plexus lesions) ; (2) Tying ankles and thighs to operating table (with risk of phlebothrombosis of veins of calf) ; (3) Apparatus to support the iliac crests (Ogier Ward, Hans) ; (4) Langton Hewer's corrugated mattress.§

Steep Trendelenburg position is now rarely necessary. Some degree of tip may, however, be preferable to deepening the level of anæsthesia or the injection of an extra dose of muscle relaxant in certain patients.

Great care is needed to prevent pressure on nerves, or stretching of nerve-trunks.

Circulatory depression, venous stagnation, and drainage of sputum from the lungs are temporarily aided in this position.

PRONE POSITION.—A pillow should be placed under each shoulder and another under the pelvis, so that breathing is not unduly interfered with and so that all pressure is completely removed

---

* Conway, C. M., Miller, J. S., and Sugden, F. L. H., *Brit. J. Anæsth.*, 1960, **32**, 219 ; Edmonds-Seal, J., and Eve, N. H., *Ibid.*, 1962, **34**, 44 ; and Thomas, E., *Ibid.*, 1963, **35**, 327.

† Friedrich Trendelenburg (1844–1924) first used his tilt in 1880 when Professor of Surgery at Rostock. This was popularized by his pupil Willy Meyer in 1884 in the U.S. Trendelenburg later occupied the surgical chairs at Bonn and Leipzig. He described a tracheotomy tube with inflatable cuff in 1869.

‡ Scott, D. B., and others, *Brit. J. Anæsth.*, 1966, **38**, 174; and Scott, D. B., and Slawson, K. B., *Ibid.*, 1968, **40**, 103.

§ Hewer, C. Langton, *Lancet*, 1953, **1**, 522.

from the abdomen and its large venous channels. A cuffed endotracheal tube is a wise precaution in case regurgitation of stomach contents should occur. Fat subjects tolerate this position badly. Anæsthetized patients stand rough movement poorly. The unconscious patient when moved can easily suffer skeletal injury.

LITHOTOMY POSITION.—When the lithotomy position is required, both legs should be moved together to avoid strain on the pelvic ligaments. If the patient is arranged while supine so that the anterior superior iliac spines are on a level with the break in the table, he will be in good lithotomy position when the legs are supported on the stirrups and will need no further pulling about, with its risk of dislodgement of intravenous needles.

LATERAL POSITION.—This handicaps the patient's breathing, and a bridge makes it still worse, so it should be used as little as possible and for a short time only. It may also be associated with hypotension.

SUPINE POSITION.—Pressure on and stretching of nerves of arm must be avoided by care of the arms. The following methods may be used during operation :—

a. Each arm can be well tucked under the buttock, palm down.

b. A draw sheet is passed under the back and over the arms, which are at the side of the body. The free ends are then firmly tucked under the buttocks, imprisoning the arms.

c. Wrist straps are firmly attached to a broad strap surrounding the table, or to the table direct.

d. Arms can be securely wrapped up at the side of the chest, with elbows flexed, in the patient's nightgown. This is useful when the gall-bladder bridge is to be employed.

e. One or both arms are abducted to a right-angle anterior to the coronal plane of the body and secured to a padded arm-table or padded board. Arm-rests unattached to the table are undesirable, as they do not move with the patient. This method is most useful if frequent estimations of blood-pressure are to be made, or if intravenous medication is likely to be necessary during the operation.

Firm fixation is especially necessary if light anæsthesia is to be employed or if the patient is to be operated on in the conscious state. In these cases, in addition, a padded strap should be passed just above the knees and firmly secured beneath the table.

Legs should be flat on the table, not crossed one over the other. The tendo Achillis must not rest on the unpadded edge of the table. A soft pad, raising heels from the table, avoids pressure on the calf veins, and so may lessen the incidence of thrombosis occurring at this site.

Effect of Posture on Respiration.—Tidal exchange is handicapped in various positions assumed during operation. Case and Stiles[*] studied changes in vital capacity of conscious subjects and estimated that compared to the sitting position tidal exchange is

---

[*] Case, E. H., and Stiles, J. A., *Anesthesiology*, 1946, **7**, 29.

Effect of Posture on Respiration, *continued.*

decreased 9 per cent in reversed Trendelenburg position ; 10 per cent in supine, prone, and left lateral positions ; 12 per cent in right lateral position ; 13 per cent with use of gall-bladder bridge ; 15 per cent with Trendelenburg (recent work casts doubts on this*); 18 per cent with lithotomy position. However, other studies† of patients anæsthetized with halothane indicate that the kidney, prone, jack-knife, and Trendelenburg positions cause 14–24 per cent reduction in ventilation; lateral, reverse Trendelenburg, and gall-bladder positions 6–10 per cent reduction. The lithotomy and prone positions caused no significant changes.

Effect of Posture on Blood-pressure.—The Trendelenburg position aids venous return to the heart and helps to ensure an adequate arterial flow to the brain. Conversely, head-up tilt may be associated with fall of blood-pressure and syncopal reactions. The venous return to the heart may be considerably embarrassed (with resultant hypotension and cardiovascular collapse): (1) During handling of organs within the abdomen; (2) insertion of abdominal packs prior to pelvic surgery; (3) raising of gall-bladder bridge; (4) in the presence of large abdominal tumours, particularly when minimal external pressure is applied.‡

Moving the Patient.—Anæsthetized patients stand moving badly : this is especially so when the blood-pressure is low. All movements should be smooth and gentle, not jerky and rough. If a canvas stretcher is not available, three people should, if possible, lift the patient, who should be rotated on to his side, face to the lifters, as soon as he is lifted from the bed or trolley.

A trolley which can maintain a head-down tilt should be used to take the patient back to bed.

Position in Bed.—The patient should lie in the semi-prone position until his reflexes return. This is maintained by a pillow between the bed and the chest ; the lower arm is placed behind the trunk ; the upper knee is flexed. This helps to maintain a free airway by causing the tongue to fall away from the posterior pharyngeal wall : it also helps to prevent aspiration of vomitus into the air-passages. The patient should not be placed in a head-up position until it is quite certain that his cardiovascular system is able to maintain an adequate circulation through the brain. Otherwise syncopal reactions and even death may occur.

About 20 per cent of the deaths associated with anæsthesia occur during the first thirty minutes after operation.

Slight elevation (10 degrees) of the foot of the bed, in the immediate post-operative period, has been shown to reduce the incidence of post-operative thrombosis and of pulmonary embolism.

* Scott, D. B., and others, *Brit. J. Anæsth.*, 1966, **38**, 174; and Scott, D. B., and Slawson, K. B., *Ibid.*, 1968, **40**, 103.
† Wood-Smith, F. F., Horne, G. M., and Nunn, J. F., *Anæsthesia*, 1961, **16**, 340.
‡ Scott, D. B., *Ibid.*, 1963, **18**, 135.

CHAPTER XIII

INTRAVENOUS ANÆSTHESIA

History.—Pierre-Cyprien Oré* (1828–1891), Professor of Physiology at Bordeaux, used chloral hydrate intravenously in 1872 in a patient suffering from tetanus, the hypodermic syringe and needle having been invented by the Frenchman, C. G. Pravaz, and the Scot, Alexander Wood, respectively, in 1853.

Intravenous hedonal was used in 1905 by Krawkow, of St. Petersburg, Russia,† and in 1912 by Max Page in London; in 1909 Burckhardt gave chloroform and ether by the intravenous route.‡

The first barbiturate was synthesized by Emil Fischer and von Mehring in 1903§: this was diethyl barbituric acid or veronal. Phenobarbitone was discovered in 1912. Somnifaine was the first barbiturate to be used intravenously; it is a combination of diethyl and diallyl barbituric acids, and was used by Daniel and G. Bardet in 1924.‖

In 1927 Bumm introduced pernocton,¶ while Zerfas, in the United States, used sodium amytal intravenously two years later.** This was soon followed by the use of nembutal (pentobarbitone) (1930).†† Magill was the first to use this clinically in Britain and Lundy in the U.S. in 1931.

Kirschner gave avertin (bromethol) intravenously in 1929.‡‡

Hexobarbitone was the first drug to make intravenous anæsthesia popular and was used by Weese and Scharpff in 1932,§§ having been synthesized by Kropp and Taub. It was first used in Great Britain by R. Jarman and L. Abel (1933).‖‖

Pentothal sodium (thiopentone) was synthesized in 1932 by Volwiler and Tabern and introduced into clinical practice by Lundy of the Mayo Clinic¶¶ and by Waters of Madison in 1934.*** First used in Great Britain by Jarman and Abel in 1935.†††

Apparatus.—Syringes of 10-ml. and 20-ml. capacity, with eccentric nozzles. Larger-bore cannula for preparing solution. Intravenous needles with short bevel. Sterile swabs and antiseptic lotion. Rubber tubing and artery forceps to use as tourniquet. Mouth

---

* Oré, P.-C., *Bull. Soc. Chirurg.*, 1872, **1**, 400.
† Krawkow, N. F., *Arch. exp. Path. Pharmak.*, 1908, Suppl., 317.
‡ Burkhardt, L., *Münch. med. Wschr.*, 1909, **2**, 2365.
§ Fischer, E., and von Mehring, J., *Ther. d. Gegenw.*, 1903, **5**, 97.
‖ Fredet, P., and Perlis, R., *Bull. et Mém. Soc. nat. de Chir.*, 1924, **50**, 789.
¶ Bumm, R., *Klin. Wschr.*, 1927, **6**, 725.
** Zerfas, L. G., and McCallum, J. T. C., *J. Ind. med. Ass.*, 1929, **22**, 47.
†† Fitch, R. H., Waters, R. M., and Tatum, A. J., *Amer. J. Surg.*, 1930, **9**, 110.
‡‡ Kirschner, M., *Chirurg.*, 1929, **1**, 673.
§§ Weese, H., and Scharpff, W., *Dtsch. med. Wschr.*, 1932, **2**, 1205.
‖‖ Jarman, R., and Abel, L., *Lancet*, 1933, **2**, 18.
¶¶ Lundy, J. S., *Proc. Staff Mtg. Mayo Clinic*, 1935, **10**, 536.
*** Pratt, T. W., Tatum, A. L., Hathaway, H. R., and Waters, R. M., *Amer. J. Surg.*, 1936, **31**, 464.
††† Jarman, R., and Abel, L., *Lancet*, 1936, **1**, 422.

Apparatus, *continued.*

gag. Pharyngeal airways. Facilities for the insufflation of oxygen into the lungs. The Mitchell (*Fig.* 23)* or Gordh needle or one of its modifications is useful if intermittent intravenous anæsthesia

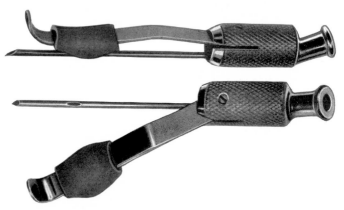

Fig. 23.—Mitchell intravenous needle.†

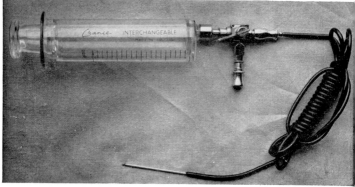

Fig. 24.—The Lee televenous apparatus for intravenous injections with the patient's arm at his side.

is contemplated, so that clotting in the intravenous needle is prevented.

---

* Mitchell, J. V., and White, G. M. J., *Anæsthesia*, 1958, **13**, 227.
† Mitchell, J. V., *Ibid.*, 1952, **7**, 258.

To give serial injections of thiopentone, relaxant, etc., with the arm at the patient's side, a needle placed into a suitable vein in the arm can be connected by a length of plastic tubing to a syringe and three-way tap (Lee)* at the head of the table. (*Fig.* 24.) Some workers prefer the arms to be folded across the chest. Serial injections can also be given into a plastic cannula introduced into a vein through (or over) a needle. If this plastic cannula becomes sheared off and disappears into the vein, it must be sought out and removed.†

Anatomy and Physiology.‡—The great majority of injections are made into the superficial veins of the hand or forearm. The veins of the forearm are superficial to the deep fascia and usually include: (1) The cephalic on the radial side ; (2) The basilic on the ulnar side ; (3) The median cubital (basilic) vein ; (4) The median antebrachial vein.

The *cephalic vein* drains the radial side of the dorsal venous network of the wrist and hand and passes up the radial side of the forearm anterior to the elbow-joint, where it lies between the brachioradialis and the biceps brachii. It gives off the median cubital vein (median basilic vein) in front of the elbow-joint and this passes medially to join the basilic vein. Passing up the arm, it lies beneath the deep fascia between the pectoralis major and the deltoid and enters the axillary vein below the clavicle, after piercing the clavipectoral fascia.

The *basilic vein* drains the ulnar side of the dorsal venous network and, running up the dorsal aspect of the forearm at first, becomes anterior below the elbow-joint. It is joined by the *median cubital vein* and passes between the pronator teres and the biceps brachii, piercing the deep fascia in the middle of the arm. It then ascends medial to the brachial artery and, at the lower border of the teres major, becomes the axillary vein.

The *median cubital vein* (median basilic or median cephalic) arises from the cephalic vein just below the lateral epicondyle and joins the basilic vein, passing upwards and medially.

The *median antebrachial vein* drains the blood from the anterior aspect of the wrist and hand. It ascends in front of the forearm and joins either the cephalic or basilic vein.

The arrangement of these veins is often irregular.

The following factors cause the blood in the veins to move proximally :—

1. Pressure transmitted from the arterial system to veins lying in the same fascial compartment and via the capillaries.
2. Massaging effect of muscles.
3. Valves preventing backflow.
4. Negative intrathoracic pressure during inspiration.

Technique of Intravenous Injection.—The easiest and most accessible vein should be chosen, and will usually be found on the dorsum

---

* Hewer, C. Langton, and Lee, J. A., *Recent Advances in Anæsthesia*, 1957, p. 97. London : Churchill.
† Annotation, *Lancet*, 1963, **1**, 762 ; and Udwadia, T. E., and others, *Brit. med. J.*, 1963, **2**, 1251 ; also Bennett, P. J., *Ibid*, 1963, **2**, 1252.
‡ Ellis, H., *Anæsthesia*, 1961, **16**, 235.

Technique of Intravenous Injection, *continued.*

of the hand.   Veins anterior to the elbow-joint should only be
used if a clean and easy venepuncture is made.   To burrow
deeply and blindly into tissues in this area is to run a danger of
injury to the median nerve or an artery.   Other possibilities are :—

1. The cephalic vein on the radial side of the forearm.
2. The internal saphenous vein, anterior to the medial malleolus.
   The skin overlying this is tough, so a specially sharp needle
   must be used.
3. Veins on the front of wrist.
4. The external jugular vein.
5. Subclavian vein—by supraclavicular puncture.*
6. A scalp vein in infants.

There is sometimes retrograde amnesia for venepuncture preceding
intravenous anæsthesia.

When the arm is chosen, the veins are made as prominent as possible
by the use of a venous tourniquet, such as a length of rubber
tubing around the arm.   If the anæsthetist is single-handed it
can be secured and released by means of an artery forceps.
Applied near the site of injection, the tourniquet steadies the
vein proximally, while the anæsthetist's finger, by stretching the
skin, steadies it distally.   This is very important in thin old
people whose veins, although prominent, very readily slip about
beneath the skin and may run away from the point of the
needle.

Aids to visualization of veins :—

1. Tourniquet—see that artery is not occluded in addition to the
   vein ;   the presence of arterial pulsation is a most useful guide
   to the position of an artery and hence to avoidance of injection
   into it.
2. Massaging of forearm in proximal direction and gentle slapping
   of tissues to promote vasodilatation.
3. Clenching of fist.
4. Holding arm downwards before application of tourniquet.
5. Application of massive hot fomentation to whole forearm for
   half an hour before injection.
6. Use of radiant heat before injection, e.g., from a portable hair
   dryer (Lundy).
7. A good and movable light.

Any form of general anæsthesia (especially halothane) will cause
dilatation of the superficial veins, and so will make venepuncture
easier.

When the skin has been well cleaned with an antiseptic, the needle
is inserted so that it comes to lie between the skin and the vein
wall ;   needle bevel can be either towards the skin or away from
it.   For this the syringe should be lying almost parallel to the
skin, unless the vein is deeply placed.   The point is now advanced and the vein wall is pierced at a different level from the
skin puncture.   This tends to prevent transfixion of the vein
and lessens hæmatoma formation when the needle is withdrawn.

---

* Yoffa, D., *Lancet*, 1965, **2**, 614.

With the needle point within the lumen of the vein it should, if possible, be advanced for a short distance to prevent slipping out. If needle becomes blocked it can often be freed by injecting a small volume of saline into it from a 1-ml. or 2-ml. syringe—not one of larger size. A few drops of procaine can be injected into the dermis with an intradermal needle before the larger needle is inserted, if necessary, to reduce pain caused by the larger needle. With the needle in the vein, the aspiration test is performed and injection can commence. After withdrawal of the needle oozing should be checked by firm pressure and elevation of the limb, if necessary.

THIOPENTONE SODIUM

(Pentothal; Thiopental; Trapanal; Penthiobarbital; Intraval; Nesdonal; Farmotal)

This is sodium ethyl (1-methyl butyl) thiobarbiturate. It is the sulphur analogue of pentobarbitone. It is 30–50 per cent more potent than hexobarbitone (evipan) and holds the field at present as the best ultra-short-acting intravenous barbiturate. Introduced commercially as pentothal sodium in 1934.

It is a yellow amorphous powder with odour resembling H_2S. It is soluble in water and alcohol and forms a 2·5 or 5 per cent solution in distilled water of pH 10·81 (pH of blood 7·4). A 2·8 per cent solution in water is isotonic. To prevent formation of free acid by carbon dioxide from the atmosphere 6 per cent sodium carbonate is added to the powder, which is prepared in an atmosphere of nitrogen. In solution it is not very stable, but can be left for 24–48 hours or longer without harm resulting on subsequent injection, provided solution remains clear. A solution which is cloudy should be discarded. The oil/water coefficient is 4·7 (of barbitone it is 0·214).

It is supplied in ampoules of 0·5, 1·0, and 5·0 g., with sterile distilled water sufficient to make a 5 per cent solution or a 2·5 per cent solution. A 2·5 per cent solution is more commonly used and is, in the writers' opinion, to be preferred.

To carry out a safe, smooth anæsthesia with this agent may prove to be more difficult than it looks. Anæsthesia with thiopentone should never be undertaken lightly.

Intravenous barbiturates may be grouped as follows :—

1. Oxybarbiturates, e.g., pentobarbitone ; amylobarbitone ; quinalbarbitone.
2. Methylated oxybarbiturates, e.g., hexobarbitone ; methohexitone.
3. Thiobarbiturates, e.g., thiopentone ; thialbarbitone ; buthalitone ; methitural (neraval) ; thiogenal ; inactin.

Pharmacology.—
  THE CENTRAL NERVOUS SYSTEM.—Like other barbiturates, it causes sedation, hypnosis, some analgesia, anæsthesia, and respiratory depression, depending on the dose injected and the rate of injection. Concentration of the drug in the plasma is not the only factor controlling the depth of anæsthesia as there is no consistent relationship between the plasma thiopentone

Thiopentone Sodium—Pharmacology, *continued.*

concentration and the depth of anæsthesia E.E.G. patterns.[*] These patterns are those of natural sleep. Cerebral oxygen consumption is lessened. This is due to interference with cerebral cellular oxygen utilization. It is an anticonvulsant and elevates the threshold of neurons to excitation. The cerebral cortex and the ascending reticular-activating system are depressed before the medullary centres. It depresses sympathetic transmission more than parasympathetic.

Thiopentone in doses insufficient to cause unconsciousness antagonizes the analgesic effects of nitrous oxide and pethidine[†] and a low concentration increases the sensitivity to pain which lasts into the post-operative period.

REDISTRIBUTION.—After a single small dose of thiopentone, its level in the plasma falls rapidly and the patient regains consciousness. This fall is due to the redistribution of the drug to other body tissues by the circulation. It used to be thought that redistribution occurred mainly to fat in which the drug is highly soluble. Recent studies,[‡] however, have shown that redistribution to fat is too slow (because of its poor blood-supply) to account for the rapid recovery from anæsthesia. Redistribution, in fact, is mostly to viscera and the lean body mass (muscles, etc.) during the first 30 minutes after intravenous injection. After a single large dose, or repeated small ones, however, the resulting equilibrium plasma level may be high enough to cause anæsthesia and because of the slow metabolism of thiopentone (10–15 per cent per hour) anæsthesia is prolonged. Anæsthesia depends not only on the concentration of the drug, but also on the length of time of exposure of tissues to the drug. It rapidly crosses the blood-brain barrier and its concentration in the cerebrospinal fluid approaches that in the plasma in 15 minutes. Equilibrium between plasma and brain is established 1 minute after intravenous injection. The initial high uptake of thiopentone by the brain accounts for the rapidity of the onset of anæsthesia.

ACUTE TOLERANCE.[§]—There is a relationship between the induction dose of thiopentone and the blood thiopentone level at which patients awake from anæsthesia. With larger induction doses the patient wakes at a higher blood level. This can be explained as the development of acute tolerance to thiopentone when given in higher dosage. A high initial concentration of thiopentone in the brain may result in an increased tolerance to supplementary doses. The greater the initial dose, the greater will be the increments of drug required to maintain surgical anæsthesia. Acute tolerance may be the mechanism whereby larger doses of thiopentone are customarily used in some hospitals than in others, with comparable duration of anæsthesia.

[*] Brand, **L.,** and others, *Brit. J. Anæsth.,* 1961, **33,** 92.
[†] Clutton-Brock, J., *Anæsthesia,* 1962, **16,** 80.
[‡] Price, H. L., *Anesthesiology,* 1960, **21,** 40.
[§] Dundee, J. W., Price, H. L., and Dripps, R. D., *Brit. J. Anæsth.,* 1956, **28,** 344.

About 70 per cent of the thiopentone in peripheral blood is bound to plasma proteins. The tissues are in equilibrium only with the unbound fraction. pH changes may affect the ratio of bound to unbound thiopentone and the equilibration between tissue and the unbound portion. A decrease in the blood pH produced by carbon dioxide retention causes a fall in the unbound plasma thiopentone level, while an increase in the pH causes a rise.* Put another way, a patient requires more of the drug if his carbon dioxide is allowed to accumulate and less if he is hyperventilated. Thus with a given dose of thiopentone the narcotic effect will last longer if he is hyperventilated than if his carbon dioxide is allowed to build up.

RESPIRATORY SYSTEM.—The chief effect is depression of the respiratory centre, depending on the dose and rate of injection. A deep breath or two, or a yawn, may precede the depression. It is because of the hypoxia produced by this depressant action that thiopentone may be dangerous from the respiratory viewpoint. The depth of breathing is related to the external stimuli and a patient may breathe adequately on the operating table only to subside into shallow respiration when left quiet and undisturbed in bed. The depth is also related to the respiratory depressant activity of drugs given for premedication. Unless, however, respiration is greatly depressed, the blood oxygen and carbon dioxide tensions undergo little change. If, after respiratory arrest, oxygen is supplied to the lungs, the rapid distribution of the drug in the tissues will usually soon occur, and spontaneous breathing will recommence. Under thiopentone the sensitivity of the respiratory centre to carbon dioxide is reduced or lost, so this gas, if in abnormal amount in the blood and tissues, will act as a further depressant. On the other hand, the carotid and aortic body reflex response to oxygen lack, resulting in respiratory stimulation, is not so easily depressed as the respiratory centre. The Hering-Breuer reflex to lung inflation is well marked during thiopentone anæsthesia, i.e., apnœa lasting 5 ₃0 seconds can be produced if the reservoir bag of an anæsthetic machine is compressed while the expiratory valve is closed, at the end of an inspiratory effort (in the absence of myoneural block). The deeper the anæsthesia, the longer the apnœa. Preliminary hyperventilation prolongs it still further. This is a useful procedure during certain radiological examinations done on the operating table, when a short period of apnœa is desirable. Reasons advanced to explain this phenomenon are : (1) Thiopentone frees the lower reflex centre from cerebral inhibition (Gordh). (2) The drug blocks the central actions of respiratory afferents in the vagus, contrary to what happens with ether or cyclopropane. (3) The drug depresses the respiratory centre to the stimulating effect of carbon dioxide, the build-up of which, during the apnœa, no longer stimulates the respiratory centre.

The parasympathetic system is depressed less than the sympathetic by thiopentone, and bronchial spasm is sometimes seen due

---

* Brodie, B. B., and others, *J. Pharmacol.*, 1950. **98**, 85.

Thiopentone Sodium—Pharmacology, *continued.*

to this cause, as well as coughing and bucking. Coughing and mild laryngospasm may occur spontaneously after injection of thiopentone, especially if the upper respiratory tract is irritable or if there is stimulation by airways, mucus, or blood.

CARDIOVASCULAR SYSTEM.—The force of the heart's contraction is weakened, and the heart dilates, but this is of no importance in normal hearts in fit patients receiving moderate doses of the drug. There is need for care when the drug is used in severe cases of cardiac decompensation as any existing coronary narrowing will result in a decrease of myocardial blood-supply. The drug is especially dangerous when the pathological condition of the heart does not allow for changes in rate or cardiac output to compensate for changes in vascular hæmodynamics, e.g., constrictive pericarditis, tight valvular stenosis, complete heart-block. The blood-pressure is depressed, depending on rate and amount of drug injected: it is probably due to dilatation of the vascular bed especially in skin and muscle, perhaps due to depression of the vasomotor centre, and the effect usually passes off with continuance of the anæsthesia. Constriction of vessels in the renal and splanchnic bed helps to counteract this. Rapid injection of too much thiopentone may have a most grave effect on the circulatory system.

Thiopentone gives no protection from vagal inhibition of the heart which may follow the use of chloroform, trichloroethylene, or cyclopropane.

Pre-existing ventricular extrasystoles may be abolished by the drug; auricular ectopic beats and auricular fibrillation are uninfluenced.

LARYNX.—Spasm is sometimes produced during thiopentone anæsthesia, either by stimuli from the site of operation, or from stimuli of the vagal nerve-endings in the larynx by mucus, blood, airways, etc., or those factors causing chronic cough. Spasm may in some cases be due to regurgitation of acid gastric contents, even in small amounts. It has also been suggested that the region of the hypothalamus controlling the parasympathetic recovers before that part controlling the sympathetic system. This effect is lessened by the pre-operative administration of atropine or hyoscine parasympathetic depressants. Laryngeal irritability is less after hexobarbitone and thiamylal than after thiopentone.

EYES.—Pupils first dilate, then contract. Sensitivity to light remains until the patient is deep enough to permit incision of the skin, and at this stage the eyeballs are usually centrally placed. During surgical anæsthesia the corneal, conjunctival eyelash and eyelid reflexes disappear. It reduces intra-ocular tension.

PREGNANT UTERUS.—Thiopentone has no effect on its tone, and so is a poor agent used alone for external version. It readily passes the placental barrier, achieving its maximal concentration in fœtal blood very soon after its injection into the mother.

FALLOPIAN TUBES.—No effect on tone of normal or abnormal tubes.

MYONEURAL JUNCTION.—A mild curariform effect, much less than that of ether. Not seen in clinical dosage.

SPLEEN.—Probably not caused to dilate, nor is hæmodilution caused.

ALIMENTARY CANAL.—Tone and motility only depressed after big doses.

EXCRETION AND METABOLISM.—It is almost completely metabolized in the body. The liver probably breaks down the drug, oxidizing its side-chains, this may be a more important factor than generally supposed in the early recovery from its effects;[*] between 10 and 15 per cent of the drug in the body is metabolized each hour: muscular tissue may help in its detoxication as may the kidneys. The degree of liver dysfunction must be considerable before a patient shows diminished tolerance to thiopentone, and tolerance is decreased only to intermittent doses given over a long period. The products of its breakdown are removed via the kidneys, but renal disease is not a contra-indication to its use, although a uræmic patient will require smaller amounts than a normal patient. A high blood-urea prolongs thiopentone narcosis. Urinary secretion is decreased during thiopentone anæsthesia due to : (a) Increased tubular resorption of water ; (b) Increased secretion of antidiuretic hormone ; (c) Hypotension ; (d) Renal vasoconstriction.

MISCELLANEOUS EFFECTS.—It passes into the cerebrospinal fluid and into the breast milk shortly after injection. The intracranial and cerebrospinal fluid pressure falls, while the blood-urea is not greatly affected. The blood-sugar rises slightly during clinical anæsthesia and varies with the degree of trauma due to the operation.[†] Disturbances in acid-base equilibrium are likely to be due to hypoventilation—not to metabolic acidosis. The barbiturates have an antagonistic action to cocaine and its derivatives. In some patients a localized muscular spasm is seen following injection. It usually takes the form of pronation of the forearm receiving the injection. Addition of nitrous oxide and oxygen usually controls it ; it occurs more frequently with 5 per cent solution than 2·5 per cent solution and can be lessened by opiates and pethidine.

Skin rashes have been very occasionally reported following its use. They may be scarlatiniform or urticarial.

Causes muscular necrosis if injected into muscular tissue.

It is a poor relaxer of the muscles of the anterior abdominal wall but usually enables a gynæcological bimanual examination to be carried out satisfactorily, and is sometimes used in small amounts to give just a little extra relaxation during closure of a laparotomy wound. A satisfactory agent used alone for the manipulation of the spine, joints, etc., if sufficient dosage is employed.

Premedication.—At the time of operation, the stomach, bowels, and bladder should be empty.

---

* Saidman, L. J., and Eger, E. I., *Anesthesiology*, 1966, **27**, 118.
† Clarke, R. S. J., *Brit. J. Anæsth.*, 1967, **39**, 518.

Thiopentone Sodium—Premedication, *continued.*

Atropine or hyoscine should usually be given to depress the vagal reflexes. A narcotic analgesic is not necessary in short operations, but is beneficial in longer ones for the following reasons:—

    1. It tranquillizes the patient, and reduces his metabolic rate.

    2. It reduces the amount of thiopentone needed and so reduces the period of post-operative depression.

    3. It helps to produce a smooth anæsthesia and reduces the incidence of muscular movements.

    4. It makes venepuncture easier.

Papaveretum, 20 mg., with hyoscine, 0·4 mg., is a favourite pre-medication. Morphine, 10–16 mg., or pethidine, 100 mg., with atropine, 0·8 mg., or hyoscine, 0·4 mg., may be substituted. Some workers prefer half these amounts. These injections should be given three-quarters of an hour before operation.

Trimeprazine, 25–50 mg. intramuscularly two hours before operation, and atropine, 0·8 mg., three-quarters of an hour before operation, are also a good combination. The use of thiopentone does not contra-indicate the use of pentobarbitone in reasonable dosage as a pre-anæsthetic sedative.

Course of Anæsthesia.—When an intravenous anæsthetic is given the following should be at hand in case of need : (1) A laryngoscope ; (2) Endotracheal tubes ; (3) Oxygen ; (4) A mask and reservoir bag ; (5) A tilting table ; (6) Suction apparatus. Guedel's classification of stages of anæsthesia does not apply. The patient is either too light (he reacts to surgical stimuli) ; he is properly anæsthetized ; or he is too deep (his respirations are very shallow, his blood-pressure depressed). The first injection should be 4–8 ml. of 2·5 per cent solution and it can be made quite rapidly in fit subjects ; more slowly in others. The concentration of the drug reaching the brain in arterial blood immediately after injection is determined by the rate of injection. If the patient counts at a uniform rate, an indication of his reaction to the drug is obtained. Just after the onset of unconsciousness, there is often a deep breath, followed by a period of respiratory depression. During this period no further injection should be given. With normal breathing re-established, further thiopentone is given according to the needs of the patient. If a little is injected at frequent intervals, observing its effects, no danger is likely to be encountered. It may be necessary to wait for surgical stimulation before the depth of anæsthesia can be ascertained for sure. A slight movement caused by the skin incision will often completely disappear once this severe stimulus has ended and is not necessarily an indication for deepening anæsthesia.

The criteria of depth are :—

    1. The activity of respiration in relation to surgical stimuli.

    2. Reflex movements of the patient in relation to such stimuli. When stimuli are severe, depth may have to be increased, e.g., when skin is incised or sutured.

Doses of thiopentone required vary from 0·1–2 g. Seldom should a larger dose be injected, and if 2·5 per cent solution is used, rarely is 1 g. exceeded. A small dose in a fit patient results in a short period of narcosis, but larger doses may be followed by prolonged sleep. Additional doses within thirty-six hours cause cumulation. A patient may respond to face slapping in the theatre, only to return to the quiet and warmth of his bed and there meet death from an unobserved respiratory obstruction. Thiopentone anæsthesia, except in the shortest and most minor operations, should always be accompanied by nitrous oxide and oxygen. Six litres per minute of the former and 2 litres of the latter is a good mixture. It enables the depth of respiration to be accurately assessed, reduces the amount of thiopentone needed by about 50 per cent, produces smoother anæsthesia, and guards against hypoxia.

Control of the airway is of primary importance in intravenous anæsthesia. A wisp of cotton-wool, held over the nares by a filament of adhesive strapping—a modification of Lundy's butterfly—gives a useful indication of the presence, rate, and depth of breathing in those few cases not receiving nitrous oxide and oxygen. In many cases respiration is free if the head is fully rotated to one side. In others, the lower jaw must be held forwards to draw the base of the tongue away from the posterior pharyngeal wall. Occasionally a pharyngeal airway or a nasopharyngeal tube is necessary, but these should only be used if the airway becomes obstructed without them, as they may stimulate pharyngeal reflexes which upset the smooth course of the anæsthesia.

A trace of trichloroethylene, or halothane, given before the pharyngeal airway is inserted, will frequently depress coughing and gagging reflexes, but should not, in the authors' opinion, be used routinely.

Respiratory obstruction and relative overdosage resulting in apnœa cause hypoxia, which, added to the depressing effect of the barbiturate, may soon inactivate the respiratory centre. The remedy for this respiratory depression or arrest is to get a free airway and to force oxygen into the lungs by pressure on the oxygen-filled reservoir bag of a gas machine, with expiratory valve shut; direct mouth-to-mouth insufflation via a face-mask; or by manual pressure on the thorax. Analeptics such as picrotoxin and nikethamide are of very secondary importance. When respiratory obstruction results from stimuli applied at too light a level of anæsthesia, the surgeon should, if necessary, be asked to wait until control of the airway is regained. The intravenous injection of a short-acting relaxant, e.g., suxamethonium, will also abolish spasm of the larynx due to this cause. Patients vary greatly in the amounts of drug they require to abolish reflex response to stimuli. Males need more than females; the fat need more than the thin; the young need more than the old.

Uses of Thiopentone.—

1. As the sole anæsthetic in very short operations; or the main agent, along with nitrous-oxide–oxygen.
2. For induction of general anæsthesia. Dose 4–6 mg./kg.

Uses of Thiopentone, *continued.*

   3. As part of the standard technique of thiopentone, relaxant, and gas–oxygen.
   4. To maintain light sleep during regional analgesia.
   5. To control convulsions, e.g., after local analgesic agents or ether.
   6. To quieten a patient rapidly who is too lightly anæsthetized.

Undesirable Effects of Thiopentone in Practice.—
   1. Respiratory depression, made worse by sedative premedication.
   2. Cardiovascular depression.
   3. Stimulation of undesirable upper respiratory tract reflexes, e.g., coughing, sneezing, laryngo- and bronchospasm.
   4. Local tissue irritation.
   5. It is a poor analgesic.
   6. Produces rather poor (prolonged) muscular relaxation.
   7. Delays recovery of full consciousness.
   8. Uncoordinated muscular movements.

Recovery from Anæsthesia.—Rate of recovery is influenced by the amount of premedication and the amount of thiopentone injected. Post-operative restlessness is rare and vomiting is infrequent. During the immediate post-operative period, the airway and the tidal exchange must be carefully watched. Out-patients should always be accompanied home after thiopentone anæsthesia.

Agents used to supplement Thiopentone.—
   1. NITROUS OXIDE AND OXYGEN.—When given as a 50 : 50 or 75 : 25 mixture, full oxygenation is assured and less thiopentone is used. It is a safety measure and is used routinely in many clinics when thiopentone is the anæsthetic, for all but short operations.
   2. PETHIDINE.—Serial injections of pethidine, e.g., 20 mg., may be used: this drug is a good analgesic, but may cause as much respiratory depression as thiopentone if given too liberally.
   3. MORPHINE.—Intravenous injection of 2–4 mg. is often helpful if a patient is taking much more thiopentone than average to obtain a level of smooth anæsthesia. After such a supplementary injection further thiopentone will often produce a profound effect. Diamorphine (1–2 mg.) has a similar action.
   4. CYCLOPROPANE, ETHER, TRICHLOROETHYLENE, AND HALOTHANE.—It is often wise to add one of these agents if a sufficiently deep plane of anæsthesia is not readily obtained with average doses of thiopentone.
      To push thiopentone may result in respiratory depression and prolonged post-operative sedation. Minimal trichloroethylene with gas and oxygen makes a specially useful supplement with a powerful depressant action on vagal reflexes, such as laryngeal spasm, cough, etc.
   5. RELAXANTS.—Most useful to prevent such reflexes as laryngeal spasm associated with, e.g., anal operations, skin incisions, orthopædic manipulations, etc. Frequently used to increase the muscular relaxation, which is not well marked when unsupplemented thiopentone is used.

6. LOCAL ANALGESIA.—A little local analgesic solution injected into the skin before its incision, and again before its suture, will enable smaller doses of thiopentone to be used, e.g., in the Trendelenburg operation for varicose veins in young men, and in hæmorrhoidectomy, etc. Topical analgesia of the pharynx and larynx, as by an amethocaine lozenge and a spray, will often prove useful before thiopentone anæsthesia in patients who are likely to need a pharyngeal airway.

Complications of Thiopentone Anæsthesia.—

1. LOCAL.—

a. PERIVENOUS INJECTION.—This may cause pain, redness, and swelling ; rarely ulceration (due to alkalinity of the solution). It may lead to median nerve injury if injection is made into the medial side of the antecubital fossa. These symptoms are less severe when the 2·5 per cent solution is used. Should solution be deposited outside the vein, 10 ml. of 1 per cent procaine can be injected into the area. This dilutes the thiopentone solution and, by promoting vasodilatation, aids absorption. The injection of 300 turbidity-reducing units of hyaluronidase dissolved in 10–20 ml. of saline also aids absorption and eases pain.

b. INTRA-ARTERIAL INJECTION.[*]—When this occurs the patient usually, but not always, feels severe burning pain down the arm and hand. It can be avoided by seeing that the artery is not occluded by the tourniquet before injection and by injecting 2 ml. of solution, and inquiring as to any pain experienced by the patient. Only if this is absent should the main injection proceed. This mishap may be dangerous and has led to necrosis and amputation of the hand. Severe pain is noticed after 2 ml. are injected, but this is not invariable. Sudden death from this cause has been reported. Presence of a pulse does not exclude the possibility that intra-arterial injection has taken place. Signs may include :—

i. A white hand with cyanosed fingers due to arterial spasm, which may be accompanied or followed by arterial thrombosis.

ii. Patches of skin discoloration, ulcer, or blisters.

iii. Œdema of forearm and hand. Œdematous areas may recover, the cause of such cases being spasm rather than thrombosis.

iv. Onset of unconsciousness may be delayed.

Accidental intra-arterial injection into arteries around the ankle and back of hand may occur.

Anatomy.—Division of the brachial artery above the elbow-joint occurs in 10 per cent of patients. When division is high, the ulnar artery reaches the forearm by running superficial to the flexor muscles and may run (i) below the deep fascia all the way down ; (ii) below the deep fascia proximally, later becoming subcutaneous ; (iii) subcutaneous

---

* Cohen, Sol., 1948, " Accidental Intra-arterial Injection of Drugs ", *Lancet*, 1948, **2**, 361 and 409.

Complications of Thiopentone Anæsthesia, *continued*.

near the elbow, later becoming deep to the deep fascia. It is this abnormal ulnar artery in its superficial position immediately deep to the median cubital vein, and without the protection of the aponeurotic tendon of the biceps, which may be accidentally punctured and used for injection.

When the brachial artery divides above elbow, the common interosseous branch of the ulnar artery is usually given off from the radial artery, so if ulnar artery is punctured its deep common interosseous branch is usually not involved.[*]

Some of the bad effects of the intra-arterial injection of drugs are due to the thrombosis of the small arteries supplying nerves, and so interfering with their conduction of motor impulses.

The *p*H of 2·5 per cent solution of thiopentone in water is 10·8 (*p*H of blood is 7·4). It is thus a strong alkaline irritant.

Pathology.—(1) The changes in *p*H of thiopentone which occur when it is mixed with blood in an artery results in precipitation of solid crystals of thiopentone which are swept along and eventually block small vascular channels at arteriolar and capillary levels. The crystals remain in the small vessels and their irritant properties cause a local release of noradrenaline with subsequent vascular spasm. Thus the greater the weight of the drug injected, the greater will be the effect—an additional argument in favour of the use of 2·5 per cent solution.[†] (2) The essential lesion is arterial thrombosis, and it may not become complete for fifteen days. (3) Intra-arterial injection of thiopentone (but not of hexobarbitone) will cause arterial spasm by releasing noradrenaline in or near the artery wall from a local store of this hormone.[‡] There is evidence that this thiopentone-induced noradrenaline vasoconstriction is potentiated by cocaine and abolished by tolazoline; it is much reduced by reserpine as this agent causes the disappearance of noradrenaline stores from the vessel walls.[§]

Treatment.—When thiopentone has been injected into the lumen of an artery during induction of anæsthesia the suggested lines of treatment are as follows: (1) Dilution of injected thiopentone; (2) Relief of arterial spasm and the pain it causes; (3) Prevention of thrombosis; (4) Later treatment of such symptoms as may arise.

If possible abandon the proposed operation and institute intensive anticoagulant therapy. Heparin, 7500–10,000 units, will double coagulation time and may need to be followed by 7500 units eight-hourly. The oral, longer-acting anticoaculants may be necessary for the 2 weeks following thiopentone injection into an artery. If postponement of

[*] McCormack, L. J., and others, *Surg. Gynec. Obstet.*, 1953, **96**, 43.
[†] Waters, D. J., *Anæsthesia*, 1966, **21**, 346; and Brown, S. S., Lyons, S. M., and Dundee, J. W., *Brit. J. Anæsth.*, 1968, **40**, 13.
[‡] Burn, J. H., and Hobbs, R., *Lancet*, 1959, **1**, 1112.
[§] Burn, J. H., *Brit. med. J.*, 1960, **2**, 414.

operation is impossible, neurectomy of the sympathetic supply to the affected limb should be performed surgically.*
The increase in blood-flow resulting will probably discourage thrombosis in the vessel damaged by thiopentone.

Additional Management.—

    i. Leave needle in the artery and inject:—

        α. Procaine hydrochloride 10–20 ml. of 0·5 per cent solution.

        β. Papaverine 40–80 mg. in 10–20 ml. of saline.

        γ. Tolazoline (priscol) 5 ml. of 1 per cent solution,† or as a continuous drip.‡

        δ. Dibenzyline, either 0·5 mg. which does not appreciably affect the general circulation, or as a drip diluted with saline 50–200 μg. per min.§

    These solutions can also be injected into the subclavian artery following a brachial plexus or stellate ganglion block.

    ii. Continue anæsthesia as an effective method of securing vasodilatation. Cyclopropane and halothane are good. Perform a brachial plexus or stellate ganglion block to remove all vasoconstrictor impulses.

    iii. Elevate limb and keep it warm; deal with such lesions as may arise.

  c. THROMBOPHLEBITIS.—This may occur in spite of a clean, aseptic venepuncture and is due to chemical irritation of the vein wall. It may follow the injection or be postponed for 7–10 days. It should be treated by heat and rest, if necessary with a plaster splint. It, too, is more common with the 5 per cent than the 2·5 per cent solution.

  d. ARTERIAL SPASM.—Is said to have followed intravenous medication, in the absence of direct injury to the artery.

  e. INJURY TO NERVES, especially the median, following injection into the medial side of the ante-cubital fossa.

  f. BROKEN NEEDLE.—As the fracture usually occurs between the hub and the shaft, at least 0·5 cm. of shaft should always be outside tissues.

2. GENERAL.—

  a. RESPIRATORY DEPRESSION.—For treatment, *see above.* Apnœa during intravenous anæsthesia may be due to : (1) Relative overdose of drug ; (2) Respiratory obstruction above the glottis, e.g., the tongue falling back ; (3) Laryngeal spasm.

  b. CIRCULATORY COLLAPSE.—This is usually due to a relative overdose causing vasodilatation and myocardial depression. Treatment : Tilt down the head end of the table ; give oxygen by intermittent positive-pressure inflation ; inject into a vein a vasoconstrictor if necessary.

  c. LARYNGEAL SPASM.—This may result from : (1) Direct local stimulation by an airway, saliva, blood, etc. ; (2) Stimulation of some remote area, e.g., anal sphincter, cervix uteri, etc. (Brewer-Luckhardt reflexes) ; (3) Part of a general anoxic

* Kinmonth, J. B., and Shepherd, R. L., *Brit. med. J.*, 1960, **2**, 939.
† Stuart, P., *Ibid.*, 1955, **2**, 1308.
‡ Waters, D. J., *Anæsthesia*, 1966, **21**, 346.
§ Duff, R. S., *Brit. med. J.*, 1956, **2**, 857.

Complications of Thiopentone Anæsthesia, *continued.*

spasm. Thiopentone predisposes to laryngeal spasm. Depth of anæsthesia should be slowly increased and oxygen administered under pressure. Intravenous injection of 20–30 mg. of suxamethonium, together with oxygen under positive pressure, may be required to relax the spasm. Occasionally, as in certain cases of asthma, a dose of thiopentone may cause intensive bronchial spasm, muscular rigidity, and reflex apnœa—an alarming condition, which usually yields to the intravenous injection of a rapidly acting relaxant, together with oxygen given under positive pressure.

d. COUGHING.—Depth should be gradually increased. Nitrous-oxide–oxygen, trichloroethylene, or other agents may be required in resistant cases. Hiccup occasionally seen.

e. SNEEZING.—May occur in eye operations, in spite of adequate topical analgesia of the conjunctival sac and nasolacrimal duct. Interruption of surgical stimuli, with slow increase of depth of anæsthesia, will often control this distressing symptom.

f. POST-OPERATIVE VERTIGO, EUPHORIA, AND DISORIENTATION.— Because of the possibility of this condition, out-patients should be accompanied home.

g. TRUE CUTANEOUS ALLERGY can occur, either in the form of a scarlatiniform rash, or as true angioneurotic œdema. Photosensitivity to thiopentone in patients recently exposed to sunlight has been reported.

h. SEVERE ANAPHYLACTIC REACTION with cyanosis, impalpable pulse, bronchospasm, and prolonged post-operative hypotension have been reported,* accompanied by a positive Prausnitz-Küstner (passive transfer) reaction and an immediate cutaneous reagin-type hypersensitivity to thiopentone.

i. INFECTIVE HEPATITIS.—Transmission of the virus of infective hepatitis, with its twelve-weeks' incubation period, if apparatus is not properly sterilized.

Advantages and Disadvantages of Thiopentone Anæsthesia.

The advantages are :—

1. Ease and rapidity of induction.
2. Absence of stage of delirium.
3. Rapid recovery (with correct dosage) and relative freedom from vomiting and post-operative discomfort, etc.
4. Absence of irritation of respiratory mucosa.
5. Ability to increase depth rapidly.

The disadvantages are :—

1. Respiratory depression.
2. Tendency to laryngeal spasm, especially following vomiting.
3. Poor abdominal relaxation with safe dosage.
4. Circulatory depression in poor-risk patients.
5. Uncoordinated muscular movements.

---

* Currie, T. T., and others, *Brit. med. J.*, 1966, **1**, 1462; and Carrie, L. E. S., and Buchanan, R. L., *Anæsthesia*, 1967, **22**, 290.

Indications.—These are legion, almost every operation in surgery having been performed under intravenous barbiturate anæsthesia. It is specially useful :—

1. For induction of general anæsthesia.
2. For short operations.
3. Under Service conditions where portability and relative ease of administration are advantages.
4. For supplementing regional analgesia.
5. In the presence of a cautery.
6. For controlling convulsions during general or local anæsthesia, eclampsia, epilepsy, tetanus, etc.
7. For narco-analysis in psychiatry, and for electroconvulsive therapy.

Thiopentone is a suitable anæsthetic for the following :—

1. Certain eye operations. Intra-ocular tension is reduced in both normal and glaucomatous eyes.
2. Minor gynæcological operations and examinations under anæsthesia.
3. Cystoscopies in patients who are not seriously uræmic or emphysematous.
4. Hæmorrhoidectomies; anal fissures, etc. (usually supplemented by a relaxant).
5. Orthopædic manipulations.
6. Encephalography and lumbar puncture under general anæsthesia.
7. Producing abdominal relaxation quickly, for a relatively short time during an operation under inhalation anæsthesia, e.g., for suturing the peritoneum, when the surgeon wants a little extra relaxation.
8. For major surgery when the balanced combination of thiopentone, gas–oxygen, and a relaxant is used.

Contra-indications.—Opinions differ as to contra-indications, some workers denying that any absolute contra-indications exist.

In the following procedures and types of case, special care is needed, and oxygen or nitrous-oxide–oxygen, half of each, must be given in addition :—

1. Children under 4 : because while their respiratory centres are easily depressed, their upper respiratory passages are relatively small, these factors predisposing to hypoxia. Moreover, children do not like needles ; while their active reflexes require large amounts of thiopentone for their subjugation, so that they sleep for long periods after operation. However, they do very well if given a sleep dose of thiopentone, followed by a relaxant, intubation, and gas–oxygen.
2. Shocked, debilitated, severely anæmic, and uræmic cases : small doses are required. The administration of pure oxygen is useful in handicapped patients before anæsthesia is induced. It also aids the removal of nitrogen from the lungs and allows nitrous oxide to exert its analgesic effects more quickly, so reducing the need for thiopentone.

There may be a dose of the drug small enough for induction of anæsthesia with safety in even the most decrepit patient,

Thiopentone Sodium—Contra-indications, *continued*.

but in the gravely ill halothane or cyclopropane has some advantages.

3. Patients with gross dyspnœa due to cardiac or respiratory disease. It should be used with extreme caution—if at all—in cases of constrictive pericarditis, tight valvular stenosis, and complete heart block.

4. Patients with respiratory obstruction.

5. Operations in which the return of reflexes immediately after operation is desirable, e.g., out-patients who have to go home alone. It is difficult to have a patient adequately anæsthetized one minute, and coughing the next, e.g., in tonsillectomy.

6. In bronchoscopy and œsophagoscopy—unless adequate topical analgesia and/or a relaxant is used also. Dangerous laryngeal spasm may be initiated.

7. Cases of acute intestinal obstruction. Aspiration of stomach contents may cause dangerous laryngeal spasm unless proper care is taken to prevent it. Also the liver in such cases is often functionally depressed.

8. Patients with acute inflammation about the mouth, jaw, and neck. Several deaths have occurred under thiopentone anæsthesia in such patients. A likely cause of death is interference with the airway associated with spasticity of the jaw due to inflammatory œdema.

9. Asthma. Attacks have occasionally been made worse by thiopentone : in other cases no adverse effect has been seen. The drug should be given slowly, the anæsthetist feeling his way cautiously. Better still, soluble hexobarbitone should be used instead.

10. Feeble, elderly patients on the brink of dementia. Recovery may be slow and associated with disorientation.

11. For external version, thiopentone is a poor relaxant. For delivery, no more than an induction dose should be used (0·25 g.).

12. In malarial patients, a little goes a long way.

13. Cases of dystrophia myotonica (J. W. Dundee). The patients react normally to curare, but abnormally to thiopentone,* and prolonged apnœa may follow injection of more than 100 mg. Myotonia is a hereditary familial disease usually seen in young adults. It may be characterized by : (*a*) Myotonia, i.e., persistence of muscular tone after its voluntary irritation ; (*b*) Muscular atrophy, most often involving the sternomastoids and facial muscles bilaterally ; (*c*) Sometimes, cataract, premature frontal baldness, thyroid adenoma, gonad atrophy, diabetes, and mental changes.

14. Addison's disease and myxœdema. Must be used with great care.

15. Myasthenia gravis. Great care necessary.

16. Patients with hepatic dysfunction. Small doses only.

---

* Dundee, J. W., *Curr. Res. Anesth.*, 1952, **31**, 257; Lodge, A. B., *Brit. med. J.*, 1958, **1**, 1043; and McClelland, R. M. A., *Brit. J. Anæsth.*, 1960, **32**, 81.

17. Porphyria,* which may be congenital or appear as acute attacks of abdominal pain somewhat resembling lead poisoning with the passage of reddish urine. Barbiturates may precipitate lower motor neuron paralysis and perhaps death, and are absolutely contra-indicated. If suspected, the urine should be tested for porphyrins.

18. Alcoholics taking disulfiram (antabuse) and patients suffering from poisoning with dinitro-ortho-cresol, a weed killer (barbiturates and D.N.C. have a synergistic depressant effect on cellular respiration†).

19. Hyperkalæmic familial periodic paralysis.‡

20. Huntington's chorea.§

21. A history of thiopentone anaphylaxis.‖

22. Patients with difficult veins. There is no excuse for subjecting a patient to the painful experience of multiple needle punctures in an effort to provide a pleasant induction of anæsthesia.

Other Methods of Thiopentone Administration.—Various types of equipment have been developed to enable thiopentone to be delivered to a vein, some by remote control.

Solution of the normal strength can be injected into the tubing of an intravenous drip by a fine intradermal needle. It can be dissolved in saline in strengths of 0·1 to 2·5 per cent and run in as a drip. Each 0·5 g. of thiopentone added to a 500-ml. bottle of intravenous fluid increases the percentage roughly 0·1 per cent. Thus 0·5 g. to 500 ml. is 0·1 per cent; 1 g. to 500 ml. is 0·2 per cent; etc. A drip rate of 40 per minute roughly equals 140 ml. per hour or 500 ml. in 4 hours; 5 per cent dextrose in water can be used. A useful method is to interpose a three-way tap between the syringe and needle and lead a saline drip to the third arm of the tap. Thus the drip ensures a patent needle, and if the tap is turned, thiopentone solution is directed from the syringe into the vein.

Description of Average Thiopentone Administration.—The arm of the patient is abducted, placed on an armboard, and built up with pads underneath so that no strain is placed on the brachial plexus. A piece of rubber tubing is fixed around the upper arm with a hæmostat and the presence of the radial pulse is verified : a second rubber tube is likewise fixed with a hæmostat surrounding the wrist and armboard. A vein is selected, preferably on the dorsum of the hand or one in the long axis of the limb away from the medial aspect of the antecubital fossa. It is cleaned with antiseptic and a small weal is raised just lateral to the vein with the finest intradermal needle, using 1 per cent procaine solution. Through the weal, a larger needle is inserted (e.g., No. 1) and it is advanced into the vein as great a distance as it will safely go. The

* Dundee, J. W., and Riding, V. E., *Anæsthesia*, 1955, **10**, 55; and Bush, G. H., *Proc. R. Soc. Med.*, 1968, **61**, 171.
† Edson, E. F., and Carey, F. M., *Brit. med. J.*, 1955, **1**, 104.
‡ Egan, T. J., and Klein, R., *Pediatrics*, 1959, **24**, 761.
§ Davies, D. D., *Brit. J. Anæsth.*, 1966, **38**, 490.
‖ Currie, T. T., and others, *Brit. med. J.*, 1966, **1**, 1462; and Anderton, J. M., and Hopton, D. S., *Anæsthesia*, 1968, **23**, 90.

Description of Average Thiopentone Administration, *continued.*

insertion of a Mitchell or other non-clotting needle through the skin weal is a preferable and more elegant technique. Thiopentone solution 2·5 per cent is injected after the anæsthetist is certain that his needle is truly intravenous : this may need aspiration of a little blood into the syringe ; 0·05 g. (2 ml.) is injected and the patient is asked if his arm is comfortable. Should pain occur in the fingers or hand, it indicates that the injection is probably intra-arterial, in which case harm is unlikely if no more is given. In the absence of hand pain, a further 5–10 ml. are injected, and when the patient loses consciousness, if a non-clotting needle has not been used, the tourniquet tubing is used to strap the syringe on to the arm : it encircles syringe, arm, and armboard and is secured with an artery forceps, not too tightly, for fear of injuring the median nerve. Nitrous-oxide–oxygen is now given (50 : 50 or 75 : 25) so that a total flow of 7–8 litres per minute is available. Just before the surgical stimulus is applied more thiopentone is injected, the amount depending on the type of patient, his reflex irritability, and the type of operation. Minimal trichloroethylene or halothane can usefully be added : (1) If the patient coughs, gags, or bucks. (2) If the insertion of an airway, being necessary, is likely to disturb the smooth anæsthesia. (3) If reflex activity (lightness) reappears after 0·75 g. of thiopentone has been injected —to prevent use of too much barbiturate. Pethidine can be used for the same purpose. (4) If an endotracheal tube is used—to prevent coughing. (5) If it is important for the patient to recover consciousness early.

Drugs Chemically Incompatible with Thiopentone.—Pethidine, alphaprodine, phenothiazine derivatives, laudexium methyl-sulphate, suxamethonium salts, nalorphine, procaine hydro-chloride, papaverine.

The following drugs form with thiopentone a slight precipitate which redissolves in an excess of the thiobarbiturate : gallamine, papaveretum, morphine, levorphan, pentolinium tartrate, trimetaphan, methyl amphetamine, methoxamine, levallorphan, lignocaine, pitressin.

METHOHEXITONE
*(Brevital ; Brietal)**

This is a methylated oxybarbiturate with the chemical name allyl-1,methyl-2-pentynyl-barbiturate. First described by Stoelting in 1957.† To each 500 mg. of powdered drug is added 30 mg. of sodium carbonate. When used in 1 per cent solution the pH is 11·1. While it is two and a half to three times as potent as thiopentone (Thomas states it is 2·75 times as potent)* complete recovery is quicker. Less irritating than thiopentone solution when injected into tissues, but intra-arterial

---

* Barron, D. W., and Dundee, J. W., *Brit. J. Anæsth.*, 1961, **33**, 81 ; Dundee, J. W., and Moore, J., *Anæsthesia*, 1961, **16**, 184 ; and Green, R. A., and Jolly, C., *Brit. J. Anæsth.*, 1960, **32**, 593.
† Stoelting, V. K., *Curr. Res. Anesth.*, 1957, **36**, 49.
‡ Thomas, E. T., *Anæsthesia*, 1967, **22**, 16.

methohexitone is as irritant and dangerous as thiopentone in the same concentration, but, of course, the 1 per cent solution as commonly used is less dangerous than 2·5 per cent thiopentone.* Causes less cardio-vascular depression than thiopentone, but more abnormal muscular movements with tremor, coughing, and hiccups; these are reduced after premedication with pethidine or opiates.† Said to be 5·2 times as potent as propanidid.‡ Dosage of the 1 per cent solution is about 5–7 mg. per stone for induction (50–120 mg.) (similar in volume to 2·5 per cent thiopentone) and this is usually followed by gas and oxygen. The aqueous solution is stable for several weeks but should not be mixed with such acid solutions as atropine sulphate, tubocurarine, and suxamethonium. Useful for induction of anæsthesia in the dental chair§ and for operations on out-patients. The only barbiturate which competes clinically with thiopentone, especially when rapid recovery is required. Has been used in a freshly prepared mixture with propanidid.||

INTRAMUSCULAR METHOHEXITONE.¶—This is reported to give satisfactory pre-anæsthetic sedation in about 85 per cent of pædiatric cases. The dose recommended is 3 mg. per lb. (6·6 mg. per kg.) in 2 per cent solution given into the upper and outer quadrant of the buttock. Sleep usually comes on in under 10 min., but if its onset is delayed, the dose can be repeated in the opposite buttock. Pre- and post-operative excitement, laryngospasm, and restlessness are not troublesome but apnœa lasting 5–10 min. is occasionally seen and requires I.P.P.V. Thus medical supervision is necessary from the time of intramuscular injection until the commencement of induction of anæsthesia. Abscesses and sloughs are said not to occur.

OTHER INTRAVENOUS ANÆSTHETICS

Buthalitone Sodium (Transithal; Baytenal; Ulbreval; Thial-butone).—This is the sodium salt of allyl-2 methyl propyl barbituric acid and was synthesized in 1936 by Miller and others in the U.S. and investigated by Weese and Koss in 1954 in Germany. It is used in 5 or 10 per cent solution which is alkaline due to the addition of 6 per cent sodium carbonate. The pH of the 2·5 per cent solution is 10·6 ; of the 5 per cent solution 10·55. Has been used to precede nitrous oxide and oxygen in the dental chair (400–600 mg.)** and in the casualty department.†† Useful, together with a relaxant, for manipulations (500–1000 mg.). Weight for weight, about half as potent as thiopentone.

Soluble Hexobarbitone (B.P.) (Evipan ; Evipan soluble ; Cyclonal sodium ; Hexanostab ; Hexanol ; Oevipana ; Oulapan).—This is sodium N methyl-c-c-cyclohexenyl methyl barbiturate. First

* Francis, J. G., *Anæsthesia*, 1964, **19**, 59.
† Dundee, J. W., and Moore, J., *Brit. J. Anæsth.*, 1961, **33**, 382.
‡ Howells, T. H., and others, *Ibid.*, 1967, **39**, 31.
§ Howells, T. H., *Ibid.*, 1968, **40**, 182.
|| Dundee, J. W., and Lyons, S. M., *Ibid.*, 1967, **39**, 957.
¶ Miller, J. R., and Stoelting, V. K., *Curr. Res. Anesth.*, 1961, **40**, 573; and *Brit. J.Anæsth.*, 1963, **35**, 68.
** Young, D. S., *Proc. R. Soc. Med.*, 1956, **49**, 735.
†† Nobes, P., *Lancet*, 1955, **1**, 797.

Soluble Hexobarbitone, *continued.*

used in 1932 by Weese and Scarpff after being synthesized by Kropp and Taub.

It is used as a 10 per cent solution (though 5 per cent is probably preferable), pH 11·3 and 11·5 respectively, its action being similar to, though less depressing to the respiration and circulation, and less irritating to the tissues than thiopentone sodium and one-half as potent. Muscular movements, twitching, sneezing, etc., are more frequent during induction than with thiopentone, but respiratory depression and bronchial and laryngeal spasm are less common. Average dose for induction of anæsthesia, 400 mg. Useful in asthmatics.

Thialbarbitone Sodium (Kemithal).—Sodium 5-cyclohexenyl-5-allyl-2-thiobarbiturate. Prepared by Carrington in 1938 in Britain but not investigated pharmacologically until 1946 (Carrington and Raventós).* Supplied in ampoules of 1 and 2 g. of dried powder. Like thiopentone, it contains a sulphur atom. Used as a 10 per cent solution, which remains stable for less than six hours, the pH of which is 10·3. In anæsthetic effect thialbarbitone 1 g. equals thiopentone 0·5 gr. Thialbarbitone is less likely to produce laryngeal spasm and respiratory depression than an equivalent anæsthetic dose of thiopentone. During recovery, especially in children, generalized muscular rigidity, unassociated with laryngeal spasm, may result from any strong stimulus.

Inactin.—This is sodium 5-ethyl-5(methyl propyl) thiobarbiturate and was first described by Tabern and Volwiler in 1935. It was introduced into clinical anæsthesia by Horatz and Sturtzbecher in 1952. It is very similar in action and duration to thiopentone but with slightly lower potency (Dundee, J. W., and Riding, J. E., *Brit. J. Anæsth.*, 1960, **32**, 206).

Methitural (Neraval ; Thiogenal).—First described by Zima and others in 1954. It is the sodium salt of methyl-thioethyl-2-pentyl thiobarbituric acid, and was used clinically by Reifferscheid and Dietmann in 1954. Dose required to produce sleep, half as much again as with thiopentone. Causes too much coughing and hiccup for routine clinical use.

Pernocton.—A 10 per cent solution of sodium butyl betabromallyl barbiturate. First used by Bumm in 1927.† The first widely used intravenous barbiturate in anæsthesia. Of historic interest only. Excretion too slow for safe routine use, but it can be used for induction, 1 ml. being given each minute until the patient is asleep. As it is stable in solution it is supplied ready dissolved.

Pentobarbitone Sodium (Nembutal ; Pentobarbital).—Sodium ethyl-methyl-butyl barbiturate. First used intravenously by Lundy in 1931.‡ It is less likely to cause laryngeal spasm than is thiopentone and has been used before endotracheal intubation on this account.

---

* Carrington, H. C., and Raventós, J., *Brit. J. Pharmacol.*, 1946, **1**, 215.
† Bumm, R., *Klin. Wschr.*, 1927, **6**, 725.
‡ Lundy, J. S., *Surg. Clin. N. Amer.*, 1931, **11**, 909.

Useful to produce sleep during operations under regional analgesia. Usual strength 7·5 per cent. Patient wakes up less confused than after thiopentone. Sodium salt used for intravenous injection.

Quinalbarbitone Sodium (Sodium seconal).—Sodium 5-allyl-5(1-methyl-butyl) barbiturate. Has a longer though less intense action than thiopentone ; has no analgesic effect. May be useful for producing sleep during a good regional block. Laryngeal spasm not very frequent.

Thiamylal Sodium (Surital sodium ; Thioquinalbarbitone ; Thioseconal sodium).—First described in 1935 by Volwiler and Tabern. Sodium 5-allyl-5-(1-methylbutyl) 2 thiobarbituric acid. It is the sulphur salt of quinalbarbitone (seconal) and is used in 2·5 per cent solution. Very similar in its action to thiopentone, slightly greater in potency and with less tendency to cause cumulation.

The electro-encephalographic monitoring of barbiturate anæsthesia in man has been described with the application of the findings to the problem of automatic control of anæsthesia (servo-anæsthesia).*

Propanidid (Epontol; FBA.1420).—This phenoxyacetic amine is a eugenol derivative with the chemical composition—propyl 4-NN-diethylcarbamoylmethoxy-3-methoxy-phenylacetate. It is a yellow oil and is prepared as a 5 per cent solution in oxyphenylated castor oil in 10-ml. ampoules. This solution is viscous but can be diluted with distilled water or normal saline and is miscible with such drugs as atropine, suxamethonium chloride, gallamine, and tubocurarine.

Following intravenous injection it may cause hyperpnœa followed by a short period of apnœa. Prolonged apnœa is not seen after clinical doses although it potentiates the effects of suxamethonium by an action on muscle-fibres and not on the motor end-plate.† It sometimes causes muscular movements and tremors and may result in vomiting, especially if it has been combined with gas–oxygen. May reduce the blood-pressure. Has no anti-analgesic effects but venous thrombosis has followed its use. No hepatoxic complications found after the usual clinical doses. Laryngeal spasm rare. Action short in duration with little hangover. May be unsuitable for use along with non-depolarizing relaxants for intubation as patient may regain consciousness during the procedure. Dose 5–10 mg. per kg. Rapidly destroyed in body, in the liver, and in plasma and not relocated to other body tissues like thiopentone. Antagonized by bemegride. Not contra-indicated in acute porphyria. Useful for very short operations and in out-patients, and can be used alone to enable blind nasal intubation to be undertaken.

Can be mixed (freshly) with methohexitone and then results in fewer side-effects than either drug used alone (propanidid 25 mg. with methohexitone 10 mg. per ml.).‡

---

* Wyke, B. D., *Anæsthesia*, 1957, **12**, 259.
† Clarke, R. J. S., and others, *Ibid.*, 1967, **22**, 235.
‡ Dundee, J. W., and Lyons, S. M., *Brit. J. Anæsth.*, 1967, **39**, 957.

Intravenous Ether.—Used in animals by Pirogoff in Russia in 1847, a year after Morton's use of ether by inhalation. Used in surgery by Burckhardt in 1909.

A 2·5 to 5 per cent solution in normal saline or glucose 5 per cent is used, 12·5 to 25 ml. of ether being well shaken up in a bottle containing 500 ml. of saline, warmed to about 90° F., not more, as the boiling-point of ether is 98·6° F. After complete solution a continuous intravenous drip is set up, slowly at first and later the fluid running as a steady stream. Once anæsthesia is induced, which may require 400 ml. of solution or more, maintenance rate is 40–60 drops per minute. A better method of induction is by thiopentone. Signs of anæsthesia are similar to those when ether is given by inhalation, although respiration is quieter. Premedication is as for ether given by inhalation. Has been recommended for oral and endoscopic procedures, e.g., tonsillectomies and bronchoscopies.*

Vomiting and respiratory irritation are less than with inhalation ether anæsthesia. A solution stronger than 5 per cent may cause hæmoglobinuria : the method is contra-indicated in renal disease. The airway needs the same attention as with any general anæsthetic. May cause thrombophlebitis.

Recovery is fairly rapid.

Emulsions of Volatile Agents.—Intravenous administration of volatile agents with a low vapour pressure and a high potency may, after further trial, prove useful. Methoxyflurane has been used in 3·5 per cent solution as an oily emulsion.†

Hydroxydione Sodium Hemisuccinate (Viadril,‡ Presuren).—This is 21-hydroxypregnane-3, 20-dione sodium succinate and is a steroid, a group of agents never used before to produce anæsthesia. Selye was the first to notice the anæsthetic properties of certain steroids in 1941. First used by Murphy§ of the University of California in 1955 at the suggestion of Laubach and his colleagues. It is a crystalline solid sold in 0·5-g. ampoules. Because of its tendency to irritate veins its popularity has been limited. Its solution is incompatible with solutions of pethidine, tubocurarine, and suxamethonium. It has no hormonal activity. It finds its chief use together with premedication, pethidine, and gas–oxygen and should not be used as the sole anæsthetic agent. When 500–700 mg. have been run in to the patient, laryngoscopy can usually be performed without causing pharyngeal and laryngeal reflex activity. Post-anæsthetic drowsiness may last for an hour or two, but vomiting is rare and the patient is said to feel better than after a comparable dose of a thiobarbiturate. Unlike the barbiturates it has an analgesic effect in low concentrations. This may explain the feeling of well-being in patients after operation.

---

* Butt, H., and others, *Curr. Res. Anesth.*, 1965, **44**, 186; and Lundy, J. S., *Surg. Clin. N. Amer.*, 1931, **11**, 909.
† Krantz, J. C., and others, *Curr. Res. Anesth.*, 1962, **41**, 257.
‡ Montgomery, F. A., and others, *Anesthesiology*, 1958, **19**, 450.
§ Murphy, F. J., Guardaghi, N. P., and De Bon, F., *J. Amer. med. Ass.*, 1955, **158**, 1412.

Abdominal relaxation poor : hypotension sometimes caused : effect on myocardium not usually serious although tachycardia has been reported. It is said to inhibit adrenaline-induced arrhythmias.* Respiratory depression less than after thiopentone. Its disadvantages are its tendency to cause thrombophlebitis and the slow onset of anæsthesia. One advantage is its benign effect on the laryngeal reflexes. Such complications as fall in blood-pressure and respiratory depression may not occur until some time after the administration of the drug has stopped.† Mostly excreted by liver, but partly excreted unchanged by kidneys. Presuren may be kinder to vein walls than Viadril. Dosage 5–8 mg. per pound. It has been recommended for the induction of anæsthesia for thyroidectomies.‡ Little used to-day.

METHODS FOR PREVENTING THROMBOPHLEBITIS (Robertson, J. D., and Wynn Williams, A., *Anæsthesia*, 1961, **16**, 389).—

1. Use of concentrated solution (5–10 per cent) in warm saline.
2. Injection into a large vein.
3. Rapid injection.
4. Injection of 5–10 per cent solution (of Presuren) in 0·25–0·5 per cent solution of procaine, through a wide-bore needle into a large vein, followed by elevation of the limb and gentle massage of arm with avoidance of elbow flexion with its risk of trapping of the solution (Galley, A. H., and Lerman, L. H., *Brit. med. J.*, 1959, **1**, 332).
5. Follow intravenous injection through the same needle immediately by 5 ml. of 1 per cent procaine solution (Morley, T. R., *Aust. N.Z. J. Surg.*, 1959, **28**, 228).
6. Employment of reactive hyperæmia following the release of an arterial tourniquet which has been in position for 3–5 min. This rapidly washes the drug out of the arm veins (Dundee, J. W., and McArdle, L. : Letter in *Brit. med. J.*, 1959, **1**, 644).

The phlebothrombosis is due to irritation of the vein wall by the drug and not its alkalinity, and it starts as an agglutination thrombosis due to stickiness of the red cells and platelets and not to a clotting mechanism.

Intravenous Paraldehyde.—This method was used first in 1913 by Noel and Souttar.§ Paraldehyde has very little respiratory depressing effect and in normal doses does not damage the liver. If a concentrated solution is injected quickly, cough and laryngeal spasm may be produced and doses of 2 ml. have been given intravenously to stimulate coughing after operation. It has been given as a 6–8 per cent mixture with isotonic glucose, at the rate of 15–20 ml. each minute. It has also been mixed with saline and ether. Paraldehyde must be fresh. To sterilize it, it can be autoclaved at 130° C. for 30 minutes, without decomposition. As a 2·5 per cent solution in normal saline intravenously, it acts as a good anticonvulsant : dosage 0·2 ml. per kg. of body-weight. It

---

* Taylor, N. R. W., and Watson, H., *Lancet*, 1958, **2**, 300.
† Hunter, A. R., *Anæsthesia*, 1957, **12**, 10; and Dent, S. J., and Wilson, W. P., *Anesthesiology*, 1956, **17**, 673.
‡ Landau, E., *Anæsthesia*, 1958, **13**, 147.
§ Noel, H., and Souttar, H. S., *Ann. Surg.*, 1913, **57**, 64.

Intravenous Paraldehyde, *continued.*

depresses the cerebral cortex. Given intramuscularly in 5-ml. doses it is useful for post-operative restlessness not due to pain.

Intravenous Diamorphine and Morphine.—The intravenous injection of morphine produces a rapid effect. It is useful:—

1. In acute pain, especially if associated with shock. Shock makes absorption from subcutaneous tissues slow and uncertain. On its reversal, sudden absorption takes place.
2. Before regional analgesia, if patient is ill at ease.
3. To supplement regional analgesia for unpleasant examinations, e.g., bronchoscopy.
4. To premedicate patients before emergency operations.

Morphine should be given slowly in dilute solution in similar dosage to that used for hypodermic injection. Like thiopentone morphine may increase laryngeal irritability.

The respiratory depressant effects of morphine (and pethidine) can be readily controlled by amiphenazole, nalorphine, and levallorphan; nausea and vomiting by cyclizine or perphenazine; and constipation by senokot.*

Pethidine.—To recapitulate its pharmacological effects, it has the following actions: (1) Morphine-like effect on pain without causing constipation. (2) Papaverine-like effect on smooth muscle, resulting in relaxation of bronchi, intestine, and uterus. (3) Atropine-like effect on heart and salivary glands. (4) Anti-histamine effect. It antagonizes the action of acetylcholine on smooth muscle.

Useful, together with local analgesia, for endoscopic examinations.†

Intravenous pethidine during anæsthesia was first used in 1947 by Neff and his colleagues in the U.S.A.‡ and by Mushin and Rendell-Baker in 1949§ in Britain.

TECHNIQUE.—Premedication may be either morphine and atropine, papaveretum and hyoscine, or pethidine 100 mg. and hyoscine 0·4 mg. After a sleep dose of thiopentone (0·25–0·75 g.) gas and oxygen are given and pethidine 10–25 mg. injected intravenously. After a short period, further pethidine (25 mg.) is given and repeated in the same dosage, roughly, every half hour. It must be given before the patient reacts to stimuli, not afterwards, as it takes some time to act. A relaxant is used as required. If veins are bad, 100 mg. can be injected intramuscularly as soon as the patient is asleep. Can be given to children in doses reduced in relation to their weight. Has been added to a continuous intravenous drip—100 mg. to 500 ml.—at a rate of approximately 1 mg. per minute.

For dressing painful burns the combination of pethidine and amiphenazole in the proportion of 3 : 1 is useful. Dose of pethidine in children 100–150 mg. ; in adults 150–250 mg.‖

* Christie, G., Gershon, S., Gray, R., Shaw, F. H., McCance, I., and Bruce, D. W., *Brit. med. J.*, 1958, **1**, 675.
† Markby, C. E. P., *Ibid.*, 1958, **1**, 1397.
‡ Neff, W. B., and others, *Calif. Med.*, 1947, **66**, 67.
§ Mushin, W. W., and Rendell-Baker, L., *Brit. med. J.*, 1949, **2**, 472.
‖ Davies, M. R., *Lancet*, 1959, **2**, 710.

For sigmoidoscopy or cystoscopy, 50–100 mg. are useful.

Pethidine has recently been combined with levallorphan (100 mg. of pethidine with 1·25 mg. of levallorphan) under the name of pethilorphan. The levallorphan is stated to have an optimal effect on respiratory depression and a minimal effect on analgesia.

Pethidine is destroyed in the liver.

ADVANTAGES.—It allows patients to be comfortably awake very soon after the end of the operation.

It relaxes the bronchi, allows easier pulmonary inflation, and depresses upper respiratory tract reflexes sometimes seen after intubation, and after thiopentone.

It reduces the rapid ventilation rate sometimes seen after even small amounts of trichloroethylene.

It postpones and reduces the need for post-operative sedation.

DISADVANTAGES.—It may cause respiratory depression and slow breathing. But this can be counteracted by the injection of nalorphine or levallorphan.

It may cause hypotension and circulatory depression due to myocardial depression and also to vasodilatation, and so anæsthesia should be started with a test dose of 10–25 mg. This effect is sometimes delayed for several hours.

It contracts the sphincter of Oddi and so may interfere with successful exploration of the common bile-duct.

In cases of severe liver dysfunction, smaller amounts of pethidine than normal are required to produce the desired therapeutic effect, before, during, and after operation.*

It may cause urticarial weals to overlie the vein into which it is injected. This is probably of no consequence.

Sometimes causes nausea and vomiting.

When given to patients taking mono-amine oxidase inhibitors it may cause alarming reactions including hypertension, convulsions, and coma, with absent tendon reflexes and an extensor plantar response. Hypotension, Cheyne-Stokes breathing, and even death may follow (*see* p. 90).

Intravenous Alcohol.—This was reported on by Marin, of Mexico, in 1929.†

The strength of 30 per cent alcohol in isotonic glucose has been used, the rate of injection being 20 ml. per minute. Anæsthesia may take 15–20 minutes to come on.

Thrombosis of the vein is the chief drawback.

Intravenous Bromethol.—First used in 1929 by Kirschner.‡ This can be given as a 1 per cent solution in saline, as a continuous drip. It is not so likely to cause laryngeal spasm as thiopentone. It causes sleep without restlessness and dilates the bronchi. It reduces the blood-pressure. Bromethol, 5 ml., can be added to 500 ml. of 5 per cent dextrose and well shaken up. The drip should run rapidly

* Dundee, J. W., and Tinckler, L. F., *Brit. med. J.*, 1952, **2**, 703.
† Marin, M. G., *The Application of Ethyl Alcohol as a General Anæsthetic, given by the Intravenous Route*, 1929. Mexico: F. Mesones.
‡ Kirschner, M., *Chirurg.*, 1929, **1**, 673.

Intravenous Bromethol, *continued.*

and sleep comes on after 75 to 250 ml. have run in. Can be used to maintain sleep during regional analgesia and is useful, together with topical analgesia, for bronchoscopy and œsophagoscopy. It is contra-indicated in liver disease. Causes thrombophlebitis in about 6 per cent of cases.

Gamma-hydroxybutyric Acid.—This is a basal anæsthetic agent, popular in France and Italy. It is derived from gamma-aminobutyric acid, a naturally occurring neurohormone which inhibits the passage of impulses across central and peripheral synapses. Its clinical effects are probably on the cortex rather than on the midbrain. Clonic movements may follow injection and accompany recovery. Sleep ensues 10–15 min. after injection and lasts 60–90 min. Respiratory and cardiovascular depression not marked.

USES.—For forceps delivery in obstetrics, in thyroid surgery, in open heart surgery, in vascular surgery, etc.

DOSE.—70 mg. per kg. intravenously.

(*See also* Laborit, H., and others, *Pr. Méd.*, 1960, **68**, 1867; Lund, L. O., and others, *Canad. Anæsth. Soc. J.*, 1965, **12**, 379; Virtue, R. W., and others, *Ibid.*, 1966, **13**, 119; Robertson, J. D., in *Recent Advances in Anæsthesia and Analgesia* (Ed. Hewer, C. Langton), 10th ed., 1967, p. 55, London: Churchill; and Vickers, M. D., *Proc. R. Soc. Med.*, 1968 (in press).

Intravenous Procaine.—First used in 1908 by Bier,[*] in an effort to produce intravenous regional analgesia, who employed a tourniquet to localize solution in a limb (*see* Chapter XV). Later used to relieve pain in endarteritis obliterans (Leriche and Fontaine, 1935), to reduce tinnitus (Barany, 1935), to relieve the itchiness of jaundice (Lundy, 1942), and to make dressing of burns painless.[†] Was used for post-operative pain (1945). Its steadying effect on the heart was investigated by Rovenstine and Burstein in 1940.

CHEMISTRY.—Procaine belongs to the alkamine ester group of drugs, which includes atropine, tubocurarine, and the antihistamines. Solutions can be sterilized by boiling, but this reduces the pH so that solution becomes more acid, more irritating, and less efficient as an analgesic. As solutions tend to oxidize on keeping with alteration of pH, they should be freshly made.

PHARMACOLOGY.—Injected intravenously, it paralyses first the parasympathetic, later the sympathetic synapses, and curarizes voluntary muscle motor end-plates perhaps by inhibiting the release of acetylcholine, these effects being antagonized by neostigmine and di-isopropylfluorphosphonate. On the other hand, procaine prevents most symptoms of neostigmine and D.F.P. toxicity. Procaine and neostigmine are antagonistic; procaine and curare are additive. The tachycardia occasionally caused by procaine will yield to intravenous neostigmine, 0·5 to 1 mg. On the central nervous system it causes muscular twitching, anxiety, disorientation, and finally convulsions. The last are

---

[*] Bier, A., *Verh. dtsch. Ges. Chir.*, 1908, **37**, 204.
[†] Gordon, R. A., *Canad. med. Ass. J.*, 1943, **49**, 478.

treated by stopping administration and injecting small doses of intravenous barbiturate, together with administration of oxygen and, if necessary, drugs to raise the blood-pressure. Reduces the irritability of the automatic conductive tissue of the heart and has a quinidine-like effect on the auricle. It causes low blood-pressure. It has an antihistamine action. When injected intravenously it becomes concentrated in œdematous, traumatized, and inflamed tissue owing to the increased capillary permeability in these situations. It is hydrolysed partly in the liver and partly in the blood-stream by plasma pseudo-cholinesterase into para-aminobenzoic acid and diethylamino-ethanol which has a digitalis-like effect on the heart, being one of the most rapidly metabolized drugs known. It is excreted by the kidneys—2 per cent as procaine, 28 per cent as di-ethylamino-ethanol, and 70 per cent as para-aminobenzoic acid. Some of the last combines with glycine to form amino-hippuric acid and some is conjugated with glycuronic acid. The comparative safety of the procaine drip lies in this rapid breakdown. The esterase which causes its hydrolysation is, like acetylcholine, inhibited by neostigmine. It may act as a sensitizing agent, causing contact dermatitis in the form of : either (1) Allergic eczema ; or (2) Pompholyx. The former disappears on withdrawal of the drug, but the latter is not so easily cured. After injection, it causes on very rare occasions urticaria or angioneurotic œdema.

True sensitivity is rare, and is proved only if the intradermal injection of 1 ml. of 1 per cent solution causes, within ten minutes, dyspnœa, agitation, and disorientation.

Liver deficiency does not contra-indicate its use but it should not be employed in patients with myasthenia gravis (it causes a mild neuromuscular block by inhibition of acetylcholine at the end-plate) or in subjects receiving full doses of digitalis or one of its congeners.

THE OPTIMAL EFFECTIVE DOSE is 4 mg. per kilo (25 mg. per stone) as 0·1 per cent solution, given in twenty minutes—this is one procaine unit (Graubard). For emergency use 10 ml. of 1 per cent solution can be given intravenously.

CLINICAL USES.—It is not to-day a drug which is used very frequently for intravenous injection.

a. To supplement general anæsthesia by thiopentone and gas–oxygen. After induction, 1 per cent procaine in saline is given as a drip, starting at 4 ml. per minute, later slowing down to half this amount. Signs of overdosage are twitchings, which subside if the drip is stopped. About 2–3 g. per hour are required by adults. The vasodilatation caused hampers the surgeon.

b. To inhibit cardiac arrhythmia during cardiac and thoracic surgery, during cyclopropane anæsthesia, etc. It is used less frequently than it was some years ago : it is after all a cardiac depressant.

c. In allergic states such as status asthmaticus, serum sickness, bronchospastic states during anæsthesia.

Intravenous Procaine, *continued.*

    d. In doses of 5–10 ml. of 1 per cent solution it increases the speed of intravenous drips (Organe and Scurr).

    e. To produce analgesia during the dressing of burns and to control post-operative pain without causing respiratory depression. Beecher[*] has advised against its use for this purpose because of its inefficiency and undesirable side-effects.

    f. To relieve certain painful trophic and vasomotor conditions, frost-bite, phantom limb, intermittent claudication, etc.

    g. To improve cases of amblyopia following retinal vascular occlusion, together with stellate ganglion block. To relieve pain and reduce intra-ocular pressure in acute glaucoma.

    h. In treatment of intractable pruritus.

    i. To relieve pain in chest injury (Rook[†]), where its use allows the application of strapping without the need for intercostal block. Cardiorespiratory embarrassment is relieved and wet lung and atelectasis are less likely to occur.

    j. To relieve pain and spasm in acute anterior poliomyelitis.

    k. To relieve orchitis and epididymitis.

    l. To improve lower nephron nephrosis with its associated oliguria.

    m. To relieve prolapsed piles.

    n. To ease labour pains.

    It should not be given along with neostigmine. As it causes a mild neuromuscular block (inhibition of acetylcholine at end-plate) it should not be given in myasthenia.

This whole subject is well discussed in Graubard and Peterson's book.[‡]

Intravenous Lignocaine.—In 0·5 per cent solution, this has been used to ease the pain of carcinomatosis and to relieve labour pains. It seems to be less toxic than procaine for a given degree of analgesia.[§] It appears that lignocaine is not broken down by pseudocholinesterase. The liver is, however, capable of breaking down the drug and diethylamino-acetic acid is one of the chief metabolites.[||] It potentiates the hypotensive effects of hexamethonium.[¶] It has been used to produce analgesia during the thiopentone–gas–oxygen–relaxant sequence when 40 mg. are injected intravenously every five minutes. A dose of 500 mg. should not be exceeded during the first hour. During the second hour the amount injected is halved. Thus used it is said to give a useful degree of analgesia both during the operation and also in the post-operative period. It causes no appreciable circulatory or respiratory depression, a low incidence of post-operative vomiting, and an early return to consciousness.[**] Intravenous lignocaine depresses the laryngeal

  * Beecher, H., and others, *J. Amer. med. Ass.*, 1951, **147**, 1761.
  † Rook, J. R., *Anæsthesia*, 1951, **6**, 4.
  ‡ Graubard, D. J., and Peterson, M. C., *Clinical Uses of Intravenous Procaine*, 1950. Oxford: Blackwell.
  § Gilbert, C. R. A., Hingson, R. A., and others, *Curr. Res. Anesth.*, 1951, **30**, 301.
  || Geddes, I. C., *Anæsthesia*, 1958, **13**, 700.
  ¶ de Clive-Low, S. G., North, J., and Gray, P. W. S., *Ibid.*, 1954, **9**, 96.
  ** de Clive-Low, S. G., and Desmond, J., *Ibid.*, 1958, **13**, 138.

reflex and has been recommended, along with thiopentone, gas–oxygen, and pethidine, for inner-ear surgery. Up to 700 mg. are given in the first hour followed by a 40 per cent decrease in each subsequent hour.* Has been used to control status epilepticus—200–400 mg. in 1 per cent solution.† The cerebral depression caused by lignocaine damps down the cough reflex and relieves laryngeal spasm, and so has been employed to produce tube tolerance in asthmatics and others. Dose 100–500 mg. of 2 per cent solution, carefully.‡ Has been used in the reversal of ventricular arrhythmias,§ especially after coronary infarction, during and after cardiac surgery, and for atrial ectopic beats. After a loading dose of 1–2 mg. per kg. a drip of 0·1 per cent solution is given.‖

The signs of acute toxicity after intravenous injection commence with hypotension and diminished tidal volume. Then come twitchings and later convulsions. A blood concentration of 5 μg. per ml. gives some general analgesia but twice this concentration causes convulsions (Bromage, P., and Robson, J. G., *Anæsthesia*, 1961, **16**, 461).

(For description of Bier's block with lignocaine, *see* Chapter XV.)

Procaine Amide Hydrochloride (Pronestyl; Procardyl).—This is procaine with an amide grouping CO.NH instead of an ester grouping CO.O. It acts for longer periods than does ordinary procaine because it is not hydrolysed by pseudocholinesterase. It is active when given by mouth. It causes no central nervous stimulation, and less hypotension than procaine, but will produce nausea and vomiting, and, in rare cases, pyrexia, agranulocytosis, allergic phenomena, and even ventricular fibrillation. It is a very weak analgesic. Peak plasma level occurs 1 hour after oral, 15 minutes after intramuscular, administration.

Used in cardiology as a substitute for quinidine, to treat paroxysmal ventricular tachycardia and ventricular extrasystoles. It is not so useful for auricular arrhythmias. The refractory period as measured by the Q–T interval is prolonged and conduction is slowed. It is not without danger, and latterly has been injected intramuscularly rather than intravenously. Excreted, mostly unchanged, by the kidneys; a small amount excreted as para-aminobenzoic acid.

In anæsthesia it is sometimes used to prevent ventricular arrhythmias arising during thoracic surgery and to reduce the incidence of arrhythmia during intubation. It potentiates hexamethonium and reduces tachycardia associated with ganglionic blocking agents. Its action in counteracting the arrhythmias associated with cyclopropane anæsthesia is inconstant, while it will not protect against the severe cardiac disturbances due to the

---

* Aldrete, I. V., and Fraser, J. G., *Canad. Anæsth. Soc. J.*, 1966, **13**, 397.
† Tavener, D., and Bain, W. A., *Lancet*, 1958, **2**, 1145.
‡ Steinhaus, J. E., *Clinical Anæsthesia. Nitrous Oxide–Oxygen*, 1964, Ch. 7. Oxford: Blackwell.
§ Southworth, J. L., and others, *J. Amer. med. Ass.*, 1950, **143**, 717.
‖ Spracklen, F. H. N. and others, *Brit. med. J.*, 1968, **1**, 89; and Jewett, D. E., Kishon, Y., and Thomas, M., *Lancet*, 1968, **1**, 266.

Procaine Amide Hydrochloride, *continued.*

combination of cyclopropane and adrenaline. Should be used with care in asthmatics and is contra-indicated during therapy with sulpha drugs.

By mouth (the preferred route in cardiology) it is given in capsules, each containing 250 mg. The intravenous dose is 3 ml. of 10 per cent solution, given over a period of 1–5 min. and cautiously repeated if required.

Intramedullary Medication.*—The bone-marrow of the sternum, or, in infants, of the tibia, is a convenient place to infuse various fluids, either for purposes of resuscitation or anæsthesia. In the absence of veins, intramedullary infusion of fluid may save lives in acute shock.

The method was popularized by Tocantins in 1941. Once the needle is in place it will not easily slip out.

Blood, saline, dextrose, and thiopentone in 0·5–2 per cent solution, can all be given via this route.

The Benzodiazepines.—These include chlordiazepoxide (librium), diazepam (valium), and nitrazepam (mogadon), and probably act by depressing the limbic system. While their chief use is in psychiatry to relieve anxiety and tension, diazepam has been used to induce anæsthesia by intravenous injection.† It is said to relieve muscle spasm. May prove useful for relieving anxiety before anæsthesia.

Its use to induce anæsthesia may be indicated in shocked patients as it is said to cause neither hypotension nor respiratory depression. Dose 1–2 mg. per kg. and up to 5 mg. per kg. in fit patients. Additional uses: (1) To relieve post-operative pain (10 mg.). (2) To reduce post-operative restlessness in old people (10 mg. i.v.). (*See also Diazepam in Anæsthesia* (Ed. Knight, P. F., and Burgess, C. G.), Bristol: John Wright, 1968; Brown, S. S., and Dundee, J. W., *Brit. J. Anæsth.*, 1968, **40**, 108; and Haslett, W. H. K., and Dundee, J. W., *Ibid.*, 1968, **40**, 250.)

Intramuscular Analgesia.—Lignocaine has been given intramuscularly to potentiate analgesia during the thiopentone–gas–oxygen sequence. The dose recommended is 75 mg. per stone in 2 per cent solution, e.g., 250 mg. before induction, after induction, and then hourly.‡ It is said to increase tube tolerance, but may cause post-operative restlessness.

---

* Dealt with here for convenience. *Also see* article by Tarrow, A. B., Turkel, H., and Thompson, M. S., *Anesthesiology*, 1952, **13**, 501.

† Brown, S. S., and Dundee, J. W., *Brit. J. Anæsth.*, 1968, **40**, 108.

‡ Dawkins, C. J. M., and Steel, G. C., *Anæsthesia*, 1957, **12**, 426.

CHAPTER XIV

NEUROLEPT ANALGESIA AND THE PHENOTHIAZINE DERIVATIVES

NEUROLEPT ANALGESIA*

This is a neologism which has been used to describe the state of a patient following the administration of one of the newer, very potent analgesic agents, such as phenoperidine or fentanyl, together with a sedative drug of the butyrophenone series such as haloperidol and droperidol. The B.M.R. is not reduced† but there is usually some respiratory depression.‡

Phenoperidine Hydrochloride (Operidine) and **Fentanyl** (Phentanyl, Sublimaze).—These are chemically related to pethidine but are much more potent. Like it they possess all the properties of narcotic analgesics such as intense analgesia, respiratory depression, small pupil, nausea and vomiting, depending on the dose used. Their effects on the cardiovascular system are minimal, while respiratory depression can be antagonized by nalorphine and its congeners. The analgesic effects of phenoperidine last from 40 to 60 min., those of fentanyl up to 30 min. Phenoperidine is metabolized and excreted in the urine in equal amounts; fentanyl is mostly destroyed in the liver and about 10 per cent excreted in the urine.

USES.—

1. As analgesics: phenoperidine 1 mg. intravenously. (Fentanyl 0·2–0·6 mg. intravenously.) Effects come on in 2–3 min., reach peak in 5 min., and wear off in 20 min. A dose of 0·5 mg. causes intense analgesia with bradycardia and perhaps some depression of breathing requiring assisted respiration; 0·2 mg. is not usually a respiratory depressant. Light general anæsthesia with or without a relaxant may be used additionally. Large doses may result in muscular rigidity, making I.P.P.V. difficult, but a relaxant will overcome this effect.

2. To produce apnœa in, e.g., chest injuries. Doses: phenoperidine up to 5 mg. and fentanyl up to 0·6 mg. intravenously.

3. Together with droperidol to produce neurolept anæsthesia. Doses: either phenoperidine 2–5 mg. or fentanyl 0·1–0·6 mg. with droperidol 5 mg. Or as thalamonal (innovar), each ml. of which contains fentanyl 0·05 mg. and droperidol 2·5 mg. Usual dose 2 ml.

Droperidol (Dehydrobenz-peridol; Droleptan).—One of the butyrophenone series of drugs which causes mental detachment, absence of voluntary movements (catatonia), a specific inhibitory effect on the chemoreceptor trigger zone controlling nausea and vomiting (apomorphine antagonism), α-adrenergic receptor block, and

* A term coined by J. Delay and P. Deneker, *Méthodes Chémiothérapeutiques en Psychiatrie*, 1961. Paris: Masson.
† Forbes, A. M., and others, *Brit. J. Anæsth.*, 1967, **39**, 851.
‡ Dunbar, B. S., and others, *Ibid.*, 1967, **39**, 861.

Droperidol, *continued.*

amphetamine antagonism. Duration of effect up to 8 hours. It acts quickly and is much more potent than haloperidol. Large doses may cause extrapyramidal disturbances which can be overcome by anti-Parkinson agents. Has little effect on liver, heart, or respiratory function. Mostly broken down in liver, but 10 per cent excreted in urine. Liver disease .calls for smaller dosage than usual.

USES.—

1. As premedication: dose by mouth 5–20 mg., intramuscularly 10 mg., intravenously 5 mg. It is effective for 8 hours. May be given as thalamonal, usual dose 2 ml. Contra-indicated in severe depression which may be made worse by the drug.
2. In certain neurosurgical operations when the patient's conscious reaction is required during the operation, e.g., in stereotactic surgery and anterolateral tractotomy.*
3. In diagnostic procedures, e.g., aortography, angiocardiography, and bronchoscopy.†
4. To provide sedation during regional analgesia.
5. In ophthalmology.‡
6. In aural surgery.
7. In general surgery together with nitrous oxide and oxygen.
8. For dressing of burns.§

(*See* good review by J. D. Robertson in *Recent Advances in Anæsthesia and Analgesia* (Ed. Hewer, C. Langton), 10th ed., 1967, p. 47. London: Churchill.)

THE PHENOTHIAZINE DERIVATIVES

This group of drugs includes, among hundreds of others:—

1. **Chlorpromazine Hydrochloride, B.P.** (2-chloro-10(3′-dimethyl-amino-*n*-propyl)-phenothiazine hydrochloride. Its synonyms are Largactil, Thorazine, Megaphen, 4560 R.P., Hibernal).

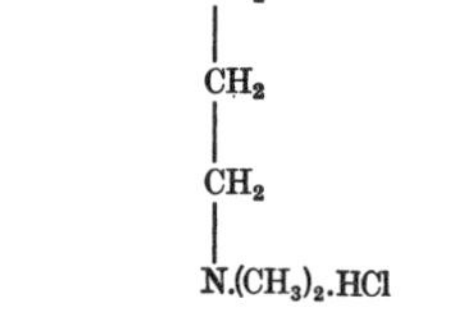

---

* Brown, A. S., *Anæsthesia*, 1964, **19**, 70; and Tasker, R. R., and others, *Canad. Anæsth. Soc. J.*, 1965, **12**, 29.
† Spoerel, W. E., and others, *Ibid.*, 1965, **12**, 622.
‡ Tait, E. C., and others, *Amer. J. Ophthal.*, 1965, **59**, 412.
§ Muir, I. F. K., and others, *Brit. J. Anæsth.*, 1966, **38**, 267.

2. **Promethazine Hydrochloride, B.P.** (N-(2-dimethylamino-*n*-propyl-) phenothiazine hydrochloride. Its synonyms are phenergan and atosil). Very useful for premedication (25–50 mg. i.m.)

3. **Promethazine-8-chlorothiophyllinate, B.P.** (Promethazine theoclate; Avomine).

4. **Diethazine Hydrochloride** (Dipacol).

5. **Ethopropazine** (Lysivane).

6. **Pecazine** (Mepazine ; Pacatal ; Lacumin).—
   ACTIONS.—Blockade of sympathetic and parasympathetic ganglia. Protects heart against the effects of cyclopropane plus adrenaline and other arrhythmia-producing stimuli. Depresses heat-regulating centre and vomiting centres and diminishes salivary and bronchial secretions. Potentiates general anæsthesia. A precipitate results if its solution is mixed with saline (not with distilled water).
   USES.—Its cardiac action makes it useful in cardiac surgery and in hypothermia (100–150 mg. intravenously). Used in labour as premedication for its sedative and drying effects. Reduces post-operative vomiting. In neurosurgery has been used to increase tube tolerance (Hunter, A. R., *Anæsthesia*, 1958, **13**, 379). Does not greatly interfere with the action of vasopressors. The hydrochloride is given by mouth, the acetate by injection.

7. **Promazine Hydrochloride, B.P.** (Sparine).—Differs chemically from chlorpromazine by the absence of a chlorine atom in the molecule, and is one-third as potent. Similar effects to the parent drug but causes less hypotension and less liver damage. Agranulocytosis has followed its use. It does not cause much pain when injected intramuscularly. Has been used by anæsthetists to make patients calm and sleepy during regional analgesia, during intra-ocular* and other types of surgery.†

8. **Perphenazine, B.P.** (Fentazin; Trilafon).—A phenothiazine derivative, five times as potent as chlorpromazine and less toxic and with fewer side-effects. Useful in treatment of nausea and vomiting

---

* Ingram, H. J., and Davison, M. Armstrong, *Lancet*, 1961, **1**, 1321; and *Proc. R. Soc. Med.*, 1963, **56**, 987.
† Swerdlow, M., and Nabi, G. F. O., *Brit. J. Anæsth.*, 1959, **31**, 543.

Perphenazine, *continued.*

associated with anæsthesia (2–4 mg. thrice daily). No evidenc that it is toxic to the liver or bone-marrow. Is a powerful centra nervous system depressant (Lind, B., *Acta anæsth. scand.*, 1960, 4 181).

9. Trifluoperazine Hydrochloride, B.P. (Stelazine).—The mos active of the derivatives of phenothiazine and is more potent tha chlorpromazine. Used as a sedative in psychiatry.

10. Trimeprazine Tartrate, B.P.C. (Vallergan).—This is the neutra tartrate of trimeprazine, 10-(3-demethylamino-2-methyl-propy) phenothiazine. In potency it lies midway between chlorproma zine and promethazine and has a strong central sedative action It is a powerful antihistaminic, anti-emetic, and spasmolytic agen and is also a good antipruritic. It does not possess the anti adrenaline properties of chlorpromazine and its effects do no last as long. Can be given in 1 per cent (or more dilute) solutior deep into the muscles in a dosage of 4 mg. per stone in adults o 5 mg. per stone in children. Does not prolong recovery perioc after operation. It is a satisfactory drug for pre-operative sedativ medication which does not add to the chances of nausea anc vomiting after operation. Can be given to children by mouth as ẽ syrup (6 mg. per ml.), dose 1·5–2 mg. per lb. (1–4 mg. per kg. 1–2 hours before anæsthesia.

Compounds (1), (2), (4), (6), and (7) are used in anæsthesia.
Compound (5) is used in the treatment of Parkinsonism.
Compounds (3) and (8) are used principally as an anti-emetic.
Compounds (1) and (9) are used in psychiatry.
Compounds (1), (2), (6) and (10) are used in premedication.
(*See also* 'Chlorpromazine and Allied Phenothiazine Deriva-tives', Rees, L., *Brit. med. J.*, 1960, **2**, 522.)
The description which follows applies primarily to chlorpromazine.

History.—Chlorpromazine was synthesized in the laboratories in France of Rhône-Poulenc-Specia by Charpentier in 1950, the summit of a prolonged research. With promethazine (synthesized in 1945) it was used in anæsthesia by Laborit and Huguenard in 1951,[*] who used the names 'potentiated anæsthesia', 'lytic cocktail', 'anæsthesia without anæsthetics', and in Britain in 1953.[†] In the same year, it was used together with surface cooling to facilitate hypothermia.[‡]

Physical Characteristics.—Chlorpromazine is a pale, crystalline powder, freely soluble in water. Ampoules are filled under nitrogen and anti-oxidants are added. Discoloured solutions should not be used. Its solutions are acid—pH of 5 per cent solution is 4·5—so it should be well diluted to avoid irritation. It is prepared in 1 per cent and 2·5 per cent solutions, which should not be exposed to light ; in tablets, each containing 10 or 25 mg. ; and as 100-mg.

---

* Laborit, H., and Huguenard, P., *Pr. Méd.*, 1951, **59**, 1329.
† Smith, A., and Fairer, J. G., *Brit. med. J.*, 1953, **2**, 1247.
‡ Dundee, J. W., Scott, W. E. B., and Mesham, P. R., *Ibid.*, 1953, **2**, 1237.

suppositories. Its solution is precipitated when mixed with thiobarbiturates, atropine sulphate, polyvidone (plasmosan), and gallamine—the precipitate is, however, dissolved in excess of gallamine. It may cause cloudiness when mixed with certain solutions of dextrose and saline. It is miscible with solutions of tubocurarine, scoline and anectine (but not all brands of suxamethonium), morphine, noradrenaline, procaine and its amide, methylamphetamine (methedrine), and, of course, pethidine and promethazine.

Pharmacology of Chlorpromazine.—It is very variable in its effect especially when taken by mouth. Its results begin to show a few minutes after intravenous injection, 15–30 minutes after intramuscular injection, and 1–1½ hours after being swallowed. It is a powerful anti-adrenaline agent but a rather weak anti-histamine drug.

1. THE CENTRAL NERVOUS SYSTEM.—It depresses the reticular formations of the brain and has an inhibitory effect on all cellular activity, the so-called narcobiotic effect (Decourt). It produces drowsiness and relieves anxiety but does not inhibit the higher psychic centres. It antagonizes drugs, other than strychnine, having a stimulating action on the brain-stem, e.g., nikethemide, nicotine, and caffeine. The E.E.G. changes are those of normal sleep and differ from those resulting from barbiturates.

2. AUTONOMIC NERVOUS SYSTEM.—It inhibits sympathetic activity centrally by depressing the centres in the diencephalon and thus prevents responses to stimuli mediated through sympathetic nerves, e.g., vasoconstriction following hæmorrhage, trauma, and shock. This central inhibition of vasomotor reflexes is one of the chief characteristics of the drug. It may also depress the heat-regulating centre in the diencephalon. It greatly reduces the effects of adrenaline on the α-receptor sites and, in a lesser degree, those of noradrenaline and acetylcholine.

3. RESPIRATORY SYSTEM.—Pulmonary ventilation may be reduced; bronchial and laryngeal reflexes and secretions are depressed. It may cause Cheyne-Stokes respiration. Has been used with success in the treatment of asthma. Increases respiratory rate depressed by pethidine.

4. CARDIOVASCULAR SYSTEM.—Chlorpromazine reduces blood-pressure by: (a) Causing peripheral vasodilatation, the result of central vasomotor depression, and (b) Peripherally antagonizing adrenaline and noradrenaline (α-blocking effect). Thus the reflex vasoconstriction following shock is not seen. The hypotension is potentiated or reduced by posturing the patient. Vasodilatation reduces peripheral resistance and cardiac output is increased. Tachycardia usually accompanies hypotension (Marey's law) but need not be long-lasting—it may be due to vagal inhibition. The skin is warm, dry, and pale with dilated veins, but the capillaries are constricted and this gives a somewhat cadaveric appearance to the patient. Whereas ordinary anæsthesia causes peripheral vasodilatation accompanied by splanchnic vasoconstriction, chlorpromazine causes both peripheral and splanchnic vasodilatation. The drug has no marked effect on the E.C.G. and protects against cardiac arrhythmia caused by cyclopropane,

Pharmacology of Chlorpromazine, *continued.*

halothane, trichloroethylene, and chloroform. If given befor the onset of shock—but not after its development—the drug prevents the intense and prolonged vasoconstriction with it accompanying visceral ischæmia. It reduces the power of adrenaline to delay absorption of local analgesic drugs.

The pressor effect of noradrenaline is not affected by chlor promazine, promethazine, or pecazine. The pressor effect of adrenaline is reversed by chlorpromazine, not affected by pro methazine or pecazine. The pressor effects of methoxamin and phenylephrine are reduced by chlorpromazine and pro methazine.

5. VOMITING.—It depresses the chemoreceptor trigger zone of Borison and Wang in the floor of the fourth ventricle, and i larger doses depresses the vomiting centre itself. It is a valuabl drug in the prevention and treatment of all types of vomiting other than that due to mechanical causes.

6. TEMPERATURE REGULATION.—
   a. Depresses the tone of muscle.
   b. May depress the heat-regulating centre.
   c. Causes peripheral vasodilatation so that the patient become strongly influenced by the surrounding temperature.
   d. Inhibits shivering by a central effect. Oxygen consumption i reduced only if the patient's temperature is made to fall.

7. OTHER ACTIONS.—Chlorpromazine is a local analgesic an also potentiates the local effects of procaine. It potentiate the effects of anæsthetics, analgesics, hypnotics, and muscl relaxants. It is not a strong antagonist of histamine nor ha it any true ganglionic blocking activity. Noradrenaline an phenylephrine are the preferred drugs, should it be desired t reverse the hypotension caused by the drug. The bradycardi usually associated with the noradrenaline drip is not seen i chlorpromazine has been given previously. The secretions o the mouth, pharynx, and upper respiratory tract are dried up It is an antipruritic.

8. SIDE-EFFECTS AND TOXIC ACTIONS.—
   a. Faintness and dizziness due to postural hypotension.
   b. Liver damage following prolonged administration, but a case following a single dose of 50 mg., has been reported; shown b an enlarged, tender liver, and jaundice of cholestatic type The kidneys are not harmed by the drug.
   c. Contact dermatitis and photosensitivity.
   d. Agranulocytosis, following prolonged administration.

9. EXCRETION.—Broken down in body into chlorpromazin sulphoxide, perhaps partly by the liver. Small amounts excrete in the urine, which may be coloured pink or purple. Interfere with the iodine, Gmelin, and Fouchet tests for bile in the urine

Promethazine Hydrochloride.—Its effects are similar to those o chlorpromazine but it has, among others, the following differences :—
   a. It has less antagonism to adrenaline.
   b. It has 100 times more antagonism to histamine.

c. It is a more potent depressant of upper respiratory tract reflexes.

d. It has slight atropine-like activity.

e. It is a powerful hypnotic in its own right and potentiates barbiturates.

f. It is said to increase sensitivity to pain.* It is supplied as 2·5 per cent solution and as tablets, 25 mg., and elixir, 5 mg. per fluid drachm.

Clinical Uses of Chlorpromazine (and Promethazine).—

1. IN ANÆSTHESIA.—

   a. As PREMEDICATION.—Various techniques have been described, including the following : Oral administration of 150 mg. the night before, with 50 mg. intramuscularly 1 hour before operation ; 25 mg. by mouth the night before, the morning before, and 4-hourly after operation for 48 hours : this has a useful anti-emetic effect ; 200 mg. as a rectal suppository, 2 hours pre-operatively ; 12·5 to 50 mg. with an equal amount of promethazine and 50–100 mg. of pethidine, intramuscularly, 1½ hours pre-operatively.

   b. As PART OF THE ANÆSTHETIC TECHNIQUE.—Again, various methods of administration have been advocated, including : (i) The slow intravenous drip of 500 ml. of dextrose containing, e.g., chlorpromazine 50–100 mg., promazine 50–100 mg., and pethidine 50–100 mg., the so-called 'lytic cocktail' which produces the state unfortunately named 'artificial hibernation'. The drip can be slowed down when the desired result has been obtained. (ii) The same amount of the three drugs can be dissolved in 20 ml. of dextrose solution and given slowly intravenously or intramuscularly before anæsthesia commences. The patient is likely to be sleepy for 5–10 hours after the administration of these amounts, and of course general anæsthetic agents will be used in smaller doses than normal.

   The authors have found the drip technique very useful in such operations as thyroidectomy, radical mastectomy, operations on the middle and inner ear, etc.,† and intra-ocular operations in young or middle-aged patients. Hypotension can be increased by tilting the table upwards and decreased by tilting it downwards. For these and other operations they prefer to use, in addition, small doses of thiopentone and relaxant for intubation, and gas–oxygen for maintenance. Straining and coughing are minimized and the long post-operative sleep may in such cases be beneficial. Chlorpromazine is more depressant than promethazine and its dose should usually be kept small.

Other anæsthetic uses include :—

   a. To produce sedation during cardiac catheterization in children, a drip is set up, containing 50 mg. of chlorpromazine

---

* Dundee, J. W., *Anæsthesia*, 1960, **16**, 61.

† Mason, S. A., *Proc. World Congress of Anesthesiologists*, 1956, 143. Minneapolis : Burgess Pub. Co. ; and Vincent, N. A., *Brit. J. Anæsth.*, 1958, **30**, 380.

Clinical Uses of Chlorpromazine (and Promethazine), *continued.*

and 100–200 mg. of pethidine and slowly run until th patient has received 1 ml. per lb. body-weight. Large amounts may be required.

b. To control hiccup during laparotomy, when 5–10 mg. ar injected intravenously and accompanied by 0·5 mg. c phenylephrine intramuscularly to prevent hypotensio The drug can be used for the same purpose in the immediat post-operative period, 50 mg. being infused as a drip kep up until the patient is comfortable.

c. To reduce labour pains ; promethazine 25 mg. with pethidin 50 mg. intramuscularly, repeated if necessary.

d. To reduce or cure post-operative vomiting.

e. To aid induced hypothermia by surface cooling.

f. To protect the patient from the serious consequences of over dosage with adrenaline or noradrenaline.

g. In the treatment of tetanus, when 25 mg. of chlorpromazin and pethidine can be given about four-hourly together wit nitrous oxide and oxygen.*

h. To aid endoscopy under local analgesia, together perhap with a barbiturate and hyoscine.

i. To control hyperpyrexia.

j. To promote sleep during operations performed under region analgesia.

k. In the presence of bronchospasm.

2. Chlorpromazine has been used in general therapeutics for :—

a. The potentiation of analgesics in inoperable carcinoma.

b. To cure vomiting due to digitalis, radiation, carcinomatosis labyrinthitis, acute alcoholism, anæmia, etc.

c. The treatment of eclampsia.

d. In organic psychoses and delirium tremens to control excite ment and relieve mental tension.

e. In management of hyperpyrexia.

See also the following reviews of phenothiazine drugs :—
Viaud, P., *J. Pharm. and Pharmacol.*, 1954, **6**, 361.
Dundee, J. W., *Brit. J. Anæsth.*, 1954, **26**, 357.
Laborit, H., and Huguenard, P., *Pratique de l'Hibernothérapie en Chirurgie et en Médecine* 1954. Paris : Masson.

Ataralgesia.—Hayward-Butt† has coined this neologism to describ a state of calmness and freedom from pain induced by the intra muscular injection of a mixture of pethidine, amiphenazole, an mepazine (pacatal). One ' unit ' consists of pethidine 100 mg. amiphenazole 25 mg., and mepazine 100 mg., and the averag adult receives 3 units three-quarters of an hour before operation minor surgery may then proceed. Occasionally thiopentone i necessary in addition.

* Bodman, R. I., Morton, H. J. V., and Thomas, E. T., *Lancet*, 1955, **2**, 230 ; and Aja Shanken, and Mehrotra, L. S., *Brit. med. J.*, 1959, **2**, 1150.
† Hayward-Butt, J. T., *Lancet*, 1957, **2**, 972.

CHAPTER XV

REGIONAL ANÆSTHESIA

History.—Modern local analgesia began with the introduction of cocaine into medical practice in 1884.*

Cocaine is the active principle of *Erythroxylon coca,* a plant grown in South America.

Schleich in Berlin (1892)† and Reclus in Paris‡ (1890) popularized infiltration analgesia, while nerve-block was described by Halsted and Hall in New York in 1884.§ The former, as a result of acting as his own guinea-pig during his researches on the new drug, became a cocaine addict. Arthur E. Barker, in 1899, with β-eucaine was using infiltration analgesia at University College Hospital.‖ Braun introduced adrenaline in 1902.¶

Substitutes for the toxic cocaine soon came. Giesel's tropococaine appeared in 1891; Fourneau's stovaine in 1904,** and Einhorn's novocain (procaine) in 1904, popularized by Heinrich Braun.††

Meischer and Uhlmann introduced nupercaine in 1929.‡‡

Lofgren and Lundqvist synthesized lignocaine in 1943, and Gordh was the first to use it in 1948.§§

The hypodermic needle was described by Rynd of Dublin in 1845,‖‖ by Pravaz of Lyon in 1853,¶¶ and by Alexander Wood of Edinburgh in 1855.*** The latter also devised a syringe and popularized hypodermic therapy.

'Regional anæsthesia' was a term first used by Harvey Cushing in 1901 to describe pain relief by nerve-block.†††

GENERAL CONSIDERATIONS

Local analgesic drugs are mostly used as the soluble hydrochlorides. It is probable that the alkalinity of the tissues frees the base and this unites with the nerve tissue. Most local analgesics are esters of aromatic acids and amino-alcohols. Cocaine and piperocaine are benzoic acid esters; procaine, amethocaine, and benzocaine are para-aminobenzoic acid esters. Cinchocaine, lignocaine, prilocaine, mepivacaine, and bupivacaine are amides. In acute inflammatory tissue, a

* Köller, K., *Klin. Mbl. Augen.,* 1884, **22**, 60.
† Schleich, K. L., *Gesellsch. f. Chir.,* 1892, **21**, 121.
‡ Reclus, P., *L'Anæsthésie localisée par la cocaine,* 1903. Paris.
§ Halsted, W. S., *N.Y. med. J.,*1884, Dec. 6.
‖ Barker, A. E., *Lancet,* 1899, **1**, 282.
¶ Braun, H., *Arch. Klin. Chir.,* 1903, **69**, 541.
** Fourneau, E., *Bull. soc. Pharmacol.,* 1904, **10**, 141.
†† Braun, H., *Dtsch. med. Wschr.,* 1905, **31**, 1667.
‡‡ Uhlmann, T., *Narkose und Anæs.,* 1929, **6**, 168.
§§ Gordh, T., *Anæsthesia,* 1949, **4**, 4.
‖‖ Rynd, F., *Dublin Med. Press,* 1845, March 12 ; and *Dublin J. Med. Sci.,* 1861, **32**, 13.
¶¶ Pravaz, C. G., *C. R. Acad. di Sci.,* 1853, **36**, 88.
*** Wood, A., *Edin. Med. Surg. J.,* 1855, **82**, 265.
††† Cushing, H. W., *Ann. Surg.,* 1902 ,**36** 321.

General Considerations, *continued.*

decreased *p*H makes these drugs less active, but the addition of adrenaline, by counteracting the vasodilatation due to inflammation will partially restore analgesic effect. Local analgesics retard or stop the propagation of nerve impulses and have a stabilizing effect on the cell membranes of nerve-fibres.

With the exception of cocaine (a vasoconstrictor) and lignocaine (no effect on vessels), local analgesic drugs are vasodilators. Vaso constricting agents such as adrenaline are usually added to local analgesic solutions to delay absorption and also to prolong their action Adrenaline keeps the solution in contact with nerve tissue for a pro longed time and also prevents the sudden flooding of the circulation with local analgesic drug.

Detoxication occurs in the liver and speed of destruction is a measure of their toxicity. Adrenaline and noradrenaline do not prolong the action of local analgesic solution applied topically.*

Liver disease may increase the toxicity of these drugs.

Other agents exhibiting local analgesic properties include : (1) Many antihistamines ; (2) Protoplasmic poisons, e.g., alcohol, phenol ammonium sulphate; (3) Cold; (4) Pressure on nerve-trunks (5) Propranolol.†

Theories of Impulse Conduction along Nerve-fibres.—Eccles describes the ionic hypothesis of nerve conduction according to which conduction is associated with the entry of sodium ions into the nerve-fibres followed by the migration of potassium ions out wards. During the interval between these events the interior of the fibres becomes positively charged relatively to the exterior— a state of reversal polarization. During recovery the ions reverse the direction of their movement. Local analgesic agents may prevent this ionic migration and so may prevent conduction of impulses. Other theories of action of local analgesic drugs include the enzymatic theory, the hormonal theory, and the Meyer Overton lipoid theory.

For recent views on this topic *see* de Jong, R., and Wagman, J. H *Anesthesiology*, 1963, **24**, 684 ; also Nathan, P. W., and Sears T. A., *Anæsthesia*, 1963, **18**, 467.

Nerve-fibres vary in their susceptibility to local analgesic solution in inverse ratio to the size of the cross-section of the fibres, e.g. small C fibres are more susceptible than the larger A fibres. (*See* p. 22.)

Site of Action.—The site of action of local analgesic drugs (and of general anæsthetics too) is at the surface membrane of cells of excitable tissues. Local analgesics affect not only nerve-fibres but all types of excitable tissue, including smooth and striated muscle e.g., in the myocardium, vessels, etc., probably by interfering with the cation fluxes across the muscle-cell membranes (as in nerve tissue).

---

* Adriani, J., and others, *Ann. Surg.*, 1963, **158**, 660.

† Singh, K. P., and others, *Lancet*, 1967, **2**, 158; and Sinha, J. N., and others, *Brit. J Anæsth.*, 1967, **34**, 887.

‡ Eccles, J. C., *The Neurophysiological Basis of Mind*, 1955. London : Oxford University Press.

Uptake.—Local analgesic drugs are lipoid-soluble bases which act by penetrating lipoprotein cell membranes in the non-ionized state. In order to make a soluble solution suitable for injection, the non-ionized base has to be converted to the ionized state.

Signs of Toxicity.—Due to : (1) Special sensitivity of the patient to the drug used (rare) ; (2) A high blood concentration of the drug from any cause. These are more common after topical analgesia of the upper air-passages than after local infiltration or nerve-block. This is because absorption from the bronchial tree is almost as rapid as from intravenous injection.

The following factors influence toxicity : (1) Quantity of solution ; (2) Concentration of drug ; (3) Presence or absence of adrenaline ; (4) Vascularity of site of injection ; (5) Rate of absorption of drug, e.g., rate is rapid from bronchial mucosa ; (6) Rate of destruction of drug; (7) Hypersensitivity of patient; (8) Age, physical status, and weight of patient.

A recent study of plasma concentrations of local analgesic drugs suggested that higher levels were reached after lignocaine than after prilocaine in equal dosage. Addition of adrenaline to the local infiltration reduced the plasma concentration of lignocaine but not of prilocaine. Higher plasma levels were found after intercostal block than after extradural injection.*

1. CENTRAL NERVOUS SYSTEM. — Convulsive-respiratory failure. Central stimulation followed by depression; restlessness, vertigo, tremor, convulsions, respiratory failure. Latent epileptics may convulse more readily than normal people. Treatment consists in: (1) Artificial ventilation with oxygen or air; (2) Intravenous injection of a pressor drug, e.g., methylamphetamine 10 mg.; (3) Intravenous injection of suxamethonium or just sufficient thiopentone to control convulsions (100–150 mg.).

2. CARDIOVASCULAR SYSTEM. — Acute collapse — primary cardiac failure.—Feeble pulse and cardiovascular collapse ; bradycardia ; pallor ; sweating ; and hypotension. This type of intoxication may be due to a rapid absorption of the drug, so that the cardiovascular system is involved before the drug has time to reach the brain.

TREATMENT.—Lower head ; give oxygen ; raise blood-pressure ; cardiac massage if necessary.

3. RESPIRATORY DEPRESSION.—This may progress to apnœa.

4. ALLERGIC PHENOMENA.—Rare : may take form of bronchospasm, urticaria, or angioneurotic œdema.† In many thousands of administrations the authors have never seen this.

Reactions to vasoconstrictor drugs may include pallor, anxiety, palpitations, tachycardia, hypertension, and tachypnœa.

Toxicity may occur as a result of simple overdosage ; by inadvertent intravenous injection ; or because of susceptibility of the patient to normal dosage. Injection with a moving needle, together with frequent aspiration testing, minimizes risk of intravenous injection.

---

* Braid, D. P. ,*Brit. J. Anæsth.*, 1964, **36**, 742.
† Noble ,D. S., and Pierce, G. F. M., *Lancet*, 1961, **2**, 1436.

Prolonging Local Analgesia.—
1. Addition of adrenaline, e.g., 1–200,000 solution.
2. Addition of 10 per cent dextran* to lignocaine and adrenaline.
3. Addition of 6 per cent dextran to amethocaine 0·15 per cent with adrenaline.†

Premedication.—Adequate premedication is essential for successful local analgesia in major surgery. A barbiturate may be given to prevent possible toxic effects from the drug used. The subject is set out in the chapter on SPINAL ANALGESIA, p. 380. While a patient under the influence of a barbiturate is partially protected from the toxic effects of local analgesic agents, he is made more susceptible to these effects if he is given ether.

The average patient does well if given pentobarbitone 200 mg. (gr. 3) two hours before operation and papaveretum 20 mg. or trimeprazine 50 mg. and hyoscine 0·4 mg. one hour before. Ill and old patients require less.

Methods of Local Analgesia.—
1. Infiltration analgesia, to abolish the pain due to surgical intervention and to ease pain associated with trauma and the injection of irritant drugs. The direct injection of drugs into the incision and wound and between bone-ends in fractures.
2. Field block. The injection of a local analgesic so as to create a zone of analgesia around the operative field.
3. Nerve-block (conduction anæsthesia). The injection of a solution of local analgesic drug into the nerve or nerves supplying the area to be operated on.
4. Refrigeration analgesia (*see* Chapter XXIX).
5. Intravenous local analgesia.
6. Intra-arterial local analgesia.
7. Topical or surface analgesia.

Syringes, etc.—Small volumes of solution can be injected with ordinary 10-ml. and 20-ml. syringes, but larger volumes require some type of self-filling syringe to expedite injection.

If a three-way tap is interposed between a 10-ml. syringe and its needle, with the third arm connected to a transfusion bottle by a length of rubber tubing, a simple home-made apparatus is at hand, the bottle acting as a reservoir for the local analgesic solution.

Useful types of apparatus have been invented by Dunn, Pitkin, and Hamilton Bailey.

PHARMACOLOGY OF DRUGS USED IN LOCAL ANALGESIA

1. **Cocaine** (Benzoyl methylecgonine hydrochloride).—A derivative of the nitrogenous base ecgonine. Cocaine is extracted from the leaves of *Erythroxylon coca*, a tree indigenous to Bolivia and Peru.

---

* Loder, R. E., *Lancet*, 1960, **2**, 346.
† Chinn, M. A., and Wirjoatjmadja, K., *Ibid.*, 1967, **2**, 835.

which the natives chew for their stimulant effect. Cocaine is soluble in water and alcohol and is now used solely for topical analgesia. It is an excellent surface analgesic and has a vaso-constrictor effect, 4 per cent being a suitable strength. It is often toxic when injected. Duration of effect, 20–30 min.

HISTORY.—Isolated in 1855 by Gaedicke. Niemann, a pupil of Wohler, purified and named the alkaloid in 1860 and its local analgesic effects were noticed in 1868 by Moreno y Maiz, surgeon-in-chief to the Peruvian Army, and also by von Anrep in 1878. Karl Koller at the suggestion of Sigmund Freud proved its use in surgery (of the cornea) in 1884 and reported his discovery on 15 Sept., 1884, at the Congress of Ophthalmology at Heidelberg. The drug was originally prepared by Merck of Darmstadt. Used by W. C. Burke of South Norwalk, Connecticut, for removal of a revolver bullet from a hand (5 minims of 2 per cent solution) in November, 1884, and also by R. J. Hall and William Stewart Halsted at the Roosevelt Hospital in New York, each of whom injected it into his own arms.*

CENTRAL NERVOUS SYSTEM.—This is stimulated from above downwards :—

On the cortex, excitement and restlessness are caused and mental powers increased. There is euphoria and a decreased sense of fatigue, hence its tendency to cause addiction.

On the medulla, increase in blood-pressure and respiratory rate and vomiting may occur. Later there may be depression, with coma or convulsions and death from respiratory failure.

It blocks nerve conduction when applied to peripheral nerve-trunks or nerve-endings, terminal nerve-fibres being blocked at a concentration of 0·02 per cent.

The sympathetic nervous system is stimulated and cocaine poten-tiates the responses of organs supplied by sympathetic nerves to adrenaline and noradrenaline. As cocaine is a powerful vasoconstrictor, adrenaline added to it is not only unneces-sary but also increases the risks of cardiac arrhythmia and ventricular fibrillation.

Depression follows stimulation. It raises body temperature by increasing muscular activity, causing vasoconstriction and so reducing heat radiation, and by its effect on the heat-regulating centre.

RESPIRATORY SYSTEM.—In small doses cocaine and procaine stimulate the respiratory rate. Larger doses may cause respira-tory arrest.

CARDIOVASCULAR SYSTEM.—Sudden cardiac standstill has occurred ; cases of severe cardiovascular collapse are also seen. Small doses increase the pulse-rate, raise the blood-pressure, and potentiate the effects of adrenaline on capillaries (dilatation or constriction). Cocaine, unlike procaine, potentiates the effect of adrenaline on the automatic conductive tissues of the heart and favours the development of ventricular fibrillation.

EYE.—Mydriasis, perhaps due to sympathetic stimulation ; there is blanching of the conjunctiva from vasoconstriction, and

---

* von Oettingen, W. F., *Ann. med. Hist.*, 1933, N.S., **5**.

Cocaine, *continued.*

clouding of the corneal epithelium, and, rarely, ulceration together with excellent analgesia. Used as 4 per cent solution for analgesia. The pupil still responds to light after it has become dilated by cocaine as the circular muscle is not paralysed, and as the ciliary muscle is not effected; accommodation remains active. Eserine counteracts the mydriatic effect of cocaine and atropine increases it. It usually reduces intra-ocular pressure but occasionally acute glaucoma results from its use.

MUSCLE.—On muscle it has a curare-like effect, even when the motor nerve has degenerated. Large doses have an effect on the heat regulating centre in the diencephalon and cause pyrexia.

ABSORPTION.—From all mucous membranes, including the urethra and bladder. There is some evidence that stronger solutions are absorbed less readily than weaker solutions, owing to the increased vasoconstriction they produce. In nose and throat surgery used in 4 per cent to 20 per cent solution.

EXCRETION.—Cocaine is detoxicated in the liver. About 10 per cent is excreted by the kidneys, unchanged.

A safe dose of cocaine for surface analgesia is 3 mg. per kg. of body-weight (20 mg. per stone), with a maximum of 200 mg (Macintosh); or 100–200 mg. in 10 per cent solution, i.e., 1–2 ml. or 4 ml. of 5 per cent solution.

ACUTE INTOXICATION.—The patient becomes restless, anxious and confused ; the pulse becomes rapid and the breathing irregular ; the pupils are dilated and there may be vomiting Convulsions and coma may precede death from respiratory failure. In other cases acute cardiovascular collapse occurs it should be treated with intravenous injection of a pressor drug, lowering of the head, and oxygen. Cardiac massage may be required. The symptoms due to nervous intoxication should be treated with suxamethonium or small doses of intravenous barbiturates and artificial ventilation with pure oxygen. The mechanism of such catastrophes is not fully understood, and is not necessarily due to over-dosage.

COCAINE SENSITIVITY TEST.—
1. Inject 10 mg. subcutaneously.
2. Count pulse-rate at five-minute intervals.
3. A rise of more than fifteen beats per minute suggests sensitivity.

2. Procaine Hydrochloride, B.P. (Novocain, Planocaine, Ethocaine, Neocaine, Allocaine, Syncaine, Kerocain, Servocaine, Scurocaine).— *p*-Aminobenzoyl-diethylaminoethanol hydrochloride. Formed by the reaction between chloroethyl diethylamine and sodium para-aminobenzoate. Soluble in water and alcohol. Synthesized by Einhorn in 1904,* it is about one-quarter as toxic as cocaine. It is useful for injection, but must be used in 20 per cent solution before it has any surface effect. Like amethocaine, it inhibits the bacteriostatic action of *p*-aminosalicylic acid and the sulphonamides. Should be stored in a cool place to retard hydrolysis.

---

* Einhorn, A. (quoted by Heinrich Braun, *Dtsch. med. Wschr.*, 1905, **31**, 1667).

For infiltration the strength used is 0·25 per cent to 1 per cent ; for nerve-block, 1 per cent to 2 per cent. Dry procaine from ampoules should be used to make up solutions before use. Maximum dose of 0·5 per cent solution, 200 ml. (1000 mg.), of 1 per cent solution, 75 ml. (750 mg.), and of 2 per cent solution, 25 ml. (500 mg.). Procaine 5·5 per cent in water is isotonic, with *p*H of 6·4.

Analgesia lasts from 45 to 90 minutes when adrenaline is added.

Toxic symptoms are referable either to the central nervous system, with convulsions, or to the cardiovascular system. Treatment as for cocaine intoxication. (*See also* p. 311.)

Was the standard local analgesic agent until the advent of lignocaine.

Novutox contains 2 per cent procaine and is prepared by a cold sterilizing process. It is made in various strengths, with and without adrenaline. *Proctocaine* contained 1·5 per cent procaine with 5 per cent benzyl alcohol and 5 per cent butyl amino-benzoate in oil, and its relatively prolonged action is probably due to its destructive action on nerve-fibres due to the presence of benzyl alcohol. It is sometimes used to prevent pain after hæmorrhoidectomy, 5–10 ml. being injected on each side of the anus.

CHLOROPROCAINE (Nesacaine).—This is a new compound, having little toxic effect, a longer duration of action than procaine with more rapid onset, together with a higher therapeutic index than any commonly used local analgesic drug.*

It is hydrolysed four times as quickly as procaine and, like it, by pseudocholinesterase. When a patient is suspected of having a low pseudocholinesterase level, e.g., in jaundice, anæmia, malnutrition, poisoning by war gas or weed killers, etc., procaine, amethocaine, and chloroprocaine should be used carefully.

3. **Lignocaine Hydrochloride, B.P.** (Xylocaine ; Duncaine ; Lido-caine).—Diethylamino-2 : 6 dimethylacetanilide, the most commonly used local analgesic agent in the U.K. to-day. A basic anilide, synthesized by Lofgren and Lundqvist in 1943 in Sweden.† First used by Gordh in 1948.‡ Very stable, not decomposed by boiling, acids, or alkalis. Its effects come on quicker and last longer than those of procaine. It seems to spread over a wider field than equal volumes of other analgesic drugs. Solutions of 0·25 to 0·5 per cent for infiltration, with adrenaline 1–250,000 ; 2 to 4 per cent for topical analgesia, in surgery of throat, larynx, pharynx, etc. For nerve-block 1·5 to 2 per cent with adrenaline, and for extradural block 1·2 to 2 per cent with adrenaline. For corneal analgesia 4 per cent; this causes no mydriasis, vasoconstriction, or cycloplegia. For urethral analgesia 1 to 2 per cent in jelly and for endotracheal tubes 5 per cent as an ointment. Toxicity not great, but cardio-vascular and central nervous symptoms of toxicity have been described. As in the case of prilocaine, the metabolism of lignocaine

* Foldes, F. F., and McNall, P. G., *Anesthesiology*, 1952, **13**, 287.
† Lofgren, N., *Xylocaine*, 1948. Stockholm: Haeggstroms.
‡ Gordh, T., *Anæsthesia*, 1949, **4**, 4.

Lignocaine Hydrochloride, *continued.*

can give rise to the formation of methæmoglobin, the average peak concentration ensuing within 4–6 hours after injection being 0·8 per cent. Cyanosis is rare.* It is not a vasodilator nor does it interfere with the vasoconstrictive action of adrenaline. It has a cerebral effect causing drowsiness and amnesia. It is metabolized in the liver diethylaminoacetic acid being the chief metabolite, and excreted renally. Duration of effect of 1 per cent solution, 1 hour; with adrenaline, 1½–2 hours. Has rapid onset. Has been given intravenously in 40-mg. doses at five-minute intervals, to potentiate the the analgesia of the thiopentone–gas–oxygen–relaxant combination, and also intramuscularly in 250-mg. doses in 2 per cent solution. Has been used in the treatment of status epilepticus,† and for ventricular arrhythmias, by intravenous injection. (*See* Chapter XIII.) Suggested maximum safe dose of lignocaine for a 70-kg. man —with adrenaline, 500 mg., i.e., 7 mg. per kg.; without adrenaline, 200 mg., i.e., 3 mg. per kg. body-weight. The following volumes are probably safe for administration:

CONCENTRATION USED	NOS. OF ML. OF SOLUTION
With adrenaline	
0·5 per cent	100
1·0 per cent	50
2·0 per cent	25
Without adrenaline	
0·5 per cent	40
1·0 per cent	20
1·5 per cent	13
2·0 per cent	10
4·0 per cent	5

For estimations of urine and blood lignocaine levels *see* Beckett, A. H., and others, *Anæsthesia*, 1965, **29**, 294; Woods, L. A., and others, *J. Pharmacol.*, 1951, **101**, 188; and Braid, D. P., and Scott, D. B., *Brit. J. Anæsth.*, 1965, **37**, 394.

4. Mepivacaine (Carbocaine).—This is a tertiary amine and was synthesized in 1956 by Ekstam and Egner.‡ Chemically it is N-methyl-pipecolic acid 2-6-xylidide. It is soluble in water and resistant to acid and alkaline hydrolysis. It is claimed to be a little less toxic than lignocaine while its local analgesic effects last rather longer. For intradural block 4 per cent solution has been used.§ When injected into the extradural space of patients in labour it passes rather rapidly into the fœtal circulation where it may cause harm.‖ It would appear to have few advantages over lignocaine.

---

* Hjelm, M., and Holmdahl, M. H., *Lancet*, 1965, **1**, 53.
† Bernhard, C. G., and others, *A.M.A. Arch. Neurol.. Psychiat.*, 1955, **74**, 208.
‡ Af Ekstam, B., Egner, B., and others, *Brit. J. Anæsth.*, 1956, **28**, 503.
§ Siker, E. S., and others, *Curr. Res. Anesth.*, 1966, **45**, 191.
‖ Morisha, H. O., and others, *Anesthesiology*, 1966, **27**, 147.

5. Bupivacaine (Marcain; LAC-43).—This is a new local analgesic drug synthesized by Ekstam and his colleagues in 1957.[*] Chemically it is 1-butyl-2,6-pipecoloxylidide hydrochloride and has the following formula:—

The base is not very soluble but the hydrochloride readily dissolves in water. It is very stable both to repeated autoclaving and to acids and alkalis, but solutions containing adrenaline should not be autoclaved more than twice. It was developed from mepivacaine, the methyl group in the piperidine ring being replaced by a butyl (C_4H_9) group. It is reputed to be four times as potent as both mepivacaine and lignocaine, so that a 0·5 per cent solution is roughly equivalent to 2 per cent lignocaine. It resembles amethocaine in its toxicity. Duration of effect is between 5 and 16 hours, the longest of any local analgesic known. Suitable dose is 2 mg. per kg. body-weight and the strength used is 0·5 per cent with adrenaline 1–200,000 which can be diluted if required. The pH of the 0·5 per cent solution with adrenaline is 3·5 and its density 0·997 g. per ml. at 37° C.

It has been used in the following situations:—

1. For prolonged extradural block, 0·5 per cent with adrenaline, 10–20 ml.
2. For brachial plexus block, the same volume and strength.
3. For sacral extradural block, as above.
4. For digital block, 1–3 ml. of 0·25 per cent solution without adrenaline.
5. Paracervical block.
6. Intercostal block.

6. Prilocaine (Citanest; Xylonest; Distanest; L 67).—A close relation of lignocaine with the chemical name:—

(±) 2-propyloamino-o-propionotoluidine.

Described by Lofgren and Tegner,[†] tested pharmacologically by Wiedling,[‡] and used clinically by Gordh in 1959.[§] A very stable compound, pharmacologically resembling lignocaine but less toxic. Whereas lignocaine is metabolized in the liver, prilocaine is metabolized in the liver and kidneys, more rapidly, partly by amidase. This rapid metabolism may account for the methæmoglobinæmia sometimes seen after its use,[||] if more than 600 mg. are injected. The condition is directly related to the dose and not to the blood picture.

[*] Af Ekstam, B., Egner, B., and Pettersson, G., *Acta chem. scand.*, 1957, **11**, 1183; *see also* Watt, M. J., Ross, D. M., and Atkinson, R. S., *Anæsthesia*, 1968, **23**, 2; and *Ibid.*, 1968, **23**, July.
[†] Lofgren, N., and Tegner, C., *Acta chem. scand.*, 1960, **14**, 486.
[‡] Wiedling, S., *Acta pharm. tox.*, Khb., 1960, **17**, 233.
[§] Gordh, T., *Acta anæsth. scand.*, 1959, Suppl. 2, 81.
[||] Scott, D. B., and Richmond, J., *Lancet*, 1964, **2**, 728; and Fujimori, M. quoted by Yutaka, Onsi, and others, *Acta anæsth. scand.*, 1965, Suppl. 16, 151.

Prilocaine, *continued.*

Methæmoglobin is continuously formed during normal red-cell metabolism but normally does not exceed 1 per cent of the hæmoglobin at any one time. The cause of this oxidation of hæmoglobin to methæmoglobin is not prilocaine itself but one of its degradation products, possible *o*-toluidine or nitrosotoluidine. Normally oxygen combines with the ferrous ions of hæmatin in hæmoglobin whereas the ferric ions of methæmoglobin will not transport the gas. The degree of cyanosis due to methæmoglobin varies in different individuals and usually disappears spontaneously in 24 hours. It is of little clinical importance unless there is severe anæmia or circulatory impairment. The oxygen-carrying capacity of the blood may be reduced 5 per cent after the injection of 600 mg. of prilocaine, while the presence of cyanosis indicates that 1·5 per cent or more of the hæmoglobin is circulating as methæmoglobin. There is an associated shift of the oxygen dissociation curve of the remaining hæmoglobin which hinders oxygen liberation at tissue level. A dose of 16 mg. per kg. or more is necessary to cause symptoms of hypoxia and is only likely to be seen after extradural block with repeated injections through a catheter. Congenital or acquired methæmoglobinæmia are probably contra-indications to the use of the agent. Treatment is by intravenous injection of 1 per cent methylene blue, 1–2 mg. per kg.

In extradural block the drug has been shown to give a slower onset and spread with a longer duration of effect and greater intensity than lignocaine, with less toxicity. A 3 per cent solution with adrenaline is excellent although 1·5 and 2 per cent solutions work well. The addition of adrenaline prolongs the duration of effect less with prilocaine than with lignocaine.[*]

It is most useful when high dosage and strong concentration are required of a local analgesic drug; when injection is into vascular areas, e.g., pudendal block and blocks about the face and neck, and for Bier's intravenous local analgesia. For topical analgesia 10 ml. of 4 per cent solution is reasonable. In excessive dosage it will, like its congeners, cause the classic signs and symptoms of stimulation and/or depression of the cardiovascular system and C.N.S. and overdose may result in respiratory arrest or in convulsions. A rough guide to dosage is to regard 10 mg. per kg. as maximal.

See review 'Citanest', ed. S. Wiedling, *Acta anæsth. Scand.*, 1965, Suppl. 16.

7. Cinchocaine Hydrochloride, B.P. (Nupercaine; Dibucain).— 2-Butoxy-N-(2-diethylaminoethyl) quinoline-4-carboxyamide. Synthesized by Meischer in 1925.[†] This is a complex amine derived from quinoline. It forms neutral solutions in water and alcohol. Solutions can be repeatedly boiled without loss of analgesic potency.

[*] Daly, D. J., Davenport, J., and Newland, M. L., *Brit. J. Anæsth.*, 1964, **36**, 737; and Bromage, P. R., *Ibid.*, 1965, **37**, 751.

[†] Meischer, K., *Helv. chim. acta*, 1932, **15**, 163; and Uhlmann, T., *Narkose u. Anæsth.*, 1929, **2**, 168.

It is precipitated from solution by alkali. It is incompatible also with hydrogen peroxide, potassium permanganate, and silver and mercury salts.

It is more toxic than cocaine and lignocaine, but also much more efficient as an analgesic. Thus its effective dose is less toxic than that of either of the two other agents, while the duration of analgesia is much longer, usually 2–3 hours although onset is slower. Detoxicated in liver.

The maximal dose depends on the concentration of the solution, but should not exceed 2 mg. per kg., or 1 mg. per kg. in highly vascular areas. Elderly or ill and feeble patients should receive less than this. Injection of 6 ml. of 2 per cent solution (accidentally) into tissues has caused death.

The usual strength used for infiltration with adrenaline is 1–1000 to 1–3000. For nerve-blocks, 1–1000. For corneal analgesia, 1–1000.

8. Amethocaine Hydrochloride, B.P. (Pantocaine, Pontocaine, Decicain, Butethanol, Anethaine, Tetracaine (U.S.P.), Pantokain, Dikain).—p-Butylaminobenzoyl-dimethyl aminoethanol hydrochloride. Belongs to cocaine, procaine group of drugs. Synthesized by Eisleb in 1928. A butyl group (C_4H_9) has been substituted for one of the hydrogen atoms of the p-amino group while two methyl groups (CH_3) replace two ethyl groups (C_2H_5) of the procaine molecule. It is a base, forming salts with acids, and melts at 150° C. Solutions prepared under sterile conditions remain sterile. Non-irritating to tissues and causes no pain on injection. It is a vaso-dilator and has a quinine-like action on the heart. Pharmacological effects similar to other local analgesic agents and has a stimulating action on the central nervous system which may later lead to depression. Like cocaine, it may cause cardiac asystole or ventricular fibrillation. It increases parasympathetic activity and inhibits the action of cholinesterase. Soluble in water and alcohol. Ten to twenty times as potent as procaine. Can be used for corneal analgesia in 0·5 per cent solution. The solution can be boiled once or twice without deterioration, but is rendered inactive by alkalis. In 0·5 per cent solution it can be used for surface analgesia, while for infiltration the usual strength is 1–2000 to 1–4000, preferably with adrenaline. Up to 400 ml. of 1–2000 solution with adrenaline can safely be used for infiltration analgesia. It is hydrolysed by pseudocholinesterase.

The maximum dose is 300 mg., or 2 mg. per lb. of body-weight, but if half this is not exceeded, toxic signs are very unlikely—apart from surface analgesia. Large doses are unwise and maximum for surface analgesia should be 8 ml. of 0·5 per cent solution given in two or three divided doses with an interval of five minutes between each dose. Absorption from the bronchial tree —when analgesia for bronchoscopy is being induced—is almost as rapid as that following intravenous injection. Cocaine is probably safer for this purpose as its vasoconstrictor action retards absorption somewhat.

Its effect lasts longer than that of procaine, but not so long as that of cinchocaine, roughly 1½ to 3 hours. Onset of analgesia slow. It is inactivated by iodine and mercuric chloride. It is mildly antiseptic. The addition of adrenaline greatly reduces its toxicity.

Amethocaine Hydrochloride, *continued.*

> Death occurs from respiratory failure, toxic signs being similar in appearance and treatment to those of cocaine.

9. Piperocaine Hydrochloride, U.S.P. (Metycaine, Neothesine).— Gamma-(2-methyl-piperidine) propyl benzoate hydrochloride. Synthesized by McElvain in 1927.* Soluble in water and alcohol. This synthetic drug is rather more toxic and lasts longer than procaine. It has a good surface effect in 2–5 per cent solution. Formerly used extensively for producing extradural sacral analgesia in 1½ per cent solution.

For chemistry of local analgesic agents, *see* Geddes, I. C., *Brit. J. Anæsth.*, 1967, **34**, 229.

Procaine and amethocaine should not be used when the patient is receiving a sulphonamide drug or *p*-aminosalicylic acid. Prilocaine, bupivacaine, lignocaine, and cinchocaine do not contain the *p*-aminobenzoic acid group.

The tricyclic antidepressants imipramine, amitryptyline, and nortriptyline, in powder form, have local analgesic effects on mucous membranes.

Long-acting Local Analgesic Solutions.—It has been shown† that the injection of 1 per cent lignocaine in 10 per cent dextran with adrenaline 1–250,000 will give analgesia for up to 10 hours. This does not hold good for extradural injection.

Autoclaving of Local Analgesic Drugs.—The commonly used agents are very stable chemical compounds. Ampoules of the hydrochloride salts of lignocaine, prilocaine, mepivacaine, and procaine can all be autoclaved (250° F. for 20–30 min.) and thereafter show no chemical change on chromatographic analysis.‡

Methods of Comparing Local Analgesics.§—

  1. For topical analgesia the drug can be tested on the human tongue, the human laryngeal reflex, the mammalian cornea, the frog's skin. The rabbit's cornea is a popular method.
  2. Tests for conduction analgesia : sciatic nerve-block in the frog, guinea-pig, or rabbit ; lingual reflex in the dog ; change in the alpha wave of the action potential of isolated nerve-fibres ; spinal analgesia—intensity and duration.
  3. Tests for infiltration analgesia : subcutaneous, intradural injection in animals and man.

As will be seen, there is no really reliable method.

DRUGS USED FOR VASOCONSTRICTION

Vasoconstrictor drugs have been used in local analgesia since Braun introduced adrenaline in 1902.

The adrenaline-induced contraction of the smooth muscle of vessel walls is modified to different degrees by the same molar concentrations

* McElvain, S. M., *J. Amer. chem. Soc.*, 1926, **48**, 2179.
† Loder, R. E., *Lancet*, 1960, **2**, 346.
‡ Katz, J., *Anesthesiology*, 1966, **27**, 835.
§ Geddes, I. C., *Brit. J. Anæsth.*, 1955, **27**, 609.

of different local analgesic agents and by different concentrations of the same agent.* The vascularity of the tissues receiving the injection is also a factor to be considered in estimating the optimal concentration in a given case. Vasoconstrictors are employed: (1) To retard absorption and reduce toxicity; (2) To prolong analgesic activity.

Adrenaline (Epinephrine).—The tartrate, which is synthetic, is used for injection, and contains a stabilizer, potassium metabitartrate, 0·1 per cent; the hydrochloride, which is of animal origin, is for topical application. For infiltration it is probably unnecessary to use a strength greater than 1–200,000. Adrenaline does not keep well in solution; discoloration indicates decomposition; it can be autoclaved once but not repeatedly. The usual amount added is 1–2 mg. to 250–500 ml. of saline, giving a 1–250,000 to 1–500,000 solution, irrespective of the strength of the analgesic solution. It is probably unwise to inject more than 0·5 mg. at one time.

Adrenaline must be used in very low dilution, if at all, in cases of thyrotoxicosis and hypertension. It may produce pallor, tachycardia, and syncope. It should not be used if chloroform or cyclopropane† is to be given as general anæsthetic in addition, lest the combination should cause ventricular fibrillation. There is also a danger when halothane is to be administered.‡ It has been suggested that, providing there is no hypercapnia or hypoxia, 20 ml. of 1–200,000 adrenaline solution can be injected with safety in any 10-min. period.§ A catechol nucleus and a primary or secondary amine are necessary in a vasoconstrictor, if it is to produce arrhythmia. Care should also be taken during trichloroethylene anæsthesia; a quantity not exceeding 0·5 mg. being used for local infiltration, with an inhaled concentration not greater than 0·6 per cent and avoidance of hypoventilation.‖ Vasoconstrictors help to produce a dry operative field. Should not be used in ring block of the digits.

Cobefrin (Corbasil).—This is 1-(3′, 4′-dihydroxyphenyl)-2-aminopropanol. A synthetic substitute for adrenaline and is used like the latter in 0·5 per cent solution instead of 1–1000 solution. It is said to be less likely to produce the minor collapse sometimes seen when adrenaline is used. Its pressor action is between one-sixth and one-half that of adrenaline, while it is more stimulating to the myocardium. It cannot safely be combined with cyclopropane. With 0·5 per cent procaine, cobefrin is used in a final strength of 1–80,000 ; with 1 per cent procaine, 1–40,000 ; with 2 per cent procaine, 1–20,000. Cannot be autoclaved.

Phenylephrine (Neosynephrine).—Used to cause vasoconstriction during local analgesia, 0·25 to 0·5 ml. of 1 per cent solution added to each 100 ml. of local analgesic solution. Causes no cerebral stimulation or tachycardia.

* Astrom, A., *Acta physiol. scand.*, 1964, **60**, 30.
† Matteo, R. S., Katz, R. L., and Papper, E. M., *Anesthesiology*, 1963, **24**, 327.
‡ Varejes, L., *Anæsthesia*, 1963, **18**, 507.
§ Matteo, R. S., Katz, R. L., and Papper, E. M., *Anesthesiology*, 1962, **23**, 360; and *Ibid.* 1962, **23**, 597.
‖ Matteo, R. S., Katz, R. L., and Papper, E. M., *Ibid.*, 1962, **23**, 156.

Noradrenaline.—This can be used to produce local vasoconstriction but is less effective than adrenaline. It is oxidized in the body more rapidly by amine oxidase than is adrenaline.

Felypressin (P.V.L.-2; Octopressin).—This is 2-phenylalanine-8-lysine vasopressin and may prove to be a useful local vasoconstrictor for use along with halothane, cyclopropane, trichloroethylene, etc. It is a synthetic derivative of the octapeptide hormone, vasopressin, from the posterior pituitary. It causes constriction of all smooth muscle but has little oxytocic or antidiuretic effect. May result in coronary arterial constriction, but has little effect on cardiac rhythm.*

Vasoconstrictors should be used very sparingly in : (1) Hypertension. (2) Thyrotoxicosis. (3) In out-patients. (4) In old age.

TOPICAL ANALGESIA†

Can be applied: (1) On gauze swabs. (2) As a liquid in a spray. (3) As a paste or ointment. (4) As an aerosol. (5) By direct instillation, e.g., conjunctival sac, nose, and trachea.

Sites.—(1) The upper air-passages, e.g., 4 per cent lignocaine, 5 ml. (2) The nasal cavities. (3) The external ear, e.g., 10 per cent lignocaine aerosol for paracentesis. (4) The conjunctival sac, e.g., 4 per cent lignocaine or 2–4 per cent cocaine or 0·5 per cent amethocaine. Stinging pain in instillation can be eased if the drug is dissolved in methyl cellulose. (5) Perineum and vagina in obstetrics, e.g., 10 per cent lignocaine aerosol for spontaneous delivery or for suture of simple lacerations. (6) Urethra, e.g., 1 per cent lignocaine gel.

INFILTRATION ANALGESIA

A weal is raised with a fine needle and through this weal a larger needle is used to inject the main bulk of solution. Procaine in 0·5 per cent solution, or lignocaine 0·25 per cent solution, is ideal for this procedure. For painless skin incisions, infiltration should be intradermal, as well as subcutaneous. A slow, gentle technique is important, and the solution should be injected while the needle is moving (the syringe-before-knife technique).

TRANSVERSE SECTION ANÆSTHESIA

A name given by Russian surgeons to a method (Vishnevsky technique) in which a transverse disk of tissue of a limb is infiltrated from skin to bone with a dilute solution of an analgesic drug such as 0·5 per cent procaine in large volume. Cinchocaine 1–5000 or 1–10,000 has also been used. In the vernacular 'the squirt-and-cut' technique.

---

* Katz, R. L., *Anesthesiology*, 1965, **26**, 619; Hugin, W., *Der Anæsthesist*, 1962, **11**, 185; Hunter, M. E., and others, *Canad. Anæsth. Soc. J.*, 1966, **13**, 40; and Katz, R. L., and Katz, G. J., *Brit. J. Anæsth.*, 1966, **38**, 712.
† Boulton, T. B., *Anæsthesia*, 1967, **22**, 101.

FIELD BLOCK OF SCALP AND CRANIUM

Anatomy.—The trigeminal nerve supplies the anterior two-thirds, the posterior divisions of cervical nerves the posterior third. (*Fig.* 25.) There are four sensory nerves in front of the ear : supratrochlear and supra-orbital, both from the first division of the fifth nerve ;

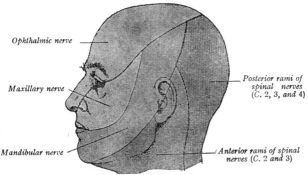

Fig. 25.—Showing the cutaneous nerve areas of the face and scalp.
(*From ' Gray's Anatomy ', by kind permission of Professor T. B. Johnston.*)

the zygomaticotemporal, from the second division of the fifth nerve ; the auriculotemporal, from the third division of the fifth nerve.

The four sensory nerves behind the ear are : the great auricular and the greater, lesser, and least occipital nerves, from the cervical plexus.

These nerves all converge towards the vertex of the scalp, so that a band of infiltration passing just above the ear through the glabella and the occiput will block them all.

Technique.—Injections must be made in three layers :—
  1. The skin.
  2. The subcutaneous tissues.
  3. The periosteum.
In addition, solution should be injected into the substance of the temporalis muscle. The dura is insensitive except at the base of the skull.

For removal of sebaceous cysts or suturing of small wounds, the area is surrounded by a zone of infiltration. Periosteal injection is only necessary if bone is to be removed.

NERVE-BLOCK FOR NOSE OPERATIONS*

Anatomy.—The nerve-supply is from the first or ophthalmic division and from the second or maxillary division of the trigeminal nerve. In more detail :—

---

* *See also* " Regional Anæsthesia for Surgery of the Nose and Sinuses ", by Loftus-Dale, H. W., *Lancet*, 1944, **1**, 562 ; and *Local Analgesia, Head and Neck*, by Macintosh, R. R., and Ostlere, M., 2nd ed., 1967. Edinburgh and London: E. & S. Livingstone.

Nerve-block for Nose Operations—Anatomy, *continued.*

The external nose is supplied by the supratrochlear branch of frontal nerve of the ophthalmic ; the anterior ethmoidal branch of the nasociliary (ophthalmic) ; the infra-orbital branch of the maxillary.

The maxillary antrum of Highmore : its lining is supplied by the maxillary nerve via the sphenopalatine ganglion.

The frontal sinus : frontal nerve ; branch of ophthalmic.

The ethmoid region : the anterior and posterior ethmoidal branches of the nasociliary.

The sensory supply of the nasal cavities—fifth nerve—is as follows :—

The anterior one-third of the septum and lateral walls by the anterior ethmoidal branch of the nasociliary nerve (division 1).

The posterior two-thirds of the septum and lateral walls by the long sphenopalatine nerves from the sphenopalatine ganglion (division 2).

Techniques.—

1. BLOCK OF MAXILLARY NERVE AND SPHENOPALATINE GANGLION.—Useful for operations on antrum (e.g., Caldwell-Luc) and on upper lip, palate, and upper teeth as far as the bicuspids.

ANATOMY.—The maxillary or second division of the fifth nerve is entirely sensory. It is given off from the middle of the Gasserian ganglion and passes forwards horizontally in the lower part of the lateral wall of the cavernous sinus until it leaves the skull through the foramen rotundum. It crosses the pterygomaxillary fissure to enter the orbit through the inferior orbital fissure and ends as the infra-orbital nerve after emerging on to the face through the infra-orbital foramen. The sphenopalatine ganglion of Meckel is situated in the pterygopalatine fossa in the upper part of the pterygomaxillary fissure, lateral to the sphenopalatine foramen. Blocking of the nerve causes analgesia in the lateral nasal, inferior palpebral, and superior labial nerves, the posterior, middle, and anterior superior alveolar nerves, and the palatal nerves which supply the skin of the upper lip, side of nose, lower eyelid and malar region, the teeth of the upper jaw and the underlying periosteum, the mucosa of the maxillary antrum and of the hard and soft palate and the posterior part of the nasal cavity.

A weal is raised 0·5 cm. below the midpoint of the zygoma, which is over the anterior border of the coronoid process, and through it a needle is introduced at right-angles to the median plane of the head until it strikes the lateral plate of the pterygoid process at a depth of about 4 cm. Set marker 1 cm. from skin surface and reinsert needle slightly anteriorly so that its point glances past the anterior margin of the external pterygoid plate and advances as far as the marker. The needle point should be in the pterygomaxillary fissure. The needle has been known to enter the pharynx or the orbit. If aspiration test is negative, 3–4 ml. of 1·5 per cent solution of lignocaine is injected and a similar amount as the needle is slowly withdrawn.

Transient paralysis of the sixth cranial nerve may result ; it soon passes off.

2. BLOCK OF ANTERIOR ETHMOIDAL NERVE (MEDIAN ORBITAL BLOCK).—This is blocked in the medial wall of the orbit as the nerve passes through the anterior ethmoidal foramen. A weal is raised 1 cm. above the caruncle at the inner canthus of the eye. A small needle is introduced along the upper medial angle of the orbit for 3·5 cm., keeping near the bone. Injection is made of 2 ml. of 1·5 per cent lignocaine.

3. BLOCK OF FRONTAL NERVE.—From the same weal as in anterior ethmoid block, the needle is introduced more laterally towards the central part of the roof of the orbit where the frontal nerve lies between the periosteum and the levator palpebræ superioris. Lignocaine, 1 ml. of 2 per cent solution, is injected in close contact with the bone.

4. BLOCK OF INFRA-ORBITAL NERVE.—The infra-orbital nerve, the terminal portion of the maxillary nerve, divides at the infra-orbital foramen into inferior palpebral, external nasal, and superior labial branches. These supply the side of the nose, the lower eyelid, the upper lip and its mucosa. The infra-orbital foramen is in line with the supra-orbital notch and canine fossa—both of which are palpable ; it is 1 cm. below the margin of the orbit, below the pupil when the eyes look forwards. The mental foramen is in the same straight line, as is also the second bicuspid tooth.

A needle is inserted through a weal 1 cm. below the middle of the lower orbital margin, a finger-breadth lateral to the ala of the nose. Lignocaine, 2 ml. of 2 per cent solution, is deposited near the nerve as it issues from the foramen, not while it is in the foramen. By this injection the upper lip and tip of nose are made insensitive.

For radical operation on the antrum, a maxillary block is indicated, together with local infiltration inside the upper lip, over the canine fossa.

For radical operation on the frontal sinus, anterior ethmoidal and frontal blocks are necessary.

For operations for dacryocystitis, anterior ethmoidal and infraorbital blocks are required.

LOCAL INFILTRATION FOR DENTAL EXTRACTION

This can be done for all teeth with the possible exception of the lower molars. Lignocaine 2 per cent with 1–80,000 adrenaline solution is commonly used. A 26-gauge needle is inserted at the junction of the adherent mucoperiosteum of the gum with the free mucous membrane of the cheek and directed parallel to the long axis of the tooth; 0·5–1 ml. of solution is injected superficial to the periosteum on the buccal and either the lingual or palatal side. Analgesia is tested for after 5 min. by pushing the needle down the periodontal membrane on each side of the tooth to be extracted. If required more solution can be injected.

Mandibular Block.—This may be required for extraction of several teeth of the lower jaw or for removal of the second or third molars. Infiltration cannot always be relied on to make these teeth

Mandibular Block, *continued.*

insensitive. A single well-placed injection makes one-half of the lower jaw and tongue analgesic, except for the central incisor which gets some nerve-supply from the other side, and the lateral buccal fold and molar buccal alveolar margin and gum supplied from the buccinator nerve. Both of these areas can be infiltrated with a small volume of solution to make them painless.

With the mouth open palpate the anterior border of the ramus of the mandible, the retromolar fossa, and the internal oblique ridge. The needle is inserted just medial to this ridge lateral to the pterygomandibular ligament for a distance of 2·5 cm. keeping the syringe parallel to the occlusal plane of the lower teeth with its barrel over the premolar teeth of the opposite side. Two to three ml. of solution are now injected.

Transient amaurosis after mandibular nerve-block has been reported[*] and may be due to intra-arterial injection of adrenaline with the local analgesic solution in patients whose orbital blood-supply is derived from the middle meningeal artery—a rare anomaly.

LINGUAL NERVE-BLOCK

The lingual nerve is the only sensory nerve supplying the floor of the mouth between the alveolar margin and the midline.

A finger in the retromolar fossa of the mandible will palpate the internal oblique line. The lingual nerve can be injected, just medial to this line, with 2 ml. of 2 per cent lignocaine. A useful method of analgesia for removing calculi from the submaxillary duct.

TOPICAL ANALGESIA OF THE NASAL CAVITIES[†]

1. The nasal cavities are first sprayed with 4 to 10 per cent cocaine, all excess solution being rejected and not swallowed. With a good light and a speculum, the cavity is now packed with gauze soaked in equal volumes of 10 per cent cocaine and 1–1000 adrenaline. Cocaine is a powerful vasoconstrictor, and so adrenaline, although beloved of rhinologists, is not really necessary. It causes, moreover, vasodilatation after the initial vasoconstriction has worn off and adds to the sympathomimetic effect of cocaine (e.g., on the heart). Adrenaline added to local analgesic solutions does not increase duration of block. Trauma must be avoided.

After ten minutes the packing is removed and the mucosa will be found to be avascular.

A wool-covered applicator is moistened with adrenaline and dipped into cocaine crystals and introduced so that it comes to lie against the sphenoid sinus, between the posterior part of the middle turbinate and the septum. A second similar applicator is placed between the septum and the anterior end of the middle turbinate. After five minutes the patient is ready for operation.

2. Use of cocaine paste. Many formulæ have been described, a useful one is : cocaine 7 g., thymol 60 mg., dried adrenal gland 1·5 g.,

* Blaxter, P. L., and Britten, M. J. A., *Brit. med. J.*, 1967, **1**, 681.
† *See* Macintosh, R. R., and Ostlere, M., *Local Analgesia, Head and Neck,* 2nd ed., 1967, 86. Edinburgh and London: E. & S. Livingstone.

liquid and soft paraffin equal parts, to make 30 g. For each patient, 2 g. of the paste are used. The nasal cavities are first sprayed with cocaine solution (4 per cent) and then the mucosa of the septum and lateral walls is lightly painted with paste, using a head mirror and light and a wool-covered probe. Paste is applied to the area of the sphenopalatine ganglion, behind the middle meatus, and also to the area of the cribriform plate, and acts on the long and short sphenopalatine nerves and the greater and lesser palatines in the first situation, and on the anterior ethmoid nerve in the second.

3. MOFFETT'S METHOD.*—The solution used is 2 ml. of 8 per cent cocaine hydrochlor.; 2 ml. of 1 per cent sod. bicarb.; 1 ml. of 1–1000 adrenaline solution. A 2-ml. syringe with bent cannula is required.

Position 1 : Patient lies on left side with pillow under left shoulder and head in lateral position at angle of 45° with vertical. One-third of solution is drawn up, half being squirted into each naris along the floor of the nose.

Position 2 : After ten minutes, second third of solution is drawn up and is similarly divided between the two sides of the nose; patient pinches nose, turns prone, lies on face for ten minutes.

Position 3 : From prone position patient rolls on to right side as in Position 1 and remains ten minutes. If the septum is to be operated on, 2 ml. of 1 per cent procaine–adrenaline should be injected into the columella and base of septum in addition, as this area is covered by squamous epithelium which will not absorb the topical agent.

The method gives good analgesia, free from the unpleasantness of gauze packing and its resulting mild trauma. A modification of this technique has been well described by E. S. Curtiss,† who finds that excellent results are obtained by simply depositing 2 ml. of the solution into the spheno-ethmoidal recess, posterior to the middle turbinate bone, on each side with the patient's neck extended until the head is upside down. Here the sphenopalatine ganglion and its branches lie and are bathed in solution occupying the superior meatus. The anterior ethmoidal nerve also becomes blocked at the same time. The procedure takes ten minutes. This has been again modified by Macintosh and Ostlere,‡ who use Moffett's angulated cannula to deposit cocaine solution (2·5 ml. of 5 per cent) on the inverted roof of the nose, after preliminary spraying. Each naris is treated and the position is maintained for ten minutes. Excess solution must not be swallowed.

A simpler method of anæsthetizing the nose has recently been described.§ Lignocaine in 1·25 per cent solution is used with 0·5 ml. of adrenaline added to each 40 ml. The head and neck of the patient are hyperextended and 20 ml. of the

* Moffett, A. J., *Anæsthesia*, 1947, **2**, 31.
† Curtiss, E. S., *Lancet*, 1952, **1**, 989.
‡ *Local Analgesia, Head and Neck*, by Macintosh, R. R., and Ostlere, M., 2nd ed., 1967. Edinburgh and London: E. & S. Livingstone.
§ Bodman, R. I., and Boyes-Korkis, F., *Brit. med. J.*, 1960, **2**, 1956.

Topical Analgesia of the Nasal Cavities, *continued.*

solution are poured into one nostril and the patient told to breathe through his mouth. The other nostril is similarly dealt with. After three minutes he sits up, blows his nose and is told not to swallow any of the solution. The entire nasal mucosa remains insensitive for at least one hour. Some nares require larger volumes of solution than others.

Cinchocaine solution, o·5 per cent, in 6 per cent glucose, as used for spinal analgesia, is a useful topical nasal analgesic.

VAGUS NERVE-BLOCK

This was described* as a method of analgesia for broncho-œsophago-scopy and in the diagnosis of pain arising in the thorax, but is now seldom used.

Anatomy.—Both motor and sensory roots spring from three nuclei (the dorsal nucleus, the nucleus ambiguus, and the nucleus of the tractus solitarius) in the medulla and leave the skull through the jugular foramen ; soon after its exit from the cranium it enlarges into a ganglion—the superior jugular ganglion—and after it is joined by twigs from the accessory nerve it again enlarges into the inferior ganglion (nodosum). It then passes down the neck in the carotid sheath, lying between the internal carotid artery and the internal vein. Then on the *right side* it passes between the first part of the subclavian artery and the right innominate vein, runs along the side of the trachea to the back of the root of the right lung, where it forms with sympathetic fibres the posterior pulmonary plexus, and is carried on to the œsophagus to form, with the left vagus, the œsophageal plexus. From this, a single cord runs posterior to the œsophagus and enters the abdomen, where it is distributed to the stomach, cœliac plexus, etc. On the *left side* the vagus enters the thorax between the left innominate vein anteriorly and between the left carotid and subclavian arteries. It crosses the left side of the aortic arch to the posterior aspect of the root of the left lung, forming here the posterior pulmonary plexus. Branches leave this to form the œsophageal plexus, after which the nerve continues into the abdomen through the œsophageal hiatus of the diaphragm, with the right vagus. The left nerve lies anteriorly and the right posteriorly at this level. The vagi terminate by giving twigs to the cœliac plexus from which they are distributed to the stomach, intestine, kidneys, and adrenals.

The pharyngeal branch, the chief motor nerve of the pharynx, and the superior laryngeal branch arise from the inferior ganglion. The recurrent laryngeal nerve arises on the left side just above the aortic arch, and winds below the aorta. On the right side it is given off in front of the first part of the subclavian artery ; while the cardiac branches arise in the neck.

Vagal stimulation may cause arterial hypotension, e.g., during pneumonectomy. The reflex may be abolished by curare.

The results of bilateral vagus block are : (1) Tachycardia ; (2) Hypertension ; (3) Aphonia ; (4) Abolition of the cough reflex. In

---

* Mushin, W. W., and Macintosh, R. R., *Proc. R. Soc. Med.*, 1945, **38**, 308.

addition, there may be signs and symptoms due to block of surrounding nerves, e.g., (a) Horner's syndrome (cervical sympathetic), (b) Falling back of the tongue (hypoglossal), and (c) Dysphagia (glossopharyngeal).

Technique.—The needle is inserted through a weal in front and slightly below the tip of the mastoid process so that its point lies on the anterior surface of the transverse process of the atlas. After aspiration, 10 ml. of solution (2 per cent procaine or 1·5 per cent lignocaine) are injected. As the hypoglossal nerve may also be blocked, flaccidity of the tongue muscles may result, and, if bilateral, may result in respiratory obstruction. A second method of vagus block at the jugular foramen is to raise a weal anterior to the mastoid process, just below the external auditory meatus. A 5-cm. needle is then inserted perpendicularly to the skin until it touches the styloid process and then slips 2 cm. behind it. Injection of a few ml. of solution may also result in block of the glossopharyngeal, accessory, and hypoglossal nerves. This block should not be lightly undertaken but has been suggested for the treatment of cardiac arrhythmia and for pain in the larynx or pharynx. Bilateral block may be used for bronchoscopy and for operations on the larynx or pharynx.

Superior Laryngeal Nerve-block.[*]—This nerve is blocked at its point of division into the internal and external laryngeal nerve, slightly below and anterior to the greater cornu of the hyoid bone. A weal is raised over the thyroid notch in the midline, the hyoid grasped between the thumb and index finger of the left hand, and displaced laterally towards the side to be injected. Through the weal, an 8-cm. needle is introduced laterally and 2 per cent procaine solution is injected as the needle is advanced to the greater cornu—but not beyond it for fear of injuring the great vessels of the neck. A further few ml. of solution are injected as the needle is withdrawn. A similar procedure is carried out on the other side, through the same weal.

This block causes analgesia of the larynx above the cords, so that food and drink must be prohibited for an adequate period depending on the drug and strength used.

It is useful, in conjunction with topical analgesia of the nose and pharynx, to enable blind nasotracheal intubation to be performed for tracheo-bronchial toilet: the coughing which results from irritation of the larynx below the cords soon passes off.

STELLATE GANGLION BLOCK[†]
(Cervico-thoracic sympathetic block)

The stellate ganglion is formed by the fusion of the lowest of the three cervical ganglia with the first thoracic ganglion. It is irregular in size and position, being usually 1 to 3 cm. long, and differs in the same individual on the two sides. Stellate ganglion block was first used for cerebral vascular accidents by Leriche and Fontaine in 1934[‡].

---

[*] Gaskill, J. R., and Gillies, D. R., *Arch. Otolaryngol.*, 1966, **84**, 654.
[†] *See* Moore, D. C., *Stellate Ganglion Block*, 1954. Springfield, Ill.: Thomas.
[‡] Leriche, R., and Fontaine, R., *Pr. méd.*, 1934, **41**, 386; and *Rev. Chir.*, 1936, **74**, 751.

Stellate Ganglion Block, *continued.*

This should be named cervico-thoracic sympathetic block, as when 10–15 ml. of analgesic solution are injected into the correct plane at the base of the neck the middle cervical, stellate, and the second, third, and usually the fourth thoracic ganglia and their rami are blocked. This results in interruption of all sympathetic fibres to most of the thorax, head, neck, and arm (except possibly the nerve of Kuntz*). Certain visceral afferent fibres are also blocked, e.g., the cervical cardiac nerves.

The stellate ganglion is often blocked by spill-over following supra-clavicular brachial plexus block.

Anatomy.—It lies in front of the head of the first rib and the seventh cervical and first thoracic transverse process, just behind the subclavian artery and origin of the vertebral artery. It lies posterior to the carotid sheath on the longus colli and longus cervicis muscles. It is anterior to the eighth cervical and first thoracic nerves, so paræsthesia involving these nerves shows, if stellate ganglion block is done from the front, that the needle is too deeply placed. On the right side the apex of the lung and the dome of the pleura are anterior relations ; on the left side these structures are 1 in. lower and so are not in such close relation-ship to the ganglion. Vasoconstrictor fibres pass from the stellate and the other cervical sympathetic ganglia to a plexus around the internal carotid artery. Twigs from the second and sometimes also from the third thoracic sympathetic ganglion often go directly to the upper extremity via the first thoracic nerve, thus by-passing the stellate ganglion (the nerve of Kuntz). But this nerve is usually blocked by spread of the analgesic solution down to the region of the fourth thoracic ganglion.

It sends grey rami to the seventh and eighth cervical nerves, gives origin to the inferior cervical cardiac nerve, and supplies twigs to the vessels in its vicinity. It may communicate with the vagus.

Physiological Effects of the Block.—

A. Horner's syndrome (miosis, enophthalmos, and ptosis). (*See* p. 340.)

B. 1. Vasodilatation in head and neck vessels and in those of arm and hand.

    2. Fall in intra-ocular pressure.

    3. Inhibition of sweating, salivary, and mucous gland secretion in the bronchi.

    4. Inhibition of cardiac pain and causalgic pain from upper extremity.

Its most frequent indication is to release vascular tone.

Indications.—Thrombosis, embolism, and spasm of vessels of the arm, head (spasm after angiography), and neck, e.g., Raynaud's disease, Sudeck's atrophy, hyperhidrosis ; causalgia of the upper limb, pulmonary embolism, status asthmaticus, angina pectoris, paroxysmal tachycardia, auriculo-temporal syndrome, tinnitus—some cases of eighth-nerve deafness, Bell's palsy,† etc. (by increas-ing blood-supply to the nerve). It was, however, shown in a

---

* Kuntz, A., *The Autonomic Nervous System*, 3rd ed., 1945. Philadelphia: Lea & Febiger.
† Korkis, F. B., *A.M.A. Arch. Otolaryng.*, 1959, **70**, 562.

controlled trial that no significant benefit resulted in cases of Bell's palsy from repeated sympathetic blockade.* Thrombosis of central retinal artery. Relief of papilloedema.† As an aid to orbital phlebography, to make angular vein easier to inject into, in cases of orbital tumour, e.g., hæmangiomata.‡ The tone of intracranial vessels is now thought to be more humoral than nervous.

Technique.—Stellate ganglion block performed on a patient with an increased bleeding time or a decreased clotting time may result in a large hæmatoma in the deep planes of the neck. Blocks for cerebrovascular accidents are done on the side opposite to that of the paralysed limbs. Long-acting drugs, e.g., 6 per cent phenol or absolute alcohol, are used chiefly to control cardiac pain. Bilateral block should not be carried out at the same time.

1. PARATRACHEAL APPROACH (Moore§).—The patient lies supine, chin forwards, neck extended without a pillow. Weal raised two finger-breadths lateral to the jugular notch and a similar distance above the clavicle, which is on the medial border of the sternomastoid overlying the transverse process of the seventh cervical vertebra. The position can be checked by palpating the tubercle of Chassaignac and the cricoid cartilage, both of which are at the level of the sixth cervical transverse process, i.e., a little higher than the weal. The needle 2 in. or 3 in. long is inserted directly backwards through the weal, while downward and backward pressure is exerted on the sterno-mastoid to draw the muscle and the carotid sheath laterally. When contact is made with bone (C.7) the needle is withdrawn 0·5 to 1 cm. so that its point lies in front of the longus colli muscle and, after careful aspiration for blood (the vertebral artery is very near) and for cerebrospinal fluid, 10 ml. of solution are injected. This will, if correctly placed, diffuse up and down in the fascial plane and will block the ganglia and rami from C.2 to T.4 inclusive. Thirty minutes may elapse before Horner's syndrome and vasodilatation of the arm appear. This technique is, in the authors' opinion, the safest.

2. ANTERIOR APPROACH (V. Apgar‖).—With the patient's head on a pillow and the face turned towards the sound side, a needle is inserted through a weal just above the clavicle and immediately lateral to the sternal head of the sternomastoid muscle. It is advanced directly backwards until it makes contact with the lateral part of the anterior aspect of the body of the seventh cervical vertebra. As the sympathetic chain lies on the longus colli muscle and not directly on the bone, the needle is withdrawn 0·5 cm., after which 5 ml. of analgesic solution are injected. Horner's syndrome may not appear for ten to fifteen minutes. The carotid and jugular vessels are lateral to this point of injection.

* Fearnley, M., and others, *Lancet*, 1964, **2**, 725.
† Foldi, M., and others, *Ibid.*, 1962, **1**, 512.
‡ James, P., *Anæsthesia*, 1965, **20**, 283.
§ Moore, D. C., *Stellate Ganglion Block*, 1954, 83. Springfield, Ill. : Thomas.
‖ Apgar, Virginia, *Curr. Res. Anesth.*, 1948, **27**, 49.

Stellate Ganglion Block—Technique, *continued.*

3. ANTERIOR APPROACH (Alton Ochsner*).—With head rotated to sound side, a weal is raised 1 cm. above and 1 cm. medial to the midclavicular point. A needle is introduced medially at an angle of 45° to the midline, avoiding a caudal inclination to miss the pleura. When the needle impinges on the body of the seventh cervical vertebra, solution is deposited. The theca, carotid, and vertebral vessels must be avoided.

4. ANTERIOR APPROACH (Leriche, Fontaine†).—Needle inserted through a weal immediately above midpoint of clavicle, and directed horizontally towards the transverse process of the first thoracic vertebra. As soon as bone is touched, direction of needle altered 30° inwards and 20° downwards. Injection is made, after the usual precautions, of 10 ml. of solution.

5. LATERAL APPROACH (Goinard‡).—From a weal just above the midclavicular point, a 10-cm. needle is introduced medially at a sharp angle and contact is made with the upper surface of the first rib. The direction of the needle is then changed until its tip is guided along the rib surface to its medial extremity, at its junction with the transverse process of the first thoracic vertebra. Here the injection is made after taking the usual most important precautions.

6. POSTERIOR APPROACH (Kappis, Läwen, Mandl, 1947 ; Labat, 1930 ; White, 1940).—Patient suitably premedicated, either sitting with head flexed, or lying prone with head flexed. Spine of seventh cervical vertebra identified and weal raised two finger-breadths laterally at a point which corresponds with tip of transverse process of first thoracic vertebra.

Ten-cm. needle introduced through weal at right-angles to skin until transverse process of first rib is touched. If distance is greater than 5 cm. direction should be slightly changed. Tip of needle manipulated caudally until it slips off lower border of transverse process. Rubber marker set at 3 cm. and needle inclined medially about 20° with median sagittal plane. A second bony contact should be made in 3 cm. If it is made at less depth, needle should be partially withdrawn and introduced at a slightly smaller angle. If contact is not yet made at depth of 3 cm., needle point must be directed slightly more towards the midline. Place a drop of solution on needle hub and ask patient to breathe deeply. A bubbling will indicate that needle tip is within pleura. When it is certain that injection will not be made into the pleura, theca, or a vessel, 10 ml. of solution are deposited in the close vicinity of the ganglion. This approach is the best one if a long-acting drug is to be used and the position of the needle should be checked radiographically. Alcohol 2·5 ml. or 6 per cent to 10 per cent phenol have given good results.

Signs of Successful Block.—

1. Horner's syndrome—miosis, enophthalmos, and ptosis.
2. Flushing of the cheek, face and neck, and arm. Enlarged veins of arm.

---

* Ochsner, A., *Surgery*, 1939, **5**, 491.
† Leriche, R., and Fontaine, R., *Pr. Méd.*, 1934, **41**, 386.
‡ Goinard, P., *Acad. di Chir.*, 1936, 258.

3. Flushing of the conjunctiva and sclera.
4. Anhidrosis of the face and neck.
5. Lacrimation.
6. Stuffiness of the nostril (Guttmann's sign).

Complications and Dangers of the Block.—
1. Pleural shock, especially on the right side.
2. Perforation of the œsophagus, with infection.
3. Intrathecal injection causing a total spinal block.
4. Intravascular injection, e.g., sending volume of solution via the vertebral artery straight up to the medulla.
5. Pneumothorax.
6. Cardiac arrest—very rare.
7. Alteration of voice from recurrent laryngeal nerve-block.
8. Phrenic nerve-block.
9. Brachial plexus block.
10. Extradural block.

Death has been reported after stellate ganglion block, so that it should not be lightly undertaken.

FIELD BLOCK FOR TONSILLECTOMY

Anatomy.—The tonsil and its immediate surroundings are supplied by the lesser palatine (from maxillary), the lingual (from mandibular) nerves, and the glossopharyngeal nerve, via the pharyngeal plexus, which gives off filaments which form a plexus called the circulus tonsillaris.

Technique.—Half an hour before the analgesia is commenced, an amethocaine lozenge 100 mg. is given, after which the mouth and pharynx should be sprayed with 4 to 10 per cent cocaine solution ; some operators object to this, preferring to keep the cough reflex active throughout.

Injections of 3–5 ml. of 1·5 per cent lignocaine and adrenaline are now made :—
1. Into the upper part of the posterior pillar.
2. Into the upper part of the anterior pillar. Both pillars must be made œdematous throughout their whole extent.
3. Into the triangular fold, near the lower pole.
4. Into the supratonsillar fossa, after drawing the tonsil towards the middle line.

The patient is sitting, well supported, in a chair. Adequate time must be given for the analgesic to act. Fainting is sometimes seen, while the depression of the tongue by the spatula may cause discomfort.

GLOSSOPHARYNGEAL NERVE-BLOCK*

Head fully rotated to opposite side with patient lying supine. At midpoint of a line joining the tip of the mastoid process to the angle of the jaw, a needle inserted vertical to the skin makes contact with the styloid process 2 cm. to 4 cm. deep. Needle partially withdrawn and reinserted 0·5 cm. deep to and posterior to styloid process. Injection

---

* Rovenstine, E. A., and Papper, E. M., *Amer. J. Surg.*, 1948, **75**, 713.

Glossopharyngeal Nerve-block, *continued*.

of 6 ml. of solution at this point will produce analgesia of posterior one-third of tongue.

Another technique for block of the glossopharyngeal nerve is to deposit solution near the jugular foramen. A 5-cm. needle is introduced through a weal just below the external auditory meatus, anterior to the mastoid process. It is advanced perpendicularly to the skin until it meets the styloid process 1·5 to 2 cm. deep and passes it posteriorly for a further 2 cm. Analgesia involves the ninth to twelfth nerves inclusive and has been maintained with a long-acting drug in cases of malignant disease in the posterior third of the tongue, and in severe cases of neuralgia. Also used in differential diagnosis between glossopharyngeal and atypical trigeminal neuralgias.

SUPRASCAPULAR NERVE-BLOCK*

This arises from the fifth and sixth cervical nerves, the upper trunk of the brachial plexus. It runs laterally beneath the trapezius and omohyoid, and enters the supraspinatus fossa through the suprascapular notch and below the superior transverse scapular ligament. It proceeds laterally deep to the supraspinatus, curves round the lateral border of the scapula to the infraspinatus fossa. It supplies twigs to the shoulder-joint, the acromioclavicular joint, and the supraspinatus and infraspinatus muscles. The nerve is the sole pathway of somatic pain from the shoulder and acromioclavicular joints and structures surrounding them. The block does not result in any skin analgesia.

Technique.—Patient should be sitting with arms to the sides and head and shoulders slightly flexed. With a skin pencil the spine of the scapula is lined in: the inferior scapular angle is located and bisected by a line which crosses the first line. A weal is raised one finger-breadth from the crossing, in the upper outer angle, and a needle inserted downwards and medially to make contact with the bone of the supraspinatus fossa, just lateral to the notch. Needle then withdrawn and reintroduced more medially until its point lies in the notch. Paræsthesiæ take the form of pain at the tip of the shoulder, and after aspiration, 10 ml. of analgesic solution are injected. The block must be at the suprascapular notch as there the nerve is accessible to a needle and no afferent branches leave it before it passes through the notch. Types of shoulder pain relieved by this block include subacromial bursitis, painful abduction of the arm; calcified deposits about the capsule of the shoulder-joint. Used for pain relief, not surgery.

CERVICAL PLEXUS BLOCK†

This is paravertebral cervical analgesia.

Anatomy.—Formed by the anterior primary divisions of the upper four cervical nerves, each one of which, after leaving the inter-vertebral foramen, passes behind the vertebral artery and comes

---

* Wertheim, H. M., and Rovenstine, E. A., *Anesthesiology*, 1941, **2**, 541.
† Rovenstine, E. A., and Wertheim, H., *N.Y. J. Med.*, 1939, **39**, 1311.

to lie in the sulcus between the anterior and posterior tubercles of the transverse process of the appropriate cervical vertebra. Each nerve lies between the scalenus medius deeply and the levator anguli scapulæ, under cover of the sternomastoid. Each of these four nerves, except the first, divides into upper and lower branches, which form three loops lateral to the transverse processes. The loops are between C.1 and C.2; C.2 and C.3; C.3 and C.4. The lower branch of C.4 joins C.5 in the formation of the brachial plexus. The upper loop is directed forwards, the lower two, backwards.

Branches are superficial (cutaneous); deep (muscular); and communicating.

SUPERFICIAL BRANCHES emerge posterior to the lateral border of the sternomastoid, near its midpoint. They are :—

1. ASCENDING BRANCHES.—Lesser occipital (C.2) and great auricular (C.2 and 3). They supply skin of the occipitomastoid region, auricle, and parotid.

2. TRANSVERSE BRANCH.—The anterior cutaneous nerve of the neck (C.2 and 3) supplying skin of anterior part of neck between the lower jaw and the sternum.

3. DESCENDING BRANCHES.—The lateral, intermediate, and medial supraclavicular nerves (C.3 and 4) supplying skin of shoulder and upper pectoral region. C.1 has no cutaneous branch.

DEEP BRANCHES of the plexus are :—

1. Phrenic nerve—C.3, 4, and 5.

2. Anterior (deep) muscular branches.

3. Posterior muscular branches to sternomastoid, levator scapulæ, trapezius, and scalenus medius.

COMMUNICATING BRANCHES are :—

1. Sympathetic—each cervical nerve receives a grey ramus from the cervical sympathetic chain—the upper four nerves from the superior cervical ganglion.

2. To vagus.

3. Branch to hypoglossal nerve from C.1 and C.2, the descendens hypoglossi which joins the descendens cervicalis (C.2–C.3) to form the ansa hypoglossi.

The posterior primary divisions of the cervical nerves supply skin and muscles of the back of the neck. Their cutaneous distribution spreads like a cape over the upper thorax and shoulders, and this area is made insensitive in cervical plexus block.

Nerve-supply of thyroid is from middle and inferior cervical sympathetic ganglion; of the œsophagus, the vagus and sympathetic; of the trachea, recurrent laryngeal and sympathetic; of the sternomastoid, the eleventh cranial, and second and third cervical nerves.

Technique.—The patient lies supine with shoulders slightly elevated and neck and head extended—as for thyroidectomy, but with his head turned away from the side to be injected. Solution used is 0·5–1 per cent lignocaine, or one of its congeners, with adrenaline.

Deep cervical block requires the deposition of analgesic solution in the region of the transverse processes of the second, third, and fourth cervical vertebræ (the sixth, seventh, and eighth nerves having no sensory branches in the neck, and the first is purely motor).

Cervical Plexus Block—Technique, *continued.*

The following weals are raised :—
1. Just below the tip of the mastoid process.
2. One finger-breadth below weal 1.
3. One finger-breadth below weal 2. Each weal is near the posterior border of the sternomastoid and corresponds with the transverse process of C.2, C.3, and C.4 respectively. The fairly easily palpable tubercle of Chassaignac—the anterior tubercle of transverse process of the sixth cervical vertebra—is a useful landmark.

Through each weal a needle is inserted in a transverse direction posterior to the sternomastoid and seeks contact with a transverse process near its tip. This is not very deeply placed (about $\frac{1}{2}$ to $1\frac{1}{4}$ in.). The needle must not be inserted deeply between, or in front of, the transverse processes for fear of piercing the dura or the carotid, internal jugular, or vertebral vessels. After a negative aspiration test for blood and cerebrospinal fluid, and while the needle is in contact with the bone, solution is injected as follows : 10 ml. through the upper and lower needles, and 5 ml. through the middle one. The chief danger is intravascular injection.

Superficial cervical block is carried out by injecting 20 ml. of analgesic solution between skin and muscle along the posterior border of the sternomastoid near its midpoint, usually just below the position where it is crossed by the external jugular vein, so as to cut off impulses from the ascending, transverse, and descending superficial branches of the plexus.

Cervical plexus block gives analgesia of the front and back of the neck, the occipital region, and a cape-like area over the shoulders to below the clavicle, the skin above the third rib anteriorly, and above the upper border of the scapula posteriorly. Its chief indication is in thyroidectomy.

Cervical plexus block has also been found useful in operations for the cure of œsophageal diverticula. Should debris be dislodged from the pouch, as the cough reflex is retained it is unlikely to soil the trachea and bronchi. Bilateral phrenic block, if it occurs, is of no clinical significance in the healthy subject.

Complications may include: (1) Phrenic block; (2) Intrathecal injection; (3) Vagus and/or recurrent laryngeal nerve-block causing aphonia; (4) Cervical sympathetic block, and Horner's syndrome.

BRACHIAL PLEXUS BLOCK[*]

History.—Halsted of New York and Crile,[†] of Cleveland, injected the plexus under direct vision in 1884 and 1897 respectively.

Hirschel injected it ' blind ', through the axilla, in 1911.[‡]

Kulenkampff, after experimenting on himself, devised the supraclavicular technique in 1912.[§]

---

[*] Fox, M., and Bunting, D. H., *Brit. J. Surg.*, 1960, **48**, 58.
[†] Crile, G. W., *Cleveland med. J.*, 1897, **2**, 355.
[‡] Hirschel, G., *Münch. med. Wschr.*, 1911, **58**, 1555 (reprinted in *Survey of Anesthesiology*, 1963 ,**7**, 281).
[§] Kulenkampff, D., *Dtsch. med. Wschr.*, 1912, **38**, 1878.

Patrick* published his modification of the Kulenkampff technique in 1940. Macintosh and Mushin† describe this method in their excellently illustrated book. The method involves blocking the plexus as it lies on the first rib, lateral to the subclavian artery.

Anatomy.—The brachial plexus is formed from the anterior primary divisions of C.5, C.6, C.7, C.8, and T.1. It forms the entire motor and almost the entire sensory nerve-supply to the arm.

It receives communicating twigs from C.4 and T.2. These nerves unite to form three trunks, which lie in the neck above the clavicle. Each trunk divides, behind the clavicle, into anterior and posterior divisions, which unite in the axilla to form cords.

The plexus is broad above and converges to the first rib.

Its anterior relations are the skin, superficial fascia, platysma, and supraclavicular branches of the cervical plexus, the deep fascia and external jugular vein; the clavicle is in front of its lower part, the scalenus anterior is in front of its upper part.

Its posterior relations are the scalenus medius and the long thoracic nerve.

Its inferior relations are the first rib, where the plexus lies between the subclavian artery anteriorly and the scalenus medius behind.

The plexus emerges from the intervertebral foramina and passes between the scalenus anterior and the scalenus medius. Close to their emergence the fifth and sixth nerves each receives a grey ramus from the middle cervical sympathetic ganglion. The seventh and eighth nerves each receives a grey ramus from the inferior cervical ganglion. The first thoracic nerve receives a grey ramus from and sends a white ramus to the first thoracic sympathetic ganglion. As the plexus converges on the first rib it is enclosed in a fibrous sheath contributed by the scalenus anterior and medius muscles.

It lies first above, and then to the outer side of, the subclavian vessels and just above the clavicle lies between the skin and the first rib, immediately behind the deep fascia.

The upper trunk is formed by the anterior rami of C.5 and C.6.

The middle trunk is formed by the anterior ramus of C.7.

The lower trunk is formed by the anterior rami of C.8 and T.1. Behind the clavicle the trunks each divide into anterior and posterior divisions, i.e., in relationship to the axillary artery.

The posterior cord is formed by the three posterior divisions.

The medial cord is formed by the lowest anterior division.

The lateral cord is formed by the upper two anterior divisions.

Branches are given off from : (1) Roots, (2) Trunks, (3) Cords.

    1. Branches from Roots.—

        The nerve to the serratus anterior (of Bell) from C.5, 6, and 7.

        Dorsalis scapulæ nerve from C.5–8.

---

* Patrick, J., *Brit. J. Surg.*, 1940, **27,** 734.

† Macintosh, R. R., and Mushin, W. W., *Local Anæsthesia: Brachial Plexus*, 4th ed., 1967. Oxford: Blackwell.

Brachial Plexus Block—Anatomy, *continued*.

    Muscular branches to the longus cervicis (C.5–8) and the three scaleni (C.5–8), the rhomboids (C.5), and a twig to the phrenic (C.5).

2. Branches from Trunks.—
    Suprascapular nerve (C.5, 6).
    Nerve to subclavius (C.5, 6).

3. Branches from Cords.—
    From lateral cord (three) : Lateral pectoral (C.5–7) ; lateral head of the median (C.5–6) ; musculocutaneous (C.5, 6, 7)
    From the posterior cord (four) : Radial (C.5, 6, 7, 8, and T.1) , circumflex (C.5, 6) ; nerve to the latissimus dorsi (C.6, 7, 8) ; upper and lower subscapular nerves (C.5 and 6).
    From the medial cord (five) : Medial head of the median ; medial pectoral ; ulnar ; medial cutaneous of the forearm (all from C.8, T.1) ; medial cutaneous of the arm (T.1).

THE SCALENUS ANTERIOR arises from the anterior tubercles of the transverse processes of the third, fourth, fifth, and sixth cervical vertebræ. It is inserted into the scalene tubercle on the inner border of the first rib. The muscle lies anterior to the plexus, being separated from it below by the subclavian artery. Its lateral border, if it is palpable, is a guide to the position of the plexus.

THE SCALENUS MEDIUS arises from the posterior tubercles of the six lowest cervical vertebræ and is inserted into the upper surface of the first rib behind the groove made by the plexus and the subclavian artery. The plexus thus lies in front of the muscle.

THE FIRST RIB lies in an almost horizontal plane, being inclined slightly downwards and forwards. It passes below the clavicle at about the junction of its inner and middle thirds. Its surfaces look upwards and downwards and its borders inwards and outwards.

    The head has a single articular facet which articulates with the body of the first thoracic vertebra. The tubercle articulates with the transverse process of the same vertebra.

    The upper surface has two transverse grooves, an anterior for the subclavian vein, and a posterior for the subclavian artery and the lowest trunk of the brachial plexus. On the inner border, between the grooves, is the scalene tubercle. The subclavius muscle originates in front of the anterior groove and the scalenus medius is inserted behind the posterior groove. The lower surface has no costal groove ; the inner border embraces the dome of the pleura ; while the outer border gives origin to the first slip of the serratus anterior.

THE SUBCLAVIAN ARTERY extends from its origin to the outer border of the first rib. The right subclavian comes from the innominate artery, the left from the aortic arch. At its highest point, each artery is about 2 cm. above the clavicle. Three parts of the artery are described, one medial, one behind, and one lateral, to the scalenus anterior.

    The relations of the third part, i.e., the part lateral to the scalenus anterior, are : Anteriorly, the skin, superficial fascia, platysma, deep fascia, descending branches of the cervical plexus, a plexus formed by the external and anterior jugular veins, and the transverse cervical and transverse scapular veins, the transverse cervical and transverse scapular arteries. Above and laterally is the plexus, while below is the first rib.

THE SUBCLAVIAN VEIN is separated from the plexus by the scalenus anterior. As it is well protected by the clavicle, it is unlikely to be punctured.

Technique (Patrick's Method).*—Patrick's aim was to infiltrate a sector of tissue lying between the midclavicular point on the skin and the first rib. He advocated starting the injections lateral to the plexus and slowly working medially, until the subclavian artery pulsations transmitted along the needle indicated that the lower trunk of the plexus had been reached. Macintosh and Mushin modified this by starting the injections into the lower trunk close to the subclavian artery and working laterally. This modification is described below. The patient should be sitting or lying supine. The head is rotated to the other side and the arm and shoulder depressed. A weal is raised 1 cm. above the midpoint of the clavicle, a position :—

a. Midway between the sternoclavicular and acromioclavicular joints.

b. Crossed by a line produced downwards from the external jugular vein, made prominent by blowing out the cheeks.

c. Just lateral to the pulsating subclavian artery, often palpable.

d. Lateral to the outer border of the scalenus anterior, sometimes palpable under cover of the sternomastoid.

A needle is inserted through the weal downwards, inwards, and backwards, so that it is pointing to the spine of the second to fourth thoracic vertebra, a finger meanwhile guarding the subclavian artery and drawing it slightly medially. A cough from the patient is a warning that the pleura is being irritated by the needle. If paræsthesia is felt, the needle is steadied and 30 ml. of solution are injected. The following nerves are blocked : the median, the musculocutaneous, the radial, the axillary, the ulnar, the medial cutaneous nerve of the arm, and the medial cutaneous nerve of the forearm.

If paræsthesiæ are not felt in the arm and hand after one or two needle thrusts, the upper surface of the first rib is contacted and the needle inserted on to it so that the pulsations of the subclavian artery are transmitted to the needle. This is at a depth of 1·2–2·5 cm. After a negative aspiration test, 10 ml. of solution are injected between the first rib and the skin. The needle is reintroduced on to the first rib, 1 cm. laterally to the first position, and 10 ml. similarly deposited. Third and fourth injections are made, each 1 cm. lateral to the last, and at each point 10 ml. are deposited between skin and rib.

Analgesia is rapid in onset if paræsthesiæ are present ; if not an interval of 20 minutes may be necessary. A feeling of warmth

---

* Patrick, J., *Brit. J. Surg.*, 1940, **27**, 734.

Brachial Plexus Block—Technique, *continued.*

and ' pins and needles ' precedes analgesia, while motor paralysis, when it occurs, follows analgesia.

An area of skin over the point of the shoulder, and another on the inner aspect of the upper arm from the axilla to its midpoint (intercostohumeral T.2), are not made insensitive. A sub-cutaneous band of injection downwards from the acromio-clavicular joint and surrounding the shoulder will render these areas analgesic.

Procaine or lignocaine 2 per cent solution will produce sensory and motor paralysis. Solution of 1 per cent will give sensory loss alone for about 1 hour. Adrenaline should be added to all solutions, so that their final strength is about 1–300,000. For prolonged operation amethocaine or cinchocaine, 1–1000, is preferred. Lignocaine 1 to 2 per cent is excellent. Nerve suturing or trimming requires the use of the stronger solutions. Toxic and ill or feeble patients should have the strength of solution and not the volume reduced.

Horner's syndrome* may or may not follow injection. It is due to paralysis of the cervical sympathetic chain and is characterized by : (1) Small pupil (paralysis of dilator pupillæ) ; (2) Ptosis (paralysis of sympathetic supply to levator palpebræ) ; (3) Enophthalmos.

It was described by Horner, a Swiss ophthalmologist (1831–86), in 1869, having been previously noted by Claude Bernard in 1862 and by François Pourfois du Petit in 1727. The constriction gives place to dilatation in the darkness, while the narrowing of the palpebral fissure is partly due to raising of the lower lid. Enophthalmos is not well marked in man. In this condition the eye becomes temporarily myopic.

There are three other signs of sympathetic paralysis :—

1. Vasodilatation of nasal mucosa, with engorgement and nasal obstruction (Guttmann's sign).

2. Absence of sweating.

3. Flushing of skin and conjunctiva.

COMPLICATIONS.—

1. Paralysis of phrenic nerve often occurs. At the level of the first rib, the phrenic nerve is separated from the brachial plexus by the scalenus anterior muscle. Higher in the neck it is in the same fascial compartment as the upper components of the plexus. Analgesic solution injected into the tissue surrounding the plexus can thus ascend to block the phrenic nerve. Such a block is harmless and causes no symptoms, even if bilateral, but if the patient has a respiratory difficulty, e.g., emphysema or kyphosis, or if a general anæsthetic is to be administered, the possibility of diaphragmatic paralysis must be borne in mind.

2. Puncture of vessels, including subclavian artery. Hæmatomata may form but cause no trouble. Intravascular injection must be avoided.

---

* Horner, J. F., *Klin. Mbl. Augen.*, 1869, **7**, 193.

3. Pneumothorax. Trouble seldom occurs. The axillary approach avoids this complication. It causes pain in the chest which may not come on for several hours. Surgical emphysema may be seen, probably due to wounding of the lung by the needle. If a radiograph shows a large area of lung collapse, air should be withdrawn from the chest. Bilateral pneumothorax may be a dangerous condition.

Pain in the chest during needling may also be due to irritation of the nerve to the serratus anterior. Silent pneumothorax is unlikely as air in the chest is usually accompanied by pain.

4. Toxic effect of drug injected. Slow injection lessens chance of this.

5. Post-operative disability following brachial plexus block is rare.*

A MODIFIED SUPRACLAVICULAR APPROACH (Ball).†—In an effort to reduce the ever-present risk of pneumothorax when the block is performed by the supraclavicular route, a simple modification has been described. The anæsthetist stands at the head of the table rather than at the patient's side. The needle is inserted at a point immediately above the clavicle and just lateral to the subclavian artery and is advanced downwards and inwards to meet the first rib. Note the absence of the ' backward ' direction. If rib contact is not achieved, the needle is withdrawn and introduced slightly more posteriorly, but still vertically downwards, so that the rib is met before it is possible to advance behind and beyond it, and on into the pleura.

Axillary Approach to Brachial Plexus.—In the axilla the nerves from the brachial plexus, together with the main artery, are enclosed in a fibrous neuromuscular bundle. The median and musculocutaneous nerves together with their sensory branches are anterior or antero-lateral, i.e., above and beyond the artery ; the ulnar nerve is inferior ; the radial nerve is postero-lateral or below and behind the vessel.

Block follows if analgesic solution is injected periarterially.

TECHNIQUE.—The patient lies supine with the arm abducted to a right-angle, the humerus externally rotated, and the elbow flexed. The skin of the axilla is shaved and cleaned and a weal is raised at the highest part of the axilla at which arterial pulsation is felt, proximal to the lower border of the pectoralis major. The pulsating vessel is identified and through the weal a 2·5–4·8 cm. needle is inserted until a click shows that the neurovascular bundle has been entered. Local analgesic solution, e.g., 5–20 ml. of 1·5–2 per cent lignocaine with adrenaline, is placed in each quadrant surrounding the vessel. To prevent dissipation of the solution downwards in the neurovascular space, a rubber tourniquet may be placed around the upper arm, close to the point of injection.‡ Occasionally the musculocutaneous nerve (C.6), which is a continuation of the lateral cord of the plexus,

* Wooley, E. J., and Vandam, L. D., *Surgery*, 1959, **149**, 53.
† Ball, Harold C. J., *Anæsthesia*, 1962, **17**, 269.
‡ Eriksson, E., and Skarby, H. G., *Nord. Med.*, 1962, **68**, 1325.

Axillary Approach to Brachial Plexus, *continued.*

is given off higher than usual and consequently escapes the effects of local analgesic solution deposited in the neurovascular space. In such cases it can be dealt with by the injection of 5 ml. of solution from a point 1 in. (2·5 cm.) distal to the crease of the elbow-joint in the cleft lateral to the tendon of the biceps where it becomes the lateral antebrachial cutaneous nerve.* Onset of analgesia takes up to 30 minutes.

EXTENT OF BLOCK BY AXILLARY APPROACH.—Complete analgesia below the elbow-joint. Good sympathetic block of arm. Shoulder-joint, supplied by the suprascapular nerve (C.5 and C.6), not made insensitive, so reductions of dislocation of this joint cannot be performed under axillary block as they can under the supraclavicular block. A subcutaneous ring injection at the level of the initial weal may be required for the painless application of a tourniquet.

ADVANTAGES.—Only one landmark, the axillary artery. No paræsthesiæ so less chance of nerve damage. No possibility of pneumothorax. No phrenic nerve-block. Less pain during injection. (*See also* Burnham, P. J., *Anesthesiology*, 1958, **19**, 281 ; Eather, K. F., *Ibid.*, 1958, **19**, 683 ; Bosomworth, P. P., and others, *Ann. Surg.*, 1961, **154**, 911; de Jong, H. R., *Anesthesiology*, 1961, **22**, 215; and Moir, D. D., *Anæsthesia*, 1962, **17**, 274.)

The Subclavian Perivascular Technique.—*See* Winnce, A. P., and Collins, J. J., *Anesthesiology*, 1964, **25**, 353.

Brachial plexus block is a most satisfactory method of analgesia though less popular since the reintroduction of intravenous regional analgesia. For dislocations of the shoulder- or elbow-joint, for tendon suture, for manipulation of fractures under the X-ray screen, for suturing of lacerations, etc., the method is excellent. A tourniquet may be applied to the upper arm even in the absence of analgesia of the inner aspect of the upper arm. It is more successful in cases with a previously painless limb than in those with an existing painful lesion, e.g., a fracture or abscess.

FIELD BLOCK FOR OPERATION ON THE FINGERS

With a fine needle an intradermal weal is raised on the dorsum of the finger near its base. From 3 ml. to 5 ml. of 1 per cent lignocaine solution are injected into the substance of the finger through this weal between the bone and the skin. Analgesia may take fifteen minutes to become established. The palmar skin is not pierced. Adrenaline should not be used. Another method of blocking the finger is to deposit 5–7 ml. of 1 per cent lignocaine solution in the interosseous spaces at each side of it, entering from the dorsal aspect and carrying the needle almost to the palmar skin. Spread of infection due to this technique is very rare, providing that solution is not injected into infected tissue.

---

* Eriksson, E., *Acta anæsth. scand.*, 1965, Suppl. 16, 291.

If a tourniquet is used, no more than 3 ml. of solution should be injected ; a tourniquet must not remain on the finger for more than fifteen minutes and not used at all in patients with Raynaud's disease.*

Hot fomentations should not be employed on anæsthetized digits. If gangrene occurs as a result of the injections treatment with heparin is beneficial.*

A similar technique—using less solution—can be employed on the toe.

WRIST BLOCK

Circular lines of intradermal and subcutaneous infiltration are carried out just above the wrist-joint.

MEDIAN NERVE (C.5–T.1).—The median nerve at the wrist lies deeply between the flexor carpi radialis laterally and the palmaris longus and flexor digitorum sublimis medially. It is injected with 5 ml. of 1 per cent lignocaine immediately lateral to the tendon of the palmaris longus. Attempts to elicit paræsthesiæ are made, but if unsuccessful the solution is injected nevertheless. The median nerve supplies the skin of the thenar eminence and of the anterior aspects of the lateral three and a half fingers together with the skin over the dorsal aspects of their terminal phalanges.

ULNAR NERVE (C.7–T.1) divides 2 in. (5 cm.) above the wrist-joint into superficial terminal and dorsal branches.

The superficial terminal branch lies between the flexor carpi ulnaris tendon and the ulnar artery. The pisiform bone is immediately medial to it. It is blocked from a weal immediately lateral to the flexor carpi ulnaris.

The dorsal branch is anæsthetized by intradermal and subcutaneous injection along a line at the level of the ulnar styloid from the medial side of the tendon of the flexor carpi ulnaris to the middle of the back of the wrist. It supplies the ulnar border of the dorsum of the hand.

RADIAL OR MUSCULOSPIRAL NERVE (C.5–T.1) is the sensory nerve of the back of the lateral part of the hand. It can be blocked by infiltrating between the skin and the bone on the postero-lateral aspect of the wrist-joint near the base of the thumb lateral to the radial artery.

Wrist block, with a finger tourniquet, is useful for surgery of the hand. For analgesia of the palm, web, and dorsum of hand, good results can be obtained by :—

1. A median nerve-block.
2. An ulnar nerve-block.
3. A subcutaneous zone of analgesia (5 ml.) across dorsum of wrist, to block branches of the radial nerve.

ELBOW BLOCK

Intradermal and subcutaneous circles of infiltration are made just proximal to the internal epicondyle.

MEDIAN BLOCK is obtained by injecting through a weal placed midway between the outer side of the tendon of the biceps and

* Bradfield, W. J. D., *Brit. J. Surg.*, 1963, **50**, 495.

Elbow Block, *continued.*

the medial epicondyle or from a weal 1 cm. medial to the brachial artery at the bend of the elbow.   The needle should be inserted in an upward direction.   If paræsthesiæ are felt, so much the better :   5 ml. of 1 per cent lignocaine are used.

RADIAL BLOCK is performed through a weal 1 cm. lateral to the tendon of the biceps, at the line of the bend of the elbow.   Alternatively a weal is raised four finger-breadths proximal to the lateral epicondyle of the humerus which overlies the point at which the nerve pierces the intermuscular septum and is close to the bone.   The needle is advanced perpendicularly to the skin towards the bone and 20 ml. of analgesic solution are deposited above and below the point of injection.

ULNAR BLOCK is performed where the nerve can be palpated behind the medial epicondyle, using 2–4 ml. of 2 per cent lignocaine.

REGIONAL ANALGESIA FOR THORACOPLASTY
(MAGILL-SEMB)

Thoracoplasty was first performed by Sauerbruch in 1911 (Sauerbruch, E. F., and Schumacher, E. D., *Technik der Thoraxchirurgie*, Springer : Berlin, 1911) and in Britain by Morriston Davies in 1912.

Premedication for operations done under regional analgesia should be fairly heavy, e.g., phenobarbitone, 200 mg. one and a half hours before operation—by mouth; omnopon, 20 mg. one hour before with an additional dose a half-hour before if necessary.   If cough is active, infection may be spread.

The technique requires two solutions, one containing procaine, 0·5 per cent, and amethocaine hydrochloride, 1–1000, in normal saline, the other containing procaine, 0·25 per cent, and amethocaine hydrochloride, 1–2000, in normal saline.   Adrenaline is added.   Many workers are now using instead 0·4–0·5 per cent and 0·2–0·25 per cent lignocaine solutions, to which adrenaline is added (1–200,000) with very good results.

The following injections are made :—

1. Supraclavicular brachial plexus block, using the stronger solution.
2. Posterior intercostal nerve-block of the upper five or six nerves, at points 1¾ in. (4·4 cm.) from the midline, using the stronger solution, 5–10 ml. for each nerve.   Paravertebral block from T.1 to T.8 (for a first-stage operation) is sometimes preferred to posterior intercostal block.
3. Infiltration of the line of incision, intradermally and subcutaneously, using the weaker solution.
4. Injection of 20–30 ml. of weaker solution under the scapula.
5. Injection into areas to receive towel clips.
6. A weal is raised 1 in. from the sternum in the first five intercostal spaces.   This blocks any fibres which may come from the other side, overlapping the middle line of the body.

Steps 1 and 6 are sometimes omitted, while the posterior intercostal block can be performed by the surgeon, under direct vision, if necessary.

The second-stage operation requires a less extensive block.

About 70 ml. of stronger and 150–200 ml. of weaker solution may be used.

Scurr has modified this technique as follows.* He uses lignocaine, 0·4 per cent for nerve-block and 0·2 per cent for infiltration. With this drug he finds that analgesia lasts for four hours, is rapid in onset, and associated with low toxicity. The solution has excellent penetrating and spreading powers, gives intense analgesia together with block of tactile sensations. He blocks the brachial plexus by the lateral or paravertebral approach, depositing solution in the region of the transverse processes of C.5, C.6, and C.7, thereby paralysing the nerve to the serratus anterior which allows easy retraction of the scapula. Diffusion of solution results in vagus block and so the reflexes usually associated with periosteal stripping are prevented.

Some advantages of regional analgesia over general anæsthesia for thoracoplasty: (1) Less hæmorrhage, because of adrenaline infiltration with the local analgesic drug; (2) Safe for diathermy; (3) Minimal respiratory movements; (4) Co-operation of patient, especially regarding cough, cough reflex retained; (5) Less upsetting to patients.

Disadvantages include: (1) Some paradoxical respiration occurs. (2) Excessive coughing may hinder surgeon. (3) Tracheal suction cannot be performed. (4) Possible toxic effects of local analgesic drug. (5) Complete analgesia is seldom obtained.

Both the operation of thoracoplasty and the regional method of analgesia for its performance are much less popular than in former days. Regional analgesia is not now widely performed for this operation (see Mansfield, R., and Jenkins, R., Practical Anæsthesia for Lung Surgery, 1967, p. 138. London: Baillière, Tindall, and Cassell).

PARAVERTEBRAL SOMATIC BLOCK

This method was introduced by Sellheim in 1906† and developed by Läwen in 1911, who called it 'paravertebral conduction anæsthesia'.‡ It involves injecting a local analgesic close to the vertebral column where the nerve-trunks emerge from the intervertebral foramina.

Macintosh and Bryce-Smith, in an excellent monograph,§ describe the paravertebral space as a wedge-shaped compartment, bounded above and below by the heads and necks of adjoining ribs; posteriorly by the superior costotransverse ligament; medially it communicates with the extradural space through the intervertebral foramen; laterally its apex leads into the intercostal space. The base is formed by the posterolateral aspect of the body of the vertebra and the intervertebral foramen and its contents.

---

* Scurr, C. F., Curr. Res. Anesth., 1952, 31, 225.
† Sellheim, H., Verh. dtsch. Ges. Gynäk., 1906, 176.
‡ Läwen, A., Münch. med. Wschr., 1911, 58, 1390.
§ Macintosh, R. R., and Bryce-Smith, R., Local Analgesia: Abdominal Surgery, 2nd ed., 1962. Edinburgh and London: E. & S. Livingstone.

Paravertebral Somatic Block, *continued.*

There is no direct communication between one paravertebral space and another, but an indirect communication exists medially through the intervertebral foramen with the extradural space. Spread from one paravertebral space to another, across the extradural space, is frequent and may involve nerves on the same or on the opposite side of the body.

When the first thoracic to second lumbar nerve-roots are blocked, their rami communicantes are blocked too.

Paravertebral cervical block is described under cervical plexus block.

Paravertebral Thoracic Block.—It is indicated for operations on the chest or abdominal wall ; for relief of post-operative, post-herpetic pain, and the pain of fractured ribs.

Anatomy.—Each thoracic nerve emerges from the intervertebral foramen and divides into anterior and posterior primary rami. The latter supplies the skin and muscles of the back in their upper portion, the former, after giving off a white and receiving a grey ramus communicans, comes to lie midway between the transverse processes. It is important to get a fixed landmark, the spine of the twelfth thoracic vertebra being a useful one. The last rib, which makes an angle of 45° with the spines of the vertebra, is traced out ; a perpendicular dropped from this rib to the middle line and measuring 5 cm. will strike the spine of the twelfth thoracic vertebra. Other fixed points are : (1) The vertebra prominens—C.7 ; (2) The spines of the scapulæ with patient sitting upright—T.3 ; (3) The angles of scapulæ with patient sitting upright—T.9 or 10. In the cervical and lumbar regions, the spinous process is on a level with the transverse process of the same vertebra. In the mid and lower thoracic regions, owing to the downward slope of the spinous processes, the tip of each spinous process corresponds to the transverse process of the vertebra below ; thus an injection at the level of the ninth thoracic spinous process will block the tenth nerve.

TECHNIQUE 1.—Weals are raised opposite the lower borders of the thoracic spines, two finger-breadths from the middle line. Through each weal a needle is thrust, perpendicular to the skin, until it strikes bone which is near the lateral extremity of the transverse process at a depth from the skin of 1–2 in. (2·5–5 cm.) The needle is partially withdrawn and directed upwards over the upper border of the transverse process, but not deep to it. At this point 5–10 ml. of solution are injected. Lignocaine, 1 to 1·5 per cent, procaine, 1 per cent, or amethocaine, 1–1000, or cinchocaine, 1–1500, is suitable. It is important to avoid puncturing the dura or a vessel : aspiration tests should be made.

TECHNIQUE 2.—Weals are raised three finger-breadths from the middle line. Through each a 10-cm. needle is inserted making an angle of 45° with the sagittal plane, until it glances off the lower border of the rib, or passes between the ribs. It is slowly advanced until at a depth of 6–7 cm. it strikes the body of a vertebra in the paravertebral space ; 10 ml. of solution are now deposited between the rib and the vertebra, taking care not to puncture the dura. The use of a sterile protractor to measure the angle has been recommended.* To avoid unnecessary needle punctures, only alternative nerves need to be injected, using 20 ml. of solution and relying on overflow, via the extradural space, to cause block of the uninjected nerves.†

Puncture of the pleura or lung, though undesirable, is not a serious error in technique, although it may lead to waste of solution and bad results. Analgesia stops 1 in. (2·5 cm.) from the midline owing to overlap from the other side. Thus, in unilateral blocks, a line of subcutaneous infiltration along the midline must be made.

Paravertebral Lumbar Block.—As the upper edge of the spinous process of a lumbar vertebra is level with the transverse process of that vertebra, weals are raised opposite this upper edge, two finger-breadths from the middle line. Through each weal a needle is introduced at right-angles to the skin surface until its point touches the long transverse process at a depth of 4–5 cm. A piece of rubber threaded on the needle as a marker is now set 3 cm. from the skin. The needle is partially withdrawn and directed slightly upwards and inwards, so that it glances off the upper border of the transverse process ; it is advanced a further 3 cm., i.e., to the marker ; and 2–10 ml. of solution are injected, after making an aspiration test. The needle is moved to and fro slightly during the injection. Care is necessary to avoid intrathecal injection.

The fifth nerve is injected through the same weal as the fourth, only the needle slides off the lower border of the transverse process of the fifth vertebra, instead of over its upper border. The needle inserted through the weal opposite the first lumbar spine blocks the twelfth thoracic nerve.

Successful paravertebral injection from T.1 to L.2 produces visceral (i.e., splanchnic) block as well as analgesia of the abdominal wall. This is because the white rami are bathed in solution. Injection can be given with the patient in the lateral, sitting, or prone positions—the last with a pillow under the abdomen.

Operations on the following regions can be performed by paravertebral block :—

Appendix, T.10–L.2.
Hernia, T.11–L.2.
Upper abdomen, T.5–12.
Lower abdomen, T.7–L.3.

The method is very useful for cases of strangulated hernia. The following organs receive their visceral nerve-supply as follows : Kidney, T.10 to L.1 ; Ureter, T.11 to L.1 ; Testis, T.10 ; Epididymis, T.11, 12 ; Bladder, T.11, 12, L.1, and S.3, 4 ; Prostate, T.10, 11, S.1 to 5 ; Ovary, T.10 ; Cervix uteri, T.11, 12, and S.1 to 4 ; Uterine body, T.10 to L.1.

Nerve-supply of adrenal glands is from the three splanchnic nerves and first and second lumbar ganglia, via cœliac, inferior

---

* Molesworth, H. W. L., *Regional Analgesia*, 1944, p. 6. London: Lewis.
† Macintosh, R. R., and Bryce-Smith, R., *Local Analgesia: Abdominal Surgery*, 2nd ed., 1962, p. 50. Edinburgh and London: E. & S. Livingstone.

Paravertebral Lumbar Block, *continued*.

phrenic, and renal plexuses ; twigs also received from vagus. Chief root value—T.10–L.2.

THORACIC SYMPATHETIC BLOCK

Block of the thoracic ganglia of the sympathetic chain by paravertebral injection of local analgesic drugs. First carried out by Sellheim (1905)* and Kappis†; alcohol first used to cause a prolonged block by Swetlow in 1926.

Anatomy.—The thoracic portion of the sympathetic chain usually consists of eleven ganglia, which, with the exception of the last two, lie against the heads of the ribs and are covered by the costal pleura ; the last two are placed on the sides of the bodies of the eleventh and twelfth thoracic vertebræ. Two rami communicantes, a white and a grey, connect each ganglion with its corresponding spinal nerve. (The cardiac afferents travel with the thoracic cardiac sympathetic fibres, enter the upper four thoracic sympathetic ganglia, and, without synapsing there, go with the corresponding white rami to the mixed spinal nerves and the posterior roots.) Stellate ganglion block will interrupt conduction along fibres from the upper four thoracic ganglia.

Site of Injection for Various Conditions.—Anatomists differ in their recommendations. Mandl, in his book *Paravertebral Block*‡ (1947), recommends the following : Angina pectoris, T.1–4 both sides ; Bronchial asthma, T.1–5 both sides ; Paroxysmal tachycardia, T.1–2 both sides ; Biliary colic, T.6–10 ; Renal colic, T.12–L.2 ; Uterine contractions (labour pains), T.11–12 ; Pancreatic pain (acute pancreatitis), T.8–10 on left side ; Upper limb, T.2 or ? T.2 and 3.

Technique.—The posterior approach is the only one possible. Patient should be either sitting with head flexed or in the lateral spinal position. Pneumothorax is a possible complication.

A weal is made two finger-breadths from the midline over the transverse process of the desired vertebra. In the upper thoracic region, owing to the obliquity of the spinous processes, the spine of a given vertebra is level with the transverse process of the vertebra below. Through the weal a 10-cm. needle is introduced at right-angles to the skin surface and contact is made with the transverse process, and then slipped inferior to it. The marker is set at 4 cm. to the skin surface, the needle inclined 20° to the median sagittal plane, and the needle is advanced until it makes contact with the body of the vertebra at a depth of about 3 cm. Into each ganglion, 5 ml. of 2 per cent procaine are injected, after it has been ascertained that the needle point is not intravascular, intrapleural, or intrathecal.

Pulmonary Plexus Block.—The pulmonary plexus is a network of autonomic fibres, akin to the cœliac plexus, lying anterior to the

* Sellheim, H., *Verh. dtsch. Ges. Gynäk.*, 1906, 176.
† Kappis, M., *Münch. med. Wschr.*, 1912, **59**, 794.
‡ Mandl, F., *Paravertebral Block*, 1928 (translated into English 1947). London: Heinemann (Medical Books) Ltd.

bodies of the upper thoracic vertebræ. Block is carried out similarly to thoracic sympathetic ganglionic block, but needle is advanced a further 1 cm. so that solution of analgesic drug comes to lie in the vicinity of the plexus. It is said to be beneficial in cases of very severe bronchospasm.

LUMBAR SYMPATHETIC BLOCK

Anatomy.—The sympathetic trunk in the lumbar region consists of four ganglia and their interconnecting fibres. It lies on the antero-lateral aspect of the bodies of the lumbar vertebræ, immediately medial to the psoas muscle, which fills the triangular space between the vertebral bodies and the transverse processes. A tendinous arch, which gives part origin to the psoas muscle, connects the upper and lower borders of each lumbar vertebra and forms a tunnel around the side of the bone in which the lumbar vessels and the grey ramus communicans run. The lumbar arteries are posterior but the veins may be anterior. The fatty tissue occupying this tunnel is an extension of that in the extradural space and it passes through the intravertebral foramina as far forward as the sympathetic chain.*

Disturbances of function of the sympathetic nervous system can produce : (1) Vasospasm ; (2) Pain ; (3) Visceral dysfunction. Sympathetic block can remedy all of these, either temporarily, for diagnosis, or permanently, by interrupting a vicious circle.

Indications.—
1. Peripheral arterial disease. This may be : (a) Vasospastic (Raynaud) ; (b) Vasospastic and organic (Buerger) ; (c) Degenerative organic (arteriosclerosis). Increased blood-supply to the limb is shown by (i) Increased surface temperature. (ii) Increased oscillations shown by an oscillometer. (iii) Increased function, e.g., later onset of claudication.
2. Traumatic vasospasm, so-called local shock.
3. Post-traumatic and post-infection œdema.
4. Acute arterial occlusion.
5. Thrombophlebitis, the symptoms of which are said to be partly due to arterial spasm in walls of veins.
6. Delayed healing of fractures.
7. Trophic ulcer, Sudeck's atrophy, traumatic osteoporosis, and Charcot's joint.
8. Causalgic states following trauma.
9. Blockade of efferent and afferent sympathetic fibres from pelvic organs.
10. Abolition of rhythmic labour pains due to uterine contractions.
11. As an aid to prognosticate the effects of surgical sympathectomy. Sympathetic block when correctly done gives more complete release of vasomotor tone than do the chemical ganglionic blocking agents.

---

* Bryce-Smith, R., *Anæsthesia*, 1951, **6**, 150.

Lumbar Sympathetic Block, *continued*.

Technique.—

POSTERIOR APPROACH.—This was described by Felix Mandl.[*]
The patient is placed in the prone position, with two pillows
flexing the lumbar spine; or in lateral spinal position with the
affected side uppermost and the spine flexed. He should be
premedicated with a barbiturate. The procedure can be carried
out in the patient's bed if necessary.

Skin weals are raised at points 5 cm. lateral to the upper borders
of the spinous processes of the 2nd, 3rd, and 4th lumbar
vertebræ. Successful injection at these points blocks all the
vasoconstrictor impulses to the lower limb. These points lie
immediately above the transverse processes of the corresponding vertebræ. A spinal needle is introduced through each weal
at right-angles to the skin for 4–5 cm. and should encounter
the transverse process; it is slightly withdrawn and directed
upwards so that it passes between the transverse processes;
it is also directed slightly inwards. After travelling 3–4 cm.
from the transverse process, the needle should make contact
with the anterolateral aspect of the body of the vertebra.
After careful aspiration to exclude both blood and cerebrospinal fluid, 20 ml. of 1 per cent lignocaine are injected at
each site. If force is required, needle tip is in anterior vertebral ligament or the psoas muscle and should be slightly withdrawn. It spreads out in the retroperitoneal tissue. The
spinal lumbar nerves run midway between the spinous processes, so if the needle point is kept in relation to the upper
border of the transverse process, pain from hitting a nerve
should be avoided. The lumbar arteries—branches of the
aorta—with their veins must also be avoided. After 5 to 20
minutes the leg becomes less painful, its temperature increases,
and it becomes dry, its superficial veins dilate, and there is
hyposensitivity to pin-prick.

See also good article by R. Bryce-Smith[†] in which he recommends
the insertion of a 12-cm. needle at an angle of 70° through a
weal three finger-breadths lateral to the superior point of the
spinous process of L.3. It should miss the transverse process
and come into contact with the body of the vertebra in the
psoas tunnel; 15–20 ml. of analgesic fluid are now injected.

LATERAL APPROACH.[‡]—The patient is placed in the lateral
position. A weal is raised at the apex of the lumbar triangle
(boundaries: lower border of last rib, superior border of iliac crest,
lateral border of paravertebral muscle group): this point is at
the level of L.2. A 6 in. (15 cm.) needle is inserted through the
weal and angulated 15° anteriorly and thrust in until bone is
struck: this should be the lateral aspect of the body of the
second lumbar vertebra. At this point 10 ml. of solution are
deposited. Withdrawal is made and the needle angulated a
further 15° anteriorly and again bone is struck and more solution

---

[*] Mandl, F., *Paravertebral Block*, 1928 (translated into English 1947). London: Heinemann
(Medical Books) Ltd.
[†] Bryce-Smith, R., *Anæsthesia*, 1951, **6**, 150.
[‡] Wallace, G., *Idid.*, 1955, **16**, 254.

injected. A third withdrawal and insertion at an additional 15° angle anteriorly is made and a third injection given. Thus the anterolateral aspect of the body of the second lumbar vertebra is well surrounded with solution.

Chemical sympathectomy should not be done in this way for fear of involving the third lumbar nerve as it leaves the intervertebral foramen.

Caudal block produces the same results but is not unilateral : it produces, in addition to sympathetic paralysis, motor paresis and analgesia which may be useful objective signs of successful sympathetic paralysis.

For chemical sympathectomy, Haxton* recommends the injection of 6 per cent phenol in water : he uses 2-3 ml. for each ganglion, after injecting 2 ml. of 4 per cent procaine which verifies the position of the needle. He employs 12-cm. needles and advances them from weals 7 cm. from the midline.

FIELD BLOCK FOR MASTECTOMY

Anatomy.—The overlying skin of the breast is supplied by the anterior and lateral branches of the 4th, 5th, and 6th intercostal nerves.

Technique.—For non-radical mastectomy, weals are raised a finger-breadth from the circumference of the breast—about eight in number. Through each weal an injection is made towards the nipple so that solution is deposited between the breast substance and the pectoral muscles. Injection should not be made into the breast substance. Finally, the circumferential weals are joined by intradermal and subcutaneous injections.

For radical mastectomy, a much more extensive procedure is required. The solution should contain one of the longer-acting drugs such as amethocaine or cinchocaine. The following procedures are necessary :—

1. Brachial plexus block.
2. Block of the first to tenth intercostal nerves, either adjacent to the vertebral column or at the posterior axillary fold for the lower ones.
3. Block of the descending branches of the cervical plexus, by infiltrating along acromion, clavicle, and sternum.
4. Infiltration of line of incision, intradermally and subcutaneously.

Induction of local analgesia for radical mastectomy is thus seen to be almost a major operation in itself. It is seldom indicated.

INTERCOSTAL NERVE-BLOCKS

The Cutaneous Nerves of the Trunk (*Figs.* 26–28).—

ANTERIORLY.—

  a. The lateral, intermediate, and medial supraclavicular branches of the superficial division of the cervical plexus (C.3–4).

  b. The anterior rami of the thoracic nerves, excluding T.1.

  c. The iliohypogastric and ilio-inguinal nerves (L.1).

POSTERIORLY.—The posterior rami of C.2, 3, 4, 5 ; T.1 to 12 ; L.1 to 3 ; the five sacral and the coccygeal nerves.

---

* Haxton, H. A., *Brit. med. J.*, 1949, **1**, 11.

Cutaneous Nerves of the Trunk, *continued.*

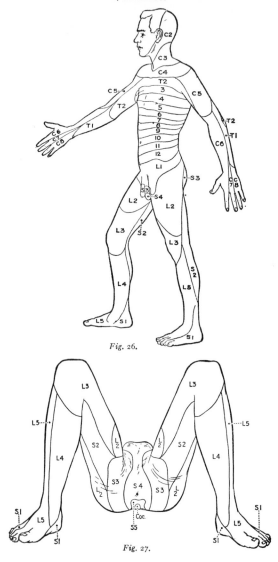

Fig. 26.

Fig. 27.

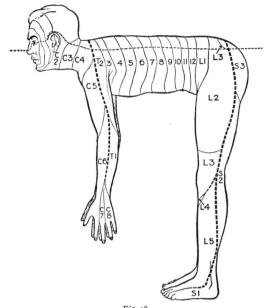

Fig. 28.

Figs. 26–28.—Distribution of cutaneous nerves. (*After* Foerster, I., *Brain*, 1933, **56**, 1.)

Anatomy of Spinal Nerves.—Typical intercostal nerves are the third
to sixth inclusive. Each nerve is formed by the union of the
anterior (motor) and the posterior (sensory) root : the latter has
a ganglion on it. The mixed spinal nerve soon divides into anterior
and posterior primary divisions (rami). The thoracic or dorsal
nerves then are distributed as follows :—

The posterior rami are smaller than the anterior. They turn backwards and divide into medial and lateral branches (except C.1,
S.4, and S.5, coccygeal) which supply the muscles and skin of
the back. Above the 6th thoracic spine the sensory nerves
come from the medial branches and emerge 1½ finger-breadths
from the middle line ; the lateral branches supplying the
muscles : below the 6th thoracic spine the lateral branches
supply the skin, emerging a hand-breadth from the middle line,
the medial branches here supplying the muscles. The first,
sixth, seventh, and eighth cervical, and the fourth and fifth
lumbar posterior primary divisions give no cutaneous branches.

The anterior rami in the thoracic region of the second to sixth nerves
are each connected to the lateral sympathetic chain by a grey
and a white ramus communicans. Each crosses the paravertebral space between the necks of contiguous ribs and then

Anatomy of Spinal Nerves, *continued.*

enters the subcostal groove where it lies below the vein and artery and between the internal and innermost intercostals (the second and third layers) as far as the anterior axillary line, at which point the nerves come into direct relationship with the pleura, as the innermost intercostal muscle terminates. It supplies muscular branches to the intercostal muscles and supplies lateral and anterior cutaneous branches to supply the skin of the chest and abdomen. The seventh to eleventh nerves pass below and behind the costal cartilages, between the slips of the diaphragm running between the internal oblique and transversus muscles (again between the second and third layers) to enter the posterior layer of the rectus sheath. They run deep to the rectus, pierce and supply it, and end as anterior cutaneous nerves.

The lateral cutaneous branch emerges in the mid-axillary line, and divides into anterior and posterior branches which supply the skin on the lateral wall of the chest as far forward as the nipple line.

The anterior cutaneous branch is the termination of the intercostal nerve ; it supplies the skin on the front of the chest, internal to the nipple line.

EXCEPTIONS.—The first nerve parts with most of its fibres to the brachial plexus and gives neither lateral nor anterior cutaneous branches, the skin over the first intercostal space being supplied by the descending branches of the cervical plexus (C.3–4). The lateral cutaneous branch of the second intercostal nerve crosses the axilla and becomes the intercostobrachial nerve supplying the skin on the medial aspect of the arm. The lateral cutaneous branch of the twelfth thoracic nerve, which does not divide into anterior and posterior branches, crosses the iliac crest to supply the skin of the upper part of the buttock as far as the greater trochanter. The twelve thoracic and first lumbar nerves supply sensory branches to the anterior chest and anterior abdominal wall, the parietal pleura, and the parietal peritoneum.

The tenth nerve—lateral and anterior cutaneous branches— supplies the area of the umbilicus.

The ninth, eighth, and seventh nerves supply the skin between the umbilicus and the xiphisternum.

The eleventh and twelfth and first lumbar nerves supply the skin between the umbilicus and the pubis.

Technique of Intercostal Nerve-block.*—

1. AT THE ANGLE OF THE RIBS (Sellheim, 1906 ;† James, 1943‡).—At this point the nerve becomes relatively superficial, lateral to the erector spinæ muscle. In this technique the rami communicantes conveying afferent impulses may be blocked by the local analgesic solution tracking medially but splanchnic analgesia may be necessary in addition. The patient is arranged

---

* Moore, D. C., and Bridenbaugh, L. D., *Curr. Res. Anesth.*, 1962, **41**, 1.

† Sellheim, H., *Verh. dtsch. Ges. Gynäk.*, 1906, p. 176.

‡ James, N. R., *Regional Analgesia for Intra-abdominal Surgery*, 1943. London: J. and A. Churchill.

in the lateral spinal position with his back well arched over the edge of the table. After swabbing with antiseptic and fixing sterile towels, two lines are drawn, one on each side four finger-breadths from the middle line, with an iodine swab ; the lines should extend from the spines of the scapulæ to the iliac crests. At a point where the lower border of the 12th rib on the patient's upper side crosses the iodine line, a needle is introduced (through an intradermal weal if necessary) until it makes contact with the rib. It is then partially withdrawn and advanced until it slips past the lower border of the rib for one-eighth of an inch : 2–3 ml. of 1·5 or 2 per cent lignocaine are then injected, while the needle point is slightly advanced and withdrawn so as to surround the nerve with analgesic solution. The intercostal nerve is thus surrounded by a zone of solution as it lies in the subcostal groove between the intercostalis internus and the internal intercostal muscles. The needle should be mounted on a syringe, so that should the pleura be punctured no air will enter the pleural cavity. The needle is then withdrawn until its point is just beneath the skin, so that it can act as a marker. The eleventh to the sixth nerves are now injected on the upper side, followed by the lower seven nerves on the patient's more dependent side. Before the sixth and seventh nerves can be injected the patient's scapulæ must be drawn laterally by crossing his arms over his chest. The needle pierces the trapezius, the latissimus dorsi, and the two intercostal muscles.

Posterior splanchnic block can be performed with the patient in the same position.

2. IN THE POSTERIOR AXILLARY LINE.—Similar injections can be carried out with the patient supine and with his arms abducted to a right-angle. In this position the ribs, and so the intercostal nerves, are not so deeply placed. A block in the mid-axillary line misses the lateral cutaneous nerve.

Blocking of the lower seven intercostal nerves on each side results in analgesia of the anterior abdominal wall from just below the nipple line to a level just above the pubic bone. In addition, it produces analgesia of the parietal peritoneum and relaxation of the muscles of the anterior abdominal wall. It is especially useful when scars from previous operations disturb the relations of the abdominal wall. For analgesia of the viscera, splanchnic analgesia is required in addition.

INTERCOSTAL BLOCK FOR RIB RESECTION IN DRAINAGE OF EMPYEMA

The surgeon is asked to mark out the position of the incision he wishes to make, and it is infiltrated intradermally and subcutaneously with 0·5–1 per cent lignocaine solution. An intradermal and sub-cutaneous line of infiltration is carried out one rib above and one below the length of rib to be removed. These lines extend 1 in. (2·5 cm.) in front and 1 in. (2·5 cm.) behind the proposed incision, and these extremities are joined by intradermal and subcutaneous infiltrations, so that a rectangle is marked out. The intercostal nerves within this rectangle are blocked at their posterior extremities with 2 per cent

Intercostal Block for Rib Resection, *continued.*

lignocaine solution. There may be slight discomfort during the stripping of the periosteum from the rib.

Local block is usually the preferred method of anæsthesia in these operations. If the patient is well enough, he should sit sideways across the table, to prevent him drowning in his own pus if the abscess ruptures into a bronchus. Otherwise he is placed in the lateral position with the head and shoulders elevated. This position is also suitable for general anæsthesia.

SPLANCHNIC ANALGESIA

Anatomy.—

SEMILUNAR OR CŒLIAC PLEXUS.—Two in number, one on each side of the midline, lying on the aorta and the crura of the diaphragm just above the pancreas, at the level of the first lumbar vertebra between the adrenal glands and behind the stomach and lesser sac. The renal vessels are inferior to the plexus while the vessels to the adrenals often pass through it. They are connected with each other and with their associated ganglia (superior mesenteric and inferior mesenteric, etc.) by a network of nerve-fibres around the cœliac axis artery. These fibres are post-ganglionic fibres of the greater and lesser splanchnic nerves. From this mass of retroperitoneal nerve tissue fibres pass with the arteries to the abdominal viscera. These plexuses also receive twigs from the right vagus and the phrenic nerves. The semilunar or cœliac ganglia with the aortico-renal and superior mesenteric ganglia together make up the solar or epigastric plexus.

GREATER SPLANCHNIC NERVE (the superior thoracic splanchnic nerve), like the lesser and the lowest splanchnic, is composed of pre-ganglionic fibres which are, in effect, elongated white rami. The majority of its fibres are myelinated. It rises from the union of four or five roots coming from the thoracic sympathetic ganglia which receive white rami from the fifth to the tenth thoracic nerves. The nerve enters the abdomen through the crus of the diaphragm on each side, with the lesser and lowest splanchnic nerves, and enters the corresponding semilunar ganglion. It also contains visceral afferent fibres. Within the abdomen the nerve lies between the diaphragm and the adrenal gland on each side.

LESSER SPLANCHNIC NERVE (the middle thoracic splanchnic nerve).—This arises from the lower thoracic ganglia of the sympathetic cord, connected with the tenth and eleventh thoracic nerves. It enters the corresponding semilunar ganglion.

LOWEST SPLANCHNIC NERVE (the inferior thoracic splanchnic nerve).—This arises from the last thoracic ganglion and enters the renal plexus and the posterior renal ganglion.

Afferent fibres from the abdominal viscera, both sympathetic and parasympathetic (vagus), pass through the cœliac ganglia. Afferent fibres from the pelvic viscera, travelling through the nervi erigentes (S.2, 3, 4), do not.

THE LUMBAR SPLANCHNIC NERVES.—Are presumably blocked when the cœliac plexus is blocked, by spreading of solution.

The first lumbar splanchnic nerve arises from the first lumbar ganglion ; the second from the second and third ganglia ; the third from the second, third, and fourth ganglia ; the fourth from the fourth and fifth ganglia. The last two join the superior hypogastric plexus.

THE HYPOGASTRIC NERVE (or pre-sacral nerves, or lumbar splanchnics).—Extends from the third lumbar vertebra to the first sacral where it ends by dividing into the right and left hypogastric nerves or plexuses. It lies in front of the lower part of the abdominal aorta, behind the peritoneum.

Afferent Pathways from Upper Abdominal Viscera.—These visceral afferents travel from sensory nerve-endings in the walls of the viscera, mesentery, etc., via the splanchnic nerves and enter cord with the white rami of the lower seven thoracic nerves, having their cell stations in the posterior root ganglia of these nerves. Afferent impulses also travel up in the vagi and the phrenics.

Nerve-supply to Adrenal Glands.—Pre-ganglionic fibres do not synapse in the cœliac or other pre-aortic plexuses, but pass directly to end around chromaffin cells of the medulla. In addition to the lesser splanchnic, fibres go to the adrenals from the tenth thoracic to the second lumbar nerves.

Nerve-supply to Testis, Kidney, and Ureter.—From each organ via perivascular nervous plexus to aortic and renal plexuses and into white rami and posterior nerve-roots from T.10 to L.1.

Technique of Splanchnic Block.—Splanchnic block can be performed before laparotomy (Wendling) or after laparotomy from the front (Braun) ; or before laparotomy from behind (Kappis). The Braun technique is usually the one performed by the surgeon.

1. BRAUN'S METHOD.*—With the abdomen opened, the liver is gently retracted upwards and the stomach is drawn to the left. The anterior aspect of the body of the first lumbar vertebra is located medial to the lesser curvature of the stomach; the aorta is retracted laterally and the long Braun needle is inserted down to the bone and 50 ml. of solution injected.

2. KAPPIS'S METHOD.†—Described in 1914. The patient is in the spinal position, sitting or lying prone. The fourth interspace is located, lying on or before the intercristal line : by counting upward, the spine of the first lumbar vertebra is identified. Weals are raised four finger-breadths from this spine, one on each side of the midline. The weals must be below the twelfth rib.

A long needle is inserted at an angle of 45° to the median plane through this weal with its bevel facing inwards. It is directed slightly upwards and thrust in until it makes contact with the body of the first lumbar vertebra. It is then partly withdrawn and its point directed more laterally until its bevel is felt to glance past the lateral aspect of the body of the vertebra. The needle is then advanced a further 1 cm. and, after a most careful aspiration test, 20–40 ml. of solution are

---

* Braun, H., *Beitr. Klin. Chir.*, 1919, **115**, 161; and Braun, H., *Die Lokal-Anæsthesie*, 1905, p. 311. Leipzig.
† Kappis M., *Zbl. Chir.*, 1930, **47**, 98.

Technique of Splanchnic Block, *continued.*

injected. The average distance between the skin and the plexus is 7–10 cm. If blood is aspirated into the syringe, the needle-point may be in the vena cava or the aorta and must be moved until it is free of these vessels. Bilateral block is probably unnecessary.

The usual strengths of solution employed are procaine or ligno-caine, 0·5 per cent ; amethocaine, 1–2000 to 1–4000 ; cincho-caine, 1–2000 to 1–4000. Adrenaline should be added.

Splanchnic block causes a profound fall in blood-pressure which can be partially controlled by ephedrine or methylamphetamine, should it be considered necessary. It produces analgesia of the abdominal viscera with the exception of the pelvic viscera, i.e., the sigmoid colon, rectum, bladder, and reproductive organs. The bowel becomes contracted and ribbon-like. The patient must be particularly well premedicated, intravenous morphine being given until his mental state is calm. The surgeon must be light handed, especially when the peritoneal cavity is being explored, as its lateral walls are not rendered insensitive either by the splanchnic block or the abdominal field block.

Therapeutically, splanchnic block is useful in the treatment of acute pancreatitis and also in fibrocystic disease of young infants, perhaps because it relaxes the sphincter of Oddi. It causes a greater blood-supply to be diverted to the pancreas. The block may be repeated if desirable. It has also been used in the terminal stages of upper abdominal cancer to relieve pain. Alcohol in saline, 50 per cent, preceded by local analgesic solution, has been employed.*

Regional analgesia for intra-abdominal surgery, requiring multiple punctures and near-toxic doses of local analgesic drugs, finds little favour to-day.

Abdominal Aortography.—This was pioneered by Dos Santos in 1929. The technique is as for Kappis's splanchnic block on the left side of the body. The patient is given a suitable sedative such as papaveretum and hyoscine and in the X-ray room is given a test dose of 1 ml. of 70 per cent diodone. If no toxic reaction is seen the patient lies prone and each lumbar spine is marked. If aortography is being performed to show the iliac vessels the injection is made opposite L.3 ; to display the renal vessels the injection is opposite L.1, while to display the cœliac axis and its branches the injection is made opposite T.12. Just before the injection is given the patient may receive 100 mg. of pethidine intravenously. The injection needle should be 16 s.w.g., 7 in. (18 cm.) in length. General or the so-called neurolept anæsthesia may be preferred but as this method of diagnosis has been known to lead to paraplegia, spinal and extradural analgesia should be avoided. With the long needle proved, by aspiration of arterial blood, to be within the aorta, 30 ml. of 70 per cent diodone are rapidly injected and radiographs quickly taken.

---

* Bridenbaugh, L. D., and Moore, D. C., *J. Amer. med. Ass.*, 1964, **190**, 877.

ABDOMINAL FIELD BLOCK

Anatomy.—The superficial fascia in the upper abdomen is a single fatty layer, but from a point midway between the umbilicus and the pubis two layers are described, the fascia of Scarpa (1809) and the superficial fascia of Camper.

Camper's fascia passes over the inguinal ligament and is continuous with the superficial fascia of the thigh. It is continued over the penis, spermatic cord, and scrotum where it helps to form the dartos muscle. In the female it is continued into the labia majora.

Scarpa's fascia is tougher. It blends with the deep fascia of the thigh and, like Camper's fascia, is continued over the penis and helps to form the dartos. From the scrotum it becomes continuous with Colles's fascia (1811) over the perineum. There is no deep fascia covering the abdomen.

EXTERNAL OBLIQUE.—The largest and most superficial of the muscles of the anterior abdominal wall. It *arises* from the external surfaces of the lower eight ribs and fans out to its attachments, which are the anterior half of the outer lip of the iliac crest and the aponeurosis which commences on a line drawn from the 9th cartilage to the anterior superior iliac spine. The aponeurosis is attached below to the anterior superior spine and to the pubic tubercle : it thus forms the inguinal ligament. In the midline it forms the linea alba which runs from the symphysis pubis to the xiphisternum. The subcutaneous or external inguinal ring is an opening in the aponeurosis.

The fibres of the external oblique pass downwards and inwards, like those of the external intercostal muscles.

INTERNAL OBLIQUE.—This is a thinner layer than the above. It *arises* from : (*a*) The lateral half of the inguinal ligament ; (*b*) The anterior two-thirds of the iliac crest ; (*c*) The thoraco-lumbar fascia.

Insertion is as follows : Fibres arising from (*a*) arch over the spermatic cord or round ligament and together with fibres from the transversus abdominis form the conjoint tendon or falx inguinalis which is attached to the pubic bone. The fibres from (*b*) and (*c*) are inserted into an aponeurosis which divides at the lateral border of the rectus into two layers which partially invest this muscle, and then fuse with the linea alba ; above, the posterior layer is attached to the lower borders of the lower six ribs and their costal cartilages.

The fibres of this muscle run upwards and inwards.

TRANSVERSUS ABDOMINIS.—*Arises* :—

a. From the lateral third of the inguinal ligament.

b. From the anterior three-quarters of the iliac crest.

c. From the thoracolumbar fascia.

d. From the inner surfaces of the lower six ribs and their cartilages interdigitating with the diaphragm.

It is *inserted* into a broad aponeurosis, the lower fibres forming part of the conjoint tendon and being inserted into the pubic bone. The remainder of the aponeurosis is inserted into the linea alba, the upper three-quarters passing behind the rectus,

Abdominal Field Block—Anatomy, *continued.*

the lower quarter passing in front of it. In the upper abdomen the aponeurosis is adherent to the peritoneum.

The fibres of the muscle run transversely. Between it and the external oblique run the lower intercostal, iliohypogastric and ilio-inguinal nerves. Below the level of the iliac crest the fibres of these three muscles are aponeurotic and run downwards and medially.

RECTUS ABDOMINIS.—Each muscle *arises* from the crest of the pubis and from the ligaments in front of the symphysis. *Inserted* into the anterior aspects of the 5th, 6th, and 7th costal cartilages and into the xiphisternum.

Three tendinous intersections cross the muscle and are firmly attached to the anterior layer of its sheath, but not to the posterior layer. One is at the level of the xiphisternum, one at the umbilicus, and the third one midway between. They represent prolongation of the 8th, 9th, and 10th ribs and are in relationship to the corresponding intercostal nerves.

The rectus sheath is not arranged in the same way throughout its length and is basically a splitting of the aponeurosis of the internal oblique and is reinforced anteriorly by the aponeurosis of the external oblique and posteriorly by the flat tendon of the transversus abdominis. It is described in three sections :—

1. From the costal margin to a point midway between the umbilicus and the pubis. Here, at the outer border of the muscle, the aponeurosis of the internal oblique divides into anterior and posterior layers ; the former fuses with the aponeurosis of the external oblique and passes in front of the rectus; the latter fuses with the aponeurosis of the transversus abdominis and passes behind the rectus. Just below the costal margin, muscular fibres of the transversus abdominis pass almost to the midline, and unless this muscle is well relaxed the peritoneum in this situation cannot easily be sutured. Where the posterior sheath ends, i.e., between the umbilicus and the pubis, it forms an arched fold, the semicircular line of Douglas. At this point the inferior epigastric artery enters the rectus sheath.

2. From the semicircular line to the pubis the aponeurosis of all these muscles passes anterior to the rectus. The fascia transversalis lies posterior to the muscle, and, with the extraperitoneal fat, separates it from the peritoneum.

3. Above the costal margin the anterior wall of the sheath is formed exclusively from the aponeurosis of the external oblique. Posteriorly the rectus is in relation to the costal cartilages of the 5th, 6th, and 7th ribs.

The rectus sheath contains, in addition to the rectus and pyramidalis muscles, the superior and inferior epigastric vessels and the terminations of the lower six intercostal nerves and vessels. The nerves pierce the lateral margin of the sheath and run in relation to its posterior wall, before they enter the substance of the muscle.

PYRAMIDALIS.—A small muscle on each side, within the rectus sheath, *arising* from the pubis and *inserted* into the linea alba. It is well developed in marsupial mammals, and serves to strengthen the linea alba.

The abdominal muscles are supplied by the lower six intercostal nerves and by the iliohypogastric and ilio-inguinal nerves.

They are accessory muscles of expiration and help to compress the abdominal viscera, as in defæcation, straining, coughing, etc. They are not muscles of normal inspiration.

TRANSVERSALIS FASCIA.—A thin membrane, continuous with the iliac and pelvic fascia. In the inguinal region it is stronger and thicker than elsewhere and through it, at the abdominal inguinal (internal inguinal) ring, passes the spermatic cord, or the round ligament.

SENSORY NERVE-SUPPLY OF ABDOMINAL WALL.—The skin in the region of the nipple is supplied by the fifth thoracic nerve.

Skin in the epigastrium is supplied by the seventh nerve.

Skin in the region of the umbilicus is supplied by the tenth nerve.

Skin midway between the umbilicus and the pubis is supplied by the twelfth nerve.

Skin of the groin is supplied by the iliohypogastric nerve (L.1).

Intercostal nerves and the last thoracic nerve pass under the costal margin between the slips of the diaphragm and run forwards between the internal oblique and the transversus abdominis before they pierce the lateral margin of the rectus sheath. After lying behind the rectus muscle, they pierce its substance and supply it, and end as anterior cutaneous nerves.

VESSELS OF THE ABDOMINAL WALL.—The only vessels likely to be injured by the anæsthetist are the superior and inferior epigastric arteries and veins. The superior artery is the termination of the internal mammary and enters the rectus sheath posterior to the 7th costal cartilage. The inferior epigastric artery arises from the external iliac artery and enters the rectus sheath behind the arcuate line of Douglas.

SURFACE MARKINGS.—The xiphoid is on a level with the body of T.9.

The subcostal plane is at L.3.

The highest part of the iliac crest is on a level with L.4.

Technique of Abdominal Field Block.—In all operations performed under field block analgesia it is necessary to infiltrate the line of incision both subcutaneously and intradermally. The injections should be commenced 15–20 minutes before the incision is to be made. Weals are raised :—

1. At the tip of the xiphisternum opposite the body of T.9.
2. One on each side at the 9th costal cartilage, where the rectus muscle crosses it.
3. One on each side at the lateral margin of the rectus, just above the umbilicus.
4. One on each side at the lateral margin of the rectus, below umbilicus—if the incision is to be prolonged.

Through weals 2, 3, and 4 a needle is inserted perpendicularly until it meets the resistance of the rectus sheath. If the patient is conscious he will experience pain when the anterior layer of the rectus sheath is pierced. The needle is advanced a further 0·5 cm. and 5 ml. of solution are injected into the sheath. After

Technique of Abdominal Field Block, *continued.*

withdrawal into the subcutaneous tissue, the needle is inclined upwards and downwards so that more solution is deposited into the rectus sheath. It is important to remember the position of the tendinous intersection so that solution is deposited between each pair to ensure even distribution of the analgesic drug. Posterior to the muscle, these intersections do not impede the spread of solution. After completion of the deep injections the weals are joined together along the lateral margin of the rectus by lines of subcutaneous injection. Similarly weal 1 is joined to each weal 2 along the costal margin. A total of 100–200 ml. of solution is used.

A costo-iliac block gives a wider zone of analgesia and relaxation than the rectus-sheath block outlined below, but is more difficult to carry out successfully. Weals are raised on each side along the costal margin and vertically downward to the iliac crest. Solution is deposited, from needles passed through these weals, into the subcutaneous and muscular layers of the abdominal wall, remembering that laterally the intercostal nerves lie between the transversalis and internal oblique. The weals are joined together by subcutaneous infiltration, as described for rectus-sheath block. In muscular subjects, in addition, solution can be injected into the rectus sheath. The volume of solution required is 150–200 ml.

Rectus-sheath block (Carl Ludwig Schleich, 1899)* is an excellent method of producing muscular relaxation when combined with a light general anæsthetic, and if the incision is to be midline or paramedian it is usual to do both sides. Perforation of the peritoneum should be avoided, but in the absence of peritonitis or adhesions no serious harm is likely to result. The anterior layer of the rectus sheath is detected by the needle throughout its whole extent, but the posterior layer only for about 3 in. above and below the umbilicus. Solution is placed posterior to the muscle so that the intercostal nerves supplying it, together with the zone of skin medial to its outer border, are blocked. If the abdomen shows the scar of a previous operation, abdominal field block may be difficult and undesirable, and intercostal block or paravertebral block may be indicated if the operation is to be performed under local analgesia.

Abdominal field block renders the abdominal wall and its underlying parietal peritoneum insensitive. To block pain impulses from the viscera and posterolateral parietal peritoneum, either light general anæsthesia or a splanchnic block is required.

FIELD BLOCK FOR REPAIR OF INGUINAL HERNIA

Anatomy.—The inguinal canal is 1½ in. long and extends from the internal inguinal ring laterally, to the external inguinal ring medially. It lies above the inner half of the inguinal ligament.

The internal or abdominal ring is just above the midpoint of the inguinal ligament : it is an opening in the transversalis fascia and just medial to it is the inferior epigastric artery.

---

* Schleich, C. L., *Schmerzlöse Operationen*, 1899, p. 240. Berlin.

The subcutaneous or external ring lies above and lateral to the pubic crest. It is an opening in the external oblique, and through it passes the spermatic cord in the male and the round ligament in the female. They lie lateral to the pubic spine.

The walls of the inguinal canal are :—

1. Anteriorly : external oblique ; internal oblique in its lateral third.
2. Posteriorly : fascia transversalis in its whole length ; conjoint tendon or falx inguinalis in its inner two-thirds ; reflected part of the inguinal ligament in its inner third.
3. The floor : inguinal ligament.
4. The roof : arching fibres of the conjoint tendon.

The contents of the inguinal canal are the ilio-inguinal nerve and the spermatic cord or the round ligament of the uterus. The spermatic cord comprises the internal and external spermatic arteries and the artery to the vas deferens ; the pampiniform plexus of veins ; the lymphatic vessels ; the autonomic nerve-fibres ; the vas deferens.

INDIRECT INGUINAL HERNIA.—This traverses the inguinal canal and is congenital. The sac is a process of peritoneum surrounded by the coverings of the spermatic cord, which are, from without inwards :—

a. The external spermatic fascia from the external oblique.
b. The cremasteric fascia from the internal oblique.
c. The internal spermatic fascia from the fascia transversalis.

DIRECT INGUINAL HERNIA.—This leaves the abdominal cavity through the triangle of Hesselbach,* the boundaries of which are : lateral, the inferior or deep epigastric artery ; medial, the outer border of the rectus ; inferior, the inguinal ligament.

NERVE-SUPPLY.—The nerve-supply of the inguinal region is from the last two thoracic and the first two lumbar nerves via the iliohypogastric, the ilio-inguinal and the genitofemoral.

The last two thoracic nerves run downwards and inwards, just above the anterior superior iliac spine, between the internal oblique and transversus muscles. They end by piercing the rectus sheath.

The iliohypogastric and ilio-inguinal nerves come from the first lumbar root. They are inferior to the last two thoracic nerves and curve round the body just above the iliac crest, gradually piercing the muscles and ending superficially : the ilio-inguinal nerve traverses the inguinal canal, lying anterior to the spermatic cord, and becomes superficial through the external ring and supplies the skin of the scrotum. The iliohypogastric nerve, after running between the internal oblique and the transversus abdominis, pierces the internal oblique just above the anterior superior iliac spine and supplies the skin over the pubis.

The genitofemoral nerve comes from the first and second lumbar nerves and divides into a genital and a femoral branch. The former enters the inguinal canal from behind, through the internal ring.

---

* Hesselbach, F. C., *Anatomisch-chirurgische Abhandlung*, 1806, Würzburg: Baumgartner.

Technique.—Three weals are made as follows :—

1. A finger-breadth internal to the anterior superior iliac spine.
2. Over the spine of the pubis.
3. Half an inch above the midpoint of the inguinal ligament.

Through weal 1 a larger needle is introduced vertically backward
until it is felt to pierce the aponeurosis of the external obliqu
with a slight click. After aspiration, 30 ml. of solution are
injected so that both the ilio-inguinal and iliohypogastric nerve
are surrounded. At this point a needle introduced perpendicula
to the skin will not pierce the peritoneum. Solution is deposite
in all layers including that small area of tissue between the wea
and the anterior superior spine.

Through weal 2 a larger needle deposits solution in the intraderma
and subcutaneous layers in the direction of the umbilicus. Thi
blocks nerve twigs overlapping from the opposite side.

Through weal 3 a needle is inserted perpendicularly to the skin unti
it pierces the aponeurosis of the external oblique. At this leve
20 ml. of solution are injected so that the genital branch of the
genitofemoral nerve is blocked.*

Intradermal and subcutaneous infiltration along the line of the
incision may be necessary to get perfect analgesia.

If the hernia is strangulated or irreducible, deeper layers should be
injected by the surgeon, under vision as he goes along.

The patient may complain of temporary discomfort while the neck
of the sac is under tension : this can often be relieved by infiltration of local analgesic solution round the neck.

Herniorrhaphy can also be performed under paravertebral nerve-
block. Injections must be made into the eleventh and twelfth
thoracic and the first and second lumbar nerves.

FIELD BLOCK FOR REPAIR OF FEMORAL HERNIA

Anatomy.—A femoral hernia passes through the femoral canal and
the saphenous opening or fossa ovalis, an opening in the deep
fascia of the thigh, $1\frac{1}{2}$ in. (3·8 cm.) below and $1\frac{1}{2}$ in. (3·8 cm.) lateral
to the pubic tubercle.

The femoral canal is the most medial of three compartments, the
most lateral containing the femoral artery and the intermediate
one the femoral vein. The femoral canal is $\frac{1}{2}$ in. (1·2 cm.) long,
and at its mouth is the femoral ring.

The femoral ring is bounded in front by the inguinal ligament and
behind by the pectineus ; laterally by the femoral vein ; and
medially by the lacunar ligament of Gimbernat (1734–1790).
Astley Cooper's (1768–1841) ligament is a backward extension
of the lacunar ligament, along the pelvic brim (iliopectineal line)
for half an inch.

The ring contains the femoral septum, or fatty pad.

The coverings of a femoral hernia are, from within outwards : the
fat from the femoral septum ; the prolongation of the fascia

---

* Macintosh, R. R., and Bryce-Smith, R., *Local Analgesia: Abdominal Surgery,* 1962, 2nd
ed., p.70 Edinburgh and London : E. & S. Livingstone.

transversalis forming the anterior wall of the femoral sheath ; the cribriform fascia of the fossa ovalis.

Technique.—The technique is similar to that for repair of inguinal hernia, with the addition that the lump in the thigh is surrounded by subcutaneous and intradermal weals.

Paravertebral block from T.10 to L.3 may also be carried out : it is a suitable procedure for operation on strangulated herniæ, both inguinal and femoral.

FIELD BLOCK FOR GASTROSTOMY

Weals are raised along the costal margin from the xiphisternum to the tip of the 10th or 11th rib—on the left side. From needles inserted through these weals the tissues between the skin and the peritoneum are infiltrated and subcutaneous infiltration is made by joining the weals together. Lastly, a line of subcutaneous infiltration between the xiphisternum and the umbilicus is made. Solution required is 50–100 ml.

ILIAC CREST BLOCK

A weal is raised 1½ in. (3·8 cm.) from the anterior superior iliac spine on a line joining this spine to the xiphisternum. A needle is inserted laterally, first just beneath the skin and then deeper until the ilium is touched. Solution is injected so that it anæsthetizes the 12th thoracic, iliohypogastric, and ilio-inguinal nerves as they lie between the internal oblique and the transversus abdominis muscles.

FIELD BLOCK FOR APPENDICECTOMY

This is most useful in interval cases, but is seldom successful in operation for acute appendicitis.

Two weals are raised, one just above and behind the anterior superior iliac spine, the second below the costal margin at the tip of the 10th rib on the right side. The tissues between the skin and peritoneum in this line are infiltrated, and subcutaneous infiltration is made between the two weals and downwards between the lower weal and the iliac bone. Thus the 10th, 11th, and 12th thoracic nerves are blocked, together with the ilio-inguinal and iliohypogastric.

Splanchnic block and bilateral somatic block are usually necessary, except in the very simplest operations on thin subjects.

FIELD BLOCK FOR SUPRAPUBIC CYSTOSTOMY

Bilateral rectus-sheath block is performed (*see* p. 362) through weals at the lateral margin of the rectus between the umbilicus and the pubis. The weals are joined by lines of subcutaneous infiltration and a similar linear weal, subcutaneous and intradermal, extends from the umbilicus to the pubis. From a weal 3 cm. above the symphysis, a needle is inserted backwards and downwards, keeping its point near the bone ; solution is then injected into the retropubic space of Retzius, using 30 ml. of analgesic solution.

REGIONAL ANALGESIA FOR PROSTATECTOMY

A useful method in the poor-risk patient, especially if not obese. Following block of the sacral nerves by extradural or low intradural analgesia, to block afferent impulses from the prostatic region, a local infiltration and field block procedure as for suprapubic cystostomy is performed. If the spermatic cord is to be ligated it can be infiltrated at the external inguinal ring.

FIELD BLOCK FOR OPERATIONS ON THE ANAL CANAL

A weal is made on each side of the anus and 1 in. (2·5 cm.) away from it. From these weals a subcutaneous rhomboidal zone of infiltration is made. Deep injections are now made from the infiltrated zone in the form of a truncated cone, a finger in the rectum preventing perforation of the mucous membrane. The nerve to the external anal sphincter is the perineal branch of the fourth sacral nerve.

FIELD BLOCK FOR CIRCUMCISION

Anatomy.—The sensory nerves of the penis are derived from the terminal twigs of the internal pudendal nerves, the dorsal nerves of the penis coming beneath the pubic bone, one on each side of the midline, lying against the dorsal surface of the corpus cavernosum. The skin at the base of the organ is supplied by the ilio-inguinal and perhaps the genitofemoral nerves. In addition, the posterior scrotal branches of the perineal nerves run para-urethrally to the ventral surface and frænum, so four nerves have to be blocked.

Technique.—An intradermal and subcutaneous ring weal is raised around the base of the penis ; the subcutaneous infiltration should precede the intradermal. The dorsal nerve is next blocked on each side by injecting 5 ml. of solution into the dorsum of the organ so that the needle point lies against the corpus cavernosum. If the needle pierces the corpus cavernosum, pain is experienced. For the ventral injection of the para-urethral branches, the penis should be pulled upwards and 2 ml. of solution injected near the base of the organ into the groove formed by the corpora cavernosa and the corpus spongiosum.

Adrenaline must not be used lest necrosis of tissue results, as the arteries of the penis are end-arteries.

FIELD BLOCK FOR TRENDELENBURG OPERATION FOR VARICOSE VEINS

Anatomy.—The great saphenous vein begins on the dorsum of the foot, ascends just in front of the internal malleolus, and joins the femoral vein about 1 in. below the inguinal ligament, after passing through the fossa ovalis. Near its termination it is joined by the superficial circumflex iliac, the superficial external pudendal, and the superficial epigastric veins. These are irregular and their number may be added to. The femoral vein is medial to the palpable femoral artery.

The sensory nerve-supply of the skin of the front of the thigh is from the first four lumbar nerves, via the lateral femoral cutaneous (L.2 and 3), the genitofemoral (L.1 and 2), the femoral (L.2, 3, and 4), the obturator (L.2, 3, and 4), and the ilio-inguinal (L.1).

Technique.—Weals are raised :—

1. Two finger-breadths below and medial to the anterior superior iliac spine.
2. Two finger-breadths external to the pubic tubercle.
3. Just below the inguinal ligament, immediately over the pulsating femoral artery.

Weals 1 and 2 are joined by a line of intradermal and subcutaneous infiltration running just above the inguinal ligament. Similar lines are extended downwards from each weal, near the inner and outer borders of the thigh, for 3–4 in. (7.5–10 cm.)

A needle is inserted perpendicularly through weal 3 so that it pierces the deep fascia and comes to lie near the femoral artery. The needle is kept moving and 20 ml. of solution are injected into this region so that the femoral nerve is blocked. This may cause some temporary weakness of the quadriceps extensor muscles of the thigh.

If sclerosing solutions are injected into the veins under general anæsthesia, lack of muscular movement may cause pooling of the solution in the deep veins, with consequent thrombosis there and sometimes pulmonary embolism. If local analgesia is used, muscular activity quickly sweeps away the sclerosant solution.

Technique of Block of Iliohypogastric and Ilio-inguinal Nerves.
—(*See* Iliac Crest Block, p. 365.)

NERVE-BLOCK AT THE UPPER PART OF THE THIGH
(*Figs.* 29–32)

Anatomy of Lumbar Plexus.—The anterior primary rami of the lumbar nerves each receive a grey ramus communicans from a lumbar ganglion, while the first and second lumbar nerves are also connected with the trunk by a white ramus.

The anterior primary rami of the first four nerves form the lumbar plexus. A branch from the fourth unites with the fifth nerve to form the lumbosacral trunk which joins the sacral plexus. It lies in the psoas major, anterior to the transverse processes of the lumbar vertebræ.

The branches of the lumbar plexus are :—

THE ILIOHYPOGASTRIC NERVE from L.1. It leaves the psoas major, crosses the quadratus lumborum, perforates the transversus abdominis, and then divides into lateral and anterior cutaneous branches. Its lateral cutaneous branch supplies the skin on the anterior part of the gluteal region after piercing the internal and external oblique muscles 5 cm. behind the anterior superior iliac spine and just above the iliac crest, while the terminal part of the nerve supplies the skin over the pubic bone after piercing the aponeurosis of the external oblique, 2 cm. medial to the anterior superior iliac spine. It does not divide into anterior and posterior branches.

Anatomy of Lumbar Plexus, *continued.*

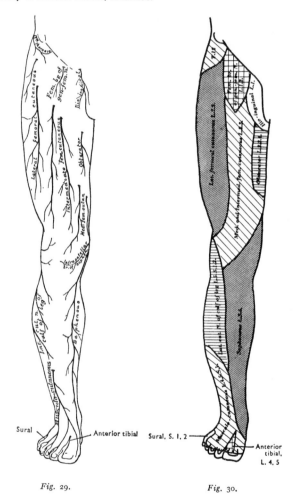

Fig. 29.

Fig. 30.

Fig. 29.—The cutaneous nerves of the right lower extremity. Anterior aspect.

Fig. 30.—The segmental distribution of the cutaneous nerves of the right lower extremity. Anterior aspect.

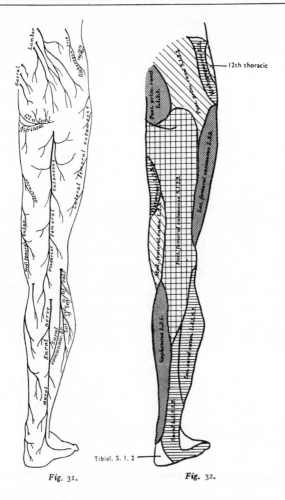

Fig. 31.   *Fig.* 32.

Fig. 31.—The cutaneous nerves of the right lower extremity.   Posterior
aspect.

Fig. 32.—The segmental distribution of the cutaneous nerves of the right
lower extremity.   Posterior aspect.

(*Figs.* 29–32 *after 'Gray's Anatomy' by kind permission.*)

15

Anatomy of Lumbar Plexus, *continued.*

> THE ILIO-INGUINAL NERVE from L.1. This accompanies the ilio
> hypogastric nerve, in its early course, lying just inferior to
> in close relationship to the iliac crest. About 2 cm. anterio
> and just below the anterior superior spine, it pierces th
> internal oblique and runs medially behind the aponeurosis
> the external oblique. It then passes with the spermatic co
> through the inguinal canal and supplies the skin of the upp
> and medial part of the thigh and the adjacent skin coverin
> the external genitals. It has no lateral cutaneous branch, unlik
> the iliohypogastric nerve, and in the inguinal canal is sensory
>
> THE GENITOFEMORAL NERVE from L.1 and 2. Its genital bran
> supplies the skin of the scrotum or labium majus, and th
> cremaster muscle. Its femoral branch supplies an area
> skin on the middle of the anterior surface of the upper pa
> of the thigh.
>
> THE LATERAL CUTANEOUS NERVE of the thigh (lateral femor
> cutaneous) from L.2 and 3 (posterior divisions). It supplies th
> skin of the anterolateral aspect of the thigh as far as the kne
> anteriorly, but laterally not quite so low after passing behir
> the inguinal ligament and the sartorius muscle, just medi
> and slightly inferior to the anterior superior iliac spine.
>
> THE FEMORAL NERVE from L.2, 3, and 4 (posterior divisions).
> It emerges from the psoas major, passes between it and th
> iliacus and enters the thigh behind the inguinal ligament ar
> just lateral to the femoral artery, from which it is her
> separated by a slip of the psoas major. It has anterior ar
> posterior divisions, the latter giving rise to the saphenor
> nerve and the medial and intermediate cutaneous nerves of th
> thigh. The femoral nerve supplies the hip- and knee-joint
> the skin of the anterior part of the thigh and the anteromedi
> part of the leg. It is motor to the quadriceps femoris, th
> sartorius, and the pectineus.
>
> THE OBTURATOR NERVE from L.2, 3, and 4 (anterior divisions
> The nerve divides into anterior and posterior branches ; th
> former supplies the adductor longus and brevis, and th
> gracilis, with a twig going to the hip-joint ; the posterior branc
> supplies the adductor magnus and the hip-joint. It suppli
> an area of skin on the medial aspect of the thigh.
>
> THE ACCESSORY OBTURATOR NERVE from L.3 and 4 (anterio
> divisions).

Anatomy of Sacral Plexus.—The anterior primary rami of the fiv
sacral and the coccygeal nerves receive each a grey ramus from th
sympathetic trunk. From the second, third, and fourth sacr
nerves white rami join the pelvic plexuses of the sympathetic, th
sacral outflow of the autonomic nervous system, or the sacr
parasympathetics.

> The sacral and pudendal plexuses are composed of the lumbosacr
> trunk (L.4 and 5) and the anterior divisions of the five sacr
> and the coccygeal nerves. They lie on the posterior wall of th
> pelvic cavity between the piriformis and the pelvic fascia ar

have in front the ureter, internal iliac vessels, and the sigmoid colon on the left.

The following branches are given off :—

Nerve to superior gemellus (L.5 ; S.1–2).

Nerve to inferior gemellus (L.4–5 ; S.1).

Nerve to obturator internus (L.5 ; S.1–2).

Nerve to quadratus femoris (L.4–5 ; S.1).

Nerve to piriformis (S.1 and 2).

Superior gluteal nerve (L.4 and 5 ; S.1).

Inferior gluteal nerve (L.5 ; S.1 and 2).

Posterior cutaneous nerve of the thigh (S.1, 2, and 3).

Great sciatic nerve (L.4 and 5 ; S.1, 2, and 3).

Perforating cutaneous nerve (S.2 and 3).

Pudendal nerve (S.2, 3, and 4).

Anococcygeal nerve (S.4 and 5 ; C.1).

THE POSTERIOR CUTANEOUS NERVE OF THE THIGH supplies the skin of the lower part of the gluteal region, the perineum, and the back of the thigh and leg.

THE GREAT SCIATIC NERVE supplies the skin of the back of the leg and sole of the foot, after dividing into medial and lateral popliteal nerves. It leaves the pelvis through the greater sciatic foramen, lying between the piriformis and the superior gemellus muscles, and occupies the space between the ischial tuberosity and the greater trochanter.

THE PERFORATING CUTANEOUS NERVE supplies the skin over the medial and lower parts of the gluteus maximus.

THE PUDENDAL NERVE leaves the pelvis through the greater sciatic foramen, crosses the ischial spine medial to the pudendal vessels, and goes through the lesser sciatic foramen. With the pudendal vessels it passes upwards and forwards along the lateral wall of the ischiorectal fossa, in Alcock's canal, a sheath of the obturator fascia. It gives off :—

a. The inferior rectal nerve supplying the external anal sphincter and the skin around the anus.

b. The perineal nerve supplying the skin of the scrotum or labium majus, and small twigs to muscles.

c. The dorsal nerve of the penis or clitoris.

d. Visceral branches supplying the rectum and bladder. From the second, third, and fourth sacral nerves. They communicate with the sympathetic pelvic plexuses. Sometimes called the pelvic splanchnic nerves of Gaskell. Homologous with the white rami communicantes of the thoracic and upper lumbar nerves. The levator ani and the coccygeus, and also the external anal sphincter, are supplied by the fourth sacral nerve.

Technique of Femoral Nerve-block.—A weal is raised a finger-breadth to the outer side of the femoral artery, just below the inguinal ligament. A needle seeks for paræsthesia and, when found, 10 ml. of 2 per cent lignocaine are injected. The nerve lies beneath the deep fascia.

Sciatic and femoral nerve-blocks in combination are useful in operations on the leg and foot from a point 5 cm. below the patella.

Technique of Femoral Nerve-block, *continued.*

Operations on or above the knee require, in addition, lateral femoral cutaneous and obturator block, the latter being difficult Manipulations of the lower half of the femur can, however, be carried out under sciatic and femoral block, and the application of a tourniquet to the thigh is painless.

Technique of Block of Lateral Cutaneous Nerve of Thigh.—A weal is raised one finger-breadth below and medial to the anterior superior spine of the ilium. A needle is inserted perpendicularly to the skin and 1 per cent lignocaine is deposited between the skin and the iliac bone and along the pelvic brim for two finger-breadth internally to the anterior superior spine : 10–15 ml. of solution are used. The nerve lies deep to the fascia lata of the thigh.

When associated with femoral block, adequate analgesia is produced for taking skin-grafts from the front of the thigh. Alternatively infiltration analgesia of skin of front of thigh can be performed using intradermal and subcutaneous injections to cover the desired area.

Technique of Obturator Block.—The obturator nerves arise from the second, third, and fourth lumbar nerves. Block is required for operations involving the knee-joint, the medial aspect of the thigh, and may be necessary to make application of an arterial tourniquet above the knee tolerable.

The anterior and posterior divisions of the nerve are blocked as they lie in the obturator canal below the superior ramus of the pubis, between the pectineus and the obturator externus.

A skin weal is raised just below the midpoint of the superior pubic ramus and a No. 1 needle introduced perpendicular to the plane of the obturator foramen and advanced just below the ramus for 1·5 cm. Paræsthesiæ should be elicited after the injection of 5 ml. of 1·5 per cent lignocaine solution.* This block is difficult and it may be preferable to perform a paravertebral somatic block of the second, third, and fourth lumbar nerves. Successful block is shown by weakness when the patient attempts to adduct the leg.

Block of the above three nerves, together with the sciatic, will produce analgesia of the lower extremity below the level of the symphysis pubis.

For insertion of a Smith-Petersen-type pin, the line of incision is infiltrated down to the bone with 0·5 per cent lignocaine or 1–1000 amethocaine. Solution is injected between the ends of the fractured neck from above the great trochanter and from a point just external to the pulsating femoral artery.

Technique of Sciatic Nerve-block.—Patient lies on sound side with hip slightly flexed. (1) A line connecting the sacral hiatus with the most prominent part of the greater trochanter is drawn and a weal raised at its midpoint. A No. 1 needle is inserted and through it 10–15 ml. of 2 per cent lignocaine with adrenaline are injected after eliciting paræsthesia.† (2) A line is traced between the upper

---

* Parks, C. R., and Kennedy, W. F., *Anesthesiology,* 1967, **28**, 775.
† Bryce-Smith, R., *Post Grad. Med. J.,* 1966, **42**, 367.

extremity of the great trochanter and the posterior superior iliac spine. From the midpoint of this line a perpendicular is dropped 3 cm. long, and at its end a weal is raised and a needle introduced at right-angles to the skin plane until it reaches the ischial spine, (5–7·5 cm.) from the skin surface. The nerve lies on this area of bone so that paræsthesiæ must be elicited before the needle strikes bone: 10–15 ml. of 2 per cent are then injected. (3) A surface marking is the junction of the medial third with the lateral two-thirds of a line joining the ischial tuberosity to the greater femoral trochanter —the needle being inserted at right-angles to the skin surface until paræsthesiæ are felt by the patient. (4) A guide to the position of the nerve is the midpoint of a line joining the posterior superior iliac spine to the ischial tuberosity.

The block is useful for reduction of fractures around the ankle. It also causes almost complete vasoconstrictor paralysis of the foot and is better, safer, and less painful than lumbar sympathetic block for this purpose. A rise in skin temperature starts in 10 minutes and is maximal in 20–30 minutes. Sciatic nerve-block gives analgesia of the whole foot with the exception of an area of skin over the medial malleolus supplied by the saphenous branch of the femoral nerve.

Technique of Sciatic Nerve-block (Anterior Approach).*—This may be useful when the patient cannot be easily moved from the supine position and when intervention on the foot or lower leg is required. Other nerve-blocks in the leg may be combined with it. With the patient lying supine the skin of the thigh is prepared and the line of the inguinal ligament trisected into equal parts. From the greater trochanter a line is drawn across the front of the thigh, parallel to the inguinal ligament. From the junction of the inner and middle third of the inguinal ligament a line is drawn perpendicular to the lower line and at this point a weal is raised. A 15-cm. needle is inserted backwards and outwards until it meets the femur. A marker is now placed 5 cm. from the skin and the needle partly withdrawn and redirected slightly medially just beyond the point where the femur was first touched until the marker lies against the skin. Injection of 20–30 ml. of 1·5 per cent lignocaine with adrenaline (1–250,000) is now made, but it must be easy and free from resistance. If this is not so on the first attempt the needle should be slightly advanced or withdrawn until ease of injection shows that the needle point lies in the neurovascular space enclosing the sciatic nerve.

For technique of lateral approach with the patient supine *see* Ichiyanagi, K., *Anesthesiology*, 1959, **20**, 601.

Technique of Perineal Block.—The perineal branch of the pudendal nerve supplies the skin of the anterior part of the perineum in front of the anus. With the patient in the lithotomy position a weal is raised on each side just internal to the ischial tuberosity. Through it a needle is advanced about 1 in. (2·5 cm.) and 10–15 ml. of 2 per cent lignocaine are injected on each side.

---

* Beck, G. P., *Anesthesiology*, 1963, **24**, 222.

Technique of Perineal Block, *continued*.

The ilio-inguinal nerve can be blocked as it curves over the tendon the adductor longus, close to the pubic bone ; the nerve suppli the skin over the symphysis or its immediate surroundings.

Pudendal Nerve-block (*See* Chapter XXV).

ANKLE BLOCK

A subcutaneous and intradermal weal are raised circumferential around the ankle just above the medial malleolus.

ANTERIOR TIBIAL NERVE is blocked by inserting a needle mi way between the most prominent points of the medial and later malleoli, on the circular line of infiltration in front of the ankl joint. It is directed medially towards the anterior border of t medial malleolus and solution is injected between the bone ar the skin; paræsthesia should be elicited if possible. Instead blocking this nerve at the ankle, its parent trunk, the later popliteal nerve can be blocked at the neck of the fibula where can be rolled under the finger—the only palpable nerve in t leg.

The amount of solution used should be 10–15 ml.

POSTERIOR TIBIAL NERVE is blocked by 10 ml. of solutic introduced through a point on the circular weal just internal the tendo Achillis, deep to the flexor retinaculum near t palpable posterior tibial artery. The needle is inserted forwar and slightly outwards towards the posterior aspect of the tibi near which the solution is deposited.

After waiting ten minutes, ankle block is suitable for operation the foot.

Posterior tibial block is useful for testing vasodilatation of the foc Following infiltration of any peripheral nerve there results vasomotor paralysis over the area of anæsthetized skin.

BLOCK FOR HALLUX VALGUS

A weal is raised near the proximal end of the first intermetatars space, superior surface, and, from this, solution is deposited betwee the two layers of skin, dorsal and plantar, as far forwards as the we between the toes. More solution is injected between the dorsal sk and the first metatarsal bone. A second weal medial to the first on on the internal aspect of the metatarsal, is raised, and injection ma between it and the bone and between the plantar skin and the bon A 10–15-minute pause is made before the operation is commence From 30 to 50 ml. of solution are used.

LOCAL ANALGESIA OF FOOT

Sole of Foot.—Supplied by posterior tibial nerve (continuation medial popliteal nerve from sciatic).

BLOCK.—Posterior tibial nerve-block. (*See above under* Ank Block.)

Dorsum of Foot.—Supplied by anterior tibial branch of later popliteal nerve.

BLOCK.—Lateral popliteal block at neck of fibula where it can be rolled under the finger. Or anterior tibial block, midway between the most prominent points of the medial and lateral malleoli, anterior to the ankle-joint. Block lateral to the third toe requires, in addition, sural block (*see below*).

Iedial Side of Foot.—Supplied by saphenous nerve from the femoral nerve. Also from anterior tibial (lateral popliteal nerve).

BLOCK.—Subcutaneous injections as it lies posterior to the vein in front of the medial malleolus.

ateral Side of Foot.—Supplied by sural nerve from the medial popliteal, goes to fifth toe and lateral side of foot.

BLOCK.—Two cm. below lateral malleolus, superficial to extensor retinaculum.

lock of Toes.—Lateral popliteal and posterior tibial nerve-blocks.

LOCAL ANALGESIA FOR REDUCTION OF CLOSED FRACTURES*

After localizing the exact site of fracture by means of X-rays, a weal raised near the fracture and a needle introduced into the hæmatoma etween the broken bone-ends. Aspiration of old blood confirms the osition and must be obtained: injection is then made of 1·5 or 2 per ent lignocaine without adrenaline. For Colles's fracture the amount quired is 15–20 ml.; injection should be made from the extensor spect of the wrist and, in addition, a few ml. should infiltrate the ulnar yloid; for Pott's fracture, 10–20 ml. of solution with hyaluronidase an be used; for fractured femur, 20–30 ml. These are high doses so ie possibility of toxic signs must be borne in mind. Cases of recent acture are the most suitable for this method of reduction, especially actures of the metatarsal or metacarpal bones. Good results are aimed for the addition of 1000 units of hyaluronidase to each 20 ml. f solution. With lignocaine, analgesia lasts two to three hours and omes on after ten minutes.

TOPICAL ANALGESIA FOR GASTROSCOPY† AND ŒSOPHAGOSCOPY‡

After pentobarbitone and atropine or other similar premedication, the patient is given a tablet of amethocaine (65 mg.), benzocaine (10 mg.), or lignocaine to suck. Too much atropine may make this difficult. The gums, tongue, palate, and pharynx are now sprayed with 4 per cent lignocaine, 4 per cent cocaine, 1 per cent amethocaine, 2 per cent butyn, or some other suitable analgesic solution. He can be given amethocaine hydrochloride 2 per cent to gargle, or Xylocaine Viscous to swallow, a 2 per cent solution in a mucilage base, very pleasantly flavoured.

TOPICAL ANALGESIA FOR BRONCHOSCOPY

The gums, tongue, palate, and pharynx are sprayed as for œsophago-scopy. After a short interval, the piriform fossæ are made

---

* Ramsey, R. H., and Pedersen, H. E., *A.M.A. Arch. Surg.*, 1957, **75**, 976.
† Williams, D. G., and others, *Brit. med. J.*, 1968, **1**, 535.
‡ Allen H. A., and others, *Curr. Res. Anesth.*, 1956, **35**, 386.

Topical Analgesia for Bronchoscopy, *continued.*

analgesic by application of swabs soaked in the solution (w
excess of it removed), applied on a curved applicator or w
Krause's laryngeal forceps. After this has been done, and af
spraying the epiglottis and the cords, a swab is gently introduc
into the glottis and held there for a short while, so that
analgesic solution completes the block of the superior laryng
nerve-endings.

In addition, the trachea must be anæsthetized by:—

1. The transtracheal method of Canuyt (1920), which consists
inserting a No. I hypodermic needle through the middle li
of the neck into the trachea. The needle should be 1½
(3·8 cm.) long so that if breakage occurs, which is usually n
the hub, the remains of the shaft can be easily remove
Aspiration of air proves its presence in the trachea. An inj
tion of 2–3 ml. of 4 per cent lignocaine or cocaine is now ma
after a deep expiration and the patient told not to cough un
the solution has trickled down the trachea into the bronch
Complications are: (1) Infection. (2) A broken needle. (
Surgical emphysema.

2. By instillation from a laryngeal syringe, holding the tong
forward, using an indirect laryngeal mirror if thought necessa

3. By passing a No. 1 endotracheal tube from the cocainized no
into the trachea and instilling down it, via a length of f
polythene tubing, a few ml. of solution near the carina.

A 10 per cent lignocaine aerosol spray is available and enables
measured dose of drug to be given with each 'squirt'. De
penetration into the bronchial tree can be achieved.

Cocaine should be used carefully in a maximum dosage of 20 n
per stone (3 mg. per kilo). Amethocaine in 0·5 per cent soluti
should not exceed 8 ml. These topical solutions should not
used on inflamed or traumatized surfaces. Lignocaine in 4 p
cent solution gives good results and is less toxic.

Cocaine Sensitivity Test.—Inject 10 mg. hypodermically, e.g., 0·25 n
of 4 per cent solution. For amethocaine sensitivity inject 2 m
e.g., 0·2 ml. of 1 per cent solution. If pulse-rate rises by mo
than fifteen beats per minute, patient is presumably sensitive
the drug.

Regional analgesia is probably safer than general anæsthesia
these examinations where there is copious sputum, airw
obstruction, or when the general condition of the patient is po
It enables the movements of the vocal cords to be seen also.

As an aid to comfortable endoscopy under local analgesia, the co
current use of divided doses of pethidine (30–100 mg.) giv
intravenously is beneficial.*

In children who may be susceptible to local analgesic drugs su
examinations are better made under bromethol or rect
paraldehyde, followed if necessary by oxygen and halothan
Ether–air, followed by trichloroethylene–air while the bronch
scope is in the air-passages, is probably as safe a technique as an
the slight theoretical risk of explosion notwithstanding.

---

* Churchill-Davidson, H. C., *Anæsthesia*, 1952, **7**, 237.

After topical laryngeal analgesia, instruction must be given to the patient not to eat or drink for at least three hours, i.e., until the sentinel of the larynx has returned to duty.

Even without the administration of extra oxygen, oxygen saturation of the blood increases during bronchoscopy performed under local analgesia.*

TOPICAL ANALGESIA OF THE URETHRA

Technique.—A useful preparation is Xylocaine Gel, a 2 per cent preparation put up in 30-ml. tubes with carboxy-methyl-cellulose. The maximum dose should probably not exceed 10 ml., i.e., 200 mg. of lignocaine. The plastic nozzle supplied by the makers of the preparation is boiled and by its aid the paste is squeezed into the urethra. A clamp is applied to the penis and the paste gently massaged into the posterior urethra. After an interval of 10–15 minutes instrumentation can begin. Toxic effects have followed the use of these fairly large doses of lignocaine† and good analgesia can be obtained with 15 ml. of 1 per cent in a jelly base. It is sometimes helpful to pass a small catheter into the urethra connected to the plastic nozzle, so as to deposit paste in the posterior urethra. Each tube contains 600 mg. of the drug.

Alternatively 30 ml. of a mixture of 0·5 per cent cocaine and 0·5 per cent sodium bicarbonate ; or 2 per cent piperocaine is instilled into the urethra with a glass urethral syringe. Sufficient volume is injected to distend the anterior urethra and allow some to be massaged back to the posterior urethra. The syringe is removed and a penile clamp applied to keep the solution in contact with the urethral mucosa. This is removed after five minutes and an applicator with cotton-wool soaked in 10 per cent cocaine is placed inside the meatus, and allowed to remain for a further five minutes.

Cinchocaine, 0·5 per cent in tragacanth paste, can be used instead, a volume of 15 ml. being injected and held by a clamp. For patients who react abnormally to ordinary analgesics, 2 per cent solution of pyribenzamine, the antihistamine, gives reasonable analgesia without toxic reactions, other than occasional drowsiness.

TRANS-SACRAL BLOCK

First performed by Pauchet (1869–1936) and Läwen in 1909, this involves blocking the sacral nerves through the posterior sacral foramina; it is usually associated with extradural sacral (caudal) block, but is frequently quite unnecessary, solution deposited in the sacral canal through the sacral hiatus usually producing excellent analgesia. It is, however, useful when an extradural sacral block is required but cannot be induced because of the difficulty of introducing a needle into the sacral canal.

Technique.—The posterior superior iliac spines are located, as the patient lies prone with his pelvis supported on a sandbag. In the

---

* de Kernfeld, T. J., and Siebecker, K. L., *Anesthesiology*, 1957, **18**, 466.
† Dix, W., and Tresidder, G. C., *Lancet*, 1963, **1**, 890.

Trans-sacral Block—Technique, *continued.*

obese, a dimple overlies the spine. The second foramen is a finger breadth caudad and a finger-breadth medial to the spine. The third, fourth, and fifth foramina are one finger-breadth apart on the same line, while the first foramen is a finger-breadth above the spine and a similar distance medial to it. The fifth foramen usually between the sacrum and the coccyx.

The foramina underlie a line a finger-breadth lateral to the median line posteriorly.

To prevent pain, caudal block should be induced a quarter of an hour before the needles for the trans-sacral block are inserted.

In intractable pain and in severe sciatica a watery solution of phenol has been injected with success into the first and second sacral foramina.

Weals are raised and needles introduced no more than half-way through each foramen. With a negative aspiration test for cerebrospinal fluid and blood, the following amounts of 0·5 per cent lignocaine, 1 per cent procaine or piperocaine are injected on each side :—

First sacral foramen, 15 ml.   Second foramen, 10 ml.
Third foramen,   4 ml.   Fourth foramen, 3 ml.
             Fifth foramen, 2 ml.

Block of the posterior divisions of the sacral nerves by long-acting agents by the trans-sacral route is said to be useful in the treatment of the hypertonic bladder in paraplegics. Block of S.3 and S.2 and S.3 on each side will enable a patient to micturate.

Analgesia of the Peritoneal Cavity by Lavage.—Amethocaine 0·1 per cent solution ; 0·5 per cent lignocaine ; 0·5 per cent or 1 per cent procaine are used. Volume 200 ml. This is poured into the peritoneal cavity and the peritoneal edges are drawn together. After 5 to 8 minutes the solution is sucked out. Results : slackening of the peritoneum, contraction of the bowel, absence of reflex response from visceral trauma. Toxic reactions are said to be rare. Good results are not seen in cases of peritonitis or when the bowel is grossly distended.

INTRAVENOUS LOCAL ANALGESIA

Involves the injection of a local analgesic solution into a vein of a limb which has been made ischæmic by a tourniquet. Most useful for operations on arms but can also be used in the leg.

Intravenous regional analgesia has recently been revived by Holmes[*] who uses the method first described by August Bier in 1908.[†] He substituted lignocaine for procaine. A Mitchell or Gordh type needle is inserted into a vein on the dorsum of the hand or foot and the limb elevated to reduce its blood content. If the limb is not painful, this can be done more efficiently by applying an Esmarch bandage.[‡]

---

* Holmes, C. M., *Lancet*, 1963, **1**, 245.
† Bier, A., *Arch. klin. Chir.*, 1908, **86**, 1007; translated in "Classical File", *Survey Anesthesiol.*, 1967, **11**, 294.
‡ Johann Friedrich von Esmarch (1832–1908). Professor of Surgery in University Kiel (when August Bier gave his first spinal block in 1898). Esmarch became, by marriage uncle of Kaiser Wilhelm II of Germany.

phygmomanometer cuff on the upper arm or thigh is inflated to prevent
arterial blood from entering the limb. An efficient arterial tourniquet
does not completely isolate the limb because of collateral circulation
through bone. The Esmarch bandage is now removed and 0·5 per cent
lignocaine solution is injected into the vein, up to 40 ml. for an arm and
up to 100 ml. for a leg. Total dose should not exceed 4 mg. per kg.*
The patient soon experiences warmth and tingling in the limb and
muscular paralysis sets in. Following the intravenous injection of
lignocaine there is a higher concentration of the agent in nerve tissue
than in other tissues.† If the patient complains of pain caused by the
phygmomanometer cuff, a circular band of local analgesic solution can
be injected above its upper margin, or a second cuff can be applied
below the first one over anæsthetized tissue and the first one removed.
Analgesia is not always perfect in skin areas supplied by the intercostobrachial, lower lateral cutaneous, and posterior cutaneous nerves of the
arm, nor in the region of the olecranon.‡ At the end of the operation the
cuff is deflated and sensation and muscular tone return in a few minutes;
toxic effects are not a problem but their possibility should be borne in
mind. The interval between injection and tourniquet release is probably
not important.§

For operations on the finger-tips in normal adults, the injected
volume of solution should be large, i.e., 50–60 ml. 0·5 per cent solution.

Signs of Toxicity on Releasing Tourniquet.—

1. Drowsiness.
2. Bradycardia.
3. Hypotension.
4. E.C.G. abnormalities (reversible asystole has been reported).‖
   Gas chromatographic assay of blood lignocaine levels after release
   of the tourniquet show the method to be reasonably safe, while
   increasing the interval between injection and the release of the
   tourniquet has little effect on blood levels of drug.§

Prilocaine in 0·5 per cent solution gives results as satisfying as
lignocaine with fewer toxic effects.¶
The site of action of the drug is on the peripheral nerve-endings.**

INTRA-ARTERIAL LOCAL ANALGESIA

Introduced by Goyanes, a Spaniard, in 1912†† and has been reintroduced recently.‡‡

A pneumatic cuff is applied to the upper arm, and a fine, short-bevel
needle, attached to a 20-ml. syringe containing 0·5 per cent lignocaine
solution, is introduced into the brachial artery near the elbow. The
cuff is then inflated until arterial pulsations are occluded and the

* Merrifield, A. J., and Carter, S. J., *Anæsthesia*, 1965, **20**, 287.
† Cotev, S., and Robin, G. C., *Brit. J. Anæsth.*, 1966, **38**, 936.
‡ Sorbie, C., and Chacha, P., *Brit. med. J.*, 1965, **1**, 957.
§ Hargrove, R. L., and others, *Anæsthesia*, 1966, **21**, 37.
‖ Kennedy, B. R., and others, *Brit. med. J.*, 1965, **1**, 954.
¶ Kerr, J. H., *Anæsthesia.*, 1967, **22**, 562.
** Fleming, S. A., and others, *Canad. Anæsth. Soc. J.*, 1966, **13**, 21.
†† Goyanes, J., *Rev. Clin. Madr.*, 1912, **8**, 401.
‡‡ Van Niekerk, J. P. de V., and Coetzee, T., *Lancet*, 1965, **1**, 1353.

Intra-arterial Local Analgesia, *continued.*

solution injected intra-arterially 5 ml. at a time until the desire
analgesic effect is obtained. The average dose in adults is 14–15 ml
considerably less than would be required in intravenous regiona
analgesia. Unsuccessful attempts at intra-arterial injection may caus
temporary vascular spasm, but no other complications were seen i
van Niekerk and Coetzee's series of 300 cases.

CHAPTER XVI

SPINAL ANALGESIA

INTRADURAL SPINAL ANALGESIA

History.—Cerebrospinal fluid discovered by Cotugno in 1764 ; it
circulation described by Magendie in 1825.

Cocaine isolated from *Erythroxylon coca* in 1860 by Niemann an
Lossen ; its analgesic properties described by Schraff in 186
and von Anrep in 1880. Introduced into medicine as loca
analgesic for ophthalmology by Karl Koller (1858–1944) an
Sigmund Freud (1856–1939) in 1884.

First spinal analgesia by J. Leonard Corning (1855–1923), New York
neurologist, in 1885. He accidentally pierced the dura whil
experimenting with cocaine on the spinal nerves of a dog. Late
he deliberately repeated the intradural injection, called it spina
anæsthesia, and suggested it might be used in surgery. "Be th
destiny of this observation what it may, it has seemed to me, o
the whole, worth recording."*

Lumbar puncture standardized as a simple clinical procedure by
Heinrich Irenaeus Quincke of Kiel† in Germany in 1891 and by
Essex Wynter in England in the same year.

First planned spinal analgesia for surgery in man performed by
August Bier (1861–1949) on 16 August, 1898, in Kiel when h
injected 3 ml. of 0·5 per cent cocaine solution into a 34-year-old
labourer.‡ Advised it for operations on legs, but gave it up
owing to toxicity of cocaine. Tuffier§ and Sicard soon afterwards
extended its scope to include the external genitals. Frederick
Dudley Tait (1862–1918) and Guido E. Caglieri (1871–1951) of
San Francisco, and also Rudolf Matas (1860–1957) of New
Orleans,‖ were its first users in the U.S. in 1899, their works
being published in the following year.

Stovaine synthesized by Fourneau (Fr., *fourneau*, stove) in 1904,¶
and novocain (procaine) described by Einhorn the following
year.**

* Corning, J. L., *N.Y. med. J.*, 1885, **42**, 483; reprinted in *Survey of Anesthesiology,*
1960, **4**, 332.
† Quincke, H. I., *Berl. klin. Wschr.*, 1891, 930.
‡ Bier, A., *Z. Chir.*, 1899, **51**, 361; translated in *Survey of Anesthesiology*, 1962, **6**, 352.
§ Tuffier, T., *C.R. Soc. Biol.*, Paris, 1899, **51**, 882.
‖ Matas, R., *Phil. med. J.*, 1900, **6**, 820.
¶ Fourneau, E., *Bull. Soc. Pharmacol.*, Paris, 1904, **10**, 141.
** Einhorn, A., *Dtsch. med. Wschr.*, 1905, **31**, 1668.

Alfred E. Barker (1850–1916) of London, the leading pioneer of spinal analgesia in Britain, was the first to realize (in 1906–7) the importance of the curves of the vertebral canal and the use of gravity in control of level of analgesia.* He and Henri Chaput (1857–1919) independently introduced heavy stovaine solutions in 1907. Babcock first to use light solution, his formula containing stovaine, alcohol, lactic acid, strychnine, etc.

Spinal analgesia little used until Gaston Labat's work in 1921.† He urged use of neocaine (procaine) crystals dissolved in cerebro-spinal fluid, together with barbotage and early Trendelenburg position. Then came George Pitkin with his light (spinocain) and heavy (duracaine) solutions and his use of the fine-bore, short-bevel needle (1927).‡

Chen and Schmidt introduced ephedrine in 1923,§ while Ocherblad and Dillon of the University of Kansas School of Medicine used it to maintain the blood-pressure in spinal analgesia in 1927.||

Meischer discovered the analgesic properties of percaine (nupercaine) in 1929, while Howard Jones published his technique in 1930.¶

Etherington Wilson's work appeared in 1934,** and Walter Lemmon's first account of continuous spinal analgesia was published in 1940.††

Lincoln Fleetwood Sise (1874–1942) of Boston in the U.S. popularized amethocaine (tetracaine)‡‡ which was synthesized by Eisleb in 1928.

In most parts of the U.K. intradural spinal analgesia is at present under a cloud, partly because of the tendency to litigation should complications follow,§§ such as the Woolley and Roe case in which paraplegia followed spinal analgesia in two patients operated on on the same day, and was thought to be due to the contamination of the analgesic solution by phenol which had entered the ampoules through minute cracks in the glass. Anxiety is made worse as the causes of some of these complications, such as adhesive arachnoiditis, are not fully understood. The method is, however, a valuable one, and if proper care is taken in the technique, it yields, in a very large proportion of cases, admirable results and satisfaction to all concerned.|||| Extradural analgesia can be substituted for intradural (spinal) analgesia in nearly every case.

ANATOMY

The Vertebræ.—The vertebral column consists of seven cervical, twelve thoracic, five lumbar, five sacral, and four or five coccygeal

* Barker, A. E., *Brit. med. J.*, 1907, **1**, 665.
† Labat, G., *Ann. Surg.*, 1921 ,**7** ,673.
‡ Pitkin, G. P., *J. med. Soc. N.J.*, 1927, **24**, 425.
§ Chen, K. K., and Schmidt, C. F., *J. Pharmacol.*, 1924, **24**, 331.
|| Ocherblad, N. F., and Dillon, T. C., *J. Amer. med. Ass.*, 1927, **88**, 1135.
¶ Jones, H. W., *Brit. J. Anæsth.*, 1930, **7**, 146.
** Wilson, W. E., *Ibid.*, 1934, **11**, 43.
†† Lemmon, W. T., *Ann. Surg.*, 1940, **111**, 141.
‡‡ Sise, L. F., *Surg. Clin. N. Amer.*, 1935, **15**, 1501.
§§ Cope, R. W., *Anæsthesia*, 1945, **9**, 249.
|||| Lee, J. A., *Ibid.*, 1967, **22**, 342.

The Vertebræ, *continued.*

vertebræ. The sacral and coccygeal vertebræ are fused in adult life.

A typical *lumbar vertebra* consists of :—

1. A body, wider from side to side than from before backwards, and kidney-shaped.

2. Two pedicles, strong and directed backwards from the upper part of the body. Each pedicle is notched, more inferiorly than superiorly and through the intervertebral foramina, formed by the two notches of contiguous vertebræ, the spinal nerves emerge. The intervertebral foramina may be accidentally entered and the dura perforated by a needle, during the induction of paravertebral analgesia.

3. Two laminæ meeting posteriorly and enclosing the vertebral foramen, which is triangular and larger than in the thoracic, but smaller than in the cervical region. The laminæ do not overlap as they do in the thoracic region.

4. The spinous process, thick, broad, and quadrilateral. It rises from the point of union of the laminæ, projects backwards, and ends in a rough uneven border.

5. Two superior and two inferior articular processes project respectively upwards and downwards from the junctions of the pedicles and laminæ. In the articulated column, the inferior articular processes are embraced by the superior articular processes of the adjacent vertebra.

6. Two transverse processes, homologous with the ribs, situated in front of the articular processes, and rising from the junction of the pedicles and laminæ in the case of the upper three, and from the pedicles in the lower two.

7. The mamillary and accessory processes on each side.

Whereas the thoracic vertebræ have articular facets for the ribs, the lumbar vertebræ have not.

The Intervertebral Fibrocartilages (Disks).—These are interposed between adjacent surfaces of the vertebral bodies. They give the vertebral column its flexibility and constitute about one-quarter the length of the column. Each is composed of :—

1. The nucleus pulposus in the centre, the remains of the notochord. A jelly-like mass existing under considerable tension.

2. The annulus fibrosus, concentric and radial fibres attached to the nucleus centrally.

3. The cartilage plates, above and below the nucleus.

In the lumbar region the disks are wedge-shaped and conform to the lumbar curve.

Nuclear retropulsion may follow a clumsy lumbar puncture. The symptoms are those of sciatica.

Infected intervertebral disk has also been reported. It leads to sinus formation.

Vertebral Column.—This has four curves, of which the thoracic and sacral are primary and are concave anteriorly. In the fœtus there is only one curve with its concavity forward. The cervical and lumbar curves are secondary and are convex anteriorly. The cervical curve is developed when the baby first holds up its head ;

the lumbar, when it begins to walk. The degree of curvature varies in different individuals and is modified by posture; thus, when the spine is fully flexed, the cervical and lumbar curves are obliterated. In the supine position the third lumbar vertebra marks the highest point of the lumbar curve, while the fifth thoracic is the lowest point of the dorsal curve. Kyphosis, lordosis, scoliosis, and hypertrophic arthritis of the spine may upset the curves and make lumbar puncture difficult.

The direction of the spinous processes determines the direction in which the spinal needle must be inserted. The spinous processes of the cervical, the first two thoracic, and the last four lumbar vertebræ are all practically horizontal and are therefore opposite the bodies of their respective vertebræ. The other spinous processes are inclined downwards, their tips being opposite the bodies of the vertebræ next below; exception, the tip of the first lumbar is opposite the intervertebral disk.

The Vertebral Canal.—Bounded in front by bodies of the vertebræ and intervertebral disks; posteriorly by arch which bears spinous processes and by ligaments between them called the interspinous; laterally by pedicles and laminæ. Size and shape vary, but is larger in cervical and lumbar regions.

CONTENTS.—
1. Roots of spinal nerves.
2. Spinal membranes with their enclosed cord and cerebrospinal fluid.
3. Structures—vessels, fat, and areolar tissue of extradural space.

The Vertebral Ligaments bounding the Canal.—
1. SUPRASPINOUS LIGAMENT, passes longitudinally over tips of spinous processes from C.7 to the sacrum.
2. INTERSPINOUS LIGAMENTS, joining spinous processes together.
3. LIGAMENTA FLAVA, running from lamina to lamina, composed of yellow elastic fibres. Half of the substance of the posterior wall of the vertebral canal is composed of the bony laminæ, half by the ligamenta flava. They become progressively thicker from above downwards.
4. POSTERIOR LONGITUDINAL LIGAMENT, within the vertebral canal on posterior surfaces of bodies of vertebræ, from which it is separated by the basivertebral veins.
5. ANTERIOR LONGITUDINAL LIGAMENT, runs along the front of the vertebral bodies to which, as also to the intervertebral disks, it is adherent.

Midline spinal puncture pierces the first three of these. In lateral approach only ligamenta flava are encountered. Bleeding may result from puncture of basivertebral veins.

The Spinal Cord.—The elongated part of the central nervous system which occupies upper two-thirds of vertebral canal and is 45 cm. long. Extent is from upper border of atlas to upper border of second lumbar vertebra, and lower still in infants. Above, continuous with brain; below, ends in conus medullaris, from apex of which filum terminale descends as far as coccyx. In fœtal life length of cord corresponds with that of vertebral canal, but the

The Spinal Cord, *continued.*

canal grows more rapidly than the cord. Thus nerve-roots which pass out transversely in early fœtal life come to be more and more oblique in direction, so that in adult life lumbar and sacral nerves descend almost vertically to meet their foramina, and are known as the cauda equina.

Spinal puncture above the L.2–3 interspace may result in cord injury, but elements of cauda equina, although they may be touched by the point of the needle, are not easily damaged seriously.

The spinal cord is ensheathed by three membranes from without inwards :—

DURA MATER.—A strong fibrous layer forming a tubular sheath attached above to margins of foramen magnum, and ending below at lower border of second sacral vertebra. Separated from bony wall of vertebral canal by the extradural space, which contains fat, areolar tissue, a venous plexus, and the anterior and posterior roots of the spinal nerves. Its main fibres are longitudinal, so the lumbar puncture needle should be introduced with its bevel separating rather than dividing these fibres. Below, the dural sac ends at the level of the second sacral vertebra.

ARACHNOID.—This is a thin transparent sheath closely applied to the dura, the subdural space being merely a capillary layer.

PIA MATER.—This is separated from the arachnoid by the sub-arachnoid space filled with cerebrospinal fluid. Here local analgesic drugs are deposited in spinal analgesia. The pia closely invests the cord and sends delicate septa into its substance. From each lateral surface of the pia mater a fibrous band, the denticulate ligament, projects into the sub-arachnoid space, and is attached by a series of pointed processes to the dura as far down as the first lumbar nerve. The pia mater ends as a prolongation—the filum terminale—which pierces the distal end of the dural sac and is attached to the periosteum of the coccyx.

There are two enlargements of the cord, one in the cervical, the other in the lumbar region, corresponding to the origins of the nerves of the arms and legs.

Spinal Segments.—The cord is divided into segments by the pairs of spinal nerves which arise from it. These pairs are thirty-one in number and are as follows : (*a*) Eight cervical ; (*b*) Twelve thoracic ; (*c*) Five lumbar ; (*d*) Five sacral ; (*e*) One coccygeal.

The nerve-roots within the dura have no epineural sheaths and are therefore easily affected by doses of analgesic drugs brought into contact with them. The cord is not transversely blocked by spinal analgesia, but it is probable that there may be some block of the longitudinal columns by penetration of the drug.

Spinal Nerves.—Thirty-one pairs, each arising from the cord by two groups of fibres called anterior and posterior roots.

Anterior root is efferent and contains fibres subserving :—

1. Motor to voluntary muscles.
2. Pre-ganglionic fibres (sympathetic) from T.1 to L.2 or 3. These later become the white rami communicantes and convey :—

   a. Dilator fibres to pupil (T.1).
   b. Vasoconstrictor fibres to salivary and lacrimal glands (T.1, 2).
   c. Accelerator and augmentor fibres to heart (T.1–4).
   d. Dilator fibres to bronchi (T.1–4).
   e. Vasoconstrictor, pilo-erector, and sudomotor fibres to skin
       of :—
         i. Head and neck (T.1–2).
        ii. Arm (T.2–T.7 to 9).
       iii. Thorax (T.2–12).
        iv. Abdomen (T.4–L.2).
         v. Leg (T.10–L.2).
   f. Inhibitory fibres to muscles of gut (T.4–L.2).
   g. Secretomotor fibres to adrenals (T.12–L.1).
   h. Motor to bladder sphincter and inhibitory to detrusor.
S.2, 3, 4 also have white rami accompanying them, the nervi
   erigentes.

Posterior root is larger than anterior. All the afferent impulses from
   the whole body, including viscera, pass into the posterior roots.
   Each posterior root has a ganglion and conveys fibres of :—
   1. Pain ⎫
   2. Tactile ⎬ These may be coarse (protopathic) or
   3. Thermal sensation ⎭ fine (epicritic).
   4. Deep or muscle sensation from bones, joints, tendons, etc.
   5. Afferents from the viscera (accompanying sympathetic).
   6. Vasodilator fibres.

Pain and temperature fibres enter the posterior horn where they
   end around cells in the grey matter ; fibres then cross to the
   contralateral side within three segments and ascend in the
   lateral spinothalamic tract to the thalamus.

Tactile impulses ascend in the ventral spinothalamic tract to the
   thalamus.

Deep or muscle sensory impulses ascend in the posterior columns
   and spinocerebellar tracts.

Vibration impulses ascend in the posterior columns.

The anterior and posterior roots unite in the intervertebral foramina
   to form the main spinal nerve-trunks, which soon divide into
   anterior and posterior primary divisions—mixed nerves. These
   are blocked only secondarily in spinal analgesia ; it is block of
   the nerve-roots which gives the effect. There is evidence, however, that analgesic drugs after subarachnoid injection can soak
   along the nerve-trunk for as much as 2 cm. beyond the intervertebral foramen. Analgesic drugs affect autonomic, sensory,
   and motor fibres in that order, while fibres which block easily
   hold the drug longest ; thus sensory block lasts longer than
   motor, and usually ascends two segments higher up the cord
   than motor block.

SEGMENTAL LEVELS (*Fig. 33*).—Perineum, S.1–4 ; Inguinal
   region, L.1 ; Umbilicus, T.10 ; Subcostal arch, T.6–8 ; Nipple
   line, T.4, 5 ; Second intercostal space, T.2 ; Clavicle, C.3–4.

The skin above the nipple line has a double innervation, from C.3
   and C.4 and from T.2, T.3, and T.4, so even with a successful
   block to C.8 there will be some sensation above the nipple

Spinal Nerves, *continued.*

line. The success of a block to T.1 is proved by the inability of the patient to hold a sheet of paper between the fingers (innervation of interossei, C.8 and T.1).

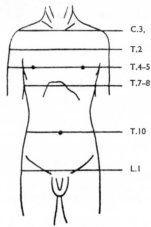

C.3,

T.2

T.4–5

T.7–8

T.10

L.1

Fig. 33.—Segmental levels.

SEGMENTAL LEVELS OF SPINAL REFLEXES.—

Epigastric, T.7, 8	Plantar, S.1, 2
Abdominal, T.9, 12	Knee-jerk, L.2–4
Cremasteric, L.1, 2	Ankle-jerk, S.1, 2

Blood-supply to Spinal Cord.—The posterior spinal arteries, two or three on each side, branch from the posterior inferior cerebellar arteries at the level of the foramen magnum. They supply the posterior columns of the cord.

The anterior spinal artery, a single vessel lying in the substance of the pia mater overlying the anterior median fissure, arises at the level of the foramen magnum from the junction of a small branch from each vertebral artery. It receives communications from the intercostal, lumbar, and other small arteries. It supplies the lateral and the anterior columns. Thrombosis of this artery causes the anterior spinal artery syndrome in which there is paralysis sparing the posterior columns (joint, position, touch, vibration sense). Communicating branches at the level of T.1 and 11 are larger than the others and help to supply the enlargements of the cord (the arteries of Adamkiewicz). The artery at T.11 supplies the cord both upwards and downwards ; that at T.1 only downwards from this level.

The Spinal Veins.—These are gathered together into anterior and posterior plexuses. They drain along the nerve-roots, through the intervertebral foramina and into the vertebral, azygos, and lumbar veins.

Nerve-supply of Meninges.—The posterior aspect of the dura and arachnoid contains no nerve-fibres and so no pain is felt on dural puncture. The anterior aspect is supplied by sinuvertebral nerves; each of these enters an intervertebral foramen and passes up for one segment and down for two segments.*

The Subarachnoid Space.—This is between the arachnoid and the pia mater and in the lumbar region it occupies more than half the anterior-posterior diameter of the vertebral canal. Communicates with the ventricular system of brain by :—

1. Foramen of Magendie, a median opening in the roof of the fourth ventricle.
2. The foramina of Luschka, two small passages in the lateral recesses of the fourth ventricle.
3. The foramina of Key and Retzius in the roof of the fourth ventricle.

The contents of the space are the spinal nerve-roots ; the denticulate ligaments ; a spongy reticulum of fibres connecting the pia to the arachnoid ; the cerebrospinal fluid.

Circulation of Cerebrospinal Fluid.—Called by Harvey Cushing the third circulation. It forms a short circuit between the arterial and venous circulations.

Fluid which is formed by the choroid plexuses in the lateral ventricles passes through, on each side, the foramen of Monro to join that formed by choroid plexuses in the third ventricle ; thence through aqueduct of Sylvius to fourth ventricle. Fluid leaves this for the subarachnoid space through the central foramen of Magendie and the lateral foramina of Luschka, Key, and Retzius and reaches the cisterna magna. It bathes the whole of the central nervous system and is absorbed into the venous sinuses through the arachnoidal villi. This circulation takes no part in spinal analgesia.

Ordinary doses of analgesic drugs injected into the spinal subarachnoid space do not reach the fourth ventricle, which contains in its floor the centres for the heart and for respiration.

The Cerebrospinal Fluid.—

SOURCE.—From the choroid arterial plexuses of the third, fourth, and lateral ventricles, by either secretion or dialysis.

REMOVAL.—Into the venous sinuses of the brain via the arachnoidal villi, and into the lymph-stream via the Pacchionian bodies (described by Antonius Pacchioni in 1705). Movement of the fluid is slow and of no importance in spinal analgesia. When injected into the subarachnoid space, drugs such as procaine are absorbed into the blood-stream.

PHYSICAL CHARACTERISTICS.—Clear and colourless with slight opalescence due to globulin. Sp. gr. at 37° C. is 1003–1009. The density is more dependent on the temperature and on the

---

* Edgar, M. A., and Nundy, S. J., *J. Neurol. Psychiat.*, 1966, **29**, 530.

The Cerebrospinal Fluid, *continued.*

contained sodium, chloride, and carbon dioxide than on the contained protein. Increased in diabetes, uræmia, and old age. Poor in cellular elements, five or less per c.mm. (lymphocytes); an increase of cells indicates meningeal irritation. Quantity, 110–150 ml. Volume of spinal cerebrospinal fluid about 25 ml., 15 ml. of which is below T.5. Pressure, 100–200 mm. of water in the lateral level position, 300–500 mm. of water in vertical position. Owing to hydrostatic pressure of column of fluid, cerebrospinal fluid drips faster from a needle in a sitting patient than from one in a lateral patient. Pressure influenced directly by intracranial venous pressure and by total amount of body fluid. Pressure increased in sleep, uræmia, alcoholism, and cerebral neoplasm ; also in cases of raised CO_2 tension, congestive heart failure, and mediastinal tumour. Factors raising venous pressure such as straining, coughing, etc., will raise the cerebrospinal fluid pressure. Decreased in wasting diseases, traumatic leakage of cerebrospinal fluid, and under the influence of large narcotic doses of barbiturates. Pressure controlled by central hypothalamic mechanism. About 500 ml. can be secreted in 24 hours if there is a free leak from the sub-arachnoid space. Changes in the osmotic pressure of the blood affect cerebrospinal fluid pressure, e.g., intravenous injection of hypertonic saline or glucose lowers cerebrospinal fluid pressure.

CHEMICAL CHARACTERISTICS.—Alkaline, pH 7·6. Protein low, 24–40 mg. per 100 ml. Sugar, 45–80 mg. per cent. Sodium chloride, 750 mg. per cent. (Sodium, 135–147 mEq./l.; chloride, 115–135 mEq./l.); urea, 10–30 mg. per 100 ml.; bicarbonate, 24 mEq./l. Antibodies, etc., not found in cerebrospinal fluid, hence great risks of infection. Drugs are not secreted into it, except urotropine and sulphonamides. After spinal analgesia both albumin and globulin increase. Alkalinity and sugar content lower, magnesium content higher, than in blood. Contains small amounts of cholinesterase, but not sufficient to inactivate such local analgesics as procaine, amethocaine, or lignocaine.

FUNCTIONS.—

1. It is a fluid cushion to protect the brain and spinal cord from trauma.

2. By its absorption and formation, according to need, it regulates the volume of the cranial contents.

3. It has a slight function in the metabolic exchanges of nervous tissue, and may take the place of lymph. Intravenous injection of large amounts of normal saline or distilled water cause a rise in pressure. Intravenous injection of hypertonic solutions, e.g., 20 per cent mannitol (1·5 g. per kg.), 50 ml. of 10 per cent saline, 100 ml. of 25 per cent glucose, or 100 ml. of 50 per cent sucrose, or 30 per cent urea in invert sugar, 1 to 1·5 g. per kg., cause a lowering of pressure.

Non-inflammatory overproduction—liquorrhœa—is seen in cases of nasal sinus infection, in otitis, at high altitudes (hypoxia), and after concussion and lumbar puncture.

The opposite condition is aliquorrhœa and may occur spontaneously in dehydration, or after lumbar puncture.

FACTORS OF SPECIAL SIGNIFICANCE

Spinal Analgesia and Respiration.—In the supine position, even high spinal analgesia (intra- or extradural) has little effect on the respiratory minute volume* perhaps because the lax abdominal wall allows easier descent of the diaphragm which compensates for intercostal paralysis. Only the diaphragm and the fifth to ninth intercostals take part in inspiration at a minute volume of less than 40 l. per min. while at rest; expiration is passive in the absence of obstruction. There is inability to cough forcefully or to raise intrapulmonary pressure.†

The pulmonary blood-volume and pulmonary blood-pressure are reduced, due to an impaired venous return to the right ventricle.

The phrenic nerve supplying the diaphragm rises from the anterior roots of C.3, 4, and 5, and should not be encroached on in spinal analgesia, but phrenic paralysis can occur. Apnœa may be due to medullary ischæmia or to a toxic effect of the drug—in extra-dural blocks.

Spinal Analgesia and Heart-rate.—The cardiac rate is accelerated by stimulation of the cardiac sympathetic nerves. White rami leave the cord with the upper four or five thoracic nerves, run up the sympathetic chain to the cervical region, and then as post-ganglionic fibres after synapsing reach the myocardium as cervical cardiac nerves ; three of these on each side, one from upper, middle, and lower cervical sympathetic ganglia. Other fibres run to corresponding ganglia of sympathetic chain and from there pass as post-ganglionic fibres to the cardiac plexus (thoracic cardiac nerves). Slowing of the heart-rate is caused if any of the anterior roots carrying these fibres is blocked, as may happen in high spinals. A further cause of slow pulse-rate is the lowering of blood-pressure in the right auricle consequent on diminished venous return (Bainbridge effect)‡ (Francis Arthur Bainbridge, 1874–1921). On the other hand, tachycardia during spinal analgesia may result from the operation of Marey's law§ (a pulse of low tension is fast) (Etienne Jules Marey, 1830–1904). Bradycardia is the more frequent effect.

Physical Factors.—Analgesic solutions injected into the subarachnoid space are influenced by :—

  a. Dispersion, i.e., mechanical mixing from force of injection.
  b. Convection, by gravity, e.g., heavy cinchocaine.
  c. Displacement of cerebrospinal fluid by large volumes of fluid (as with hypobaric cinchocaine).
  d. Diffusion, gradual intermingling by osmotic tension, of no practical importance.

Factors influencing Height of Analgesia in Intradural Block.—
  1. POSITION OF PATIENT DURING INJECTION.—Sitting : hyperbaric solutions tend to fall, and hypobaric solutions to rise.

---

  * Moir, D. D., and Mone, J. G., *Brit. J. Anæsth.*, 1964, **36**, 380; and Moir, D. D., *Ibid.*, 1963, **35**, 3.
  † Egbert, L. D., and others, *Anesthesiology*, 1961, **22**, 882.
  ‡ Bainbridge, F. A., *J. Physiol.*, 1914, **48**, 332; and *Ibid.*, 1915, **50**, 65.
  § Marey, E. J., *C.R. Acad. Sci.*, Paris, 1861, **53**, 95.

Height of Analgesia in Intradural Block, *continued.*

Lateral position : unilateral analgesia is more pronounced than bilateral, if injections are made slowly and patient remains on side during fixation of the drug. Gradual spread to the other side usually results.

2. INTERSPACE CHOSEN.—The higher the interspace chosen for injection the higher will be the resulting analgesia, leaving other factors out of account. A good rule is to choose L.2–3 interspace for upper abdominal cases ; L.3–4 interspace for lower abdominal and leg operations ; and the L.4–5 interspace for perineal procedures. In the very tall a space higher is sometimes advantageous, while in the very short, one space lower may be chosen.

3. VOLUME OF FLUID INJECTED.—Height of analgesia is directly proportional to amount of fluid injected.

4. BARBOTAGE (Fr. *barboter*, to dabble, to paddle, to mix, a name given to the method by Le Filliatre in 1920).*—A method of mixing the solution with a greater volume of cerebrospinal fluid than the syringe will hold, and of increasing dispersion. It decreases the concentration and specific gravity of the solution and so lessens the effects of gravity after injection. E.g., if syringe contains 2 ml., withdraw 1 ml. and inject 1·5 ml., withdraw 1 ml. and inject 1·5 ml., withdraw 1 ml. and inject 1·5 ml., etc.

5. DOSE OF DRUG INJECTED.—Nerve tissue absorbs local analgesic drugs as blotting-paper absorbs ink ; a limited amount of nerve tissue can only absorb so much drug, the surplus being available for convection or absorption into the blood-stream. The greater the concentration, the longer will its effect last.

6. FORCE AND RATE OF INJECTION.—Height is directly proportional to this. A slow, gentle injection is necessary to get full benefit of specific gravity differences, as in unilateral blocks.

7. SPECIFIC GRAVITY OF SOLUTION.—The specific gravity of injected solutions should always be known, and they should be classed as hyperbaric, hypobaric, or isobaric. In the case of the first two, subsequent posture has a great influence on the level of analgesia. It requires but a few points difference for the effect of specific gravity to be shown. It is impossible to add any soluble solid to cerebrospinal fluid without raising its specific gravity.

8. POSTURE OF PATIENT AFTER INJECTION.—

If patient remains on the side, curves of spine are without effect, and gravity of solution controls side of analgesia.

If patient is supine :—

a. Hyperbaric solutions pass to the bottom of sacral and dorsal curves ; some of it to both, if injection is made at apex of lumbar curve. Lowest point of dorsal curve coincides with the 6th thoracic vertebra, so upward spread of a reasonable volume of a heavy solution will not occur unless a steep Trendelenburg position is assumed. Similarly, hyperbaric

---

* Le Filliatre, G., *Précis de Rachianesthésie Générale*, 1921. Paris: Librairie Le François.

analgesic fluid placed in the sacral curve cannot spread upwards over the hollow of the back, without a head-down tilt. Thus, for blocks above the perineum with these solutions, the head of the patient should be slightly inclined downwards during injection.

   b. Hypobaric solutions gravitate to the top of the lumbar curve, but few solutions are truly hypobaric.

   c. Isobaric solutions are uninfluenced by gravity, and their maximum effect is at point of injection.

In the lithotomy position lumbar curve is obliterated. In Trendelenburg's position hypobaric solutions travel caudad, while hyperbaric solutions move cephalad. The normal spinal curvature limits this movement. Raising the head and shoulders accentuates the dorsal curve and tends to prevent spread of hyperbaric solutions to the cervical area with its phrenic roots.

As an analgesic solution travels it leaves some of its drug behind fixed to nerve tissue, and thus gradually becomes more dilute. This is the so-called ' brake action '.

Duration of Analgesia.—Depends on the drug used. The upper end of an abdominal incision regains sensation before the lower end. Cinchocaine, bupivacaine* and amethocaine last longer than lignocaine and procaine.

Fixation Time.—For lignocaine about five minutes. For procaine, 3–15 minutes. Amethocaine and cinchocaine take longer. These drugs are eventually absorbed into the blood-stream, ascend via the azygos vein, and are destroyed in the liver.

DRUGS USED TO PRODUCE INTRA- AND EXTRADURAL SPINAL ANALGESIA

(For Pharmacology, *see* Chapter XV)

Cocaine Hydrochloride, B.P.—This was the first drug used, followed by tropacocaine, stovaine, procaine, cinchocaine, amethocaine, piperocaine, and lignocaine.

   Procaine, cinchocaine, amethocaine, and lignocaine are the chief drugs used to-day. Cocaine is now given up entirely for this purpose.

Amylocaine (Stovaine).—First used in spinal analgesia by Henri Chaput in 1905. Was popular for many years, but is now known to be irritating and has lost much of its popularity. It was put up in 2-ml. ampoules containing 5 per cent stovaine in 5 per cent glucose, sp. gr. 1025, dose 1–2 ml.; this is Barker's formula. Chaput's solution was supplied in 1-ml. ampoules containing 10 per cent stovaine in 10 per cent sodium chloride, sp. gr. 1080, the dose being 0·6–1 ml. Contains no *p*-aminobenzoic radical.

Procaine Hydrochloride, B.P. (Ethocaine; Novocain; Neocaine; Syncaine; Scurocaine; Planocaine; Kerocain, etc.).—Synthesized by Einhorn in 1904† and advocated by Braun.‡ Put up in ampoules

---

* Watt, M. J., Ross, D. M., and Atkinson, R. S., *Anæsthesia*, 1968, **23**, 2.
† Einhorn, A., *Dtsch. med. Wschr.*, 1905, **31**, 1668.
‡ Braun, H., *Ibid.*, 1905, **31**, 1667.

Procaine Hydrochloride, *continued.*

containing dry crystals in amounts varying from 50 to 300 mg.; and in solutions of 5 per cent and 10 per cent. Can be autoclaved.* The crystals are dissolved in cerebrospinal fluid and injected, while the 10 per cent solution is usually diluted with an equal volume of cerebrospinal fluid before injection. In 5 per cent strength or less, procaine is not irritating to nervous tissue and meninges. Analgesia lasts from forty to eighty minutes with procaine.

Amethocaine Hydrochloride, B.P. (Tetracaine, U.S.P.; Anethaine; Decicain; Pantocaine; Pontocaine; Butethanol).—Was synthesized in 1928 by O. Eisleb.† Can be autoclaved although it loses some potency,‡ or boiled on one or two occasions but is inactivated by alkalis. Of slower onset, but of longer duration, than procaine, lasting $1\frac{1}{2}$–$2\frac{1}{2}$ hours. Put up in ampoules containing 20 mg. of dried powder, also in solution 1 per cent, each ml. containing 10 mg. Spinal D is a 0·5 per cent solution in 6 per cent glucose, with sp. gr. 1025; spinal D-isotonic is 0·4 per cent amethocaine in 4·6 per cent glucose and distilled water to make up 5 ml., sp. gr. 1018 and pH 5.§ The maximum intrathecal dose is 20 mg. A long-acting drug for extradural block (1–1000 to 1–2000) together with lignocaine 1·5 per cent. Usually combined with dextrose solution to make it hyperbaric.

Cinchocaine Hydrochloride, B.P. (Nupercaine; Percaine; Dibucain, U.S.P.).—This is 2-butoxycinchoninic acid 2-diethylamino ethylamide hydrochloride. Introduced in 1929 by Meischer, is not a cocaine derivative, but it is allied to quinoline. It, too, has a slower onset, but more lasting effect, than procaine, and may give analgesia for $1\frac{1}{2}$–3 hours. Like amethocaine, it is easily destroyed by traces of alkali, so that needles, syringes, etc., should be washed through with cinchocaine solution which is subsequently discarded.

---

* Katz, J., *Anesthesiology*, 1966, **27**, 835.
† Eisleb, O., *Arch. exp. Path. Pharmak.*, 1931, **160**, 53.
‡ Whittet, T. D., *Anæsthesia*, 1952, **9**, 271.
§ Dinsdale, T., *Ibid.*, 1947, **2**, 17.

Alkali causes visible precipitation and cloudiness, which disappears on the addition of weak acid.   Weight for weight it is highly toxic, but not dose for dose.   Can be boiled or autoclaved without decomposition on one or two occasions (autoclaved at 115° C. at 10 lb. pressure for 30 minutes).

Ampoules are of three types :—

a. The 20-ml. ampoule of hypobaric solution, 1–1500 cinchocaine in 0·5 per cent saline, with sp. gr. 1·0036 at 36° C.   Each ampoule contains 13·3 mg. cinchocaine.

b. The 3-ml. ampoule containing 1–200 cinchocaine with 6 per cent glucose, sp. gr. 1024 at 37° C., hyperbaric solution (Silverton, 1934).   Each ampoule contains 15 mg. of cinchocaine.

c. 2-ml. and 3-ml. ampoules of isobaric cinchocaine 1–200 in buffered solution, with sp. gr. 1006 (Keyes and McLellan, 1930).

Lignocaine Hydrochloride, B.P. (Xylocaine; Duncaine; Lidocaine, U.S.P.).—This is ω-diethylamino-2, 6-dimethylacetanilide and was synthesized by Lofgren and Lundqvist in 1943.* It is non-irritating, is stable to autoclaving, and relatively non-toxic. For spinal analgesia has been used in a strength of 5 per cent with dextrose 3·1 per cent, the specific gravity being 1018 and the pH 6·5: 1·5 ml. of this solution gives about 2 hours of good analgesia up to the umbilicus.†

Osmolality of Intradural Spinal Analgesic Solutions.—The normal range of osmolality of c.s.f. is between 257 and 305 milliosmoles per litre at 37° C. It is reasonable to use solutions of local analgesic agents which have an osmotic pressure close to that of c.s.f. to prevent damage to neural tissue. Hyperbaric (0·5 per cent) nupercaine and 1 and 2 per cent lignocaine in saline are in this respect reasonable, but both 5 per cent procaine and 5 per cent lignocaine are (from this point of view only) too concentrated.

---

* Lofgren, N., *Studies on Local Anæsthetics: Xylocaine, a New Synthetic Drug*, 1948. Stockholm: Haeggstroms.
   † Adams, B. W., *Anæsthesia*, 1956, **11**, 297.

Adrenaline.—Added to a solution of local analgesic before injection into the theca it prolongs its action by 50 per cent or more. A recent series of 11,000 cases bears this out.[*] Dosage 0·25 ml. of 1–1000 solution (Braun, 1902). Phenylephrine has also been used successfully for this purpose.[†] Many workers avoid intrathecal adrenaline because of the danger of possible neural ischæmia. Serial injections will also prolong the effect. When adrenaline is added (1–200,000) to lignocaine solution for high extradural blocks the peripheral resistance and mean arterial blood-pressure are decreased: this causes a rise in cardiac output.[‡]

PRELIMINARY MEDICATION

Inadequate premedication during spinal analgesia shows callous unconcern for the patient. It may also wreck the smoothness of an otherwise correct technical procedure.

The rapidly acting barbiturates, pentobarbitone and quinalbarbitone, in doses of 100–200 mg. given 1½–2 hours before operation, are reliable and effective. Because of vasodilatation, they may cause a slight fall in blood-pressure. In addition, morphine, 8–16 mg., with atropine, 0·4–0·8 mg., or with hyoscine, 0·4 mg., are usually given one hour before operation. The ampoule of papaveretum, 20 mg., with hyoscine, 0·4 mg. (or half ampoule), is convenient for this purpose. In patients over 60 hyoscine may cause excitement and is better avoided. Patients who come to the theatre in an anxious state of mind should be helped by further intravenous doses of morphine.

Many anæsthetists prefer to give only light premedication, such as morphine, 10 mg., with hyoscine, 0·4 mg., and to produce sleep during the operation by thiopentone in small doses, supplemented by gas and oxygen or light cyclopropane if necessary.

The phenothiazine drugs give good pre-operative, together with prolonged post-operative sedation, but cause, in addition, hypotension which may require a pressor drug for its control. The authors have found trimeprazine tartrate 25–50 mg. a useful agent for this purpose.

ARMAMENTARIUM

Sterilization is most important and the whole outfit should be dry sterilized by gamma radiation or autoclaved. All-glass syringes are ideal while plastic disposable syringes are excellent. Sterile distilled water must be regarded with suspicion unless it comes from a fresh, previously unopened container. Ampoules should not be stored in spirit or other antiseptic solution, as minute faults in the glass may result in contamination of the contents with untoward results.[§] If the autoclave is used the hydrochloride salts of lignocaine, prilocaine, mepivacaine, and procaine show no chemical change on gas chromatography.[‖] Boiling for

[*] Moore, D. C., and Bridenbaugh, L. D., *J. Amer. med. Ass.*, 1966, **195**, 907.
[†] Meagher, R. P., Moore, D. C., and de Vries, J. C., *Curr. Res. Anesth.*, 1966, **45**, 134.
[‡] Bonica, J. J., and others, *Acta anæsth. scand.*, 1966, Suppl. 23, 429.
[§] Cope, R. W., *Anæsthesia*, 1945, **9**, 249 (description of the "Woolley and Roe Case").
[‖] Katz, J., *Anesthesiology*, 1966, **27**, 835.

five minutes in water cannot be relied on to kill spores. Dry heat is not suitable for ordinary glass and metal syringes. Light and heavy cinchocaine solutions show decreased potency if autoclaved for more than two hours while amethocaine is rather less stable.*

The lumbar puncture needle should be of fine gauge (20–22 gauge) and have a short bevel.

TECHNIQUE OF LUMBAR PUNCTURE
FOR INTRADURAL BLOCK

The lumbar puncture must be done in a good light on a table which can be tilted.

Lumbar puncture is contra-indicated in patients with papilloedema or cerebral oedema, especially as the result of tumours in the posterior fossa.

Puncture in Lateral Position.—The patient should be supported by a nurse and positioned as follows :—

Back to be at edge of table and parallel to it.

Knees to be flexed on to abdomen.

Head to be brought down to knees.

Hips and shoulders to be vertical to table to avoid rotation of vertebral column.

Sudden movement to be avoided.

In unilateral operations patient should lie on diseased side when hyperbaric solutions, on the sound side when hypobaric solutions, are to be used. In the obese the median crease sags downwards sometimes as much as 1 in., so point of needle should be inserted above crease in these cases.

The line joining the highest points of the iliac crests crosses either the spine of the fourth lumbar vertebra or the interspace between L.4 and L.5. Precise identification of the lumbar spines may be impossible, but this does not matter so long as the first lumbar interspace (and those above this level) are avoided. When the chosen interspace is located the intradermal needle is inserted after careful palpation, midway between the two spines, and a small weal of local analgesic solution is raised. The hands of the anæsthetist have been scrubbed up and he has donned a sterile gown and gloves. The back has been painted over a large area with antiseptic and towels arranged suitably. While the skin weal is taking effect, a syringe is filled with analgesic solution. A small incision is made in the skin with a large skin needle to prevent a tough skin from grasping the spinal needle tightly and to prevent a core of skin being carried into the intra- or extradural space with the lumbar puncture needle.†

Some prefer to use a Sise or a Rowbotham introducer as a cannula through which to introduce the spinal needle. The needle is then slowly pushed forwards parallel to the floor and at right-angles to the back, with its bevel in the plane to separate and not to divide the longitudinal fibres of the dura. If bone is

* Whittet, T. D., *Anæsthesia*, 1954, **9**, 271.
† Charlebois, P. A., *Canad. anæsth. soc. J.*, 1966, **13**, 585.

Puncture in Lateral Position, *continued.*

met, withdraw and slightly alter direction either upwards or downwards. The extradural space can be identified in many cases if a drop of analgesic solution is left on the hub of the needle as it is pushed inwards: the negative pressure of the space causes the drop to be indrawn.* From this point, the dura is only a millimetre or two away. When the dura is pierced a click can often be felt. A successful puncture is followed by a free flow of cerebrospinal fluid on withdrawal of the stylet. Flow must be free, not an occasional drop. Rotation of needle and pushing it in an extra millimetre will often ensure a free flow. Blood-stained cerebrospinal fluid is of no importance and usually becomes clear after a few ml. have leaked away. Withdrawal of pure blood shows that needle point is probably in a vein, and another puncture must be made. A dry tap is sometimes, but not always, due to failure to introduce the needle into the subarachnoid space.

Median approach easier than the lateral, but if latter is preferred needle is inserted ½ in. from the midline directly opposite the centre of the interspace, and the needle is inserted at an angle of 25° to the midline. With this approach, flexion of the back is not so important, it is said to cause minimal pain, and tough ligaments are avoided, and so the sense of touch and needle control are more accurate. Sometimes it is successful when attempts using median approach have failed. In very fat patients bony landmarks may be impalpable, and in such cases it is a good plan to raise three weals in the midline 1 cm. apart. If bone is struck when needle is inserted through one weal a successful puncture may be made if the others are used in turn. Another method to facilitate puncture in obese patients has been described,† the needle entering the relatively large space between the fifth lumbar vertebra and the sacrum. A weal is raised 1 cm. medial and 2·5 cm. superior to the medial superior aspect of the posterior superior iliac spine : this point is 1·5 cm. lateral to the midpoint of the lumbosacral interspace and from it a needle is advanced 25° to the midline. This approach may also be used for lumbar extradural blocks. If the needle touches a root of the cauda equina the patient will complain of pain, probably in the leg ; usually no harm results from this, but if injection of the drug causes pain the position of the needle should be slightly altered. It shows that the needle point is within the vertebral canal and has pierced the ligamentum flavum. If failure results from puncture in one interspace it can often be made successfully if an adjacent interspace is used.

Puncture in the Sitting Position.—Many workers find this easier than the lateral. Patient is placed across the table with his feet resting comfortably on a stool ; spine should be flexed with chin pressed on to sternum. Flexion of the spine rather than flexion

---

* Gutierriez, A., *Rev. Cirug., B. Aires*, 1932, **12**, 665.
† Surks, S. N., and Wood, Paul, *Anesthesiology*, 1951, **12**, 239.

of the hips is the aim. Puncture in this position is required for Etherington Wilson's technique with hypobaric solutions, while it is convenient when block of the sacral roots is to be done, although this latter block can be done equally well if the puncture is made with the patient in the lateral position, provided that the caudal end of the patient is tipped downwards.

Puncture in the lumbar region requires no after-treatment other than a dab with antiseptic to the skin. Infection does not occur in the skin and subcutaneous tissues.

INJECTION OF THE ANALGESIC DRUG

The prepared solution is drawn up in correct amount into a suitably graduated syringe. It is beneficial to rinse out the syringe first with some of the solution, which is later discarded. When crystals are used, cerebrospinal fluid is allowed to drip into the ampoule, and, after solution has taken place, the fluid is re-injected. During injection, occasional aspiration of a small quantity of cerebrospinal fluid confirms that all of the solution reaches the subarachnoid space. The needle should remain in situ for a few seconds after injection to prevent leak of analgesic solution through the dural puncture hole.

If the height of analgesia is to be controlled by the time a patient remains tilted, levelling off should take place when sensory loss reaches two spinal segments below the desired level. This allows for a little spread with advancing time. For almost any work inside the abdominal cavity, except with the most gentle surgeons, analgesia should reach to the subcostal arch (T.6–8), so that the table can be levelled when analgesia reaches the umbilicus (T.10). Upper abdominal procedures require block to T.2–5. The cough test is useful in estimating height of analgesia. The patient is asked to cough : the relaxed part of the abdomen bulges out, and any segment not relaxed remains firm and rigid. Disappearance of the knee-jerks shows block at least up to L.2.

SERIAL OR CONTINUOUS SPINAL (INTRADURAL) ANALGESIA

Introduced by Lemmon, a Philadelphia surgeon, in 1940.* The method is very useful when either the scope or the duration of the operation is uncertain. It enables minimal dosage to be given without fear of inadequate analgesia, and so is desirable in the aged, the very young, and the physically handicapped. In ill patients, a short-acting agent such as procaine hydrochloride 5 per cent, dissolved either in cerebrospinal fluid or saline, is useful.† Over 2000 consecutive cases were reported by Lemmon, with only one of them requiring supplementary anæsthesia. Originally, the needle remained in situ during the operation and projected into a gap in a specially designed mattress. Tuohy modified the technique.‡ He inserted a special lumbar puncture

* Lemmon, W. T., *Ann. Surg.*, 1940, **111**, 141.
† Lee, J. A., *Lancet*, 1943, **2**, 156.
‡ Tuohy, E. B., *Surg. Clin. N. Amer.*, 1945, **111**, 141.

Serial Spinal Analgesia, *continued.*

needle which is very slightly angulated at its point (Huber poin
Through it he put in a plastic catheter and directed it either caud
or cephalad by means of the direction of the angulation of the need
When an inch or two of catheter was inside the theca, the needle w
withdrawn over it and a syringe connected to the other end of t
catheter by a fine needle. No special mattress is required. The effec
of the analgesic can be rapidly removed by saline irrigations of t
subarachnoid space.

SPECIMEN TECHNIQUES

1. Heavy Cinchocaine.—

Before injection the cinchocaine solution may be diluted with
equal or greater volume of cerebrospinal fluid in the syringe.

a. LOW SPINAL.—A small volume of hyperbaric solution spre
by gravity and inclination of spine.

Block of S.2–S.5 (piles, anal fissure, etc.).—Lumbar puncture
L.4–5 interspace ; patient sitting or lying lateral with defini
caudad tilt; injection of 0·6 ml. with an equal volume of c.s
slowly, so that it trickles slowly into the bottom of the su
arachnoid space. After one minute patient can lie supine,
lumbar curve prevents spread upwards.

Block of S.1–S.5 (urethra, bladder-neck, prostate, etc.).—Lumb
puncture, L.3–4 interspace ; patient sitting or lying on sid
with caudad tilt; injection of 1 ml. with an equal volume
c.s.f. slowly, and patient lies level after one minute.

Block of L.1–S.5, i.e., of lumbar and sacral plexuses.—For un
lateral analgesia, sound side upwards ; puncture in L.3-
interspace ; patient in lateral position with spine leve
Inject 1·4–1·6 ml. with an equal volume of c.s.f. slowly ar
maintain lateral position for five to fifteen minutes. Unilater
analgesia gradually spreads to the other side unless patie
is maintained in lateral position throughout operatio
Suitable for operations on leg.

For bilateral blocks make injection with spine tilted 5°, hea
down, to prevent solution from accumulating in sacr
curve. Immediately after injection turn patient on
back and level table.

b. MID-SPINAL.—For lower abdominal analgesia (T.7–8 to L.4
Puncture, L.3–4 interspace ; patient in lateral position wit
spine showing 5° head-down tilt. Inject 1·4 to 1·8 ml. with a
equal volume of c.s.f. solution and maintain position for fiv
minutes for unilateral cases. For bilateral and intra-abdomin
cases patient turned supine after injection and tilt maintained

c. HIGH SPINAL.—For upper abdominal analgesia (T.2–5 to L.4
Puncture, L.2–3 interspace ; patient in lateral position with
head-down tilt of spine. Inject 2 ml. with an equal volume
c.s.f. solution using a little barbotage. After injection, patie
turned supine and tilt maintained. No steep tilt allowed fc
15 minutes after injection. Any excess solution pools at botto
of thoracic curve opposite roots of T.5.

2. Hypobaric Cinchocaine.—

    a. HOWARD JONES'S TECHNIQUE.*—Depends on displacement of cerebrospinal fluid by a large volume of analgesic solution, plus gravity to keep the solution in the desired place. Height of analgesia largely dependent on volume of solution injected. Cinchocaine and syringe should be warmed to body temperature. Patient lateral with affected side uppermost. Puncture, L.2–3 or L.3–4. Inject solution slowly, withdrawing a drop after each 3 ml. to see that needle point is still in place. To calculate dosage, measure spine from C.7 (vertebra prominens) to inter-cristal line. It varies between 15 in. and 20 in. In males, this distance in inches, minus 4, gives number of ml. to be injected to give analgesia to T.5. In females, subtract 6 from the figure in inches. Thus, 18 ml. is maximum dose. A rough guide is to inject 10–12 ml. for block to T.10 ; 12–14 ml. for block to T.7–8 ; 15–18 ml. for upper abdominal block T.2–5. For block of sacral nerves alone inject 6 ml. at L.4–5 interspace. The needle is withdrawn after injection and patient is turned on to face to ensure soaking of posterior nerve-roots. He is returned to supine position after six minutes, with table in slight Trendelenburg position, which is maintained throughout operation. If spine is kyphotic, tilt must be more pronounced. For sacral block, prone position is unnecessary.

Macintosh† gives good reasons for assuming that the 1–1500 solution of cinchocaine should be regarded as isobaric at room temperature and advises that it can be injected unheated with the patient in any posture, after which he is positioned for operation. He believes it acts purely by volumetric displacement if this technique is followed.

    A good result follows fairly rapid injection of the solution, with immediate assumption of supine position with slight head-down tilt. Good analgesia for upper abdominal operations is accompanied by inability to sit up or to cough effectively. There is loss of sensation as far as the nipple line or just above it.

    b. ETHERINGTON-WILSON'S TECHNIQUE.‡—Depends on timing the ascent of the light solution up the vertebral canal with the patient sitting upright. A standard dose of 13–14 ml. is injected at the L.4–5 interspace. A measurement between the spine of T.4 and the interiliac line is made with patient vertical ; this gives the high spinal run. It is simpler to measure from C.7 to the interiliac line and then subtract 4 in., the average distance between the spines of C.7 and T.4. Having got the high spinal run in inches, multiply it by the factor 5, and the resulting number is the time in seconds that the patient remains sitting after the start of the injection. This gives analgesia to T.5 or a little above. Injection must take 15 seconds, timing it by a stop-watch, and the patient is turned to the supine position smoothly but swiftly, with an 8° head-down tilt,

  * Jones, H., *Brit. J. Anæsth.*, 1930, **7**, 99.

  † Macintosh, R. R., *Lumbar Puncture and Spinal Analgesia*, 1951. Edinburgh : E. & S. Livingstone.

  ‡ Etherington-Wilson, W., *Proc. R. Soc. Med.*, 1933, **27**, 323 ; and *Ibid.*, 1944, **38**, 109.

Hypobaric Cinchocaine, *continued.*

immediately at the conclusion of the calculated number
seconds. After lumbar puncture, the flexed back is exten
so that the patient sits bolt upright. The solution is warn
to body-heat before injection.

For mid-spinals (T.10) patient remains sitting for three-quart
of the time for high block, while for low blocks the figur
divided by one-half. Thus, if distance between C.7 and L.
is 20 in., 20 minus 4 gives a high spinal run of 16. T
multiplied by factor 5 gives a time of 80 sec. for a high spin
three-quarters of 80, i.e., 60 sec., for a mid-spinal ; half
80, i.e., 40 sec., for a low block. The author of this techni
claimed for it 85 per cent of perfect results.

c. LAKE TECHNIQUE.*—This with the Howard Jones a
Etherington Wilson techniques are seldom used to-day.

UNILATERAL ANALGESIA WITH HYPOBARIC CINCH
CAINE.—Patient placed in lateral position, side to be opera
on uppermost. Warmed (105° F.) cinchocaine solution, 12-
ml., injected in L.2-3 interspace. Lateral position maintai
with slight head-down tilt. This method was described
Harris and Rink in 1937† and was recommended for operati
on the kidney. Flaccidity of gluteal muscles of upper butt
indicate a successful result.

3. Amethocaine Hydrochloride.—This is used as crystals dissol
in cerebrospinal fluid ; as 1 per cent solution either alone or mi
with 10 per cent glucose ; as 1 per cent solution in 6 per c
glucose, when it can be treated for dosage like hyperbaric cincl
caine (Silverton's solution). When 1 per cent solution is mi
with one and a half parts of 10 per cent glucose, sp. gr. of mixt
is 1013. Popular in the U.S.A.

a. SISE'S TECHNIQUE.‡—Draw correct amount of 1 per cent so
tion into 5-ml. syringe (1 ml. = 10 mg.) and add 3 ml. 10
cent glucose solution. Puncture in L.3-4 interspace and
jection made in 30 seconds. Table put into 10° Trendelenbu
and patient turned supine ; one minute from time injection w
started, lessen tilt to 5°. In a further minute, table levelled
and height of analgesia tested. Patient's head and neck rais
on sandbag throughout proceedings. If, on testing, level is t
high or too low, alter tilt accordingly for a minute and re-t
before levelling off. Never leave patient in a tilted position f
more than one minute without testing level of analgesia. F
blocks of lumbar and sacral nerves alone, after patient is turn
on to back, table is put into reverse Trendelenburg tilt of 3-
and there maintained. Dosage is based on size and conditi
of patient. Small dose for frail, old, small patient ; large do
for tough, tall, young patient ; medium dose for average patien
For operations on anus : amethocaine, 8, 7, 6 mg. (according
type).

* Lake, N. C., *Lancet*, 1938, **2**, 241 ; and *Ibid.*, 1958, **1**, 387.
† Harris, T. A. B., and Rink, E. H., *Guy's Hospital Reports*, 1937, **87**, 1.
‡ Sise, L. F., *Surg. Clin. N. Amer.*, 1935, **15**, 1501.

For operations on perineum, bladder, legs, vagina : 14, 12, 10 mg.

For hernia and appendix operations : 16, 14, 12 mg.

For lower abdominal operations : 18, 16, 14 mg.

For upper abdominal operations : 20, 17, 14 mg.

b. Amethocaine crystals dissolved in cerebrospinal fluid make a slightly hyperbaric solution. Dosage is one-tenth that of procaine.

c. SPINAL " D " HEAVY.—Ampoules of 3 ml. of 0·5 per cent amethocaine with 6 per cent glucose ; sp. gr. 1035.

For perineal block—1·5 ml. injected with caudal end of theca below head end.

For lower abdominal block—2 ml. injected in lateral position with head end of spine tilted slightly downward (8°). Patient placed in supine position with tilt maintained, but with head raised on pillow.

For upper abdominal block—2·5 ml. injected in lateral position with head end of spine tilted slightly downward. Patient then placed supine with tilt maintained and head raised on pillow.

d. SPINAL " D " ISOTONIC.*—Amethocaine 0·4 per cent, dextrose 4·6 per cent, and water to 5 ml. Sp. gr. 1018 and pH 5.

4. Lignocaine.—Solution of 5 per cent with dextrose 3·1 per cent has a pH of 6·5 and sp. gr. of 1018 and is a satisfactory agent for spinal analgesia with rapid onset and two hours' duration. Should be diluted with cerebrospinal fluid before injection. Has been recommended for endoscopic prostatectomy, given with the patient sitting, in a dose of 1·5 ml. when analgesia should extend to about T.10.† The 5 per cent solution is more potent than 0·5 per cent cinchocaine solution and it tends to give a higher block because of diffusion within the subarachnoid space. It may result in a complete and unpleasant numbness with absolute loss of the sense of touch.‡

Total Spinal Analgesia.—This was used by Le Filliatre in 1921§ and by Koster in 1928‖ and was re-introduced by Griffiths and Gillies of Edinburgh¶ as a method of providing the surgeon with an almost bloodless operation field. The technique causes block of all the vasoconstrictors (T.1–L.2) together with analgesia and relaxation. Procaine 150–200 mg. dissolved in 4 or 5 ml. of cerebrospinal fluid with a steep head-down tilt, or heavy cinchocaine, are the drugs used and general anæsthesia is induced by thiopentone and maintained with nitrous oxide and plenty of oxygen, allowing spontaneous respiration to be a guide to the oxygenation of the medullary centres. It is stated that the generalized vasodilatation and full oxygenation prevent either tissue or parenchymatous organ damage, including the kidneys and heart. Posture is

* Dinsdale, T., *Anæsthesia*, 1947, **2**, 17.

† Adams, B. W., *Ibid.*, 1956, **11**, 297.

‡ Walker, O., *Brit. J. Anæsth.*, 1957, **29**, 512.

§ Le Filliatre, G., *Précis de Rachianesthésie Générale*, 1921. Paris: Libraire Le François.

‖ Koster, H., *Amer. J. Surg.*, 1928, **5**, 554.

¶ Griffiths, H. W. C., and Gillies, J., *Anæsthesia*, 1948, **3**, 134.

Total Spinal Analgesia, *continued.*

employed : (1) to ensure adequate blood-supply to the brain the head down-tilted ; (2) to allow drainage of blood into depen parts, such as the lower limbs.

Contra-indications to total spinal analgesia might include :—

1. Conditions interfering with coronary blood-flow : (*a*) Coro disease ; (*b*) Aortitis ; (*c*) Aortic valvular disease ; (*d*) Cer cases of congenital heart disease.
2. Severe anæmia.
3. Conditions associated with low blood-volume : (*a*) Sho (*b*) Malnutrition ; (*c*) Toxic states.
4. Conditions interfering with oxygenation : (*a*) Respira obstruction ; (*b*) Severe emphysema.
5. Conditions causing decrease in cerebral blood-flow—arte sclerosis.

A pressor drug to raise the blood-pressure should be given* if t is :—

1. Alteration in rate or rhythm of respiration.
2. Increase in the arteriolar-capillary refill time.
3. Sudden fall in blood-pressure after stabilization.
4. Cyanosis in the presence of adequate respiration.

While this technique was an important advance in its day it is sel employed now.

CONDUCT OF THE ANALGESIA

The patient should usually be lightly asleep, if not he should be m comfortable on the table. Blood-pressure apparatus to be fixed arm. The oscillometer is very useful as no stethoscope is needed, v its tendency to slip out of place. During the procedure the patient r require his lips moistened or his face fanned. Nausea may someti be controlled by deep mouth-breathing. If analgesia ascends high the body, consciousness may be lost, as afferent impulses reaching cortex become fewer and fewer. Apparatus for general anæsthesia for oxygen therapy should be at hand, as also should suitable pres drugs. *There must always be an open vein.* It is the duty of the anæsthe to exercise constant vigilance—of the circulation and of the respirati

COMPLICATIONS IN THE CONSCIOUS PATIENT DURING SPINAL ANALGESIA

(1) Nausea. (2) Vomiting. (3) Headache. (4) Precordial discomf (5) Paræsthesiæ in the limbs. (6) Difficulty in phonation. (7) Hy tension. (8) Restlessness.

EFFECTS OF SPINAL ANALGESIA, BOTH INTRA- AND EXTRADURAL

Nervous System.—

ORDER OF BLOCKING NERVE-FIBRES.—(1) Autonomic p ganglionic B fibres. (2) Temperature fibres—cold before wa (3) Pinprick fibres. (4) Fibres conveying pain greater t pinprick. (5) Touch fibres. (6) Deep pressure fibres. (7) Som

---

* Griffiths, H. W. C., and Gillies, J., *Anæsthesia,* 1948, **3,** 134.

motor-fibres. (8) Fibres conveying vibratory sense and proprioceptive impulses.

During recovery, return of sensibility is in the reverse order.

For work on the susceptibility of nerve-fibres to analgesic solution *see* Nathan, P. W., and Sears, T. A., *Anæsthesia*, 1963, **18**, 467.

Phantom limb pain can occur in patients who have suffered from such pains and may require morphine or even general anæsthesia for its relief. The pain finally eases off when numbness disappears. Painless phantom sensations are not uncommon.* They are related to the position of the limb at the time of the motor blockade, and do not occur if the patient is supine with outstretched limbs at this time. Spinal analgesia may also exacerbate pain in patients who have a severe pain in a limb, e.g., sciatica (Gwendolen Harrison, 1951,† and Leatherdale‡). In spinal analgesia, entirely adequate for surgery of a lower limb, a patient may complain of pain due to the tourniquet. A concentration of a solution of local analgesic drug may give excellent analgesia for ordinary sensation, conveyed by small nerve-fibres, but may not be adequate to block transmission in larger fibres transmitting pressure-pain sensation. An increased concentration will avoid this. Another explanation of bizarre pains occurring during otherwise adequate low spinal analgesia may be that some pain fibres pass in sympathetic nerves to reach the cord at a higher level.§

Injection of local analgesic solution into the extradural space may cause headache and vertigo. Absorption of drug from this solution or its direct intravascular injection may result in disorientation, psychic abnormalities, and twitching or convulsions. The last should be treated by intravenous barbiturate.‖

Cardiovascular System.—There are four different ways in which spinal block can influence the cardiovascular system: (1) Vasodilatation of resistance and capacitance vessels; (2) Block of cardiac efferent sympathetic fibres from T.4 to T.1 resulting in bradycardia and interference with cardiac output; (3) Depression of vascular smooth muscle and β-adrenergic blockade of myocardium with fall in cardiac output, following systemic absorption of the local analgesic drug; (4) Adrenaline effect (if present) following absorption, resulting in β-stimulation and associated rise in cardiac output and reduction in peripheral resistance.

The chief effect is hypotension due to pre-ganglionic block of sympathetic fibres running with the anterior roots across the subarachnoid or extradural space. The resulting vasodilatation markedly reduces the peripheral resistance in accordance with the law of Poiseuille.¶ This states that in laminar flow in tubes the flow-rate is directly proportional to the perfusion pressure but

* Prevoznik, S. J., and Eckenhoff, J. E., *Anesthesiology*, 1964, **25**, 767.
† Harrison, G., *Anæsthesia*, 1951, **6**, 115.
‡ Leatherdale, R. A. L., *Ibid.*, 1956, **11**, 249.
§ de Jong, R. H., and Cullen, S. C., *Anesthesiology*, 1963, **24**, 628.
‖ Mark, L. C., and others, *J. Clin. Neurophysiol.*, 1964, **16**, 280.
¶ Poiseuille, J. L. M., *C. R. Acad. Sci., Paris*, 1840, **11**, 1041.

Cardiovascular System, *continued.*

proportional to the fourth power of the diameter. Small variations in vessel calibre can compensate in individual organs. The tone of the myocardium and the blood-volume are not altered by the block.

Pulse-rate usually slowed, associated with hypotension (Bainbridge reflex). Sometimes due to block of cardiac sympathetic (accelerator) fibres, T.1–T.4. Hypotension sometimes causes tachycardia via the sinus reflex, but if block is high, efferent pathway of this reflex arc is paralysed.

Blood-pressure fall is usually shown in the first twenty minutes after injection. Spinal analgesia, by reducing the venous return to the heart, results in a reduction of blood to the coronary vessels which, if they are atheromatous, may prove serious.

THEORIES OF CAUSATION OF FALL IN BLOOD-PRESSURE.—

a. Diminished cardiac output consequent on reduction of venous return to heart, due to muscular paralysis and lack of muscular propulsive force on veins and to quiet breathing due to intercostal paralysis and consequent lack of activity of thoracic pump.

b. Dilatation of post-arteriolar capillaries due to paralysis of vasoconstrictors. It is seen in entire vascular area, somatic and visceral, where anterior roots are paralysed, together with their sympathetic vasoconstrictor fibres. Compensatory vasoconstriction takes place in areas not anæsthetized via sinus reflexes. In high spinal blocks, majority of vasoconstrictor fibres—including those to arm (T.2–10)—are paralysed, hence low blood-pressure. As a concentration of solution (e.g., procaine 0·2 per cent) less than that required to cause muscular relaxation or analgesia will produce sympathetic block, vasoconstrictor paralysis is often complete even if sensory block is only up as high, say, as T.4. The warm, dry arm with dilated veins is often seen in cases of high spinal analgesia.

c. Splanchnic dilatation.

d. Paralysis of sympathetic nerve-supply to adrenal glands (splanchnic nerves), with consequent catecholamine depletion.

e. Absorption of drug into circulation. This is much more likely to be a cause of hypotension after extradural than after intradural analgesia because of the larger amount of analgesic drug injected.

f. Ischæmia and hypoxia of vital centres.

Spinal analgesia may not cause much fall in blood-pressure in the absence of surgical stimuli or bodily movement. Blood-pressure drop below 80 systolic and 60 diastolic should be taken notice of, while systolic blood-pressure below 50 is unsatisfactory. Blood-pressure and pulse-rate usually fall together. There is no hæmoconcentration as in true shock. A palpable superficial temporal artery is a reassuring sign, while a palpable carotid pulse accompanied by adequate tidal exchange indicates that the patient is not gravely collapsed.

TREATMENT OF LOWERED BLOOD-PRESSURE (If thought to be necessary).—Intravenous fluid; oxygen inhalations;

Trendelenburg position; injection of pressor drug; elevation of the legs. When there is bradycardia, atropine 0·2 mg. alone will often elevate blood-pressure. When hypotension is accompanied by bradycardia, phenylephrine and methoxamine are probably better avoided, unless accompanied by atropine. Some or all of these should be used prophylactically in high blocks and other cases judged to be doubtful risks. It has been recently suggested that ephedrine, to increase the cardiac output and venous return, is a more satisfactory drug than methoxamine, etc.* Blood-pressure and pulse-rates should be charted on record cards at frequent intervals during the operation.

The vasoconstrictor reflex produced by hæmorrhage is abolished by spinal block, in proportion to the height of the block, so that the patient is unable to protect himself against this stress.

Respiratory System.—During spinal analgesia, breathing always becomes slow and shallow, depending on the extent of motor block. Intercostal paralysis is compensated for by increased descent of the diaphragm which is made easier by the lax abdominal walls. Formerly this was thought to be accompanied by hypoxia and accumulation of carbon dioxide in the tissues. Recent work has not supported this.† Falls of mean expiratory reserve volume up to 48 per cent after intradural and up to 21 per cent after extradural block have been reported, while mean inspiratory capacity was little affected.‡ If there is any effect on the phrenic roots, patient cannot talk, but can whisper. Such a condition requires oxygen immediately. Oxygen therapy is beneficial in high block as it decreases heart-rate and cardiac output and increases total peripheral resistance.§ Breathing is quiet and in bronchospastic conditions there is some reflex bronchodilatation from stimulation of pressor receptors in the aorticocarotid sinuses by hypotension. There is decreased pulmonary blood-volume and pulmonary arterial blood-pressure from reduced venous return to the right heart. In extradural block there may be hypopnœa passing imperceptibly into apnœa, perhaps a toxic manifestation of the injected local analgesic drug. Should respiratory paralysis occur, efficient artificial respiration must be started, using the anæsthetic machine, a mechanical respirator, or mouth-to-mouth breathing.

Post-operatively, respiratory function is better if the pain of the operation is relieved by spinal block, rather than by centrally acting analgesics. There is less alveolar collapse and consequent physiological shunting which may arise from shallow breathing.

Gastro-intestinal System.—No effect on the œsophagus, the innervation of which is vagal. The small gut is contracted as the sympathetic dilator impulses are removed, the vagus being all-powerful.

* Cain, W. E., and Hamilton, W. K., *Anesthesiology*, 1966, **27**, 209.
† Moir, D. D., *Brit. J. Anæsth.*, 1963, **35**, 3; Moir, D. D., and Mone, J. G., *Ibid.*, 1964, **36**, 380; Askrog, V. F., and others, *Surg. Gynec. Obstet.*, 1964, **119**, 563; de Jong, R. H., *J. Amer. med. Ass.*, 1965, **191**, 698; and Ward, R. J., Bonica, J. J., and others, *Ibid.*, 1965, **191**, 275.
‡ Freword, F. G., and others, *Anesthesiology*, 1967, **28**, 834.
§ Ward, R. J., and others, *Curr. Res. Anesth.*, 1965, **45**, 140.

Gastro-intestinal System, *continued.*

Sphincters are relaxed and peristalsis is active although not mor frequent. Handling of the small bowel by the surgeon may caus it to dilate, as may the injection of atropine before operation Nausea and vomiting due to the hypotension may occur an usually come on in waves lasting a minute or so and then passin; away spontaneously. The spleen enlarges two or three times i; high block, when its sympathetic efferent fibres (splanchnic nerves are paralysed. Stimuli arising in the upper abdomen may ascen along the unblocked vagi and perhaps the phrenics, and caus discomfort if the patient is conscious. Para-œsophageal infiltration of local analgesic solution will prevent this. It blocks vaga afferents.

THEORIES OF CAUSATION OF NAUSEA AND VOMITING.—
  a. Hypotension.
  b. Increased peristalsis.
  c. Traction on nerve-endings and plexuses, especially via vagus.
  d. Presence of bile in stomach due to relaxation of pyloric an bile-duct sphincters.
  e. Morphine or pethidine (premedication).
  f. Psychic factors.
  g. Hypoxia.

TREATMENT consists in attending to the hypotension and hypoxia if present; deep breathing through the mouth; reassurance anc attention to general comfort; supplementary anæsthesia witl thiopentone and nitrous-oxide–oxygen, or cyclopropane, etc., i; the condition persists or if the surgeon's work is being interfered with.

Endocrine System.—Whereas operations under general anæsthesia cause a rise in the blood steroids and an eosinopenia, this is not sc under block analgesia. (After operation the blood steroids rise equally in the two cases.) This may be because afferent impulses from the site of operation are prevented by the block from reach-ing the neurosecretory centre in the ventral hypothalamus which controls the release of ACTH from the anterior pituitary, and sc an increased level of 17-hydroxycorticosteroids does not occur.*

Does this suggest that block protects the patient against the stress of operation?

Genito-urinary System.—Sympathetic supply to kidneys from T.11 to L.1, via the lowest splanchnic nerves.

Effects due to hypotension. Below 80 mm. Hg renal flow is reduced but does not cease until blood-pressure has fallen to about 15 mm. Hg. These changes are transient and disappear when blood-pressure rises again. Not known how low blood-pressure can be allowed to fall without permanent damage. Sphincters of bladder not relaxed, so soiling of table by urine is not seen, and tone of ureters not greatly altered. The penis is often engorged and flaccid due to paralysis of the nervi erigentes (S.2 and 3); this is a useful positive sign of successful block.

* Virtue, R. W., and others, *Surgery*, 1957, **41**, 549; and Hammond, W. G., and others, *Ann. Surg.*, 1958, **148**, 199.

Spermatorrhœa is sometimes seen. Block of the nerves from T.11 downwards results in painless labour.

The tone of the uterus is not greatly altered after spinal analgesia in pregnancy, so that this and extradural block are not contra-indicated then.

In late pregnancy, smaller doses of analgesic solution are required.*

Body Temperature.—Vasodilatation favours heat loss; absence of sweating favours hyperpyrexia in hot environments. Catecholamine secretion is depressed, hence less heat is produced by metabolism.

Broken Needles.—If a needle breaks, the proximal part and the stylet should, if possible, be left in place to serve as a guide to distal part. If proximal part has already been removed, another needle is thrust along the track of the first one for purposes of localization. Removal should be attempted at once. With patient prone, a portable X-ray may be helpful.

DIFFICULTIES AND COMPLICATIONS

The Intradural Spinal that does not take.—Usual cause is failure to deposit all of the analgesic solution in the proper part of the subarachnoid space. May be due to difficulty with lumbar puncture; displacement of needle point, after successful puncture, by the syringe, movement, etc.; use of a long-bevelled needle which allows part of the solution to be injected inside, part outside, the sub-arachnoid space; faults in the use of gravity, tilts, dosage, etc., to control level of block; faults in the solution, alkalinization, etc.; idiosyncrasy, or the so-called rachi-resistance. This last is a definite entity. It may be impossible to aspirate cerebrospinal fluid from a needle, the point of which is truly in the subarachnoid space, the patient being in the lateral position.

If an *extradural block* does not come on after the injection of a reasonable amount of local analgesic solution, the injection has gone astray.

Treatment of Collapse during Spinal Analgesia (Intradural and Extradural).—Turn patient on to back (except in patients in advanced pregnancy or with large abdominal tumours which may cause pressure on the vena cava and interfere with venous return to the heart—in these cases a bolster placed under the right flank may relieve pressure on the vessel). The anæsthetist, the assistant, and the surgeon each has a task to perform. The anæsthetist must see that adequate amounts of oxygen get into the alveoli. The assistant, after lowering the head of the table, gets an intravenous drip going, and administers a pressor drug intra-venously. Lowering head of table raises central blood-pressure and increases venous return to heart, while elevation of the legs increases the volume of circulating blood. The surgeon confirms the absence of the heart-beat, applies external cardiac massage, if necessary, and if the abdomen is open he massages the heart through the left diaphragm using a strong compression and a

* Bromage, P. R., *Brit. J. Anæsth.*, 1962, **34**, 161.

Treatment of Collapse, *continued.*

quick release if no aortic pulsation or cardiac activity is palpa
Transthoracic cardiac massage is preferable and should not
delayed if after one minute the transabdominal massage fails
restore cardiac activity.

The causes of mortality in spinal analgesia are :—

a. Lowering of blood-pressure to point where coronary arteries
not adequately perfused.

b. Hypoxia of vital centres.

c. Progressive upward paralysis of respiratory mechanism. Ha
should not occur as intermittent positive-pressure ventilat
will carry the patient on until the paralysis wears off.

d. Occasional toxic reaction to drugs injected in extradural blc

Sequelæ.—

1. HEADACHE.—Only seen after intradural block, never a
extradural. This is the most frequent after-effect, occurr
in 3–20 per cent of patients. Never present during the ope
tion, usually coming on in first three post-operative da
Usually worse in sitting position and frequent after sm
operations such as piles. Often occipital and associated w
pain and stiffness in neck ; may be vertical or frontal. He
aches are not rare after simple lumbar puncture. Sicard f
suggested in 1902 that cause might be leakage of cerebrospi
fluid into extradural space. A patent needle track has b
shown in dura at necropsy eleven days after puncture. L
of up to 10 ml. of fluid during lumbar puncture probably l
no effect on subsequent headaches.

Puncture with an unflexed back may reduce the incidence of he
aches as the dural hole is not stretched open.

DIAGNOSIS.—A post-spinal headache is probably caused by
method of analgesia if:—

a. It is different from any headache previously experienced
the patient.

b. It is initiated or made worse by adoption of the sitting
erect posture.

c. It has occipital and nuchal components.

d. It is relieved by abdominal compression—which raises
venous pressure.

THEORIES OF CAUSATION.—

a. Low cerebrospinal fluid pressure. The theory which is m
popular to-day is that the choroid plexus is unable
secrete sufficient fluid to maintain the cerebrospinal fl
pressure, and this is made worse by all conditions produc
fluid loss, e.g., hæmorrhage, vomiting, sweating, lactati
etc. The rate of leakage of cerebrospinal fluid exceeds
rate of formation, and this results in changes in the hyd
dynamics of the fluid, with loss of cushioning of the br
and pressure or traction on vessels and sensitive br
structures, basal dura, tentorium, etc. Pain arising fr
the tentorium cerebelli is transmitted by the fifth ner
that from structures on or below the inferior surface of

tentorium is transmitted by the ninth and tenth cranial and upper three cervical nerves. The negative pressure in the extradural space may draw cerebrospinal fluid from the subarachnoid space. In cases of traumatic leakage of cerebrospinal fluid, the choroid plexus can form 500 ml. per day. Patients who develop spinal headaches have a lower cerebrospinal fluid pressure than controls who have received a spinal but do not complain of headaches. Yet again, cerebrospinal fluid pressures taken before spinal analgesia show that those patients who have a low value do not necessarily get headaches. Schaltenbrand considers that post-spinal headache is due to reflex aliquorrhœa—reduction of cerebrospinal fluid formation by the choroid plexuses, resulting from physiological trespass.

 b. High cerebrospinal fluid pressure—a response to meningeal irritation. This is the mechanism of headache caused by chemical or bacterial invasion. The pressure of cerebrospinal fluid bears no constant relationship to systemic arterial blood-pressure, but varies directly with the intracranial venous pressure. Queckenstedt's test eases pain if applied to patients with low-pressure headache, makes it worse in those with high-pressure headache.[*]

TREATMENT.—This is prophylactic and combative. For the former the elimination of neurotic and unsuitable patients before operation, including those with a history of frequent severe headaches ; the use of a small needle (Antoni, 1923), or of the Vienna or Duttner double needle in which the outer larger needle is put into the extradural space and a fine-bore needle inserted through it into the theca ; or one with a conical tip ; separation rather than cutting of longitudinal fibres of dura, by situation of needle bevel (Greene, 1926) ; surgical and chemical cleanliness ; blocking foot of bed for 12–24 hours post-operatively ; avoidance of strong light and also reading during this time. Low-pressure headache is ameliorated by posture, and by analgesics.

Treatment of established headache depends on cerebrospinal fluid pressure ; if this is thought to be low the following measures may help : frequent long drinks, a tight abdominal binder, injection of normal saline, 25–50 ml., into either the sacral or lumbar extradural space (injection of saline into the sacral canal has recently been found not to raise the cerebro-spinal fluid pressure significantly[†]); intrathecal injection of 30 ml. warm saline or 1 per cent glucose; intravenous injection of 20–50 ml. distilled water. Posterior pituitary extract has also been recommended because of its antidiuretic power, and dihydroergotamine 1 ml., intravenously or intramuscularly, perhaps repeated, or hydergine, sublingually, may be beneficial. Oxygen inhalations may do good while carbon dioxide increases the cerebral blood-flow. Deutsch[‡] has had good

* Queckenstedt, Hans, *Dtsch. Z. Nervenheilk.*, 1916, **55**, 325.
† Usbiaga, J. E., and others, *Curr. Res. Anesth.*, 1967, **46**, 293.
‡ Deutsch, Enoch V., *Anesthesiology*, 1952, **13**, 496.

Sequelæ, *continued.*

results after the intravenous injection, spread over three an[ ] half hours, and repeated if required, of 5 per cent ethyl alco[ ] in 5 per cent glucose in water. This is said to increase cereb[ ] vasodilatation and stimulate the choroidal plexuses to secr[ ] more cerebrospinal fluid. If cerebrospinal fluid pressure thought to be high : lumbar puncture ; fluid depletion, int[ ] venous glucose, 50 per cent in normal saline, 50–200 m[ ] magnesium sulphate, 50 per cent enema given per rectu[ ] 6 oz. ; caffein sodium benzoate, $7\frac{1}{2}$ gr., intravenous, repeat[ ] Simple analgesics, short-wave diathermy, etc., may also helpful. Tolazoline, 25–30 mg., intravenously or by mou[ ] 8-hourly for several days, has recently been recommended

2. BACKACHE.—Probably not much more common after spir[ ] than after general anæsthesia The less traumatic the pu[ ] ture the better. A small pillow under the lumbar region redu[ ] incidence of post-operative backache irrespective of method anæsthesia. Damage to intervertebral disk by the needle h[ ] been reported.

3. RETENTION OF URINE.—A little more common after spir[ ] than after general anæsthesia. Usually yields to carbach[ ] 0·5–1 mg. intramuscularly, repeated if necessary, or neostigmi[ ] 0·5 mg. intramuscularly. Very occasionally prolonged retenti[ ] due to spasm of vesical sphincter consequent on spinal analge[ ] is seen.

4. MENINGITIS.—Usually due to faulty asepsis, but can occ[ ] with a seemingly flawless technique. Distilled water, gumm[ ] ampoule labels, should be viewed with suspicion. Contaminati[ ] with chemical antiseptics, detergents, concentration of the dr[ ] and variations in pH have all been blamed. Autoclaving of t[ ] whole pack is the ideal to be aimed at, and disposable, p[ ] sterilized syringes, etc., are excellent. If all-glass syringes a[ ] used, they can be placed, with their needles, in a hot-air oven 160° C. for one hour before use. Infection with *B. pyocyane[ ]* has been reported and infection can occur with certain Gra[ ] negative bacilli, difficult to cultivate on routine examinati[ ] of the cerebrospinal fluid. The authors have never seen a case meningitis following extradural block in many thousands of cas[ ]

5. PARALYSIS OF SIXTH CRANIAL NERVE, palsy of extern[ ] rectus causing diplopia. Rare and usually disappears spo[ ] taneously in a few weeks. Onset usually between fifth a[ ] eleventh post-operative days and associated with headache. is only seen when the patient gets out of bed. May be delay[ ] for three weeks, while simple lumbar puncture without injecti[ ] of analgesic solution can cause it. Has been said to occur about 1 in 300 cases of spinal analgesia. Paralysis is nev[ ] complete and is a different entity from the total paraly[ ] associated with such conditions as skull fracture.

Other possible causes are : (*a*) Mechanical, due to upset of hydr[ ] dynamics of cerebrospinal fluid pressure causing stretching

---

* Peelen, M., *New Eng. J. Med.*, 1967, **277**, 987.

the abducens nerve. Harvey Cushing pointed out that as the sixth nerve runs forwards from the posterior margin of the pons it is crossed by either the anterior inferior cerebellar or the internal auditory artery, or by both, so that if slight displacement of the cerebellum occurs, these arteries are stretched, and being fixed below to the basilar artery, may cut into the nerve like a tight band. (b) Inflammatory, low-grade meningitis. (c) Toxic, due to specific action of drug used acting on an unstable binocular vision mechanism, phylo-genetically a recently acquired one; a similar condition is seen in acute alcoholic intoxication.

When severe headache occurs, steps must at once be taken to prevent diplopia. The patient must be sent back to bed and rehydrated both orally and parenterally. The antidiuretic hormone in posterior pituitary extract may be useful.

While the condition persists, dark glasses should be worn, with the outer one-third of glass of affected eye made opaque. About 50 per cent of cases recover within a month. If after two years, spontaneous recovery of function has not occurred, operative cure may be considered. About 25 per cent of the cases show bilateral nerve involvement.

Paralysis of every cranial nerve except the first and tenth has been reported after spinal analgesia, and transient deafness or tinnitus is not uncommon. Diplopia has been reported following general anæsthesia and after the use of relaxants and may then persist for some time.

6. OTHER NERVE LESIONS.—Permanent neurological sequelæ first reported by Koenig in 1906.[*] Transient lesions of cauda equina causing abnormalities of leg reflexes, incontinence of fæces, retention of urine, loss of sexual function, sensory loss in lumbosacral distribution, and temporary paralysis of peroneal nerve. Most of these clear up spontaneously. Radiculitis, ascending myelitis, adhesive arachnoiditis, meningo-encephalitis, and bulbar involvement have all been reported. Their cause is not fully understood nor is it always due to the method of pain relief.[†] It may well be the result of the drug injected, while the low pH of a large volume of injected solution has also been blamed. Six grave cases of severe central nervous system sequelæ are reported by Bergner,[‡] four of these ending fatally, with incubation periods varying from 24 hours to 18 days. These analgesias appear to have been expertly managed with all right and proper precautions having been taken. Electro-myographic studies enable lesions of the lower motor neuron type due to spinal analgesia to be differentiated from other neurological and myopathic conditions.[§] Paralysis of the eighth nerve has been reported.

Anterior spinal artery syndrome (*see Lancet*, 1958, **2**, 515; and Wells, C. E. C., *Proc. R. Soc. Med.*, 1966, **59**, 790) is a motor

* Greene, N. M., *Anesthesiology*, 1961, **22**, 682.
† Lee, J. A., *Anæsthesia*, 1967, **22**, 342.
‡ Bergner, R. P., and others, *Anesthesiology*, 1951, **12**, 717.
§ Marinacci, A. A., *J. Amer. med. Ass.*, 1959, **168**, 1337; and *Bull. Los Angeles neurol. Soc.*, 1960, **25**, 170.

Sequelæ, *continued.*

neuron paralysis without involvement of the posterior columns of the spinal cord, subserving joint position sense, touch, and vibration sensibility. It has followed spinal analgesia. (*See* Annotation, *Lancet*, 1967, **2**, 143.)

A constricting pachymeningitis may develop some time after subarachnoid block. Sequelæ may not be seen until many months after the performance of the block.*

There is at present some emphasis on the serious neurological sequelæ of spinal analgesia and the pendulum of popularity has swung away from the method.† On the other hand, the technique is not without its strong supporters, who, after most careful post-operative assessment, are not able to blame it for the production of significant neurological sequelæ. Among these may be mentioned Vandam, L. D., and Dripps, R. D., *Surgery*, 1955, **38**, 463, and *J. Amer. med. Ass.*, 1956, **161**, 586 ; Lake, N. C., *Lancet*, 1958, **1**, 387 ; Ochsner, Alton J., *Southern Med. J.*, 1957, **50**, 1156; Arner, O., *Acta chir. scand.*, 1952, Suppl. 167; and Moore, D. C., and Bridenbaugh, L. D., *J. Amer. med. Ass.*, 1966, **195**, 907.

Neurological complications following spinal analgesia are not necessarily due to the method,‡ while such complications following surgical operations may be seen in patients who have had general anæsthesia.§

(*See* article " Complications of Spinal Analgesia " by Greene, N. M., *Anesthesiology*, 1961, **22**, 682.)

THE CHOICE OF SPINAL INTRA- AND EXTRADURAL ANALGESIA

Advantages.—Prevents the tough, strong patient from being soaked with muscle relaxant and preserves spontaneous respiration ; cheap ; ideal for fit patients who object to being put to sleep ; lessens risk of vomiting causing pulmonary aspiration in patients with full stomach ; quiet relaxed abdomen together with small contracted intestines and spontaneous breathing helps surgeon ; shock from surgical trauma lessened ; upset of body chemistry minimal ; intestinal function returns early ; risk of explosion absent ; wound bleeding reduced. Since the advent of muscle relaxants, the need for spinal analgesia has decreased, but it is still a useful method which has stood the test of time. Can be employed deliberately to produce hypotension and so less bleeding during operation.

Disadvantages.—Operative mortality is slightly higher, at least in high spinals, than after general anæsthesia ; it puts more of a strain on the cardiovascular system than a general anæsthetic by

---

* Rosenbaum, H. E., Long, F. B., Hinchly, T. R., and Trufant, S. A., *Amer. med. Ass. Arch. Neurol. and Psychiat.*, 1952, **68**, 783.

† Kennedy, F., and others, *Surg. Gynec. Obstet.*, 1950, **91**, 385 (reprinted in *Survey of Anesthesiology*, 1964, **8**, 273).

‡ Leatherdale, R . A. L., *Anæsthesia*, 1959, **14**, 274.

§ Hewer, C. Langton, and Lee, J. A., *Recent Advances in Anæsthesia and Analgesia*, 1957, 8th ed., p. 135. London: Churchill; and Lett, Z., *Brit. J. Anæsth.*, 1964, **36**, 266.

tending to cause hypotension ; some patients do not like the idea of it; the incidence of post-operative headache (in intradural block). It does not reduce the incidence of post-operative chest complications.

Indications.—These vary greatly with different surgeons and anæsthetists. Specially indicated in strong muscular patients, too tough for general anæsthesia. Useful in cases of acute bronchitis, active pulmonary tuberculosis, and bronchiectasis because of lack of the supposed pulmonary irritation still erroneously thought to be caused by even a skilfully given general inhalation anæsthetic ; myasthenia and some other disorders involving muscles, to avoid the use of relaxants or deep general anæsthesia; kidney, liver disease, and diabetes because body chemistry is not interfered with. Acute cases with a full stomach may be less dangerous under spinal than general anæsthesia (stomachs cannot always be emptied by a stomach tube).

Amputations through thigh or hip ; intestinal obstruction in the absence of acute distension or grave toxæmia ; paralytic ileus in the absence of acute peritonitis ; transurethral manipulations and in some cases of prostatectomy, especially if done per urethram ; hæmorrhoids when the surgeon requires an atonic sphincter. In operative obstetrics.* For ligation of the inferior vena cava in cases of acute cor pulmonale. Five special indications are : (1) When a bloodless field is especially desirable. (2) When a contracted bowel (not seen with relaxants) is required, e.g., abdomino-perineal resection of rectum, Hartmann's operation, etc. (3) In abdominal gynæcological operations in fat patients. (4) For amputations in old, arteriosclerotic, or diabetic patients. (5) In operative obstetrics because of its benign effect on the fœtus and its protection of the mother from inhalation of gastric contents.

Contra-indications to Intra- and Extradural Block.—Should not, without a good reason, be pushed on to unwilling or uncooperative patients, including young children. Often unwise in the following groups without careful consideration:—

a. CARDIOVASCULAR.—Severe shock; hypovolæmia; dehydration; hypotension, with blood-pressure below 80–90 systolic; hypertension when associated with myocardial weakness; patients unable to do reasonable physical work because of obesity, senility, myocardial degeneration, toxæmia. Patients with a recent history of cardiac infarction should not receive a high spinal. If coronary disease is present, a reasonable blood-pressure is required to force blood into the coronary arteries. Such patients need special care. Cerebral atheroma.

b. MECHANICAL.—Patients with a splinted diaphragm which interferes with breathing, such as hydramnios, large ovarian and uterine tumours, e.g., pregnancy; ascites, omental obesity ; hypoxia is always a risk in these cases, and oxygen should be given from the commencement of the analgesia if a spinal is

* Hillman, K., *Canad. Anæsth. Soc. J.*, 1965, **12**, 398.

Contra-indications to Intra- and Extradural Block, *continued.*

used, employing intermittent positive-pressure ventilation if necessary. Dosage should be reduced in such patients.

c. RESPIRATORY.—Patients who are breathless from any cause ; these may become hypoxic, especially if level of analgesia is high. On the other hand, patients with emphysema or broncho-spasm often do surprisingly well after spinal block.

d. ABNORMALITIES OF THE CENTRAL NERVOUS SYSTEM. —Spinal analgesia should not be given to a patient with an abnormality of the central nervous system, whether it be congenital or acquired, infective or degenerative, active or inactive or healed. Any subsequent symptoms may be blamed on the spinal. Patients who are chronic sufferers from head-aches will in all probability get a headache of moderate severity after operation following intradural block. If it is suspected on the history (headache, vomiting, blurred vision) or the physical signs (papilloedema, bradycardia, drowsiness) that the patient has an expanding cerebral lesion, a tumour, cyst, or abscess, which may, if the intracranial pressure is suddenly altered, cause obstruction to the cerebrospinal fluid or blood-circulation (the pressure cone) (intradural block).

e. GASTRO-INTESTINAL PERFORATIONS.—Contraction of the gut adds to the soiling of the peritoneum in these cases.

f. GENITO-URINARY.—Patients who may have an enlarged pros-tate (which is not the reason for the surgical procedure). Bladder difficulty may be complained of after operation and blamed on the method of pain relief.

If kidney function is poor, the low blood-pressure associated with spinal analgesia may result in temporary oliguria which may upset the subnormal renal function.

g. CASES WITH DEFORMED BACKS.—Because of difficulty in the performance of lumbar puncture.

h. SKIN SEPSIS in lumbar region.

i. NEUROLOGICAL OPERATIONS.—In operations for lesions of the spinal cord or cauda equina, on medico-legal grounds.

Many anæsthetists, however, favour the use of extradural block for laminectomy for prolapsed disk. (Thorne, T. C., personal communication.)

j. PATIENTS WITH DISORDERS OF BLOOD CLOTTING.— Hæmorrhage from puncture of extradural veins may be un-desirable.

k. IN CASES OF DEHYDRATION.—These are bad risks and a much smaller dose of drug than usual is required.

SPINAL INTRADURAL ANALGESIA IN NON-SURGICAL CONDITIONS

Therapeutic.—Patients with autonomic imbalance of the alimentary canal such as *megacolon*, etc. Relief of the condition by spinal block is an indication that sympathectomy may be helpful. The serial spinal technique of Lemmon is excellent for this high block. In megacolon, block should reach to T.5. Patients with *eclampsia* are sometimes benefited by a high spinal block up to T.8, which reduces their blood-pressure. Patients with *acute pulmonary œdema* due to left ventricular failure are said to have been successfully treated by spinal block, which produces a bloodless phlebotomy caused by vasomotor paralysis. The vasodilatation results in a decreased venous return to the right heart and hence to the lungs, relieving left ventricular failure. *Renal anuria* has been successfully treated by high spinal block, which results in dilatation of renal vessels and increased secretion of urine.

Reactionary hæmorrhage from prostate bed has been stopped by spinal analgesia to S.1, which leaves intact the fibres producing vasoconstriction and contraction of the prostatic bed (L.1 and 2), blocking those fibres (S.2, 3, 4) causing dilatation of the vessels and prostatic capsule.

In cases of *embolism of the lower extremity*, continuous spinal analgesia has been successfully employed, a block to T.10 removing the vasoconstrictor fibres from the whole leg. By this means, a block has been maintained for 50–60 hours. Continuous spinal analgesia lasting for fourteen days has been reported, and that without serious complications.[*] In such cases, continuous extradural analgesia would be better. If, after many hours, an analgesic drug loses its effect, substitution of another drug should be tried.

For the treatment of *paraplegic clonus* in patients who have already lost sexual function and bladder control, 5–10 ml. of absolute alcohol should be injected, after 5 ml. of 5 per cent procaine solution. This also helps to establish the automatic bladder.[†]

SPINAL ANALGESIA IN INTRACTABLE PAIN.[‡]—Subarachnoid alcohol injection, which was recommended by Dogliotti in 1931 and by G. Todd in 1937, is sometimes helpful in incurable cases of malignant disease with severe pain below the groin and iliac crests, i.e., in the lumbar and sacral distribution. The patient is placed in the semi-prone position with diseased side uppermost and head tilted downwards. Alcohol (absolute), which must be previously autoclaved, is injected between T.11 and T.12, or T.12 and L.1, the dose being 0·5 ml. The semi-prone position ensures a greater effect on the posterior roots than on the anterior with this hypobaric solution. The position must be maintained for one hour. The beneficial effect may not be fully apparent for a week. About 10 per cent of patients get rectal or bladder disability, or weakness of the legs, but this is an improvement on the results after chordotomy. Headache may follow, but subarachnoid adhesions are not produced. The procedure may have to be repeated.

When sympathetic fibres alone need to be blocked, a weak analgesic solution can be used, e.g., 0·2 per cent procaine or 0·05 per cent amethocaine hydrochloride in distilled water which is hypobaric. A suitable dose of the latter is 6–12 ml. (6–12 mg.) which usually gives a sympathetic block up to about T.8.

---

* Ansbro, F. P., *Anesthesiology*, 1954, **15**, 569.
† Evangelow, M., and Adriani, J., *Ibid.*, 1955, **16**, 594.
‡ Hay, R. C., *Curr. Res. Anesth.*, 1962, **41**, 12.

Therapeutic, *continued.*

Hypothermic irrigation of the subarachnoid space has been use
for the treatment of intractable pain,* using 10 ml. of norm.
saline at 2–4° C. The good effects may, however, be due 1
hyperosmolarity rather than hypothermia.

Intrathecal ammonium sulphate 6 per cent in buffered solution wit
a *p*H of 7·2 is said to block the C type fibres carrying pai
impulses from root irritation by metastatic growths in the cord
3·5 ml. of the 6 per cent solution should be mixed with cerebr
spinal fluid and slowly re-injected.†

Phenol (5 per cent) in glycerin and (7·5 per cent) in myodil hav
been injected intrathecally for the treatment of painful refle
spasms and spasticity. Not very effective in long-standin
paraplegias with contractures. These injections may cau
bowel and bladder disturbances and sensory loss and should t
confined to bedridden patients. Both solutions are hyperbar
and careful positioning is necessary. Preliminary injection of
local analgesic or of a radio-opaque material‡ will act as a guid
to correct technique. The dose of the two solutions varies fro
1 to 3 ml. (*See* articles by Nathan, P. W., and Scott, T. G
Lancet, 1958, **1**, 76; Nathan, P. W., *Ibid.*, 1959, **2**, 109
Liversedge, L. A., and Maher, R. M., *Brit. med. J.*, 1960, **2**, 3
Maher, R. M., *Lancet*, 1960, **1**, 895.)

R. M. Maher§ has recommended 2 per cent solution of chlorocres
in glycerin, which he has found to be more manageable tha
phenol for relieving pain in cancer. The initial dose is 0·75 m
and this may have to be repeated.

Diagnostic.—

1. INTESTINAL OBSTRUCTION.—Can be differentiated int
organic and functional by spinal analgesia ; if functional, con
traction of the gut, with relaxation of sphincters, results i
passage of gas and fæces within twenty minutes. Differenti
spinal block using 0·2 per cent procaine solution can be used
This concentration will give paralysis of the sympathetic fibre
running to the splanchnics, without any sensory (or motor) effec
(Large-bowel nerve-supply : *parasympathetic*, vagi, and S.2, 3
4—motor ; *sympathetic*, T.5–L.3—inhibitory.) Neither opiate
nor atropine should be given to these patients, as both drug
inhibit the gut.

2. THROMBO-ANGIITIS OBLITERANS.—If the vasoconstricto
fibres supplying the lower limbs which come from T.10–L.2 ar
blocked there is an increase in skin temperature of as much a
8° C. in normal legs and in the vasospastic types of this disease
in the thrombotic types this increase does not take place an
further surgery is not likely to be beneficial.

3. DIAGNOSIS OF THE CAUSE OF PAIN IN THE INFERIOF
EXTREMITY, BACK, AND TRUNK.—Injection at 10-min
intervals of:—

---

* Hitchcock, E., *Lancet*, 1967, **1**, 1133.
† Judovitch, B. D., Bates, N., and Bishop, K., *Anesthesiology*, 1944, **5**, 341.
‡ Mark, V. H., and others, *New Engl. J. Med.*, 1962, **267**, 589.
§ Maher, R. M., *Lancet*, 1963, **1**, 965.

a. Ten ml. of isotonic saline (placebo).
b. Ten ml. of 0·2 per cent procaine in saline (sympathetic block).
c. Ten ml. of 0·5 per cent procaine in saline (sensory block).
d. Ten ml. of 1 per cent procaine in saline (motor block).
The changes produced are assessed and evaluated as an aid to diagnosis.*

SPINAL INTRADURAL ANALGESIA IN CHILDREN

Risk of circulatory depression minimal because of elasticity of their cardiovascular systems. Puncture should be in L.3–4 interspace because cord extends lower in children than in adults. Dosage for analgesia to T.8 is 10 mg. of procaine for each year; some prefer to use 1 mg. procaine per lb. of body-weight. For a newborn baby, 1–2 ml. of 1–1500 cinchocaine has been successfully used, injected through an intravenous needle. For pyloric stenosis in babies, 20 mg. of procaine in 1 ml. cerebrospinal fluid. Specially indicated in shocking procedures, such as open operations on hip-joint; useful for operations in the presence of acute respiratory infection, intestinal distension, or a full stomach. Also in hot humid atmosphere, to prevent ether convulsions. Lack of co-operation is chief drawback, so premedication must be adequate. Small doses of morphine, repeated as necessary, make a good sedative. The technique is seldom employed in Britain.
See also articles by Slater† and by Berkawitz.‡

SPINAL INTRADURAL ANALGESIA IN OBSTETRICS

Certain physiological changes occur during late pregnancy. There is a rise of 30 per cent in the cardiac output, and maternal blood-volume increases by 10–15 per cent. Blood-pressure drops towards the end of pregnancy. By pressing on the pelvic veins and vena cava the gravid uterus obstructs venous return and this is worse in the supine position (hypotensive supine syndrome of late pregnancy).
A given dose of a local analgesic solution will ascend higher in extradural§ and in intradural block in a pregnant than in a non-pregnant patient, so doses should be kept small. (This view has been denied.‖) It may be because there is a smaller volume of cerebrospinal fluid due to the greater space taken by the dilated extradural veins because of the venous obstruction.
Block analgesia is excellent for the delivery of premature infants, and is suitable for delivery in diabetes and toxæmia. *Severe post-partum hæmorrhage* has been relieved ; spinal analgesia increases uterine tone in labour.
For Cæsarean section, method is unpopular as unexplained deaths have occurred, especially after the use of procaine. Reason for these deaths may be that the supine hypotensive syndrome adds to the hypotension caused by the block or that the pregnant uterus splints the diaphragm, so that hypoxia is the dangerous factor. There is

* Ahlgren, E. W., and others, *J. Amer. med. Ass.*, 1966, **195**, 813.
† Slater, H. M., and Stephen, C. R., *Anesthesiology*, 1950, **11**, 709.
‡ Berkawitz, S., and Greene, B. A., *Ibid.*, 1951, **12**, 376.
§ Bromage, P. R., *Brit. J. Anæsth.*, 1962, **34**, 161.
‖ Kalas, D. B., and others, *Curr. Res. Anesth.*, 1966, **45**, 848.

Spinal Intradural Analgesia in Obstetrics, *continued.*

evidence, too, that smaller doses are required by women in labour than in normal patients. Oxygen inhalations (100 per cent) from the beginning of the analgesia should avoid this danger. Advantages are that the baby is completely unaffected by the drug, crying immediately after delivery, while the uterine muscle contracts excellently owing to paralysis of sympathetic dilator fibres. Premedication should consist only of atropine; supplementary anaesthesia can be given after the delivery of the baby, should it be necessary. Analgesia must reach to the ninth thoracic dermatome. The authors and their associates* have had considerable satisfaction from this method and recommend it. They use 1·6 ml. of hyperbaric cinchocaine in the average case.

Because of its lack of effect on the foetus, and its power of producing absolute relaxation of the pelvic-floor muscles, spinal block to S.1 is excellent for forceps delivery, 1 ml. of heavy cinchocaine being injected below L.4 with back level during and after injection.

In patients in labour, the blood-pressure must not be allowed to fall below 85 mm. Hg so that very frequent estimations of the blood-pressure must be taken throughout the operation and before it begins. Administration of pressor drugs, however, does not necessarily result in increased blood-supply to the foetus (*see* Chapter XXV).

Collapse from Spinal or Extradural Analgesia during Pregnancy.†—This may be due to two factors :—

1. Increased sensitivity of vasomotor system to block by local analgesics.

2. Tendency of some patients to develop hypotension if kept lying on the back in late pregnancy (hypotensive supine syndrome of late pregnancy) due to interference with venous return and caused by pressure of uterus on inferior vena cava. If this postural hypotension is present before labour, legs should be raised or patient should be placed on her side.

SPINAL INTRADURAL ANALGESIA IN PREGNANCY

Spinal and extradural block in pregnancy do not materially increase the uterine tone and do not harm the foetus.‡

SPINAL INTRADURAL ANALGESIA IN UROLOGY

Very useful in cystoscopies and transurethral procedures. If retrograde pyelography is to be done soon after cystoscopy, block must not ascend higher than the roots of L.2, otherwise overfilling of the renal pelves will not be prevented by the patient feeling pain. For transurethral resection of the prostate, 1·5 ml. of lignocaine (5 per cent), given in the sitting position, gives good results.§ In suprapubic

* Thorne, T. C., *Proc. R. Soc. Med.*, 1954, **47**, 301.
† Williams, B., *Anæsthesia*, 1958, **13**, 448.
‡ Ruppert, H., *Proc. World Congress of Anesthesiologists*, 1956, 161. Minneapolis: Burgess Pub. Co.
§ Adams, B. W., *Anæsthesia*, 1956, **11**, 297.

prostatectomy some surgeons appreciate the relaxation and freedom from toxic effects obtained with spinal analgesia. Others fear that reactionary hæmorrhage may arise with the patient back in bed and his blood-pressure returning to normal as the block passes off. For nephrectomy or nephrolithotomy, done with the patient in the lateral position, hypobaric solutions should be used ; fat, heavy patients kept in this position for any length of time tend to become hypoxic from interference with their respiration, and thus often do better with general anæsthesia, or spinal block accompanied by 100 per cent oxygen inhalations.

SPINAL ANALGESIA IN THORACIC SURGERY

This is seldom, if ever, used to-day, although thoracic extradural block is sometimes used for pain relief. A negative pressure test is used for locating the extradural space in this region.

SUPPLEMENTARY ANÆSTHESIA
(For Intradural and Extradural Analgesia)

No patient should receive a spinal injection without having an open vein, e.g., a Mitchell or Gordh needle or a drip. This is to enable acute hypotension or convulsions to be rapidly reversed.

Supplementary anæsthesia may be : (1) Planned from the beginning, and may be given either before or after the spinal injection. (2) Given during the course of the operation because of the partial failure, wearing off, or extension of scope of the operation ; because of the emotional discomfort and anxiety of the patient ; because of persistent vomiting or restlessness.

1. Intravenous, inhalation, or a combination of the two, may be used. In a similar manner, light halothane or light cyclopropane can be given before the spinal injection, and some workers, before embarking on a prolonged operation, prefer their patients to be intubated. By use of these methods, the patient need never know that he has had a spinal analgesic.

Alternatively, the spinal is given in the usual way and allowed to become fixed. When it is ascertained that its height is adequate, general anæsthesia is induced, and carried to a light plane. For operations below the umbilicus, thiopentone makes an excellent supplement, but for higher blocks an inhalation agent is preferred by many. It has the advantage that oxygenation can be increased.

2. If the patient requires a general anæsthetic during the course of the operation it is important to avoid a stage of delirium during the induction, and this is best done by a little intravenous thiopentone. Then gas and oxygen, a volatile supplement, or cyclopropane can be added.

The authors prefer to use minimal thiopentone in 2·5 per cent solution, injected as necessary into a non-clotting needle: to this is sometimes added nitrous oxide, 6 l. per minute, and oxygen, 2 l. per minute. An endotracheal tube may be desirable: (a) If the airway is difficult to maintain without it; (b) If the operation is likely to last a long time, especially if it

Supplementary Anæsthesia, *continued.*

takes place in the upper abdomen. If the tube is used, cyclopropane or gas–oxygen and pethidine, halothane, or trichloroethylene are suitable supplements.

Intravenous heroin, 1–4 mg., may be sufficient to settle a nervous patient down if there is a little return of sensation towards the end of an operation. Intraperitoneal swabbing with 100 ml. of ½ per cent procaine will also have a beneficial effect if mild pain stimuli are worrying the patient. During a hernia operation, pulling on the sac may disturb the patient; pain from this can often be abolished by injection of a little procaine into the neck of the sac. Similarly, infiltration of the peri-œsophageal branches of the vagus, at the cardiac end of the stomach, will do much to prevent sensations of nausea and faintness from worrying the patient in upper abdominal operations, if he is conscious, and to prevent hiccup if he is not.

The use of phenothiazine derivatives such as chlorpromazine and promethazine, 25 mg. of each, with pethidine 50 mg. in the premedication, will usually result in a calm and drowsy patient, but fall in blood-pressure extending into the postoperative stage is a disadvantage and may be a danger.

EXTRADURAL BLOCK

Definition.—Blockage of nerve-roots outside the dura. A method giving reflex flaccidity of muscles, analgesia, a degree of hypotension, and consequent ischæmia secondary to sympathetic blockade while allowing intercostal respiration to continue relatively unimpaired.

History.—Introduced by Corning, and used in dogs by Cathelin[*] and Sicard (1872–1929)[†] in 1901, and applied in clinical surgery by Pagés in 1921 (Pagés, F., *Rev. Sanid. Milit. (Madrid)*, 1921, **11**, 351[‡]) and by Dogliotti in 1931 (Dogliotti, A. M., *Zbl. Chir.*, 1931, **58**, 3141). Popularized in Britain by Massey Dawkins (Dawkins, C. J. M., *Proc. R. Soc. Med.*, 1945, **38**, 299). The publications and researches of Bromage have led to a reappraisal of many opinions formerly held concerning the physiology and pharmacology of the method.[||]

Anatomy.—The spinal dura mater represents the meningeal layer of the dura mater of the brain: the periosteum lining the vertebral canal represents the outer layer of the cerebral dura. Between the spinal dura and the vertebral canal is the extradural (epidural, peridural) space. Its average diameter is 0·5 cm. and it is widest in the midline, posteriorly in the lumbar region.

Its boundaries are: superiorly the foramen magnum and inferiorly the sacrococcygeal membrane; posteriorly the anterior surfaces of the laminæ and their connecting ligaments, the roots of the vertebral spines and the ligamenta flava;

[*] Cathelin, F., *C. R. Soc. Biol., Paris*, 1901, **53**, 452.
[†] Sicard, J.-A., *Ibid.*, 1901, **53**, 396.
[‡] Translated in *Survey of Anesthesiology*, 1961, **5**, 326.
[||] Bromage, P. R., *Brit. J. Anæsth.*, 1962, **34**, 161; and *Anesthesiology*, 1967, **28**, 592.

anteriorly the posterior longitudinal ligament covering the vertebral bodies and the disks ; laterally the pedicles and intervertebral foramina. The interspinous ligaments and the ligamenta flava, dense gristly tissue, are important in locating the extradural space.

The contents include the dural sac and the spinal nerve-roots, the extradural plexus of veins and the spinal arteries, lymphatics and fat. The veins become distended when the patient strains or coughs, i.e., during bouts of increased intra-thoracic pressure. The veins form a network which runs in four main trunks along the space. They communicate with venous rings at each vertebral level, with the basivertebral veins on the posterior aspect of each vertebral body, and with the ascending and deep cervical, intercostal, ilio-lumbar, and lateral sacral veins. These veins have no valves and constitute the valveless vertebral venous plexus of Batson.* They connect the pelvic veins below with the intracranial veins above, so that air or local analgesic solution injected into one of them will ascend straight to the brain. They drain into the inferior vena cava via the azygos vein, so that when there is obstruction to vena caval flow, as with large abdominal tumours, advanced pregnancy, etc., they become distended. There are fifty-eight inter-vertebral foramina and the degree of their patency is an important factor in controlling the height of analgesia a given volume of analgesic solution will produce. They tend to be more permeable in the young than in the old, so that a given volume of solution tends to cause a higher block in the old than in the young.

The dura mater is attached to the margins of the foramen magnum, but this does not prevent the passage of analgesic drug into the cranial cavity. It is also attached to the second and third cervical vertebræ and to the posterior longitudinal ligament. It ends at the lower border of the second sacral vertebra, a point corresponding in level with the posterior superior iliac spines. Prolongations of the dura surround the spinal nerve-roots and fuse with the epineurium of the complete spinal nerves, as they traverse the intervertebral foramina. Extradural block includes blocking of the sympathetic fibres travelling with the anterior or ventral roots, which soon become the white rami. Usual distance between skin and extradural space 4–5 cm.

Causes of Negative Pressure in Extradural Space.—There is usually a negative pressure in the extradural space; this is increased when the back is fully flexed but soon returns to normal.† Janzen (1926)‡ thought it was due to dimpling of the dura, Heldt and Moloney (1928)§ described an inherent negative pressure. Macintosh and Mushin have pointed out that the extradural

---

* Batson, O. V., *Amer. J. Roentgenol.*, 1942, **48**, 715.
† Odom, C. B., *Amer. J. Surg.*, 1936, **34**, 547.
‡ Janzen, E. J., *Dtsch. Z. Nervenheilk.*, 1926, **94**, 280.
§ Heldt, H. J., and Moloney, C. J., *Amer. J. med. Sci.*, 1928, **175**, 371.

Causes of Negative Pressure in Extradural Space, *continued.*

space communicates with the paravertebral spaces which share the general intrathoracic negative pressure during inspiration.* Negative pressure in extradural space is not the same at all levels and in the sacral canal it is absent.

This negative extradural pressure may account for the leakage of cerebrospinal fluid into the extradural space after lumbar puncture. In 20 per cent of cases there is no negative pressure in the space.

Pressure in the cervico-thoracic extradural space reflects pressure in the superior vena cava, and that in the lumbar extradural space reflects pressure in the inferior vena cava. Changes in the abdominal or thoracic cavities can be transmitted to the extradural space directly through the intervertebral foramina or indirectly through the superior or inferior vena cava. A rise in pressure may favour spread of local analgesic solution.†

Site of Action.—When a solution of a local analgesic is injected into the extradural space it may exert its effect: (1) On the nerve-roots in the extradural space; (2) On the nerve-roots in the paravertebral spaces after they have shed their dural sheaths;‡ (3) On the nerve-roots in the intradural or subarachoid space after inward diffusion of the drug across the dura;§ (4) Diffusion into the subperineural and subpial spaces from the so-called "ink-cuff" zone‖ where the anterior and posterior nerve-roots fuse. Analgesic drug may eventually pass centripetally and reach the substance of the cord and diffuse out from this into the cerebrospinal fluid, where, however, its concentration is too low for much pharmacological activity.¶ Injected solution can thus spread up and down the space, especially in the elderly; laterally into the paravertebral space, especially in the young, and centripetally into the neuraxis along the subpineural (subperineural) spaces.

Factors influencing spread of solution.—(1) The volume of solution injected ; (2) The age of the patient, the old requiring less than the young ; (3) The force of injection—fast injection spreads the solution thinly over a wide area and may give an incomplete but extensive zone of analgesia ; (4) The drug used—lignocaine appears to spread more widely than procaine, etc. ; (5) The level at which an injection is given ; (6) Gravity—a head-down tilt aids upward diffusion of the solution and vice versa, while an injection given in the sitting position will not reach as high as the same volume given in the lateral position ; (7) The length of the vertebral column ; (8) Full-term pregnancy or abdominal tumours. One-third to one-half normal doses required;** (9)

* Macintosh, R. R., and Mushin, W. W., *Anæsthesia*, 1947, **2**, 100.
† Usubiaga, J. E., and others, *Brit. J. Anæsth.*, 1967, **39**, 612.
‡ Flowers, C. F., *Ibid.*, 1954, **19**, 146.
§ Usubiaga, J. E., and others, *Anesthesiology*, 1964, **25**, 752.
‖ Brierly, J. B., *J. Neurol. Psychiat.*, 1950, **13**, 203.
¶ Bromage, P. R., *Brit. J. Anæsth.*, 1962, **34**, 161.
** Hehre, F. W., and others, *Curr. Res. Anesth.*, 1965, **44**, 89; and Bromage, P. R., *Canad. med. Ass. J.*, 1961, **85**, 1136.

Concentration of local analgesic solution.* A given volume of a high concentration will spread further than an equal volume of a lower concentration.* (10) In diabetes and in occlusive arterial disease less solution is required.* The height of analgesia produced by a given volume of solution is one of the great uncertainties of anæsthesia. Four segments on each side of the point of injection are said to be effected by the extradural injections of 10–15 ml. of analgesic solution.

Local Analgesic Solutions Used.—

Lignocaine 1 to 2 per cent which has a rapid onset in about ten minutes and gives good relaxation; 10 mg. per kg. with adrenaline, by single injection, is a guide to safe dosage. Duration of effect $1\frac{1}{2}$ to 2 hours—depending on strength of solution employed: 0·8 per cent solution gives good sensory without motor block. The writers have had very considerable experience of the use of 1·5 per cent solution for surgical work and find it most satisfactory. In very muscular patients, 2 per cent solution may produce more intense muscular relaxation.

Amethocaine hydrochloride can be added to lignocaine solution, e.g., 50 mg. added to 50 ml. giving a 0·1 per cent strength. It increases the duration of analgesia by about 50 per cent.

Prilocaine is excellent for extradural blockade and lasts longer than lignocaine in the same concentrations. Concentrations of 1·5,† 2,‡ and 3§ per cent, with adrenaline 1–200,000, have been recommended. It is a little less toxic than lignocaine.

Bupivacaine (marcain) is a new long-acting drug which has been used in 0·5 per cent concentration with adrenaline (1–200,000), giving analgesia for period up to 8 hours.‖ Volumes in excess of 20 ml. need to be given with great care.

Cinchocaine, 1–1200, maximum dosage, 60 ml. Analgesia is slow in onset—up to 20 minutes—but prolonged in effect—3 to 4 hours. Piperocaine, 1·5 per cent solution.

Adrenaline is added in the usual strength, i.e., 0·1–0·25 ml. to 50 ml. of solution. It produces inotropic and chronotropic effects on the heart.¶ Some workers omit this as they fear the combined effect of hypotension and vasoconstriction on the nerve tissue.

Potentiation of Local Analgesic Solutions.—

1. Combination of local analgesic bases with CO_2 to form bicarbonate salts. Rapid conversion of the bicarbonate to undissociated free base takes place after injection as the partial pressure of the CO_2 falls to that of the tissues. These salts are said to combine low toxicity, rapid onset, and sensory and motor block of intense degree.**

* Bromage, P. R., *Brit. J. Anæsth.*, 1962, **34**, 161.
† Wendl, H. K., *Acta anæsth. scand.*, 1965, Suppl. 16, 249.
‡ Scott, D. B., *Ibid.*, 1965, Suppl. 16, 111.
§ Bromage, P. R., *Brit. J. Anæsth.*, 1965, **37**, 753; and Scott, D. B., *Proc. R. Soc. Med.*, 1965, **58**, 420.
‖ Watt, M. J., Ross, D. M., and Atkinson, R. S., *Anæsthesia*, 1968, **23**, 2 and *Ibid.*, 1968, **23**, July, and Ekblom, L., and Widman, B., *Acta anæsth. scand.*, 1966, Suppl. 21, 33.
¶ Bonica, J. J., and others, *Ibid.*, 1966, Suppl. 23, 429.
** Bromage, P. R., *Ibid.*, 1965, Suppl. 16, 55.

Potentiation of Local Analgesic Solutions, *continued.*

2. Addition of 1 per cent potassium chloride to the solution, equal to a potassium concentration of 128 mEq./l., causes a shortened latency and more intense degree of sensory block. Contamination of the subarachnoid space with the potassium salt will cause, however, severe depolarizing muscular spasms.*

Method of Location of Extradural Space.—Before any block is attempted, an open vein must be guaranteed (Mitchell needle, Gordh needle, drip, etc.). No block must be attempted without this supremely important precaution. The extradural space can be entered from the midline or laterally, with the patient on his side or sitting. *For the midline approach,* meticulous care must be taken to insert the needle in the sagittal plane. The back should be painted with antiseptic solution and not obscured by sterile towels. The type of lumbar puncture needle selected

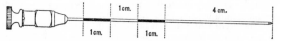

Fig. 34.—The Lee marked needle (Medical & Industrial Equipment Ltd.).

varies with the anæsthetist; some workers prefer the standard spinal needle of 20 S.W.G., others favour a needle of larger bore, e.g., 16 or 18 S.W.G. A thin-wall 18-S.W.G. needle serves well. The needle should be suitably marked to enable the depth of the point to be instantly recognized† (*Fig.* 34). Full flexion of the spine should be employed for the insertion of the needle into the interspinous ligament, but this position stretches the dura and makes it more liable to puncture. The back should therefore be slightly deflexed as the needle is advanced towards the space from the interspinous ligament. The level from which the block is made is not very important and any easily palpable interspace should be chosen although a high space is preferable for a high block and vice versa.

For the *lateral approach* a weal is raised 1 cm. from the midline opposite the lower edge of the spinous process. The needle is then inserted at right-angles to the back until the bony lamina is touched and the depth of this noted. The needle is next withdrawn as far as the muscle sheath and re-inserted at an angle of 10° upwards and 10° medially. When the needle lies at the depth of the laminæ, the stylet is withdrawn and the loss of resistance test applied.

Both the midline and the lateral entry into the space may be performed with the patient in the sitting position, and this may be the easier way in obese and in some arthritic cases, and also for thoracic puncture, using a negative-pressure method.

An easily palpable interspace should be selected, if possible a high one above L.2 for a high block and a lower space for a low block.

* Bromage, P. R., and Burfoot, M. F., *Brit. J. Anæsth.,* 1966, **38**, 857.
† Lee, J. A., *Anæsthesia,* 1960, **15**, 186.

Injection in the thoracic region is more difficult, and for it the patient should either be sitting up and a negative pressure test employed or the loss of resistance test used.

The following points suggest that the needle is in the extradural space :—

1. Sudden lack of resistance to advancing needle.

2. Sudden ease of injection of a little air from a syringe attached to needle, or injection of a little local analgesic solution. If point is in interspinous ligament plunger rebounds : if it is in the space, plunger can be pushed in easily. (Sicard and Forestier, 1922 ; Dogliotti, 1931.*) In the authors' opinion this is by far the best method in the lumbar region. It is the "loss of resistance to injection" test, the medium being injected can be air (preferably), local analgesic solution, saline, or distilled water.† A method making use of the negative pressure is preferable in thoracic injections, during which the patient should be sitting up.

3. Withdrawal of hanging drop of saline on hub of needle. Gutiérrez's sign.‡

4. Movement of bubble on Odom's indicator§ (a glass tube with fine bore containing saline and an air-bubble) which can be attached to hub of spinal needle—or Brooks's modification of this.‖

5. Macintosh's extradural space indicator—a small rubber balloon attached to an adaptor which is connected to the needle when it lies in the interspinous ligament. With a fine hypodermic needle, air is injected into the thick rubber of the neck of the balloon, and when the extradural space is entered, the small balloon diminishes in size.¶

6. The Macintosh spring loaded needle,** devised by R. H. Salt.††

7. The Iklé syringe.‡‡ Both these last two automatically indicate, by the release of a spring, when the extradural space with its low resistance has been entered.

8. The Drip Indicator.§§

In the unconscious patient the rapid injection of liquid into the extradural space is accompanied by an increase in the rate and depth of respiration. This test is not always positive in conscious patients, if injection is made slowly, or if injection is made into subarachnoid space. (Durrans's sign.)‖‖ The injection of 5 ml. of distilled water will cause some discomfort to the patient if it is placed in the extradural space—an additional help in localization (Lund).†

---

* Dogliotti, A. M., *Zbl. Chir.*, 1931, **58**, 3141.
† Lund, P. C., *Int. Anæs. Clin.*, 1964, **2**, 471.
‡ Gutiérrez, A., *Rev. Cirg., B. Aires*, 1932, **12**, 665; and *Ibid.*, 1933, **13**, 255.
§ Odom, C. B., *Amer. J. Surg.*, 1936, **34**, 547.
‖ Brooks, W., *Anæsthesia*, 1957, **12**, 227.
¶ Macintosh, R. R., *Ibid.*, 1950, **5**, 98.
** Macintosh, R. R., *Brit. med. J.*, 1953, **1**, 398.
†† Salt, R. H., *Anæsthesia*, 1963, **18**, 404.
‡‡ Iklé, A., *Brit. J. Anæsth.*, 1950, **22**, 150.
§§ Dawkins, R. J. M., *Anæsthesia*, 1961, **16**, 108; and *Ibid.*, 1963, **18**, 66.
‖‖ Durrans, S. F., *Ibid.*, 1947, **2**, 106.

Method of Location of Extradural Space, *continued.*

Injection must only commence when position of needle point is certain.

An initial test injection of 5 ml. is made and, if in 5 minutes there is no evidence of subarachnoid block such as inability to move feet, the remainder of the solution is slowly injected, frequent aspiration tests being made to avoid risk of subarachnoid or intravenous injection. Many workers of experience omit this test dose.

The patient is then turned on the back with slight head-down tilt.

PROCEDURE IF DURA IS PIERCED.—The choice is as follows (1) Leave needle in theca so that it occludes the dural puncture and attempt to locate the extradural space from a higher or lower level. Withdraw first needle after injection through the second needle into the extradural space. (2) Convert the block into an intradural (subarachnoid) one. (3) Abandon the method and use general anæsthesia.

A pressor drug may be given, as there is likely to be some fall in the blood-pressure, but the ischæmia which results from this block may well be one of its most desirable features with which it might be inadvisable to interfere. The authors use a pressor agent with decreasing frequency, as vasocontriction may cause tissue anoxia and metabolic acidosis, from under-perfusion.

Onset of complete analgesia may require 10–20 minutes and can be checked by : (1) Disappearance of anal tone (S.4–5) ; (2) Disappearance of knee-jerks (L.2–4) ; (3) Disappearance of tone of abdominal muscles (T.8–L.1); (4) Disappearance of ankle-jerk (S.1–2); (5) The existence and extent of skin analgesia.

The maximal concentration of lignocaine in the blood-stream after extradural block occurs, on average, 18 minutes after injection and after a shorter period if adrenaline is not used.[*]

Delayed extension of the block (and even delayed apnœa) may be due to medial spread of the local analgesic solution in nerve trunks from the extradural space into the spinal cord itself (intraneural spread). Delay may be as long as 40 minutes.[†]

Absorption into the intraneural spaces and centripetal spread is said to occur from the region of the junction of the anterior and posterior nerve-roots.[‡]

Continuous Extradural Analgesia.[§]—Greater control over duration and extent of analgesia can be gained if instead of a single injection of solution, repeated injections are made through a plastic catheter introduced into the extradural space. The plastic catheter of 1 mm. bore, made of nylon, or polyvinyl chloride, is passed through a large needle (e.g., Tuohy),[||] the slightly angulated tip of which is accurately placed in the extradural space. The angle at the tip carries the catheter either up or down within the space according to the direction it is turned. This special needle, though rather large

[*] Bromage, P. R., and Robson, G., *Anæsthesia*, 1961, **16**, 461.
[†] Morrow, W. F. K., *Brit. J. Anæsth.*, 1959, **31**, 359.
[‡] Bromage, P. R., *Ibid.*, 1962, **34**, 161.
[§] Curbelo, M. M., *Curr. Res. Anesth.*, 1949, **28**, 13.
[||] Tuohy, E. B., *J. Amer. med. Ass.*, 1945, **128**, 262.

in bore (16–18 gauge), is relatively easy to insert and many workers use it routinely, even for 'one-shot' injections. The catheter, however, does not always travel in the desired direction.*

The insertion of a catheter into the extradural space is especially useful: (1) When the extent of the operation is uncertain; (2) When the duration is uncertain; (3) When the time of commencement is uncertain—the catheter can be put in at leisure and the injection given when necessary; (4) In handicapped patients, to enable small doses to be given and later increased.

VOLUMES OF SOLUTION OF 1·5 PER CENT LIGNOCAINE REQUIRED.—For prostatectomy 10–20 ml.; for vaginal and perineal repair 20–40 ml. ; for herniæ, appendicectomies, etc., 25–35 ml. of solution are required ; for hysterectomies, etc., 25–35 ml. ; for upper abdominal operations, 35–40 ml. For Cæsarean section 15–25 ml., taking care to control the blood-pressure. In infants 5–6 ml. of 1 per cent lignocaine has been reported to give good results (or 1 ml. per 2 lb. body-weight).†

Those workers who regard the mass of solute as more important than the volume of solution in judging dosage suggest that 35 mg. per spinal segment to be blocked at age 20, decreasing to 15 mg. per segment at age 80, when using solutions between 2 and 5 per cent, is a suitable guide. Adrenaline is added (1–200,000) to the lignocaine solution.‡

Indications for Extradural Block.—

1. IN UPPER ABDOMINAL OPERATIONS.—A block to T.4 or T.5 is required and this obtunds all afferent impulses conveyed to the posterior root ganglia from upper abdominal viscera. It does not obtund impulses conveyed up the vagus or phrenic nerves and so reflex disturbances, hiccoughs, nausea and retching, and laryngeal spasm (Brewer-Luckhart reflex) may cause trouble. The method is seen at its best in fit young patients. Greater control is obtained if an endotracheal tube is passed before or after the extradural injection, and this allows unimpeded spontaneous respiration of gas–oxygen and a trace of supplement, e.g., halothane, trichloroethylene, or cyclopropane, to prevent coughing on the tube. In the presence of emphysema or a tendency to bronchospasm, it may be preferable to omit the tube.

2. IN LOWER ABDOMINAL OPERATIONS.—The method is seen to its best advantage in these cases. Muscular relaxation, contracted bowels, wound ischæmia with adequate spontaneous respiration combine to give excellent conditions for surgery.

3. IN HERNIA REPAIRS.—An excellent method unless the patient is grossly obese, arthritic, or unfit.

4. IN OPERATIONS ON THE LOWER LIMBS.—Extradural block is seldom really necessary in these operations but never-theless gives excellent results in relatively fit patients.

5. OPERATIONS ON THE VERTEBRAL COLUMN.—In lamin-ectomies the injection of a full dose of solution produces wound ischæmia which many surgeons find most welcome. Experienced

---

* Sanchez, R., and others, *Brit. J. Anæsth.*, 1967, **39**, 485.
† Ruston, F. G., *Canad. Anæsth. Soc. J.*, 1954, **1**, 37; and *Ibid.*, 1964, **11**, 12.
‡ Bromage, P. R., and others, *Brit. J. Anæsth.*, 1964, **36**, 342.

Indications for Extradural Block, *continued.*

workers employ volumes up to 40 ml. of 1·5 per cent lignocaine with adrenaline in fit patients.*

6. OBSTETRIC ANALGESIA.†—Bupivacaine may have a use here.‡
Skill and care in the selection of patients of older age-groups for extradural block is very necessary.

Management of the Patient during Extradural Block.—The general effects on the patient are similar to those described in the section on spinal analgesia. Management of the patient on the operating table is the same as in intradural block (*see* pp. 402 and 419.

The blood-pressure is likely to be higher in a conscious than in an unconscious patient. Most anæsthetists have their patients drowsy, under the influence of an intravenous thiobarbiturate, or under general anæsthesia, e.g., gas and oxygen, halothane, or cyclopropane. The blood-pressure can be controlled as outlined below, the actual degree of hypotension depending on the amount of ischæmia thought desirable and the general condition of the patient. The proponents of total spinal analgesia believe that, given adequate ventilation and oxygenation, a systolic blood-pressure of 35 mm. Hg is adequate as it is greater than the sum of the venous pressure and the osmotic pressure of the plasma, always provided that peripheral resistance is abolished by the vasodilatation consequent on sympathetic block§. The blood-pressure of the authors begins to rise if that of their patients descends very much below 60 mm. Hg. During periods of hypotension a head-down tilt should, if possible, be adopted and maintained into the postoperative period until the blood-pressure rises satisfactorily. Breathing pure oxygen causes a decrease in heart-rate and cardiac output and an increase in total peripheral resistance, i.e., a decreased myocardial work-load without decrease in oxygen transport to the tissues. It is beneficial for patients with a high block.‖ The phenothiazine drugs will increase hypotension, given before or during the operation.

Breathing during extradural block is generally quieter and easier than under general anæsthesia. There may be a reflex broncho-dilatation initiated by baroreceptors stimulated by low blood-pressure, in the aorticocarotid sinuses, or it may be due to relative ischæmia of the mucosæ of the bronchi consequent on the low blood-pressure in their supplying vessels, the bronchial arteries. During high extradural block the respiratory minute volume, the tidal volume, blood gas estimations, and the vital capacity are not greatly altered.¶

COMPLICATIONS.—

1. Inadequate block : this must be covered by some convenient form of general anæsthesia.

* Thorne, T. C., personal communication.
† Brandstater, B., *Proc. 2nd Eur. Cong. Anæsth.*, 1966, **3**, 345.
‡ Duthie, A. M., Wyman, J. B., and Lewis, G. A., *Anæsthesia*, 1968, **23**, 20.
§ Griffiths, H. W. C., and Gillies, J., *Ibid.*, 1948, **3**, 134.
‖ Ward, R. J., and others, *Curr. Res. Anesth.*, 1966, **45**, 140.
¶ Moir, D. D., *Brit. J. Anæsth.*, 1963, **35**, 3; and Moir, D. D., and Mone, J. G., *Ibid.*, 1964, **36**, 480.

2. Hypotension : this should be dealt with *secundum artem*. Posture, pressor drugs, intravenous infusions, atropine in the presence of severe bradycardia.
3. Hypopnœa : this will need careful attention to the airway and may call for assisted respiration. It may progress to frank apnœa, and this need not be due to either total spinal or to total extradural block. It well may be a sign of toxicity of the analgesic drug. It usually lasts about 1 hour and need not interrupt the operation providing respiration is controlled.
4. Nausea and vomiting : this can be managed by additional intravenous or inhalation anæsthesia.
5. Spasmodic muscular movements of the arms and shoulders: these may be seen in patients kept lightly asleep with thiopentone or soluble hexobarbitone. Intravenous heroin, pethidine, more barbiturate, or light general anæsthesia may be required.
6. Total spinal analgesia : the possibility of this must always be present in the mind of the anæsthetist performing an extradural block. If this has occurred the patient is likely to show, within 3 minutes of injection of the analgesic drug : (*a*) marked hypotension, (*b*) apnœa, (*c*) dilated pupils. He is in grave danger of death from asphyxia. Management : turn patient into the supine position, ventilate the lungs, inject a pressor drug into the open vein, set up an intravenous drip. This will in most cases rescue the patient from imminent death. Later, a tube can be passed and ventilation can be controlled with equal volumes of oxygen and nitrous oxide. The operation can in most cases proceed and breathing will probably recommence within the hour. Unpleasant sequelæ are unlikely.
7. Toxicity due to the injected drug ; this may occur after rather small amounts of drug, e.g., 150 mg. of lignocaine in 1·5 per cent solution, but is not common. It can follow intravascular or extradural injection, that is the subsequent block may be absent or good. The signs are disorientation going on to twitching, convulsions, and perhaps apnœa. Management consists of injecting a barbiturate (e.g., thiopentone, 150 mg.) into the open vein (to inject into the vein of a violently convulsing patient may be impossible) ; the administration of oxygen by I.P.P. if necessary ; protection of the patient's teeth and tongue from the trauma of the fits ; injection of 50 mg. of suxamethonium. In the authors' experience the last has never been necessary.

ADVANTAGES claimed for the method as against spinal analgesia are :—
1. Less danger of meningitis and neurological sequelæ.
2. Absence of post-operation headache and urinary retention.
3. Prolonged post-operation analgesia—up to 6 or 8 hours after bupivacaine, cinchocaine, or amethocaine.

ADVANTAGES, as compared with general anæsthesia :—
1. Protection of the patient from the afferent impulses of the operation.
2. Maintenance of spontaneous respiration.

Management of the Patient during Extradural Block, *continued.*

3. Provision, by one injection of analgesia, of relaxation, ischæmia and contracted bowels.
4. Very suitable in certain patients with asthma, bronchitis, or emphysema.
5. Can be employed in patients who are not suitable for muscle relaxants, e.g., in myasthenia.

DISADVANTAGES are :—

1. Difficulty of being sure of position of needle point, with risk of subarachnoid injection of a large volume of solution. If a massive spinal injection (subarachnoid) is given by mistake artificial respiration with oxygen must be efficiently carried out, with the use, if necessary, of a pressor drug.
2. Time taken over the block.
3. Time taken before onset of analgesia.

Contra-indications.—These are similar to those set out on p. 413 for intradural block.

Patients who are over 65, and those with large abdominal tumours, arteriosclerosis, and diabetes need especial care.

Sequelæ.—

1. Paraplegia*—a rare occurrence. In a recently reported series of 50,000 blocks, 2 patients developed paraplegia, 1 of whom had metastatic carcinoma.† The senior author of this book, in over twenty-five years of active employment of extradural block, has only seen 1 case.
2. Anterior spinal artery syndrome.‡ Paraplegia not involving the posterior column of the cord, so that joint, position sense, touch and vibration sense are spared. This was first described in 1909 by Miller (*J. nerv. ment. Dis.*, 1909, **36**, 601). An extremely uncommon occurrence.
3. Intra-ocular hæmorrhage has been reported after the injection of 120 ml. of solution§ and even after the rapid injection of 30 ml.|| This may raise the cerebrospinal fluid pressure with resulting subhyaloid bleeding.
4. Occasional backache caused by the needle.¶

Therapeutic Uses of Extradural Block.—

1. Post-operative pain relief and for prevention of post-operative chest complications. Insertion of an extradural catheter into the upper thoracic region, either by the midline or by the lateral route, between T.1 and T.4 will enable local analgesic solution (e.g., 0·5–1·5 per cent lignocaine, 8–10 ml.) to be deposited in the region where afferent fibres from the abdominal wall enter the posterior roots. Puncture in the upper thoracic region, using a hanging drop test in the sitting position, is easier than a

---

* Braham, J., and Saia, A., *Brit. med. J.*, 1958, **2**, 657.
† Hillmann, K., *Canad. Anæsth. Soc. J.*, 1965, **12**, 4.
‡ Annotation, *Lancet*, 1958, **2**, 515 ; and Davies, A., and others, *Brit. med. J.*, 1958, **2**, 654.
§ Evans, W., *Lancet*, 1930, **2**, 1225.
|| Kelman, H., *Amer. J. Surg.*, 1944, **64**, 183 ; and Clark, C. J., and Whitwell, J., *Brit. med. J.*, 1961, **2**, 1612.
¶ Wolfson, B., and Ingram, C. G., *Brit. J. Anæsth.*, 1959, **29**, 514.

mid-thoracic approach, owing to the obliquity of the spinous processes. In this way analgesia of the wound and anterior abdominal wall is produced so that the patient can be encouraged to cough and breathe deeply without the severe pain usually caused by such activity. Analgesia lasts about 90 minutes and fresh injections can be given as frequently as necessary. If the patient is kept flat for 20 or 30 minutes thereafter he can then get up and walk about without much fall in blood-pressure.* Respiratory function is restored much more efficiently by afferent blockade than by narcotic analgesics.†

2. This technique may also be used in the management of closed chest injuries. Single-shot or continuous extradural block has also been used to control the severe pain of acute pancreatitis, and dissecting aneurysm. It has also been used in eclampsia as a method of deliberate hypotension, and in status asthmaticus.

3. Treatment of circulatory disturbances after poliomyelitis. Block of the pre-ganglionic fibres supplying the lower limbs (T.10 to L.2 or 3) improves the circulation and may need to be repeated. Cinchocaine 1–1500 gives sympathetic block without sensory involvement. Dose : for small child 16 ml., and for an adult 40 ml.‡

4. In causalgia, Sudeck's atrophy, thrombophlebitis, traumatic vasospasm, acute and chronic arterial occlusion, renal calculi (to aid passage of the stone),§ sciatica, and post-spinal headache. Alcohol injected into the space requires general anæsthesia as it causes severe pain.

The whole subject of extradural block is fully and most competently discussed by Lund, P. C., *Peridural Analgesia and Anesthesia*, 1966. Springfield: Thomas.

EXTRADURAL SACRAL BLOCK (CAUDAL BLOCK)

This method of analgesia was introduced by Cathelin‖ and Sicard¶ in 1901 and was used by Schlimpert of Freiburg in 1913, and in obstetrics by Stoeckel** in 1909, who was the first to report painless vaginal delivery following injection of the recently discovered agent procaine into the extradural space, and by Läwen,†† who potentiated his solution by the addition of sodium bicarbonate. Hingson of Cleveland has been a pioneer and proponent of the method.‡‡ Has been used in animals, especially in cattle, since 1925. Very suitable for block of the sacral and lumbar nerves. For higher block the lumbar approach to the extra-dural space is preferable as less solution will thereby be used.

---

* Simpson, B. R., Parkhouse, J., Marshall, R., and Lambrechts, W., *Brit. J. Anæsth.*, 1961, **33**, 628; Cole, P. V. C., *Anæsthesia*, 1964, **19**, 526; Scott, D. B., and Walker, L. R., *Ibid.*, 1963, **18**, 82; and Green, R., and Dawkins, R. J. M., *Ibid.*, 1966, **21**, 372.

† Bromage, P. R., *Brit. J. Anæsth.*, 1967, **39**, 721.

‡ Allison, R. C., *Anæsthesia*, 1958, **13**, 157.

§ Lloyd, J. W., and Carrie, L. E. S., *Proc. R. Soc. Med.*, 1965, **58**, 634.

‖ Cathelin, F., *C.R. Soc. Biol., Paris*, 1901, **53**, 452.

¶ Sicard, M. A., *Ibid.*, 1901, **53**, 396.

** Stoeckel, W., *Zbl. Gynäk.*, 1909, **31**, 1.

†† Läwen, A., *Zbl. Chir.*, 1910, **37**, 708.

‡‡ Hingson, R. A., and Southworth, J. L., *Amer. J. Surg.*, 1942, **58**, 92; and Hingson, R. A., and Edwards, W. B., *J. Amer. med. Ass.*, 1943, **121**, 252.

Anatomy of Sacrum.—A large triangular bone formed by the fusion of the five sacral vertebræ, articulating above with the fifth lumbar vertebra and below with the coccyx.

Pelvic surface is concave from above downwards and from side to side. It is crossed by four transverse ridges, at the lateral extremities of each being an anterior sacral foramen, directed forward and laterally. Each foramen opens into the sacral canal and transmits an anterior primary ramus of one of the upper four sacral nerves.

Posterior surface is convex and down its middle line runs the median sacral crest with its three or four rudimentary spinous processes. The laminæ of the fifth and sometimes of the fourth sacral vertebræ fail to fuse in the midline ; the deficiency thus formed is known as the sacral hiatus. The tubercles representing the inferior articular processes of the fifth sacral vertebra are prolonged downwards as the sacral cornua. These cornua, with the rudimentary spine of the fourth vertebra above, bound the sacral hiatus. Four posterior sacral foramina correspond with the anterior foramina. Each transmits a sacral nerve posterior ramus and communicates with the sacral canal.

Lateral surfaces are broader above than below and are ear-shaped. Each articulates with the ilium. In the female the articular surface extends to S.2, in the male to S.3.

Base of the sacrum is directed upwards and forwards and articulates with the fifth lumbar vertebra. The central portion forms the sacral promontory, this being flanked by the sacral ala on each side. The body of the first sacral vertebra is not as wide in the female as in the male. The ala represents the transverse and costal processes of the first sacral vertebra.

Apex is directed downwards and articulates with the coccyx.

Coccyx represents four rudimentary vertebræ—sometimes three or five.

Female sacrum is shorter and wider than the male sacrum : it is directed more obliquely backward, thus increasing the size of the cavity of the pelvis.

SACRAL CANAL is a prismatic cavity running throughout the length of the bone and following its curves. Superiorly it is triangular on section and is continuous with the lumbar vertebral canal. Its lower extremity is the sacral hiatus, closed by the posterior sacrococcygeal membrane. Fibrous strands sometimes occur in the canal and divide the extradural space into compartments. These may account for some cases of failure to produce uniform analgesia. Its anterior wall is formed by fusion of the bodies of the sacral vertebræ ; its posterior wall, by fusion of the laminæ. The hiatus results from lack of fusion of the laminæ of the fifth sacral vertebra. On each lateral wall of the canal, four foramina are present, which divide in the form of a Y into anterior and posterior sacral foramina. The contents of the sacral canal are :—

    1. The dural sac which ends at the lower border of the second sacral vertebra, on a line joining the posterior superior

iliac spines.   The pia mater is continued as the filum terminale.

2. The sacral nerves and the coccygeal nerve, with their dorsal root ganglia.

3. A venous plexus formed by the lower end of the internal vertebral plexus.   These vessels are more numerous anteriorly than posteriorly and so needle point should be kept as far posteriorly as possible.

4. Areolar and fatty tissue—more dense in males than females.
Each sacral nerve is provided with a thick sheath from the dura.

The sacral hiatus is a triangular opening, caused by failure of the fifth (and sometimes of the fourth) laminar arch to fuse, with apex upwards formed by the fourth sacral spine, and a sacral cornu on each side below and laterally.   (But this is so in only 35 per cent of sacra.*)   It is covered over by the sacrococcygeal ligament which is pierced by the coccygeal and fifth sacral nerves.   It is superior to the sacrococcygeal junction, usually about 1½–2 in. from the tip of the coccyx and directly beneath the upper limit of the intergluteal cleft.   *Anatomical abnormalities* of the sacrum are not uncommon.   They include : (1) Upward and downward displacement of the hiatus. (2) Pronounced narrowing or partial obliteration of the sacral canal, making needle insertion difficult. (3) Ossification of the sacrococcygeal membrane. (4) Absence of the bony posterior wall of the sacral canal, due to failure of fusion of laminæ.

The average capacity of the sacral canal is 34 ml. in males and 32 ml. in females.   Its average length is 3 to 4 in.

When a local analgesic solution is injected into the sacral canal it ascends upwards in the extradural space for a distance proportional to the volume of solution, the force of injection, the amount of leakage through the intervertebral foramina and the consistency of the connective tissue in the space.   While the first two are controllable, the last are not, so precise placement of the solution is impossible and sometimes leads to unexpected results.   As the extradural space communicates through the intervertebral foramina with the paravertebral spaces (which are not themselves intercommunicating), extradural block affects : (1) Anterior nerve-roots ; (2) Posterior nerve-roots and root ganglia ; (3) The mixed spinal nerves ; (4) The ganglia of the sympathetic chain ; (5) The grey and white rami communicantes ; (6) The visceral afferent fibres accompanying the sympathetic fibres.

Technique of Injection.—A needle, e.g., a Mitchell or a Gordh, is inserted into a vein.   The patient is in the prone position with hips slightly flexed over two pillows.   To prevent tensing of the gluteal muscles the patient should be asked to abduct his legs and

---

* Trotter, M., and Letterman, G. S., *Surg. Gynec. Obstet.*, 1944, **78**, 418.

Technique of Injection, *continued.*

turn his toes in. Other positions are the lateral, knee–chest, and knee–elbow. After cleaning and towelling, the tip of the coccyx is identified and the triangular sacral hiatus palpated about $1\frac{1}{2}$–2 in. (3·8–5 cm.) above it. The hiatus must be clearly visualized. Its anatomy is not constant; sometimes it is larger, sometimes smaller, than normal. It is difficult to feel in fat patients. If necessary, a dose of thiopentone can be injected into a Mitchell needle just before the block is commenced.

A weal is raised over the hiatus, using no more than 2 drops of solution, as œdema obscures the landmarks. A needle, such as a number 1, is inserted through the sacrococcygeal membrane so that it makes an angle of about 20° with the line drawn at right-angles to the skin surface. Once through the membrane the needle is depressed a further 45° towards the intergluteal cleft and the needle is inserted into the sacral canal, keeping in the midline. The point must not ascend higher than the line joining the posterior superior iliac spines lest the dura, which ends at this level, be entered. Occasionally the dural sac extends lower down than the level of the second piece of the sacrum. The mean distance between the apex of the hiatus and the dural sac is 4·5 cm. In many cases the needle used for the skin weal can be used to enter the sacral canal.

After aspiration tests for blood and cerebrospinal fluid have been proved negative, a test dose of 8 ml. of solution can be injected if thought necessary. Should *blood* flow through the needle, its position must be slightly altered. Should *cerebrospinal fluid* appear, the method of analgesia must be abandoned and sub-arachnoid injection substituted for it in suitable cases, the proper amount of drug being introduced into the theca through the sacral needle.

Five minutes after the test injection, movement of the toes is called for : if this is present, a subarachnoid block has not resulted and the needle point is not in the theca ; further injection can then be proceeded with. When the needle is correctly placed, injection is easy, no great force being required to depress the plunger of the syringe. Should the needle be *posterior to the canal*, a tumour is raised over the sacrum as the injection proceeds. Injection of a few ml. of air will produce surgical emphysema with its crepitus, if the needle is superficial to the canal. If the needle point comes to lie *between periosteum and bone* the force needed for injection will be great—a sure sign of an incorrect position. Young males, because of the tough nature of their peridural fat, require larger doses, injected with greater force, than females, while 2 per cent solution of lignocaine gives better results than 1·5 per cent solution in these patients.

Drugs.—Lignocaine 1 to 1·5 per cent solution is excellent, giving a rapid onset and a profound degree of analgesia. Its effects can be prolonged if amethocaine powder is added to make a strength of 0·1 per cent or 0·2 per cent. Piperocaine in 1·5 per cent solution in normal saline or Ringer's solution is very satisfactory. Prilocaine in 1·5 or 2 per cent solution is excellent and bupivacaine shows

great promise, especially where a prolonged action is required.*
Procaine, 2 per cent in normal saline, can be used, while if a
prolonged effect is wanted cinchocaine, 1–500 in normal saline, or
0·15 per cent amethocaine hydrochloride in saline, can be employed,
with a maximal dosage of 50–60 ml. Adrenaline should be added.

DOSAGE.—Level of analgesia is governed by :—
1. Quantity of solution.
2. Speed of injection.
3. Gravity.
4. Age of patient.

Poor-risk cases require a smaller dose by at least 20 per cent.

Low Block, i.e., up to L.2 to L.4, for operations on anus, rectum,
perineum, or urethra, circumcision, vaginal plastics, etc. :
inject 30 ml. of 1 per cent or 1·5 per cent lignocaine slowly.
In 10 minutes analgesia will develop and will last one hour ;
20 ml. of solution is sufficient for the average case of hæmorrhoids or anal fissure.

Mid Block, i.e., up to T.10, for operation on lower limbs, pelvic
organs, hernia, etc. : inject 30 ml. with table in slight
Trendelenburg tilt. In 5 minutes inject a further 10–20 ml.
fairly rapidly. For operations on lower extremities the tilt
can be reversed.

High Block, i.e., up to T.4–5, for operations on upper abdomen :
inject 30 ml. and pause 5 minutes. Then tilt the table and
inject a further 30 ml. After a second similar pause inject a
third dose of 10 ml. High block may take half an hour to
develop and should last a further 60–90 minutes. Motor
block is not marked, but as the reflex arc is broken no reflex
rigidity of the muscles of the anterior abdominal wall results
from stimuli. The rami communicantes are paralysed and
the blood-pressure falls, though not so suddenly as after
subarachnoid block. A pressor drug should be at hand, to
be used in suitable cases.

Toxic reactions to the drugs used are sometimes seen, as dosage
is fairly large. An occasional twitch requires no treatment,
but convulsions should be combated with intravenous hexobarbitone or thiopentone. Collapse due to cardiovascular
depression consequent on reduction of the blood-pressure is
treated on the usual lines by elevating the lower limbs and
injecting a pressor drug.

The extent of analgesia is not by any means related only to the
volume of solution injected, but also to the volume which
leaks through the sacral foramina and the intervertebral
foramina and to the degree of the lumbo-sacral angle.† The
best control of the height of analgesia is obtained by the use
of the continuous technique.

Sacral Extradural Block in Infants and Children.—Perhaps
because of their healthy cardiovascular systems, young children
stand this form of analgesia well. It may be necessary occasionally
to provide light general anæsthesia for the injection.

---

* Herbring, B. G., *Acta anæsth. scand.*, 1966, Suppl. 21, **45**.
† Bryce-Smith, R., *Anæsthesia*, 1954, **9**, 203.

Sacral Extradural Block in Infants and Children, *continued.*

Solution to be used—1 per cent lignocaine with adrenaline 1–200,000. Dose: 10 mg. per kg. for block up to T.12; 12·5 mg. per kg. for block up to T.10. Infants less than 3 months old require 10 mg. per kg. of a 0·5 per cent solution. Close watch must be kept on ventilation and pulse.*

Advantages.—
1. Absence of post-operative headaches.
2. Less cardiovascular depression than with subarachnoid analgesia.
The method is excellent for cystoscopies, hæmorrhoidectomies, and gynæcological plastic operations and is highly recommended by the present authors.
It is also most useful for forceps deliveries in obstetrics, owing to the excellent relaxation of the cervix, and pelvic floor and perineum.
It can be used for orthopædic operations on the foot, for ligation of varices, and for the prolonged relief of post-operative pain after, e.g., hæmorrhoidectomy : in this case a plastic catheter is left in the sacral canal and through it doses of 12 ml. of local analgesic solution can be injected as required.
Its therapeutic indications include low backache ; sciatica ; vasospastic disease of the lower limbs ; white leg ; acute anuria, sometimes ; and intractable pelvic pain using up to 60 ml. of proctocaine.†

Disadvantages.—
1. Length of time taken for development of analgesia.
2. Lack of accurate control of height of analgesia.
3. Muscular relaxation not maximal in mid and high blocks, although it is excellent in low blocks.
4. Technical difficulty.
5. Risk of inadvertent subarachnoid injection.
6. Hypotension and possible signs of drug toxicity.
7. It produces complete flaccidity of the anal sphincters, a condition unpopular with some surgeons doing such operations as cure of fistula-in-ano.

CONTINUOUS CAUDAL (EXTRADURAL SACRAL) BLOCK

This is chiefly used to produce painless labour. Single extradural sacral injections have been used for many years in obstetrics (Stoeckel, 1909 ; Schlimpert, 1913), but the continuous technique was introduced in 1942 by Edwards and Hingson,‡ who used a needle connected to rubber tubing. Manalan substituted a uteric catheter.§

Autonomic Nerve-supply of Uterus.—
1. Visceral efferent sympathetic (motor to upper uterine segment). The middle thoracic segments from T.3 downwards, perhaps as

---

* Fortuna, A., *Brit. J. Anæsth.*, 1966, **39**, 165.
† Kenny, M., *Brit. med. J.*, 1947, **2**, 862.
‡ Edwards, W. B., and Hingson, R. A., *Amer. J. Surg.*, 1942, **57**, 459 ; and Hingson, R. A., and Edwards, W. B., *Curr. Res. Anesth.*, 1942, **21**, 301.
§ Manalan, J. A., *J. Indiana med. Ass.*, 1942, **35**, 564.

low as L.2, via splanchnic nerves and cœliac, aortic, renal, and hypogastric plexuses, and thence with blood-vessels to the great cervical ganglion of Frankenhauser. In addition, some of the motor supply of the body of the uterus may come from below the sensory supply, i.e., T.11, L.2. The inferior hypogastric plexus, pelvic plexus, or plexus of Frankenhauser is situated on each side of the rectum in the base of the broad ligament. The cervix and lateral vaginal fornix are medial relations. Each plexus is a thin sheet. The parasympathetic roots are the pelvic splanchnic nerves, while the pre-ganglionic sympathetic roots come from cells in the last three thoracic and first two lumbar segments of the cord.

2. Visceral afferent sympathetic (sensory to uterus). Block of these eases pain of the first stage of labour, with exception of those near the end of this stage. Eleventh and twelfth thoracic (and possibly first lumbar). Fibres go from uterus (ganglion of Frankenhauser) via sympathetic nerves to pelvic, hypogastric, and aortic plexuses, enter the sympathetic chain at the level of L.5 and ascend in the chain, entering the cord via the white rami of T.11 and T.12, and the eleventh–twelfth posterior thoracic roots and thence up posterior columns of cord (J. G. P. Cleland, 1933). The fibres then cross over to the spinothalamic tract on the opposite side of the cord and ascend to the thalamus and thence to the frontal and parietal areas of the cortex. Block of the sympathetic chain between L.5 and T.12 gives the same freedom from first-stage labour pains as block of the eleventh–twelfth thoracic ganglia.

3. Visceral afferent and efferent parasympathetic (inhibitory to uterus ; sensory and motor to cervix ; sensory to upper birth canal). Second, third, and fourth sacral nerves, directly to great cervical ganglion of Frankenhauser.

Somatic Afferent Nerves of Lower Birth Canal.—

The inferior rectal, perineal, and dorsal nerve of the clitoris—from the pudendal nerve (S.2, 3, 4).

The ilio-inguinal (L.1) and the genitofemoral (L.1, 2).

There are twenty nerves transmitting labour pains, viz.—(a) The visceral afferents of the eleventh and twelfth thoracic—pain of uterine contraction ; (b) The posterior roots of the second, third, and fourth sacral nerves, carrying pelvic afferents (Hy. Head) —pain of cervical dilatation ; (c) The rectal, perineal, and pudendal branches of the sacral plexus—pain of perineal stretching ; (d) The ilio-inguinal and genitofemoral branches of the lumbar plexus.

In labour the method should be commenced : (1) When presenting part is engaged ; (2) When cervix is dilated to the size of half-a-crown (in primiparæ) ; (3) When contractions are occurring regularly at not more than five-minute intervals and are of half-minute duration.

Technique.—

With patient in the lateral, knee–elbow, or knee–chest position, a malleable spinal needle is inserted into the sacral canal for 1–2 in. (2·5–5 cm.). To this is attached a closed system

Continuous Caudal Block—Technique, *continued.*

comprising a length of fine-bore, plastic or thick-walled rubber tubing, a syringe, and a reservoir containing the analgesic solution. The needle is taped between the buttocks and the patient turned on her back. Injections are not begun until labour is well established.

Solutions used :—

1. Lignocaine, 1 to 1·5 per cent 20 ml. This gives a block up to T.11 in most cases, patients in labour showing a higher level of analgesia than normal women. Repeated injections have a decreasing effect.
2. Prilocaine in similar dosage.
3. Procaine, 2 per cent in normal saline.
4. Piperocaine, 1·5 per cent in normal saline, or Ringer's solution.

If 0·15 per cent amethocaine is used, probably one or two separate injections will carry the patient through the latter part of her labour, avoiding the need for the continuous technique.

Test dose, 8 ml. of solution, i.e., lignocaine or prilocaine, 80–120 mg., piperocaine, 120 mg., or procaine, 160 mg.

Initial dose, 30 ml. injected in 60 seconds if test dose shows after 10 minutes no evidence of subarachnoid injection having been given. This usually produces freedom from pain in 10 to 15 minutes.

To maintain this, subsequent doses of 20 ml. are given on an average every 30–40 minutes.

Labour is retarded if analgesia rises higher than half-way between the pubis and the umbilicus, i.e., higher than or including the tenth thoracic segment, as it will affect motor fibres supplying the upper uterine segment. Unilateral analgesia may occur.

The following modifications have been suggested :—

1. Introduction of a ureteric catheter or plastic tube into the sacral canal, through a wide-bore needle (e.g., Tuohy*) which is afterwards withdrawn over the catheter (Manalan, 1942 ; Block and Rochberg, 1943 ; and later Adams, Lundy, and Seldon, 1943). This is less traumatic than an indwelling needle and less likely to break or slip into the theca.
2. Maintenance of analgesia by a continuous drip instead of repeated injections. A rate of 8–12 per minute is average. Speeding of drip suggests slipping of needle into theca.
3. Addition of adrenaline to solution to prolong its effect (1–200,000). Some workers avoid adrenaline because of its relaxing effect on the uterus.
4. Addition of a barbiturate in early labour to minimize toxic effect of analgesic drugs and for its sedative effect.

For Cæsarean section 1 per cent lignocaine is used. After test dose of 10 ml., a primary dose of 20 ml. is injected, followed by 20 ml. every ten minutes until analgesia reaches to the costal margins. The operation must not be begun until a proper height of analgesia has been obtained. The method demands freedom from rush and absence of adherence to a time schedule. For ' one shot ' injection, 30–35 ml. of 1·5 per cent lignocaine is

---

* Tuohy, E. B., *J. Amer. med. Ass.*, 1945, **128**, 262.

usually safe and adequate. An intravenous drip should be routine and it is desirable to maintain the blood-pressure above 80 mm. Hg. Oxygen inhalation (100 per cent) should be given before and during the operation.

Results.—In ideal cases labour is not retarded ; the perineum is relaxed from the outset ; the first and third stages are shortened, although the second stage is prolonged, frequently requiring forceps delivery—which is rendered easy by the relaxation of the pelvic floor and perineum, analgesia being adequate for the forceps extraction and episiotomy ; respiration of the fœtus is spontaneous at birth ; there is some fall in blood-pressure ; there is complete freedom from pain, throughout labour. Hingson claims that in 90 per cent of cases pain at the end of the first stage, second-stage pain, and pain from repair of perineal tears can be abolished completely. It should not be used for early pain of the first stage.

Limitations and Dangers of Continuous Caudal Analgesia.—

1. Fœtal hypoxia due to hypotension of mother. Maternal blood-pressure must not be allowed to fall below 80 mm. Hg systolic : fall in blood-pressure must be treated by pressor drugs, posture, elevation of the legs, and intravenous fluids. The signs of hypoxia in the fœtus : (*a*) Bradycardia. (*b*) Increased movements. (*c*) Increased meconium.
2. Broken needles or plastic tubing.
3. Arrested or prolonged labour, due to too high spread of solution, or its leakage through the anterior sacral foramina on to the ganglion of Frankenhauser.
4. Increased incidence of occipito-posterior positions.
5. Increased incidence of operative deliveries.
6. Massive spinal analgesia. If this occurs, patient becomes pale and blue and later apnœic. The chief danger is anoxia, circulatory collapse being some minutes away. Routine resuscitation is as follows :—
   a. Rhythmical inflation with oxygen.
   b. Give blood-pressure-raising drug.
   c. Turn patient on to side and withdraw 20–40 ml. of cerebrospinal fluid.
   d. Give intravenous drip.
7. Infection.
8. Drug susceptibility on part of the mother, and also of the fœtus from transplacental contamination.
9. Maternal hypotension and circulatory depression. Elevation of the legs to a right-angle results in an efficient autotransfusion.
10. Fœtal bradycardia. Can be reversed by atropine, i.v. to mother.*

In spite of these dangers the stillbirth and neonatal death-rates are quoted as being less in cases delivered under continuous caudal analgesia than in cases delivered under other forms of analgesia and anæsthesia, or under none at all.

Special Indications.—

1. In patients with cardiac disease.
2. In patients with nephritis.

---

* Parker, J. R. B., *Proc. R. Soc. Med.*, 1965, **58**, 634.

Continuous Caudal Block—Special Indications, *continued.*

3. In patients with toxæmia. It lessens hypertension and water retention and is sufficient for painless delivery either per via naturales or by Cæsarean section.
4. In patients with pulmonary disease.
5. In breech extractions.
6. For premature labour.
7. In cases of rigid, slowly dilating cervix, and uterine inertia.
8. For forceps delivery—by one shot, rather than continuous technique.
9. In emergency Cæsarean section when the patient has a full stomach.

Contra-indications.—
1. Patients who have quick, easy labours.
2. Unstable, neurotic, or frightened patients who will not co-operate —e.g., in second stage, patients must be told when to bear down and must help themselves in this respect.
3. Deformity of sacral region—it is impossible to enter the sacral canal of some patients. In expert hands, failures occur in about 10 per cent of cases.
4. Disease of the central nervous system.
5. Obesity—because of difficulty in inserting needle.
6. Local infection.
7. Gross anæmia.
8. Placenta prævia and accidental hæmorrhage, because of the relaxation the method produces in the lower uterine segment.
9. Severe disproportion.
10. When intra-uterine manipulations are anticipated—because of the increase in uterine tone.
11. Susceptibility to local analgesic drugs.
   During the labour a close watch must be kept on the fœtal heart and the maternal condition, especially the blood-pressure. The technique must only be employed in well-equipped hospitals and by experienced anæsthetists and obstetricians. Facilities for the treatment of collapse—oxygen, intravenous fluids, etc.— must be at hand. Ready access to a vein must be present from the start of the procedure.

Uses in Therapeutics of Caudal and Continuous Caudal Block (Hingson*).—
1. To control eclampsia. It reduces the blood-pressure, stops convulsions, relieves blurred vision and headaches, diminishes pulmonary œdema, relieves failing heart, increases renal output, and abolishes labour pains.
2. To relieve oliguria and anuria associated with reflex renal ischæmia.
3. In post-operative paralytic ileus and distension.
4. In arterial embolism of lower limbs.
5. In thrombophlebitis of lower limbs.
6. To aid prognosis of sympathectomy in essential hypertension.
7. For prolonged relief of post-operative or post-traumatic pain.

---

* Hingson, R. A., *Brit. med. J.*, 1949, **2**, 777.

8. For facilitating removal of rectal fæcal impaction.

9. For treatment of renal colic by block up to T.8 and forcing fluids.

Caudal block gives good results in cases of chronic cold feet, phlegmasia alba dolens, vasospastic disease of the legs, and diabetic neuropathy. Although the effects of single injections are transitory, the relief of symptoms frequently last a considerable time, owing to the interruption by the block of a self-perpetuating vicious circle. The drug used is usually proctocaine and the amount about 50 ml., which should be warmed before injection into the sacral canal. The types B and C fibres are more susceptible to blocking than the A type fibres.*

The injection of up to 50 ml. of proctocaine into the sacral canal of patients who complain bitterly of intolerable pain due to malignant disease of the pelvis has been recommended. The bladder and anal sphincters are unlikely to be permanently paralysed by the technique. Pain relief is not always perfect.

CHAPTER XVII

ANALEPTICS,† ANTAGONISTS, AND PRESSOR AGENTS

ANALEPTICS AND ANTAGONISTS

The chief action of these drugs is to stimulate respiration and to reverse narcotic activity of sedative drugs. When given in large doses they are mostly convulsants. Their stimulating action on respiration is greatest in non-anæsthetized or lightly anæsthetized patients. In conditions of respiratory arrest their use comes far behind that of oxygen and I.P.P.V.

Classification.—

Drugs acting directly on medullary centres, e.g., nikethamide ; amiphenazole ; picrotoxin ; vanillic acid diethylamide ; cardiazole ; micoren (prethcamide).

Drugs acting reflexly through aortic and carotid bodies, e.g., lobeline ; nicotine ; cyanide ; also nikethamide and vanillic acid diethylamide.

Drugs improving cerebral blood-flow, e.g., carbon dioxide.

Drugs stimulating vital centres and increasing blood-flow, e.g., ephedrine and methamphetamine.

Amiphenazole.—This is 2 : 4-diamino-5-phenylthiazole hydrochloride and goes under the trade name of daptazole or D.A.P.T. and was investigated by Shaw and Bentley in 1949.‡ It is soluble in water but decomposes if allowed to stand for more than twenty-four hours (or up to seven days in a refrigerator). The dry powder is stable and it is usual to dissolve 30 mg. in 1·5 ml. of saline (or

---

* Galley, A. H., *Proc. R. Soc. Med.*, 1952, **45**, 748; and *Ibid.*, 1954, **47**, 304.
† From the Greek : ana = again ; lepsis = the act of taking, i.e., a restorative.
‡ Shaw, F. H., and Bentley, G., *Med. J. Aust.*, 1949, **2**, 868.

Amiphenazole, *continued.*

morphine solution).   When injected into a patient whose breathing has been depressed by morphine, pethidine, alphaprodine, methadone, etc., considerable increase in the depth of breathing rapidly takes place, but dose may have to be large (150–300 mg. intravenously).*   It has no effect on normal, undepressed respiration.

$$C_6H_5\!-\!\!\!\overset{\displaystyle C\,-\!\!\!-\!\!\!-\!\!\!-\,S}{\underset{NH_2-C\diagdown_{}\diagup C-NH_2.HCl}{}}$$

As well as counteracting respiratory depression in the morphinized patient, amiphenazole also : (1) Reduces vomiting. (2) Lessens constipation. (3) Restores the cough reflex.   In clinical doses the drug apparently does not reduce the depth or duration of sensory depression.   Given with bemegride it acts as a respiratory stimulant in cases of overdosage with barbiturates.

The use of the drug with morphine, to control the depressant effects while allowing the analgesic effects to remain, has been reported† and has given good results in the treatment of patients with chronic severe pain and in the alleviation of post-operative pain. An initial dose of 15–30 mg. of morphine is given accompanied by amiphenazole 25 mg. intramuscularly given from one syringe. This is repeated when the pain returns, the aim being to keep the patient completely free from discomfort.   Should the rate of respiration be less than eight per minute, or should any cyanosis appear, 20 mg. of amiphenazole are given intravenously and repeated at 10-minute intervals until the respiratory depression has been overcome.   The average patient shows no signs of toxicity from 200–300 mg. of the drug.   A rough guide as to dosage is to give equal amounts of amiphenazole and morphine.

THERAPEUTIC USES.—

1. With bemegride for treatment of acute poisoning by barbiturates, glutethamide, etc.   Somewhat outmoded therapy.

2. In treatment of acute poisoning by opiates and their respiratory depressant congeners.   Dose 15 mg. intravenously every 5 min. until patient recovers normal respiration.

3. In treatment of respiratory depression in newborn.   Dose 3 mg. in 1 ml. saline into umbilical vein.

4. In the treatment of carbon dioxide narcosis in respiratory failure in chronic bronchitis and emphysema.   Dose 150 mg. intravenously hourly or as continuous drip.   Can be taken by mouth, 100-mg. tablets, two, 4-hourly.

5. To enable large doses of opiates to be given in severe chronic pain (*Brit. med. J.*, 1959, **2**, 1018).

6. Along with opiates in treatment of post-operative pain when the side-effects, including respiratory depression, are lessened.

In recent years this agent has lost favour.

---

* Gershon, S., and others, *Brit. med. J.*, 1958, **2**, 366.
† McKeogh, V., and Shaw, F. H., *Ibid.*, 1956, **1**, 142 ; and Christie, G., Gray, R., Shaw, F. H., McCance, I., and Bruce, D. W., *Ibid.*, 1958, **1**, 675.

Bemegride (Megimide ; N.P. 13).—This is β-ethyl-β-methyl glutarimide and has the structural formula :—

$$CH_3 \diagdown \atop CH_3CH_2 \diagup C \diagup{\displaystyle CH_2-CO} \diagdown \atop {\displaystyle CH_2-CO} NH$$

It is similar in basic structure to the barbiturates.

It was first used in 1955 in the treatment of barbiturate overdosage,
in medical patients* and after intravenous thiobarbiturate
anæsthesia.† Has lost its former popularity.

It appears that the drug acts as a central cerebral stimulant and
stimulant of the reticular activating system, and not as a
specific barbiturate antagonist and so is unlike nalorphine in
its reversal of morphine overdosage, but it alters the E.E.G.
pattern of barbiturate intoxication. It does not increase the
rate of excretion of barbiturate nor does it decrease the duration
of coma, but it produces a relatively safe state where respiration
and reflexes are no longer depressed and when blood-pressure,
pulse-rate, and muscle tone are nearly normal. Untoward
effects include vomiting and convulsive movements and a toxic
psychosis resembling mescaline or lysergic acid intoxication.
For the reversal of thiobarbiturate anæsthesia the intravenous
injection of 10 ml. of 0·5 per cent solution is recommended but
larger doses may be required. Patients so treated may fall
asleep again but can be thereafter readily aroused.‡ Should be
avoided in epilepsy as it may stimulate fits. It has been stated
to reverse the hypnotic effects of the following drugs: glutethamide, dolitrone, carbromal, chlorbutol, methyl-pentynol, chloral
hydrate, propanidid, paraldehyde, hydroxydione.§

Vanillic Acid Diethylamide (Vandid ; Ethamivan).—This is a central
and reflex (carotid body) respiratory stimulant, similar in its
action, but fifteen times more powerful than nikethamide (nicotinic
acid diethylamide). It is rapidly metabolized in the tissues:
and when injected intravenously to an adult has given good results
in poisoning by barbiturates, morphine, alcohol, and coal gas,

$$HO \diagdown \hspace{-1em} \bigcirc \hspace{-1em} {}^{CH_3.O} -CO.N \diagdown {}^{C_2H_5}_{C_2H_5}$$

when dose should be 5–10 ml. of 5 per cent solution. Has been
used to shorten recovery time after intravenous barbiturate

* Shulman, A., Shaw, F. H., Cass, N. M., and Whyte, H. M., *Brit. med. J.*, 1955, **1**, 1238 ;
and Gershon, S., and Shaw, E. H., *Ibid.*, 1957, **2**, 1509.

† Harris, T. A. B., *Lancet*, 1955, **1**, 181.

‡ Wyne, B. D., and Frayworth, E., *Ibid.*, 1957, **2**, 1025 ; and Waine, T. E., and Dinmore,
P., *Anæsthesia*, 1958, **13**, 324.

§ Shulman, A., and Laycock, G. M., *Brit. med. J.*, 1958, **1**, 871.

Vanillic Acid Diethylamide, *continued.*

anæsthesia. Convulsions have occurred after the intravenous injection of 500 mg.* Has been used as a "chemical respirator" in 0·1 per cent solution intravenously in a dose of 0·05–0·07 mg. per kg. per minute in chronically hypoventilating patients.† Well absorbed from mucosa of mouth and tongue in neonates in a dose of 0·5 ml.‡ For neonates the dose is 0·2 ml. of 5 per cent solution intramuscularly. Supplied in 5-ml. ampoules of 5 per cent solution and in 20-mg. tablets, and as intravenous infusion 0·6 per cent rendered isotonic with saline in 540-ml. bottles.

Nikethamide, B.P. (Coramine; Anacardone; Corvotone; and Nikamide).—Nicotinic acid diethylamide; a pyridine derivative put up in 25 per cent solution. Allied to nicotinic acid.

First synthesized in 1923. It stimulates the respiratory centre and the carotid and aortic bodies. It slightly improves the circulation and produces peripheral vascular dilatation, but has no direct stimulant action on the heart. There is a wide margin between its therapeutic and its toxic doses. Convulsions follow overdosage, and these are succeeded by depression. A drug gradually falling from favour.

$$
\begin{array}{c}
\text{HC} \overset{\displaystyle\text{C}}{\underset{\displaystyle}{\Big\|}} \overset{\text{H}}{} \quad \overset{\text{O}}{} \\
\end{array}
$$

Used to combat respiratory depression following barbiturates, bromethol, and volatile anæsthetics. Supplied in 1·7-ml. and 5·5-ml. ampoules.

Given intravenously in 3- to 5-ml. doses, which can be repeated. Additional intramuscular injection prolongs its effect. Used in asphyxia neonatorum, when it can be injected into the umbilical vein. It may do good when infant is depressed due to pre-partum narcotic medication of mother; 0·5 ml. dropped on to the tongue may exert a useful stimulant effect in neonates.‡

Has been added (1 ml. to 1 g.) to intravenous barbiturates to prevent respiratory depression which is probably a useless procedure.

Sometimes used during neurosurgical operations to arouse patients sufficiently for them to co-operate in mapping out anæsthetic and hyperæsthetic areas.

A dose of 5 ml. given rapidly intravenously, perhaps preceded by 0·1 g. of thiopentone, will often cause an explosive cough and aid in clearing the airway in cases of threatened atelectasis. Paraldehyde 2 ml. intravenously has a similar effect.

It has been recommended as a treatment for reversal of apnœa to shake up a muddled respiratory centre (Nosworthy),§ and to act like a self-starter to the respiratory engine. Has also been

* Locket, S., *Brit. med. J.,* 1960, **2,** 1805.
† Dechene, J., *Canad. Anæsth. Soc. J.,* 1965, **12,** 173.
‡ Barrie, H., Cotton, D., and Wilson, B. D. R., *Lancet,* 1962, **2,** 742.
§ Nosworthy, M. D., *Anæsthesia,* 1958, **13,** 111.

used as an intravenous drip in the treatment of carbon dioxide retention occurring during exacerbations of chronic bronchitis.[*] Convulsions are said not to occur when nikethamide is used under these circumstances.

It is converted, before excretion, into a close derivative of nicotinamide, and is related to the antipellagra vitamins.

While thirty years ago, for a patient to die without benefit of nikethamide almost amounted to malpractice, to-day it is seldom used.

Tetrahydroaminacrine (Tacrine hydrochloride; T.H.A.; Romotal).[†]— This was first synthesized in 1945 by Albert and Gledhill and was used by Shaw and Bentley in 1949. Its chemical name is 1 : 2 : 3 : 4 : tetrahydro-5-aminoacridine and its structural formula:—

Like amiphenazole it is a partial antagonist to morphine, in contradistinction to nalorphine and levallorphan which are complete antagonists.

PHARMACOLOGY.—(1) A reliable central respiratory stimulant. (2) Arouses patients after barbiturate anæsthesia. (3) Has an anticholinesterase effect and antagonizes tubocurarine and gallamine at myoneural junctions. (4) Potentiates the action of suxamethonium at myoneural junctions. (5) Reduces incidence of ventricular fibrillation after digitalis and electric shock. (6) Causes hypersecretion only after large doses. (7) Is stable in solution and can be used in same syringe as morphine.

CLINICAL USES.—(1) For intractable pain in conjunction with morphine and its congeners. A dose of morphine of 15 mg. with a similar amount of tacrine will prevent the depression often seen with morphine alone. Is said to prevent addiction and symptoms of withdrawal of morphine. (2) For postoperative pain relief along with morphine, but when given with morphine it increases the dizziness and nausea both pre- and post-operatively.[‡] A further report[§] has shown that it causes the level of consciousness to be lighter when given with morphine than when morphine is given alone, and the patient is more alert. (3) As a decurarizing agent, dose being 30–60 mg. Atropine is necessary if larger doses are employed. (4) To potentiate and prolong neuromuscular block produced by suxamethonium.[‖] After premedication with atropine, tacrine 15 mg. is given intravenously followed by 20 mg. of suxamethonium (the patient

* McNichol, M. W., and others, *Brit. med. J.*, 1963, **1**, 646.
† Stone, V., and others, *Ibid.*, 1961, **1**. 471.
‡ Clarke, R. S. J., and Dundee, J. W., *Brit. J. Anæsth.*, 1965, **37**, 779.
§ Simpson, B. R., Seelye, E., Clayton, J. I., and Parkhouse, J., *Ibid.*, 1962, **34**, 95.
‖ Gordh, T., and Wahlin, A., *Acta anæsth. scand.*, 1961, **5**, 55; and Barrow, M. E. H., and Smethurst, J. R., *Brit. J. Anæsth.*, 1963, **36**, 465.

Tetrahydroaminacrine, *continued.*

being anæsthetized beforehand). The resulting relaxation lasts 10 min. and may be maintained by further amounts of the relaxant at 6–7-min. intervals, e.g., 10 mg. If more suxamethonium is needed at intervals of less than 6 min. then an additional dose of tacrine should be injected. Recovery is rapid and complete in 5–10 min.

Picrotoxin.—An old drug, the use of which as an analeptic was re-introduced in 1931 by Maloney, Fitch, and Tatum. The most potent of this group of analeptics. A non-alkaloidal extract of the bean *Cocculus indicus*. Not much used now.

It stimulates the cortex, having an antinarcotic action, which becomes a convulsant action with toxic doses ; also stimulates midbrain and the medulla and thus respiration. It has no effect on the distribution, metabolism, or excretion of thiopentone.

Used in 0·3 per cent solution, the dose being 1–2 ml. (3–6 mg.) intravenously, and repeated after an interval if necessary. Muscular twitching is a sign of overdosage. It antagonizes effects of the overdosage of morphine, bromethol, ether, and barbiturates. The greater the depression, the less satisfactory is the drug as an antidote. Has a latent period of 10 min. after intravenous injection.

Doxapram Hydrochloride (Stimulexin).[*]—This is a non-specific respiratory stimulant with a high ratio between effective stimulation and convulsant activity. Partly metabolized and partly excreted unchanged in urine. Can be given intravenously as a single injection or as a drip containing 3 mg. per hour.

In a recent double-blind trial doxapram was found to be the most efficient respiratory stimulant of five tested (nikethamide, prethcamide, amiphenazole, and ethamavan). Ethamavan came second.[†]

Methyl Phenidate (Ritalin).—This is alpha phenyl-*d*-pyridyl-2-acetic acid methylester monohydrochloride and was first used by Schmidt and Drassdo in Germany in 1954. It is a non-specific respiratory stimulant and can be given intravenously, intramuscularly, or by mouth. Shortens recovery time from thiopentone and pethidine[‡] Dose: 0·1–0·2 mg. per kg. intravenously.[§] The intravenous injection of 20 mg. has been recommended for the treatment of hiccup during anæsthesia.[||]

PRESSOR AGENTS

Pressor drugs act : (1) Peripherally ; (2) Centrally, on the heart. Factors to be considered : Mode of action, on vessels or heart ; duration of pressor effect ; effectiveness of repeated doses ; presence or

[*] Steele, A. D., and Rodman, T., *Amer. Rev. resp. Dis.*, 1966, **94**, 600; and Stephen, C. R., and Talton, I., *Curr. Res. Anesth.*, 1964, **43**, 628.
[†] Edwards, G., and Leszcynski, S. O., *Lancet*, 1967, **2**, 226.
[‡] Graham, R., *Ibid.*, 1957, **2**, 599.
[§] Gale, A. S., *Anesthesiology*, 1958, **19**, 521.
[||] Macris, S. G., and others, *Curr. Res. Anesth.*, 1963, **42**, 440; and Vasiloff, N., and others, *Canad. Anæsth. Soc. J.*, 1965, **12**, 306.

absence of side-effects. Drugs of this nature should not be used routinely, but only when a severe fall of blood-pressure is anticipated or actually occurs.

Blood-pressure is maintained by : (1) The force of cardiac output. This may be reduced because of a weakening of cardiac action or because of a diminished venous return. (2) Impulses passing from the vaso-motor centre in the medulla via the anterior spinal roots and white rami from T.1 to L.3 and the grey rami to the muscular tissue in the walls of the vessels. In spinal intradural and extradural analgesia these impulses are blocked by paralysis of the pre-ganglionic fibres in the anterior nerve-roots.

While pressor effects may follow the injection of drugs at certain times and in certain situations (digitalis, atropine, calcium, neostig-mine, steroids) the pressor drugs related to adrenaline may be used after intradural or extradural block and during general anæsthesia. These sympathomimetic amines may be grouped in several ways, none of them completely satisfactory, e.g.,

A. 1. Agents whose vasoconstrictor effects depend on the integrity of the sympathetic nerves : ephedrine and methylamphet-amine.

2. Agents whose vasoconstrictor effect is not diminished by sympa-thetic denervation :—

a. Noradrenaline and phenylephrine which constrict the smooth muscle in vessel walls.

b. Metaraminol and methoxamine when the action is partly direct on the vessel walls and partly due to liberation of noradrenaline from stores in nerve-endings or chromaffin cells. Their effect is diminished by reserpine.

B.* 1. Drugs showing a decreased pressor response following a noradrenaline infusion, and giving a powerful action in reserpine-treated subjects : noradrenaline, adrenaline, and phenylephrine.

2. Drugs showing a reduced pressor response following nor-adrenaline infusion and a moderate response in reserpine-treated subjects : metaraminol and methoxamine. This is an intermediate group.

3. Drugs depending for their action on the presence of noradrena-line in the vessel walls and having little effect on subjects treated with reserpine : methylamphetamine, ephedrine, and mephentermine.

C. A pressor amine acts: (1) Directly, by stimulating the α receptors of vascular smooth muscle, e.g., adrenaline, noradrenaline, methoxamine, phenylephrine, and metaraminol. (2) Indirectly, by causing release of noradrenaline from post-ganglionic neurons, which then excites the α receptors, e.g., methyl-amphetamine and mephentermine. Ephedrine has a mixed action. The mode of action of these agents is partly dependent on their chemical structure.†

---

* Burn, J. H., and Rand, M. J., Brit. med. J., 1959, 1, 394 ; and Benazon, D., Anæsthesia, 1962, 17, 344.
† Dingle, H. R., Ibid., 1966, 21, 151.

Pressor Agents, *continued.*

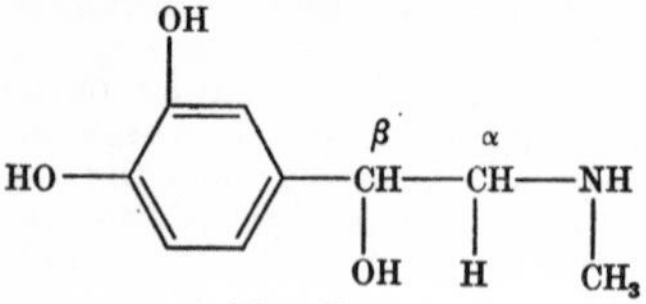

Adrenaline

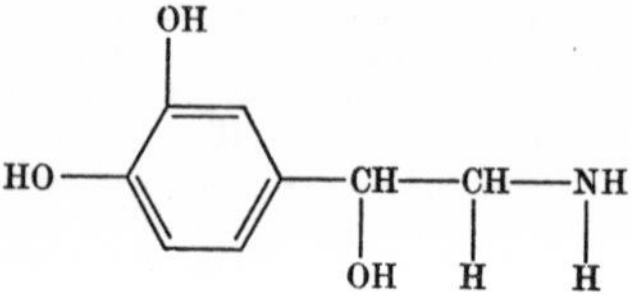

Noradrenaline

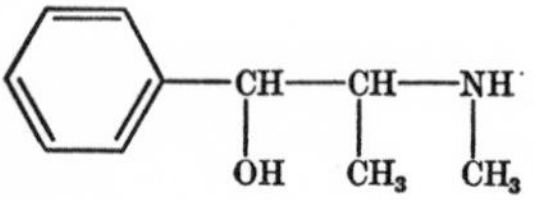

Ephedrine

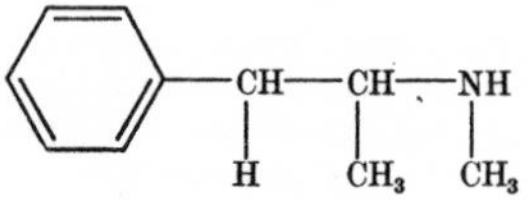

Methylamphetamine
(methedrine)

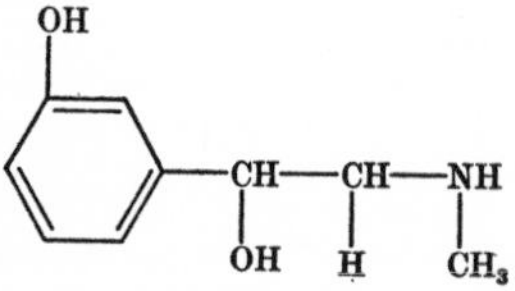

Phenylephrine

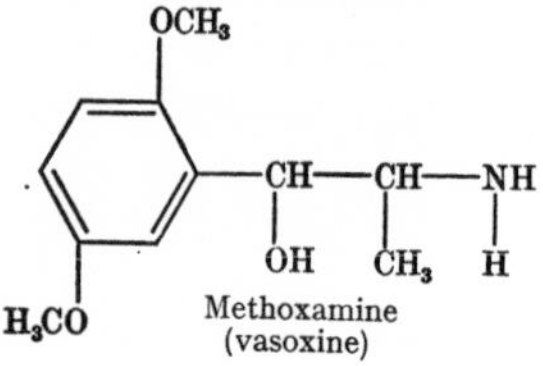

Methoxamine
(vasoxine)

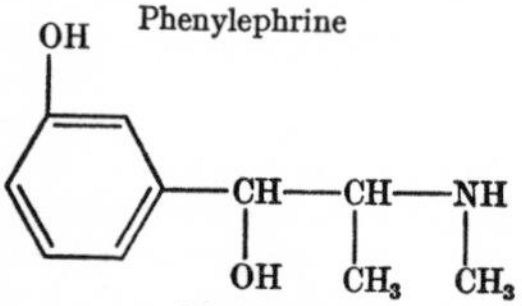

Metaraminol
(aramine)

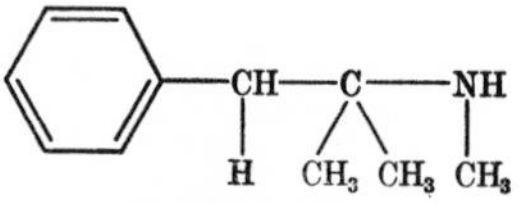

Mephentermine
(mephine)

Distribution of α and β Receptors in the Body.*—

Heart $<$ Rate — β
Force — β

Blood-vessels $<$ Skin, Kidney — α
Skeletal muscle — β

Bronchi — β
Uterus — α and β
Gastro-intestinal tract — α and β
Bladder — β

Adrenaline, B.P. (Epinephrine).—

HISTORY.—Isolated by Oliver and Schäfer in 1894† and produced in crystalline form by Takamine‡ and Aldrich, independently, in 1901, the first hormone to be synthesized (Stolz, 1905). It is derived from noradrenaline which is synthesized in the body from tyrosine; dopa and dopamine being intermediate stages.

---

* Ahlquist, R. P., *Amer. J. Physiol.*, 1948, **153**, 586.
† Oliver, G., and Schäfer, E. A., *J. Physiol.*, 1904, **16**, 1.
‡ Takamine, J., *Therapeutic Gaz.*, 1901, **27**, 221.

PHARMACOLOGY.—General effects similar to those resulting from stimulation of adrenergic nerve-endings, but ultimate action is chiefly on effector cells. Stimulates both α and β receptors. It is formed in the adrenal medulla, where it is stored in intracellular granules and at adrenergic nerve-endings, and is liberated by acetyl choline (humoral transmitter) by impulses from the autonomic pre-ganglionic fibres supplying the medullary cells. Ampoules of adrenaline can be autoclaved once or twice without loss of potency.*

CARDIOVASCULAR SYSTEM.—Its main effect is to increase the stroke volume, rate, and cardiac output. It increases the incidence of arrhythmias, by making the automatic conducting system more irritable. Adrenergic blocking agents do not prevent direct stimulation of myocardium, although they do prevent arrhythmias. The systolic blood-pressure rises, but the diastolic is not greatly altered. After the blood-pressure rises there comes a short period of hypotension ; the drug has a biphasic reaction causing secondary vasodilatation, e.g., in the nasal mucosa following constriction due to adrenaline. Vessels in different situations react to adrenaline in different ways. While the vessels of the skin, mucosæ, subcutaneous tissues, splanchnic area, and kidneys are constricted (α effects), those in muscles are relaxed after small doses (β effects), constricted after large doses. While the cerebral and pulmonary arteries are constricted, the coronaries vary; angina pectoris may be precipitated in patients with coronary disease, because of the augmentation of cardiac work on top of narrowed vessels. The overall action of adrenaline on vessels is one of dilatation, the increase in cardiac output being responsible for the rise in blood-pressure. The peripheral venous pressure is increased. Following intravenous infusion, the effects of adrenaline last longer than do those of noradrenaline. The most potent drug known to stimulate an arrested heart, but its transient and rather violent effect and the danger of ventricular arrhythmias limit routine use as a pressor agent.

THE RENAL BLOOD-FLOW.—This is decreased because of the constriction of the renal vessels.

THE RESPIRATORY SYSTEM.—The bronchi are relaxed, following both topical (1–100 solution in atomizer) and systemic administration. This may increase the tidal volume even in normal patients. Depth of respiration slightly increased, and irregular breathing sometimes seen. If a large dose is injected, the rise in blood-pressure may produce a reflex from the carotid and aortic pressoreceptors, causing temporary apnœa.

THE ALIMENTARY CANAL.—While the muscle of the gut is relaxed, the pyloric and ileocolic sphincters are contracted (both α and β effects). The spleen contracts and empties its cells into the circulation. The secretion of the intestinal glands is inhibited. Sweating and pilomotor activity not much stimulated in man. Dilates the pupil when carried to the eye in the blood-stream, but not (in health) when instilled into the conjunctival sac.

---

* Thomas, D. V., *Anesthesiology*, 1956, **17**, 752.

Adrenaline, *continued.*

Glycogen is mobilized from the liver, giving rise to an increase i the blood-sugar level. There is very little stimulating effec on the central nervous system. Large doses stimulate small clinical doses inhibit uterine tone in labour. I elevates the pain threshold. Adrenaline is a mild ganglion blocking agent but does not cause increased secretion of the adrenal cortex even though it may result in a short perio of eosinopenia after injection.

Following injection, untoward reactions may includ anxiety, restlessness from mild cerebral stimulation, throb bing headache, vertigo, pallor, and palpitations; hyper thyroid and hypertensive patients are specially liable t these.

Discoloration of adrenaline indicates decomposition with the formation of adrenochromes. Potassium metabisulphit (0·1 per cent) is added to the commercial product to preven this.

It must be used with the greatest care when the patient i inhaling chloroform, trichloroethylene, halothane, or cyclo propane, because of the risk of the production of ventricula fibrillation. In the presence of thyrotoxicosis and o hypertension, it must be given with great caution. Shoul not be used with local analgesics in ring block of the digit or of the penis.

It is mostly degraded by conjugation with glycuronic and sul phuric acids and excreted in the urine. A smaller part i oxidized by amine oxidase and inactivated by o-methyl transferase.

Total dose should not exceed 0·5 mg. (i.e., 0·5 ml. 1–1000 solution)

CLINICAL USES.—(1) To produce vasoconstriction in local analgesi and in the skin and subcutaneous tissues before incisions, e.g. in thyroidectomy (1–200,000 to 1–500,000). (2) To dilate bronch in asthma, given intramuscularly, intravenously, by spray, o by aerosol. (3) To treat allergies, e.g., hay fever, urticaria incompatible blood transfusion, etc.

Noradrenaline Acid Tartrate, B.P. (l-Arterenol; Norepinephrine Levophed) (*nor* = nitrogen *ohne radikol*—German).—A primary catecholamine differing from adrenaline in having no methy group attached to its nitrogen atom. Concerned in the humora transmission of adrenergic nerves. Synthesized in the body from dietary protein (tyrosine → dopa → dopamine). It is formed a adrenergic nerve-endings, where most of it is destroyed by amine oxidase and o-methyl-transferase very quickly. Fresh human adrenal glands contain four times as much adrenaline as nor adrenaline. It can be synthesized commercially. When blood calcium level is high, noradrenaline release is high, and vice versa Should be stored away from light. Should be infused in dextrose 5 per cent solution, not in saline, blood, or plasma, which favour its decomposition and loss of potency.

HISTORY.—Humoral transmission of nerve impulses described by Elliott in 1905 and proved by Otto Loewi in 1921.* Properties of racemic noradrenaline described by Barger and Dale in 1911. Modern interest in the drug stimulated by von Euler (1946),† who showed that noradrenaline is present in extracts of sympathetic nerves. The lævo-isomer is the more active.

PHARMACOLOGY.—A powerful α-receptor site stimulator. Probably the major pressor amine found at post-ganglionic adrenergic nerve-endings responsible for reflex vascular effects, adrenaline being mainly responsible for metabolic activities. The amount of noradrenaline released by a sympathetic impulse is increased when a slow intravenous infusion of noradrenaline is given. It thus appears that the noradrenaline present in sympathetic fibres is not only synthesized there, but also accumulates as a result of uptake from the blood-stream.‡

CARDIOVASCULAR SYSTEM.—No influence on cardiac output, as bradycardia (antagonized by atropine or ganglionic blocking agents) counteracts the increase in force of contraction. In animals and man§ dilates coronary vessels. The most powerful vasoconstrictor in common use, acting on all vessels except possibly the coronaries. The blood-pressure, both systolic and diastolic, rises. Heart-rate sometimes slowed, a reflex activated by hypertension on the presso-receptors in the aortic and carotid sinuses. Should only be used with great care in patients receiving chloroform, trichloroethylene, cyclopropane, or halothane as it may precipitate arrhythmias. Unlike adrenaline it does not stimulate the cortex of the brain.

May cause gastro-intestinal ischæmia when given by infusion.

RENAL BLOOD-FLOW.—Reduced owing to constriction of renal vessels. It stimulates uterine contractions, unlike adrenaline, which in clinical doses inhibits them.

The dextro-isomer acts primarily on the smooth muscle of the bronchi ; the lævo-isomer acts primarily on the smooth muscle of the vessels. The drug is less toxic than adrenaline. While adrenaline is the flight or fright hormone, noradrenaline is the pressor hormone. Its pressor activity is potentiated by the alkaloids of ergot, ergotamine, ergotoxine, and ergometrine (ergonovine).

It is put up as the bitartrate in 1–1000 solution, each ml. containing 1 mg. of noradrenaline. It is to be given diluted by intravenous infusion. For direct injection in an emergency a special solution 1–10,000 can be used in a dosage of 50–75 microgrammes (½–¾ ml.).

ADMINISTRATION OF NORADRENALINE (AND OTHER PRESSOR DRUGS).—If 2 ml. of 1–1000 solution are added to 500 ml. of dextrose, or blood, the resulting solution contains 4 µg. per ml. This solution has been used as a continuous intravenous

* Loewi, O., Pflüg. Arch. ges. Physiol., 1921, **189**, 239.
† von Euler, U. S., Acta physiol. scand., 1946, **12**, 73.
‡ Burn, J. H., Brit. med. J., 1961, **1**, 1623.
§ von Euler, U. S., Lancet, 1955, **2**, 151.

Noradrenaline, *continued.*

drip, starting at a rate of 2 ml. per minute (8 µg.). The speed
is later adjusted according to the blood-pressure reading. The
solution should be made up freshly for each case, and obviously
the reduction in the rate of drip must be gradual, and must be
controlled by frequent blood-pressure readings. Extravasation
of the drip fluid into the tissues has caused necrosis.

Should be run directly, or via a plastic catheter, into a large proximal
vein, to prevent tissue sloughing. Blanched and ischæmic skin
areas can sometimes be prevented from sloughing by injection of
acetylcholine 100–200 mg. using a fine needle, or of phentolamine solution 5 mg. in 10 ml. of saline. Once a drip is started
it must not be stopped suddenly for the following reasons
(1) It eventually depresses the vasomotor centre ; (2) It eventually depresses ganglionic transmission ; (3) It may, with a metabolite, form a new vasodilating substance ; (4) Receptor cells or
muscles in arterial walls become saturated with noradrenaline
and so lose their ability to react to sympathetic stimulation or
to additional exogenous noradrenaline. The patient can be
weaned from a noradrenaline drip by substituting a drip of
mephentermine, methylamphetamine, or ephedrine. Methoxamine, phenylephrine, and metaraminol drips do not show this
tachyphylaxis. Before the infusion is finally stopped, transmission must be given time to recover.[*]

INDICATIONS.—

1. Following removal of chromaffin-cell tumours such as phæo-
chromocytomata.

2. During operations on patients with coronary or cerebral ischæmia, to maintain the blood-pressure at near normal levels
In the former, arrhythmias may occur and may require E.C.G.
monitoring. Unlike adrenaline it causes no cerebral stimulation ; it causes some cerebral vasoconstriction.

3. To counteract blood-pressure fall after the too rapid injection
of intravenous barbiturates 0·25–1 ml. of the 1–10,000 solution
should be used.

4. To sustain the circulation after massive hæmorrhage while
waiting for blood and possibly to enable economy in the
amount of blood transfused in severe shock.

5. To maintain the circulation during intradural and extradural
analgesia, for although the chief fall in pressure in these cases
is due to reduced cardiac output (from reduced venous return)
there is at the same time reduced peripheral resistance.

6. To reverse grave hypotension caused by ganglionic-blocking
drugs, phenothiazine drugs, opiates, pethidine, etc.

7. In cases of peripheral circulatory collapse. Its place here is not
yet determined and sound arguments in favour of the production of vasodilatation and hence of increased tissue
perfusion have been advanced. Infusion of toxic doses may
cause acute pulmonary œdema. The vessels gradually lose

[*] Burn, J. H., *Brit. J. Anæsth.*, 1956, **28**, 459, and *The Autonomic Nervous System*, 1903.
Oxford : Blackwell Scientific Publications.

SUMMARY OF EFFECTS OF ADRENERGIC DRUGS

DRUG	RECEPTOR SITE STIMULATION	CARDIAC OUTPUT	SYSTOLIC BLOOD-PRESSURE	DIASTOLIC BLOOD-PRESSURE	PULSE-RATE	CARDIAC IRRITABILITY	CORONARY ARTERY FLOW	PERIPHERAL VASCULAR SYSTEM	CENTRAL NERVOUS SYSTEM
Adrenaline	Alpha; beta	Increased	Increased	Unchanged or reduced	Increased	Increased	Increased	Overall vasodilatation	Stimulated
Noradrenaline	Alpha	No change or reduction	Increased	Increased	Slowed	Increased	Increased	Overall vasoconstriction	No effect
Ephedrine	Alpha; beta	No change or increase	Increased	Increased	Slowed	Increased	Increased	Overall vasodilatation	Stimulated
Phenylephrine	Alpha	Reduced	Increased	Increased	Slowed	Increased	Increased	Overall vasoconstriction	No effect
Methylamphetamine	Alpha; beta	Increased	Increased	Increased	Increased	Increased	Increased (?)	Overall vasodilatation	Stimulated
Methoxamine	Alpha	Reduced	Increased	Increased	Slowed	Little change	Little change	Overall vasoconstriction	No effect
Mephentermine	Alpha	Increased	Increased	Increased (?)	Increased	Increased	Increased (?)	Overall vasodilatation	Stimulated
Metaraminol	Alpha; beta	No change or reduction	Increased	Increased	Slowed	Increased	Increased	Overall vasoconstriction	No effect

Noradrenaline, *continued.*

their responsiveness to physiologically released or artificially infused noradrenaline during periods of prolonged low blood-pressure, so active resuscitation must be started early with this drug if it is to be used at all. Should not be used in patients with oliguria as it reduces renal flow.

8. To treat the shock associated with coronary thrombosis.
9. To raise blood-pressure and stimulate the myocardium thereby in cases of cardiac standstill.* The special solution 1–10,000 should be used (0·25–0·75 ml.).

CONTRA-INDICATIONS.—Hypertensive patients are especially sensitive to the effects of the drug and so the speed of drip must be slow until the patient settles down. Cyclopropane, halothane or trichlorethylene must be given very cautiously and never to deep planes of anæsthesia while the drug is being infused.

Ephedrine, B.P.—An α and β adrenergic stimulator. Introduced into Western medicine in 1924 by Schmidt and Chen.† The active principle (isolated in 1885 by Yamanashi) of ma huang, a Chinese plant. Chemically allied to adrenaline. Manufactured artificially. Its pharmacological action was formerly thought to inhibit amine oxidase, a tissue enzyme which destroys adrenaline (Gaddum and Kwialkowski, 1938)‡ and this action is akin to that of neostigmine which inhibits cholinesterase—one protects and spares adrenaline the other acetylcholine. More recently it has been suggested that it releases stored noradrenaline from nerve-endings in the vessel walls.§ It does not act directly on the effector cells but is a potent sympathetic stimulant, raising blood-pressure, stimulating the myocardium, constricting arterioles, relaxing smooth bronchial and intestinal muscle, dilating the pupil and stimulating the cortex and medulla. Probably dilates the coronary arteries and overcomes the coronary constriction caused by pituitary extract. Its vasopressor effects are not reversed by adrenergic blocking agents—unlike those of adrenaline. It dilates the vessels of skeletal muscles. It is not oxidized by amine or phenol oxidase but is excreted unchanged by the kidneys completely in 24 hours. Used in states of hypotension, asthma, heart-block, urticaria, narcolepsy, and enuresis. Gives some relief in cases of myasthenia. The lævorotatory form is the more active. It thus delays the rate of destruction of adrenaline and so maintains a high blood-adrenaline level. Its direct vasoconstrictive action on the vessels is a secondary effect. The rate and also the force of cardiac contraction are increased. Duration of effect is prolonged, from 30 to 40 minutes after intramuscular injection, but repeated doses not as effective as initial dose (tachyphylaxis). Cerebral stimulation results in a subjective feeling of apprehension, trembling, and discomfort. It increases the tone of the bladder sphincter and this may be one cause of postoperative retention. It may tend to produce wakefulness, either

* McMillan, I. K. R., Cockett, F. B., and Styles, P., *Thorax*, 1952, **7**, 205.
† Chen, K. K., and Schmidt, C. F., *J. Pharmacol.*, 1924, **24**, 339.
‡ Gaddum, J. H. and Kwialkowski, H.,, *J. Physiol.* (*Lond.*), 1938, **94**, 87.
§ Burns, J. H., and Rand, M. J., *Lancet*, 1958, **1**, 673.

during or after operation—an action shared by methylamphetamine. It has a local analgesic effect. Has recently been advocated in the treatment of hypotension due to spinal block as it increases cardiac output and venous return.[*] Put up in ampoules of 30 mg. Dose: 15–30 mg. ($\frac{1}{4}$–$\frac{1}{2}$ gr.).

Methoxamine Hydrochloride, B.P.C. (Vasoxine, Vasoxyl).—This is a synthetic vasopressor which is chemically β-hydroxy β (2,5-di-ethoxyphenyl) isopropylamine. It can be autoclaved, is non-irritating, and is a potent agent with a rather prolonged effect which comes on two minutes after intravenous injection and may last up to an hour.

It has little effect on cardiac output, and causes an increased peripheral resistance, and a rise in the right auricular and ventricular pressure and in peripheral venous mean pressure. Its action is peripheral on the arteries and veins (α stimulator). Pulse-rate slowed, an effect blocked by atropine. This may be a carotid and aortic sinus effect. Gives rise to no cardiac arrhythmia and seems to be safe in the presence of cyclopropane and halothane. Does not stimulate the higher centres. Pilomotor effect marked and causes desire to empty bladder. It reduces the urinary volume by depressing the glomerular filtration rate and constricting the renal artery. Must be used carefully in cases of hypertension, cardiac disease, and hyperthyroidism. Rarely can act as a partial β blocker[†] and induce ectopic beats.

Dosage must be kept small : 5–20 mg. intramuscularly ; 2 mg. intravenously. Before repeat doses are given, important to see that effects of earlier injection have worn off. Delayed hypertensive effects have been observed. Put up in 1-ml. ampoules containing 20 mg.

Phenylephrine Hydrochloride, B.P. (Neosynephrine, Neophryn).—An α stimulator. First described in 1931 by Kuschinsky and Oberdisse.[‡] It acts partly by releasing stored noradrenaline from post-ganglionic neurons and so is moderately potentiated by mono-amine oxidase inhibitors. Abnormally high blood-pressure due to this combination may be treated by phentolamine or chlorpromazine, α blockers. It causes reflex bradycardia, and little improvement in the force of cardiac contraction. Chief effect is to cause vasoconstriction by direct action on vessel walls, and so can be used in place of adrenaline, together with local analgesics for infiltration. Does not stimulate the cerebral cortex nor markedly relax the bronchi. Effect lasts 10–15 minutes, but repeated injections have the same action as the first one. Can be given in a continuous drip, 1 ml. (10 mg.) in 500 ml. of 5 per cent glucose, the rate of drip varying from 50 to 200 drops a minute. Has no effect on conducting tissue of heart, but may cause bradycardia from vagal stimulation, so that bradycardia, together with heart-block, are contra-indications to its use. Does not constrict coronary

---

[*] Cain, W. E., and Hamilton, W. K., *Anesthesiology*, 1966, **27**, 209.
[†] Karim, S. M. M., *Brit. J. Pharmacol.*, 1965, **24**, 365.
[‡] Kuschinsky, G., and Oberdisse, K., *Arch. exp. Path. Pharmak.*, 1931, **162**, 46.

Phenylephrine Hydrochloride, *continued.*

vessels but does constrict renal and cerebral arteries. Dilates th
pupil; relieves nasal congestion. There are no side-effects. Dosage
0·2–0·5 ml. of 1 per cent solution intravenously. Sensitizes th
heart to catecholamines so that if cyclopropane or halogenate
volatile anæsthetics are being used, initial dose should not excee
0·1–0·2 mg. intravenously.* If added to spinal analgesic solutio
(dose 2–3 mg.) will prolong action of latter. Does not elevate blood
sugar. It inhibits uterus and gut. It cannot be autoclaved.

Methylamphetamine Hydrochloride, B.P. (Methamphetamine
Methedrine, Pervitin, Desoxyephedrine, Desoxyn, Norodin).—
Allied to amphetamine (benzedrine); structurally is *d*-n-methyl
amphetamine hydrochloride. Described in 1909 by Ogata an
used clinically in 1943.† Increases cardiac rate and force o
contraction and output (β stimulator, with very little α-stimulating
effect). May cause bradycardia via vagal effect. Increases blood
flow through kidneys. Produces vasoconstriction by direct action
on vessels. Also stimulates respiration. Action long-lasting, and
effective in repeated doses. Maximal effect $8\frac{1}{2}$ minutes after
intravenous injection. Compared with noradrenaline, onset of its
effects delayed, but it lasts longer. It elevates mood, reduces
appetite, and stimulates cortex, having a mild analeptic effect
Has been used successfully to antidote acute barbiturate poisoning.
It reduces post-operative vomiting and is said to lessen nausea and
vertigo after fenestration operations. Ampoules contain 20 mg. per
ml. Dosage, as prophylactic, 15–20 mg. intramuscularly. If blood-
pressure falls unduly, 5–10 mg. intravenously with 15–20 mg.
intramuscularly. Blood-pressure should be checked before repeat-
ing dosage. It may be dangerous in thyrotoxicosis and in heart
disease.

Metaraminol Bitartrate (Aramine).—This is *l*-1-(m-hydroxyphenyl)-
2-amino-1-propanol. An α stimulator with slight β-stimulating
effects. It stimulates the myocardium without producing arrhythmia and is a peripheral vasopressor. It raises both the systolic and
diastolic plood-pressures. Its effect on vessels is similar to that of
methoxamine and is not diminished by sympathetic denervation.
Its action is partly direct on the vessel walls and partly due to the
liberation of noradrenaline from stores in nerve-endings or
chromaffin cells. Previous administration of reserpine diminishes
the effect. No effect on cerebral cortex. After intramuscular
injection, 10 minutes elapse before its action is seen; after intravenous injection, 2 minutes. Duration of effect 20 to 60 minutes.
Its use with cyclopropane is suspect.

Dosage: intramuscularly 2–10 mg.; intravenously 0·5–5 mg.; by
infusion, 15–100 mg. in 250–500 ml. as a substitute for the
noradrenaline drip.

Supplied in 1-ml. ampoules of 1 per cent solution.

---

* McIntyre, J. W. R., *Canad. Anæsth. Soc. J.*, 1965, **12**, 634.
† Dodd, H., and Prescott, F., *Brit. med. J.*, 1943, **1**, 345.

Mephentermine Sulphate, B.P. (Mephine, Wyamine).—This is n-methylphenyl tertiary butylamine sulphate. It is similar in effect to ephedrine, but causes no ventricular arrhythmia and has no direct effect on the myocardium. No increase in heart output but blood-pressure raised. Does not increase heart-rate and may slow it because of hypertensive effect on the aorticocarotid baroceptors. Does not stimulate the cortex. Increases renal blood-flow. No danger of cumulative effect. Can be given intramuscularly when effect comes on in 10–15 minutes and lasts for 1–2 hours. Effect after intravenous injection is immediate and lasts for 30 or 45 minutes. Dose intravenous—3–5 mg. slowly, repeated when necessary, 20–35 mg. intramuscularly; as infusion 150 mg. in 500 ml. 5 per cent dextrose. Has been stated to prevent adrenaline-induced ventricular fibrillation during cyclopropane anæsthesia.*

Felypressin (Octopressin).—This is 2-phenylalinine-8-lysine vaso-pressin, a synthetic derivative of the octopeptide hormone vaso-pressin from the posterior pituitary. Causes contraction of all smooth muscle—including coronaries—but has little oxytoxic or antidiuretic effect. On injection causes local vasoconstriction without secondary vasodilatation as adrenaline does. Little effect on cardiac rhythm and may be relatively safe in patients receiving halogenated volatile anæsthetics or cyclopropane. Dose—up to 5 pressor units.† Used for intradermal and subcutaneous injection to produce ischæmia.

If pressor agents are required in patients inhaling halogenated vapours or cyclopropane, methoxamine or mephentermine would appear to be safest.

Ether and cyclopropane at light planes will raise the blood-pressure slightly during spinal analgesia. Oxygen is most helpful and may be given, either alone, or combined with 50–70 per cent nitrous oxide. Trendelenburg's position is most helpful, provided a hyperbaric solution has not just been injected intradurally. Elevation of the legs empties their blood into the circulation—auto-transfusion. Finally, intravenous fluid, by helping the venous return to the heart, is of paramount importance.

Vasopressor drugs acting centrally are useless in high spinal anal-gesia, as the effector pathways (the anterior roots of the spinal nerve) are out of action. Such a drug is carbon dioxide.

Gross hypertension may follow the use of ergot preparations given intravenously if the patient has already received a sympatho-mimetic amine, as ergometrine (ergonovine), ergotamine, and ergo-toxin may cause contraction of the muscular wall of blood-vessels.

Following intra- or extradural sympathetic blockade, hypotension is best treated by posture, intravenous fluid, and either phenyl-ephrine or methoxamine. Both cause peripheral vasoconstriction and do not cause cerebral stimulation which might awaken a sedated patient. To combat hypotension due to myocardial failure, methylamphetamine, metaraminol, and mephentermine,

---

* Lynch, P. R., Webber, D. L., and Oppenheimer, M. J., *Anesthesiology*, 1955, **16**, 632.
† Hugin, W., *Der Anesthesist*, 1962, **11**, 185; and Hunter, M. E., and others, *Canad. Anæsth. Soc. J.*, 1966, **13**, 40.

Pressor Agents, *continued*.

as they stimulate cardiac output and cause vasodilatation, ar
useful.

(*See also* Symposium on Adrenergic Drugs and their Antagonists
Brit. J. Anæsth., 1966, **30**, 665 et seq.)

INFLUENCE OF OTHER DRUGS ON PATIENTS GIVEN PRESSOR AMINES

1. **Reserpine.**—This reduces the amount of noradrenaline stored in
sympathetic post-ganglionic fibres, so that the effects of sympa
thetic stimulation are diminished. It also releases 5-hydroxy
tryptamine from the brain and the intestine. Patients under it:
influence show a diminished response to those pressor amine:
which act by releasing stores of noradrenaline in the vessel walls
ephedrine, methylamphetamine, mephentermine. This effect may
last for two weeks after reserpine has been discontinued. It cause:
an increased response to noradrenaline. Hypotensive effects o
reserpine can be reversed by those agents acting directly on the
smooth muscle of vessel walls, e.g., adrenaline, noradrenaline
phenylephrine, or methoxamine; not by those having an effect du
to the liberation of catecholamines, e.g., ephedrine, methyl
amphetamine, and mephentermine.

2. **Guanethidine** (Ismelin).—Its hypotensive effects are probably
achieved in the same way as those following reserpine except that
it does not deplete the catechol amines in the brain or adrenal
gland.

3. **Chlorpromazine and Promethazine.**—These cause the pressor
activity of injected adrenaline to be reversed. They do not greatly
affect the pressor activity of noradrenaline. They reduce the
pressor activity of methoxamine and phenylephrine.

USE OF PRESSOR DRUGS IN ANÆSTHESIA

1. In hypotension produced by drugs, e.g., ganglionic blocking agents,
phenothiazines, opiates, pethidine, barbiturates, halothane, etc.
2. In hypotension due to diminished circulatory volume pressor drugs
are harmful, reducing tissue perfusion and increasing acidosis: may
also result in renal ischæmia and cardiac overload.
3. In hypotention due to posture.
4. In hypotension due to a threatened coronary circulation. Vasopressin
and angiotensin, coronary constrictors both, should not be used.
5. Following removal of phæochromocytoma.
6. To maintain renal function and urinary output (along with generous
fluid replacement). Methylamphetamine increases renal blood-flow.
Tachyphylaxis often causes trouble when pressor agents are
used, e.g., the bad reputation of the noradrenaline drip (embalming
fluid!)

Adrenergic Blocking Agents.—

ALPHA BLOCKERS.—These can be separated into the following
groups:—

1. THE IMIDAZOLINES.—(*a*) Tolazoline, B.P. (priscol) antagonizes
the vasoconstrictive effects of the catecholamines and in
addition has a direct vasodilating effect on blood-vessels. Can

be injected into an artery to relieve spasm (25–30 mg.).
(b) Phentolamine methanesulphonate and hydrochloride, B.P.
(regitine, rogitine). This drug, not used much now, has an
atropine-like effect on the heart and is a direct stimulant of
cardiac muscle. Effects last a quarter of an hour after intravenous injection. Was used to control the blood-pressure
during operations for the removal of phæochromocytomas as
well as in the diagnosis of this tumour. For the former
purpose, dose is 5 mg. intravenously repeated as required.
Dose for adrenaline overdose: 5–10 mg. intravenously.

2. THE BENZODIOXANS.—Piperoxan hydrochloride, B.P.C. Has a
rapid action and short duration of effect. Similar uses to
phentolamine and dose is in the order of 20 mg. intravenously.

3. THE CHLORO-ETHYLAMINES.—(a) Phenoxybenzamine hydrochloride, B.P. (dibenyline, dibenzyline). The blocking effects
of this agent are slow in onset and are irreversible: they last
until the drug is excreted. Used in phaeochromocytoma
surgery and to antagonize the vasoconstriction associated with
shock (together with fluid replacement). Can be given either
by mouth or by drip intravenously, 0·5–2 mg. per kg.
(b) Dibenamine.

4. THE ERGOT ALKALOIDS.—Ergotamine and certain dehydro-
genated derivatives have a feeble anti-adrenaline effect but
may potentiate the effects of other pressor agents especially
in hypertensive patients, e.g., during labour.

5. THE PHENOTHIAZINES.—Chlorpromazine and certain other
related compounds have an α-blocking effect.

BETA BLOCKERS.—Although dichloro-isoprenaline (DCI) and
pronethalol (alderlin)* fall into this group, only propranolol
(inderal) is now used. Pronethalol, one-tenth as potent as
propranolol, has been shown to be carcinogenic in mice and so
has been withdrawn. It was first used in 1962. Propranolol† is a
crystalline solid soluble in water and alcohol. It has the following
effects:—

CARDIOVASCULAR SYSTEM.—

1. Slows the heart by direct action on cardiac sympathetic β
receptors. Abolishes the tachycardia caused by isoprenaline
injection. Does not depress the vagus.
2. Decreases contractile force and blocks positive inotropic
effects of isoprenaline, but not those of digitalis or calcium.
3. Prevents fall in blood-pressure following isoprenaline injection.
4. Potentiates the pressor effects of adrenaline.
5. Peripheral vascular resistance first temporarily decreased,
then increased for a prolonged period.

NERVOUS SYSTEM.—No marked effect. Is a powerful local analgesic.
6 ml. of 0·4 per cent solution is efficient and non-toxic.‡

MYONEURAL JUNCTION.—Augments action of depolarizing and
reduces action of non-depolarizing agents.§

* Black, J. W., and Stephenson, J. S., *Lancet*, 1962, **2**, 331.
† Black, J. W., and others, *Ibid.*, 1964, **1**, 1080, and *Brit. J. Pharmacol.*, 1965, **25**, 547.
‡ Sinha, J. N., and others, *Brit. J. Anæsth.*, 1967, **39**, 887.
§ Wislicki, L., and Rosenblaum, I., *Ibid.*, 1967, **39**, 939.

Adrenergic Blocking Agents, *continued.*

RESPIRATION.—Causes bronchial constriction, especially in asth
matic and bronchitic patients, an effect reversed by iso
prenaline and atropine.

METABOLISM.—Probably reduces the free fatty acid and bloo
glucose levels caused by adrenaline.

CLINICAL USES IN ANÆSTHESIA.—Protects the heart from adrer
ergic stimulation associated with anxiety, atropine, surgica
stimulation, injected adrenaline, thyrotoxicosis, phæochromo
cytoma, and hypercapnia, and so reduces arrhythmias. Ha
been used to abolish arrhythmias associated with the use o
halothane* and cyclopropane and hypothermia. To potentiat
hypotension caused by ganglionic blocking agents; it prevent
tachycardia.†

DOSAGE.—Intravenously, 1–5 mg. very carefully.

(*See also* Johnstone, M., *Brit. J. Anæsth.*, 1966, **38**, 516.)

CHAPTER XVIII

THE USE OF
MUSCLE RELAXANTS IN ANÆSTHESIA

It is usual to classify muscle relaxants used in anæsthesia as : (1) Non
depolarizing (or antidepolarizing) agents, e.g., tubocurarine, gallamin
triethiodide, laudexium methylsulphate, nor-allyl-toxiferine, benzo
quinonium chloride (tachycurares), and: (2) Depolarizing agents, e.g.
decamethonium, suxamethonium, suxethonium halides, hexamethylene
carbaminoylcholine bromide (imbretil) (leptocurares). Under certai
circumstances the depolarizing drugs can exert an antidepolarizin
effect, the so-called dual or biphasic block. Other factors have to b
considered, such as the ionic cell environment, the tissue blood-flow
and the interaction together of different drugs.

History.—

1596. Sir Walter Raleigh mentioned the arrow poison in his book
Discovery of the Large, Rich, and Beautiful Empire of Guiana.

1811–1812. Sir Benjamin Collins Brody (1783–1862) experimented
with curare (*Phil. Trans.*, 1811, **101**, 194; and *Ibid.*, 1812, **102**,
205).

1825. Curare introduced into Europe by Charles Waterton (1783–
1865)—*Wanderings in South America.* He described a classic
experiment in which he kept a curarized she-ass alive by artificial
ventilation with a bellows through a tracheostomy.

1850. Claude Bernard (1813–1878),‡ the great French physiologist,
stimulated by Magendie, showed that curare acts by paralysing the
myoneural junction. He proved that in frogs, after curarization,

---

* Hellewell, J., and Potts, M. W., *Anæsthesia*, 1965, **20**, 269.
† Hewitt, P. B., Lord, P. W., and Thornton, H. L., *Ibid.*, 1967, **22**, 82.
‡ Bernard, C., *C. R. Soc. biol.*, Paris, 1851, **2**, 195; and *Leçon sur les Effets des Substances
Toxiques et Médicamenteuses*, 1851. Paris: Baillière.

there is no failure of conduction along motor nerves, nor is there failure of the curarized muscles to respond to direct electrical stimulation. This led to his discovery of the concept of the motor end-plate.

1862. Curare used by Chisholm in the American Civil War.

1872. Curare used by Demme in the treatment of tetanus.

1894. R. Boehm, the German pharmacologist, separated curare into "pot", "gourd", and "tube" curare according to the method used for storing it by the South American Indians.

1912. Curare used by Arthur Läwen of Leipzig* in an effort to reduce the amount of ether employed in abdominal surgery.

1935. King,† of London, working in Sir Henry Dale's laboratory, isolated *d*-tubocurarine chloride from the crude drug, and Ranyard West used it in the treatment of tetanus.‡

1938. Gill popularized its use in the U.S.A. in his book *White Water and Blue Magic*, 1940, New York.

1939. H. Palmer and Bennett employed curare to modify electro-convulsive therapy. Curare came to anæsthesia via psychiatry (electroplexy).§

1942. Harold R. Griffith and Enid Johnson used curare (the commercial preparation intocostrin) deliberately to give relaxation during surgery on 23 Jan. in Montreal, Canada. A famous day in the history of anæsthesia.‖

1943. Extraction of tubocurarine from *Chondrodendron tomentosum* by Wintersteiner¶—the source of the drug as used to-day. First publication of Cullen, a U.S. pioneer of its use.**

1944. Earliest mention of the use of curare with unsupplemented nitrous oxide and oxygen by Waters;†† also by Harroun.‡‡

1946. T. C. Gray and his colleagues established the position of curare in Britain.§§

1947. Bovet described gallamine triethiodide. This was used clinically in France by Huguenard and Boué in 1948 and by Mushin in 1949 in Britain. Influential article describing use of gas, oxygen, pethidine and curare by Neff.‖‖

1948. Decamethonium described by Barlow and Ing and by Paton and Zaimis. Used clinically by Organe in 1949.

1951. Suxamethonium first used in anæsthesia by von Dardel in Stockholm and by Mayerhofer in Vienna. Scurr introduced it into Britain.

1954. Sensational article by Beecher and Todd suggesting that the use of relaxants increased deaths due to anæsthesia nearly sixfold.¶¶ This has, of course, been completely disproved.

---

* Läwen, A., *Beitr. Klin. Chir.*, 1912, **80**, 168.
† King, H., *J. Chem. Soc.*, 1935, **57**, 1381.
‡ West, R., *Lancet*, 1936, **1**, 12.
§ Palmer, H., *J. ment. Sci.*, 1946, **92**, 411; and Bennett, A. E., *J. Amer. Med. Ass.*, 1940, **14**, 322.
‖ Griffith, H. R., and Johnson, G. E., *Anesthesiology*, 1942, **3**, 418.
¶ Wintersteiner, O., and Dutcher, J. D., *Science*, 1943, **97**, 467.
** Cullen, S. C., *Surgery*, 1943, **14**, 261.
†† Waters, R., *Anesthesiology*, 1944, **5**, 618.
‡‡ Harroun, P., and others, *Ibid.*, 1944, **7**, 24.
§§ Gray, T. C., and Halton, J. A., *Proc. R. Soc. Med.*, 1946, **39**, 400.
‖‖ Neff, W. B., and others, *Cal. Med.*, 1947, **66**, 67.
¶¶ Beecher, H. K., and Todd, D. P., *Ann. Surg.*, 1954, **140**, 2.

History, *continued.*

> (*See* Thomas, K. Bryn, *Curare. Its History and Usage*, 1954. London:
> Pitman.)

The Physiology of Muscular Contraction.—It was shown by S
Henry Dale, in 1936,[*] that a motor nerve liberates acetylcholin
at the myoneural junction on the arrival of a nerve impulse
It becomes fixed at anionic sites or the end-plate membrane an
permits entry of sodium which causes a sudden depolarization
The motor end-plate is specifically sensitive to acetylcholine an
becomes depolarized (made electrically negative) by it (the moto
end-plate potential). This current of depolarization excites th
adjacent part of the muscle-fibre (muscle action potential) an
passes along the membrane of the muscle-fibre and is the fina
stimulus for causing the contraction of the contractile part of th
muscle-fibre. The released acetylcholine is meanwhile hydrolyse
by the true acetylcholinesterase in the region of the motor end
plate, the two substances combining together so that when th
excited muscle-fibre has come out of its refractory state it will no
become excited again by a depolarized end-plate unless a new
nerve impulse has arrived and released a new supply of acety
choline.

The synthesis of acetylcholine takes place chiefly at the moto
nerve-endings by transfer of acetyl groups from co-enzyme A
under the influence of the enzyme choline acetylase. Afte
synthesis the acetylcholine is received on the end-plate an
then destroyed, a complex process.

Recent work indicates that acetylcholine is released as groups o
packets of molecules which have been named ' quanta ' an
each of which contains several hundred molecules. The arriva
of one quantum at the receptor is signalled by small (0·5 mV
and transient depolarization of the post-junctional membrane
In the absence of motor nerve activity such small potentia
changes may be observed as random occurrences. When th
action potential travels down the axon, several hundred quant
may be released and the amplitude of post-junctional membran
potential change may be 100 mV. of duration 1 millisecond
The output of quanta is affected by changes in the calcium t
magnesium ratio.

    See also review by Roberts, D. V., *Brit. J. Anæsth.*, 1963, **35**, 51c

Neuromuscular Block.—

    1. NON-DEPOLARIZERS OF THE MYONEURAL JUNCTION.
    2. DEPOLARIZERS OF THE MYONEURAL JUNCTION.
    3. AGENTS WHICH INTERFERE WITH THE FORMATION
       OF ACETYLCHOLINE, e.g., procaine, excess of magnesium
       and phosphate ions, deficiency of calcium ions, the toxin o
       the *B. botulinus*, and the triethyl analogue of choline.[†] Thi
       third group of drugs is not of great importance to anæsthetists

---

[*] Dale, H., Feldberg, W., and Vogt, M., *J. Physiol.*, 1936, **86**, 353.
[†] Laurance, D. R., and Webster, R. A., *Lancet*, 1961, **1**, 481.

4. DUAL,* DESENSITIZATION,† OR BIPHASIC BLOCK.‡—
While a single dose of a depolarizing drug causes pure depolarizing
(phase 1) block (except in myasthenia and in normal infants in
the first few weeks of life, when it causes a mixed block at the
first injection) repeated doses can cause a change in response
of the motor end-plate so that non-depolarizing (phase 2) block
follows the original depolarizing block. Changes in the reverse
direction never occur. If this dual block is present it is, of
course, theoretically increased by non-depolarizing drugs and
decreased by anticholinesterases, e.g., edrophonium. It may
rarely follow a single injection of suxamethonium (e.g., 50 mg.).
    Further developments in this interesting branch of physiology
are likely to take place and will eventually link up with the
aetiology of myasthenia gravis.

5. MIXED BLOCK.—Following injection of depolarizing and non-
depolarizing drugs into the patient simultaneously. The
division of relaxants may not be as well defined as at first
thought. All relaxants may pass through a phase of depolarization to be followed sooner or later by one of non-depolarization.
With tubocurarine the depolarization is transient and non-
depolarization develops early. With suxamethonium the depolarizing phase is prolonged and non-depolarization possibly
delayed.§

Action of Muscle Relaxants.—Neuromuscular blocking agents
compete with acetylcholine for cholinergic receptors at the end-
plate and prevent the access of acetylcholine to these receptors.
After adsorption to the receptor protein, the depolarizing and
non-depolarizing drugs behave differently.

1. The non-depolarizing or antidepolarizing agents (formerly called
substitution blockers or competitive inhibitors of acetylcholine, e.g., tubocurarine, gallamine, laudexium) prevent
access of acetylcholine to the receptor protein so that no depolarization, no change in resting potential of the motor end-
plate, and no muscular contraction—with consequent paralysis
—take place. They do not cause muscular fasciculation when
given intravenously. The paralysis is *increased* by : (1) additional non-depolarizing drugs ; (2) ether ; (3) cyclopropane ;
(4) procaine ; and is *decreased* by : (1) anticholinesterase drugs
(e.g., neostigmine) ; (2) depolarizing drugs ; (3) adrenaline ;
(4) acetylcholine ; (5) lowering of temperature.

RESPONSE TO ELECTRICAL STIMULATION (in the absence of
complete paralysis).—Both single (twitch) (1–10 per sec.)
and tetanic (10–20 per sec.) rates of stimulation lead to a
successive fade in the response. Following a volley of
tetanic stimuli, a single-twitch stimulus causes an increased
response, i.e., post-tetanic facilitation. In contrast, with
depolarizing agents there is a well-sustained response
to successive stimuli following both a single-twitch stimulus
and fast tetanic stimuli. The response to a single-twitch

* Zaimis, E. J., *Nature, Lond.*, 1952, **170**, 617.
† Thesleff, S., *Acta physiol. scand.*, 1955, **34**, 218.
‡ Jenden, D. J., and others, *J. Pharmacol.*, 1951, **103**, 348.
§ Payne, J. P., *Brit. J. Anæsth.*, 1961, **33**, 285.

Action of Muscle Relaxants, *continued.*

stimulus after a series of tetanic stimuli is not increase
i.e., there is no post-tetanic facilitation.

These responses can be shown, either electromyographi
ally or mechanically, following the application of a supr
maximal current (in the absence of complete myoneur
block) to the ulnar nerve, either at the elbow or just abo
and medial to the pisiform bone at the wrist by a nerv
stimulator.* Such a small piece of apparatus can b
inexpensively produced.†

2. The depolarizing drugs (e.g., decamethonium and suxameth
nium) cause depolarization of the end-plate like that cause
by acetylcholine which in this case persists. The depolariz
tion spreads to the muscle-fibres, making them electricall
unresponsive to subsequent stimuli, even after repolarizatic
is complete: the repolarization phase of normal neur
muscular transmission is interfered with. Flaccid paralysi
preceded by transient stimulation, results in normal ma
(but not in myasthenic man and in some other species
Depolarizing relaxants cause fasciculation after intravenou
injection. Their effect is *increased* by : (1) acetylcholine an
anticholinesterase agents ; (2) lowering of temperature
(3) additional depolarizing drugs. Their effect is *decrease*
by : (1) non-depolarizing agents ; (2) ether and cyclopropan

**Differences between Depolarizing and Non-depolarizing Re
laxants.—**

A. DEPOLARIZING AGENTS.—

1. They produce fasciculation on intravenous injection.
2. They are potentiated by anticholinesterase drugs and lowerin
of body temperature.
3. They are antagonized by non-depolarizing relaxants.
4. Single-twitch and tetanic electrical impulses produce no fad
in response ; after a burst of tetanic stimuli there is n
increase in response to a single-twitch stimulus (no post
tetanic facilitation).

B. NON-DEPOLARIZING AGENTS.—

1. They do not cause muscular fasciculation on intravenou
injection.
2. Their effects are reversed by anticholinesterase drugs, and b
lowering the temperature.
3. Single-twitch and tetanic electrical impulses produce a gradua
fade in response ; after a volley of tetanic stimuli, there i
an increased response to a single-twitch impulse (post-tetani
facilitation).‡

TUBOCURARINE CHLORIDE, B.P.

Source of Curare.—From the bark, leaves, and vines of the tropica
plant *Chondrodendron tomentosum*, growing near the upper reache
of the Amazon. Has long been used by natives of S. America t

---

* Christie, T. H., and Churchill-Davidson, H. C., *Lancet*, 1958, **1**, 776.
† Cohen, A. D. *Anæsthesia*, 1963, **18**, 534.
‡ Churchill-Davidson, H. C., *Brit. J. Anæsth.*, 1959, **31**, 290.

poison the heads of their arrows. They transport it in bamboo tubes, hence the name tubocurarine. It is a quaternary alkaloid.

Pharmacology.—The drug has neither anæsthetic nor analgesic properties when given in clinical doses.

EFFECT ON MOTOR END-PLATE.—It is the classic non-depolarizing myoneural blocking agent and acts by preventing the adsorption of acetylcholine to the cholinergic receptors and so prevents the changes in the end-plate which cause muscular tone and contraction. Therapeutic doses produce the following effects in sequence : ptosis, imbalance of extra-ocular muscles with diplopia (which rarely may last several days), relaxation of muscles of the face, jaw, neck, and limbs. It is possible to paralyse the limb muscles without greatly reducing the respiratory minute volume. Relaxation of the anterior abdominal wall muscles, the intercostals, and the diaphragm are the last muscles to be paralysed (except occasionally the levatores palpebræ superiores), their weakness giving rise to diminished respiratory movements and finally to apnœa. Muscular power returns in from fifteen to fifty minutes.

CEREBRAL EFFECTS.—None in clinical doses. The electrical activity of the brain is first increased, later decreased. Intracisternal injection into animals has caused convulsions. Large doses have been suspected of causing depression of the medullary centres and this may be one cause of prolonged apnœa following its use,* especially if complicated by depletion of intracellular potassium.

EFFECTS ON AUTONOMIC NERVES.—These are due to substrate competition with acetylcholine for cholinergic receptors of autonomic ganglia, and result in autonomic block without preliminary ganglionic stimulation : the block is not complete, but diminishes vascular tone and may help to prevent shock. The alkaloid has a greater effect on sympathetic ganglia than the other relaxants, and a greater effect on pre- than on post-ganglionic neurons.

EFFECTS ON RESPIRATION.—It paralyses the muscles of respiration ; the diaphragm, being less sensitive than other muscles, is usually the last one to be paralysed. Bronchospasm, perhaps due to histamine release (aided sometimes by thiobarbiturates), is sometimes seen, especially in patients with a tendency to asthma who are subjected to upper respiratory tract stimulation. Usually pharyngeal, laryngeal, and bronchial reflexes are depressed so that endotracheal intubation and irritant anæsthetic vapours are well tolerated.

EFFECTS ON CIRCULATION.—In ordinary doses there is no effect on the heart. There may be slight hypotension due to sympathetic ganglionic blockade together with histamine release. The clotting time is not altered. There is an antifibrillatory action on the ventricles and a decreased likelihood of arrhythmia. Hypertension (not due to hypercapnia) has also been reported.

GASTRO-INTESTINAL SYSTEM.—The effect on the stomach and intestine is variable. The cardiac sphincter is probably not relaxed.

---

* Foster, P. A., *Brit. J. Anæsth.*, 1956, **28**, 448.

Tubocurarine—Pharmacology, *continued.*

ABSORPTION AND EXCRETION.—Absorbed when administered intravenously, intramuscularly, subcutaneously, intraperitoneally, sublingually, and per rectum. In practice, nearly
always given intravenously, occasionally intramuscularly. It
is excreted via the kidneys, some of it being first altered in the
muscles. About 30 per cent can be recovered unchanged from
the urine. The liver probably does not destroy the drug. Plasma
proteins have the power of binding tubocurarine and this may
influence its fate in the body,* and there seems to be a positive
correlation between the tubocurarine requirements and the
serum level of gamma-globulin.† Some is retained in the tissues
in an inactive state after its pharmacological effects have
worn off.

OTHER ACTIONS.—It has been recommended for the control of
certain reflexes which give rise to hypotension and bradycardia,
e.g., carotid sinus, cœliac plexus, pelvic reflexes : it acts in
these cases by depressing parasympathetic ganglia. It releases
histamine from the tissues and heparin from the liver and is
perhaps not the first choice for use in patients with severe
bronchospasm. It crosses the placental barrier but only in
small amounts and does not affect the fœtus clinically when the
dosage is reasonable. It may increase the uterine tone. Patients
with liver disease may require more tubocurarine than usual, to
compete with the increased amount of acetylcholine resulting
from the poor supply of cholinesterase and pseudocholinesterase.
Neither diabetes nor renal disease contra-indicates its use.

After intravenous injection effect commences within ten seconds
and is at its maximum within three minutes. After intramuscular injection, effect is seen after ten to fifteen minutes.
After oral administration it is inactive unless taken in excessive
dosage.

Tubocurarine is generally supplied in 1·5-ml. ampoules containing
15 mg. and this is usually miscible with solutions of thiobarbiturates.
Tubadil is a suspension of tubocurarine in oil, 25 mg. per ml., and is
said to have an effect lasting up to twenty-four hours. It is used to
relieve pain due to muscular spasm, e.g., after hæmorrhoidectomy.

It is advised that a uniform strength of solution should be used,
i.e., 3 mg. per ml. It is simple to add 1·5 ml. of tubocurarine solution
to 3·5 ml. of saline in a 5-ml. syringe, which gives the recommended
strength.

Dosage.—6–10 mg. causes limb paralysis without greatly reducing
respiratory efficiency. 15–20 mg. causes paralysis of abdominal
muscles. 20–30 mg. is required for intubation of the larynx.
These are average doses.

Duration of Effect.—Twenty to thirty minutes. After repeated
dosage, a cumulative effect may occur.

---

* Aladjemoff, L., and others, *J. Pharmacol.*, 1958, **123**, 43.
† Baraka, A., and Gabal, F., *Brit. J. Anæsth.*, 1968, **40**, 89.

Clinical Uses of Tubocurarine Chloride and Gallamine Tri-ethiodide.—

1. To make endotracheal intubation by the direct route relatively easy and atraumatic, by removing the tone of the cords and neck muscles. It is inferior to suxamethonium in this respect.
2. To aid muscular relaxation during light anæsthesia.
3. To lessen laryngeal spasm and quieten upper respiratory reflexes during anæsthesia.
4. To facilitate control of respiration by producing respiratory paralysis.
5. To facilitate bronchoscopy, œsophagoscopy, etc.
6. To reduce the intensity of muscular contractions in electroconvulsive therapy, but suxamethonium is the better drug for this purpose.
7. To prevent shivering during induction of hypothermia.
8. To prevent straining during spontaneous respiration : this may even increase tidal volume.

Tubocurarine 3 mg. and gallamine 20 mg. are equipotent.

Technique.—Because of the occasional patient who is susceptible to the drugs, some workers advise that a trial dose should be given intravenously to the conscious patient and its effects watched. They give 5 mg. and wait four minutes ; the normal response of this dosage may be lassitude and difficulty in keeping the eyes open, with some diplopia. The susceptible patient will show ptosis not under voluntary control, dysphagia, dysarthria, and difficulty in breathing. Development of any of these signs calls for a reduction of subsequent dosage.

Following this trial injection in the ordinary abdominal operation, a further 10–25 mg. of tubocurarine chloride are injected and followed immediately by the injection into the same needle of 4 to 10 ml. of 2·5 per cent thiopentone solution. The face-mask is now applied and a gas–oxygen mixture is gently forced into the lungs (during inspiration, if the patient is breathing). After two or three minutes, the larynx is exposed, sprayed with a topical analgesic solution, if thought necessary, and intubated under direct vision through a laryngoscope. Assisted or controlled breathing is maintained, and additional doses of thiopentone, perhaps pethidine, and tubocurarine are given as required. An anæsthetic vapour may also be added.

The inhalation agent or agents can be given in the closed circuit (if trichloroethylene is not used) or in the semi-closed circuit. Assisted or controlled respiration must always be used if the tidal exchange is reduced in volume, an almost invariable occurrence when proper abdominal relaxation is produced by tubocurarine chloride or gallamine.

During thiopentone–gas–oxygen–tubocurarine anæsthesia, the following signs often indicate the need for extra relaxant :—

1. Hiccup, due to contraction of the periphery of the diaphragm.
2. Rigidity of the abdominal wall.
3. Increased resistance to inflation of the lung (in the absence of respiratory obstruction), i.e., decreased compliance.
4. Bucking or coughing on the endotracheal tube.

Tubocurarine Technique, *continued.*

5. Increased amplitude of respiration in the absence of controlled respiration.

Extra analgesic is (in the opinion of some workers) required if (1) The patient moves his skeletal muscles in response to the surgical stimulus, e.g., face, limb, or neck muscles. (2) The pulse rate rises. (3) Sweating, unexplained by other causes, occurs (4) There is reflex response to surgical stimuli, e.g., hiccups.

Whenever muscle relaxants are used, it is of paramount importance to see that the patient is breathing reasonably deeply before he leaves the operating table. Respiratory depression at the end of the operation should be treated either by inflation until the tidal volume becomes normal, or, more usually, by the injection of neostigmine with atropine.

OTHER METHODS.—There are many other techniques of using the muscle relaxants, and the following may be mentioned :—

1. Induction and maintenance with an intravenous barbiturate together with inhalation of gas–oxygen. Additions of relaxant just before skin incision and again if necessary before the abdomen is explored, with further additions as required.

2. Maintenance with cyclopropane, with relaxant given when required, in small doses.

3. Maintenance with gas–oxygen–ether, or gas–oxygen–halothane, with relaxant given as required in smaller dosage than average.

4. Maintenance with a general anæsthetic with injection of a large dose (in several separate amounts) sufficient to produce apnœa ; this must be followed by controlled breathing.

5. Among others, the Liverpool school of anæsthetists rely on an initial dose of thiopentone for induction followed by tubo-curarine and inflation with gas and oxygen, intubation with a cuffed tube, and controlled breathing employing definite hyperventilation with its resulting hypocapnia or respirator alkalosis, e.g., 20 ml. per kg. with a maximum of 20 litres per minute, in adults. No more thiopentone is ordinarily given, but additional doses of relaxant are freely used to provide proper operating conditions, e.g., to abolish returning respiratory movements, returning muscle tone, reflex response, hiccups, etc. Neostigmine and atropine at the end of the operation enable normal respiration to be resumed before the patient leaves the operating room.

The light levels of general anæsthesia used with the relaxants are not accompanied by vasomotor depression, hence shock is lessened.

Since the use of the relaxant drugs became general, the need (although not the employment) of endotracheal intubation has decreased. The average lower abdominal operation of moderate duration should seldom call for intubation, as reflex laryngeal spasm is rare, always provided that the stomach and œsophagus contain no vomitable material. Assisted or controlled respiration can be performed without an endotracheal tube, and inflation of the stomach with anæsthetic gases can be prevented by maintaining a clear airway and avoiding excessive inflation pressure. Many anæsthetists of experience, however, intubate all their abdominal cases.

Infants and children tolerate the drugs well if the dosage is suitably adjusted to their general condition and body-weight. An average initial dosage is 2 mg. per stone of tubocurarine or 1 mg. per lb. of gallamine.

The drugs have been used, without general anæsthesia in small doses, for cataract extraction. They have an early and selective action on the extra-ocular muscles when given in small doses.

Dosage bears no relationship to age, sex, or weight.

Tubocurarine in Neonates.*—Although neonates up to six weeks old are roughly twice as sensitive to non-depolarizing relaxants as adults, the view has recently been expressed that tubocurarine can be a safe and satisfactory muscle relaxant in neonatal anæsthesia. The dose should be small (0·05 mg. in premature babies and 0·5 mg. in the full-term neonate in 0·05 per cent solution as an initial dose, subsequent doses being in the order of 0·125 mg. to 0·25 mg. respectively). Neostigmine should be used routinely 0·036 mg. per lb. with atropine 0·008 mg. per lb. Causes of trouble may be due to: (1) Overdosage; (2) Use of additional respiratory depressant drugs; (3) Unintentional hypothermia; (4) Use of neomycin and streptomycin ; (5) Supplementation by ether.

Advantages and Disadvantages.—With tubocurarine and its congeners, profound muscular relaxation can be produced quickly while the patient is under very light general anæsthesia. This combination of relaxant and light anæsthesia is relatively non-toxic, while it does not add to operative shock. The relaxing effects on the muscles of the larynx remove the worrying symptoms of spasm which have marred so many otherwise smooth anæsthesias.

Reduced tidal exchange or frank apnœa may readily be produced, and unless remedied will seriously harm the patient. *Emphasis must be placed on the danger of the patient returning to bed with a poor tidal exchange which will not only cause oxygen lack and carbon dioxide excess, but will also predispose to the formation of patches of collapse of the lungs.* Inspiratory stridor, due to atony of the vocal cords, has been described following the use of relaxants.

Occasionally some residual paresis of the muscles of accommodation persists for twenty-four hours after operation, making reading difficult.

The drugs must be used with special care if given to the same patient on two occasions within twenty-four hours, as a cumulative effect may occur.

They must not be used in patients suffering from myasthenia gravis except for purposes of diagnosis, when minute doses are given.

Tubocurarine potentiates the hypotension caused by halothane, so care is necessary if the two drugs are used together.

---

* Bush, G. H., and Stead, A. L., *Brit. J. Anæsth.*, 1962, **34**, 721 ; and Bush, G. H., *Ibid.*, 1963, **35**, 552; and Churchill-Davidson, H. C., and Wise, R. P., *Canad. Anæsth. Soc. J.*, 1964, **11**, 1.

Tubocurarine—Advantages and Disadvantages, *continued.*

So potent are tubocurarine chloride and gallamine, and so likely a[ ]
they to cause respiratory depression, that their use should l[ ]
restricted to experienced anæsthetists who are fully competer[ ]
to institute and maintain efficient artificial respiration in a[ ]
types of patient.

In cases of liver damage, Dundee and Gray* have experience[ ]
abnormal resistances to tubocurarine. This may be associate[ ]
with a lowered serum pseudocholinesterase, and increase[ ]
sensitivity to acetylcholine at the end-plate.

Other Uses of Tubocurarine and Gallamine.—They have bee[ ]
used in the treatment of tetanus, spasticity and rigidity associate[ ]
with neurological disease, orthopædic conditions, myositis, arthriti[ ]
and strychnine poisoning. Unfortunately, voluntary power [ ]
abolished as well as spasticity. Tremor is not improved.

As a diagnostic test for myasthenia gravis, 0·1 to 0·2 mg. per ston[ ]
of tubocurarine is slowly injected intravenously. If myastheni[ ]
is present, a marked exaggeration of its symptoms is produce[ ]
in a minute or two. These can be dissipated by the immediat[ ]
intravenous injection of neostigmine and atropine (1·5 mg. an[ ]
0·6 mg.).

Electroconvulsive therapy† was formerly modified by tubocurarine[ ]
The shorter-acting relaxants are now commonly used to softe[ ]
the convulsions of E.C.T.

GALLAMINE TRIETHIODIDE (FLAXEDIL), B.P.

A synthetic curarizing agent producing non-depolarizing neuro[ ]
muscular block, first prepared by the Frenchmen, Bovet and Halpern[ ]
in 1947. First clinical report on its use in anæsthesia by Huguenar[ ]
and Boué‡ in France and by Mushin and others (*Lancet*, 1949, **1**, 726[ ]
Chemically it is 1,2,3 tri-(β-diethylaminoethoxy)-benzene-triethyl iodid[ ]

Physical and Chemical Properties.—Before solution it is a whit[ ]
amorphous powder prepared synthetically with a melting-point [ ]
145–150° C. Dissolves in water and alcohol to form stable solu[ ]
tions compatible with thiopentone. Supplied in 4 per cent solutio[ ]
in ampoules containing 2 ml. (80 mg.) and 3 ml. (120 mg.). (2 per cen[ ]

---

* Dundee, J. W., and Gray, T. C., *Lancet*, 1953, **1**, 16.
† First performed by Cerletti, N., and Bini, L., *Arch. Neurol. Psychiat.*, 1938, **19**, 266.
‡ Huguenard, P., *Brux. Méd.*, 1949, **27**, 2059.

solution is used in France.) Opinions vary as to its relative strength compared with 15 mg. of tubocurarine chloride ; 80 mg. is perhaps a fair estimate.

Pharmacology.—Duration of effect shorter than that of tubocurarine (15–20 minutes against 20–30 minutes). Gallamine has a curariform action on the neuromuscular mechanism (i.e., it interferes with the action of acetylcholine), and previous doses of tubocurarine chloride sensitize the patient to it. Its action is antagonized by the anticholinesterases (e.g., neostigmine) more efficiently than is tubocurarine. It has less effect on the sympathetic ganglia than tubocurarine chloride (and so can be used with halothane) but shows an atropine-like vagal blocking effect on the postganglionic nerve-endings of the heart which results in tachycardia, even with small doses, e.g., 20 mg.* This outlasts the relaxant effect and makes it very suitable for use with halothane. In some patients receiving cyclopropane, this tachycardia is absent, because of the action of the gas on the sino-auricular node and conductive tissues of the heart. It often causes a slight rise in blood-pressure. It is said to be less liable to release histamine than tubocurarine. It depresses the respiratory function, and will produce apnœa if dosage is pushed. Allergic reactions have been reported following its use.† It passes the placental barrier and perhaps should not be used in obstetrics routinely, although many workers have found it satisfactory in clinical obstetrical practice. It does not influence uterine contractions. Excretion is by the kidneys, and it should be used carefully in patients with decreased renal filtration rate, e.g., in hypotension or circulatory depression, and in renal disease, in case prolonged curarization results. Hypocapnia, following hyperventilation, potentiates its effects.‡

Clinical Uses.—Similar to those of tubocurarine chloride, 20 mg. being the equivalent of 3 mg. of tubocurarine. Given intravenously the first dose usually loses its effect in half an hour. To relax the peritoneum in an average patient, a dose of from 60 mg. to 160 mg. is needed. Children tolerate larger relative doses, e.g., 1 mg. per lb. Very useful for direct vision intubation (120–160 mg.). More accurate doses can be given if it is diluted with saline to 2 per cent so that each ml. contains 20 mg. Can be used intramuscularly with hyaluronidase (the ampoule of powder dissolved in the gallamine solution) in doses about 50 per cent greater than would be required by the intravenous route.

It is possibly better avoided : (1) When there is pre-existing tachycardia : any condition exaggerating sympathetic activity makes gallamine undesirable as the heart loses its protective vagal response; (2) When there is renal impairment: there is a relationship between the duration of action of the drug and renal excretion. Prolonged apnœa due to the defective renal excretion of the drug may be treated by artificial diuresis or by dialysis.§

* Doughty, A. G., and Wylie, W. D., *Proc. R. Soc. Med.*, 1951, **44**, 375.
† Walmsley, D. A., *Lancet*, 1959, **2**, 237.
‡ Walts, L. F., Lebowitz, M., and Dillon, J. B., *Brit. J. Anæsth.*, 1967, **39**, 845.
§ Churchill-Davidson, H. C., Way, W. L., and de Jong, R. H., *Anesthesiology*, 1967, **28**, 540.

Gallamine Triethiodide—Clinical Uses, *continued.*

If there is inadequate renal excretion due either to pre-existing renal disease or to renal inadequacy consequent on the operation (e.g., left heart failure or shock), recurarization may result after reversal with neostigmine. This may require additional doses of the anti-cholinesterase drug during the first twenty-four hours after operation ; (3) In obstetrics, where doses should not be large.

Dosage.—Test dose 20–30 mg. 50 mg. will paralyse muscles of limbs without greatly affecting respiration. 80–100 mg. will usually cause apnœa. 120–160 mg. is required for smooth intubation.

Duration of Effect.—About twenty minutes.

DIALLYL NORTOXIFERIN (ALLOFERIN; ALCURONIUM CHLORIDE)

This is derived synthetically from toxiferin,* an alkaloid of calabash curare. It is a medium-acting non-depolarizing relaxant the effects of which come on 3–4 minutes after injection and last for 15–20 minutes. Is miscible in the same syringe with methohexitone but not with thiopentone. No effect on pulse-rate. Said to be twice as potent as tubocurarine as regards onset of action and duration of effect in children[†] and in adults,[‡] while a dose of 10 mg. is said to give good conditions for intubation and for abdominal relaxation in adults.[§]

Suggested dosage: 1 mg. per stone (0·16 mg. per kg.) and double this for intubation.[||] In children, 0·125–0·2 mg. per kg.

Its effects are reversed by neostigmine provided an overdose of the relaxant is avoided.

DIMETHYL TUBOCURARINE IODIDE (METUBINE, D.M.E.) ;[¶] BROMIDE (DIAMETHINE) ; AND CHLORIDE (MECOSTRIN)

Prepared by King and Dutcher (1935). Pharmacological properties described by Collier in 1948.[**] This non-depolarizing relaxant is 2–2 times as potent as tubocurarine ; its action does not last as long, and there is less histamine release and autonomic blocking action than is seen after tubocurarine. Its onset is more rapid than and its duration half that of tubocurarine, and it is more sparing of the diaphragm. Most of the drug is excreted in the urine. The average paralysing dose is 1 mg. per stone, and it is said to be often possible to maintain adequate spontaneous respiration together with good relaxation, at least in lower abdominal operations. Prepared in 3-ml. ampoules, 2 mg. per ml. It is

---

* Frey, R., and Seeger, R., *Canad. Anæsth. Soc. J.*, 1961, **8**, 99.

† Bush, G. H., *Brit. J. Anæsth.*, 1965, **37**, 540.

‡ Baraka, A., *Ibid.*, 1967, **39**, 624.

§ Venn, P. H., *Ibid.*, 1965, **37**, 213.

|| Hunter, A. R., *Ibid.*, 1964, **36**, 466.

¶ *See* articles by Wilson, H. B., Gordon, H. E., and Raffan, A. W., *Lancet*, 1950, **1**, 1296 and Bullough, J., *Proc. World Congress Anæsthesiologists*, 1956, 251. Minneapolis : Burgess Publ. Co.

** Collier, H. O. J., and others, *Nature, Lond.*, 1948, **161**, 817; and Collier, H. O. J., *Brit. med. J.*, 1950, **1**, 1293.

aid to enable inflation of the lung to be performed more easily than vhen other relaxants are used. Now seldom used.

LAUDEXIUM METHYL SULPHATE (LAUDOLISSIN)*

This is a heterocyclic decamethylene *bis*-quaternary ammonium ompound, synthesized by Taylor and Collier in 1949.† It is a true ion-depolarizing myoneural blocking agent, one half as potent as ubocurarine, not always completely antagonized by neostigmine, icting longer than tubocurarine (45–50 minutes), and having no indesirable side-actions. Its effects are potentiated by ether and intagonized by small doses of suxamethonium. It does not release iistamine. Maximal effect comes on five minutes after injection. It s not miscible with thiopentone or pethidine, gallamine, atropine, or iuxamethonium chloride. A test dose of 10 mg. should be given. *See* articles by Bodman, R. I., Morton, H. J. V., and Wylie, W. D., *Lancet*, 1952, **2**, 517; Dundee, J. W., Gray, T. C., and Riding, J. E., *Brit. J. Anæsth.*, 1954, **26**, 13.)

ANTAGONISTS TO NON-DEPOLARIZING RELAXANTS

NEOSTIGMINE.—The clinical antagonist is neostigmine methyl-sulphate (prostigmine) which was synthesized by Aeschlimann and Reinert in 1931‡ and which is twice as powerful as physo-stigmine, isolated in 1864 from the calabar bean, the anticurare action of which was discovered by Pal in 1900,§ and used in animal experimentation in 1909.‖ Neostigmine is an anti-cholinesterase. It is partly broken down by pseudocholinesterase and partly excreted unchanged by the kidneys. Tubocurarine combines with the receptor protein without causing depolariza-tion and thereby prevents acetylcholine from combining with the receptor and causing depolarization. If now the acetylcholine can be raised by increasing the amount of anticholinesterase (e.g., neostigmine) present to a level at which the excitation threshold of the end-plate is reached, then neuromuscular block will be overcome.

$$N(CH_3)_3SO_4.CH_3$$

COO . N(CH_3)_2

Neostigmine, besides being an anticholinesterase, is also a de-polarizer and can cause on its own a depolarizing type of block. This is due to the build-up of acetylcholine, following the inhibition of cholinesterase. Phase 2 block can eventually result. The amount needed to cause paralysis by persistent depolarization is much greater, normally, than that required to antagonize an effective dose of tubocurarine or gallamine.

* No longer available in Britain.
† Collier, H. O. J., and Taylor, E. P., *Nature, Lond.*, 1949, **164**, 491.
‡ Aeschlimann, J. A., and Reinert, M., *J. Pharmacol.*, 1931, **43**, 413.
§ Pal, J., *Zbl. Physiol.*, 1900, **14**, 255.
‖ Meltzer, S. J., and Auer, J., *J. Exp. Med.*, 1909, **2**, 622.

Neostigmine, *continued.*

Depolarizing blocks due to the following are not alway reversed by neostigmine:—

1. That due to neomycin.
2. That due to phase 2 blocks following suxamethonium.
3. Sometimes, that following diallyl nortoxiferin.*

When injected into a conscious patient it may caus muscular fasciculations. In addition, it is a direct stimulant cholinergic effector cells. It has nicotinic effects and has direct stimulant effect on muscle. In small doses it stimulate and in larger doses it depresses autonomic ganglia. It also ha muscarinic effects (from *Amarita muscaria*) which are blocke by atropine, e.g., bradycardia, intestinal peristalsis and spasm bronchial and salivary secretion and bronchospasm, stimu lation of the sweat-glands, contraction of the pupil, an contraction of the bladder. It induces menstruation in certai cases of delay and may cause decreased coronary flow. I potentiates morphine analgesia. Dose 0·5 mg. carefull repeated up to a total of 5 mg., with atropine 1·3 mg. ($\frac{1}{50}$ gr. For injection the methylsulphate is used: for oral adminis tration, the bromide.

EDROPHONIUM (Tensilon).—This is 3-hydroxy phenyl dimethy ethyl ammonium chloride, and is supplied in 1 per cent solutior It has, like neostigmine, anticholinesterase, depolarizing, an direct stimulating effects on the motor end-plate. Muscarini effects are present but are not as severe as those of neostigmine nevertheless atropine may be required to combat them. It actions come on quicker, but do not last as long as those c neostigmine, consequently hypoventilation and recurarizatio may follow an initial stimulant effect on the respiration. Dos is 10 mg., carefully repeated : this is equivalent in immediat effect to 1·25 mg. of neostigmine. Because of its short-actin decurarizing action it should be used only to diagnose th presence (or absence) of dual or biphasic block in a patient wit prolonged apnœa after depolarizing muscle relaxants have bee used.

PYRIDOSTIGMINE† (Mestinon) is the dimethyl carbonic ester c *n*-methyl pyridium bromide. It has one-quarter the potenc of neostigmine but a longer duration of action and a slowe onset. It is not as reliable as neostigmine as an antagonis to tubocurarine. Dose 10 mg., the equivalent of 2·5 mg. o

* Hunter, A. R., *Brit. J. Anæsth.*, 1964, **36**, 466.
† Brown, A. K., *Anæsthesia*, 1954, **9**, 92.

neostigmine. Recent work* suggests that it is equal to neostigmine and superior to edrophonium, causing less oropharyngeal secretion than the former, with less bradycardia.

These three drugs are used also in the diagnosis and treatment of myasthenia gravis.

Clinical Uses of Neostigmine.—

1. The muscarinic effects, especially bradycardia, must be prevented by atropine (1·3 mg. ($\frac{1}{50}$ gr.) for each 2·5 mg.) which can be given before, or with, the neostigmine—good reasons are advanced for each of these times. Simultaneous injection of the two drugs appears to be safe.†

2. The maximal dose should probably seldom exceed 5 mg. as neostigmine can itself cause myoneural block of a depolarizing type.

3. As both gallamine and, to a less extent, tubocurarine block the vagal ganglia, neostigmine is safer in curarized than in non-curarized patients.

4. Cyclopropane, halothane, thiopentone, jaundice, and duodenal ulcer may all be associated with vagotonia and so call for extra care if neostigmine is used.

5. Neostigmine may cause bronchial constriction and secretion and so may predispose to atelectasis ; may be undesirable in severe asthma.

6. Edrophonium is not a very satisfactory antidote to curarizing agents. It acts quickly, but only for a short time, so that re-curarization has been seen.

Many workers always give neostigmine if a non-depolarizing relaxant has been used. Before it is injected, the patient should be in a state of hypo- or normocapnia,‡ and have a normal Po_2.§

In the average case, towards the end of the operation, hyperventilation should give place to normal ventilation. Atropine and neostigmine are given in small and if necessary repeated doses of 0·5 mg. of neostigmine. Breathing can be stimulated by moving the tube within the trachea and by application of a suction catheter to the carina. Very rarely, 5 ml. of nikethamide or 2 ml. of vanillic acid diethylamide can be injected into a vein to rouse what Nosworthy called a muddled respiratory centre. I.P.P.V. must be carried out until the patient can ventilate adequately himself.

Adrenaline, potassium, calcium, guanidine, depolarizing relaxants, Evans blue, and Congo red are antagonistic to curare, but are not used clinically.

* Katz, R. L., *Anesthesiology*, 1967, **28**, 528.
† Kemp, S. W., and Morton, H. J. V., *Anæsthesia*, 1962, **17**, 170.
‡ Riding, J. E., and Robinson, J. S., *Ibid.*, 1961, **16**, 346.
§ Baraka, A., *Brit. J. Anæsth.*, 1968, **40**, 27.

Clinical Uses of Neostigmine, *continued.*

Signs of decurarization after injection of neostigmine for inadequat
respiration :—

1. Return of normal tidal exchange measured either by an anemo
   meter or by the flow-meters of the anæsthetic machine usin
   a Ruben or other non-rebreathing valve.
2. Effective coughing on endotracheal tube.
3. Ability to open eyes and keep them open.
4. Presence of tone in the masseters.
5. Ability to raise the head from the pillow.

Signs of incomplete decurarization :—

1. Persistence of chin or tracheal tug (sometimes) : this may b
   associated with intercostal paralysis.
2. Ineffective coughing on tube.
3. Ptosis.
4. General fidgeting, jerky movements.

Deaths have occurred following the use of neostigmine and atropine
possible causes are : (1) Cardiac inhibition ; (2) Adrenergic effect
of neostigmine and atropine causing ventricular fibrillation
(3) The atropine itself causing arrhythmia, especially in th
presence of hypercapnia.* There is evidence that harm fron
neostigmine is only likely if it is given while the patient ha
hypercapnia or hypoxia.† Respiratory alkalosis seems t
protect the heart.‡ It is of fundamental importance that th
patient should not be left until he is able to ventilate himsel
adequately.

DECAMETHONIUM IODIDE§

This is *bis*-methylammonium decane di-halide and was originall
known as C.10. It was introduced by Barlow and Ing‖ and by Pato
and Zaimis in 1948¶ and used in anæsthesia by Organe in the followin,
year.** Prepared commercially as Eulissin, decamethonium di-iodide
each ml. of solution containing 2 mg.

$$(CH_3)_3—N—(CH_2)_{10}—N—(CH_3)_3$$
$$\quad\ \ | \qquad\qquad\qquad |$$
$$\quad\ \ I \qquad\qquad\qquad I$$

Chemistry.—In its pure form is a white, crystalline salt, soluble i
water, neutral in solution, stable, and resistant to heat. Th
solution mixes well with thiopentone and alkaloids, and is non
irritant to tissues.

Pharmacology.—

MUSCULAR SYSTEM.—It causes neuromuscular block by pro
longed depolarization of the motor end-plate in skeletal muscles

* Pooler, H. C., *Anæsthesia*, 1957, **12**, 198.
† Baraka, A., *Brit. J. Anæsth.*, 1968, **40**, 27.
‡ Riding, J. E., and Robinson, J. S., *Anæsthesia*, 1961, **16**, 346.
§ *See* articles by Organe, G., *Canad. Anæsth. Soc. J.*, 1956, **3**, 5 ; and by Hunter, A. R., *Brit
J. Anæsth.*, 1950, **22**, 218.
‖ Barlow, R. B., and Ing, H. R., *Nature, Lond.*, 1948, **161**, 718.
¶ Paton, W. D. M., and Zaimis, E. J., *Ibid.*, 1948, **162**, 810.
** Organe, G. S. W., Paton, W. D. M., and Zaimis, E. J., *Lancet*, 1949, **1**, 21.

the intercostals and diaphragm being affected less intensely. In addition its action extends to the muscle-fibres themselves on each side of the end-plate and makes them unexcitable. It acts like acetylcholine, which cannot be hydrolysed. It prevents the access of acetylcholine to the cholinergic receptors of the end-plate. Muscular twitching may be seen soon after its injection, an effect made worse by a high blood-adrenaline level. The subsequent muscle pains differ from those caused by suxamethonium, being largely confined to the jaw and calf muscles. It is not antagonized by the anticholinesterases such as neostigmine (which, by causing acetylcholine to persist, may increase the paralysing effect of decamethonium), but by the compound pentamethonium iodide, when given in 10–100 times the dose of decamethonium iodide. This effect is too dangerous to make clinical use of, because of the resulting hypotension. Repeated use may lead to the depolarizing effect at the end-plate giving place to a non-depolarizing effect, the so-called phase 2 block,* and this, if present, can be reversed by edrophonium or neostigmine. It explains the tachyphylaxis seen on repeated dosage —one is really giving a depolarizing drug to a patient whose myoneural junctions are depressed by non-depolarization and this creates an antagonism. Ether anæsthesia, together with the presence of adrenaline in the circulation, tends to lessen its action—the opposite effect to that seen when non-depolarizing relaxants are used. Its action on muscles varies with the amount of blood circulating in them.

Patients with myasthenia gravis are said to be less affected by the drug than are normal people and a single injection results in dual block which is antagonized by edrophonium and neostigmine.

CARDIOVASCULAR SYSTEM.—Little or no effect.

CENTRAL NERVOUS SYSTEM.—Little or no effect with clinical dosage. There may be slight depression of autonomic ganglia. May dilate pupils.

HISTAMINE RELEASE.—Very slight. Bronchospasm does not occur.

PLACENTAL BARRIER.—Probably does not reach fœtus. No effect on uterus.

EXCRETION.—Excreted mainly unchanged in urine : not hydrolysed, hence its longer duration of action than suxamethonium.

Dosage.—3 mg. is roughly equipotent to 15 mg. of tubocurarine. Maximum dosage, 10 mg.

Duration of Effect.—About 15 minutes—rather less than gallamine.

Clinical Uses.†—The drug causes a depolarizing block which is active but does not last long. It gives place to a non-depolarizing block, which, although incomplete, is longer lasting : with increasing amounts the non-depolarizing block becomes more complete. The average dose to relax the abdomen is 3 mg., and its maximal effects

---

* White, D. C., *Brit. J. Anæsth.*, 1953, **25**, 82.
† Organe, G., *Canad. Anæsth. Soc. J.*, 1956, **3**, 5; and Lawson, J. I. M., *Brit. J. Anæsth.*, 1958, **30**, 240.

Decamethonium Iodide—Clinical Uses, *continued.*

on muscles is seen 3–4 minutes after injection; 4–5 mg. will produce apnœa for 10 or 20 minutes, and, very shortly after the recommencement of respiration, the ventilation is back to normal again. For intubation it can be mixed in the same syringe with suxamethonium. For abdominal surgery repeat doses may be required in 10 to 40 minutes after the initial dose. If sufficient is given to enable an easy closure of the peritoneum, there is a good chance that the patient will be moving a reasonable tidal exchange at the end of the operation. It can be used to facilitate intubation when combined with thiopentone, but is not a good inhibitor of the cough reflex, making the drug unreliable in thoracic surgery. The patient may pass from apnœa to breathing disturbed by cough, very rapidly—a highly inconvenient occurrence. In other cases, prolonged apnœa has been reported. It is stated to have, possibly, some vagal inhibitory effect. It has been successfully used for Cæsarean section.

The drug should be confined to those operations expected to last less than ninety minutes and 10 mg. should not be exceeded. If the operation is nearing its end, suxamethonium 10–20 mg. may be given and repeated : otherwise it is better to finish the operation with gallamine 10 mg., repeated if required. A useful relaxant for short operations in patients who are thought to be better without neostigmine, e.g., those with asthma.

Patients who develop prolonged apnœa after repeated doses of decamethonium may be given edrophonium followed perhaps by neostigmine, if it is suspected that a dual block has developed and this has been electrically confirmed.

It has been shown that, as in the case of suxamethonium, second and subsequent doses of decamethonium may cause cardiac slowing.* Not often used now.

SUXAMETHONIUM HALIDES

History.—Prepared in 1906 by Hunt and Taveau.† In 1949 Bovet and his colleagues‡ and Castillo and de Beer§ described the paralysing action of the *bis*-choline esters of succinic acid, showing that they produced muscular paralysis of short duration and rapid onset. The first clinical use was reported from Sweden (von Dardel and Thesleff),‖ from Austria (Brücke and Mayerhofer),¶ and from Italy in 1951, and in the same year Scurr published his experiences with a small sample of suxamethonium iodide.**

Chemistry.—The active part of the molecule is the cation, formed by the succinic radicle with a quaternary ammonium group at each end of the molecular chain. If these end-groups contain three

---

* Williams, R. T., and Gain, E. A., *Canad. Anæsth. Soc. J.*, 1962, **9**, 263.
† Hunt, R., and Taveau, R. de M., *Brit. med. J.*, 1906, **2**, 1788.
‡ Bovet, D., and others, *R. C. Ist. sup. Sanit.*, 1949, **12**, 107.
§ Castillo, J. C., and de Beer, E. J., *J. Pharmacol.*, 1950, **99**, 458.
‖ von Dardel, O., and Thesleff, S., *Nord. Med.*, 1951, **46**, 1308; and *Acta chir. scand.*, 1952, **103**, 321 (translated in 'Classical File', *Survey of Anesthesiology*, 1967, **11**, 176).
¶ Brücke, H., Mayerhofer, O., and Hassfurther, M., *Wien. Klin. Wschr.*, 1951, **47**, 885.
** Scurr, C. F., *Brit. med. J.*, 1951, **2**, 831.

methyl groups (CH_3), the substance is a suxamethonium compound ; if two methyl and one ethyl (C_2H_5), then it is an ethonium compound—hence suxamethonium and suxethonium. The cation is combined with one of the halogens, chlorine, bromine, or iodine, which forms the anion, and this fact leads to the difference in the molecular weights in the different compounds. As the halide ion is inactive, the cation, identical in each case, is the active moiety and its weight should be regarded as the weight of active drug used. Thus 100 mg. of suxamethonium chloride contains 80 mg. of active cation, while 120 mg. of suxamethonium bromide contains 80 mg. of active cation. Solutions deteriorate in hot environments.

$$\begin{matrix} Br. & CH_3 \\ or\ Cl. & CH_3 \\ or\ I. & CH_3 \end{matrix} \Bigg\rangle \overset{+}{N}.CH_2.CH_2.O.\underset{\underset{O}{\|}}{C}.CH_2.CH_2.\underset{\underset{O}{\|}}{C}.O.CH_2.CH_2.\overset{+}{N} \Bigg\langle \begin{matrix} CH_3 & Br. \\ CH_3 & or\ Cl. \\ CH_3 & or\ I. \end{matrix}$$

The following compounds have been prepared :

SUXAMETHONIUM CHLORIDE, B.P. (Succinylcholine chloride, Scoline, diacetyline choline, succinyl-dicholine chloride, Anectine, Lysthenon, Paranoval, Brevidil M. (in solution), Quelicin, Tachycuraryl, Midarine).—Scoline is put up in 2-ml. ampoules each containing 100 mg. of the drug in 5 per cent solution, equal to 40 mg. of active cation per ml., and in 10-ml. bottles containing 500 mg. of the drug or 400 mg. of active cation.

SUXAMETHONIUM BROMIDE, B.P. (Succinylcholine bromide, Brevidil M. in powder).—Each ampoule contains 60 mg. of dry powder equivalent to 40 mg. of active cation.

SUXAMETHONIUM IODIDE (Celocurine, Succinylcholine iodide).

SUXETHONIUM BROMIDE (Brevidil E.).—Each ampoule contains 150 mg. of dry powder.

SUXETHONIUM IODIDE (I.S.362).—First prepared in Rome by Bovet in 1949.

Suxamethonium solution is unstable when mixed with alkalis, and loses activity when mixed with thiopentone. It should be stored in a refrigerator.

It is destroyed in the body by pseudocholinesterase (Bourne, J. G., Collier, H. O., and Somers, G. F., *Lancet*, 1952, **1**, 1225).

Pharmacology.—

MUSCULAR SYSTEM.—These compounds, like acetylcholine, act by depolarizing the motor end-plate. They prevent the access of acetylcholine to the cholinergic receptors of the end-plate. They also influence the muscle-fibres adjacent to the end-plate, making them unexcitable. This depolarization causes the fasciculation of muscle bundles, especially in the neck and limbs, seen after rapid injection of a small initial dose followed by larger subsequent doses, and an appreciable interval between the first and subsequent doses.* It causes post-operative aching especially

---

* Harrison, G. A., *Brit. J. Anæsth.*, 1965, **37**, 129.

Suxamethonium Halides—Pharmacology, *continued.*

in ambulant patients,* which may last for several days.†
Thiopentone has a protective effect against this pain and stiffness
but protection is of short duration and thiopentone should—in
this context—be given *immediately* before the relaxant. Unlike
acetylcholine, however, the drugs are not almost instantaneously
hydrolysed, so that depolarization remains and the muscle-fibres
become no longer electrically excitable and are in fact paralysed.

On rapid intravenous injection there is muscular twitching,
especially noticed in the head and neck. This very soon passes off
and gives place to muscular relaxation, which persists for three
to five minutes, and then in almost all cases rapidly disappears.
If a relatively large amount is given either intermittently or
by intravenous drip, a phase 2 block may occur. Generalized
hypertonicity of muscles has been reported following the
injection of this relaxant and may progress to hyperpyrexia and
even death.‡ The suxethonium compounds have an even more
evanescent action.

RESPONSE TO ELECTRICAL STIMULATION.—Following the application of a supramaximal current, in the absence of complete
myoneural block, there is a well-sustained response to successive stimuli following both a single (twitch) stimulus and fast
tetanic stimuli. The response to a single-twitch stimulus,
after a series of tetanic stimuli, is not increased, i.e., there
is no post-tetanic facilitation and no fade. These responses
are seen after the use of both mechanical nerve stimulators
and after electromyography.

CARDIOVASCULAR SYSTEM.—No effect on myocardium. While
the injection of a single dose of the drug does not greatly interfere
with the heart-rate and may increase it, repeated injections
cause slowing and even transient cardiac standstill, owing to
interference with cardiac excitation and conduction. It is
related to the size and not to the number of repeated injections
and is a muscarinic response. Atropine prevents these potentially
dangerous effects,§ and is usually advisable before the injection
of this relaxant. Suxamethonium may cause a rise in blood-
pressure, perhaps due to stimulation of autonomic ganglia, a
nicotinic response.

CENTRAL NERVOUS SYSTEM.—In clinical doses, none. The
drug may show muscarinic effects.

ALIMENTARY SYSTEM.—There may be an increase in salivary
and gastric secretions, due to muscarinic effects, especially if
atropine is not used. In liver deficiency, a reduced pseudocholinesterase value may be a cause of prolongation of effect of
suxamethonium and of resistance to the non-depolarizing
relaxants. An increase in intragastric pressure of more than
20 mm. H_2O has been reported, associated with the fasciculations

* Churchill-Davidson, H. C., *Brit. med. J.*, 1954, **1**, 74.
† Craig, H. J. L., *Brit. J. Anæsth.*, 1964, **36**, 612.
‡ Relton, J. E. S., *Canad. Anæsth. Soc. J.*, 1967, **19**, 22; and Hall, L. W., and others, *Brit. med. J.*, 1966, **2**, 1305.
§ Lupprian, K. G., and Churchill-Davidson, H. C., *Brit. med. J.*, 1960, **2**, 1774.

following injection.* The cricopharyngeal sphincter loses its tone.†

PLACENTAL BARRIER.—The drug in a dosage of less than 500 mg. does not reach the fœtal circulation so is excellent for operative obstetrics and Cæsarean section. Increase in uterine tone has been reported, with consequent harm to the fœtus from interference with placental blood-flow.‡

HISTAMINE RELEASE.—Less than with tubocurarine. True anaphylaxis has been reported following its intravenous injection§ with signs and symptoms of tachycardia, bronchospasm, hypotension, pharyngeal and facial œdema, and a positive passive transfer (Prauznitz-Küstner) reaction.

SERUM POTASSIUM.—Potassium is released from muscle tissue, following injection of suxamethonium, and this raises the serum potassium level. This may give rise to arrhythmia.‖

EFFECT ON INTRA-OCULAR PRESSURE.—An intubation dose raises the pressure an average of 7 mm. Hg but this soon returns to normal and need not contra-indicate the use of the drug in intra-ocular surgery. The first dose should not, however, be injected during the operation while the eye is open.¶ The cause of this rise is uncertain and may be due to vascular changes within the eyeball. Temporary enophthalmos may follow intravenous injection.** Severe glaucoma may contra-indicate the use of the drug.

HYDROLYSIS AND EXCRETION.—

1. IN THE NORMAL PATIENT.—Suxamethonium is hydrolysed into choline and succinic acid. This occurs in two stages. In the first stage, plasma or pseudocholinesterase breaks down suxamethonium (or succinyldicholine) into succinyl monocholine quite rapidly. True cholinesterase from the red cells plays no part in this. In the second stage succinyl monocholine is converted into choline and succinic acid six times more slowly. As succinyl monocholine is itself a depolarizing relaxant (with one-twentieth the potency of the dicholine), large amounts of it can cause a prolonged apnœa after suxamethonium has been given, but only if the dose is 1 g. or more. Both true and pseudocholinesterase take part in this second hydrolysis. Some succinyl monocholine as also some suxamethonium is excreted in the urine.

In addition, alkaline hydrolysis of suxamethonium (in the absence of respiratory or metabolic acidosis) takes place in the plasma in the complete absence of pseudocholinesterase, but only to the extent of 5 per cent per hour.

2. IN THE ABNORMAL PATIENT.—It has been stated that about one in every three thousand of the population carries an abnormal

* Andersen, N., *Brit. J. Anæsth.*, 1962, **34**, 363.
† Davies, D. D., *Ibid.*, 1963, **35**, 219.
‡ Felton, D. J. C., and Goddard, B. A., *Lancet*, 1966, **1**, 852.
§ Jerums, G., and others, *Brit. J. Anæsth.*, 1967, **39**, 73.
‖ List, W. F., *Ibid.*, 1967, **39**, 480.
¶ Dillon. J. B., and others, *Anesthesiology*, 1957, **18**, 44.
** Björk, A., and others, *Acta anæsth. scand.*, 1957, **1**. 41.

Suxamethonium Halides—Pharmacology, *continued.*

pseudocholinesterase gene which is liable to cause prolonged apnœa if normal doses of suxamethonium are injected.[*] Lehmann recommends that in patients receiving suxamethonium for the first time the dose should be restricted to 30 mg. This will not prevent prolonged apnœa but will restrict it to a relatively safe degree. The normal pseudocholinesterase level (Warburg) is 60–120 units.

3. IN DISEASE.—An acquired deficiency of pseudocholinesterase may exist in very ill patients, in those under treatment for malignant disease with AB 132, in malnutrition, in those with dehydration and electrolytic imbalance, and in those suffering from anæmia, parenchymatous liver disease, obstructive jaundice, carcinomatosis, organophosphorus poisoning, and therapeutic radiation. A low serum albumin concentration (in the absence of albuminuria), and a very high SGOT or SGPT level in the serum indicating possible liver damage, call for great care in the use of suxamethonium.

Cholinesterase.—Cholinesterases are enzymes which catalyse the hydrolysis of choline esters with the production of choline and the corresponding acid.

1. True cholinesterase : i.e., specific cholinesterase, acetylcholinesterase, red-cell cholinesterase. (Described in man by Vahlquist, B., *Skand. Arch. Physiol.*, 1935, **72**, 133.) It is found not only in red cells but also in motor and sensory nerves, sympathetic and parasympathetic nerves, brain, and muscle. Acetylcholinesterase is found in red cells and at cholinergic synapses and myoneural junctions—where it hydrolyses acetylcholine.

2. Pseudocholinesterase (acylcholine acylhydrolase (A.C.A.H.)—distinguished from the above by Allen, G. A., and Hawes, R. C., *J. Biol. Chem.*, 1940, **133**, 375): i.e., non-specific cholinesterase, plasma or serum cholinesterase. Pseudocholinesterase has little effect on acetylcholine at physiological concentrations but will hydrolyse other compounds. Both enzymes are inhibited by neostigmine, the anticholinesterase, but pseudochlinesterase is not inhibited by substrate excess. Pseudocholinesterase is a mucoprotein formed in the liver and normally the serum contains 60–120 units. A level less than 25 is low. There is a high value in early childhood, and as age advances it gets less. Its amount is one measure of hepatic function. A unit of pseudocholinesterase is defined as the amount of enzyme which will produce 1 microlitre of CO_2 by hydrolysis of acetylcholine in a bicarbonate buffer; or 1 unit of enzyme activity is defined as that which hydrolyses 1 micromole of acetylcholine per minute per ml. of serum at 37° C.[†] A stable enzyme, well preserved in freeze-dried plasma.

Low pseudocholinesterase levels may occur: (1) After therapeutic radiation.[‡] (2) After contamination with organic phosphorus

[*] Lehmann, L. H., *Brit. med. J.*, 1961, **2**, 705.
[†] Rose, L., Davies, D. A., and Lehmann, H., *Lancet*, 1965, **2**, 563.
[‡] Belfrage, P., and Schildt, B., *Acta anæsth. scand.*, 1927, **11**, 65.

insecticides. (3) In hyperpyrexia. (4) In cardiac failure. (5) In uræmia (albuminuria has no effect). (6) In liver disease. (7) In malnutrition. (8) In severe anæmia. (9) In very ill and handicapped patients. (10) Following treatment of carcinoma with cyclophosphamide* or of glaucoma with ecothiopate iodide (phosphorline iodide) eyedrops.† (11) In the second half of pregnancy, labour, and the early post-partum days.‡ (12) As a familial abnormality in about 1–3000 of the population. Procainamide and quinidine both potentiate the neuromuscular blocking effect of suxamethonium.§

High pseudocholinesterase levels occur: (1) In obesity. (2) In toxic goitre. (3) In nephrosis. (4) In depressed states with anxiety. (5) In psoriasis. (6) In alcoholism.

Two varieties of pseudocholinesterase apparently exist, the common or normal type and the rare abnormal type.‖ The common variety is able to hydrolyse suxamethonium at concentrations which are impossible for the rare variety. Ordinary plasma pseudocholinesterase estimations will not differentiate between the common and the rare varieties of the enzyme in the blood-stream, but the differentiation can be carried out by estimation of the dibucaine (i.e., cinchocaine or nupercaine) number.¶ This is the percentage inhibition of the enzyme by a 10^{-5} molar concentrate of cinchocaine (U.S. dibucaine) and is known as the dibucaine number or D.N. of the serum. The abnormal enzyme, which is cinchocaine-resistant, occurs in about 1–3000 of the population, the D.N. is about 20 per cent, and the reaction is prolonged. This small group is homozygous and its serum contains only abnormal enzyme. In 97 per cent of the population the average D.N. is about 80 per cent and the reaction to suxamethonium is normal, while in the remaining 3 per cent it is about 62 per cent. They synthesize equal amounts of normal and abnormal enzyme and are not unusually sensitive to the relaxant. There is a group of patients with congenital absence of all types of pseudocholinesterase. Other small groups with 'silent' genes have been postulated, while fluoride has been employed as an enzyme inhibitor.**

If otherwise unexplained apnœa lasts for more than 15 minutes after a reasonable dose of suxamethonium, the serum of the patient (and also that of his blood relatives) should be examined for abnormal pseudocholinesterase. If this is present, the individuals concerned should be informed about it and instructed to pass on the information in the event of subsequent anæsthetics being necessary.

* Mone, J. G., and Mathe, W. E., *Anæsthesia*, 1967, **22**, 55.
† McGavi, D. D. M., *Lancet*, 1965, **2**, 272.
‡ Shnider, S. M., *Anesthesiology*, 1965, **26**, 335; and Robertson, G. S., *Brit. J. Anæsth.*, 1966, **38**, 361.
§ Cuthbert, M. F., *Ibid.*, 1966, **38**, 775.
‖ Kalow, W., and Davies, R. O., *Biochem. Pharmacol.*, 1958, **1**, 183.
¶ Kalow, W., and Genest, K., *Canad. J. Biochem. Physiol.*, 1957, **35**, 339.
** Harris, H., and Whittaker, M., *Nature, Lond.*, 1961 **191**, 496.

Cholinesterase, *continued.*

A test paper (acholest) can be used to estimate the pseudo cholinesterase level of the serum, but it will not differentiate the typical from the atypical enzyme.*

Pharmacogenetics of Pseudocholinesterase.†—A population may contain : (1) Normal homozygotes with two normal genes and a D.N. of 75–80 ; (2) Heterozygotes with a normal and an abnormal gene and a D.N. of 50–65 ; (3) Abnormal homozygotes with two abnormal genes and a D.N. of 16–25. The molecular structure and hence the pharmacological activity, of pseudocholinesterase is determined by a pair of non-dominant, allelomorphic, autosomal genes.

The abnormal homozygotes are likely to cause trouble clinically as in addition to an abnormal type of enzyme there is often a decrease in the total amount of enzyme so that they are unusually sensitive to suxamethonium. The persistence of the drug in the blood-stream due to delayed hydrolysis may well result not only in prolongation of the block but in its change from a depolarizing to a dual block. (*See also* Vickers, M. D., *Brit. J. Anæsth.*, 1963, **35**, 1528.)

There are four allelic genes which control the inheritance of pseudo cholinesterase. (For terminology *see* Mone, J. G., and Mathie, W. E., *Anæsthesia*, 1967, **22**, 55; and Kalow, W., 'Pharmaco genics and Anæsthesia—a Review', *Anesthesiology*, 1964, **25**, 377.

Foldes and his colleagues (*Science*, 1953, **117**, 383) have demonstrated substrate competition for pseudocholinesterase between esters of benzoic acid (and lignocaine) and suxamethonium. The use of procaine in conjunction with suxamethonium may cause delayed hydrolysis of the latter, as both drugs appear to be hydrolysed by pseudocholinesterase.

Clinical Uses of Suxamethonium Halides.—Atropine is often given before suxamethonium to control any muscarinic effects produced. While suxamethonium is usually given by intravenous injection preferably in weak solution—1 per cent or less to minimize muscular fasciculations—it can be injected intramuscularly in dose of 2 mg. per kg., or with the addition of hyalase in a dose of 1 mg. per kg. This may be useful in children before intubation; in patients with poor veins and as a deliberate route of administration to smooth the transition from apnœa to spontaneous respiration and reduce the incidence of laryngeal spasm, cough, etc.

A single intravenous dose of 50 mg. of suxamethonium chloride lasts from two to four minutes ; apnœa lasting longer than ten minutes after such a dose in an adequately oxygenated patient is evidence of abnormal response.

FOR INTUBATION.—As the muscular twitches are quickly produced and painful, the patient should first be put to sleep and then given the relaxant. Suitable dose is 24–80 mg. of

---

* Churchill-Davidson, H. C., and Griffiths, W. J., *Brit. med. J.*, 1961, **2**, 994; and Wang R. L. H., and Henschel, E. O., *Curr. Res. Anesth.*, 1967, **46**, 281.
† Liddell, J., *Proc. R. Soc. Med.*, 1968, **61**, 168; and Bush, G. H., *Ibid.*, 1968, **61**, 171.

active cation, e.g., 30–100 mg. of suxamethonium chloride. To overcome acute laryngeal spasm, 50 mg. of suxamethonium should be injected followed by rapid inflation or intubation.

FOR BRONCHOSCOPY.—Serial doses are given as required under general anæsthesia, e.g., by thiopentone : the first before the introduction of the endoscope ; subsequent ones as required. Oxygen should be given concurrently either down the side-tube of the bronchoscope or via a long and narrow endotracheal catheter at a flow-rate of at least 5 l. per min.

FOR ORTHOPÆDIC MANIPULATIONS.—A moderate dose of thiopentone, followed by 50 mg. of suxamethonium, will result in a state of profound relaxation for a short period.

FOR ABDOMINAL CLOSURE.—Doses can be given serially during the suture of the peritoneum with the full expectation that normal breathing will have returned as the skin stitches are completed. Should the patient in such a case still be partly curarized from gallamine or tubocurarine used during the operation to maintain relaxation, it is unwise to give neostigmine at the end of the operation to completely overcome the effects of the former drugs, neostigmine being a pseudocholinesterase inhibitor and likely to delay hydrolysis of suxamethonium.

FOR ANÆSTHESIA DURING DRESSING OF BURNS.—There is evidence (Bush, G. H., and others, *Brit. med. J.*, 1962, **2**, 1081, and Finer, B. L., and Nylen, B. O., *Ibid.*, 1959, **1**, 624) that cardiac arrest due to increased vagal tone is a definite risk during induction of anæsthesia with suxamethonium in patients burnt 2–7 weeks previously. This may be preventable by atropine intravenously.

The neonate, up to 6 weeks of age, is resistant to the relaxant but may early develop a phase 2 block and so may be better managed by very small doses of non-depolarizing agents.

FOR ELECTROCONVULSIVE THERAPY (*see* p. 491).

The *continuous suxamethonium drip* is used as a controllable and rapid method of maintaining relaxation of different degrees during abdominal and other surgical procedures. Various strengths have been described, a popular one containing 10 ml. (500 mg.) of suxamethonium chloride in 500 ml. of saline, giving a dilution of 0·1 per cent. If this amount of drug is added to 400 ml. of saline then the strength is 0·1 per cent of active cation.

The solution is run in from a standard drip set at a rate of 30 drops per minute until muscle weakness develops. No twitching is seen at this slow rate, and undue sensitivity to the drug is quickly noticed. Thiopentone is then injected (0·25–0·5 g.) and the drip speeded up to 60 drops a minute. If ventilation fails it is assisted, and when the jaw is fully relaxed, the laryngoscope is used in the ordinary way. During mainten-ance of anæsthesia it is desirable, in the view of some workers,* to maintain some respiratory movements, otherwise it is difficult to ascertain if the patient is receiving too much drug. Many other workers abolish respiration and allow it to return

---

* Foldes, F. F., *Muscle Relaxants in Anesthesiology*, 1957, 119. Springfield, Ill. : Thomas.

Clinical Uses of Suxamethonium Halides, *continued.*

occasionally during the operation, but this may result in intermittent relaxation. Assisted or controlled breathing must of course be carried out. The amount used varies between 4 and 10 mg. of the cation per minute. When the peritoneum is sutured, the drip may be stopped. Average rate of drip, 30 to 60 drops a minute or 150 to 400 ml. each hour. If after a prolonged suxamethonium drip the patient is requiring increasing amounts of drug, i.e., is probably developing a dual block, it may be better to give a small dose of a non-depolarizing relaxant to maintain block and to avoid accumulation of succinyl monocholine. Such small doses last a long time and can be reversed by neostigmine.

A disadvantage of the suxamethonium drip is that although respiration may return easily enough at the end of the operation it may be somewhat depressed in volume. Some workers prefer serial injections given at carefully judged intervals to the continuous drip.

Muscle Pains after Suxamethonium.—The bromide and the chloride of the active cation are equally guilty of causing pain and there is no difference in the incidence of pains following suxamethonium and suxethonium halides. A preliminary injection of tubocurarine 3–5 mg.[*] or of gallamine 5–20 mg.[†] reduces the incidence but may contribute to post-operative apnœa. Lignocaine has been suggested for this purpose too. After the injection of thiopentone, lignocaine 2–6 mg. per kg. (say 300 mg.) is injected and in 3 minutes the relaxant follows.[‡] This also prolongs the period of apnœa.[§] There appears to be no direct relationship between the fasciculations and actual muscle pains. Pains more frequent in women and middle-aged patients than in those at the extremes of age and in men. The longer the interval between the injection of an intravenous barbiturate and the suxamethonium, the more intense the post-operative pains. Pains may be delayed until the third or fourth post-operative day.[||]

It is suggested that the muscle-cell injury—as shown by the creatinine phosphokinase level—is produced by suxamethonium given intermittently, especially if the patient is receiving halothane.[¶] Pain is less frequent in patients who are muscularly 'fit' than in the 'unfit'[**] and when the injection is given slowly.

The Potentiation of Suxamethonium by the Use of Extenders.— Duration of effect increased by a factor of 2 with neostigmine, by a factor of 3–4 with tacrine, and by a factor of 8–10 by hexafluorenium.

[*] Morris, D. D. B., and Dunn, C. H., *Canad. Anæsth. Soc. J.*, 1957, **1**, 383.
[†] Glauber, D., *Brit. J. Anæsth.*, 1966, **38**, 541.
[‡] Wikinski, R., and others, *Anesthesiology*, 1965, **26**, 3.
[§] Usubiaga, J. E., and others, *Curr. Res. Anesth.*, 1967, **47**, 225.
[||] Burtles, R., and Tunstall, M. E., *Brit. J. Anæsth.*, 1961, **33**, 24 ; and Burtles, R., *Ibid.*, 1961, **33**, 147.
[¶] Tammisto, T., and others, *Brit. J. Anæsth.*, 1966, **38**, 510.
[**] Newman, P. J. F., and Louden, J. M., *Ibid.*, 1966, **38**, 533.

1. By *tacrine hydrochloride* B.P.C. (Romotal, T.H.A., tetrahydro-aminacrine).—Chemically this is 5-amino-1,2,3,4,-tetrahydro-acridine, and it was introduced into clinical medicine in 1949 by Shaw and Bentley, of Melbourne.* Peripherally it acts as an anticholinesterase to reverse the myoneural blocking effects of tubocurarine, but does not perform this function efficiently in man. It has also been employed to potentiate and prolong the block produced by suxamethonium.† If 50 mg. of suxa-methonium are injected into the unconscious patient and the effect on respiration noted, a similar dose can be given followed immediately by 10 mg. of tacrine. This will prolong the effect of the second and subsequent doses of the relaxant about three times so that the development of a dual block from excess suxamethonium is rendered less likely and succinyl monocholine will not build up in the blood-stream. Relaxation is more continuous, and the incidence of muscle pains reduced.‡ Its use should be preceded by atropine to prevent bradycardia. Dual block has, however, been reported to occur frequently and can be demonstrated by post-tetanic facilitation in response to electrical stimulation of the ulnar nerve at the wrist.§

The drug also has a stimulant effect on both the cortex and the medulla and acts as a partial antagonist to morphine (not very efficiently) (*see* p. 445).

2. By *hexafluorenium* (Mylaxen).—This is a *bis-quaternary* ammo-nium compound which was synthesized by Cavallito in 1954.‖ On injection it potentiates and prolongs the neuromuscular blocking effect of suxamethonium and suxethonium halides by inhibiting the activity of plasma cholinesterase. In addition, it has a mild non-depolarizing neuromuscular effect which poten-tiates the action of ether and tubocurarine and antagonizes that of decamethonium.¶ It also prevents the muscular twitching seen after the injection of suxamethonium. Its muscarinic effects, unlike those of neostigmine, are not marked, while tachycardia, reversible with propranolol, has been reported.** The dose suggested is 0·5 mg. per kg., followed shortly by suxamethonium either as a drip infusion or as a single-shot injection—anæsthesia having been induced by thiopentone. This results in a five- to sevenfold decrease in the amount of suxamethonium required for a given operation.†† Thus, following the dose of hexa-fluorenium, the intravenous injection of 0·2 mg. per kg. of suxamethonium will give apnœa and good muscular relaxation for about 20 minutes. The block can be continued by injection of subsequent doses of 0·15 mg. per kg. of suxamethonium for 1–1½ hours.

* Shaw, F. H., and Bentley, G. A., *Med. J. Aust.*, 1949, **2**, 868.
† Gordh, T., and Wahlin, A., *Acta anæsth. scand.*, 1961, **5**, 55 ; and Barrow, M. E. H., and Smethurst, J. R., *Brit. J. Anæsth.*, 1963, **35**, 465.
‡ Smart, J. F., *Anæsthesia*, 1964, **19**, 524.
§ Macdonald, D. J. F., *Brit. J. Anæsth.*, 1967, **39**, 629.
‖ Cavallito, C. J., and others, *Anesthesiology*, 1956, **17**, 547.
¶ Torda, T. A. G., Foldes, F. F., and others, *Ibid.*, 1967, **28**, 1010.
** Van Hemert, V. R., and Pearce, C., *Brit. J. Anæsth.*, 1965, **37**, 585.
†† Foldes, F. F., and others, *Anesthesiology*, 1960, **21**, 50.

Potentiation of Suxamethonium, *continued*.

It has been stated that patients taking trifluoperizine (stelazine) are resistant to the action of suxamethonium. Doses of 1–2 mg. intramuscularly have caused a reversal of apnœa caused by the relaxant.* Propanidid potentiates depolarizing relaxants.†

Prolonged Apnœa following the Use of Muscle Relaxants.—This has occurred and has proved fatal following the use of non-depolarizing relaxants,‡ depolarizing relaxants, and the combination of the two. (It has also been seen after intra- and extra-dural blocks, and in medical patients with chronic hypercapnia who have been given a high oxygen atmosphere to breathe.) It must always be treated in the first place by I.P.P.V.

1. PROLONGED APNŒA AFTER THE USE OF NON-DEPOLARIZING RELAXANTS.§—Evidence is accumulating that the non-depolarizing relaxants may have abnormal effects if *the potassium metabolism is disordered* as in dehydration and electrolyte depletion. One of the abnormal effects may be a central depressant action on the medullary centres leading to respiratory and circulatory failure. It may be associated with an initial resistance to the relaxant—depolarizing or non-depolarizing. Non-depolarizing relaxants should be used most carefully in ill and handicapped patients and in those with electrolyte imbalance and intracellular potassium depletion, e.g., in dehydration, starvation, vomiting, diarrhœa, metabolic disturbances, acidosis, diabetic coma, and after the use of cortisone (*see* p. 495). The intravenous infusion of 0·3 per cent potassium chloride (which contains 40 mEq. per l.), 100–200 ml., may be helpful.‖ This should be controlled by E.C.G. which, with potassium excess, will show tall, peaked T-waves, going on to ventricular fibrillation. On the other hand, 500 ml. during 1 hour is unlikely to be dangerous unless renal excretion is seriously impaired. A normal blood potassium level (3·7–5·6 mEq. per l.) does not exclude a reduced intracellular potassium content, especially when dehydration is present. *Hyponatræmia* may prolong apnœa and demands infusion of 5 per cent sodium chloride solution. If reasonable doses of neostigmine, i.e., up to 5 mg., fail to restore normal breathing 30–60 mg. of ephedrine should be injected intramuscularly. This diminishes the rate of adrenaline destruction, thereby potentiating neostigmine (adrenaline has of course an anti-curarizing action) and also helps to maintain the high potassium level of the muscle-fibres. In addition, ephedrine helps to maintain the blood-pressure.¶

2. PROLONGED APNŒA AFTER THE USE OF DEPOLARIZING RELAXANTS.—After a single dose of suxamethonium the commonest causes are :—

* Ruddell, J. Shegog, *Lancet*, 1963, **1**, 889.
† Doenicke, A., and others, *Brit. J. Anæsth.*, 1968, **40**, 415.
‡ Hunter, A. R., *Brit. med. J.*, 1956, **2**, 919.
§ Foster, P. A., *Brit. J. Anæsth.*, 1956, **28**, 488.
‖ Foldes, F. F., *Clin. Pharmac. Therap.*, 1960, **1**, 345.
¶ Burn, J. H., *Brit. J. Anæsth.* 1957, **29**, 242.

a. Atypical pseudocholinesterase. A rapid screening test is described by Swift and La Du.* Homozygotes for the atypical gene show this.

b. Dehydration and electrolyte imbalance leading to the development of dual block at a very early stage.

c. A low serum pseudocholinesterase level. There is no relationship between the blood-enzyme level and the duration of apnœa in this acquired condition.†

Other factors are :—

a. An over-dosage with the relaxant drug, i.e., more than 1 g. in an infusion. It is interesting to remember in this connexion that in order to prevent over-dosage of suxamethonium, Foldes‡ advises that with a continuous drip, apnœa should never be allowed to occur and assisted rather than controlled respiration is employed.

b. A low pseudocholinesterase level in the blood (i.e., less than 25 units, Lehmann). This seldom causes prolonged apnœa if 50 mg. is not exceeded, a dose adequate for most patients requiring a single injection, e.g., for intubation or E.C.T.† It is unlikely to be the cause of apnœa prolonged beyond 20–30 minutes, and if the pseudocholinesterase level is more than 25 units. A low pseudocholinesterase level may occur in liver disease, severe anæmia, malnutrition, starvation, electrolyte imbalance, and contamination with those organic phosphorus insecticides which are pseudocholinesterase inhibitors and include hexaethyl tetraphosphate (HETP) ; tetraethyl pyrophosphate (TEPP) ; parathion ; pestox 3 ; isopestox ; and AB 132 used in the chemotherapy of cancer. The level may be reduced following the regular ingestion of some contraceptive pills,§ while promazine has also been blamed for causing prolonged apnœa.‖ Apnœa due to a low pseudocholinesterase value may be reversed by a blood transfusion as even stored blood contains 30 units of pseudocholinesterase in each ml. and retains 80 per cent of its pseudocholinesterase activity after storage for 25 days at 6° C. One pint of fresh blood restores the serum pseudocholinesterase level by 10 units per ml.; 1 pint of stored blood restores it by 5 units per ml. Reconstituted plasma is also useful as it contains 36–40 units per ml.

c. An excessive formation of succinyl monocholine. In 1952 Whittaker and Wijesundera¶ pointed out that the hydrolysis of succinylcholine takes place in two stages, succinyl monocholine being the intermediate product. This has between $\frac{1}{20}$ and $\frac{1}{50}$ the relaxing effect of the parent compound,** but

* Swift, M. R., and La Du, B. N., *Lancet*, 1966, **1**, 513.
† Hunter, A. R., *Anæsthesia*, 1966, **21**, 337.
‡ Foldes, F. F., *Muscle Relaxants in Anesthesiology*, 1957. Springfield, Ill. : Thomas.
§ Robertson, G. S., *Lancet*, 1967, **1**, 1232.
‖ Regan, A. G., and Aldrete, J. A., *Curr. Res. Anesth.*, 1967, **46**, 315.
¶ Whittaker, J. P., and Wijesundera, S., *Biochem. J.*, 1952, **52**, 475.
** Lehmann, H., and Silk, E., *Brit. med. J.*, 1953, **1**, 767.

Prolonged Apnœa after Muscle Relaxants, *continued.*

as it is hydrolysed rather slowly by both true and pseudo-cholinesterase, it may accumulate in the blood-stream, but only if relatively large amounts of suxamethonium (1·5–2 g.) have been used, e.g., as a drip infusion.

d. A dual block, a phenomenon described by Zaimis[*] in 1953. According to this theory, the end-plate can, under certain circumstances, react in such a way that the initial depolarizing block gives way to a non-depolarizing block, which is antagonized by such anticholinesterase agents as edrophonium and neostigmine. Dual block is very rarely seen after single doses of either decamethonium or suxamethonium but may be the cause of confusion after repeated doses, e.g., the suxamethonium drip or multiple doses of decamethonium. Depolarizing block will usually, but not always, turn eventually to non-depolarizing block. Dual block appears to occur more readily when suxamethonium is given intermittently than when it is infused at a constant rate.[†]

e. The myoneural blocking effect of the normal product of suxamethonium breakdown, choline, if large amounts of suxamethonium, e.g., 400–500 mg., have been injected.[‡]

Other Causes of Prolonged Apnœa.—

1. Central depression of the respiratory centre by morphine or its congeners; thiopentone; cyclopropane; or other volatile anæsthetics.

2. Hypocapnia: in this case respiration will recommence if the blood carbon dioxide level is allowed to rise. Provided the respiratory centre is not depressed and the mucosa of the upper respiratory tract is not analgesic, spontaneous respiration will usually start when the relaxant is reversed, even in the presence of a low arterial Pco_2,[§] if the carina or bronchi are stimulated.

3. Hypercapnia: prolonged hypoventilation or deficient carbon dioxide elimination from the anæsthetic circuit can poison the respiratory centre and cause apnœa. It can sometimes be overcome by vigorous hyperventilation using either fresh soda-lime or a non-rebreathing circuit.

4. Depression of the Hering-Breuer mechanism during controlled respiration. This will usually yield to more gentle inflation together with the addition of a little carbon dioxide for short periods.

5. Reflex laryngeal apnœa. Due to the presence of an endotracheal tube. Removal of the tube leads to restoration of spontaneous respiration.

6. Moribundity (Paton).[‖] There are some gravely ill patients who breathe again only with difficulty once they become apnœic. In such patients it may be wise not to abolish voluntary respiration at all.

[*] Zaimis, E., *J. Physiol.*, 1953, **122**, 238.
[†] White, D. C., *Brit. J. Anæsth.*, 1963, **35**, 305.
[‡] Burn, J. H., *Ibid.*, 1957, **29**, 242.
[§] Utting, J. E., and Gray, T. C., *Ibid.*, 1962, **34**, 785.
[‖] Paton, W. D. M., *Anæsthesia*, 1958, **13**, 253.

7. Metabolic acidosis can cause a clinical picture similar to that of myoneural block.*
   (*See also* Utting, J., *Brit. J. Anæsth.*, 1963, **35**, 521.)

Diagnosis of the Cause of Prolonged Apnœa.—
1. Electrical stimulation of a peripheral nerve to differentiate central depression from neuromuscular block (for apparatus *see* Christie, T. H., and Churchill-Davidson, H. C., *Lancet*, 1958, **1**, 776).
2. Examination of an arterial blood specimen—taken without air contact—to assess Pco_2 and pseudocholinesterase level.
3. Edrophonium, to exclude dual block once shallow respiration has commenced. (*See also* Paton, W. D., *Anæsthesia*, 1958, **13**, 253.)

Differential Diagnosis between Hypopnœa due to Central Depression and that due to Peripheral Paralysis.†—
a. CENTRAL DEPRESSION.—Breathing slow, reasonably deep. No tracheal tug ; no pause at end of inspiration.
b. PERIPHERAL PARALYSIS (Myoneural Block).—Breathing jerky, shallow, and of normal rate. Pause after inspiration and again after expiration (Morton's rectangular breathing). Tracheal tug.
Electrical stimulation of the ulnar nerve, always supposing that myoneural block is not complete, should settle any doubt.

Treatment of Prolonged Apnœa.—
1. Patiently maintain intermittent positive-pressure ventilation with about 8 litres per minute of nitrous oxide and oxygen (at least 30 per cent), carefully avoiding both over- and under-ventilation.
2. Use nerve stimulator to determine whether apnœa is central or peripheral in origin, and, if possible, whether it is of the depolarizing or the non-depolarizing type.
3. Treat non-depolarizing block with neostigmine and atropine (*see above*).
4. Treat depolarizing (or unknown type of) block by administration of 400–800 ml. of triple strength plasma or blood, as rapidly as the circulation will allow, to increase pseudocholinesterase level of the plasma.
5. When some spontaneous respiration has started, and not before, give 10 mg. of edrophonium, and if this causes improvement it can be followed by atropine and neostigmine very carefully in repeated small doses. Cases of dual block which are not reversed by neostigmine have been reported.

Use of Relaxants in Electroconvulsive Therapy (Electroplexy).—
Convulsions were first used in psychiatry in 1934 by Meduna; Cerletti and Bini inducing them electrically in 1938; Bennett used curare in 1940‡ and Holmberg and Thesleff used suxamethonium in 1951.§
The stomach and bladder must be empty and the patient reassured. Thiopentone is given intravenously, the dose varying from

---

* Brooks, D. K., and Feldman, S. A., *Anæsthesia*, 1962, **17**, 161.
† Bourne, J. G., *Brit. J. Anæsth.*, 1953, **25**, 116.
‡ Bennett, A. E., *J. Amer. med. Ass.*, 1940, **114**, 322.
§ Holmberg, A. G., and Thesleff, S., *Nord. med.*, 1951, **46**, 1567.

Use of Relaxants in Electroconvulsive Therapy, *continued*.

o·2 to o·4 g. Most workers give atropine, o·8 mg., routinely ; others avoid it. The authors prefer to give it combined with the thiopentone. Suxamethonium chloride 40–50 mg. in 1 per cent solution (to reduce the incidence of post-operative muscular pain) is now injected. When the twitching ceases and the chest has been inflated two or three times with oxygen, the patient is ready for the attention of the psychiatrist. After the convulsion, it is usually necessary to inflate the lungs with oxygen or air. Damage to the teeth and lips is a real danger and is likely to occur during the passage of the current rather than during the modified convulsion. Inflation of the chest with oxygen during the convulsion prolongs it. After the current is passed, a modified convulsion is likely if: (1) There is a pilomotor reaction.[*] (2) The pupil fails to contract when inspected. When teeth are present, they should be separated by firm rubber tubing or other suitable bite block.

There is evidence that patients suffering from depression with anxiety have an abnormally high pseudocholinesterase level.[†]

Modifications of this technique include giving 50 mg. of chlorpromazine by mouth two hours before the procedure as a tranquilliser (and a venous dilator !) ; substituting gallamine 30–60 mg. for suxamethonium, with or without the addition of neostigmine after the convulsion; and substituting propanidid for thiopentone, injecting it with atropine and suxamethonium in the same syringe.[‡] Psychiatrists vary in the amount of paralysis they require and are like surgeons in this respect! Some believe that a certain amount of healthy jerking is beneficial to their patients, and so smaller doses of relaxants (and greater risk of fractures) will be the order of the day.

As both the systolic and diastolic blood-pressures and the heart-rate rise and as the adrenaline and noradrenaline levels in the blood are increased during the treatment, patients with hypertension or cardiac hypertrophy will need careful assessment before being subjected to this heroic but very effective form of treatment. The omission of atropine may result in a period of asystole for 2 or 3 seconds.[§]

Use of Relaxants in the Treatment of Tetanus.—Mild cases require only careful nursing and sedation. All of the commonly used relaxants have been used to control the spasms of tetanus at one time or another and so has chlorpromazine.[‖]

Mephenesin given into the stomach by Ryle's tube, because it is a local analgesic of the pharynx, has been successfully used in mild cases. In the more severe ones the initial dose should be 1 g. given intravenously, well diluted, followed by one or two

---

* Edridge, A., *Proc. R. Soc. Med.*, 1952, **45**, 869; and Thomas, E., and others, *Brit. med. J.*, 1953, **2**, 97.
† Rose, L., Davies, D. A., and Lehmann, H., *Lancet*, 1965, **2**, 563.
‡ Jackson, P. W., and Woodhead, Z., *Anæsthesia*, 1967, **22**, 704.
§ Graventstein, J. S., and others, *Brit. J. Anæsth.*, 1965, **37**, 833.
‖ Bodman, R. I., Morton, H. J. V., and Thomas, E. T., *Lancet*, 1955, **2**, 230 ; and Adrian, J., and Kerr, M., *Sth. med. J.* (*B'ham, Ala.*), 1955, **48**, 858.

ounces of the elixir into the stomach, and repeated as may be necessary. The drug can be given also intramuscularly.

Chlorpromazine is useful in mild cases. It depresses basal ganglia and internuncial neurons of the cord. It will control mild convulsions without producing deep unconsciousness or respiratory depression. Dosage 100–150 mg. intramuscularly four- to six-hourly.* When reasonable doses of chlorpromazine fail to control convulsions, the use of muscle relaxants and I.P.P.V. must be considered.

In severe convulsive tetanus, the plan should be to induce flaccid paralysis and maintain artificial respiration (*see* Chapter XXXV). (*See* articles by Shackleton, P., *Lancet*, 1954, **2**, 155; Honey, G. E., Dwyer, B. E., Smith, A. C., and Spalding, J. M. K., *Brit. med. J.*, 1954, **2**, 442; Galloway, W. H., and Wilson, H. Bruce, *Anæsthesia*, 1955, **10**, 303; Woolmer, R., *Brit. med. Bull.*, 1958, **14**, 1, 54; Robinson, J. S., *Brit. J. Anæsth.*, 1963, **35**, 570.)

Use of Different Relaxants in the Same Patient.—The effects of tubocurarine, gallamine, and laudexium are additive and so are those of decamethonium and suxamethonium. In general, depolarizers should not be used after non-depolarizers. Only if the effects of the first drug have worn off should one of the other group be used. Before a depolarizing drug is able to relax muscles after a non-depolarizing drug has been given, it first has to overcome the inhibition of the physiological depolarization caused by the non-depolarizing drug. Thus larger doses of a depolarizer are required to produce relaxation in a patient recovering from a non-depolarizing drug, e.g., large doses of suxamethonium (i.e., at least 50 mg. to 100 mg.) must be given at the end of an operation for peritoneal closure in a patient recovering from tubocurarine or gallamine, and apnœa, once achieved, may be prolonged and difficult to reverse. It is a reasonable practice to use a single dose of suxamethonium for intubation, followed by a non-depolarizing relaxant during the operation, provided the effects of the suxamethonium are allowed to wear off before the non-depolarizing drug is given. Prolonged administration of a depolarizing relaxant with production of phase 2 block sensitizes the end-plate to the effects of the non-depolarizers and decreases end-plate sensitivity to additional depolarizer. A block caused by a small dose of a non-depolarizer given after prolonged administration of a depolarizer can be readily antagonized by a small dose of neostigmine.

MEPHENESIN (MYANESIN)

First described by Berger and Bradley in 1946 (Berger, F. M., and Bradley, W., *Brit. J. Pharmacol.*, 1946, **1**, 265). Chemically it is α= β-dihydroxy Y (2 methyl-phenoxy)-propane. Barnett Mallinson wrote the first clinical account of the drug in 1947 (Mallinson, F. B., *Lancet*, 1947, **1**, 98). Known in the U.S.A. as tolserol and lissaphen and atensin. A drug very little used to-day.

Supplied in 10-ml. ampoules of 10 per cent solution, dissolved in equal volumes of propylene glycol and ethyl alcohol.

---

* Kelly, R. E., and Laurence, D. R., *Lancet*, 1956, **1**, 118.

Mephenesin, *continued.*

Pharmacology.—Has a strong anti-strychnine and anti-tetanus effect probably acting on the basal ganglia and reducing the excitabilit of spinal cord reflexes by depressing the internuncial neuron between the anterior and posterior horn cells. It does not interfer with the passage of impulses across the myoneural junction, conse quently anticholinesterases do not antagonize its effects. It i absorbed slowly from the alimentary canal, and when suitabl dissolved can be injected intramuscularly. Is not very good as relaxant of the larynx. In its present form it is liable to caus thrombosis of the vein, together with destruction of red cells hæmoglobinuria, and oliguria. Cases of death have been reported following its use, presumably due to uræmia consequent on the blocking of renal tubules with products of red-cell destruction, a effect probably due to the propylene glycol in which it is dissolved More recent work tends to show that if the drug is given in strength of 2 per cent or less, red-cell destruction does not occur. It i the strength of solution which is important rather than the total amount injected.

Clinical Uses.—Is used more for the control of spastic states such a mild cases of tetanus, strychnine poisoning, status epilepticus than as a relaxant in anæsthesia, where it now has few uses. It is stated to give relaxation of the muscles of the abdominal wal without the simultaneous production of respiratory depression, but it is inferior to tubocurarine chloride, gallamine, etc.

Average dose is up to 1 g. (50 ml. of 2 per cent solution) given shortly before the peritoneum is opened. Effect lasts twenty to thirty minutes, and can be repeated. Can be given as an elixir, 1 g in half an ounce, or as tablets (0·5 g.).

Because it depresses the thalamus it has been used in psychiatry for ' pharmacological leucotomy '.

BENZOQUINONIUM CHLORIDE (MYTOLON)

Synthesized in the U.S.A. in 1950 by Cavallito and co-workers (Cavallito, C. J., and others, *J. Amer. Chem. Soc.*, 1950, **72**, 2661). It is a red crystalline solid, sparingly soluble in water. Used in 0·3 per cent solution (3 mg. per ml.). It is not reversed by edrophonium or neostigmine although it obtains its effect by non-depolarization. It has anticholinesterase properties, about one-quarter those of neostigmine. It is not very rapid in onset, its maximal effects coming on in ten to fifteen minutes, afterwards gradually passing off. It has no effect on the cardiovascular system, gives no evidence of hista- mine release such as bronchoconstriction, and does not affect transmission of autonomic impulses. It is a powerful vagotonic drug and causes salivation, bradycardia, and colic. Atropine antagonizes these effects. Respiratory depression does not last long.

Dose for intubation 4·5–9 mg., for maintenance, 4·5–6 mg., every twenty to thirty minutes. With ether, less is needed.

Not yet decided whether it is a depolarizer or a true curariform drug, i.e., a competitive myoneural blocking agent. (*See* articles by

Arrowood, Julia, *Anesthesiology*, 1951, **12**, 753 ; and Dundee, J. W., Gray, T. C., and Rees, G. Jackson, *Anæsthesia*, 1952, **7**, 134.)

DIOXAHEXADECANIUM BROMIDE (PRESTONAL)

This was synthesized by Girod and Haefliger in 1952, and first used in clinical anæsthesia by Rudolf Frey in Heidelberg in 1956.* It causes a type of myoneural block, having some of the attributes of both depolarizing and non-depolarizing agents. The apnœa caused by its injection is not readily reversed by anticholinesterase drugs. It is relatively short-acting and does not cause either muscular pains or fasciculations. On injection it causes tachycardia and flushing, perhaps due to histamine release, and should be given slowly. It has found no clinical usefulness in Britain (Jolly, C., *Anæsthesia*, 1957, **12**, 3).

EXCRETION OF RELAXANTS

1. Decamethonium, gallamine, and benzoquinonium are excreted by the kidney unchanged.
2. Tubocurarine and its dimethyl compound are mostly excreted by the kidneys.
3. Suxamethonium is almost completely hydrolysed.

SOME FACTORS INFLUENCING NEUROMUSCULAR BLOCK

1. IN DISEASE.—
   a. *Myasthenia gravis* (*see* Chapter XXVI). Patients abnormally sensitive to non-depolarizers and resistant to depolarizers.
   b. *Myasthenic syndrome.* Neuropathy in carcinoma falls into several main groups: (1) The neuromuscular group; (2) Cerebellar degeneration; (3) Sensory neuropathy; (4) Motor neuron disease; (5) Encephalomyelitis; and (6) The myasthenic syndrome. Patients with carcinomatosis, especially if the primary tumour is in the bronchus, may have latent myasthenic reactions and so may be extremely sensitive to depolarizing (Phase 2 block) and to non-depolarizing relaxants. This may be one cause of the so-called neostigmine-resistant curarization. A test dose of tubocurarine or gallamine is advised if such patients give a history of any muscular weakness.† The latent myasthenic response may also be seen in patients with thyroid disease, polyarteritis nodosa, polymyositis, dermatomyositis, systemic lupus erythematosus ; symptoms of muscular weakness should be inquired about and liver function assessed if such patients are to receive relaxants.‡
   c. Patients with *liver deficiency* may show, because of a low value for pseudocholinesterase, abnormal sensitivity to suxamethonium and abnormal resistance to tubocurarine and

---

* Frey, R., *Proc. World Congress of Anesthesiologists*, 1955, 262. Minneapolis: Burgess Pub. Co.
† Croft, P. B., *Brit. med. J.*, 1958, **1**, 181 ; and Henson, R. A., and others, *Brain*, 1954, **77**, 82.
‡ Potts, M. W., and Thornton, J. A., *Brit. J. Anæsth.*, 1961, **33**, 405.

Some Factors influencing Neuromuscular Block, *continued.*

gallamine.* It may be partly due to alteration in the albumin/globulin ratio in the plasma. Obstructive jaundice, without liver damage, may, on the other hand, require smaller doses of non-depolarizers than normal.

d. Patients with *kidney disease*, especially when the filtration rate is reduced as in shock, hypotension, and circulatory depression, may excrete gallamine and decamethonium more slowly than normal.

e. Patients with *electrolyte imbalance*. Hypokalæmia produces oversensitivity to non-depolarizing relaxants while potassium has anti-curare effects.

The magnitude of the end-plate potential can be considered to bear a direct relationship to the ratio of intracellular to extracellular potassium concentration.

i. Relative fall in extracellular potassium. It is the ratio of intra- to extra-cellular potassium which is important, not the absolute value of either. Cell membrane is hyperpolarized with resistance to the action of acetylcholine. Non-depolarizers are potentiated, depolarizers antagonized. Response to neostigmine normal.

ii. Relative rise in extracellular potassium. Resting membrane potential is lowered—less highly polarized. Increased sensitivity to depolarizers, resistance to non-depolarizers.

iii. Fall in both intracellular and extracellular potassium. The commonest situation in clinical practice. Resting membrane potential relatively unaffected, and response to muscle relaxants normal. The danger lies in the lack of reserve, a relatively small shift of potassium into the cells may precipitate symptoms of hypokalæmia (e.g., metabolic and respiratory acidosis, administration of glucose).

It has been suggested that in conditions of potassium imbalance, muscle relaxants may penetrate the blood/brain barrier.† Also that the blocking action of tubocurarine on the sympathetic ganglia might be enhanced (to account for the hypotension observed terminally in cases of ' neostigmine-resistant curarization ').‡

iv. Metabolic and respiratory acidosis produce signs resembling partial curarization.

(*See also* Feldman, S. A., *Brit. J. Anæsth*, 1963, **35**, 546.)

f. Patients with *collagen diseases*, e.g., systemic lupus erythematosus, polymyositis, dermatomyositis, etc., may show increased sensitivity to non-depolarizing relaxants, as in myasthenia.

g. Patients *with asthma*. There is no real evidence that tubocurarine increases bronchospasm. The muscarinic effects of neostigmine must be well suppressed by atropine.

2. EFFECT OF DRUGS.—

a. *Antibiotics.*—Neomycin (first report Pridgen, J. E., *Surgery*, 1956, **40**, 571), streptomycin, kanamycin, polymixin, and

---

* Dundee, J. W., and Gray, T. C., *Lancet*, 1953, **2**, 11.
† Foster, P. A., *Brit. J. Anæsth.*, 1956, **28**, 488.
‡ Gray, T. C., *Brit. med. J.*, 1956, **2**, 1365.

colistimethate, if given parenterally or intraperitoneally, may cause a non-depolarizing block which will be potentiated by tubocurarine and gallamine, and by ether and cyclopropane even if given 24 hours before. It is reversed by neostigmine.* The membrane potential of the end-plate is dependent on the presence of calcium ions and this is reduced by the antibiotics. Intravenous calcium chloride or gluconate may have both a prophylactic and a therapeutic use in these cases.† Tetracycline and penicillin show no neuromuscular blocking activity.

b. *Ganglionic Blocking Agents.*—Hexamethonium, trimetaphan, and phenactropinium all produce neuromuscular block. Preliminary curarization reduces the dose of hypotensive drug needed to obtain a certain effect. Neostigmine antagonizes the effects of hexamethonium and phenactropinium but potentiates those of trimetaphan.‡

c. *Oxytocin.*—Prolonged intravenous infusion of oxytocin modifies the action of suxamethonium. Fasciculations are minimal or absent and normal doses are ineffectual in causing apnœa. Non-depolarizing block does occur, however, rather slowly, and may be prolonged if not reversed by neostigmine.§ Other work has contradicted this.‖ The occasional case of prolonged apnœa in labour following suxamethonium may be due to the low maternal level of pseudocholinesterase in late pregnancy and the puerperium.

d. In the fully *digitalized* patient, although there is no alteration in the muscle relaxation produced by suxamethonium, this relaxant may result in ventricular arrhythmias: these can be abolished by tubocurarine (as can the arrhythmias of digitalis intoxication). Thus in fully digitalized patients, e.g., in cardiac surgery, there is an argument against the use of suxamethonium. The transmembrane flux of potassium may be implicated in causation.¶

e. *Quinidine.***—The *d*-stereo isomer of quinine, potentiates both depolarizing and non-depolarizing relaxants.

3. BLOOD-FLOW.—The greater the blood-flow in a muscle, the sooner the onset and the quicker the recovery from myoneural block.

4. BODY TEMPERATURE.—With depolarizing agents, low temperature prolongs block. With non-depolarizing drugs, a low temperature decreases the degree of block, but not its duration.

5. CARBON DIOXIDE.—In the cat, carbon dioxide opposes the action of suxamethonium, decamethonium, and gallamine, but increases the activity of tubocurarine.†† In man hypercapnia potentiates and hypocapnia diminishes the action of tubocurarine.

* Pittinger, C. B., and others, *Curr. Res. Anesth.*, 1958, **37**, 276.
† Corrado, A. P., *Ibid.*, 1963, **42**, 1.
‡ Deacock, A. R., and Davies, T. D. W., *Brit. J. Anæsth.*, 1958, **30**, 217.
§ Hodges, R. J. Hamar, and others, *Brit. med. J.*, 1959, **1**, 413.
‖ Ichiyanagi, K., and others, *Brit. J. Anæsth.*, 1963, **35**, 611.
¶ Dowdy, E. G., and Fabian, L. W., *Curr. Res. Anesth.*, 1963, **4**, 501.
** Miller, R. D., Way, W. L., and Katzung, B. G., *Anesthesiology*, 1967, **28**, 1036.
†† Payne, J. P., *Brit. J. Anæsth.*, 1958, **30**, 208.

Some Factors influencing Neuromuscular Block, *continued.*

With gallamine the reverse occurs.* This probably is not of grea
clinical importance.† The addition of carbon dioxide to th
inhaled atmosphere antagonizes gallamine and slightly poten
tiates suxamethonium block.‡

Respiratory acidosis prolongs and alkalæmia reduces the effec
of myoneural block due to tubocurarine in man. Respirator
acidosis decreases the myoneural blocking effect of gallamine.§

Changes in blood pH within the clinical range have little effec
on the plasma distribution of tubocurarine.||

6. AGE.—Neuromuscular transmission in infants differs from tha
in adults.¶ In infants:—

   a. Depolarizing drugs produce many of the changes seen in adult
   after non-depolarizing agents (early Phase 2 block).

   b. Prolonged apnœa after the use of depolarizing drugs can b
   reversed by anticholinesterase agents (providing the type c
   block is proved to be the non-depolarizing variety).

   c. No fasciculations are seen after the injection of depolarizin
   relaxants.

   d. There is great sensitivity to non-depolarizers, but these agent
   are well tolerated in small dosage.

   A change to the normal adult type of reaction occurs at th
   5th to 6th week.

7. EXERCISE.—Fatigue prolongs non-depolarizing block.
8. DIFFERENTIAL EFFECT ON VARIOUS MUSCLE GROUPS
   —The higher the cholinesterase content of a muscle, the mor
   sensitive is it to non-depolarizing relaxants. The external ey
   muscles, the diaphragm, and the heart have cholinesterase i
   decreasing amounts.

CHAPTER XIX

HYPNOSIS : ELECTRICAL ANÆSTHESIA

HYPNOSIS

History.—Anton Mesmer (1734–1815) introduced ' animal magnet
ism ' and successfully treated a child with hysterical blindness i
1777. A commission appointed in 1784 by the French Academy o
Science at the request of Louis XVI, and including Benjami
Franklin, Dr. Guillotin (of guillotine fame), and Lavoisier amon
its members, reported unfavourably on the method in 1784
James Braid (1765–1860), a Manchester surgeon, experimente

---

* Walts, L. F., Lebowitz, M., and Dillon, J. B., *Brit. J. Anæsth.*, 1967, **39**, 845.
† Bridenbaugh, P. O., Churchill-Davidson, H. C., and Churcher, M. D., *Curr. Res. Anesth.*
1966, **45**, 804.
‡ Baraka, A., *Brit. J. Anæsth.*, 1967, **39**, 786.
§ Baraka, A., *Ibid.*, 1964, **36**, 272.
|| Cohen, E. H., and others, *Anesthesiology*, 1965, **26**, 727.
¶ Churchill-Davidson, H. C., and Wise, R. P., *Ibid.*, 1963, **24**, 271.

with the method and introduced the name 'Hypnosis'. Cloquet (1790–1883) in 1829 performed a mastectomy under mesmeric sleep and following this several surgeons operated painlessly by the same method. The chief advocate of hypnosis in England was Elliotson (1791–1868), first professor of medicine at University College Hospital, London, around 1838, while James Esdaile (1808–1859), a Scotsman, used hypnosis for many surgical operations in India (1846).

The introduction of inhalation anæsthesia following 1846 led to the abandonment of hypnosis in surgical practice. Of recent years interest has been rekindled. Reports on hypnosis have been published by the British Medical Association in 1892 and 1955, and by the American Medical Association in 1958.

The Hypnotic State.—This is a state of altered consciousness characterized by heightened suggestibility, narrowed awareness, selective wakefulness, and restricted attentiveness. We may consider the stages of hypnosis as follows :—

1. HYPNOID STATE.—A relaxed, drowsy, pre-hypnotic state.
2. LIGHT TRANCE.—Susceptible to post-hypnotic suggestion.
3. MEDIUM TRANCE.—Production of analgesia and amnesia. Glove anæsthesia for minor operations. Increased susceptibility to post-hypnotic suggestion.
4. DEEP TRANCE.—A state of complete anæsthesia and total amnesia. Can usually only be achieved in a patient who has been hypnotized on a number of previous occasions.

About 10–15 per cent of individuals are not susceptible to hypnosis. About 40–50 per cent can be taken to the hypnoid and light trance stage, 20–25 per cent to medium trance, and 15–20 per cent to deep trance. Children are the most susceptible, and individuals over 55 years of age are less easy to hypnotize. Intelligent people are more susceptible and mental defectives almost impossible to hypnotize. Deafness or language barriers make hypnosis difficult.

Technique of Hypnosis.—A trance is usually brought about with the help of repetitive stimuli, auditory, visual, or tactile. The aim is a reduction of sensory intake to one or two monotonous stimuli. For details of technique the reader is referred to the various monographs on the subject.* Plenty of time may be necessary. It may be of help to combine suggestion with the use of sedative drugs.

Mechanism of Hypnosis.—This is not understood. There have been suggestions that the site of block may be the first sensory synapse, the thalamic region, and the reticular system. Recent work suggests, however, that there is no diminution of the evoked potential arriving at the cortex.†

---

* Ambrose, G., and Newbold, G., *A Handbook of Medical Hypnosis*, 1956. London: Baillière, Tindall & Cox; Schneck, J. M., *Hypnosis in Modern Medicine*, 1963. Springfield, Ill.: Thomas; Marmer, M. J., *Hypnosis in Anesthesiology*, 1959. Oxford: Blackwell.
† Mason, A. A., in *General Anæsthesia* (Ed. Evans, F. T., and Gray, T. C.), 2nd ed., 1965, Vol. 2, Ch. 33, 'Hypnotism'. London: Butterworths.

Advantages of Hypnosis.—The patient may be kept awake or asleep and pain-free. There is no danger of the toxic side-effects of chemical agents. Post-hypnotic suggestion may be valuable in the post-operative period.

Disadvantages of Hypnosis.—It is difficult and time-consuming to accomplish in a high proportion of cases. It is too unreliable compared to chemical anæsthesia. There is a possibility that hypnosis may occasionally release underlying psychiatric disorders.

Indications for Hypnosis.—

1. May be useful for simple operations, when the ordinary technique of general or regional anæsthesia might be considered dangerous.
2. In obstetrics. Has been used for relief of pain during labour.
3. For repeated dressing of burns in children.
4. For painful fillings in the dental chair.
5. For relief of painful conditions, in selected patients.

Contra-indications.—

1. Refusal of the patient to be hypnotized.
2. When the patient is under psychiatric care.
3. When the patient is in a state of extreme anxiety which prevents him giving full attention to the hypnotist.
4. When quiet surroundings, time, and an experienced hypnotist are not available.

In spite of the increased attention given to hypnosis in recent years, the practical utility of this method of pain relief is very limited.

ELECTRICAL ANÆSTHESIA

First shown to be possible by d'Arsonval, a French physicist (1851-1940), in 1890. Since then various attempts have been made to produce general, spinal, and local anæsthesia by passage of an electric current. In recent years there has been increased interest in the method.

When an electric current is passed through the head the result may be: (1) Electrical sleep, a condition in which the patient can be roused by appropriate stimuli (which may have an application in space travel). (2) Electrical anæsthesia, a condition in which it is not possible to rouse the patient and in which surgical operations can be performed.

Experimental work has been carried out *in animals*. Various effects are obtained according to the nature of the current and the site of electrodes. Direct current is not easy to manage. Large surface electrodes are required because of polarization and there is a danger of burns. Alternating current is more satisfactory. The electrodes can be hypodermic needles placed under the scalp in contact with the periosteum. They are usually fronto-occipital, but may be bi-temporal or multiple. The main body of the brain must be between the electrodes. Various wave-forms have been used, sine, square, and triangular.

A frequency is chosen which causes the least movement of the animal. It is important to increase the current slowly. The animal eventually falls over and appears to be anæsthetized. If the current is switched off there is immediate recovery and the animal can be led away. The only after-effect is some residual analgesia. Should the current be interrupted unintentionally, the animal recovers, and it is necessary to restart the process with a low current.

The state produced by the electrical current differs considerably from the conventional picture of chemical anæsthesia. There are species variations in response. The cow is much easier to anæsthetize with electricity than the horse. Throughout anæsthesia there may be some movement of the animal and conditioned reflexes may persist into deep electrical anæsthesia. Muscular relaxation is produced, satisfactory for laparotomy, but areas such as the snout, genitals, and paws may still respond to stimulation. There may be changes in respiration and heart action in deep electrical anæsthesia. It is possible to use the electro-encephalogram with the help of filters.* This shows mainly an increase in slow-wave activity, which is not necessarily indicative of unconsciousness.

The applications of this technique to humans require a good deal of further work. Undesirable side-effects have been common in such studies as have been undertaken. These include skin burns at the site of application of the electrodes, cardiac irregularities, tonic muscle spasms, respiratory stridor, laryngospasm, and salivation. It would seem necessary to use light general anæsthesia and a muscle relaxant to obviate them.

Electrical anæsthesia is thus not yet a satisfactory clinical method in humans, although a series of veterinary operations (including organ transplantation) has been reported on. It may be that in the future it will become possible to administer electrical anæsthesia without the need for covering chemical anæsthesia and muscle relaxants. If so, the method might become advantageous because of the lack of chemical toxicity and the immediate reversal on switching off the current.

(*See also*: Langley, E. O. J., *J. ment. Sci.*, 1949, **95**, 1; Van Poznak, A., *Anesthesiology*, 1963, **24**, 101; Smith, R. H., *Electrical Anesthesia*, 1963. Springfield, Ill.: Thomas; Knutson, R. C., Tichy, F. Y., and Reitman, J. H., *Anesthesiology*, 1956, **17**, 815; Hardy, J. D., and others, *J. Amer. med. Ass.*, 1961, **175**, 599; Clutton-Brock, J., *Anæsthesia*, 1966, **21**, 101; Knutson, R. C., First International Symposium on Electro-sleep Therapy and Electroanesthesia, *Curr. Res. Anesth.*, 1967, **46**, 333.)

CHAPTER XX

CHOICE OF ANÆSTHETIC, AS INFLUENCED BY TYPE OF OPERATION

UROLOGY

No general anæsthetic should be given if uræmic coma is imminent. Ether has a toxic effect on diseased kidneys. Normal operative procedures cause no change in the renal circulation. Under anæsthesia the blood-pressure is a poor guide to the renal circulation but function is seriously impaired with pressures below 60 mm. Hg. During anæsthesia,

---

* Knutson, R. C., and others, *Anesthesiology*, 1963, **24**, 728.

Urology, *continued.*

methylamphetamine increases, while noradrenaline and adrenaline decrease renal blood-flow. Thus cyclopropane, ether, and thiopentone reduce renal blood-flow probably by vasoconstriction. The effect of halothane is less marked. Blood-loss of up to 1500 ml. does not cause renal damage unless it is prolonged and especially if associated with hypotension: so blood-loss must be replaced if it is excessive. Total renal ischæmia of more than 30 minutes' duration is likely to result in damage to the tubules.

When the filtration rate of the renal tubules is greatly reduced, e.g. shock, cardiovascular depression, gallamine should only be used with care because it is excreted by the kidneys.

Many patients undergoing urological operations are old, atheromatous, and suffering from disease of the kidneys and cardiovascular system. A high blood-urea may be associated with a decreased tolerance towards intravenous barbiturates, which should be used especially carefully in cases which show this abnormality. For example, moderate doses of thiopentone may cause very prolonged sleep in a uræmic patient. The blood-urea seldom rises above normal until the glomerular filtration rate has fallen to about 25 per cent of normal. When this is reduced to 5 per cent of normal the blood-urea may reach 300 mg. per 100 ml. Symptoms due to uræmia rare until the blood-urea approaches 150 mg. per 100 ml. Vomiting, if severe and persistent, may result in hypokalæmia and this may prolong the effects of non-depolarizing relaxants, while hyponatræmia may cause similar trouble. Old patients are usually more placid and philosophical than young patients, so are often good subjects for regional analgesia. Premedication should be minimal and, when necessary, atropine used in all patients over the age of about 60, rather than hyoscine.

1. Nephrectomy.—

NERVE-SUPPLY TO KIDNEY.*—The *renal plexus* arises by numerous small roots from the semilunar, superior mesenteric, and aortico-renal sympathetic ganglia, which in their turn derive supply from the three splanchnic nerves—predominantly from lowest splanchnic. All arise in the tenth, eleventh, and twelfth thoracic segments. The vagus probably takes no part in renal innervation. This bundle of nerve-fibres is grouped into upper, lower, and posterior renal nerves, which are in relationship to the renal artery. From the posterior renal nerve is given off the superior nerve to the ureter. Ureteric afferents ascend in T.11 and T.12 and L.1 and L.2. Pain may be referred to the distribution of the genito-femoral nerve.

Lateral position throws strain on respiratory efficiency of patient, for although perfusion of the alveoli is increased, ventilation is decreased. Nevertheless, oxygen uptake from the lower lung is always greater. A reduction of minute volume of 9 per cent occurs in the lateral position with spontaneous breathing; breaking the table reduces this still further. Use of kidney bridge increases this strain, and further predisposes to hypoxia and post-operative atelectasis of contralateral lower zone.

---

* Oldham, J. B., *Ann. R. Coll. Surg. Engl.*, 1950, **7**, 222.

Endotracheal gas–oxygen, with a thiobarbiturate and a relaxant and perhaps pethidine, makes a useful combination with I.P.P.V., and so does halothane and oxygen with either spontaneous or assisted respiration.

Unilateral intradural analgesia with 12–14 ml. of hypobaric cincho-caine is useful when patient is fit and muscular (*see* p. 400). Owing to the discomfort of the lateral position, light general anæsthesia is often a useful supplement. Analgesia must ascend to T.8. Extradural block is useful in experienced hands. Neither method greatly influences the tone of the ureters.

Rarely, the pleura is damaged during kidney operations; the resulting collapse of the upper lung may, in association with the handicapped lower lung, prove dangerous unless I.P.P.V., preferably through an endotracheal tube, is employed. An under-water drain in the early post-operative period may be required.

Transplantation of the ureter requires maximal relaxation, obtained either by extradural analgesia or by a muscle relaxant with light general anæsthesia. Intra- and extradural analgesia, by causing a tonic, small, and contracted colon, have been known to interfere with the ureterocolic anastomosis.

Patients who have undergone a ureterosigmoidostomy may develop a hyperchloræmic acidosis due to reabsorption of chloride from the bowel, and a hypokalæmia, the latter giving rise to muscular weakness and even respiratory paralysis.* Serum electrolytes should be checked daily and normal saline infusions avoided. Treatment includes potassium replacement and, if necessary, assisted respiration. These electrolyte changes do not occur with transplantation into an ileal loop.

2. Suprapubic Cystostomy.—

THE INNERVATION OF THE URINARY BLADDER.—The bladder, lower ends of the ureters, and the prostate are supplied by filaments of the inferior hypogastric plexus. This is formed from: (1) The sympathetic L.2 and L.3 roots and ganglia T.12–L.3. (2) The parasympathetic—S.2, S.3, and S.4. Fibres from the sources pass first to the pre-sacral or superior hypogastric plexus and from here fibres pass to the inferior hypogastric plexus. Stimulation of the sympathetic component causes contraction of the bladder neck and of the prostatic and seminal vesicular musculature and the ureteric orifices. The sympathetic is inhibitory to the detrusor muscle. The parasympathetic is motor to the detrusor and inhibitory to the internal sphincter. The external sphincter is innervated by the internal pudendal nerve—this nerve conveys sensation from the posterior urethra and the sphincter. *Visceral afferent* fibres from the bladder pass with: (1) sympathetic fibres to the dorsal roots of the second and third or first and second lumbar nerves via the hypogastric plexus and the upper lumbar sympathetic ganglia; (2) para-sympathetic fibres to the sacral roots 1 to 3.

---

* Annotation, *Lancet*, 1959, **7**, 837.

Suprapubic Cystostomy, *continued.*

In poor-risk cases, regional block. Analgesia and relaxation of the anterior abdominal wall may be obtained by regional analgesia including rectus sheath block* (*see* p. 362). In average cases where relaxation is not required, halothane and oxygen, thiopentone (with or without pethidine) with gas and oxygen, light cyclopropane, or light ether. In stout patients, the addition of a muscle relaxant may be necessary. Intra- or extradural analgesia (up to T.10) is very seldom necessary.

3. **Suprapubic and Retropubic Prostatectomy.**—Relaxation is required and considerable hæmorrhage may occur. *Extradural analgesia* using 7–20 ml. of 1·5 per cent lignocaine, with or without light general anæsthesia, gives good results, especially if emphysema and bronchospasm are also present. *Spinal analgesia* to T.10, obtained by 1–1500 cinchocaine (10–12 ml.); 1·4 to 1·6 ml. of hyperbaric cinchocaine, or procaine, 100–150 mg., provides relaxation and reduces hæmorrhage, but like extradural analgesia it causes a fall in blood-pressure which may embarrass the cardiovascular system and mask hæmorrhage; bleeding may then occur when the patient is back in bed with a blood-pressure returned to near normal. The blood-pressure can, in these cases, be maintained by suitable drugs, e.g., methylamphetamine or methoxamine, should this be thought necessary. Methylamphetamine does not have the effect of causing constriction of the renal vessels. Blood-pressure-raising drugs should be given carefully to hypertensive patients, and only after it is known that the block has acted successfully. This ensures against undue rise in pressure which might harm the inelastic vascular system.

Many workers prefer for prostatectomy a *general anæsthetic*, e.g., halothane and oxygen, thiopentone with gas–oxygen–trichloroethylene; cyclopropane; light ether (in the absence of diathermy). Relaxation can be produced or increased by a suitable muscle relaxant. Arrangements should be made to have intravenous dextrose and blood to hand in these cases.

HYPOTENSIVE ANÆSTHESIA gives good results in experienced hands, with a low morbidity and mortality.† The blood-pressure is reduced by pentolinium tartrate (5–10 mg.), hexamethonium or trimetaphan. Halothane and oxygen can also be employed to produce wound ischæmia (*see also* 'Prostatectomy and Hypotensive Anæsthesia', *Proc. R. Soc. Med.*, 1967, **57**, 1179).

EPSILON-AMINOCAPROIC ACID.‡—The urine contains a soluble plasminogen activator, urokinase, which converts plasminogen to plasmin: this can dissolve the fibrin in the clot, causing bleeding. Urokinase is specifically inhibited by epsilon-aminocaproic acid with reduction of post-prostatectomy hæmorrhage. Its use does not increase the incidence of post-operative thromboembolism.§ Recommended dosage, 5 g. intravenously, 4–5 times

---

* Ellis, H., and Leatherdale, R. A. L., *Lancet*, 1958, **2**, 1189.
† Sheppard, N. L., and Grace, A. H., *Proc. R. Soc. Med.*, 1961, **54**, 1127.
‡ Andersson, L., *Acta chir. scand.*, 1965, **130**, 393; Gans, H., *Ann. Surg.*, 1966, **163**, 178; and *Brit. med. J.*, 1967, **4**, 725.
§ Vinnicombe, J., and Shuttleworth, K. E. D., *Lancet*, 1966, **1**, 232.

daily, starting on the operating table, during first 3 post-operative days; thereafter 3 g. by mouth for several days.

4. Transurethral Prostatectomy.—If *general anæsthesia* is used the explosion hazard must be remembered. Halothane and oxygen or thiopentone–gas–oxygen and trichloroethylene are suitable.

Low intradural spinal is very satisfactory and needs to extend up to S.1. To render the dome of the bladder insensitive to distension, block must be to T.10 and skin analgesia must reach the umbilicus. If, in addition, the vasa are to be tied, a little local infiltration may be required in addition; this small operation demands a block up to T.12.

Suitable techniques are 1·2 ml. of heavy cinchocaine; 1·5 ml. of 5 per cent lignocaine with dextrose given in the sitting position (in each case diluted at least half-and-half with cerebrospinal fluid), 1 ml. of 1 per cent amethocaine (10 mg.) with 1 ml. 10 per cent glucose given in sitting position.

Extradural lumbar or sacral block may be used for these cases, while both it and low intradural spinal block can be accompanied by minimal thiopentone if the patient is anxious.

Isotonic saline should be used for irrigation as ordinary water may be absorbed into the vascular system and result in: (1) Hæmolysis with subsequent renal damage; (2) Bacterial contamination; (3) Water intoxication which results when a greatly increased volume of water enters the circulation. It causes a dilutional hyponatræmia which may lead to prolonged action of non-depolarizing relaxants,* cerebral or pulmonary œdema, raised blood-pressure, acute left ventricular failure, nausea, vomiting, headache, and possibly convulsions and coma. Intravenous sodium chloride 5 per cent solution may be helpful in treatment.†

5. Cystoscopy.—Topical analgesia is fairly satisfactory, e.g., lignocaine 1 or 2 per cent jelly, but should not be used after recent instrumentation or in the presence of bleeding from the urethra (*see* p. 377); a 2 per cent solution of pyribenzamine (tripelennamine), the antihistaminic drug, can be used successfully in these patients as an analgesic. Cases with gross cystitis are often unsuitable for local analgesia as the distension of the bladder with irrigating fluid causes painful spasm. Women will frequently tolerate this examination without general anæsthesia if simple sedatives are given.

If a *general anæsthetic* is used for cystoscopy, the anæsthetist must provide: (1) Complete loss of sensation; (2) Relaxation of bladder sphincters and abdominal wall; (3) Quiet breathing through a patent airway; (4) Freedom from hazard of explosion. In the authors' opinion, this anæsthetic procedure can be difficult to accomplish smoothly, e.g., in emphysematous old men with bronchitis. It should never be undertaken lightly and may require endotracheal intubation. Even in experienced hands, anæsthesia for cystoscopy is often inelegantly given. Halothane and oxygen is an excellent choice.

---

* Jacobson, J., *Anæsthesia*, 1965, **20**, 329.
† Marx, G., and Orkin, L., *Anesthesiology*, 1967, **23**, 802.

Cystoscopy, *continued.*

Thiopentone with gas and oxygen together with a relaxant is a suitable anæsthetic, but prolonged recovery may interfere with pyelography. In patients with uræmia, thiopentone dosage must be kept very low.

Extradural sacral block is very satisfactory, but care must be taken to prevent analgesia from involving the renal pelvis, if pyelo graphy is contemplated, and therefore it must not involve the eleventh and twelfth thoracic nerves.

Low intradural spinal is also satisfactory, e.g., cinchocaine, 0·5 per cent solution, 1 ml.; procaine, 60–90 mg., in 2 ml. of cerebro spinal fluid given in sitting position. Block up to T.9 is required to obtund completely the discomfort of bladder distension.

6. Circumcision.—*In babies,* open ether. Ethyl chloride should be avoided, induction being more safely carried out with V.A.M. (vinesthene anæsthetic mixture) Babies easily develop laryngeal spasm, sometimes necessitating interruption of the operation until the airway is patent again. Adequate depth of anæsthesia before the infliction of surgical trauma will usually prevent what may be a very dangerous complication. Other workers prefer halothane, cyclopropane, or, if experienced in infant anæsthesia, intravenous barbiturate, suxamethonium, intubation and gas–oxygen given by I.P.P.V. *In children,* general anæsthesia; *in adults* thiopentone, with gas and oxygen, and perhaps halothane or trichloroethylene, extradural sacral block, or regional block (*see* p. 366).

7. Renal Homotransplantation.*—As non-depolarizing relaxants are largely excreted by the kidneys, these drugs must be used very carefully. Bilateral nephrectomy may precede transplantation Renal dialysis may cause a fall in the plasma cholinesterase level The post-transplant patient may develop a diuresis so that fluid and electrolyte replacement must receive attention.

ABDOMINAL SURGERY

Essentials of Good Technique.—Good technique must provide :—
a. Safety.
b. Good relaxation of the muscles of the anterior abdominal wall and peritoneum. As the rectus and the transversus muscles are accessory muscles of respiration, their tone persists in planes of third-stage anæsthesia which produce complete flaccidity of the muscles of the limbs. The posterior fascial sheath of these two muscles is fused with the peritoneum in the upper abdomen so they must be well relaxed when the peritoneum is sutured Relaxation is aided by flexing the head and neck, and by raising the knees 6 in. from the table.
c. Quiet breathing. With ether, when intercostal paralysis is complete, the diaphragm compensates by increased and sometimes jerky movement : this is not seen with halothane or cyclopropane, which produces quieter breathing (although at a greater

---

* Strunin, L., *Brit. J. Anæsth.*, 1966, **38**, 812. *See also Proc. R. Soc. Med.*, 1968, **61**, in press.

risk of causing respiratory acidosis). Most abdominal operations are now performed under some type of intermittent positive-pressure respiration although operation on the lower abdomen can often be well conducted using halothane and oxygen with spontaneous (sometimes assisted) respiration.

d. Protection from shock and circulatory depression.

e. Minimal disturbance of respiratory function after operation from chemical irritation of the mucosa, from prolonged hypoventilation of the lungs, with alveolar collapse, disturbance of the ventilation perfusion mechanism and consequent hypoxia, or from prolonged depression of the cough reflex. Upper abdominal relaxation can only be produced coincidently with intercostal paresis, so that tidal exchange is always reduced when this relaxation is present unless breathing is assisted or controlled.

f. Minimal interference with body chemistry.

g. Protection of the airway from aspiration of gastric contents (*see* p. 510). The risk of such aspiration is not of course confined to abdominal operations. If it is suspected that vomitable material is present in the stomach, the successful passage of a stomach tube will make certain, and through it liquid can be aspirated. The Ryle tube has three markings on it corresponding to the average distance between the upper teeth and the pylorus, the fundus, and the cardia, respectively. A more efficient tube is the semi-stiff œsophageal tube (e.g., size 12, 7 mm. diameter), through which can be sucked a larger volume of fluid, together with small solid particles.

h. Pleasant induction and relative freedom from post-operative sequelæ.

For producing relaxation of the anterior abdominal wall, subarachnoid block, although it is not at present popular, is the most efficient technique. Next comes extradural block, followed closely by the use of a muscle relaxant. The contraction of the gut associated with the sympathetic paralysis is often advantageous, whereas the lack of cardiovascular depression is one of the strongest points favouring the use of the muscle relaxants. Then follows the use of deep ether, and some way after that halothane and cyclopropane. Thiopentone and vinesthene cannot be relied upon for this purpose, while trichloroethylene and nitrous-oxide–oxygen are quite inadequate, if used alone.

Agents and Methods.—These include: (1) Light general anæsthesia with a relaxant; (2) Deep general anæsthesia; (3) Light general anæsthesia with regional block; (4) Regional block alone. The occasional anæsthetist will produce the best results with *ether*, using either an open mask or a gas machine. The E.M.O. inhaler is very useful for maintaining ether anæsthesia. Ether is well tolerated by most patients, while its margin of safety is wide; muscular relaxation is good and breathing can be made reasonably quiet. As it is a respiratory stimulant, the blood carbon-dioxide level is not so likely to rise as is the case with some other anæsthetic agents. Gas and oxygen can be used for induction. The semi-closed or closed circuit may be used for maintenance. Unfortunately ether has many well-known disadvantages.

Abdominal Surgery—Agents and Methods, *continued.*

Halothane when used with oxygen* in a concentration of 2–10 per cent into a partially rebreathing system will often give most satisfactory operating conditions, especially for interventions in the lower abdomen. The use of small doses of gallamine or of assisted respiration may sometimes be necessary.

Cyclopropane is most useful in experienced hands. It produces quiet breathing and less post-operative chest complications than ether. Relaxation cannot be guaranteed, but can be produced by the addition of a muscle relaxant, minimal ether, or regional analgesia. With slow deepening of anæsthesia in patients of moderate musculature, cyclopropane is often adequate when used alone, and if controlled breathing is employed. Preliminary examination of the patient's abdominal wall will tell the experienced anæsthetist what agent or technique will be necessary to produce good relaxation.

A large endotracheal tube is of great help in upper abdominal operations and many lower interventions.

Thiopentone is only suitable for abdominal operations in thin asthenic patients in operations of short duration. It should be accompanied by gas and plenty of oxygen. It is not a good agent for the production of abdominal relaxation, but is excellent when combined with a relaxant. It can be used, however, in a dose of 100–250 mg. to produce extra relaxation for a short time, e.g., while the peritoneum is being sutured in patients under inhalation anæsthesia.

Extradural lumbar block is a neglected but, in the authors' opinion, an excellent method of providing for the surgeon a patient who is completely relaxed, has contracted bowels, and in whom afferent impulses are blocked. Lignocaine 1·5 per cent solution —with adrenaline—is used in doses of 20–45 ml. For prolonged operations an extradural catheter should be inserted, and serial injections given or bupivacaine 0·5 per cent with adrenaline can be used.†

Spinal intradural analgesia finds its most useful field in abdominal operations. The higher the level of analgesia obtained, the less safe does it become. Thus it is safer for lower abdominal section —to T.9 or 8—than for upper laparotomies, T.5 or 4.

High spinal is useful in fit, sthenic, muscular individuals. The quiet breathing, complete relaxation, and contracted bowels produce good operating conditions.

Mid-spinal, i.e., to T.9 or 8, is safe for patients who are reasonably fit.

It is usually preferable to combine intra- or extradural analgesia with light general anæsthesia, either with thiopentone, gas and oxygen, halothane, or cyclopropane. A safety factor is to have the patient breathe an oxygen-rich atmosphere. A supply of pressor drugs and atropine, and an open vein into which to inject them, must always be to hand.

---

* Johnstone, M., *Brit. J. Anæsth.*, 1961, **33**, 29.
† Watt, M. J., Ross, D. M., and Atkinson, R. S., *Anæsthesia*, 1968, **23**, 2; and *Ibid.* 1968, **23**, July.

The *muscle relaxants* are most useful to produce relaxation. They can be combined with thiopentone (with or without pethidine) and inhalation agents.

Good results follow the combination of thiopentone induction (up to 0·5 g. of 2·5 per cent solution), gas and oxygen (at least 30 per cent), intravenous injections of 10–25 mg. of pethidine as required, and a muscle relaxant such as tubocurarine or gallamine, or a drip of suxamethonium. Another useful technique involves a sleep dose of thiopentone, a muscle relaxant followed by hyperventilation with nitrous oxide and oxygen, with flows up to 20 litres per min. The resulting hypocapnia potentiates the analgesia and reduces the amount of relaxant needed. Patients so treated awaken soon after operation and do not require analgesic drugs for several hours. As pethidine takes some minutes to act, it must be given well in advance of its need. The average patient requires about 1 mg. per minute. Signs of too light a plane of anæsthesia are: (1) Small movements of hands, face, head, or hips and knees. (2) Increasing resistance to inflation. (3) A rising pulse-rate.

Regional analgesia in expert hands performed on thin patients gives good results. It can take the form of intercostal block (*see* p. 354) or abdominal field block (*see* p. 359), combined with either posterior or anterior splanchnic block (*see* p. 357). Light general anæsthesia can be combined with regional analgesia, the latter producing the necessary relaxation.

Post-operative Analgesics.—There is some evidence that diacetyl morphine (heroin) 2·5–5 mg. causes less post-operative nausea and vomiting than morphine. Morphine may also cause a high intracolic pressure which may give rise to rupture of the bowel in cases of acute diverticulitis and bowel anastomosis. In such cases pethidine is to be preferred.* (*See also* the Symposium on Post-operative Pain, *Brit. J. Anæsth.*, 1967, **39**, Sept.)

Preparation for Emergency Operations.—Fluid and electrolyte balance must be attended to.

The problem of regurgitation and vomiting is not confined to obstetrical and emergency abdominal operations.

A Ryle's tube (6–12 gauge, 4–7 mm. diameter) should be passed through the nose, or an œsophageal tube (gauge 12) passed through either the nose or mouth. The stomach should then be aspirated with the patient supine and on each side in turn. When there is retroperistalsis, e.g., in acute intestinal obstruction, the stomach may refill from the duodenum between the time of emptying and the introduction of the endotracheal tube (*see also* p. 217 *et seq.*).

The Hydrodynamics of Regurgitation.—The normal intragastric pressure is 5–7 cm. H_2O and double this in advanced pregnancy. This is well below the pressure required for reflux through the cardia.† Even when the stomach is distended the pressure is unlikely to be greater than 18 cm. H_2O, unless there is contraction of the abdominal muscles.‡

* Painter, N. S., *Proc. R. Soc. Med.*, 1963, **56**, 800.
† Spence, A. A., and others, *Anæsthesia*, 1967, **22**, 249.
‡ Mullane, E. J., *Lancet*, 1954, **1**, 1209.

The Hydrodynamics of Regurgitation, *continued.*

If the glottis is maintained at a height in centimetres above the cardia greater than the intragastric pressure in cm. H_2O, i.e., with a head-up tilt of 40–45°, and if the abdominal muscles are prevented from contracting, then regurgitation is unlikely.[*]

Measurements of intragastric pressure during the fasciculation following injection of suxamethonium are usually not greatly increased,[†] but in about 12 per cent of patients a rise greater than 19 cm. H_2O occurs.[‡] This evidence might suggest that suxamethonium should not be used for intubation in such patients even with a high head-up tilt, as gastric contents could be forced up to the glottis by the increase in intragastric pressure. The question needs clarification as reported pressure measurements are not in agreement.[†‡]

Vomiting is an active reflex action controlled by a centre in the medulla. Regurgitation is a passive flow of gastric contents and is made more likely by gravity acting on an inefficient cardia[§] or a cardia made inefficient by the presence of an indwelling tube. This can usually be prevented by a head-up tilt.

Methods of Induction of Anæsthesia when the Stomach may not be Empty.—Before induction, the following equipment must be checked to see that it is present and correct. A tilting table, laryngoscopes, cuffed endotracheal tubes with syringe to inflate cuff, sucker with catheters, and bronchoscope with suitable suction tubes.

The indwelling stomach or Ryle's tube should usually be removed after aspiration and just before anæsthesia is induced so as not to interfere with the integrity of the cardiac sphincter. If necessary the tube can be reinserted during the operation.

1. In the head-down position with a slow careful induction with the avoidance of coughing, using gas–oxygen and a volatile agent and a little carbon dioxide to maintain the urge to breathe. In this method one relies on gravity, suction, and the presence of an active laryngeal reflex to prevent aspiration of gastric contents ; vomiting may occur. In very ill patients the laryngeal reflex may not be very active. This is probably the best method for occasional or inexperienced anæsthetists or for patients in whom intubation is likely to be difficult and therefore time consuming (on anatomical grounds).[||]

2. In the lateral position (left) with the table tilted head downwards. Induction with halothane 2–4 per cent in pure oxygen, 6 l. per min., followed by suxamethonium and intubation in this same lateral position.[¶]

3. In the head-up position with a 40–45° tilt. A footpiece must be used to prevent the patient slipping onto the floor, and the

[*] Snow, R. G., and Nunn, J. F., *Brit. J. Anæsth.,* 1959, **31**, 493.
[†] Spence, A. A., and others, *Anæsthesia,* 1967, **22**, 249.
[‡] Roe, R. B., *Ibid.,* 1962, **17**, 179.
[§] Dinnick, O. P., *Proc. R. Soc. Med.,* 1957, **50**, 547.
[||] Inkster, J. S., *Brit. J. Anæsth.,* 1963, **35**, 160.
[¶] Bourne, J. G., *Anæsthesia,* 1962, **17**, 379.

anæsthetist may require a stool to stand on. In ill patients, the table can be arranged so that he is really sitting as in the dental chair. Following pre-oxygenation, anæsthesia is induced by either thiopentone or a half-and-half mixture of cyclopropane and oxygen, followed rapidly by either suxamethonium or gallamine 80–160 mg. With the former relaxant, muscle fasciculations may occasionally increase the intragastric pressure, and with the latter, intubation may take rather longer but is less likely to be accompanied by the appearance of gastric contents near the glottis.*

It has been suggested that pressure over the cricoid during induction will prevent regurgitation by compressing the œsophagus.† This could be combined with any of the other methods.

Once the endotracheal tube is in the larynx and its cuff inflated, danger from aspiration of gastric contents during induction is past.

Perforated Peptic Ulcer.—The operation is usually short; the patient is usually shocked; he is very liable to post-operative chest complications. Cases with this condition are usually acute emergencies, i.e., their stomachs are likely to contain vomitable material. Moreover, the surgeon is likely to handle and compress the stomach, expelling some of its contents into the œsophagus. For these reasons a cuffed endotracheal tube should usually be passed, to protect the air-passages from contamination. Precautions must be taken to prevent aspiration of gastric contents during induction of anæsthesia and these will in many cases include the passage of a Ryle's or œsophageal tube beforehand. The experienced anæsthetist may care to pass the cuffed tube with the head of the table tilted upwards 45° using either cyclopropane and oxygen in equal proportions, or in stronger and less handicapped patients, thiopentone, following withdrawal of the stomach tube and consequent restoration of the function of the cardiac sphincter. In either case a relaxant will probably be used. Beginners might be wiser to use gas–oxygen–ether with the table tilted downwards and with an efficient suction catheter near at hand in case of vomiting during induction. It must be remembered that a stomach tube can lie unresisted in the trachea of an ill patient, so before such a tube is used for irrigation, its accurate position must be verified. Most workers now prefer the pre-oxygenation, thiopentone, relaxant, nitrous oxide, hyperventilation technique described on p. 467. Intercostal block with splanchnic block is an elegant, but more difficult technique. (*See* pp. 354, 357.)

Acute Intestinal Obstruction.—Factors to be considered are :—

1. The degree of shock present.
2. The presence or absence of regurgitation or vomiting. The former is a passive process requiring no muscular force : the

* Snow, R. G., and Nunn, J. F., *Brit. J. Anæsth.*, 1959, **31**, 493.
† Sellick, B. A., *Lancet*, 1961, **1**, 404.

Acute Intestinal Obstruction, *continued.*

latter is a muscular reflex act. The former is aided by a head-down tilt and rendered less likely if the head is tilted upwards 45°.

3. The degree of distension.

4. The degree of electrolyte imbalance.

In both normal people and those with intestinal obstruction, much fluid is excreted by the proximal small intestine, only to be reabsorbed lower down. In high obstruction this subsequent reabsorption is prevented, hence vomiting, and interference with fluid balance. Low obstruction gives rise to distension. Vomiting causes loss of chlorides and alkalosis, and consequently great fluid loss and dehydration. Distension causes interference with circulation of the bowel wall, and pressure on the great veins causes reduced venous return to the heart, a low blood-pressure, and interference with cardiac action.

Biochemical changes in intestinal obstruction include : (1) Hæmoconcentration ; (2) Reduction of fixed base in serum ; (3) Diminution of plasma chlorides ; (4) Increased blood-urea and non-protein nitrogen ; (5) Increase in carbon-dioxide combining power of plasma ; (6) Acid urine, with perhaps ketone bodies and low urinary chloride.

The stomach should always be emptied by either a Ryle's or a wider bore œsophageal tube, preferably the latter. Either of these can be passed through the nose after preliminary cocainization. It should be introduced in the conscious patient, such introduction being made a little less unpleasant by sedative premedication, together with instructions for the patient to suck an amethocaine lozenge beforehand. Grave illness does not make this any less necessary. The tube should be taken out before induction of anæsthesia but may be reintroduced after induction and retained until the return of the reflexes. A patient with increasing cyanosis, tightly clenched jaws, and fæculent material issuing from the nose is a truly terrifying sight, and one which carries a bad prognosis. That which cannot be easily treated had better be prevented.

Intra- and extradural analgesia produces good relaxation, contracts the bowel, and does not interfere with the cough reflex although the efficiency of coughing may be greatly reduced in high blocks. It produces circulatory depression and is dangerous in shocked and debilitated patients, e.g., where systolic blood-pressure is below 100 mm. Hg. General anæsthesia is safer in ill subjects. The actual agents and techniques used to produce general anæsthesia vary with different workers. The following may be used : Cyclopropane ; thiopentone with gas–oxygen, trichloroethylene, halothane, or ether. A muscle relaxant will almost certainly be necessary.

Spinal analgesia will not reduce distension due to ileus associated with peritonitis.

Operations associated with Hæmorrhage.—Cyclopropane and halothane are very good for these cases. While the former maintains the blood-pressure, the latter increases tissue perfusion. Intradural and extradural block are seldom indicated. Full oxygenation through a patent airway is most important. Blood, or plasma volume expander in its absence, must be transfused, and hydrocortisone may be helpful.

Abdominoperineal Resection of Rectum.—Maximal relaxation is necessary and contracted intestines an advantage. Extra- or intradural analgesia with light general anæsthesia, or a muscle relaxant with light general anæsthesia, is suitable. As there is often considerable hæmorrhage, blood-drips, etc., must be set up. An endotracheal tube is desirable.

The writers prefer—in the usual patient who is submitted to this operation (i.e., an oldish, rather handicapped patient)—either a combination of thiopentone, pethidine, relaxant, and gas–oxygen, given through a large orotracheal tube with controlled respiration, or a continuous or single injection extradural block combined with oxygen and halothane given through an endotracheal tube with spontaneous (or occasionally assisted) respiration. A blood-drip is set up in a vein. If an extra length of plastic tubing is used, the arm can be secured to the table as it lies against the side of the patient. Intravenous drugs can be given either into the tubing or more elegantly into a televenous apparatus (*see* Chapter XIII).

Rectosigmoidectomy.—Heavy cinchocaine, 1·2 ml. diluted with cerebrospinal fluid, injected with patient's head elevated, followed by the level supine position, together with light general anæsthesia ; or low lumbar (or sacral) extradural block with light general anæsthesia. Patients do equally well with light general anæsthesia together with a relaxant.

Ventral Hernia.—General anæsthesia, together with a muscle relaxant, is suitable. Bucking and coughing on the endotracheal tube during extubation, with consequent strain on suture lines, should be prevented.

For fit adult patients, extra- or intradural analgesia can be used, to facilitate wound closure by contracting the bowels.

Operations for Portal Hypertension.*—These may include portacaval anastomosis, splenorenal anastomosis, and proximal gastric transection (isolation and ligation of the vascular connexions of the œsophagus and stomach together with excision of the portion of the stomach containing varices). Hæmatemesis may require œsophagotomy and ligation of varices as an emergency measure. The approach may be transthoracic.

PRE-OPERATIVE EVALUATION is important as liver function may be impaired. Hunt considers that operation is contraindicated where the serum albumin is less than 3·2 g. per cent. Serum pseudocholinesterase is of interest to the anæsthetist who contemplates use of suxamethonium, but it is uncommon

---

* Hunt, A. H., and others, *Lancet*, 1956, **1**, 881 ; and Bowen, R. A., *Anæsthesia*, 1960, **15**, 3.

for the value to be below the critical level of 25 units when prolonged apnœa is likely.

PREMEDICATION should not be heavy. *Induction* with a sleep dose of thiopentone is recommended, though larger doses may interfere with liver function.* Suxamethonium can be used for intubation if the possibility of a low serum pseudocholinesterase is borne in mind. Nitrous-oxide–oxygen–tubocurarine or oxygen–cyclopropane–with small doses of tubocurarine can be used for maintenance. The total dose of tubocurarine used may be high, since these cases often exhibit a resistance to the drug.

The patient should be fixed to the table in such a position that the incision can, if necessary, extend far laterally on each side, and so that venograms can be taken. The patient's arms are flexed and raised so that the hands rest on the opposite shoulders, where they are supported. The position is similar to that adopted at the commencement of the hornpipe dance.

It is vital to have a good intravenous drip and blood readily available. Bleeding is often considerable, owing to the raised venous pressure and blood should be started early during the operation. Swab weighing helps the anæsthetist to keep pace with blood-loss.

Gastrectomy.—Before operation, many surgeons like the patient to swallow a Ryle's tube, so that the stomach can be aspirated and kept empty. This is a most unpleasant experience for the patient. Other surgeons favour the passage of a Ryle's or an œsophageal tube after anæsthesia has been induced.

PASSAGE OF RYLE'S TUBE IN CONSCIOUS PATIENT.—The patient sits up and a well-lubricated tube (glycerin or liquid paraffin) is inserted into a patent naris, which has been cocainized. The patient sips water while the tube is advanced with each act of swallowing. It should be inserted until the third mark is at the naris. A tube which is too soft should be discarded, as it must not collapse when subjected to the negative pressure of the sucker. Distance from incisor teeth to cardia averages 17 in. (43 cm.). A Ryle's tube may be in the trachea without either the patient or the anæsthetist being aware of it. Plastic tubes are usually preferable to those made of rubber.

PASSAGE OF RYLE'S TUBE IN UNCONSCIOUS PATIENT.— Steen recommends the following excellent method for the passage of a rubber tube. (A plastic tube can frequently be introduced into the stomach 'blind'.) A well-lubricated Ryle's tube is inserted into a No. 6 Magill nasotracheal tube so that its tip is just within the lumen of the larger tube near the bevelled end. This is then passed blindly or with the aid of a laryngoscope into the œsophagus from the nose. The Ryle's tube is now inserted well into the stomach through the Magill tube. When aspiration of stomach contents shows its correct position, the

---

* Dundee, J. W., *Thiopentone and Other Thiobarbiturates*, 1956, 174. London and Edinburgh: E. & S. Livingstone.

Magill tube is withdrawn and the Ryle's tube held firmly against the posterior wall of the pharynx as the larger tube leaves the nose. Intermittent suction is kept up during the operation.

The authors generally use one of the following techniques : A. (1) The intravenous injection of 0·3 to 0·5 g. of thiopentone in 2·5 per cent solution through the televenous apparatus (*see* Chapter XIII) or through a Mitchell non-clotting needle. (2) Through the same needle, injection of suxamethonium 50–100 mg. (perhaps preceded by gallamine 20 mg. in order to avoid the muscular fasciculation of suxamethonium). (3) Inflation with mixture of nitrous oxide 6 l. and oxygen 2 l. (4) Spraying of cords with 4 per cent solution of lignocaine, via a Macintosh laryngeal spray and a laryngoscope. (5) Insertion, under direct laryngoscopic vision, of a large (size 8–12) Magill rubber endotracheal tube with inflatable cuff. (6) Maintenance with additional doses of muscle relaxant, and pethidine, together with the gas and oxygen mixture in a semi-closed circuit. B. (1) Induction with thiopentone 200–250 mg. (2) Injection of gallamine 120–160 mg. or tubocurarine 20–30 mg. (3) Inflation of the lungs with gas and oxygen. (4) Intubation with a large cuffed tube, followed by controlled respiration, and hyperventilation (up to 20 l. per min.), with gas and oxygen and such additional doses of relaxant as may be necessary to keep the patient still, relaxed, and free from reflexes. Slight flapping of the abdominal wall (hiccups) is the usual signal that more relaxant is needed and this should generally be gallamine 40 mg. or tubocurarine 6 mg. (5) Neostigmine and atropine to restore normal ventilation.

The recommencement of spontaneous respiration after controlled apnœa requires, in addition to reversal of the relaxant, an active respiratory centre and an excitatory stimulus applied to the upper air passages which is not obturated by local analgesia of the mucosa. Hence sedative drugs, e.g., opiates and pethidine, and local analgesic sprays and ointment should be used sparingly in such cases.

The passage of a cuffed endotracheal tube is advisable, as the surgeon may expel blood-clot or other material from the stomach, up into the œsophagus and pharynx, even in the presence of a freely patent Ryle's tube.

Alternative techniques are :—

1. Cyclopropane, muscle relaxant, intubation.
2. Thiopentone, gas–oxygen–ether.
3. Extra- or intradural analgesia with light general anæsthesia. This method is less satisfactory in upper than in lower abdominal operations because of the hypotension and hiccuping which may occur.
4. Intercostal block, splanchnic block, light general anæsthesia.
5. Halothane and oxygen, with small doses of relaxant when required.

The depth of anæsthesia needs to be greatest :—

1. During the incision of the skin.
2. During the initial abdominal exploration.
3. While the cardiac end of the stomach is under tension.
4. During the closure of the peritoneum.

Gastrectomy, *continued.*

The aim should be to have the patient breathing deeply, moving about the bed, and coughing as soon after the end of the operation as possible.

The Cœliac Plexus Reflex.—Mechanical stimulation of the cœliac plexus (by retractors, packs, the gall-bladder bridge, etc.) may result in sudden reflex arterial hypotension. This autonomic reflex may be obtunded by curare.*

Hiccup is a troublesome reflex, too often associated with present-day methods of light anæsthesia. Its exact cause is ill understood, but it is likely to be associated with a high nervous tone, and light anæsthesia. The best method of prevention and treatment is the use of adequate amounts of a relaxant drug. It may also yield to: (1) Inhalation of amyl nitrite. (2) Inhalation of concentrated ether vapour for a few breaths. (3) Inhalation of ammonia. (4) Intravenous injection of methylamphetamine. (5) Increased depth of general anæsthesia. (6) Block of vagus nerves near cardia. This also has prophylactic value. (7) Intravenous injection of methyl phenidate (ritalin), 20 mg.†

Anæsthesia for Complete Vagotomy.—If the surgeon wants to ensure complete section of the vagi according to the technique of Burge and Vane whereby gastric contractions can be recorded by stimulating the abdominal vagus nerves with an electrode which encircles the œsophagus,‡ care must be taken not to depress the vagi pharmacologically. Thus belladonna alkaloids must be entirely avoided. In a series of 150 patients undergoing this operation for peptic ulcer, there were no untoward cardiovascular effects due to uninhibited vagal activity.§

Operations on the Biliary Tract.—Vitamin K analogue should be given before operation. Anæsthetic technique is similar to that used for gastrectomy. High elevation of a gall-bladder bridge may cause hypotension by interfering with venous return by obstructing the vena cava. The dynamics of the biliary ducts must be considered in connexion with pre- and post-operation pain relief in patients with biliary disease. Normally the increase in intrabiliary pressure required to overcome the tone of the sphincter of Oddi does not cause pain. Analgesics (e.g., morphine and pethidine) may, by stimulating this sphincter to contract, increase the intrabiliary pressure up to 20 cm. of water, and thus produce pain. Parasympathetic stimulators have a similar effect. To relieve biliary colic, therefore, the dose of analgesic must be great enough to cause cerebral depression. The following drugs lower intrabiliary pressure by relaxing the sphincter: (1) Amyl nitrite; (2) Nitroglycerin 1 mg.; (3) Papaverine 150 mg. Atropine, even up to 2 mg., is disappointing in this respect.

* Burstein, C. L., *Fundamental Considerations in Anesthesia*, 2nd ed., 1955, Ch. 7. New York: Macmillan.
† Vasiloff, N., *Canad. Anæsth. Soc. J.*, 1965, **12**, 306.
‡ Burge, H., and Vane, J. R., *Brit. med. J.*, 1958, **1**, 615.
§ Riddoch, M. E., and Clark, C. G., *Brit. J. Anæsth.*, 1962, **34**, 464.

Cases of *acute hæmorrhagic pancreatitis** are bad anæsthetic risks no matter what agent and method are used, so that obscure abdominal emergencies should have serum amylase tests done, and operation can be avoided. Intravenous trasylol has been recommended.† For description of anæsthesia for *excision of islet-cell tumours of pancreas* see Hargadon, J. J., and Ormston, T. O. G., *Brit. J. Anæsth.*, 1963, **35**, 807.

Sigmoidoscopy.—If *general anæsthesia* is required for this, successful administration may not be without difficulty. The patient is usually required to lie on his side. A suitable technique is halothane and oxygen, or thiopentone, a relaxant, and gas–oxygen. Dilatation of the anal sphincter may cause laryngeal spasm or other respiratory difficulty, unless the reflex mechanism is subdued, and in certain cases, endotracheal intubation may be desirable. *Extradural sacral block* is satisfactory in these cases too but may not relieve pain due to the injection of air.

Anæsthesia for Leaking Aortic Aneurysm.‡—This condition carries a high mortality. Patients are usually in poor general condition and may be suffering from shock, ileus due to retroperitoneal hæmatoma, or hæmatemesis from leakage into the duodenum of the aneurysm. Large volumes of blood may be required with the usual risks which may follow massive transfusion, such as failure of clotting mechanism, and calcium and potassium imbalance requiring intravenous calcium. Metabolic acidosis may occur and must be suitably treated by intravenous infusions of 2·74 per cent sodium bicarbonate solution.§

If the lesion is above the origin of the renal arteries the outlook is especially grave as the application of an aortic tourniquet is likely to cause renal and spinal cord ischæmia with irreversible damage.

Before induction of anæsthesia, inflatable tourniquets should be placed high up on the thighs, to be blown up and let down gradually after the aortic clamp has been released.

The technique of general anæsthesia should provide endotracheal intubation free from the risk of aspiration of stomach contents with induction preferably in the head-down position because of the associated shock. Maintenance should be light general anæsthesia with non-depolarizing relaxants as required. The patient may be in a critical shocked condition. It may be necessary to proceed with operation without waiting for resuscitative measures. Blood transfusion should be started as quickly as possible. Coughing and straining are to be avoided lest the aneurysm should rupture. It may therefore be wise to avoid pre-operative passage of an œsophageal tube, and to use a muscle relaxant to avoid any danger of coughing on the endotracheal tube.

ANÆSTHESIA FOR RUPTURED THORACIC AORTA.‖—This may be required for surgical repair following trauma in road traffic accidents. Cardiopulmonary bypass may be necessary.

---

* Fleming, L. B., *Brit. med. J.*, 1968, **1**, 813.
† *Ibid.*, 1966, **2**, 1580.
‡ Knight, P. F., *Anæsthesia*, 1963, **18**, 151; and Elliott, J., *Ibid.*, 1967, **22**, 406.
§ Brooks, D. K., and Feldman, S. A., *Ibid.*, 1962, **17**, 161.
‖ Roberts, J. C., and Lord, P. W., *Ibid.*, 1967, **22**, 415.

Bilateral Adrenalectomy.—This may be combined with bilateral extirpation of the ovaries and may be completed in one or two stages ; it may be done for carcinoma of the breast or prostate or Cushing's syndrome. Patients suffering from secondary carcinomatosis may require special care directed to their bones, their blood-picture, and their pleura—in case of effusion. Pre-operatively, a salt-free diet, diuretics, digitalis, sedatives. Cortisone 100 mg. should be given one hour before operation and four times daily on the first, three times daily on the second post-operative day, and then in gradually decreasing amounts until it can be taken by mouth. Intravenous phenylephrine or noradrenaline during operation may be required and may be needed in the postoperative few days. Later sodium chloride must be increased. During operation thiopentone and pethidine are not usually needed in large amounts whereas doses of gallamine and tubocurarine are apt to be greater than normal, perhaps because of the deficient pseudocholinesterase in the blood of these usually ill patients. General anæsthesia with good muscular relaxation is suitable, while extradural block is often satisfactory.

Phæochromocytoma.*—This is a tumour of the adrenal medullary cells of chromaffin origin, which, although it may be histologically benign, may be dangerous because of excessive secretion of adrenaline and noradrenaline. The growth may not be confined to the adrenal but may occur wherever chromaffin tissue is found, e.g., in the paravertebral spaces, near the great vessels of the abdomen, in the organ of Zuckerkandl near the aortic bifurcation, and in the cœliac plexus. The patient exhibits hypertension, either paroxysmal or continuous, hyperhidrosis, and elevated basal metabolic rate with some fever perhaps. Some cases of hypotension have also been described.† The operation is to remove the tumour, usually by the retropleural or retroperitoneal route. The condition is diagnosed by clinical examination ; estimation of urinary catecholamines which may be 100–300 micrograms daily (normal 20–40) ; certain radiological investigations, and by pharmacological agents, e.g., phentolamine, 5 mg. intravenous, causing a fall in blood-pressure or histamine, 0·05 mg., causing a rise (this may be dangerous).

Pre-operative care : Perhaps intravenous dibenamine, 5 mg. per kg. or other sympatholytic drugs to control blood-pressure, together with sodium chloride. Pre-operative blood-volume studies have been found useful.

Anæsthetic technique must cater for : (1) Good relaxation—gallamine is not the best drug to use because it may cause tachycardia ; (2) The possibility of accidental pneumothorax ; (3) The effects of excess adrenaline or noradrenaline during

* Goldfien, A., *Anesthesiology*, 1963, **24**, 462 ; Thompson, J. E., and Arrowood, J., *Ibid.*, 1954, **15**, 658 ; Helps, E. P. W., *Lancet*, 1955, **2**, 267 ; Mushin, W. W., *Anæsthesia*, 1957, **12**, 15 ; Gebbie, D. M., and others, *Canad. Anæsth. Soc. J.*, 1967, **14**, 39 ; Robertson, A. I. G., *Proc. R. Soc. Med.*, 1962, **55**, 432 ; and Englebert, E. R., and others, *Canad. Anæsth. Soc. J.*, 1966, **13**, 598.

† Richmond, J., and others, *Lancet*, 1961, **2**, 904 ; Hamrin, B., *Ibid.*, 1962, **2**, 123 ; and Ramsey, J. D., and Longlands, J. H. M., *Ibid.*, 1962, **2**, 126.

operation when the tumour is manipulated (propranolol may be useful here to block β-receptors); (4) Circulatory depression when tumour is removed. Hypoxia which stimulates medullary secretion must be avoided, as also must cyclopropane. Excessive hypertension may be controlled by the intravenous injection of piperoxan hydrochloride 20 mg. or phentolamine (rogitine, regitine) 5 mg., while a continuous intravenous drip of nor-adrenaline 4 mg. per litre (which is not inactivated by phentol amine) or of phenylephrine 20 mg. per litre may be needed during the first post-operative days. Angiotensin has also been found useful in maintaining blood-pressure in the post-operative period (2 μg. per min. for up to 2½ min.);* (5) Massive blood transfusion may be necessary; (6) Careful monitoring is also advised—in particular of central venous pressure, because of the sudden changes in cardiovascular hæmodynamics which may occur.

Halothane has been suggested as the agent of choice for these operations.

(*See also* Rollason, W. N., *Brit. J. Anæsth.*, 1964, **36**, 251; Murphy, M., Prior, F. N., and Joseph, S., *Ibid.*, 1964, **36**, 813; Schnelle, M., and others, *Surg. Clin. N. Amer.*, 1965, **45**, 991; de Blasi, S., *Brit. J. Anæsth.*, 1966, **38**, 740; and Engelbrecht, E. R., Hugill, J. T., and Graves, H. B., *Canad. Anæsth. Soc. J.*, 1966, **13**, 598.)

Neuroblastoma.—This is a catecholamine-secreting malignant tumour arising from the sympathetic nervous system in infants and children, situated in the retroperitoneal or retropleural region. It may secrete catecholamines during surgery and should be managed like a phæochromocytoma with α-adrenergic blocking agents, phentolamine, and blood transfusion.†

Hernia.—The anæsthesia depends on the degree of relaxation demanded by the surgeon. *Extradural block*, using 25–30 ml. of 1·5 per cent lignocaine solution, is suitable in fit subjects. If *spinal analgesia* is used, block to T.9 is necessary and is obtained by, for example, light cinchocaine, 10–12 ml.; 0·5 per cent cinchocaine, 1·6 ml.; procaine, 150 mg. There may be discomfort when the sac is under tension : this can be eased by the injection of a little procaine into the neck of the sac. Where much relaxation is not required, light *general anæsthesia* is indicated, and should the surgeon wish it, a muscle relaxant can be injected, together with such a combination as gas, oxygen, and thiopentone ; halothane ; cyclopropane ; gas–oxygen and ether. Thiopentone, pethidine, gas and oxygen, and gallamine or tubocurarine is also a very good combination.

Paravertebral block of T.10–L.2 is excellent for cases of strangulated hernia (*see* p. 347), and regional block is also favoured in normal cases by some surgeons and anæsthetists (*see* p. 362).

Post-operative chest complications frequently follow these operations, especially in fit young men who smoke cigarettes, no matter what anæsthetic agent is used. They should, consequently, be

---

* *Brit. med. J.*, 1966, **1**, 1353.
† Farman, J. V., *Brit. J. Anæsth.*, 1965, **37**, 866.

Hernia, *continued.*

advised to avoid smoking for the month preceding operation, and be taught how to breathe deeply and how to cough effectively. In addition they will require vigorous 'shake-up' treatment after operation.

Operations for incisional hernia require profound relaxation.

The chief danger in operation for strangulated hernia is from aspiration of stomach contents into the chest during induction of anæsthesia. *See also under* ACUTE INTESTINAL OBSTRUCTION (p. 511).

Hæmorrhoidectomy.—The choice is between :—

1. *Light general anæsthesia* with a muscle relaxant.

2. *Extradural sacral block*—15–20 ml. of 1·5 per cent lignocaine or 0·5 per cent bupivacaine* with adrenaline (*see* p. 431).

3. *Thiopentone* (0·5 to 1 g.) and a relaxant (e.g., gallamine, 40–100 mg.) ; gas and oxygen should be given at the same time. Occasionally the complication of laryngeal spasm will require, in addition to the use of a muscle relaxant, halothane, cyclopropane, ether, or trichloroethylene. If this troublesome accident shows itself, it may well be prudent to ask the surgeon to interrupt his highly stimulating manipulations until control of breathing has once again been obtained.

4. *Low intradural spinal* (S.4–5), e.g., procaine, 60 mg., or cinchocaine, 0·5 per cent, 0·6 ml. diluted with cerebrospinal fluid, between L.4 and L.5 with patient sitting. In men of prostate age, spinal analgesia is better avoided, so that it will not be blamed for any disorders of micturition which may arise post-operatively.

5. *Local infiltration* with lignocaine or procaine. From a point 1 in. (2·5 cm.) posterior to the anus, with the index finger of the left hand in the rectum, 1·5 per cent lignocaine–adrenaline solution is injected: total amount, 25 ml. Only one site of injection used, and anus and anal canal are ensheathed by a cylinder of procaine solution.

6. *Presacral block.*—This consists in depositing 8 ml. of local analgesic solution in front of the fourth sacral foramen on each side. With the left index finger in the rectum, palpating the fourth foramen, a 12-cm. needle is inserted through the ischiorectal fossa until its point is near the finger-tip; the solution is now injected, and soon the sphincter relaxes. During the injection—which is, of course, bilateral—the patient can be lightly anæsthetized. Post-operative pain is said to be greatly reduced.†

Proctocaine, which is frequently used after anal operations, contains butyl-*p*-aminobenzoate (butesin) 6 per cent, benzyl alcohol 5 per cent, procaine base 1·5 per cent in sterile almond oil. It should be warmed before use to make it less viscous and should not be injected immediately beneath the mucosa.

Injection into the area of 1 per cent lignocaine in 10 per cent dextran (Loder's solution) is useful in relieving post-operative pain.‡ Xyloproct suppositories can also be used.

---

* Watt, M. J., Ross, D. M., and Atkinson, R. S., *Anæsthesia*, 1968, **23**, 2; and *Ibid.*, 1968, **23**, July.
† Bracey, D. W., *Brit. med. J.*, 1965, **2**, 880.
‡ Willis, J. H., *Ibid.*, 1965, **2**, 1002.

The first post-operative bowel action can be made more tolerable by the self-administration of gas and oxygen, equal parts, or trichloroethylene-air.

Ventilation Failure in Injuries of the Chest and Abdomen.—

CENTRAL VENTILATION FAILURE.—Due to depression of the respiratory centre by morphine, alcohol, anæsthetics, brain damage, and circulatory failure. There is likely to be depressed breathing without dyspnœa and it may be overlooked.

PERIPHERAL VENTILATION FAILURE.—Due to : (1) Pain ; (2) Paradoxical respiration ; (3) High paralysed diaphragm (perhaps occurring reflexly due to pain) ; (4) Lung compression from pneumothorax, hæmothorax, gastro-intestinal ileus, or ruptured diaphragm; (5) Airway obstruction due to secretions, blood, vomit, pulmonary œdema transudate ; (6) Traumatic pneumonopathy (traumatic wet lung). Œdema of lung resulting from neurogenic, mechanical, circulatory, and chemical factors. All of these are made worse by difficulty in coughing. (*See* Barrett, N. R., *Lancet*, 1960, **1**, 294 ; and Harley, H. R. S., *Proc. R. Soc. Med.*, 1961, **54**, 558.)

EAR, NOSE, AND THROAT SURGERY*

In throat and nose surgery, the problems of anæsthesia are related to the fact that the operations are carried out on the upper respiratory tract. The anæsthetist must preserve a clear airway, while allowing the surgeon adequate access, and must take steps to prevent soiling of the trachea and bronchial tree with blood and debris. The problems are most evident during operations on the larynx itself.

Ear surgery is associated with the performance of delicate manœuvres under microscopic vision. The patient's head must remain immobile and blood must not be allowed to obscure the very small surgical field.

The following factors should be considered when surgery is to be carried out on the upper respiratory tract:—

1. Premedication must be adequate, but not heavy enough to cause a sluggish cough reflex after operation.
2. Smooth induction will reduce the incidence and degree of hæmorrhage.
3. No topical analgesic should be applied to the larynx or trachea, as the cough reflex must be brisk after operation.
4. Entrance of blood and debris into the chest must be prevented by the use of an inflatable cuff on an endotracheal tube and/or efficient pharyngeal packing.
5. The use of a slight reversed Trendelenburg position minimizes venous oozing.

Induction with thiopentone, intubation under a relaxant, and maintenance with gas, oxygen, and trichloroethylene, with or without pethidine, can usually be relied on to provide a safe and smooth technique. Halothane and oxygen are also satisfactory.

Intranasal Operations.—If topical or regional analgesia is not used, general anæsthesia should be maintained through an orotracheal

---

* *See also* Ballantine, R. I. W., and Jackson, I., *Anæsthesia*, 1955, **10**, 279.

Intranasal Operations, *continued.*

tube sealed off with a cuff or a pharyngeal or nasopharyngeal pack. These packs should not be removed until the return of the patient's cough reflex. Forgetfulness to remove a pharyngeal pack on the other hand is one of the easiest mistakes for an anæsthetist to make and it can readily prove fatal. Connexions to the tube can conveniently be led down over the patient's chest. In this position, particularly if the surgeon asks for flexion of the neck, there is a liability for the tube to kink—a non-kinking tube, such as a flexometallic or Oxford tube, is advantageous. Muscle relaxants will aid intubation, but care must be taken to see that the cough reflex is active at the end of the operation. General anæsthesia may be combined with topical application of vasoconstrictors to the nose (e.g., cocaine 4–10 per cent) to reduce bleeding (*see* p. 326).

Tonsillectomy in Children.—

PREMEDICATION.—Provision of the right psychological atmosphere is of the greatest value in obtaining smooth induction of anæsthesia without tears. Sedative premedication must be given carefully because of possible depressant effect on the cough reflex. When the facilities of a recovery room are available and the nursing supervision before and after operation is skilled and alert, heavy basal narcosis can be prescribed so that the child arrives in the anæsthetic room asleep. This may be by rectal thiopentone 1 ml. of 2 per cent solution per lb. body-weight; or oral trimeprazine (vallergan) 1·5 mg. per lb. body-weight given 2 hours pre-operatively. Other recommended premedication routines include methylpentynol,* 500 mg. for ages 2–4, 750 mg. ages 4–8, and 1 g. ages 8–10, 1 hour before induction of anæsthesia. Morphine and atropine or hyoscine can be given by injection in dosage on a weight basis, or (as a rough measure), according to age, 1 minim per year plus 1, of the standard ampoule containing papaveretum 20 mg. and hyoscine 0·4 mg. in 1 ml.

Atropine or hyoscine can be given by injection once oral or rectal sedative medication has had its effect. The authors prefer hyoscine 0·2 mg. intramuscularly. Otherwise hyoscine 0·4–0·8 mg. can be given by mouth.

Where skilled nursing facilities do not exist it is safer to avoid all sedative premedication and use atropine or hyoscine alone for premedication. This is especially true before guillotine tonsillectomy when rapid return of reflexes is essential.

DISSECTION TONSILLECTOMY.—Many anæsthetists prefer an endotracheal tube which may be nasal or oral. An oral tube may be kept clear of the operative field if a Doughty blade is used.† The use of a tube allows the plane of anæsthesia to be more easily maintained, reduces oozing, and obviates respiratory obstruction. I.P.P.V. can be combined with it or the patient allowed to breathe spontaneously. The alternative is endopharyngeal insufflation using the Boyle-Davis gag, in which case the patient should be taken well down into Plane 3 before

---

* Gusterson, F. R., *Lancet*, 1955, **1**, 940.
† Doughty, A. G., *Ibid.*, 1957, **1**, 1074.

the mouth is opened and the operation commenced. If this is not done it may be difficult to maintain adequate anæsthesia until the end of the operation.

Nitrous-oxide–oxygen–ether, halothane, or thiopentone and relaxant are satisfactory techniques. Ethyl chloride can be used for blind intubation. The aim should be to have the patient coughing within a minute or two of the completion of the operation.

Adenoids can be curetted either with the endotracheal tube in situ or after its withdrawal when the cough reflex has returned.

The patient should be returned to the ward in the tonsil position (semi-prone, prevented from rolling on to his face by a pillow beneath the chest, and prevented from rolling supine by bringing the lower arm behind the body) and remain in this position until full consciousness is regained.

GUILLOTINE TONSILLECTOMY.—Nitrous-oxide–oxygen induction, open ethyl chloride, divinyl ether, or trichloroethylene, followed, if necessary, by a little diethyl ether. It is necessary to produce relaxation of jaw muscles—the masseters, pterygoids, and temporales to allow easy insertion and opening of the gag ; relaxation of the palatoglossus in the anterior pillar and of the palatopharyngeus in the posterior pillar, and of the superior constrictor of the pharynx : the pharyngeal reflex must be absent, but coughing must return quickly.

Premedication is atropine alone. The teeth are examined and any loose ones noted : if these are disturbed they must be accounted for. A Doyen gag is inserted and if possible opened while the child is conscious and he is then anæsthetized, preferably commencing with gas and continuing with open ethyl chloride. Children over five may require in addition a little ether. The tonsils are removed in the supine position with the child breathing air and he is then immediately turned on to his side while the adenoids are curetted. He returns to his bed in the tonsil position, a welter of blood, sweat, and tears, but in skilled surgical and anæsthetic hands, the results can be good.

ANÆSTHESIA FOR POST-TONSILLECTOMY HÆMORRHAGE can be a grave responsibility. The patient is likely to have a stomach full of blood clot and to be shocked. After atropine premedication and with the patient on his side in the Trendelenburg position, anæsthesia is perhaps most safely induced with gas, oxygen, trichloroethylene, and ether. The patient is then turned on his back ; his pharynx is sucked clear of blood and an oral endotracheal tube is passed. A nasal tube after adenoid curettage might not be welcomed by the surgeon. Post-operative suction and *blood transfusion* are both *likely to be necessary* while vomiting of blood after operation must be expected and care taken to prevent its aspiration into the trachea.* (*See also* Gorham, A. P., *Anæsthesia*, 1964, **19**, 565.)

Mortality of tonsillectomy in children about 1 in 1800.†

* Davies, D. D., *Brit. J. Anæsth.*, 1964, **36**, 244.
† Alpert, J. J., Peterson, O. L., and Colton, T., *Lancet*, 1968, **1** , 1319.

Tonsillectomy in Adults.—

LOCAL ANALGESIA.—*See* p. 333.

GENERAL ANÆSTHESIA.—A nasotracheal tube is generally mos convenient, though an oral tube can be used. The anæsthetic technique should provide quiet respiration without straining but with return of pharyngeal reflexes at the end of operation Spontaneous or I.P.P.V. can be employed.

Anæsthesia for post-tonsillectomy hæmorrhage in the adult is simila to that for acute intestinal obstruction and a tube must be inserted into the trachea without the aspiration of blood or vomitus.

Laryngectomy.*—The available methods are :—

1. With no pre-existing tracheostomy. A cuffed endotracheal tube is passed, and a tracheostomy performed towards the end of the operation.

2. Tracheostomy performed immediately before the operation under general or local analgesia—the insertion of a cuffed tube through the opening.

3. Anæsthesia through a pre-existing tracheostomy opening.

ANÆSTHETIC MANAGEMENT.—It is important to assess the likelihood of narrowing of the laryngeal aperture by growth When there is obvious respiratory difficulty, it is wise to perform a preliminary tracheostomy under local analgesia. If there is any doubt, it is better to omit respiratory depressant drugs and give atropine or hyoscine alone for premedication. Otherwise pethidine and hyoscine make a good combination.

During induction of anæsthesia care must be taken that control of the airway is maintained. In some cases where there is respiratory obstruction it is difficult to inflate the lungs using a bag and mask. Distortion of the normal anatomy by tumour or œdema may render intubation difficult. In these circumstances the authors prefer to give a sleep dose of thiopentone through an indwelling Mitchell needle or televenous apparatus. Nitrous oxide and oxygen are given, and ability to inflate the lungs tested by manual compression of the reservoir bag. If this is readily achieved suxamethonium follows, the larynx sprayed with 4 per cent lignocaine, and a large-size cuffed endotracheal tube passed. (Occasionally it is only possible to pass a small tube, and a range of tubes should be available.) Anæsthesia is continued with nitrous oxide and oxygen, supplemented by trichloroethylene or halothane. The aim is to secure quiet respiration with laryngeal reflexes obtunded. Forced inspiration may lead to a negative pressure in neck veins with the danger of air embolism.

When the larynx is severed from the trachea, the endotracheal tube is removed. The surgeon inserts a sterile tube via the tracheostome. The authors have found a cuffed flexometallic endotracheal tube useful for this purpose. It can be led down over the sternum and the connexions kept clear of the surgical field.

---

* Coffin, S., *Anæsthesia*, 1955, **10**, 289.

An intravenous drip should be set up. Blood transfusion may be required, particularly if block dissection of the neck is undertaken.

For *laryngofissure,* a cuffed tube is inserted from the mouth while the early dissection is done. After a planned tracheostomy a smaller (number 5 or 6) cuffed, sterile short tube is placed in the trachea by the surgeon and connected to the anæsthetic machine.

PHARYNGOLARYNGECTOMY WITH COLONIC REPLACE-MENT.—*See* Gorham, A. P., Baskett, P. J. F., and Clement, J. A., *Anæsthesia,* 1965, **20,** 279.

Laryngoscopy.—Local analgesia (as for Bronchoscopy,* *see* p. 375) General anæsthesia (as for Bronchoscopy, *see* p. 574). The anæsthetist should be on the watch for respiratory obstruction due to a laryngeal growth (as for laryngectomy).

Anæsthesia for Perfusion with Cytotoxic Drugs in Cancer of the Head and Neck.†—Operation consists of exposure of the common carotid, its bifurcation, and the branches of the external carotid artery, and injection into the correct vessel (tested by the prior injection of the dye Disulphine blue) of the cytotoxic drug. Difficulties arising may be : (1) Inability to use facepiece ; (2) Difficulty in intubation ; (3) Artificial cyanosis due to the dye ; (4) Fall in B.P. due to the cytotoxic drug; (5) Acute respiratory obstruction following injection of drug; thus, routine tracheostomy is required if the neoplasm involves larynx, pharynx, or tongue.

Operations on the Middle Ear.—

MASTOID OPERATIONS.—Endotracheal anæsthesia in association with any standard anæsthetic is satisfactory provided that coughing and straining are avoided and every care taken to avoid oozing.

OPERATIONS FOR OTOSCLEROSIS.—Operations on the stapes require delicate surgical manipulations under microscopy. It is therefore important that there should be a dry surgical field. This may be achieved by:—

1. Use of local analgesia—lignocaine and adrenaline.
2. Scrupulous anæsthetic technique. Avoidance of coughing, straining, etc. A reinforced latex endotracheal tube ensures a clear airway.
3. Head-up tilt to assist venous drainage from the head.
4. Smooth quiet respiration can be achieved using agents such as the phenothiazine derivatives, halothane, chloroform.
5. Deliberate hypotension, e.g., trimetaphan.

PARACENTESIS OF DRUM.—Myringotomy for release of pus requires a short general anæsthetic, e.g., nitrous oxide, oxygen, halothane. Suction clearance of a collection of fluid in the middle ear under microscopy requires a quiet patient and tracheal intubation is often advisable.

---

* Orr, D., and Jones, I., *Anæsthesia,* 1968, **23,** 194.
† Condon, H. A., *Brit. J. Anæsth.,* 1963, **35,** 438.

ORTHOPÆDIC OPERATIONS

Manipulations, requiring good relaxation for a short time, are conveniently done under thiopentone or methohexitone, a relatively large dose being given just before the surgeon is ready to produce his trauma. A relaxant can be added if required.

Children who may require several operations, e.g., talipes, should be well premedicated.

Leg amputations may be done under unilateral intradural spinal analgesia, a method well tolerated in old people undergoing amputation for gangrene: care must be taken to keep the block unilateral, by maintaining the lateral position for 20–30 minutes after subarachnoid injection. Otherwise thiopentone, gas–oxygen with or without a relaxant, trichloroethylene, halothane, or cyclopropane; refrigeration analgesia can be used.

For operations on the limbs, more use should be made of various techniques of regional analgesia, including intravenous regional analgesia, sciatic nerve, and wrist and finger block, etc.

Brachial plexus block is most useful for operation on the upper limb, including reduction of shoulder dislocations (p. 336).

For insertion of the Smith-Petersen type pin, thiopentone with gas–oxygen and, if necessary, minimal trichloroethylene or halothane is also a satisfactory technique. Other workers employ relaxants and controlled respiration for hip operations in old patients. Unilateral spinal analgesia up to T.12 gives good relaxation, e.g., cinchocaine, 0·5 per cent, 1·4 ml. or procaine, 100–120 mg. The patient usually tolerates being turned on to his injured side quite well. Extradural analgesia also gives good results in experienced hands.* The operation can be done under local infiltration analgesia with careful premedication. Amethocaine, 1–2000, is infiltrated from the skin to the bone in the line of incision. An attempt is made to deposit solution between the fractured bone-ends from above the great trochanter, and also from a point just external to the femoral artery, located by its pulsation. Blood replacement is important. Ventilation is often made easier if an endotracheal tube is passed. In elderly patients, amount of thiopentone should be kept as small as possible.

Anæsthesia for Calf Muscle Denervation for Intermittent Claudication.—The operation is performed to divide branches of the medial popliteal nerve with the patient in the prone position. Mechanical stimulation of the nerves is necessary for their identification, so no myoneural blocking agents should be active at this time.

THYROID OPERATIONS

Diagnosis of Hyperthyroidism.—

1. Clinical observation.
2. Plasma protein-bound iodine estimation—a difficult test.
3. Uptake of radio-iodine.
4. B.M.R. estimation.

---

* Hill, P., Wharton, L., and Delaney, E. J., *Brit. J. Anæsth.*, 1962, **34**, 107.

Pre-operative Preparation.—The patient must be made safe for surgery by the physician, especially if suffering from hyperthyroidism. This must always be maximally controlled before operation. Rest in bed, full diet, sedatives, iodine, digitalis, and antithyroid drugs may be necessary, e.g., propyl methyl thiouracil 200 mg. q.h. or carbimazol 5 mg. q.h. or potassium perchlorate. The vascularity caused by the thiouracil drugs can be reduced if Lugol's solution (iodine 5 per cent in 10 per cent potassium iodide) is given 10 minims 4-hourly, during the 7–10 days before operation. The last agents will sometimes produce a basal metabolic rate lower than normal in the thyrotoxic patient by inhibiting the production of thyroid hormone, and if this is so, pre-operative sedation and basal narcosis must be prescribed with the fact of hypometabolism in mind. It is important to check the possibility of respiratory obstruction from retrosternal goitre, compression of the trachea or its deviation by examination of the radiographs.

Bad signs are : (1) Failure of pulse-rate to become less than 100 ; (2) Auricular fibrillation : this does not contra-indicate operation ; (3) History of previous heart failure ; (4) Failure to gain weight under medical treatment ; (5) Prolonged existence of disease ; (6) Vomiting, diarrhœa.

Premedication.—Full doses of sedatives (e.g., opiates, pethidine, barbiturates, phenothiazine drugs) may be required in nervous and anxious patients.

Anæsthetic Agents.—All the commonly used agents have their advocates : Gas–oxygen, gas–oxygen and ether, gas–oxygen and tricholoroethylene, gas–oxygen and thiopentone with or without intravenous pethidine and relaxant. Some use cyclopropane routinely : others fear it in the presence of cardiovascular abnormality. Intermittent doses of thiopentone or pethidine can be injected into the ankle veins, during the operation, if the patient is not settling well. Oxygen and halothane gives good results, while the chlorpromazine–promethazine–pethidine combination causes prolonged post-operative sedation which may be considered advantageous after these operations.

Airway.—Most anæsthetists are in favour of endotracheal airways ; some are against them. Endotracheal airways avoid respiratory obstruction and hypoxia, with oozing ; without their use post-operative tracheitis and mucus collection are lessened and a lighter plane of anæsthesia is tolerated.

A tube is almost essential : (1) If, on examination of the radiograph, the trachea is deviated or compressed ; (2) If goitre is retrosternal ; (3) If malignancy is suspected ; (4) If the vocal cords are functioning abnormally when viewed through a laryngeal mirror in husky, stridulous patients ; (5) In recurrent cases.

If in doubt it is better to intubate before the operation than during its course. The authors use a tube routinely.

Where pre-operative stridor is present, intubation should be performed under topical laryngeal analgesia, preceded by a period of inhalation of 100 per cent oxygen.

Thyroid Operations—Airway, *continued.*

Stimulation of the recurrent laryngeal nerve causes spasm of the corresponding cord, with a high-pitched crowing sound, when patient is not intubated. If nerve is divided, the cord first becomes abducted and flaccid ; later it assumes the cadaveric position between abduction and adduction. Later still, some voluntary control is gained.

Techniques of Intubation.—(1) Intravenous injections of thiopentone, a muscle relaxant (e.g., suxamethonium 30–100 mg.), and followed by direct vision oral intubation. (2) In anatomically difficult patients. After 0·2 to 0·4 g. of 2·5 per cent thiopentone solution is injected, the nose, pharynx, and larynx are efficiently sprayed with a topical analgesic, e.g., 4 per cent cocaine. The tube is passed into the nasopharynx and gas and oxygen and, if desired, a little trichloroethylene or halothane are given. Then tube is slipped into trachea. Failure can be followed by re-application of mask and a further attempt.

A cuffed tube is likely to cause more post-operative tracheitis than an uncuffed one and in the absence of I.P.P.V. is quite unnecessary.

TECHNIQUE FOR INTUBATION UNDER TOPICAL ANALGESIA.*—In patients with severe tracheal deviation or obstruction, it may be better to attempt intubation under topical analgesia. The patient should be premedicated and given an amethocaine lozenge to suck. He should then sit on a chair facing the anæsthetist, with a nurse supporting his head. A Eustachian catheter is slid over the back of the tongue to the epiglottis, the anæsthetist's finger acting as a guide. Lignocaine, 4 per cent solution, is now injected down the catheter in 1-ml. doses during inspiration, and after an interval the patient is placed supine and intubation of the larynx is performed.

Conduct of Anæsthesia.—The eyes should be oiled and protected from the mask, towels, etc. Hyperextension of the neck is unnecessary and should be avoided. A head-up tilt is said to reduce venous oozing. Infiltration of the skin and subcutaneous tissues in the zone of the incision reduces oozing in the skin flaps. Injection of 1–200,000 to 1–500,000 adrenaline-saline should precede the incision by 15 min. Cardiac arrhythmia may follow the administration of halothane, trichloroethylene, or cyclopropane in a patient into whose tissues adrenaline-saline has been infiltrated.†

The authors prefer a semi-closed circuit with a non-rebreathing valve. The arms and legs of the patient should be firmly secured to prevent inconvenient movement during the operation at the light plane of anæsthesia necessary. During the operation the blood-pressure and pulse-rate should be charted. The curve of the latter is more important than the actual rate, which increases on intubation, while the incision is being made, and during mobilization of the gland. If all is well, the rate decreases towards the end of operation. The trachea and pharynx

---

* Barron, D. W., *Anæsthesia*, 1959, **14**, 339.
† Rosen, M., and Roe, R. B., *Brit. J. Anæsth.*, 1963, **35**, 51.

should be aspirated with a sucker at the conclusion of the operation but vigorous coughing immediately after operation is to be avoided as it may contribute to reactionary hæmorrhage. If 20–50 mg. of suxamethonium are given before extubation and the patient then inflated with oxygen, the cords can be examined at the time when respiration returns, to see that they move normally.

The carotid sinus syndrome is occasionally seen (Heymans and others, 1933). Irritation of a carotid sinus produces sudden effects which may be: (1) Vagal; cardio-inhibitory, with bradycardia —atropine being the remedy; (2) Vasodepressive, the remedy being a pressor drug. The operation should be temporarily stopped, the head of the table lowered, artificial respiration instituted, and 10 ml. of 1 per cent procaine injected near the bifurcation of the common carotid artery of the side being operated on. The intravenous injection of atropine, 0·6 mg., may help, while good results have followed the intravenous injection of curare (Burstein).*

Recently the authors have been using the phenothiazine drugs with satisfactory results. After routine premedication the patient is placed on the operating table with a head-up tilt. Chlorpromazine, promethazine, and pethidine in a dosage of about 50 mg. of each is injected intravenously, preferably slowly via a drip. A small dose of thiopentone or hexobarbitone is now given, followed by suxamethonium in a dose of 50–100 mg. The patient is oxygenated by intermittent pressure on the reservoir bag of the anæsthetic machine and his trachea, cords, and pharynx are sprayed thoroughly with 4 per cent lignocaine. A large tube is then inserted, well lubricated with xylodase paste. Inflation is continued, and soon spontaneous respiration takes place of a mixture of nitrous-oxide–oxygen (70–30) with a flow rate of about 8 l. per minute, using a non-return semi-closed circuit connected to the endotracheal tube (see p. 119).

The technique reduces bleeding and attention is focused on: (1) The head-up tilt; (2) Intubation without any straining; (3) Large patent airway; (4) Adequate respiratory minute-volume; (5) Absence of carbon dioxide rebreathing.

The endotracheal tube can remain in situ post-operatively until it is resented by the patient.

Halothane and oxygen is another most satisfactory combination in thyroid operations.

Regional Analgesia.—Regional analgesia may include bilateral deep and superficial cervical plexus block (see p. 334) together with intradermal and subcutaneous infiltration of t he line of incision.

E. S. Rowbotham preferred to solve the problem as follows: Intradermal weals are made: (1) In the suprasternal notch; (2) Just above the midpoint of the clavicles (farther out, if the goitre is very large); (3) On each side of the neck, opposite the greater

---

* Burstein, C. L., *Fundamental Considerations in Anesthesia*, 2nd ed., 1955, 78. New York: Macmillan.

Regional Analgesia, *continued.*

cornua of the hyoid bones. From each of these five points, deep and superficial infiltration is carried out, the superficial injections resulting in a layer of solution covering the whole area. Injections are made throughout with a moving needle and after negative aspiration tests before the deep injections. These, given through the same weals, are designed to deposit solution—(a) on each side of the trachea, (b) laterally to the goitre, (c) around the superior poles, (d) near the ansa hypoglossi. Using the upper cervical weal, the needle is advanced 2 in (5 cm.) parallel to, but beneath, the anterior border of the sterno-mastoid, beneath which lies the carotid sheath, the ansa being anterior to the sheath—5 ml. of solution are injected on each side as the needles are withdrawn. Rowbotham used no more than 150 ml. of 1–4000 amethocaine with 1–400,000 adrenaline solution.*

Respiratory Obstruction after Thyroidectomy.—The causes may be :—

1. REACTIONARY HÆMORRHAGE.—This may cause pressure on the trachea and requires immediate evacuation of the hæmatoma.
2. ŒDEMA OF THE LARYNX, which is usually seen on the second or third day after operation. Diagnosis is by indirect laryngoscopy and if stridor becomes troublesome a tracheostomy will be required, the tube being removed about five days later. As a temporary measure, endotracheal intubation may be useful and a tube can be left in place for from 1 to 3 days.
3. RECURRENT LARYNGEAL NERVE INJURY.—This is most likely to occur after operations for recurrent thyroidectomy. It may be temporary, due to bruising, or permanent, due to nerve division—the former may last up to six weeks. Paralysis of one recurrent nerve may or may not cause obstruction ; paralysis of both cords will make a tracheostomy necessary. Even slight obstruction may prove fatal in handicapped patients, e.g., cardiac cases, and tracheostomy is always better done early than late. Its delay is the most frequent cause of death after thyroidectomy.
4. COLLAPSE OF TRACHEA.—This is rare unless the actual tracheal cartilage is removed in malignant cases. When this condition is suspected the following conditions must be first excluded : œdema of larynx, recurrent laryngeal nerve injury, or hæmorrhage under the strap muscles. Treatment is intubation, followed if necessary by tracheostomy.
5. INJURY TO THE SUPERIOR LARYNGEAL NERVE.—This is rare but can be suspected if there is : (a) A change in the voice ; (b) Difficulty in swallowing. The former is due to cricothyroid paralysis, the latter to sensory paralysis. The condition soon improves.

Obstruction to respiration severe enough to cause insomnia requires either tracheostomy or intubation.

---

* Rowbotham, E. S., *Anæsthesia in Operations for Goitre,* 1945, p. 64. Oxford: Blackwell; and *Proc. R. Soc. Med.,* 1949, **42**, 115.

Routine examination of the larynx before and after thyroidectomy
has shown that one-third of cases of unilateral paralysis resulting from trauma to the recurrent nerve are symptomless and in
nearly all of these a normal voice is re-established whether the
paralysis disappears or not : treatment is unnecessary.*

Complications of Operation.—
1. Hypothyroidism.
2. Recurrence of hyperthyroidism (in toxic cases).
3. Hypoparathyroidism.
4. Laryngeal nerve damage.

Post-operative Care.—Fowler's position ; morphine when required ;
aspirin for the muscular pain in the neck. The patient should be
kept cool. Thyroid crises, which are now rare, and characterized
by delirium, restlessness, mania, sweating, and tachycardia, and
atrial fibrillation, progressing to heart failure, are best treated
with oxygen. The patient should be cooled and he may be
benefited by chlorpromazine, corticosteroids, digitalis, anti-thyroid
drugs and iodine given either per rectum or intravenously, reserpine,
trimetaphan,† oxygen, and intravenous saline.

Anæsthesia for Patients with Cut Throat.—*See* Ellis, F. R.,
Anæsthesia, 1966, **21**, 253.

GYNÆCOLOGY

Abdominal operations often do well with lumbar extradural analgesia
(20–35 ml. of 1·5 per cent lignocaine), combined with minimal
thiopentone or gas–oxygen.‡ The authors use this method extensively.
Light cinchocaine 10–12 ml. or heavy cinchocaine 1·4–1·7 ml. are very
satisfactory if spinal (intradural) analgesia is contemplated. The abdominal pack to cover the intestines should be inserted gently to avoid
initiating reflexes from the upper abdomen. If general inhalation
anæsthesia is used, breathing must be quiet and relaxation good. The
combination of a muscle relaxant with light general anæsthesia is very
satisfactory, but it does not produce the contracted bowels seen after
intradural and extradural analgesia. Halothane and oxygen will also
give satisfactory results with relaxation sometimes aided by gallamine.
Endotracheal intubation will usually be necessary for those patients
thought likely to develop respiratory difficulty, e.g., those with a short
fat neck or an underdeveloped lower jaw. Obese, hypertensive patients
do not always tolerate an extreme Trendelenburg position without
some hypoxia if breathing spontaneously. They are improved if
30–40 per cent of oxygen is given during the operation and the breathing
is assisted or controlled.

Anæsthesia in patients with *Meigs' syndrome*§ may present problems.
Ovarian tumours are associated with pleural effusion, usually on
the right side, and ascites. This may result in a reduced vital

---

* Ellis, M., *J. Laryng.*, 1946, **61**, 286.
† Malers, E., and others, *Lancet*, 1963, **2**, 641.
‡ Loudon, J. D. O., and Scott, D. B., *J. Obstet. Gynæc. Brit. Emp.*, 1960, **67**, 561; and
Lee, J. A., *Int. Anesthesiol. Clin.*, 1964, **2**, 499.
§ Meigs, J. V., and Cass, J. W., *Amer. J. Obstet. Gynec.*, 1937, **33**, 249.

Gynæcology, *continued.*

capacity with hypoxæmia and hypercapnia. Tapping should
be done immediately before surgery to prevent refilling. The
ascites may be associated with hiatus hernia with its potential
dangers (*see* Chapter XXVI). A partially collapsed lung may
require expanding.*

The Trendelenburg position is unphysiological and should be maintained for as short a time as possible. The less steep it is the
better for the patient's respiratory and cardiovascular function
Levelling of the table should be gradual. Recent work has
shown that in patients undergoing major gynæcological surgery
under extradural lumbar block and light general anæsthesia,
and operated on in either the horizontal, head-down, or lithotomy
positions, no significant effects of posture were detected as
measured by minute volume and blood-gas estimations.†

Vaginal operations can be performed under extradural lumbar or sacral
block (*see* Chapter XVI), spinal analgesia, or general inhalation
anæsthesia. Stretching of the cervix or trauma to the perineum
may produce laryngeal spasm, requiring a deeper plane of anæsthesia or a small dose of a muscle relaxant. The authors prefer
lumbar extradural block for vaginal repair operations. It
combines afferent block, muscular relaxation, and moderate
hypotension and ischæmia.‡ The dosage of 1·5 per cent lignocaine solution used is 20–30 ml. Light thiopentone sleep can
be employed if thought desirable, or heavy premedication may
suffice. Some workers prefer to use induced hypotension by
ganglionic blockade for vaginal surgery.§ Other surgeons infiltrate the tissues with adrenaline-saline (1–250,000 to 1–500,000).
For dilatation and curettage, thiopentone, with gas and oxygen,
or gas–oxygen–trichloroethylene is excellent. While suxamethonium may occasionally be necessary, its routine employment is unwarranted because of the muscular after-pains which
sometimes develop. In problem patients, a small dose of a
long-acting relaxant may help to smooth out difficulties. The
barbiturate should be in the blood-stream at the exact time
that the surgical stimulus is applied.

Autonomic reflexes arising in the pelvis may be: (*a*) Pelvicardiac,
causing bradycardia and hypotension; (*b*) Pelvilaryngeal,
causing adduction of the cords (Brewer-Luckhart).

EYE SURGERY

In intra-ocular surgery, a sudden rise in intra-ocular tension from
the normal 15–25 mm. Hg following coughing, vomiting, contraction
of the orbicularis oculi, or straining may cause a severe disturbance, and
so in the past these operations have been usually performed under
local analgesia. (It was, in fact, the poor quality of the general
anæsthesia available in Vienna in the 1880's that stimulated Karl
Koller to seek practical means of producing local analgesia of the

---

* Donnelly, P. B., *Anæsthesia*, 1966, **21**, 216.
† Scott, D. B., and Slawson, K. B., *Brit. J. Anæsth.*, 1968, **40**, 103.
‡ Moir, D. D., *Ibid.*, 1968, **40**, 233.
§ Linacre, J. L., *Ibid.*, 1961, **33**, 45.

eye, and to employ cocaine for this purpose—so initiating the whole concept of local analgesia in surgery.) More recently, following modern improvement in general anæsthetic technique,* cataract operations have been done under careful general anæsthesia, taking great pains to avoid coughing and similar disturbances. Ocular ischæmia is aided by a flawless anæsthetic technique, a tilted table, and the instillation of adrenaline into the conjunctival sac. Intra-ocular tension is reduced by the use of non-depolarizing relaxants, by lowering the blood-pressure, and by deep anæsthesia. A lowered intra-ocular tension may be required for intra-capsular lens extraction and for some other intra-ocular operations; a normal tension for extracapsular lens extraction.

Local Analgesia.—*See* Duncalf, D., and Rhodes, D. H., *Anesthesia in Clinical Ophthalmology*, 1963. Baltimore: Williams & Wilkins.

ADVANTAGES.—(1) Safer ; (2) Less post-operative nausea and vomiting ; (3) Early ambulation and feeding ; (4) Less bleeding ; (5) Less risk of pulmonary embolism ; (6) Less upset of biochemical processes ; (7) Less post-operative restlessness ; (8) Less post-operative lung pathology ; (9) Less post-operative coronary or cerebral thrombosis.

TECHNIQUE OF ANALGESIA OF CORNEA AND CONJUNCTIVAL SAC.—If local analgesia is to be used, 4 per cent cocaine should be instilled into the conjunctival sac every two minutes on five occasions. This will give analgesia of the cornea and conjunctiva, but not of the iris or ciliary body : nor will it produce analgesia in a glaucomatous eye. It has the disadvantage that it produces dilatation of the pupil (bad in glaucoma), while it irritates and dries the corneal epithelium. Amethocaine 0·5 or 1 per cent, when combined with adrenaline, does not have these effects and can also be used for tonometry. Halocaine, butyn, and piperocaine—all in 1 per cent solution—have also been used and 4 per cent lignocaine solution is popular and efficient. If the local analgesic drug is dissolved in methyl cellulose, stinging of the eye will not result when instillation into the conjunctival sac takes place.

Propranolol in 0·25–0·4 per cent solution is reported to be a safe and efficient analgesic for use in the conjunctival sac.† Systemic effects are unlikely if the dose is restricted to 6 ml.

Local Analgesia for Surgery of Lacrimal Sac.‡—Local analgesia reduces bleeding if adrenaline is added to any suitable analgesic solution, e.g., 1 per cent procaine or 1 per cent lignocaine. The nerve-supply of the lacrimal sac is from : (1) The infratrochlear branch of the first division of the fifth nerve. (2) The anterior superior alveolar branch of the second division of the fifth nerve. (*a*) A weal is raised 5 mm. above the inner canthus at the orbital margin and through this, solution is injected just within the orbit to block the infratrochlear nerve. (*See* p. 325—anterior ethmoid block.) (*b*) The needle is partially withdrawn and solution is

---

* Zorab, E. C., *Brit. J. Ophthal.*, 1961, **45**, 614.
† Singh, K. P., and others, *Lancet*, 1967, **2**, 158; and Sinha, J. H., and others, *Brit. J. Anæsth.*, 1967, **39**, 887.
‡ Philps, A. S., *Proc. R. Soc. Med.*, 1951, **44**, 169.

Local Analgesia for Surgery of Lacrimal Sac, *continued*.

injected subcutaneously over the lacrimal sac, avoiding the angular vein. (*c*) The anterior superior alveolar nerve is blocked from a point 10 mm. below the inner canthus. (*d*) From the first weal over the inner canthus, a deep zone of infiltration is made, to give hæmostasis. (*e*) The naris on the bad side is sprayed with cocaine solution and then packed with cocaine gauze or painted with cocaine paste (p. 326). For excision of a chronically infected lacrimal sac, infratrochlear nerve-block and infiltration of the line of incision are all that is required.

For dacryocystorhinostomy :—

1. The nasociliary nerve is blocked within the orbit (anterior ethmoidal block, p. 325).
2. The line of incision is infiltrated and this extends into the zone of skin supplied by the infra-orbital nerve.

The operation can also be performed under general anæsthesia, using adrenaline–saline infiltration or ganglionic blocking agents to provide ischæmia.

Retro-ocular Block.—This must be done before operation under local analgesia on the globe of the eye. After topical analgesia of the cornea and conjunctival sac, the long and short ciliary nerves and ciliary ganglion are blocked within the muscle cone. Retro-ocular block reduces intra-ocular pressure and makes prolapse of the vitreous less likely. Hyaluronidase (6–10 turbidity-reducing (T.R.) units to each ml. of solution) aids diffusion and enables rather larger volumes of solution to be injected—up to 3 ml. The injection should also paralyse the extra-ocular muscles. Two per cent lignocaine is a suitable solution.

Retro-ocular or retrobulbar block may be :—

1. Superior,* through the superior rectus, with the patient looking downwards, from a weal just above the middle of the tarsal plate. A 5-cm. needle is used and is inserted 3–4 cm. backwards, slightly inwards and downwards. During movement of the needle, injection is continuous as a safeguard against injuring veins.
2. Infero-lateral, from a weal at the infero-lateral margin of the orbit.† A 5-cm. needle is inserted backwards along the floor of the orbit, until its tip is posterior to the eye at the apex of the orbit: 1–2 ml. of solution are injected. A transconjunctival approach may also be employed. Deposition of a little solution is also necessary in the superior rectus.

To immobilize the lids, prevent screwing up the eyes and so raising intra-ocular pressure, twigs of the facial nerve are blocked in the parotid gland by injecting 3 ml. of 1 per cent lignocaine on to the neck of the mandible, just below the zygoma. If the eyeball is to be opened, paralysis of the orbicularis oculi so produced is necessary, to prevent squeezing of the globe.

---

* Macintosh, R. R., and Ostlere, M., *Local Analgesia, Head and Neck*, 2nd ed., 1967, 121. Edinburgh and London; E. & S. Livingstone.

† Atkinson, W. S., *Anesthesia in Ophthalmology*, 1955, 41. Springfield, Ill.: Thomas ; and Duncalf, D., and Rhodes, D. H., *Anesthesia in Clinical Ophthalmology*, 1963, p. 54. Baltimore: Williams & Wilkins.

Another method of making the eyelids insensitive and immobile, so that a speculum can be introduced, is to inject a little procaine from a weal over the external palpebral ligament, along the margin of each eyelid. From the same weal, the needle should be directed backwards towards the ear, to block the fibres of the facial nerve supplying the orbicularis oculi.

General Anæsthesia

It is important that intra-ocular pressure should not be unduly raised by anæsthesia.

Intra-ocular pressure is lowered by: (1) Hyperoxæmia, (2) Hypocapnia, (3) Hyperventilation, (4) Volatile anæsthetics and cyclopropane, (5) Non-depolarizing relaxants, (6) Narcotic analgesics, e.g., morphine and pethidine.

It is raised by: (1) Hypoxæmia, (2) Hypercapnia, (3) Coughing, sneezing, straining, and other causes of venous obstruction in the head and neck, (3) Suxamethonium, (4) Atropine (in narrow-angle glaucoma only).

When the blood-pressure rises, the intra-ocular pressure does not greatly alter but when it is less than 85 mm. Hg the intra-ocular pressure falls.

Drainage of the anterior chamber is increased by contraction of the ciliary muscle, e.g., eserine; decreased by relaxation, e.g., atropine.

Advantages of General Anæsthesia.—

1. Co-operation of patient ceases to become a problem.
2. No risk of retrobulbar hæmatoma from injection of local analgesic drug.
3. Less of an ordeal for the patient.
4. Quieter atmosphere in theatre facilitates delicate surgery.

Anæsthetic Drugs in Ophthalmic Surgery.—

ATROPINE.—This raises the intra-ocular pressure only in the presence of glaucoma with a narrow angle between the cornea and iris. Pilocarpine drops, 1 per cent, overcome this danger. It dilates the pupil.

ADRENALINE.—Does not dilate the pupil if instilled into the conjunctival sac but will do so if injected intravenously.

MORPHINE.—Contracts the pupil from stimulation of the third cranial nerve nucleus.

SUXAMETHONIUM.—This increases intra-ocular tension* but the rise is probably confined to the period of apnœa and so is no reason for banning this useful aid to intubation.† Its cause is probably an intra-ocular vascular one, comes on in 30 sec., is maximal at 2 min., and has disappeared in 5 min. after injection. It should not be used for the first time during an operation when the eye is already open, for fear of precipitating vitreous prolapse.

---

* Dillon, J. B., and others, *Anesthesiology*, 1957, **18**, 44 and 439; and Lincoff, H. A., and others, *Am. J. Ophthalmol.*, 1947, **43**, 440.
† Taylor, T. H., Mulcahy, M., and Nightingale, D. A., *Brit. J. Anæsth.*, 1968, **40**, 113.

Anæsthetic Drugs in Ophthalmic Surgery, *continued.*

The intravenous injection of acetazolamide, 500 mg., immediately before induction of anæsthesia, largely prevents rise in intra ocular pressure due to suxamethonium. It is a carbonic anhydrase inhibitor and interferes with the secretion o aqueous.* It has no effect on either the pupil size or the drainage from the eye. Mannitol, 0·5–1·5 g. per kg., or urea 1 g. per kg. body-weight, has also been advocated.† A case of cholestatic jaundice, hepatitis, and death has been reported following the ingestion of 13 g. of acetazol .mide over a period of 26 days.‡

TUBOCURARINE.—Useful for reducing the tone of extra-ocula muscles and for producing apnœa.

Repeated small doses of *dimethyl ether of tubocurarine* have been recommended§ for cataract surgery. The drug is given unti ocular palsy shows itself. It causes general and local muscula relaxation, allays apprehension, and limits ocular movements preventing vitreous prolapse without much respiratory depression.

GALLAMINE.—Has the same attributes as tubocurarine but, in addition, blocks the vagal reflexes (causing bradycardia, arrhyth mias, and even cardiac standstill) occasionally seen when the extra-ocular muscles, especially the internal rectus, are unde tension.‖

THIOPENTONE.—Useful for the induction of anæsthesia, for main tenance of anæsthesia, and for premedication per rectum in children. Reduces the tension in normal and glaucomatous eyes.

BROMETHOL.—Lowers intra-ocular tension and is useful for pre medication in children.

PHENOTHIAZINE DRUGS.—Chlorpromazine, promazine,¶ and promethazine combinations produce anti-emesis, endotracheal tube tolerance, anæsthetic potentiation, and post-operative seda tion. They may be combined with pethidine, e.g., chlor promazine, promethazine, and pethidine, 50 mg. of each in 250 ml. of dextrose given slowly intravenously, followed by thiopentone, relaxant, intubation, and gas–oxygen. In olde patients this may cause too much fall of blood-pressure.

HALOTHANE.—When given with oxygen in a concentration o 2–8 per cent delivered into a partially closed circuit with spon taneous respiration, this is an excellent agent for intra-ocula operations which is well recommended by the authors. I causes little post-operative vomiting, aids ischæmia, and lower tension inside the eye, especially if the blood-pressure falls below about 85 mm. Hg.

---

* Carballo, A. S., *Canad. Anæsth. Soc. J.*, 1965, **12**, 486.
† Duncalf, D., and Rhodes, D. H., *Anesthesia in Clinical Ophthalmology*, 1964. Baltimore: Williams & Wilkins.
‡ Kristinsson, A., *Brit. J. Ophthal.*, 1967, **51**, 348.
§ Agarwal, L. P., *Ibid.*, 1953, **37**, 558.
‖ Deacock, A. R. de C., and Oxer, H. F., *Brit. J. Anæsth.*, 1962, **34**, 451.
¶ Ingram, H. V., and Davison, M. H. Armstrong, *Lancet*, 1961, **1**, 1321; and *Proc. R. Soc Med.*, 1963, **56**, 987.

I.P.P.V.—When this method is employed, using tubocurarine and an endotracheal tube, the intra-ocular pressure rises if the inflating pressure is more than 10 cm. water, but not if the inflating pressure is below this.*

ECOTHIOPATE IODIDE (phosphorline iodide).—Depressed levels of pseudocholinesterase can occur within a few days of commencing the use of drops of this agent in the treatment of glaucoma.†

HYPOTENSIVE ANÆSTHESIA IN OPHTHALMIC SURGERY.—See Edridge, A., Proc. R. Soc. Med., 1963, **56**, 985.

Some Suitable General Anæsthetic Techniques.—

1. For squint in children. Sedative premedication, e.g., rectal thiopentone, 1 ml. of 2 per cent solution per lb. of body-weight. Then intravenous thiopentone, suxamethonium, endotracheal tube, and gas–oxygen through a non-rebreathing circuit with spontaneous respiration. Other workers prefer the thiopentone, gas–oxygen, relaxant, controlled breathing technique through an endotracheal tube. To prevent vagal reflexes, the intravenous injection of atropine or gallamine (10–20 mg.) should be employed. Gallamine also relaxes the extra-ocular muscles. Retro-orbital block of 2 ml. of 2 per cent lignocaine is also effective.

2. Squint in adults. No special problems occur other than the prevention of vagal reflexes by atropine or gallamine.

3. Intra-ocular operations. In children as for squint. In fit adults, chlorpromazine, promethazine, and pethidine followed by intubation and gas–oxygen. If the larynx is likely to be irritable as in heavy smokers or in infection, additional pethidine, thiopentone, or halothane or trichloroethylene. In older or less fit patients, endotracheal oxygen and halothane preferred by the authors gives satisfactory results. The techniques should aim at enabling extubation to be carried out without the production of coughing, and so topical analgesia of the larynx and trachea with 4 per cent solution of lignocaine is in most cases helpful. Post-operative tracheal suction is better avoided in most patients for the same reason. There are workers of experience who only insert an endotracheal tube in especially difficult patients in both children and adults.‡

The combination of local analgesia with heavy sedation for intra-ocular operations has been recommended ; promazine, promethazine, and pethidine are given in divided doses followed in 60–90 min. by intravenous phenazocine, 1·2–3 mg., and then by retrobulbar block.§ The so-called neurolept analgesia, produced by droperidol and fentanyl or phenoperidine, now has an increasing number of advocates.‖ Yet another method combines sedation by oral methylpentynol, intramuscular

---

* Marretta, P. V., and Dossi, F., Min. Anesthesiol., 1962, **29**, 94.

† McGavi, D. D. M., Lancet, 1965, **2**, 272; Pantuck, E. J., Brit. J. Anæsth., 1966, **38**, 406; and Gesztes, T., Ibid., 1966, **38**, 408.

‡ Verner, I. R., Proc. R. Soc. Med., 1967, **60**, 1280; and Edridge, A. W., Ibid., 1967, **60**, 1283.

§ Ingram, H. V., and Davison, M. H. Armstrong, Lancet, 1961, **1**, 1321 ; and Proc. R. Soc. Med., 1963, **56**, 987.

‖ Bryn Thomas, K., Proc. 2nd Eur. Cong. Anæsth., 1966, **2**, 229.

Some Suitable General Anæsthetic Techniques, *continued.*

chlorpromazine and intravenous pethidine, and small doses of gallamine (not exceeding 40 mg.). Nitrous-oxide analgesia is then produced by allowing 6 litres of gas per minute to fall near the patient's nose, underneath the towels. No endotracheal tube is used in this technique, which is, of course, accompanied by local analgesia of the eye.*

Special Points.—(1) All disturbances causing movement, cough, or contraction of the orbicularis oculi must be avoided as they may increase the intra-ocular tension with resulting iris prolapse or vitreous prolapse. (2) Post-operative vomiting and coughing should be minimized for the same reason. (3) Post-operative restlessness often yields to intramuscular paraldehyde, 5 or 10 ml., or to chlorpromazine, 20–50 mg. (3) Congenital cataract may be associated with dystrophia or with diabetes. (4) For examination of the fundus oculi in babies, rectal thiopentone or halothane is suitable. (5) Before intra-ocular operations the pressure in the eye can be reduced by the intravenous injection of acetazolamide, 500 mg., or urea. (6) A variety of stimuli arising in or near the eye cause abnormalities of the rate or rhythm of the heart.† Anæsthesia appears to make the heart vulnerable to increased vagal tone, especially in the young.‡ Cardiac standstill is the danger, preceded by bradycardia, especially following traction on the internal rectus, or pressure on the eyeball so that adequate cardiac monitoring, be it only a finger on the radial pulse, should accompany these interventions. Gallamine and atropine intravenously are useful preventives, but retrobulbar injection of local analgesic solutions is not as efficient.§ (7) A large drop of 1 per cent atropine may contain 1 mg. of the drug; of adrenaline 1–1000, 0·1 mg., and of phenylephrine 10 per cent, 10 mg. These may have systemic effects. For removal of sutures, halothane and oxygen is excellent.

(*See* discussion, *Proc. R. Soc. Med.*, 1967, **60**, 1273.)

MASTECTOMY

An endotracheal tube coupled with adequate ventilation minimizes oozing as also does a table tilt with head raised. By the use of topical analgesia and short-acting relaxants, a smooth intubation, free from coughing and straining, should be carried out and this too will reduce the tendency to bleed. Only light general anæsthesia is required. Gas and oxygen, with minimal intermittent thiopentone and pethidine, is a good combination, with or without the addition of a little trichloroethylene and spontaneous breathing. Halothane and oxygen is favoured by the authors, and this can frequently be given without an

---

* Ives, J., *Brit. med. J.*, 1959, **1**, 821.

† Aschner, B., *Wien. klin. Wschr.*, 1908, **21**, 1529.

‡ Howland, W. S., and Papper, E. M., *Anesthesiology*, 1952, **13**, 343; and Mendelblatt, F. I., and others, *Amer. J. Ophthalmol.*, 1967, **53**, 506.

§ Bosomworth, R. P., Zeigler, C. H., and Jacoby, J., *Ibid.*, 1958, **19**, 7 ; and Walton, F. A., *Canad. Anæsth. Soc. J.*, 1957, **4**, 414.

See also good review *Proc. R. Soc. Med.*, 1963, **56**, 979, and Kenny, S., *Brit. J. Anæsth.*, 1963, **35**, 317.

endotracheal tube, while others prefer the intravenous barbiturate relaxant, intubation, and nitrous-oxide–oxygen by the I.P.P.V. technique.

ANÆSTHESIA FOR OUT-PATIENT TREATMENT OF HERNIA AND VARICOSE VEINS, ETC.*

Patients who are to leave hospital soon after the end of these relatively major operations require anæsthetic management which allows rapid recovery, free from sickness. Premedication, if necessary at all, might well be perphenazine (fentazin) 5 mg. intramuscularly. If a second similar dose is given several hours after operation, nausea is reduced still further. If intravenous induction is necessary, then propanidid or methohexitone is preferable to thiopentone. Anæsthesia may be maintained by gas–oxygen with trichloroethylene or halothane or halothane and oxygen. Post-operative pain can often be controlled by one or more tablets containing butobarbitone, phenacetin, and codeine (sonalgin), or similar combintaion.

GENERAL ANÆSTHESIA FOR AMBULANT PATIENTS

This presents problems which may be most difficult to solve. Factors to be considered are the need for rapid recovery and the lack of preparation of the patient, e.g., his full stomach. As in operations for major surgery, anæsthesia should provide a quiet, relaxed, and unconscious patient. The relatively unskilled anæsthetist may find cyclopropane and oxygen, half of each, useful, given from a 6-litre bag, followed, if necessary, by gas and 20 per cent oxygen. Unconsciousness lasting from one and a half to two minutes can be produced in all patients by 10–15 breaths of the oxygen–cyclopropane mixture. Vomiting is the disagreeable complication and is worse in children than in adults. Nitrous oxide and oxygen alone, or supplemented with trichloroethylene or halothane, can be used. Regular intake of alcohol is the great enemy of unsupplemented gas–oxygen anæsthesia. Intravenous barbiturates are useful, especially methohexitone (5–15 mg. per stone in 1 per cent solution). Propanidid is preferred by some anæsthetists, since the patient is able to leave the hospital earlier than after intravenous barbiturates. (*See also* Chapter XXIV.) Local analgesia is most rewarding in suitable cases, e.g., brachial plexus or sciatic nerve-block; finger block or intravenous regional analgesia (*see* Chapter XV).

ANÆSTHESIA IN UPPER RESPIRATORY TRACT OBSTRUCTION†

This may occur : (1) At the lips ; (2) In the mouth ; (3) In the nose ; (4) In the pharynx ; (5) In the larynx ; (6) In the trachea.

Signs.—Stridor ; dilating alæ nasi ; rib and intercostal retraction ; use of accessory muscles, e.g., scalenes and sternomastoids ; indrawing over clavicles ; perhaps cyanosis.

Symptoms.—Dyspnœa ; anxiety ; restlessness ; inability to sleep.

* Sutherland, J. S., and Horsfall, G. L., *Lancet*, 1961, **1**, 1044.
† Verrill, P. T.. *Brit. J. Anæsth.*, 1963, **35**, 237.

Anæsthesia in Upper Respiratory Tract Obstruction, *continued.*

Diagnosis.—Inspiratory stridor suggests obstruction at or above cords ; expiratory stridor suggests obstruction in bronchial tree ; inspiratory with expiratory stridor suggests tracheal obstruction. These cases present difficulties because of possible :—

1. Trismus, e.g., in Ludwig's angina.*
2. Voluntary use of accessory muscles of respiration to overcome respiratory obstruction associated with the lesion : if this is present, fatal hypoxia may follow loss of consciousness. Thus tracheostomy under local analgesia may be necessary before the induction of general anæsthesia. Blind nasal intubation in the conscious patient after spraying the nares and larynx with local analgesic solution (cocaine 4 per cent in the nares) may be the method chosen by experienced workers in some cases. The inhalation of a mixture of helium 79 per cent and oxygen 21 per cent has a density of 330 as against 1000 for air. A volatile agent, or cyclopropane, can be added to this mixture and fairly readily inhaled with much less distress to the patient than he experiences with air. Premedication should be non-depressing to respiration, e.g., a phenothiazine derivative.

A peritonsillar abscess can be opened under lignocaine or cocaine topical analgesia with the head low.

In severe upper respiratory obstruction, tracheostomy may be necessary before induction of general anæsthesia, or even during induction in emergency.

Before inducing general anæsthesia in a patient with an acute infection of the neck, who is hypoxic, 100 per cent oxygen should be given for ten minutes, followed by a smooth gas–oxygen–halothane or trichloroethylene induction. Early passage of a nasopharyngeal tube will remove any respiratory obstruction due to trismus, or the presence of a bulky or œdematous tongue or pharynx. Blind nasal intubation, helped by topical analgesia, can then be carried out. A rather small tube, e.g., size 6·5 or 7, is easier to insert than a larger one, and is permissible for short operations.

It is probable that thiopentone is not responsible for any excitation of carotid sinus reflexes in these cases. Thus, in small doses for induction, it is probably safe.

If the abscess is superficial it can be opened under refrigeration anæsthesia, i.e., application of ice to the part for 45–60 minutes.

BURNS†

These can often be cleaned and dressed under pethidine or morphine, given slowly by intravenous injection so that the minimal effective dosage can be ascertained. The intravenous injection, via a drip, of 1 g. of procaine dissolved in 500 ml. of 5 per cent glucose saline has been advocated. After a time, painless dressing of burns will usually be permitted. Alternatively, neurolept analgesia—a combination of droperidol and phenoperidine (or fentanyl)—can be used.‡

---

* Garland, J. M. B., *Anæsthesia*, 1963, **18**, 29.

† *See* Rook, J. M., *Lancet*, 1953, **1**, 1214 ; Shannon, D. W., *Ibid.*, 1955, **1**, 111 ; and Middleton, H. G., and Wolfson, L. J., *Brit. med. Bull.*, 1958, **14**, 1, 42.

‡ Muir, I. F. K., *Brit. J. Anæsth.*, 1966, **38**, 267.

For dressing of burns, gas and oxygen analgesia is also useful.

The danger of suxamethonium and endotracheal intubation in anæsthesia for burns has been pointed out.* Cardiac arrest, perhaps due to increased vagal tone, would seem to be a definite danger in such cases, especially if the initial burns occurred between three and seven weeks before the anæsthesia. Intravenous atropine should reduce the risk of cardiac arrest. Serum pseudocholinesterase may be low.†

SKIN-GRAFTS

Skin-grafts can often be removed painlessly from the thigh after block of the lateral femoral cutaneous and, if necessary, the femoral nerves, or by intradermal and subcutaneous infiltration of skin of anterior part of thigh. Work has also been done on superficial freezing of donor areas by ice-bags.

* * * *

Choice of anæsthetic is always dependent on the skill and experience of the anæsthetist and on the preferences of the surgeon and the patient. Every form of anæsthesia has its disadvantages and complications and is responsible for a certain morbidity and mortality. To everything there is a season.

It is relatively easy to acquire techniques, but judgment in their use is the reward of clinical experience, carefully garnered (Walsh).

There is no general anæsthetic which can be called ' the best ', and an anæsthetist is likely to benefit his patient most when he uses the technique and drugs with which he is familiar. For the tiro there are few absolute contra-indications to ether, which remains after 122 years the safest all-purpose anæsthetic.

Skilfully managed, any one of a number of agents and techniques can usually be applied, the final solution often being a matter of individual preference.

CHAPTER XXI

ANÆSTHESIA FOR NEUROSURGERY‡

Special Problems involved.—
  1. Raised intracranial tension.
  2. The poor general condition of some patients.
  3. The length of operation.
  4. Maintenance of the airway. Inaccessibility of the endotracheal tube and connexions during long operations, coupled with the strict necessity of maintaining an absolutely free airway with

---

* Bush, G. H., and others, *Brit. med. J.*, 1962, **2**, 1081 ; and Finer, B. L., and Nylen, B. O., *Ibid.*, 1959, **1**, 624.

† Bush, G. H., *Anæsthesia*, 1964, **19**, 231.

‡ See also Ballantine, R. I. W., and Jackson, I., *A Practice of General Anæsthesia for Neurosurgery*, 1960. London: Churchill; Ballantine, R. I. W., in *Recent Advances in Anæsthesia, and Analgesia*, 9th ed., Ch. V (Ed. Hewer, C. Langton), 1963. London: Churchill; Hunter, A. R., *Neurosurgical Anæsthesia*, 1964. Oxford: Blackwell; and Gilbert, R. G. B., Brindle, G. F., and Galindo, A., *Anæsthesia for Neurosurgery*, 1966. London: Churchill.

Special Problems involved, *continued.*

    absence of straining or coughing. The need to suck out the trachea in some patients.

5. Posture. Head-up, sitting, lateral, or prone positions may be required throughout a lengthy operation. There may be greater danger to the patient through imperfect positioning.

6. Surgical trauma may produce hæmorrhage and/or cerebral ischæmia. Vital structures are often very near the area of surgical manipulation. The anæsthetist must keep a close watch on the vital signs.

7. Use of diathermy requires non-explosive technique.

8. Air embolism may occur in head-up positions.

Cerebral Hæmodynamics.—Though cerebral blood-flow, cerebral vasculo-resistance, and cerebral metabolic rate are factors which can be measured, their relationship and significance are not fully understood. The brain should probably be regarded as several organs within a compact structure with separate functional needs and separate patterns of regional blood-flow, not necessarily reflected in total measurements.

    Intracranial contents may be considered as comprising: solids in brain tissue 24 per cent, water in brain tissue 60 per cent, cerebral blood-volume 3–5 per cent, cerebrospinal fluid 11–13 per cent. The intracranial contents are restricted inside a rigid indistensible chamber, the skull, although some volume changes can occur via the foramen magnum to the spinal cord, subarachnoid and extradural spaces.

CEREBRAL BLOOD-FLOW IS REGULATED BY.—

    1. Arterial Blood-pressure.—If the other factors controlling cerebral blood-flow are kept within normal limits, cerebral blood-flow does not alter greatly with blood-pressures between 90 and 180 mm. Hg. In the supine position the healthy brain receives between 750 and 900 ml. of blood per minute or about 15 per cent of the left ventricular output.

    2. Venous Pressure.—This may be influenced by: (*a*) Gravity; (*b*) Intrathoracic pressure; (*c*) Intra-abdominal pressure; (*d*) Blood-volume; (*e*) Circulatory efficiency; (*f*) Venous tone.

    3. The Blood CO_2 Tension.—A $Paco_2$ of 60–80 mm. Hg increases cerebral blood-flow by 100 per cent, while a decrease to 26 mm. Hg reduces blood-flow by 30 per cent.

    4. Cerebrospinal Fluid Pressure.

    5. Oxygen Tension.—Inhalation of 85–100 per cent oxygen reduces cerebral blood-flow by one-fifth and under hyperbaric conditions by even more. A reduction of oxygen inhalation to 10 per cent increases cerebral blood-flow by 30 per cent.

    6. Cerebrovascular Resistance.—This depends on the average radius of the cerebral vessels and on the viscosity of the blood.

    7. Vasomotor Factors.—These have little effect on cerebral blood-flow, as the autonomic fibres to vessels have little or no influence on the regulation of their diameter.

    8. Temperature.—Heat causes cerebral vasodilatation while cold has the reverse effect.

9. DRUGS.—Cerebral vasodilatation is produced by halothane, ether, and chloroform.

The anæsthetist can reduce bleeding during intracranial operations by strict attention to carbon-dioxide homeostasis and to intracerebral venous pressure.

The critical value for cerebral flow rate is 30 ml. per 100 g. brain per min. (normal 53 ml. per 100 g. per min.). Where cerebro-vascular disease and marginal cerebral blood-flow pre-exist, abrupt rises in venous pressure during straining or coughing may produce symptoms of insufficiency, especially if there is an associated fall in arterial pressure (e.g., during induction of anæsthesia). Where there is an increased intracranial pressure, increase in resistance would produce fall in flow but for compensatory mechanisms. But above 450 mm. Hg, compensation lags and fall below 40 ml. per 100 g. per min. results. Even though this figure is higher than in a patient without raised pressure, coma may result.*

Cerebrospinal Fluid.—*See* p. 387.

Intracranial Pressure.—Normal intracranial pressure is between 60 and 150 mm. of C.S.F., measured in the horizontal position with the spine and external occipital protuberance in the same line.

DECREASED INTRACRANIAL PRESSURE.—This may occur : (*a*) Following blood loss ; (*b*) Following dehydration ; (*c*) Post-operatively, after removal of a space-occupying lesion. Its significance to the anæsthetist is not great. Occasionally, following removal of a subdural or extradural hæmatoma it may be desirable to lower the head of the table and transfuse fluid intravenously in order to re-expand the brain.

RAISED INTRACRANIAL PRESSURE.—This may occur physio-logically as a result of coughing, sneezing, straining at stool, etc. Pathologically raised intracranial tension may occur :—

1. By pressure from outside. A bony tumour or craniostenosis.
2. By presence of a space-occupying lesion. Neoplasm, abscess or hæmatoma.
3. In hydrocephalus.
4. With venous obstruction.
5. With arterial dilatation.
6. With cerebral œdema, which in turn may be due to inflamma-tion, neoplasm, trauma, hypoxia, venous obstruction, etc.
7. With head-down position.

Raised intracranial pressure may be aggravated by general anæs-thesia if hypoxia, hypercapnia, coughing or straining are allowed to occur.

EFFECTS OF RAISED INTRACRANIAL PRESSURE.—

1. A clinical picture of headache, vomiting, altered conscious-ness.
2. Papillœdema.
3. Third nerve paralysis. This nerve is stretched when supra-tentorial pressure rises. Complete paralysis results in

---

* *See* Rosomoff, H. L., *Brit. J. Anæsth.*, 1965, **37**, 246.

Intracranial Pressure, *continued.*

ptosis, external strabismus, and pupil dilatation. Partial paralysis with pupillary dilatation only is more usual.

4. Restriction of normal circulation of C.S.F. Flow may be impeded through the foramina of Majendie and Luschka to set up a vicious circle.

5. Interference with normal blood-supply to pons, medulla, and hypothalamus. Stimulation of the vital centres causes a rise of systolic blood-pressure, fall of diastolic pressure, bradycardia, and respiratory irregularities leading to depression and apnœa. These changes are of particular concern to the anæsthetist as they may occur during the course of anæsthesia and represent a dangerous rise in intracranial pressure requiring immediate steps to protect the patient.

Methods of lowering intracranial pressure during operation are discussed on p. 548.

ANÆSTHETIC TECHNIQUE

Local Analgesia.—The added risks of general anæsthesia in the presence of raised intracranial tension, coupled with the insensitivity of most of the intracranial structures to painful stimuli, suggest the advantages of local techniques. Premedication may be phenobarbitone, 200 mg. intramuscularly, 1½ hours before operation.

The skin and scalp may be infiltrated with 0·5–1·0 per cent procaine, 0·25–0·5 per cent lignocaine, or 1–2000 amethocaine or cinchocaine. Adrenaline should be added in strength of between 1–250,000 and 1–500,000. Adrenaline cuts down oozing in a vascular area and limits blood-loss, which may be significant when a large flap is raised. Other vasoconstrictors are sometimes used.

The bone is only slightly sensitive, and drilling, though uncomfortable, is usually tolerable. The contents of the cranium are insensitive with a few exceptions. Sensitive regions are : (1) The dura mater at the base of the skull ; (2) The area around the middle meningeal artery ; (3) The nervus spinosus ; (4) The trigeminal ganglion.

During operation careful watch on the patient's general condition is mandatory, just as in general anæsthesia. Alterations in levels of consciousness may also be observed. Sometimes a patient will need restraint. Oxygen blown under the towels near the mouth will prevent a feeling of suffocation. The anæsthetist should be prepared to intervene to provide an artificial airway should the level of consciousness deteriorate.

ADVANTAGES OF LOCAL ANALGESIA.—

1. Avoidance of further rise of intracranial pressure which may occur with general anæsthesia, especially if coughing or straining is allowed.

2. The airway is well maintained in the conscious patient and respiration is often quieter than can be obtained with general anæsthesia.

DISADVANTAGES OF LOCAL ANALGESIA.—
1. Unsuitable for children.
2. Unsatisfactory for uncooperative adults. If there is impairment of consciousness, restraint will be needed to prevent movements of the limbs and head.
3. Long operations are a strain for the conscious patient.

INDICATIONS FOR LOCAL ANALGESIA.—
1. The presence of raised intracranial pressure where the operative intervention is relatively slight, e.g., ventriculography, burhole biopsy, etc.
2. When the patient's co-operation is required at some stage in the operation, e.g., localization of subjective phenomena.
3. For some emergencies, where a rapid rise of intracranial tension may make general anæsthesia particularly hazardous, e.g., middle meningeal hæmorrhage.
4. Where facilities for skilled administration of general anæsthesia are not available.
5. When the general condition of the patient is a contra-indication to general anæsthesia.

General Anæsthesia.—

PREMEDICATION.—Sedative drugs, particularly morphine or pethidine, should be withheld in the presence of :—
1. Raised intracranial pressure.
2. Head injury.
3. The prone, sitting, or steep head-up position.

Atropine or hyoscine should be given in sufficient dosage to prevent salivation. This is particularly important as endotracheal suction is not simple once the operation has begun. Phenothiazine derivates are sometimes given for their sedative or anti-emetic action, e.g., promethazine or perphenazine.

INDUCTION.—Induction should be smooth and avoid coughing or straining or undue central depression. To this end the anæsthetist should commence in good time and perform an unhurried induction watching carefully throughout in order to forestall coughing or bucking on the endotracheal tube. After an episode of coughing, it may take half an hour for the central venous pressure to return to normal.*

THE AIRWAY.—Intubation is essential to ensure maintenance of a clear airway in intracranial surgery or in laminectomy. The cords and trachea should be sprayed with topical analgesic and the tube lubricated with analgesic ointment to help prevent coughing. The tube should be of the largest size consistent with atraumatic introduction—usually 10–12 mm. internal diameter. Precautions should be taken to prevent kinking. A flexometallic tube is the best available for this purpose. It is helpful to remove the soft bevel of these tubes so that it cannot cause respiratory obstruction by approximating to the tracheal wall. A cuffed tube should be used if there is any danger of regurgitation of stomach contents (e.g., prone position, emergency cases, etc.); a pharyngeal pack is advisable if hæmorrhage

---

* Scott, D. B., *Anæsthesia*, 1963, **18**, 135.

General Anæsthesia, *continued.*

into the airway is a possibility (e.g., frontal craniotomy with open frontal sinus, fractured base of skull, etc.). The endotracheal connexions should be wide bore and avoid turbulent flow. The expiratory valve should be sited as near to the patient as possible and its diaphragm should be lightly mounted to prevent resistance to expiration; when spontaneous respiration is allowed it is often better to remove the spring, or to lift the diaphragm of the valve with a safety-pin. The use of a T-piece has also been recommended, especially in children.

THE COURSE OF ANÆSTHESIA.—Rebreathing should be avoided by maintaining a high gas flow. Non-rebreathing valves can be used, though they must be reliable as access to them during operation may be difficult. Use of soda-lime may increase resistance to respiration and is not generally recommended except with controlled respiration. Only light planes of anæsthesia are required, such as to prevent coughing or straining on the endotracheal tube. Topical analgesia to the larynx helps to prevent this. An intravenous drip is advisable for all major cases, so that blood transfusion can be given if necessary.

MONITORING.—Readings of blood-pressure, pulse-rate, and respiratory rate should be taken at least every 10 minutes. Any changes not obviously related to anæsthesia should be reported to the surgeon as they may be caused by intracranial manipulations or by a sudden rise in intracranial pressure. An œsophageal stethoscope is a useful aid, while an electrocardiogram acts as an excellent pulse monitor. Some anæsthetists who favour hyperventilation techniques perform hourly estimations of arterial Pco_2, Po_2, pH, bicarbonate and buffer base.[*] Hewer has developed a simple method of spirometry for use during spontaneous respiration.[†] Characteristic patterns may give early warning to the surgeon. For example, ischæmia of the brain-stem results in a sudden deep breath followed by a series of shallow respirations.

AIR EMBOLISM.[‡]—This is a particular danger in the sitting or steep head-up position, especially when respirations are controlled with a resulting fall in venous pressure. Many of the veins in the fibro-fatty tissues of the back of the neck do not collapse readily after they have been divided, but are held open. The mastoid emissary vein is a particularly common site for air entry. Portals of entry within the dura are relatively uncommon. Warning of air embolism may be given by fall of blood-pressure, pulse irregularities, respiratory irregularities, apnœa, or circulatory arrest. During that part of the operation when embolism is likely to occur, a pulse monitor is valuable and jugular compression may be applied. An œsophageal or precordial stethoscope may enable the anæsthetist to hear the

---

[*] Gilbert, R. G. B., Brindle, G. F., and Galindo, A., *Anæsthesia for Neurosurgery*, 1966. London: Churchill.

[†] Hewer, A. J. H., *Proc. R. Soc. Med.*, 1966, **60**, 362.

[‡] *See also* Hunter, A. R., *Anæsthesia*, 1962, **17**, 467.

characteristic sounds of air passing through the heart. If air embolism is suspected, the following measures may be useful: (1) Jugular compression; (2) Flood the wound with saline; (3) Lower the head and put the patient in the left lateral position; (4) Cardiac compression if heart action ceases, after aspiration of air from the heart.*

AGENTS AND TECHNIQUES.—

HYPERVENTILATION.†—I.P.P.V. with hyperventilation is becoming an increasingly popular technique during intracranial surgery.‡ The advantages are:—

1. The moderate rises of arterial Pco_2 (over 55 mm. Hg) which are common in light general anæsthesia with spontaneous respiration are avoided. Such rises cause an increase in cerebral blood-flow and cerebrospinal fluid pressure.

2. Resulting cerebral vasoconstriction leads to an excellent surgical field.

3. Minimal quantities of anæsthetic agents are required.

The anæsthetic agents used are thiopentone, nitrous oxide and oxygen, muscle relaxant, and full topical analgesia to the larynx and trachea. Volatile supplements, halothane or methoxyflurane, are sometimes given in the initial stages. Tubocurarine, the relaxant most frequently employed, is given in full doses to increase overall compliance which allows ventilation with minimal elevation of mean airway pressure. A mechanical ventilator ensures that ventilation is uniform. It may be combined with a negative phase and periodic hyperinflation to prevent miliary atelectasis. Some units monitor blood gases and adjust ventilation accordingly. There is no indication for lowering $Paco_2$ below 25–30 mm. Hg, at which level the cerebral blood-flow has been reduced about 50 per cent. Levels below 20 mm. Hg may lead to E.E.G. changes and an increase of anaerobic metabolism of glucose in the brain.§

Other workers have used the neurolept agents. Premedication with droperidol and atropine, then intravenous phenoperidine, 5 mg., after which the patient must be reminded to breathe. Then thiopentone, suxamethonium, intubation, nitrous oxide, oxygen, I.P.P.V. with tubocurarine to reduce inflation pressures to a low level.||

CONTROLLED VENTILATION WITH NORMAL $Paco_2$.†— Respiratory alkalosis may be undesirable:—

1. In the sitting position, when hypotension may occur.

2. During hypothermia, when there is likelihood of cardiac arrhythmias.

In these circumstances, it may be desirable to keep $Paco_2$ within normal limits. This can be accomplished if serial blood gas estimations are made.

---

* See also Marshall, B. M., Canad. Anæsth. Soc. J., 1965, **12**, 255.
† See also Gilbert, R. G. B., Brindle, G. F., and Galindo, A., Anæsthesia for Neurosurgery, 1966. London: Churchill.
‡ Furness, D. N., Brit. J. Anæsth., 1957, **29**, 415.
§ Wollman, H., and others, Anesthesiology, 1965, **26**, 329; and Alexander, S. C., and others, Ibid., 1965, **26**, 624.
|| Brown, A. S., Horton, J. M., and MacRae, W. R., Anæsthesia, 1963, **18**, 143.

General Anæsthesia, *continued.*

SPONTANEOUS RESPIRATION.—This is now less popular than formerly, since, even with impeccable technique, small rises of Paco$_2$ occur with resultant increase in cerebral blood-flow and cerebrospinal fluid pressure. Spontaneous respiration may have advantages in posterior fossa explorations, when the surgeon is working near the brain-stem. Sudden changes in respiratory pattern may then indicate ischæmia of the vital centres and serve as a warning mechanism to the surgeon. Techniques include:—

1. Thiopentone (sleep dose), nitrous oxide, oxygen, trichloro-ethylene. Suxamethonium for intubation. Small dose (10 mg.) of pethidine to control tachypnœa.

2. Thiopentone (sleep dose), nitrous oxide, oxygen, halothane, or oxygen–halothane. Suxamethonium for intubation. Small doses of pethidine to control tachypnœa.

3. Nitrous oxide, oxygen, halothane in small children.

4. Thiopentone, nitrous oxide, oxygen, pethidine. Care must be taken to avoid respiratory depression.

Reduction of Intracranial Tension.—A raised intracranial tension produces a tight dura and brain and makes exploration difficult. There are various methods of reducing intracranial tension :—

1. Ventricular tap. The surgeon needles the lateral ventricle and removes fluid until the pressure falls.

2. Spinal drainage. Controlled withdrawal of C.S.F. via a catheter put into the subarachnoid space in the lumbar region. Fluid is not withdrawn until the dura is open to prevent coning.

3. Use of hypertonic solutions intravenously: (*a*) *Mannitol** ($C_6H_{14}O_6$) is a hexahydric alcohol closely related to the hexose sugars and isomeric with sorbitol. Solutions can be sterilized by auto-claving. Dose of the intravenous solution, 20 per cent, is 50–100 g. Little is metabolized and only small amounts reabsorbed by the renal tubules. Does not irritate the tissues. Causes a brisk osmotic diuresis, and small 'rebound' increase in brain volume; (*b*) *Urea*, 30 per cent solution in 10 per cent invert sugar in water, run in intravenously over 1–2 hours at a rate of 60 drops per minute; it is eventually distributed to the brain and owing to the reverse osmotic gradient results in a rebound increase in brain volume; (*c*) 100 ml. 50 per cent *sucrose*; (*d*) Triple strength *plasma*, 1–1·5 g. per kg. body-weight.

Note that the solution of urea is very irritant to the tissues so that necrosis may occur if the solution is allowed to leak extravascularly and thrombosis of the vein itself may occur. Urea can also be given by mouth (post-operatively) in a dose of 12 g. in 100 ml. water flavoured with milk or orange, 3 times a day. Urea also has a diuretic effect, so it is important to watch out for bladder distension.

4. Increasing head-up tilt.

5. Lowering blood-pressure. Use of ganglionic blocking drugs.

---

* *Brit. med. J.*, 1963, **2**, 239; and Wise, B. L., and Chater, N., *Arch. Neurol., Chicago*, 1961, **4**, 200.

6. Hypothermia.
7. Hyperventilation.
8. Use of muscle relaxants to reduce intra-abdominal pressure and hence venous pressure.
9. Use of steroids. Dexamethasone, 60 mg. daily, has been advocated for treatment of post-operative œdema.*

Use of Hypothermia in Neurosurgery.—This has a definite place : (1) It allows important vessels to be temporarily occluded during removal of vascular tumours or aneurysms ; (2) It produces a reduction in cerebrospinal fluid pressure ; (3) It may make hypotensive techniques safer ; (4) It is useful in the treatment of some cases of head injury. The temperature should not be taken below 30° C., since it is difficult to institute immediate cardiac massage in the middle of a neurosurgical operation should ventricular fibrillation supervene.

The technique used is almost always surface cooling. Premedication with chlorpromazine and promethazine may help to promote heat loss via the skin (*see also* Chapter XXIX). Attempts have been made at selective cooling of the brain by returning cooled blood to the internal carotid artery but such work is still in its trial stages.

It has been suggested that temperatures lower than 30° C. may be reached with safety† : (1) With very slow cooling ; (2) If adequate blood-pressure is maintained to facilitate coronary artery perfusion ; (3) Using intravenous alcohol to counteract shivering and vascular spasm without reduction of blood-pressure ; (4) If hypercapnia is avoided.

PROFOUND HYPOTHERMIA IN NEUROSURGERY.—Surgical repair of intracranial aneurysms has been performed under profound hypothermia (15° C.). At this temperature some form of extracorporeal circulation is necessary. This involves thoracotomy for insertion of cannulæ, etc. (*see* p. 586).

Recently neurosurgical operations have been carried out under profound hypothermia using a closed-chest extracorporeal technique.‡ Cannulæ are placed in femoral veins and the femoral artery, and blood taken through a pump oxygenator and heat exchanger. Flow rates are lower than with open chest perfusion so temperature falls more slowly. During rewarming external defibrillators are used to restore cardiac rhythm. Pulmonary vascular damage is a potential hazard due to persistent bronchial blood-flow and rise of pulmonary venous pressure. The presence of patent ductus, coarctation of the aorta, or aortic insufficiency is a contra-indication to the method.

Controlled Hypotension.—This is particularly useful in the removal of hæmorrhagic tumours (e.g., meningioma) and in the surgery of

---

* Ramusan, T., and Gulati, D. R., *J. Neurosurg.*, 1962, **19**, 535; and Shenkin, H. A., Goliboff, B., and Haft, H., *Ibid.*, 1962, **19**, 897.
† Hewer, A. J., *Brit. med. J.*, 1963, **2**, 240.
‡ Michenfelder, J. D., Terry, H. R., Daw, E. F., MacCarty, C. S., and Uihlein, A., *Anesthesiology*, 1963, **24**, 177.

Controlled Hypotension, *continued*.

intracranial aneurysms. It also produces a reduction in intra
cranial tension. The technique of controlled hypotension is dis
cussed in Chapter XXVIII.

Anæsthesia for Craniotomy.—Careful anæsthetic technique is re
quired along the lines already indicated. Remember that fronta
craniotomy may involve opening of the frontal sinuses wit
hæmorrhage into the respiratory tract. Parietal craniotomy ma
demand acute flexion of the neck so that the danger of a kinke
endotracheal tube is correspondingly greater. Some tumours (e.g.
meningioma) are particularly vascular and may involve sever
blood-loss.

POSTERIOR FOSSA CRANIOTOMY.—This may be performed i
the prone, lateral, or sitting position. Surgical manipulation
near the brain-stem may interfere with the vital centres causin
respiratory or pulse irregularities.* Air embolism is a particula
hazard in the sitting position and so is hypotension. The latte
may be counteracted by: (1) Pressor drugs; (2) Bandaging o
the lower extremities to prevent venous pooling; (3) Applicatio
of a G-suit.† The sitting position may also be employed fo
operations on the cervical spine. Most anæsthetists do not emplo
controlled respiration which would mask respiratory signs.

Intracranial Aneurysms.—Surgical treatment may be difficult an
carry a high risk depending on the general condition of the patient
the level of consciousness, the site of the aneurysm, and its relatio
to adjacent structures. Hypotension (60–80 mm. Hg arteria
pressure) has been used with or without moderate hypothermia
but there is a danger of retractor anæmia, and local brain ischæmi
as a result of low perfusion pressure and local vascular spasm
Profound hypothermia has been used (p. 549) in an effort to reduc
the harmful effects of ischæmia. Profound and easily reversibl
hypotension has been tried. A cardiac pacemaker is used to rais
the rate to between 200 and 250 beats per min. Cardiac outpu
falls virtually to zero, and arterial and venous pressures approximate
to 20 mm. Hg. This is only allowed for 4 or at the most 6 min
Provided the myocardium is healthy, brief profound hypotensio
of this order is probably safe. External defibrillation must be
available in case of ventricular fibrillation.‡

Operations on the Spinal Column.—Laminectomy often requires
the prone position. Tumours of the spinal cord may interfere
with intercostal nerve-supply or even the phrenic nerve-roots
Operations for prolapsed intervertebral disk may be carried out ir
the lateral or prone position. In any event careful positioning is
essential to allow free respiratory movement and avoid back-
pressure on veins and increased vascularity at the operation site.§

* *See also* Whitby, J. D., *Brit. J. Anæsth.*, 1963, **35**, 624.
† Gardner, W. J., and Dohm, D. F., *J. Amer. med. Ass.*, 1956, **162**, 774.
‡ Brown, A. S., and Horton, J. M., *Proc. 2nd Eur. Cong. Anæsth.*, 1966, **1**, 665.
§ Taylor, A. R., Gleadhill, C. A., Bilsland, W. L., and Murray, P. F., *Brit. J. Anæsth.*,
1956, **28**, 213; and Pearce, D. J., *Proc. R. Soc. Med.*, 1957, **50**, 107.

Bleeding from the extradural veins is the chief trouble. Pressure on the chest or abdomen, coughing and straining squeeze blood out of the abdominal and thoracic veins into the vertebral veins, so distending them. The ideal position (if the surgeon cannot be persuaded to operate with the patient on his side) is the jack-knife position with the prone patient's pelvis supporting his weight. This allows the extradural veins to collapse. The field of operation should be the highest point on the operating table. A head-down position is contra-indicated if a myelogram has been recently performed. The use of a cuffed endotracheal tube gives control of the airway and prevents aspiration of stomach contents. A muscle relaxant, by reducing intra-abdominal pressure, will reduce bleeding. Adrenaline 1–250,000 in saline can be infiltrated into the skin and muscles.

For laminectomy in the lumbar region, a light general anæsthetic given through an endotracheal tube is usually employed, otherwise an extradural spinal analgesic can be used.* This may require the injection of large volumes of solution, e.g., lignocaine 1·5 per cent solution with adrenaline, 35–40 ml. in young fit patients, if bleeding is to be reduced.† The patient may be semi-prone or fully prone, in the so-called 'Mohammedan praying position'.‡ If a general anæsthetic is given and the operation performed with the patient prone, a stomach tube should be passed to avoid aspiration of stomach contents into lungs, as regurgitation may follow pressure on the patient's lumbar region. In these cases, a well-padded rest should be placed beneath each shoulder, and beneath the pelvis, so that a small space separates the patient's chest from the table. This will aid respiration and reduce bleeding by preventing an increase in the abdominal and hence in the extradural venous network. Also it will prevent circulatory depression resulting from pressure on the inferior vena cava.

When the surgeon places special value on wound ischæmia, hypotension can be produced by: (1) Intradural block; (2) Extradural block; (3) Ganglionic blocking agents,§ (4) Halothane, with‖ or without I.P.P.V.

Anæsthesia for Carotid Artery Surgery.—Two problems present themselves in these cases: (1) The prevention of anoxic brain damage during periods of arterial occlusion; (2) The management of a group of patients, many of them elderly with generalized arterial disease.

Surface cooling to 30° C. with gas–oxygen and halothane in a semi-closed circuit has been advised.¶ Hypercapnia has been used to promote blood-flow to the brain through collateral vessels during occlusion of the carotid artery.** Cervical plexus block has also been advocated.††

* Matheson, D., Canad. Anæsth. Soc. J., 1960, 7, 149.
† Thorne, T. C., personal communication.
‡ Lipton, S., Anæsthesia, 1950, 5, 208.
§ Holmes, F., J. Bone Jt Surg., 1956, 38, 846.
‖ Sleath, G. W., and Archer, L. T., Canad. Anæsth. Soc. J., 1967, 14, 407.
¶ Knight, P. F., Brit. J. Anæsth., 1961, 33, 40.
** Wells, B. A., Keats, A. S., and Cooley, D. A., Surgery, 1963, 54, 216; and Homi, J., Smart, J. F., and Wasmuth, C. E., Proc. 2nd Eur. Cong. Anæsth., 1966, 1, 629.
†† McCrory, C. B., Rainer, G., Feiler, E. M., and Bloomquist, C. D., Ibid., 1966, 2, 43.

Anæsthesia for Diagnostic Procedures.*—

CEREBRAL ANGIOGRAPHY.—This was popularized by Egas Moniz, of Portugal—of leucotomy fame—in 1927,† and developed by Engeset in 1944 and by Lindgren in 1947. It is usually done through the intact skin, when 40 per cent diodone or 60 per cent urografin is injected into a carotid artery : average dose about 30 ml. Local analgesia is usually satisfactory, though there may be subjective symptoms of flushing, heat, and retro bulbar pain. General anæsthesia is indicated in children or in uncooperative adults, or when surgery is to follow immediately after radiography. Some favour general anæsthesia for all cases believing that the vasodilatation produced is of value.‡ Brown§ has described a hypotensive response due either to vascular spasm from the irritant effect of the dye on hypersensitive vessels or to temporary cerebral œdema resulting from damage to vascular endothelium. Note that patients may have had a recent subarachnoid hæmorrhage and may be gravely ill with effects of direct cerebral damage, vascular spasm, or cerebral œdema.

ARTERIAL CATHETERIZATION.—Percutaneous femoral or brachial arterial catheterization may be requested by the neuro radiologist. Neurolept analgesia gives good results.‖

VENTRICULOGRAPHY.—Two bur holes are made, one on each side of the skull. A cannula is passed into each lateral ventricle Cerebrospinal fluid is withdrawn and replaced by oxygen. The outlines of the ventricular system are then seen on radiographs The investigation is often performed on patients with raised intracranial pressure.

Local analgesia is satisfactory in adults, unless it is anticipated that craniotomy will follow radiography. General anæsthesia is required in children. The patients must be carefully watched for several hours after completion of the investigation.

PNEUMO-ENCEPHALOGRAPHY.—Air is introduced to the ventricular system from below. There is a danger of herniation of the medulla and air embolism. The investigation should not be carried out in the presence of raised intracranial pressure. The patient is placed in a sitting position.

1. Cisternal injection. With neck flexed, a needle is introduced into the cisterna magna ; fluid removed ; and air introduced.
2. Lumbar injection. Lumbar puncture ; fluid removed ; air introduced.

When the air has reached the ventricular system, radiographs are taken. These investigations are often very unpleasant when performed under local analgesia. Symptoms include headache, nausea, vomiting, sweating, and vasomotor collapse. Headache may last for hours or days. General anæsthesia is usually preferred.

---

* See also Wylie, W. D., and Churchill-Davidson, H. C., A Practice of Anæsthesia, 1960, p. 778. London: Lloyd-Luke; and Boulton, T. B., in Recent Advances in Anæsthesia and Analgesia, Ch. VII, 9th ed. (Ed. Hewer, C. Langton), 1963. London: Churchill.
† Egas Moniz, Rev. neurol., 1027, 2, 42.
‡ Brindle, G. F., Gilbert, R. G. B., and McGrath, J. J., Curr. Res. Anesth., 1965, 44, 565.
§ Brown, A. S., Anæsthesia, 1955, 10, 346.
‖ Gilbert, R. G. B., and others, Internat. Anesthesiol. Clinics, 1966, 4, 771.

ANÆSTHETIC TECHNIQUE.—The principles of technique do not differ from those of neurosurgical operations in general. Thiopentone, nitrous oxide, oxygen with trichloroethylene or halothane is usually satisfactory. A flexometallic tube is recommended to ensure a clear airway at all times. Local analgesia to the larynx together with a sufficient depth of anæsthesia to prevent coughing on the tube is advisable. The head and neck may be moved for radiographs. Take care that anæsthetic connexions do not block the radiological field ; if necessary the patient may be disconnected from the machine during exposure.

Anæsthesia in Head Injuries.*—Anæsthesia may be required for elevation of a depressed fracture, suture of widespread lacerations, etc. Anæsthesia may also be required for treatment of some other surgical condition in the presence of a head injury.

Each case needs individual assessment. Look for : (1) Evidence of an acute rise of intracranial pressure (e.g., middle meningeal hæmorrhage, dilated fixed pupil on one side, slow breathing or apnœa, hypertension, tachycardia, etc.); (2) Level of consciousness and maintenance of airway; (3) Evidence of bleeding into airway (e.g., fracture base of skull); (4) Associated injuries (e.g., pneumothorax, ruptured spleen, fractured femur); (5) Shock; (6) Full stomach.

A cuffed endotracheal tube is usually indicated especially in comatose patients, when it may be passed after the injection of suxamethonium and topical analgesia. The operation can then be performed under local analgesia or light general anæsthesia. Tracheostomy may be required. Careful observation is necessary. Blood transfusion may be indicated. Local analgesia may suffice. Cerebral damage may follow an additional rise in intracranial tension due to induction of anæsthesia.

Thermocoagulation of the Globus Pallidus.—This is carried out for Parkinson's disease. The operation involves : (1) Stereotaxic radiological localization of the globus pallidus ; (2) Craniectomy ; (3) Insertion of electrodes so that their tips lie in the calculated position ; (4) Heat coagulation ; (5) Closure. The patient should be conscious during the actual coagulation so that the effect of the lesion can be observed as it is being made. This operation may therefore be carried out under local analgesia. Hurter† has described a technique which provides anæsthesia while air is injected into the ventricular system and during craniectomy, but allows rapid recovery of consciousness before coagulation. Premedication, atropine 0·85 mg. ($\frac{1}{75}$ gr.), sleep dose of thiopentone, suxamethonium 100 mg., topical spray 4 per cent lignocaine to larynx and trachea, flexometallic oral endotracheal tube, nitrous oxide–oxygen, pethidine 10–20 mg., halothane. Local analgesia is used in the scalp. Anæsthesia is discontinued on completion of the craniectomy and the endotracheal tube withdrawn when consciousness returns. Other workers omit all premedication since atropine may interfere with postoperative assessment. Methohexitone is used in an intravenous drip (about 2·4 mg. per minute)

---

* See also Hart, S. M., Brit. J. Anæsth., 1965, **37**, 189.
† Hurter, D. G., Ibid., 1960, **32**, 160.

Thermocoagulation of the Globus Pallidus, continued.

together with small doses of gallamine where tremor is severe.
Rapid recovery of consciousness occurs when the drip is discontinued.*

Neurolept analgesia has been used successfully.† It offers sedation with suppression of physical and mental discomfort, while
the patient's full co-operation is maintained. The subject is given
droperidol, 2–4 mg., slowly intravenously, followed by phenoperidine, 2–3 mg., slowly, taking care that respirations are not
unduly depressed. The patient appears to sleep, but responds to
questions and is co-operative. This state comes on after 15 minutes
and lasts for about 3 hours, during which time surgery is carried
out under local analgesia.

Hydroxydione has also been advocated as the anæsthetic agent of
choice as it is said to induce light anæsthesia with preservation
of synaptic responses, that is to say, thalamic activity is unchanged.‡

CHAPTER XXII

ANÆSTHESIA IN THORACIC SURGERY§

Development.—In trying to avoid atelectasis, Sauerbruch (1875–1951)
in Breslau in 1904 did his early thoracotomies in an airtight
chamber with atmospheric pressure reduced by 7 mm. Hg, while
the patient's head and the anæsthetist were outside, in atmospheric
air (negative-pressure breathing).|| He later advocated positive-
pressure breathing. Elsberg obtained the same effect in 1910 by
insufflating anæsthetic gases into the trachea at a positive pressure
of 20 mm. Hg. The first use of endobronchial (one lung) anæsthesia
was described by Gale and Waters,¶ while a bronchus blocker was
described by Archibald, at the suggestion of Harold R. Griffith, in
1935.** Crafoord, of Stockholm, reported his method of artificial
respiration by means of Frenckner's mechanical spiro-pulsator††
in 1938,‡‡ and this was developed and simplified by Nosworthy
(1941)§§ who advocated controlled breathing by intermittent
pressure on the reservoir bag of a closed circuit, using cyclopropane.
This technique had previously been introduced by Guedel and
Treweek, in 1934, using ether.|||| Cyclopropane had a great
popularity during the decade following 1935, but is now on the

* Coleman, D. J., and de Villiers, J. C., *Anæsthesia*, 1964, **19**, 60.
† Brown, A. S., *Ibid.*, 1964, **19**, 70.
‡ Vourc'h, G., Hardy, J., and Denarit, M., *Brit. J. Anæsth.*, 1963, **35**, 208.
§ *See also Thoracic Anæsthesia* (Ed. Mushin, W. W.), 1963. Oxford : Blackwell.
|| Sauerbruch, F., *Zbl. Chir.*, 1904, **31**, 146; and *Mitt. Grenz. Med. Chir.*, 1904, **13**, 399.
¶ Gale, J. N., and Waters, R. M., *J. thorac. Surg.*, 1931, **1**, 432.
** Archibald, E., *Ibid.*, 1935, **4**, 335.
†† Frenckner, P., *Acta Otolaryngol.*, 1934, Suppl. 20, 100.
‡‡ Crafoord, C., *Acta chir. scand.*, 1938, Suppl. 54.
§§ Nosworthy, M. D., *Proc. R. Soc. Med.*, 1941, **34**, 479.
|||| Guedel, A. E., and Treweek, D. N., *Curr. Res. Anesth.*, 1934, **13**, 263.

decline in chest surgery because of its effect on the automatic conducting tissue of the heart, and because of the increasing use of diathermy with the risk of explosion. The use of muscle relaxants has made it relatively easy to control respiration.

The Problem of Open Pneumothorax.—Normally, the lungs are kept inflated by :—

1. The atmospheric pressure acting on the alveoli.
2. The adhesion of the two layers of the pleura due to the surface tension of the thin layer of fluid separating them. When the chest is opened, atmospheric pressure becomes equal on the alveolar and pleural surfaces and the elastic recoil causes collapse of the lung.

When one side of the chest is opened, negative pressure is lost. The larger the hole, the more pronounced the effect. The lung on the affected side collapses, due to recoil of its elastic tissues. The mediastinum, unless fixed by adhesions, is deviated to the sound side and presses on the sound lung. If the lung is adherent to the chest wall, these effects may not be marked. If the condition is not soon checked, death from cardiorespiratory depression follows.

RESPIRATION is affected by :—

1. Collapse of the lung, and retraction of the mediastinum.
2. PARADOXICAL BREATHING. (Sometimes called internal paradoxical respiration, to distinguish it from external paradoxical respiration seen in respiratory obstruction or in fourth plane anæsthesia, when the chest and abdomen move paradoxically, the chest contracting during inspiration.)—When lung tissue is unsupported by a rigid chest wall, it tends to move in response to pressure changes in the bronchi, which is high during expiration and lower during inspiration. These changes are minimal during quiet breathing, increase during deep or partially obstructed breathing, and are maximal during coughing. The partially collapsed lung on the affected side is emptied still more with each inspiration as air is drawn from it into the sound lung. During expiration, as chest cavity gets smaller, sound lung squeezes some of its vitiated air into the collapsed lung. (The remainder of its air enters the trachea.) Thus affected lung expands during expiration and collapses during inspiration, and, owing to the amount of vitiated air drawn from the affected lung into the sound one, the latter cannot interchange gases efficiently (increased dead space effect).

The air passing from one lung to the other is sometimes called the pendulum air.

3. MEDIASTINAL FLAP.—If the mediastinum is mobile and an open pneumothorax exists, its structures tend to move across to the sound side, drawn by the negative pressure there : effect is greater during inspiration than expiration. The result is pressure on the sound lung and interference with its efficiency. Respiration is stimulated both in rate and depth by the collapse of the lung and by hypoxia and hypercapnia, and the hyperpnœa which follows this stimulation makes the mediastinal movement worse. If the mediastinum is fixed by

The Problem of Open Pneumothorax, *continued.*

inflammatory adhesions, its movement is less marked ; nevertheless the sound lung has to take over the whole of the tidal exchange, eventually causing muscular exhaustion and hyper capnia.

The result is OXYGEN LACK AND CARBON DIOXIDE EXCESS.

CIRCULATION is affected by :—

1. ABSENCE OF NEGATIVE INTRATHORACIC PRESSURE which normally aids filling of the auricles : the venous return and cardiac output are thus reduced.

2. MEDIASTINAL FLAP, due to respiration ; causing intermittent obstruction of the superior and inferior venæ cavæ, and consequent tachycardia and hypotension.

3. REFLEX DISTURBANCES AND CHANGES DUE TO POSTURE.— Infiltration with local analgesic solution of the pulmonary plexus at the hilum of the lung, or of the vagus nerves in the neck, minimizes reflex disturbances.

The result is a CLINICAL PICTURE OF SHOCK.

The hazards of open pneumothorax are lessened if hyperpnœa is avoided.

Solution of the Problem of Open Pneumothorax

Controlled Respiration (which may start off as assisted respiration) —This has become standard practice in British anæsthesia since important papers by Guedel[*] and Nosworthy[†] in the early 1940's who utilized cyclopropane. The introduction of muscle relaxants has allowed easy control of pulmonary ventilation without deep general anæsthesia. By manual or mechanical pressure on the reservoir bag during inspiration only, both paradoxical breathing and mediastinal flap are abolished. It is really intermittent positive-pressure anæsthesia. Expiration should be allowed to take at least twice the time given to inspiration. In this way complete deflation of the chest with proper carbon dioxide elimination is ensured, while the number of heart-beats occurring during the period of normal intrathoracic pressure will be greater than the number taking place during the phase of abnormally high intrathoracic pressure when the venous return is smaller than normal. Before the chest is opened, the pressure needed to inflate the lungs is about 20–30 cm. H_2O. After thoracotomy it is about 10 cm. H_2O and during controlled respiration the intrabronchial pressure varies between atmospheric and $+$ 10 cm. H_2O. It is difficult to build up more than 20–30 cm. H_2O using a thin rubber bag.

Apnœa may result from one or more of the following : (*a*) Peripheral muscular paralysis by a relaxant. (*b*) Hypocapnia. (*c*) Central depression from drugs. (*d*) Reflex inhibition of the respiratory centre due to distension of the lungs. (*e*) A mixture of the above.

The advantages of controlled breathing are :—

1. Paradoxical breathing and hypoventilation are corrected.

* Guedel, A. E., *Anesthesiology*, 1940, **1**, 13.

† Nosworthy, M. D., *Proc. R. Soc. Med.*, 1941, **34**, 479.

2. Mediastinal flap is abolished.
3. Control of the operative field is facilitated and movement can be made to suit the surgeon.
4. Work done by the patient is reduced.
5. The feel of the reservoir bag aids the anæsthetist in his assessment of anæsthetic depth.

During intrathoracic surgery, most anæsthetists in Britain employ controlled breathing from the start of the operation. This may be manual or mechanical. Before the chest is open, a negative phase increases the venous return to the heart and is specially beneficial when the circulating blood-volume is low. After the chest is opened, a negative phase does not benefit the circulation significantly.

The disadvantages of controlled respiration are :—
1. Risk of rupture of emphysematous bullæ.
2. By reversing the intrathoracic pressures during the respiratory cycle the venous return is hindered.
3. Absence of respiration as a guide to anæsthetic depth.
4. Possibility of production of alkalosis from hyperventilation. Of little clinical importance in most cases.

Ventilatory Capacity.—The functional reserve of the lungs may be limited by lung disease. This may be obvious clinically or may be found by application of lung function tests (*see* p. 49). These factors play a considerable part in the pre-operative evaluation of the patient and help to determine the advisability and extent of surgical removal of lung tissue. They are also important in the post-operative period because a superadded lung collapse or infection may prove very serious.

It is important that lung operations be postponed if there is evidence of recent acute infection of the respiratory tract. Such operations are usually carried out under an antibiotic umbrella. Pre- and post-operative physiotherapy and nursing care are of extreme importance.

Pulmonary Secretions

Since the introduction of antibiotics and postural drainage, the patient with excessive secretion is becoming uncommon, but wet cases still occur in bronchiectasis, lung abscess, bronchopleural fistula, and associated with new growths when obstruction to a bronchus may cause a pool of infected secretions to lie peripherally. Methods for controlling the spread of secretions include :—

1. Pre-operative preparation : postural drainage and antibiotic therapy and measures to improve the general health of the patient and dry up secretions.
2. Regional analgesia during which the cough reflex is not lost—in thoracoplasty, empyema, etc.
3. Posture during operation. When the patient is tilted head-down 35° for left thoracotomy, 55° for right thoracotomy, and is on his side, secretions from the upper—diseased—lung will flow by gravity into the trachea and can be aspirated, thus preventing contamination of the healthy lung. Similarly if the patient is prone, necessitating a posterolateral incision, secretions can be

Pulmonary Secretions, *continued.*

aspirated. (Overholt* (requiring a special table) ; Parr
Brown.†) Useful position in children too small for the use o
blockers, who are undergoing lobectomy ; and in upper lob
ectomies in adults. When the patient is in the prone position
the table should be tilted head down by 10° and secretions ca:
either be aspirated from a cuffed endotracheal tube or allowe
to gravitate around a non-cuffed tube into the pharynx and
mask, from which they can be sucked intermittently. Anæs
thesia in the prone position keeps the weight of the mediastinum
off the sound lung and nearly always does away with the nee
for balloons, except in very wet cases, to prevent pus from th
lower lobe contaminating the upper lobe Alternatively, secre
tions can be retained in the diseased lobe by suitable posture
e.g., the sitting position for lower lobectomy in bronchiectasis
An empyema is also often drained with the patient sitting
especially if there is any chance of bronchopleural fistula with
its risk of the patient drowning in his own secretions.

4. Endotracheal suction. Listen to the corrugated tubing—secre
   tions are usually heard if present and can be removed by suction
   catheter. In wet cases routine suction every 10 minutes may
   be advisable. Secretions are likely to move into the main
   bronchi after changes in position and after manipulation of the
   lung.

5. Ask the surgeon to apply the bronchial clamp as soon as possible
   when the chest is open.

6. Endobronchial intubation and blocking with inflatable cuffs.

Endobronchial Instrumentation.—Isolation of one lung or major
lobe has the following advantages :—

1. Secretions and blood can be confined to the diseased lung or lobe
2. The lung to be operated upon can be made quiet and collapsed.
3. A bronchopleural fistula can be isolated.

Methods include :—

1. Bronchial tamponage (Crafoord,‡ 1938).
2. Intubation of the sound bronchus (Gale and Waters, 1931 ; Magill
   1936 ; Vellacott, 1954 ; Gorden and Green, 1955 ; Macintosh
   and Leatherdale, 1955 ; Green, 1958 ; Machray, 1958).
3. Use of bronchial blocker (Magill, 1934, 1936 ; Vernon Thompson
   1943).
4. Use of a double-lumen tube (the Carlens catheter (1949) and its
   modifications ; Bryce-Smith, 1959 ; Bryce-Smith and Salt
   1960 ; White, 1960).

BRONCHIAL TAMPONAGE.—Under direct vision through a
bronchoscope, the bronchus is packed with ½-in. gauze, moistened
with topical analgesic. A disadvantage is that the lung does
not collapse at thoracotomy and may hinder the surgeon.
Seldom used now.

BRONCHIAL BLOCKERS.—These are cuffed suction catheters
They are placed in position under direct vision through a

---

* Overholt, R. H., *J. thorac. Surg.*, 1946, **15**, 384.
† Brown, A. I. Parry, *Thorax*, 1948, **3**, 161.
‡ Crafoord, C., *Acta chir. scand.*, 1938, **81**, Suppl., 54.

bronchoscope. It is important to check the apparatus first :
(a) To make sure the blocker will pass through the bronchoscope ; (b) To determine how much air or water is required to
inflate the cuff ; (c) To check that the introducer is lubricated
and straight to make for easy withdrawal ; (d) To mark the
catheter, so that it will be known when the balloon has just
passed through the bronchoscope.

The bronchoscope is passed under topical or more usually
light general anæsthesia with relaxant, and the carina and major
landmarks identified. Then the tip of the bronchoscope is
placed just proximal to the position desired for the blocker. The
blocker is introduced to the mark already made and the cuff
inflated with an amount of air or water already determined.
Use a small clip to retain the air or water so that the bronchoscope can be withdrawn over it. Then withdraw the introducer
and bronchoscope gently. Check the position of the balloon
by auscultation. The catheter can be used to remove secretions
distal to the balloon by suction. This will also produce collapse
of the lung as the chest is opened.

BRONCHIAL INTUBATION.—An endobronchial tube is passed into
the main bronchus on the sound side. This may be a Machray
modification of the standard Magill endotracheal tube, which is

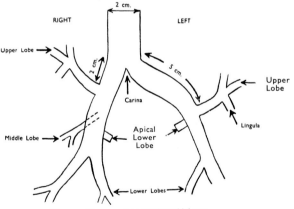

Fig. 35.—Diagram of tracheobronchial tree.

longer and has a smaller cuff than usual.* Such a tube is satisfactory in the left main bronchus, but on the right side it is
likely to occlude the upper lobe bronchus which originates close
to the carina (*Fig.* 35). Endobronchial tubes for use in the
right main bronchus therefore require special construction.

The tube may be passed blind, but this may not be easy,
especially if the normal anatomy of the carina is distorted by

* Machray, R., *Tuberc. Index*, 1958, **13**, 172.

Endobronchial Instrumentation, *continued.*

disease.   Concavity of the tube should be towards the side of
the bronchus to be intubated.   Careful auscultation of the lung
zones for air entry will confirm the position.   A tube of internal
diameter 8–9 mm. is suitable.

The tube may be passed under direct vision over a bronchoscope.   The Magill bronchoscope (*Figs.* 36 and 37) has been

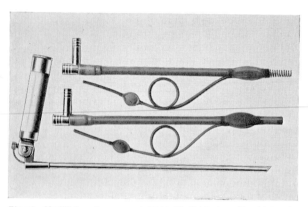

Fig. 36.—Magill's bronchoscope, and right (with distal wire coil) and left endobronchial tubes.   (Medical & Industrial Equipment Ltd.)

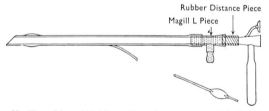

Fig. 37.—Magill's endobronchial tube and bronchoscope, prepared for introduction into
the patient.   Medical & Industrial Equipment Ltd.)

specially designed for this procedure.   It is a thin instrument
(8 mm.) and is passed inside the endobronchial tube, as an introducer.   Both the bronchoscope and the tube require lubrication,
and it is important to check the length and the bevel so that the
bronchoscope reaches to the end of the endobronchial tube.
The whole is then used as a bronchoscope and carefully placed
in position.   The cuff is inflated and the bronchoscope withdrawn.   Check the accuracy of position by auscultation for air
entry.

Types of Endobronchial Apparatus.—

THE VERNON THOMPSON BRONCHUS BLOCKER* (*Fig.* 38).—
The rubber balloon is covered with nylon to provide a rough
surface. It is then less likely to become dislodged.

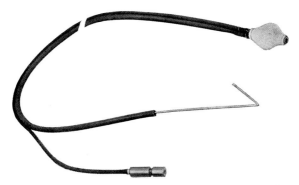

Fig. 38.—Vernon Thompson bronchus blocker. (Medical & Industrial
Equipment Ltd.)

THE MAGILL BRONCHUS OCCLUDER† (*Figs.* 39 and 40).—

Smaller than the Thompson blocker. It will go down the
Magill (8 mm.) bronchoscope and can be used in older children,

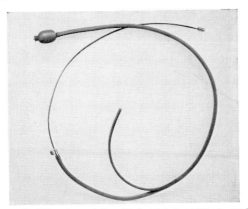

Fig. 39.—Magill bronchus occluder. (Medical & Industrial Equipment Ltd.

* Rusby, L. N., and Thompson, V. C., *Post grad. Med. J.*, 1943, **19**, 44.
† Magill, I. W., *Proc. R. Soc. Med.*, 1935, **29**, 643.

Types of Endobronchial Apparatus, *continued.*

or to occlude a secondary bronchus in adults. More likely to slip than the Thompson instrument.

MAGILL ENDOBRONCHIAL TUBES* (*Figs.* 36 and 37).—Similar to Magill endotracheal tubes but of greater length to reach the

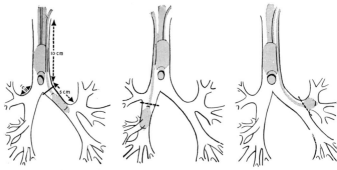

Fig. 40.—Magill blocker and cuffed endotracheal tube in place.

main bronchus. For left lung anæsthesia Machray's modification with a short cuff is satisfactory. For right lung anæsthesia the distal inch of the tube is a spiral wire with no rubber covering to allow aeration of the right upper lobe.

CARLENS'S DOUBLE-LUMEN CATHETER† (*Fig.* 41).—Designed for differential bronchospirometry in 1949, this is a moderately rigid double-lumen rubber catheter, with two inbuilt curves and two inflatable cuffs : it has a rubber hook just above the lower curve which engages the carina and ensures a correct position. The distal part lies in the left main bronchus and has an inflatable cuff so that the left main bronchus can be made gas-tight without obstruction of the left upper lobe bronchus. Just above the carinal hook the right half of the tube has its orifice facing the right main bronchus and above this again is an inflatable tracheal cuff. Pilot bags are fitted to the two inflating tubes. Produced in three sizes, 37, 39, 41 (French), each lumen approximating to Magill sizes 5, 6, and 7. During a left pneumonectomy, closure of the left main bronchus is carried out (after aspiration) following the deflation of the balloons and withdrawal of the tube for 5 cm. The proximal cuff is reinflated and the apparatus then used as a single-lumen endotracheal tube. When there is stenosis or obstruction of the left main bronchus, the tube cannot be used. It is passed blindly through a laryngoscope, and adequate air entry into the lungs confirms

---

* Magill, I. W., *Proc. R. Soc. Med.*, 1935, **29**, 649.

† Carlens, E., *J. thorac. Surg.*, 1949, **18**, 742; Björk, V. O., and Carlens, E., *Ibid.*, 1950, **20**, 151; and Björk, V. O., Carlens, E., and Friberg, O., *Anesthesiology*, 1953, **14**, 60.

the correctness of its position. The relatively small size of the lumina results in underventilation if respiration is spontaneous, but this does not occur if a mechanical respirator is used. The tube is not unduly traumatic.

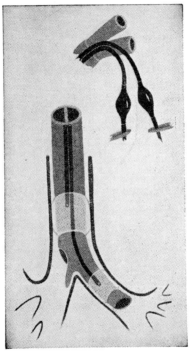

Fig. 41.—Carlens's double-lumen intrabronchial tube. (*Björk, Carlens, and Friberg*, '*Anesthesiology*', 1953.)

THE MACINTOSH AND LEATHERDALE TUBES* (*Figs*. 42, 43).
—Two tubes have been designed for insertion into the bronchi through a laryngoscope : (*a*) A left endobronchial tube with inflatable cuffs designed to lie in the left main bronchus and in the trachea : a small side-channel is provided, used either to aspirate secretions from the non-functioning lung or to distend it. (*b*) A combined endobronchial cuffed suction blocker and endotracheal tube with inflatable cuff. For left lung surgery,

---

* Macintosh, R. R., and Leatherdale, R. A. L., *Brit. J. Anæsth.*, 1955, **27**, 556.

Types of Endobronchial Apparatus, *continued.*

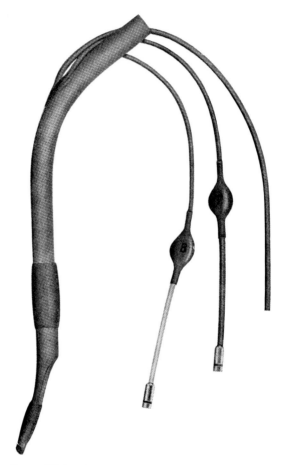

Fig. 42.—M.L. bronchus blocker. (Medical & Industrial Equipment Ltd.)

tube (*b*) is used. It is angulated so that it will blindly enter the left main bronchus. When the cuff on the blocker is inflated, the left lung is isolated, respiration taking place through the right lung only. For right lung surgery the tube (*a*) is passed into the left main bronchus until it is stopped at the carina by its angulation. The endobronchial, and if necessary the endo-tracheal cuff is now inflated, while through the small side-tube oxygen can be supplied to the right lung or secretions sucked from it. In some cases a rubber director aids insertion.

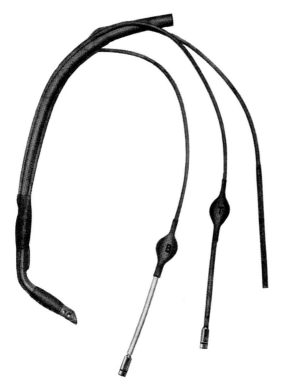

Fig. 43.—M.L. bronchus tube.   (Medical & Industrial Equipment Ltd.)

THE GREEN-GORDON TUBE (*Fig.* 44).—For surgery on the left lung, involving right lung anæsthesia, the Green-Gordon tube can be employed.* This is a tube provided with two inflatable cuffs. The lower 4 cm. of the tube (Magill sizes 8 and 9) is angulated at 15° and on the angulated portion is a lateral slot 2 cm. × 3 cm. wide, with an inflatable cuff attached to the

---

* Green, R., and Gordon, W., *Anæsthesia*, 1957, **12**, 86.

Types of Endobronchial Apparatus, *continued.*

margins of this aperture and surrounding the remainder of the tube. A stiff rubber hook projects from the tube, opposite, and 1 cm. above the slot. The tracheal cuff has its lower margin 2 cm. above the hook. A wire stilette is used during its insertion through the laryngoscope. It is passed blindly into the right bronchus, under topical or general anæsthesia, through the mouth, and comes to rest when its hook catches on

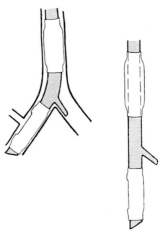

Fig. 44.—The Green-Gordon tube. (*By courtesy of White, G., and the Publishers of the* '*British Journal of Anæsthesia*'.)

the carina. The upper (tracheal) cuff is now inflated, followed by the lower cuff in the right bronchus. The presence of breath-sounds in the right lung and its upper lobe shows correct placing. In size the tubes correspond with Magill sizes 8 and 9.

It is useful in high stenosis of the left main bronchus; neoplasm high up in the left main bronchus; fistula involving the left main bronchus; plastic operations on the left main bronchus.

THE BRYCE-SMITH–SALT TUBE* (*Fig.* 45).—This is a double-lumen tube which may be regarded as a right-sided version of the Carlens catheter. The endobronchial section is directed at an angle of about 17° and carries a cuff with an anterolateral slot to fit against the right upper lobe orifice. The tube is inserted through the glottis with the aid of a laryngoscope and then advanced blindly until it lies in position. The cuffs are inflated, the correct siting of the tube confirmed by auscultation, and any necessary adjustments made. There is no carinal hook.

* Bryce-Smith, R., and Salt, R., *Brit. J. Anæsth.*, 1960, **32**, 230.

THE BRYCE-SMITH TUBE.*—A modification of the Carlens's
double-lumen (left endobronchial) tube. Made in three sizes.
WHITE'S TUBE† (*Fig.* 46).—This is a double-lumen tube for
intubation of the right main bronchus. The slotted cuff on

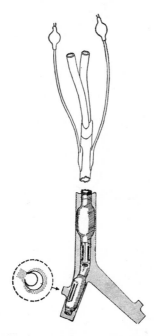

Fig. 45.—Right-sided double-lumen tube in position. Inset shows a section
(×2) of the slotted cuff in relation to the upper lobe orifice. (*By courtesy of Bryce-
Smith, R., and Salt, R., and the Publishers of the ' British Journal of Anæsthesia '.*)

the endobronchial section allows aeration of the right upper
lobe. A carinal hook helps to maintain its position. It is
passed through the glottis with the aid of a laryngoscope and
then advanced blindly. Correct positioning must be confirmed
by auscultation.
ROBERTSHAW'S   LOW-RESISTANCE,   DOUBLE-LUMEN
TUBES‡ (*Fig.* 47).—These are modifications of the Carlens
catheter, designed to have the maximal possible size of lumen
and hence a lower resistance to gas flows. Right- and left-sided

* Bryce-Smith, R., *Brit. J. Anæsth.*, 1959, **31**, 274.
† White, G. M. J., *Ibid.*, 1960, **32**, 232.
‡ Robertshaw, F. L., *Ibid.*, 1962, **34**, 576.

Types of Endobronchial Apparatus, *continued.*

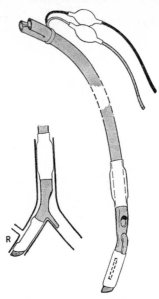

Fig. 46.—White's double-lumen right endobronchial tube. (*By courtesy of White, G., and the Publishers of the 'British Journal of Anæsthesia'.*)

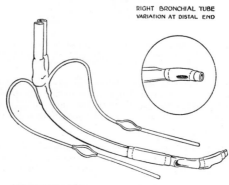

RIGHT BRONCHIAL TUBE
VARIATION AT DISTAL END

LEFT BRONCHIAL TUBE

Fig. 47.—Left-sided double-lumen tube (Robertshaw). Inset shows the slotted bronchial cuff on the right-sided tube. (*By courtesy of the Publishers of the 'British Journal of Anæsthesia'.*)

versions have been developed. The former follows the principles of Green-Gordon and has a slotted endobronchial cuff to allow inflation of the right upper lobe. There is no carinal hook.

Summary of Endobronchial Apparatus.—

1. ENDOBRONCHIAL BLOCKERS.—
    a. Vernon Thompson for left main bronchus. Cuff covered with woven net.
    b. Magill for left main bronchus and secondary bronchi.
    Both must be introduced under direct vision through a bronchoscope. Ventilation is by endotracheal tube.

2. COMBINED BRONCHUS BLOCKER AND ENDOTRACHEAL TUBES.—
    a. Macintosh-Leatherdale.
    b. Stürtzbecher.*
    Both are passed blindly through a laryngoscope. Each has an inflatable cuff on the tracheal part and on the endobronchial blocker.

3. ENDOBRONCHIAL TUBES.—
    a. Magill left. Magill right, with wire coil.
    b. Machray left-sided, with short cuff.
    c. Green-Gordon right-sided tube, with slot to avoid occlusion of the right upper lobe bronchus. Has carinal hook.
    d. Macintosh-Leatherdale, left-sided with inflatable cuffs on tracheal and bronchial parts.
    e. Brompton (Pallister†), left-sided with one cuff on tracheal part and two cuffs (one inside the other) on bronchial part (in case of rupture).
    f. Vellacott,‡ right-sided, for sealing off the right upper lobe, allowing ventilation of the left lung and the middle and lower lobes of the right lung.
    g. The Green right-sided for sealing off right upper lobe. Has carinal hook. Allows ventilation of the left lung and the middle and lower lobes of the right lung.
    The Magill, Machray, Brompton, and Vellacott endobronchial tubes are threaded over a bronchoscope for insertion. The Gordon-Green and Macintosh-Leatherdale tubes are passed blindly through a laryngoscope. The Gordon tube can be passed either way. Pallister's modification of the Gordon-Green can be passed over a bronchoscope.

4. DOUBLE-LUMEN TUBES.—
    a. Carlens, with carinal hook, into left bronchus.
    b. Bryce-Smith, no hook, into left bronchus.
    c. Bryce-Smith–Salt, into right main bronchus, allowing for ventilation of right upper lobe. No carinal hook.
    d. White, into right main bronchus, allowing for ventilation of right upper lobe ; has carinal hook.
    e. Robertshaw low-resistance tubes for insertion into right and left main bronchi.

---

* Stürtzbecher, F., *Anæsthetist*, 1953, **2**, 151.
† Pallister, W. K., *Thorax*, 1959, **14**, 55.
‡ Vellacott, W. N., *Brit. J. Anæsth.* 1954, **26**, 442.

Summary of Endobronchial Apparatus, *continued.*

Bronchoscopes are, of course, not needed for the insertion of an
of these double-lumen tubes.

(*See also* an account of the evolution of endobronchial intubation
White, G. M. J., *Brit. J. Anæsth.*, 1960, **32**, 235.)

Choice of Anæsthetic Technique.—Some anæsthetists prefer to us
endobronchial techniques almost routinely.   But *the majority c
lung resections can be carried out very satisfactorily with ordinar
endotracheal anæsthesia, controlled respiration, and intermitter
suction.*   The decision to use an endobronchial instrument wi'
depend on the nature of the operative procedure, the pathologica
processes present in the lungs, the equipment available, and th
anæsthetist's experience.   The use of double-lumen endobronchia
tubes for 'one lung' anæsthesia results in a fall in arterial oxyge:
tension, and this must be compensated for by using a gas mixtur
containing at least 33 per cent oxygen,* while some author
recommend 50 per cent oxygen.†

PREMEDICATION.—Standard premedication may be used, bearin
in mind the general condition of the patient.   An opiate ma
help to facilitate controlled respiration, provided undue depres
sion is avoided.

ANÆSTHETIC AGENTS.—

1. The thiopentone–relaxant–nitrous-oxide–oxygen technique, witl
   or without pethidine, and with controlled respiration, i
   popular and works well.   Smaller doses of relaxant are ofte
   required for thoracotomy than for upper abdominal relaxation

2. Cyclopropane–oxygen, with small doses of supplementar
   relaxant.   This is, however, an explosive mixture whic
   precludes the use of diathermy.   Where frequent suction i
   required, it is difficult to keep up the cyclopropane concentra
   tion in a closed circuit.

3. Halothane and oxygen.   Blood-pressure must be carefull
   watched.   Controlled respirations may be dangerous unles
   the inspired concentration is known, and the pulse and blood
   pressure carefully monitored.   The majority of worker
   would prefer that the vaporizer should be outside the circui
   of a rebreathing absorption system.   Halothane is advan
   tageous in that it facilitates controlled respiration and is non
   explosive.

BLOOD TRANSFUSION is often required and it is a good genera
rule to set up an intravenous drip before any thoracotomy o
major thoracoplasty.

SOME TECHNICAL POINTS.—

1. As the pleural cavity is opened, slacken pressure in the breathing
   system to allow the lung to fall away from the chest wall.

2. Bronchial suture.   This is usually performed with a bronchia'
   clamp in place and presents no problem.   Occasionally it is
   advantageous to remove the bronchial clamp before inserting
   sutures.   This may mean inability to inflate the lungs for a

---

* Seed, R. F., *Proc. R. Soc. Med.*, 1967, **60**, 750.
† Edwards, E. M., and Hatch, D. J., *Anæsthesia*, 1965, **20**, 461.

few minutes because of the large leak. When this is to be done hyperventilate with oxygen beforehand and watch the condition of the patient carefully during the apnœic period. If cyanosis or untoward signs develop ask the surgeon to plug the leak with a gauze swab while the lungs are hyperventilated.

3. After suture of the bronchial stump is completed the anæsthetist may be asked to test for leaks. This is done by tightening the expiratory valve and increasing the pressure temporarily. It may be necessary to withdraw an endo-bronchial tube first into the trachea. Leaks are usually self-evident. Be careful not to maintain an unduly high pressure in the bronchial tree for too long.

4. Closure of the chest. Make sure that the lungs are fully expanded before closure. During closure keep the lungs up as near to the chest wall as possible, but be careful not to push the lungs up on to the suture needle. It is wise to stop ventilation at the moment of insertion of the needle.

Residual air in the pleural cavity can be removed :—

a. Without drainage. The chest wall is closed except for a small tube communicating with the pleural cavity. The lung is fully expanded by bag pressure, the tube withdrawn and its small hole sutured.

b. A wide-bore needle is inserted into the pleural cavity after its closure, and connected to a sucker, then pulled out when all the air is evacuated.

c. An intra-pleural drainage tube is used and connected to an underwater seal. The method usually adopted.

d. The Heimlich flutter valve. This is a disposable valve which can be used in place of an underwater seal. It allows drainage outwards, but air cannot pass back into the chest. The valve moves with the patient's respiration.

PNEUMONECTOMY.—It is easier to place instruments in the left main bronchus because of the greater distance between the carina and the upper lobe orifice on that side. A blocker in the left main bronchus is generally satisfactory for left pneumonectomy. The cuff is deflated and withdrawn into the trachea immediately before the bronchial clamp is applied. It is best not to attempt to withdraw it past the endotracheal tube as it may become wedged in the glottis. A left endobronchial tube is generally best for right pneumonectomy. It can be withdrawn into the trachea to test for air leaks in the bronchial suture line before closure of the chest.

A blocker cannot be passed into the left main bronchus when growth has filled the lumen. One of the types of right endo-bronchial tubes may then be indicated.

Most pneumonectomies can be performed under ordinary endo-tracheal anæsthesia. But remember that a collection of pus can be squeezed from behind an obstructive carcinoma.

UPPER LOBECTOMY.—It is not easy to block the upper lobe orifice leaving a clear airway to the lower lobe. Attempts to introduce such instruments frequently meet with failure. Upper lobectomy for tuberculosis is seldom associated with copious secretions since the advent of chemotherapy.

Choice of Anaesthetic Technique, *continued.*

UPPER LOBECTOMY WITH SLEEVE RESECTION.—Upper lobectomy is sometimes carried out for carcinoma along with a segment of the main bronchus. This means that the main bronchus will be open for some time and the large air leak may make inflation of the lungs impossible. Endobronchial anæsthesia to the sound lung overcomes these difficulties.

LOWER LOBECTOMY.—This operation may be performed for bronchiectasis, and the volume of sputum may be large. A blocker can be passed below the upper lobe orifice to block the lower lobe on the left side or the middle and lower lobes on the right side. Many of these operations are performed in children. In older children a Magill blocker may be useful. In young children with copious sputum the sitting position should be considered.

SEGMENTAL RESECTION.—Resection of part of a lobe, usually for isolated tuberculous disease. Endotracheal anæsthesia is satisfactory. There may be considerable alveolar air leak afterwards. Occasionally negative pressure must be applied to the drain to keep the lungs expanded post-operatively.

THORACOPLASTY.—Usually carried out in the treatment of advanced tuberculosis with cavitation. Sometimes to reduce the pneumonectomy space after pneumonectomy.

Local analgesia has been advocated so that the patient remains awake and retains a cough reflex. Prolonged coughing is, however, a nuisance to the surgeon and may in fact not be effective in the presence of chest-wall deficiency due to removal of ribs. Note also that the spontaneously breathing patient has a degree of paradoxical respiration during thoracoplasty.

General anæsthesia with an endotracheal tube allows removal of secretions by suction catheter. Controlled respiration prevents paradoxical respiration (which may be important in those with extensive disease and minimal respiratory reserve). Injection of weak adrenaline solution in the paravertebral space and in the line of incision and under the scapula helps to reduce bleeding.

Local analgesia combined with light general anæsthesia (thiopentone–nitrous-oxide–oxygen) has been advocated. It may, however, give the worst of both worlds—abolition of cough mechanism, poor facilities for suction, and a degree of paradoxical respiration. (*See also* p. 344.)

BRONCHOPLEURAL FISTULA.*—This produces two complications :—

1. A leak allowing gases to escape during thoracotomy and which may make inflation of the lungs impossible.
2. A collection of fluid in the pleural cavity or post-pneumonectomy space may escape through it to flood the bronchial tree.

The best solution is the isolation of the fistula by use of an endobronchial tube to the opposite lung. There is some danger

---

* Ryder, G. H., Short, D. H., and Zeitlin, G. L., *Brit. J. Anæsth.*, 1965, **37**, 861.

in the use of a bronchial blocker in the bronchial stump, as it may easily be pushed through the weakened suture line, converting a small fistula into a large one.

DRAINAGE OF EMPYEMA OR PNEUMONECTOMY SPACE INFECTION.—An empyema is usually drained under local anæsthesia in the sitting position. General anæsthesia may be dangerous in the presence of unsuspected bronchopleural fistula and so should not be undertaken lightly. General anæsthesia is, however, necessary for operations more extensive than simple drainage and in children, and then the technique to be used should be carefully considered in the light of a possible bronchopleural fistula.

LUNG ABSCESS.—May be caused by a breaking-down carcinoma or inhalation of infected material. A tuberculous cavity with a fluid level presents similar anæsthetic problems. Pre-operative postural drainage, physiotherapy, and antibiotics may reduce the amount of infected material and change its character. Endobronchial instrumentation may be used to prevent accidental flooding of the bronchial tree during surgery.

LUNG CYSTS.—Large lung cysts cause compression of surrounding lung tissue. They may have a communication with the main bronchus which allows gases to pass in much more easily than out. Intermittent positive pressure may therefore cause a rise in tension in the cyst and may cause further collapse of surrounding tissue with deterioration in the patient's condition. Induction must be carefully carried out in such cases. The tracheobronchial reflexes are often hypersensitive. If coughing is allowed to occur it may result in further rise of tension in the cyst. Spontaneous respiration should be maintained until the cyst has been isolated by an endobronchial instrument or a bronchial clamp. It may be wise to carry out full topical analgesia of the tracheobronchial tree before induction of general anæsthesia. Halothane is a useful agent since smooth quiet respiration can usually be obtained.

Pulmonary hydatid cysts are common in Middle East countries. They may be bilateral and multiple and may require surgical removal if they become large. They may erode into the bronchial wall and become infected. Accidental rupture of cyst contents into the bronchial tree may occur during surgery with the risk of flooding of the airway and dissemination of the disease. Endobronchial instrumentation is often indicated.[*]

ACCIDENTAL PNEUMOTHORAX.—This may occur during operations close to the pleura (e.g., cervical sympathectomy, thoracoplasty, nephrectomy, thyroidectomy), as well as a complication of local blocks (e.g., brachial plexus block, intercostal block). Accidental pneumothorax on the contralateral side can occur during thoracotomy with mediastinal dissection. When it occurs during general anæsthesia the lungs should be held inflated to blow off all possible air while the hole is closed. Accidental pneumothorax may be suspected by reason of altered

---

[*] Al-Enaizi, A., *Proc. 2nd Eur. Cong. Anæsth.*, 1966, **2**, 235.

Choice of Anæsthetic Technique, *continued.*

pattern of spontaneous respiration and confirmed by absence of breath-sounds on auscultation. The air must then be aspirated.

ACUTE MASSIVE PULMONARY EMBOLUS.—This has been successfully treated using cardiopulmonary bypass.* Symptoms and signs may include sudden chest pain, dyspnœa, cyanosis, tachycardia, hæmoptysis, accentuation of the second heart-sound to the left of the sternum, E.C.G. suggestive of cor pulmonale, enlarged proximal pulmonary segments, oligæmia of lung fields, and confirmation can be by pulmonary angiography. Inhalation anæsthesia is required with full oxygenation. Muscle relaxants are required, but thiopentone should be given with extreme caution.

BRONCHOSCOPY.—

1. TOPICAL ANALGESIA.—*See* section in chapter on REGIONAL ANALGESIA (p. 375). Topical analgesia is safer than general anæsthesia if the patient has respiratory obstruction or is expectorating large amounts of blood or pus. It enables also the surgeon to assess the movements of the vocal cords. This cannot be accurately done if the patient is anæsthetized.

2. GENERAL ANÆSTHESIA.—Patient premedicated according to general condition. Whatever method of general anæsthesia is used, many authorities believe that it is best combined with topical spray to larynx and trachea to prevent laryngospasm and undue straining under light anæsthesia.

   a. Topical spray with 4 per cent cocaine or 4 per cent ligno-caine after thiopentone and suxamethonium. After respira-tion returns, bronchoscopy is performed. Supplementary doses of thiopentone are given as required.†

   b. The apnœic oxygenation technique: Thiopentone and suxa-methonium combined with topical spray. As soon as respiration returns supplementary doses of suxamethonium are given to maintain apnœa during bronchoscopy. During apnœa the patient can be kept oxygenated according to the principles of *aventilatory mass flow.* Oxygen is taken up from alveolar gases at a much faster rate than carbon dioxide is eliminated. Gases therefore move down the bronchial tree to occupy the space. If the bronchial tree and upper airways can be kept rich in oxygen by endo-tracheal or pharyngeal insufflation, the patient remains well oxygenated, although Pco_2 rises. Oxygenation is maintained by: (1) oxygen insufflation with a high flow using a separate tube or catheter lying alongside the bronchoscope and inserted beforehand;‡ (2) oxygenation utilizing the side-tube of the bronchoscope though this may be less effective when the bronchoscope is inserted into one of the main bronchi. Oxygenation can be maintained, but hypercarbia occurs and the method should not be used for

---

* Cooley, D. A., Beall, A. C., and Alexander, J. K., *J. Amer. med. Ass.,* 1961, **177**, 283.
† Macintosh, R. R., *Anæsthesia,* 1954, **9**, 77.
‡ Cheatle, C. A., and Chambers, K. B., *Ibid.,* 1955, **10**, 171.

longer periods than 15–20 minutes, watching the pulse. The incidence of arrhythmia appears to be no higher with this technique than with others. Sinus tachycardia is the commonest abnormality.* With this technique it is also possible for the patient to regain consciousness during the paralysis with suxamethonium, so additional small doses of thiopentone may be required, or a non-flammable adjuvant added to the oxygen.

   c. Alternatively, efforts can be made to maintain gas exchange: (1) By a cuirass to compress the chest;† (2) By intermittent ventilation, using an endotracheal tube pushed into the mouth of the bronchoscope;‡ (3) By orotracheal nitrous-oxide–oxygen with I.P.P.V.;§ (4) By using a ventilating bronchoscope, which is of special construction to allow I.P.P.V. at the same time as the operator visualizes the bronchial tree through a window.‖

   d. Deep inhalation anæsthesia, performing bronchoscopy as anæsthesia lightens. Ether in air can be used in children. Also nitrous-oxide–oxygen–trichloroethylene or halothane.

Any method should be used so as to allow rapid return of reflexes at the end of the procedure. The patient should be placed in the lateral position afterwards to allow drainage of blood, etc.

If massive hæmorrhage occurs from the pulmonary artery during biopsy, a bronchus blocker or an endobronchial tube should be passed at once. These instruments should always be available during bronchoscopy.

Contra-indications to general anæsthesia for bronchoscopy may include :—

   1. Respiratory obstruction, e.g., due to growth. Dyspnœa.

   2. Poor general condition of patient, e.g., cyanosis at rest.

   3. Large amounts of sputum.

BRONCHOGRAPHY.—Lipiodol (originally introduced as an anti-syphilitic by Lafay in 1901) was used as a contrast medium in 1922 by Sicard and Forestier. About 10–15 ml. are needed to fill one adult lung ; a child takes 6–8 ml. for a single side. ' Dionosil ' has advantages over lipiodol as it is cleared from the lungs in 8 hours and very little enters the alveoli. But dionosil is more likely to provoke coughing.

In wet cases postural drainage helps to clear the bronchial tree before bronchography. This results in better bronchograms and makes the procedure safer.

Local Analgesia is satisfactory in adults and co-operative children. Little local analgesia is needed. An amethocaine or lignocaine lozenge may be sucked beforehand and local

---

* Jenkins, A. V., *Anæsthesia*, 1966, **21**, 449.
† Pinkerton, H. H., *Brit. J. Anæsth.*, 1957, **29**, 422.
‡ Churchill-Davidson, H. C., *Anæsthesia*, 1953, **8**, 128.
§ Borman, J. B., and others, *Brit. J. Anæsth.*, 1964, **36**, 233.
‖ Heron, R. A. C., *Anæsthesia*, 1950, **5**, 40; Mathewson, H. S., *Anesthesiology*, 1956, **17**, 623; Kovacs, S., *Ibid.*, 1957, **18**, 335; and Berquo, G., and Ficho, P. C., *Curr. Res. Anesth.*, 1960, **39**, 523.

Choice of Anæsthetic Technique, *continued.*

analgesic solution sprayed into the larynx. It is not generally necessary to anæsthetize the trachea or bronchial mucosa. The contrast medium is introduced through a catheter passed via the nose or over the back of the tongue or by direct injection through the cricothyroid membrane.

GENERAL ANÆSTHESIA is necessary in small children (below 6 years) or in the uncooperative. Bronchography performed in small children with severe bronchiectasis, copious sputum, and diminished respiratory reserve may be a hazardous procedure. A skilled team of radiologist, anæsthetist, and nurses is required. The actual anæsthetic agents used are not so important provided the following points are observed :—

1. Endotracheal anæsthesia should be employed using a suction angle piece. A narrow catheter can then be inserted down the lumen of the endotracheal tube to inject the oil. A gum elastic catheter is satisfactory, marked so that the radiologist knows when it has just passed the tip of the endotracheal tube.*

2. Suction must be available to clear the bronchial tree : (a) before injection of the radio-opaque oil ; (b) at the conclusion of the procedure ; (c) as an emergency at any time.

3. Apnœa must be maintained from the time of injection of the oil until the radiographs are taken. This helps to prevent alveolar filling. It means that the whole team must be ready to carry out their duties quickly, e.g., (a) inject suxamethonium and hyperventilate with oxygen ; (b) inject radio-opaque medium ; (c) hold the head during positioning of the patient to fill the various lobes and radiography ; (d) ventilate with oxygen. Other relaxants (e.g., gallamine) can be used in place of suxamethonium.

4. Keep the child under close observation afterwards. The anæsthetic technique should provide for a rapid return of reflexes, but cyanosis may still occur associated with coughing, breathholding, laryngospasm or movement of secretions within the bronchial tree. The lateral position and head-down tilt may be advantageous.

5. Another technique which has been recommended is ether anæsthesia to Stage III, plane 3. The child then breathes air. Oil is poured over the back of the tongue (20 ml.). Spontaneous respiration is maintained, the oil is aspirated into the bronchial tree, and films taken.

(*See also* Parkhouse, J., *Brit. J. Anæsth.*, 1957, **29**, 447 ; and Boulton, T. B., in *Recent Advances in Anæsthesia and Analgesia*, 9th ed., p. 188 (Ed. Hewer, C. Langton), 1963. London : Churchill.)

ŒSOPHAGOSCOPY.—An endotracheal tube should be passed through the nose or (cuffed) through the mouth. An armoured tube is less likely to be compressed by the œsophagoscope. It is necessary to provide relaxation of the post-cricoid sphincter

---

* Macintosh, R. R., and Mushin, W. W., *Brit. med. J.*, 1950, **1**, 1319.

and this may be achieved using muscle relaxants or deep anæsthesia. In obstructive lesions, e.g., carcinoma, it is possible for a dilated œsophagus above the lesion to contain food, etc., which may be regurgitated. Suction should therefore always be available. Œsophagoscopy may produce trauma and bleeding may occur after biopsy or in the presence of œsophageal varices. The anæsthetic technique should allow rapid return of reflexes. At the end of the procedure make sure the pharynx is cleared of blood, etc., and turn the patient on the side.

Suggested techniques :—

1. Thiopentone–suxamethonium–nitrous-oxide–oxygen. Intermittent doses of suxamethonium as required.

2. Thiopentone → inhalation technique ; nitrous-oxide–oxygen–trichloroethylene or nitrous-oxide–oxygen–halothane, supplemented by small doses of gallamine as required.

3. Oxygen–halothane.

This examination can also be performed under topical analgesia (*see* p. 375).

ŒSOPHAGECTOMY.—The patient's general condition is often poor due to lack of nutrition. Pre-operative assessment and treatment to correct nutritional and electrolyte deficiencies are therefore important. The operation may be long and blood transfusion is usually required. The abdomen may be opened as well as the thorax.

THYMECTOMY.—Pioneers in the operation of thymectomy for myasthenia gravis have been Blalock* and Keynes.† The disease, which was described in 1895 by Jolly,‡ causes muscular weakness involving the extra-ocular muscles, or those of the larynx and pharynx, hand, etc. It is subject to spontaneous remissions and exacerbations. There are many theories as to its causation ; one postulates the formation of a toxin with a curare-like action by the thymus. Neostigmine and edrophonium may be used for diagnosis, as also may the anti-depolarizing relaxants together with electromyography. The operation for the relief of myasthenia gravis involves splitting of the sternum. One or both pleural cavities may be opened.

Cases should be carefully assessed pre-operatively with particular reference to muscular weakness and treatment with neostigmine. It is usually wise to maintain neostigmine dosage up to the time of operation, if necessary it may be given intramuscularly 1·5 to 2·5 mg. Pre-operative medication with atropine should be generous to avoid excessive salivation.

Induction may be with a small dose of thiopentone, with oxygen–cyclopropane, or with oxygen–halothane. Intubation can usually be performed easily without the aid of muscle relaxants. Controlled respiration is facilitated by the judicious administration of cyclopropane, halothane, or pethidine. Muscle relaxants are seldom required. Non-depolarizing

* Blalock, A., and others, *J. Amer. Med. Ass.*, 1945, **128**, 189.
† Keynes, G., *Lancet*, 1954, **1**, 1197; and *Ann. R. Coll. Surg., Engl.*, 1953, **12**, 88.
‡ Jolly, Friedrich, *Neurol. Zbl.*, 1895, **14**, 34.

Choice of Anæsthetic Technique, *continued.*

relaxants are contra-indicated as they prolong muscular weakness by interfering with the action of acetylcholine at the end-plate and causing apnœa of many hours' duration. Depolarizing relaxants may act like non-depolarizing relaxants in this disease and may be reversible by anticholinesterases : they may, too, prolong muscular weakness, but small doses of decamethonium or suxamethonium used for intubation, or to obtain control of respiration, are unlikely to cause prolonged respiratory depression. Some patients have an abnormal resistance to their action.

Undue respiratory depression is to be avoided in the post-operative phase. Neostigmine and atropine may be administered if the respirations are shallow, but if there is no response to ordinary doses the patient should be respired with an artificial ventilator and all drugs withheld until the pharmacological picture becomes clarified. (*See also* Chapter XXVI.)

Special post-operative risks include :—

1. Atelectasis—owing to interference with coughing because of muscular weakness and interference with the physics of the thorax.

2. Excessive mucus secretion due to neostigmine or pyridostigmine : this is controllable by atropine.

3. Pneumothorax due to surgical accidents.

If respiration remains inadequate the patient should be treated like a case of bulbospinal poliomyelitis, by tracheostomy, a cuffed tube, and intermittent positive-pressure ventilation.[*]

CRUSH INJURY OF THE CHEST.—This may cause painful breathing or subsequent hypoxia and cardiorespiratory embarrassment. Injury (and operation) to the chest wall is likely to interfere with the patient's ability to rid the tracheobronchial tree of secretions. Moisture accumulates in areas of lung underlying the traumatized area.

To help the patient to breathe and cough extradural block via an indwelling catheter in the thoracic region is invaluable.[†] Otherwise intravenous procaine—500 ml. of 0·2 per cent solution—is useful.[‡] It will often prevent the development of traumatic wet lung. Adequate strapping and intercostal block may also be helpful. A patent airway must be maintained using suction, endotracheal intubation, or tracheostomy. The control of paradoxical movements of the chest wall may be managed by stabilizing a portion of the thoracic cage by skeletal traction. A device called the ' limpet '[§] has also been used to hold out the flail area of chest while plaster-of-Paris is applied to form an intact exoskeleton. This can usually be done without general anæsthesia. Severe

* Chang, J., and others, *Canad. Anæsth. Soc. J.*, 1957, **4**, 13; and Pennington, G. W., and Edwards, F. R., *Thorax*, 1960, **15**, 262.
† Collie, J. A., and Lloyd, J. W., *Anæsthesia*, 1967, **22**, 392.
‡ Rook, J. R., *Ibid.*, 1951, **6**, 221.
§ Schrire, T., *S. Afr. med. J.*, 1963, **37**, 170 ; and Editorial, *Lancet*, 1963, **2**, 871.

cases are probably best managed by intermittent positive-pressure respiration, after a tracheostomy has been performed (to aid suction and to reduce dead space), apnœa being induced by hyperventilation. This method has given good results in recent series of cases.*

(*See also* Mansfield, R., and Jenkins, R., *Practical Anæsthesia for Lung Surgery*, 1967. London: Baillière, Tindall, and Cassell.)

ANÆSTHESIA FOR CARDIAC OPERATIONS

The first operation for relief of mitral stenosis by digital dilatation through the left atrial appendage was carried out by Souttar at the London Hospital in 1925.† The first successful operation using cardio-pulmonary by-pass was carried out by Lillehei in 1955.‡

Surgery of the heart raises a number of problems for the anæsthetist :

1. Open pneumothorax. *See* p. 555.
2. Diminished cardiac reserve. Cardiac output may be reduced to the point where compensation for a sudden fall in peripheral resistance cannot take place. Anæsthetic drugs must therefore be administered with particular care. Full oxygenation must always be maintained.
3. Blood-loss and replacement. Be careful not to overload the circulation with saline or blood. Blood-loss may occur suddenly and rapidly during operation. Blood for transfusion must be instantly available with the means for rapid administration.
4. Surgical manipulations of the heart. These may cause ectopic beats or other arrhythmias. The force of ventricular contraction may diminish with hypotension and even asystole can occur. During such manipulations it is essential to watch carefully, so that they may be interrupted if necessary to allow the heart a period of rest and recovery.
5. Open heart surgery. If the heart is to be isolated from the circulation provision must be made to prevent irreversible brain damage. Protection for short periods is provided by hypothermia. Longer periods require the use of cardiopulmonary by-pass, perhaps in association with hypothermia.

Anæsthetic Technique.—The need is for a perfect technique providing quiet, smooth, light anæsthesia without hypoxia.

1. Premedication with morphine and atropine or hyoscine—reduced dosage in the poor risks. Some anæsthetists fear the tachycardia produced by atropine and omit it. Pre-oxygenation—then minimal intravenous thiopentone to provide a smooth induction but without undue depression. A sleep dose only is required; remember that slow circulation time may be responsible for a delayed response. Intubation using a muscle relaxant and cuffed Magill's tube. Maintain controlled respirations with nitrous-oxide–oxygen–relaxant. Many prefer suxamethonium (30–50 mg.) for intubation which can then be carried out

* Avery, A. A., *J. thorac. Surg.*, 1956, **32**, 291 ; Windsor, H. M., and Dwyer, B., *Thorax*, 1961, **16**, 3 ; and Griffiths, H. W. C., *Lancet*, 1963, **1**, 1108.
† Souttar, H. S., *Brit. med. J.*, 1925, **2**, 903.
‡ Lillehei, C. W., and others, *Surg. Gyn. Obstet.*, 1955, **101**, 447.

Cardiac Operations—Anæsthetic Techniques, *continued.*

atraumatically in a light plane of anæsthesia, followed by tubocurarine chloride (12–20 mg.) once the effect of suxamethonium has worn off. Supplementary doses of tubocurarine can be given if required.

A slow intravenous drip of 5 per cent glucose is set up before surgery commences and blood must be ready in the theatre and for immediate transfusion at a rapid rate. Blood-pressure and pulse-rate should be charted. The electrocardiogram is a valuable monitor for the diagnosis of arrhythmias ; but remember that it is an index of electrical activity of the heart and not of functional efficiency.

During manipulations of the heart, such as exploration of the mitral valve, increase oxygen in the anæsthetic mixture up to 100 per cent. At the same time observe the heart function closely to look for evidence of the effect of such manipulations : (a) watch the heart directly ; (b) palpate the radial pulse, which may become weak or disappear for a time ; (c) blood-pressure ; (d) arrhythmias. A finger blocking the mitral orifice may cause multiple ectopic beats, absence of radial pulse, and deterioration of ventricular beat. The heart action usually returns to normal if the finger is withdrawn ; if not it indicates more severe effects on the heart which should be allowed a rest period. Bradycardia with an inefficient ventricular beat is a serious sign requiring a short period of rest (unless massage is indicated) and full oxygenation. Cardiac asystole or ventricular fibrillation should be treated on the usual lines (*see* Chapter XXXIV). The use of procaine (0·2 per cent solution in 5 per cent glucose) to prevent arrhythmias has fallen out of favour. It has been found unnecessary in most cases, and has the disadvantage that it is itself a myocardial depressant.

Make sure that the lungs are fully expanded before the chest is closed. At the end of operation reverse any residual effects of relaxant drugs with atropine and neostigmine. Full tracheobronchial toilet is advisable prior to extubation. The patient should be returned from theatre breathing oxygen from a portable apparatus attached to the head of the bed.

2. One technique* recommended employs only nitrous-oxide–oxygen and a relaxant, with the idea that possibly such drugs as thiopentone may in some cases handicap the circulation. Premedication is, e.g., promethazine 50 mg. and atropine 0·6 mg. The patient is given pure oxygen which in three minutes displaces most of the nitrogen from the lungs. Nitrous oxide 8 l. and oxygen 2 l. per minute are now given and after two minutes —or less if delirium ensues—a dose of tubocurarine is given sufficient to cause apnœa, e.g., 25–30 mg. A large cuffed tube is now passed. Respiration is controlled using a Waters circuit and a flow-rate of nitrous oxide 2 l. and oxygen 1 l. per minute. A machine is not used to ventilate the patient.

---

* Gray, T. C., and Riding, J. E., *Anæsthesia*, 1957, **12**, 129.

At the end of the operation atropine 1·3 mg. and, when that has caused tachycardia, neostigmine 2·5 to 5 mg. are injected.

3. Oxygen and cyclopropane. This method is favoured in some clinics in North America. An induction dose of thiopentone can be given carefully with a short-acting muscle relaxant to facilitate intubation. Respirations can usually be controlled with small concentrations of cyclopropane, particularly if morphine has been used as part of the premedication. If there is any difficulty in controlling respiration, a small dose of muscle relaxant is given rather than an increase of cyclopropane concentration. This technique gives excellent results in skilled hands. Arrhythmias are no commoner than with nitrous oxide if full oxygenation is maintained, hypercarbia avoided, and the concentrations of cyclopropane kept minimal. This of course precludes the use of diathermy.

4. Halothane. Halothane can be used with oxygen or nitrous-oxide–oxygen. It facilitates controlled respiration. It must, however, be used very carefully. Most anæsthetists believe that the vaporizer must always be outside the rebreathing circuit and arranged so that minimal concentrations can be administered. Clinical administration should be particularly directed at the avoidance of hypotension, which may sometimes become severe during cardiac manipulations. A technique only for those thoroughly familiar with the drug in controlled respiration.

Mitral Valvotomy, Aortic Valvotomy.—Anæsthesia along the lines indicated above is satisfactory for cardiac surgery that does not require the special techniques of hypothermia or cardiopulmonary by-pass.

Patent Ductus Arteriosus.*—The ductus is a wide channel between the distal part of the aortic arch and the pulmonary artery in fœtal life, when it conveys blood from the right side of the heart to the aorta, by-passing the functionless lungs. When the lungs expand after birth, the ductus gradually closes (completely in four weeks), being replaced by the ligamentum arteriosum. If closure does not occur, blood flows from the high-pressure aorta to the low-pressure pulmonary artery, a reversal of the direction from intra-uterine life. The results are: (1) Increased intrapulmonary pressure; (2) Right ventricular hypertrophy to deal with it; (3) Small volume of blood passing down aorta, with low diastolic blood-pressure and high pulse-pressure—these pressures become normal when the ductus is tied; (4) Hypertrophy of left ventricle. Cyanosis is not marked unless other congenital abnormalities exist also. There is a loud systolic and diastolic murmur, the former being more pronounced. Endocarditis frequently coexists and greatly adds to the risks of operation.

A slow drip should be set up as grave haemorrhage may take place while ductus is being cleared. Tying the ductus results in increase in the peripheral blood-volume, so drip must be slow.

Optimum time for operation is 5–12 years of age. In its absence, expectation of life is halved.

* Gross, R. E., *Ann. Surg.*, 1939, **110**, 321.

Coarctation of Aorta.*—Induced hypotension, e.g., with trimetapha has a useful place in anæsthesia for this condition. It reduc blood-loss from the enlarged vessels in the chest wall and mak the actual suturing of the aorta easier. The blood-pressure shou be rising again when the clamps are taken off the aorta, otherwis at this stage circulatory collapse may occur. The technique general anæsthesia should present few special problems and th generally employed method is thiopentone, relaxant, oxyge inflation, insertion of a cuffed tube, controlled respiration wit nitrous oxide and oxygen.

Pericardectomy.—Constrictive pericarditis limits diastolic expansio of the heart. A rise in atrial pressure follows which in turn lead to venous congestion and peripheral œdema. Advanced cas present as poor risks for anæsthesia and surgery. Cardiac outpu may be reduced to the point where compensation for a sudden fa in peripheral resistance cannot take place. The surgical procedur involves considerable manipulation of the heart. Arrhythmia and fall of blood-pressure are likely to occur, and it may be neces sary to pause from time to time to allow the heart to recove Intravenous transfusion may be dangerous because of the ris of overloading the circulation. At the same time hæmorrhage ma occur and blood should be accurately replaced.

It has been stated many times that thiopentone is contra-indicate in the presence of constrictive pericarditis.‡ Many anæsthetis are, however, prepared to use the drug carefully. It should b given slowly in dilute solution. Otherwise induction can be b an inhalation method, providing hypoxia or excitement is nc allowed to occur.

These cases are poor risks and require very careful handling. The usually need only small doses of drugs and the anæsthetis should be on his guard against overdosage. Watch carefull the general condition of the patient, so that the surgeon ma be warned to allow the heart to rest.

Open Heart Surgery under Moderate Hypothermia.—If the perio of cardiotomy and circulatory arrest is limited to 2 minutes or les and the patient is well oxygenated beforehand, normal bod temperature is satisfactory. Hypothermia to 30° C. allow circulatory arrest for an operation which can be completed in to 7 minutes. This is satisfactory for closure of atrial septa defects of the ostium secundum type and operations for pulmonar stenosis. The time limits set by ' conventional ' hypothermia d not allow more elaborate operations on the open heart to b undertaken with safety. Hypothermia may be achieved b surface cooling or by extracorporeal methods. It is losing it popularity. *See* Chapter XXIX.

Open Heart Surgery using Extracorporeal Circulation.—This i indicated when the surgical procedure needs circulatory arrest fo

---

* Crafoord, C., and Wylin, G., *J. thorac. Surg.*, 1945, **14**, 347.
‡ Parry Brown, A. I., and Sellick, B. A., *Anæsthesia*, 1953, **8**, 4; and *Brit. med. Bull.*, 1955 **11**, 174.

a period longer than the 5 to 7 minutes which is normally considered safe under conventional hypothermia. Operations include surgical correction of atrial and ventricular septal defects, Fallot's tetralogy, pulmonary stenosis, aortic stenosis, mitral incompetence, and prosthetic operations on the heart valves.

The use of an extracorporeal circulation allows circulation of the vital organs (the brain) while the heart is isolated from the circulation. It has been made possible by the discovery of heparin and its use in preventing clotting of the blood, and by the role of protamine in restoring the coagulation mechanism. At the same time considerable research into the construction of apparatus was necessary before the technique could be safely applied to human patients.

The extracorporeal circulation must incorporate a pump or pumps to provide circulation and an oxygenator for gaseous exchange. At the same time it is important that the blood is not damaged, and the apparatus must be capable of sterilization.

Lillehei has employed a human donor (father or mother) to supply arterial blood to a child, and this method has worked in clinical practice, although there are ethical and other problems, so that attention has been turned to the development of machines.

The perfusion flow rate is usually calculated as 2400 ml. per min. per sq. metre body surface, or as 70–80 ml. per min. per kg. body-weight. The oxygenator must be capable of providing efficient gas exchange at the required flow rate and the venous and arterial cannulæ must be capable of carrying this blood-flow. The arterial cannula is usually inserted into the femoral artery and venous blood taken from the right atrium or superior and inferior venæ cavæ. Heparin is given in a dosage of 2–3 mg. per kg. body-weight or 90 mg. per sq. metre surface area and, in addition, the pump must be primed with sufficient heparinized blood or blood and low molecular weight (40,000) dextran mixture. The dosage of protamine at the end of perfusion should be 2–3 mg. per kg. Hexadimethrine ('Polybrene') is also used to neutralize heparin in a 1 : 1 ratio. Both drugs require to be given intravenously over a period of minutes. Otherwise hypotension may occur as a result of intense pulmonary artery constriction.

PUMPS are of three main types :—

1. Roller pumps. The tubing is squeezed by an arm rotating in a circle (e.g., DeBakey pump).*

2. Sigmamotor pumps. Progressive squeezing of succeeding parts of the tubing in a consecutive manner.

3. Compression pumps. Even compression of the tubing along a length. Requires a valve system to ensure unidirectional flow.

Any pump for use with the extracorporeal circulation should be completely reliable, should not damage the blood, should have tubing with smooth internal surfaces, and should be controllable at flow rates between zero and 5 l. per min.

---

* DeBakey, M. E., *Med. surg. J.*, 1934, **87**, 386.

Open Heart Surgery using Extracorporeal Circulation, *continued.*

OXYGENATORS.—

1. LILLEHEI-DE WALL BUBBLE OXYGENATOR.*—Venous blood f. the patient enters the bottom of a long upright cylin together with a stream of oxygen. Bubbles of gas are sep ated from blood as it flows back through a helix to the re voir. A drawback is that it can only operate with relativ low blood-flows.

2. THE GIBBON PUMP-OXYGENATOR.†—This has been modified the Mayo Clinic.‡ Blood flows as a thin film over a num of vertical screens made of stainless-steel wire mesh measuring 18 × 12 in. Each screen is capable of oxygenat 165 to 250 ml. blood per min. Between 4 and 14 screens be used ; requirements are calculated according to surf area of the patient (2400 ml. per min. per sq. metre).

3. THE MELROSE PUMP.§—A large cylindrical tube is inclined an angle of 20° with the horizontal. Inside are rows of el tical plastic disks which carry a thin film of blood. When cylinder rotates at 120 rev. per min. the available surf area exposed for oxygenation is about 120 sq. metres oxygen can be introduced at rates of 100 ml. per litre per m

4. DISPOSABLE BUBBLE OXYGENATORS are now availab Portable apparatus has also been designed.¶

5. MEMBRANE OXYGENATORS.—These are being developed in hope that there will be less damage to the blood which be separated from direct contact with the gases.

6. USE OF THE PATIENT'S OWN LUNGS IN SITU.—Two separ extracorporeal circulations are used to replace the right a left sides of the heart. This method has been used w profound hypothermia (15° C.).**

High flows of oxygen must be delivered to the oxygenators. In Gibbon and Melrose machines this is about 10 l. per m Such flows would normally displace too much carbon dioxi A mixture of 2·5–3·5 per cent carbon dioxide in oxygen therefore used to keep the arterial carbon dioxide tension wit normal limits.

During cardiotomy the venous return to the heart is occlud There is, however, loss of blood which is returned to the hea (1) from the coronary circulation ; (2) from the bronch arteries via the pulmonary veins (may be considerable in con tions such as Fallot's tetralogy) ; (3) from incompetent aor valves. Such blood may be removed by suction and retra fused. Conventional suckers, however, entrain a large volu of air with frothing and damage to red cells. A special l

* De Wall, R. A., Lillehei, C. W., and others, *Surg. Clinic. N. Amer.*, 1956, **36**, 1025.
† Gibbon, J. H., *Arch. Surg.*, 1937, **34**, 1105.
‡ Kirkbin, J. W., and others, *Proc. Mayo Clin.*, 1955, **30**, 201 ; and *Thorax*, 1957, **12**, 93
§ Aird, I., Melrose, D. G., Cleland, W. P., and Lynn, R. B., *Brit. med. J.*, 1954, **1**, 12 and Melrose, D. G., *Ibid.*, 1953, **2**, 57.
‖ Gott, V. L., and others, *Thorax*, 1957, **12**, 1 ; Arnfred, E., and others, *Ibid.*, 1961, **16**, 3 and Gunning, A. J., Hodgson, D. C., and Burrows, P., *Lancet*, 1965, **1**, 584.
¶ Pareth, M., *Ibid.*, 1964, **2**, 1291.
** Drew, C. E., and others, *Ibid.*, 1959, **1**, 745 and 748.

pressure (DeBakey) sucker may be used, and the blood returned to the venous reservoir after de-bubbling.

Methods designed to reduce the loss of blood from the open heart include : (1) Arrest of coronary circulation by a clamp across the root of the aorta combined with elective cardiac arrest (2 ml. 25 per cent potassium citrate injected into the coronary circulation). Allows up to 20 minutes, and is reversed when removing the clamp washes out the potassium from the coronary circulation. (2) Hypothermia to 15° C. when cell metabolism is so low that coronary circulation can be safely arrested. Local hypothermia may be achieved by coronary perfusion of cold dextran.

ANÆSTHETIC TECHNIQUE.—This does not differ substantially from anæsthesia for cardiac operations without extracorporeal circulation. Thiopentone, nitrous oxide, oxygen, relaxant anæsthesia is satisfactory. It is wise to give an extra dose of muscle relaxant before perfusion starts to prevent sudden respiratory movements. Note that blood in the pump reservoir may have a higher Pco_2 than the blood in the patient who has been hyperventilated. Halothane has also been used (in low concentrations), and this may be continued during the by-pass procedure by inserting a Fluotec (0·5 to 1 per cent setting) in the oxygen lead to the oxygenator. During by-pass some anæsthetists fill the lungs with 80 per cent helium and 20 per cent oxygen to prevent collapse and congestion.

Monitoring during extracorporeal circulation may include :—

1. Venous pressure. A rise in pressure suggests obstruction or malposition of the venous lines. A fall, with inadequate flow to the machine, suggests concealed blood-loss. At the end of operation high pressure may be caused by over-transfusion or myocardial insufficiency ; low pressure by inadequate transfusion.

2. Arterial pressure. Usually measured by cannulation of the radial artery.

3. E.E.G. Gives an indication of the adequacy of cerebral perfusion. It may give warning before irreversible damage is done.

4. E.C.G. Gives warning of inadequate coronary flow, of injury to conducting mechanism of heart, etc.

5. Blood-loss. Swab weighing and measurement of suction bottles should be charted at regular intervals. Blood can be transfused via the arterial line of the pump or through a separate intravenous drip. Other guides to blood-loss include the reservoir of the pump, the venous pressure, the arterial pressure. Weighing of the whole patient before and after operation gives a good estimate of overall loss and replacement.

6. Arterial pH, Pco_2, and the standard bicarbonate. Metabolic acidosis may occur due to tissue hypoxia with low perfusion rates. Carbon dioxide is an important factor in the control of cerebral blood-flow. Respiratory alkalosis may therefore be harmful if the cerebral perfusion is only just adequate during the extracorporeal circulation or the post-perfusion period. Some authorities believe that controlled respiration

Open Heart Surgery using Extracorporeal Circulation, *continued.*

should be maintained by large doses of muscle relaxants ra⟨ than by hyperventilation.

7. Arteriovenous oxygen difference. Determines the adequacy tissue perfusion.

8. Temperature recording.

9. Urine flow. A simple index of adequate renal perfusion.

BLOOD REPLACEMENT.—(1) *Preperfusion period.* It is import to keep pace with measured blood-loss, and desirable to trans⟨ an excess of some 50–250 ml., depending on the size of patient. (2) *Perfusion period.* The proportion of blood in patient and in the extracorporeal system varies somewhat v⟨ vascular tone. The central venous pressure is the most reli⟨ indication that the correct amount of blood is in the patie⟨ circulatory system at the end of perfusion. (3) *Post-perfus⟨ period.* Blood should be transfused according to blood-loss ⟨ central venous pressure. A reading of 5–10 cm. water may considered satisfactory. (4) *Post-operative period.* Blood n⟨ need to be given if bleeding occurs.

EXCESSIVE BLEEDING.—This may occur after perfusion, ⟨ may be due to: (1) Inadequate neutralization of heparin; Fibrinogen depletion (less than 100 g. per cent). Fibrino⟨ 4–6 g. may need to be given; (3) Reduction in platelets; Failure of surgical haemostasis.

LUNG CHANGES.*—These may arise due to: (1) Overloading the pulmonary vessels during surgery; (2) The post-perfus⟨ lung syndrome: perivascular œdema and hæmorrhage, congest⟨ and thickening of inter-alveolar walls, patchy collapse, int⟨ alveolar hæmorrhage, venous admixture disturbance of ver⟨ lation–perfusion relationships, presence of cells resembl⟨ immature plasma cells.

POST-OPERATIVE CARE.—Respiratory and metabolic acid–b⟨ changes must be carefully monitored and corrected if necessa⟨ Sometimes elective tracheostomy is performed to allow I.P.P⟨ Oxygen is given to correct hypoxæmia. Intravenous fluids n⟨ careful regulation.

(*See also*, for excellent review, Beard, J., *Thoracic Anæsthesia* (⟨ Mushin, W. W.), 1963, Ch. 15. Oxford: Blackwell.)

Open Heart Surgery with Profound Hypothermia.—As the bo⟨ temperature falls below 28° C. there is a period of ventricu⟨ fibrillation which quietens into cardiac standstill as the tempe⟨ ture falls further. Such low temperatures cannot, however, achieved safely without the use of an extracorporeal circulati⟨ A heat exchanger is incorporated in the arterial line of the pu⟨ and body temperature may then be allowed to fall to 15° Temperature gradients occur and measurements should be ma⟨ from various sites of which the most important are œsophag⟨ (approximating to cardiac) and nasopharyngeal (approximati⟨ to brain temperature).

---

* Kolff, W. J., Effler, D. B., and Groves, L. K., *Brit. med. J.*, 1960, **1**, 1149; and Neb⟨ R. A., Melrose, D. G., Sykes, M. K. and Robinson, B., *Lancet* 1965, **2**, 251, 254.

Drew* has developed a technique using the patient's own lungs as the oxygenator and providing separate extracorporeal circulations for the left and right sides of the heart. Left heart by-pass is from left atrium to femoral artery. Then cooling is begun. When temperature of the heart approaches 30° C. or when cardiac action becomes inadequate right heart by-pass is started from the right atrium to the pulmonary artery. The lungs are then ventilated with oxygen by I.P.P.V. When the brain temperature is estimated to reach 15° C., circulation and ventilation are discontinued. The surgeon has then a period of about one hour to operate on a dry still heart. Then the circulation is restarted and the heat exchanger used for warming.

Cardiac Catheterization.†—First performed by Forsmann—on himself—in 1929; awarded the Nobel Prize in 1956. The examination entails passing a small catheter from the forearm vein into the right heart and pulmonary artery, under radiographic control. Pressures are taken, and also samples for blood–gas analysis. The patients are often in poor general condition and the investigation is not without risk. Ventricular extrasystoles may be induced and fatal ventricular fibrillation has been recorded. Continuous E.C.G. monitoring is usually employed. Cardiac catheterization should be avoided in the presence of Ebstein's malformation of the tricuspid valve, when it is known to be particularly dangerous.

In adults and older children the procedure is usually carried out with local infiltration for insertion of the catheter in the vein. In young children heavy sedation or full general anæsthesia may be required. There has been dispute about the best methods of achieving a solution to the following requirements : (1) The child must be still for a prolonged period ; (2) There must be no interference with blood–gas analysis, especially oxygen ; (3) There must be no significant disturbance of hæmodynamics ; (4) Conditions must be achieved in near complete darkness for radiographic screening ; (5) Non-explosive techniques are advisable in the X-ray room.

Thus oxygen should not be utilized in an anæsthetic mixture for inhalation. Severe respiratory depression is to be avoided and the technique used should maintain a ' steady state ' for a reasonable length of time.

Some suggested techniques :—

1. RECTAL THIOPENTONE.—Suggested by Smith.‡ Rees§ recommends a combination of drugs for children under 5 years of age : quinalbarbitone (by mouth) 15 mg. per stone ; morphine (subcutaneously) 1·5 mg. per stone ; atropine (subcutaneously) 0·3 mg. per stone ; thiopentone (rectal) 140 mg. per

* Drew, C. E., Keen, G., and Benazon, D. B., *Lancet*, 1959, **1**, 745 ; Drew, C. E., and Anderson, I. M., *Ibid.*, 1959, **1**, 748 ; and Drew, C. E., *Brit. med. Bull.*, 1961, **17**, 37.
† *See also* Boulton, T. B., in *Recent Advances in Anæsthesia and Analgesia*, 9th ed., p. 176 (Ed. Hewer, C. Langton), 1963. London : Churchill.
‡ Smith, J. A., *Brit. med. J.*, 1950, **1**, 705.
§ Rees, G. J., and Hay, J. D., in *General Anæsthesia* (Ed. Evans, F. T., and Gray, T. C.), 1959. London : Butterworths.

Cardiac Catheterization, *continued.*

stone. Inglis* supplements rectal thiopentone with intravenou
pethidine.

2. RECTAL BROMETHOL.—(Fieldman† and Norris.‡) Dos
120 mg. per kg.

3. ' LYTIC COCKTAIL '.—Smith§ uses a solution containing chlor
promazine 50 mg., promethazine 50 mg., and pethidine 200 mg.
in a volume of 8 ml. 1 ml. of this solution is injected intra
muscularly for every 20 lb. body-weight (0·7 ml. per 20 lb. i
cyanotic children).

The above methods provide a level of basal narcosis. The cathete
may then be inserted under local analgesia. The patien
breathes air. Disadvantages include the unpredictable deptl
and duration of narcosis, the possibility of sudden movement
the likelihood of cardio-respiratory depression if supplementar
doses have to be given intravenously, and the fact that the
airway is not assured.

4. INHALATION METHODS.—Oxygen-rich mixtures cannot be
used without interfering with blood-gas analysis. Trichloroethylene–air (Keats‖) produces a high incidence of tachypnœa. Halothane–air or halothane–ether azeotrope and air
(Adams and Parkhouse¶) is more satisfactory. It is wise to
pass an endotracheal tube. Respiratory depression will interfere
with oxygenation, but this may be obviated by controlling
respiration. The E.M.O. inhaler or a Fluotec and Ambu bag is
satisfactory.

Angiocardiography.—May be performed at the same time as catheterization. A large amount of 70 per cent sodium acetrizoate is
injected rapidly into a large vein to result in a radio-opaque bolus
passing through the heart and great vessels. This is followed by
high-speed serial radiography.

The injection may result in bronchospasm, laryngospasm, coughing,
and even vagal inhibition of cardiac rhythm. The investigation is more dangerous than catheterization (mortality under
1 per cent in experienced hands). The procedure is unpleasant
for the patient and general anæsthesia is necessary in children.

The anæsthetic technique is simpler than for catheterization since
oxygen can be used in an inhalation mixture. It is common to
paralyse the patient with suxamethonium or other relaxant and
to ventilate with nitrous oxide and oxygen via an endotracheal
tube. It has been recommended** that intrathoracic pressure
should be raised just prior to injection and released as it is made.
This helps to draw the radio-opaque bolus to the right side of

* Inglis, J. M., *Anæsthesia*, 1954, **9**, 25.
† Fieldman, E. J., Lundy, J. S., DuShane, J. W., and Wood, E. H., *Anesthesiology*, 1955,
16, 868.
‡ Norris, W., *Brit. J. Anæsth.*, 1963, **35**, 358.
§ Smith, C., Rowe, R. D., and Vlad, P., *Canad. Anæsth. Soc. J.*, 1958, **5**, 35.
‖ Keats, A. S., Telford, J., Kurosu, Y., and Latson, J. R., *J. Amer. med. Ass.*, 1958, **166**, 215.
¶ Adams, A. K., and Parkhouse, J., *Brit. J. Anæsth.*, 1960, **32**, 69.
** Rees, G. J., in *General Anæsthesia*, Vol. 2 (Ed. Evans, F. T., and Gray, T. C.), 1959, p. 202.
London: Butterworths.

the heart and provide good angiocardiograms. Maintenance of high oxygen of the arterial blood throughout the procedure helps to prevent dangerous reactions.

Insertion of Indwelling Pacemakers.—The small transistorized pacemaker is implanted into the abdominal wall. Wires lead through the diaphragm to the ventricular muscle. The procedure involves thoracotomy and abdominal incision and demands general anæsthesia. The patient usually suffers from Stokes-Adams attacks due to complete heart-block which has not responded to drug treatment. This may have included a course of steroid therapy. Ventricular asystole or fibrillation is a possible hazard at any stage. The heart may or may not be already adequately paced by an external or intravenous catheter pacemaker.

Scrupulous care is necessary. Howat* recommends premedication with atropine to prevent salivation (it has no action on heart-rate in the presence of heart-block), and morphine or pethidine in suitable dosage. Where the heart is already adequately paced, induction is with thiopentone (100–150 mg.), suxamethonium, hyperventilation with 100 per cent oxygen, thorough topical anæsthesia to larynx and trachea, cuffed endotracheal tube, nitrous oxide, and oxygen. Maintenance is with nitrous oxide, oxygen, and halothane. Muscle relaxants are avoided since muscle twitches due to imperfect positioning of the electrodes are masked by them. Where pacing is faulty or absent he recommends avoidance of intravenous induction and uses nitrous oxide, oxygen, suxamethonium drip. After the pacing is satisfactory suxamethonium is discontinued and halothane used in low concentration.

An external pacemaker should always be at hand and ready for emergency use, and an assistant should be standing by to apply external cardiac compression if necessary. Continuous electrocardiographic monitoring is essential throughout.

Anæsthesia for the Electrical Reversal of Atrial Fibrillation.†—Anæsthesia is necessary as the shock is painful. A similar technique to that used in electropexy may be adopted. If quinidine sulphate is injected as part of the treatment, suxamethonium apnœa may be prolonged. Other workers have dispensed with muscle relaxants, light halothane anæsthesia being used following an induction dose of thiopentone or methohexitone.‡

(*See also Anesthesia for Surgery of the Heart* (Ed. Keown, K. K.), 2nd ed., 1963. Springfield, Ill.: Thomas; and *Thoracic Anæsthesia* (Ed. Mushin, W. W.), 1963. Oxford: Blackwell; and Feldman, S., *Recent Advances in Anæsthesia and Analgesia*, 10th ed., Ch. 6 (Ed. Hewer, C. Langton), 1967. London: Churchill.)

---

* Howat, D. D. C., *Lancet*, 1963, **1**, 855.
† Oram, S., and others, *Ibid.*, 1963, **2**, 159 ; Grogono, A. W., *Ibid.*, 1963, **2**, 1039.
‡ Gilston, A., Fordham, R., and Resnekov, L., *Brit. J. Anæsth.*, 1965, **37**, 533; and McClish, A., Desprès, J. P., and Déchêne, J. P., *Canad. Anæsth. Soc. J.*, 1965, **12**, 288.

CHAPTER XXIII

PÆDIATRIC ANÆSTHESIA

The Neonate.—Defined as an infant during the first 28 days of life. The mature 7-lb. infant is normally one-third the length, has one-ninth the body surface, and one-twentieth the weight of the average adult. The head is large compared with the body, and the neck muscles are inadequately developed to maintain it in position without support.

Respiration.—In comparison with adults, neonates have a larger proportion of dead space in their lungs. Their ribs are nearly horizontal in the position of deep inspiration, while the diaphragm is pushed up by the large liver, hence respiration is rapid, diaphragmatic, and may easily become deficient. To compensate for this, the infant's trachea is relatively wider in proportion to lung volume than is the adult's trachea, so his shallower inspirations are facilitated. Deep inspiration is anatomically impossible in infants. The lungs are much less efficient ventilating organs than they eventually become, with a respiratory surface per unit weight one-third that of adults. To compensate for this, the respiratory rate is increased in infants—up to about 40 per minute. Bucking does not occur in the first three months of life, although the laryngeal reflexes are very active as the child is living on fluids. In infants, the tongue is often pushed against the palate, causing respiratory obstruction.

The respiratory pattern of the neonate may be one of three types: (1) *Regular.* Inspiration and expiration taking equal time in the cycle with no expiratory pause; (2) *Cogwheel.* A definite and extended respiratory pause following a lengthened expiratory phase; (3) *Periodic.* Bouts of regular pattern, interrupted by apnœic intervals or groups of shallow respirations. Periodic respiration may be seen in premature infants, or as a result of birth injury or hypoxia of the respiratory centres. Because of the variations seen in respiratory patterns it is difficult to measure a 'normal' rate in the neonate, though average figures of 34 per minute have been found.* Average tidal volumes for the neonate are 20 ml.

The child's larynx differs from the adult larynx in being:† (1) Higher up: the rima glottidis is opposite the third–fourth cervical interspace in the infant, in adults one interspace lower. (2) The epiglottis is relatively longer, being V- or Y-shaped, instead of flat as in the adult. It makes an angle of 45° with the anterior pharyngeal wall while in adults it lies closer to the base of the tongue. The Macintosh laryngoscope blade is not the best for infants as it does not flatten out the curvature of the epiglottis. (3) The narrowest part of the larynx may be at the level of the

---

* Smith, C. A., *The Physiology of the Newborn Infant*, 3rd ed., 1958. Oxford: Blackwell.
† Eckenhoff, J. E., *Anesthesiology*, 1951, **12**, 401.

cricoid cartilage, which is not distensible, as are the cords, the narrowest part in adults: thus an endotracheal tube may be squeezed through the glottis, but be held up at the cricoid causing there trauma and œdema. If this occurs, a smaller tube should be substituted. Laryngeal trauma may be dangerous in infants and œdema may result either from clumsy intubation or from irritation due to too large a tube being left too long in the larynx. In children under 3, both main bronchi come off the trachea at an equal angle, unlike the arrangement in adults. At birth the trachea is 4 cm. long and 6 mm. wide. Calculation for length of endotracheal tube—distance from teeth to carina is age divided by 2 plus 12 cm.; for diameter of tube *see* p. 594.

In infants, a negative pressure is sometimes created in the stomach during inspiration, and gas may be sucked in. To relieve this a catheter should be used as a stomach tube if the abdomen is distended or if breathing is laboured.

The Cardiovascular System.—*In the fœtus* the left ventricle drives blood through the aorta to the body tissues and to the placenta in the proportion of one-third to two-thirds. Oxygenated blood from the placenta mixes with venous blood in its return to the heart. About half of this mixed blood passes through the foramen ovale to the left heart. The other half flows to the right heart for the pulmonary circulation, though a variable part of this passes through the ductus arteriosus to the aorta.

At birth, when the umbilical cord is tied, systemic arterial resistance rises because blood passing formerly to the placenta now has to pass through the arterial system to the body tissues. At the same time, as regular respiration is established, there is a profound fall in pulmonary vascular resistance, and an increase in blood-flow to the lungs. Pressure in the pulmonary artery falls and a reversal of flow occurs in the ductus arteriosus. The lumen of this vessel decreases in size over the next 7–10 days and is usually finally obliterated. The foramen ovale also closes.

The blood-volume of the neonate is about 300 ml. (or 84 ml. per kg.), and this doubles by 1 year of age. Normal blood-pressure is 80/60 mm. Hg. Normal pulse-rate 120–140 per minute. Cyanosis may reflect the high hæmoglobin content of the neonate.

Premedication.—Some anæsthetists aim to give heavy premedication so that the child arrives in the theatre suite asleep ; they can then be anæsthetized by gravity nitrous oxide or cyclopropane without the patient regaining consciousness. Other anæsthetists prefer to establish rapport with the child and to provide an environment without fear; light premedication is given and the child 'talked' to sleep, anæsthesia being induced by inhalation or intravenous routes.

ROUTES OF PREMEDICATION.—

1. ORAL.—Some anæsthetists do not like this method because of the danger of vomiting and because absorption of drugs from the alimentary tract is uneven. Others find it a satisfactory method, acceptable to the child.

2. RECTAL.

3. INTRAMUSCULAR.

Premedication, *continued.*

MORPHINE.—1·5 mg. can be given for each stone of body-weight. If 15 mg. are diluted in 10 ml. of water in a syringe, 1 ml. is the dose for each stone. Similarly, if an ampoule of papaveretum, 20 mg., and hyoscine, 0·4 mg., is diluted to 10 ml., 1 ml. can be injected for each stone of body-weight.

Morphine is badly tolerated by newly born infants, but over the age of 6–12 months they do well with the drug. It is well tolerated between the ages of 5 and 8 years.

NEPENTHE.—Contains 0·91 per cent of total opium alkaloids or 0·84 per cent of anhydrous morphine. For injection it is prepared in ½-oz. containers, and the dosage is 1 minim per year in children.

PETHIDINE.—10 mg. per stone.

PENTOBARBITONE (NEMBUTAL).—This is well tolerated by children.

By mouth the dosage can be 40 mg. per stone, with 200 mg. as the maximum. Quinalbarbitone (seconal) has a similar dosage. Both drugs may be associated with post-operative restlessness.

By rectum, 60 mg. per year of age is adequate, with a maximum dose of 400 mg. The drug is given either in suppository or the capsules, pierced at each end with a pin, can be inserted into the rectum three hours before operation.

RECTAL THIOPENTONE.—1 g. of thiopentone to be dissolved in 50 ml. of tap water (2 per cent solution) ; the dose being 1 ml. per lb. weight. Also put up in special ready-mixed emulsion and in suppositories of 125 mg., 250 mg., 500 mg., and 750 mg. A very reliable way to ensure that a child is asleep when brought to the anæsthetic room.

CHLORAL HYDRATE.—$CCl_3.CH(OH)_2$. Prepared in 1832 by Liebig and used as a soporific in 1869. It is changed in the body into trichlorethanol CCl_3CH_2OH and trichloracetic acid. This, when given by mouth, is a safe and efficient pre-operative sedative. Dose, 10–20 mg. per lb. For use in infants before operation under local analgesic ; dose is 20 mg. per lb.

TRIMEPRAZINE TARTRATE.*—This is related to chlorpromazine and promethazine and like them is a central sedative, antihistaminic, anti-emetic, and spasmolytic. It has none of chlorpromazine's anti-adrenaline properties. Its side-effects may include dryness of the mouth, vertigo, depression, and fainting. Put up in a palatable syrup as Vallergan Forte (6 mg. per ml.), dose 1·5–2 mg. per lb. 1½ hours before anæsthesia. It does not prolong the period of recovery and is a useful and convenient drug to give children before operation. Can be given by intramuscular injection 5 mg. per stone in children under 12, and 4 mg. per stone in older children and in adults, 1½ hours before operation.

For Minor Procedures in Children.—For dressing of burns, changing of dressings, proctoscopy, removal of sutures, etc., intravenous

---

* Cope, R. W., and Glover, W. J., *Lancet*, 1959, **1**, 858.

pethidine 100–150 mg. between the ages of 4 and 14 ; over 14, 150–200 mg. Amiphenazole 30 mg. should be added to each 75 mg. of pethidine.*

ATROPINE AND HYOSCINE.—These drugs are well tolerated by children and are necessary since salivation is often profuse.

SUGGESTED DOSAGE OF ATROPINE AND HYOSCINE.—

Weight	Atropine	Hyoscine
0–25 lb.	0·2 mg. ($\frac{1}{300}$ gr.)	0·15 mg. ($\frac{1}{400}$ gr.)
25–50 lb.	0·3 mg. ($\frac{1}{200}$ gr.)	0·2 mg. ($\frac{1}{300}$ gr.)
50–100 lb.	0·4 mg. ($\frac{1}{150}$ gr.)	0·3 mg. ($\frac{1}{200}$ gr.)
Over 100 lb.	0·6 mg. ($\frac{1}{100}$ gr.)	0·4 mg. ($\frac{1}{150}$ gr.)

During the first 2 or 3 days of life the infant rarely needs any drying agent, since there is virtually no respiratory tract secretion.†

The classic method of anæsthesia in infants and children has been spontaneous respiration of various mixtures of anæsthetic gases and vapours. In recent years, largely under the influence of the Liverpool school of anæsthetists,‡ this has been giving place to intravenous induction of anæsthesia with a sleep dose of thiopentone, followed by a relaxant, intubation, and intermittent positive-pressure ventilation with a gas–oxygen mixture. This new method has been extensively applied to all pædiatric operations from the simplest circumcision or tonsillectomy to the most major abdomino-thoracic interventions. It gives excellent results in the hands of those skilled in its use but requires a degree of manual dexterity and considerable experience. In the authors' opinion, the older techniques may well be safer when applied by the occasional anæsthetist.

Open Drop Technique.—Can be used for diethyl ether anæsthesia, although smoother quicker induction may be obtained with divinyl ether, vinesthene anæsthetic mixture, or ethyl chloride (although this agent is less popular than it was formerly).

Bag and Mask Anæsthesia.—A suitable method of induction is to allow nitrous oxide to flow from a mask held 2 in. above the patient's face. About 10 l. per min. are required for this. When consciousness is lost, the mask is applied to the face, the gas flow reduced and oxygen added. Cyclopropane can be used for induction in a similar manner. Care must be taken that dead space is not too high when small children and infants are anæsthetized by these methods. An adult-size reservoir bag is undesirable because in a large bag it is difficult to assess respiratory movements of low volume, while the thick rubber may offer resistance to respiration. A bag of 500 ml. capacity is suitable.

---

* Davies, M. R., *Lancet*, 1959, **2**, 710.
† Digby, Leigh M., and Belton, M., *Pediatric Anesthesiology*, 1960. New York : Macmillan.
‡ Rees, G. Jackson, *Modern Trends in Anæsthesia*, Ch. 12 (Ed. Evans, F. T., and Gray, T. C.), 1958. London: Butterworths; Rees, G. Jackson, *Brit. J. Anæsth.*, 1960, **32**, 132; Booth, A., and others, *Anæsthesia*, 1960, **15**, 361 ; and Bush, G. H., *Brit. J. Anæsth.*, 1963, **35**, 552.

Bag and Mask Anæsthesia, *continued.*

The closed circuit should not be used unless specially designed apparatus is available to minimize dead space such as the absorber of Cope and that of Sandiford.*

The tidal exchange in a newborn baby may be as little as 20 ml., so even with a tiny mask, dead space must be greatly increased unless oxygen is run under it to carry away excess carbon dioxide.

Insufflation Techniques.—Oropharyngeal insufflation can be carried out by means of a mouth hook in the corner of the mouth or by use of the Boyle-Davis gag. Since the gas mixture is diluted with air it is wise to get the child to Stage III, plane 3 before commencing insufflation. This technique may be used in tonsillectomy.

Endotracheal Intubation (*see also* p. 264).—Intubation is more frequently employed than it was before the use of relaxants made it relatively easy to perform. Many pædiatric anæsthetists feel that advantages gained far outweigh the disadvantages.

ADVANTAGES.—
1. Patency of the airway ensured.
2. Dead space reduced.
3. Pulmonary ventilation readily controlled.
4. Secretions can be removed from the respiratory tract.
5. The anæsthetist is removed from the immediate operative field.

DISADVANTAGES.—
1. Obstruction to air flow unless a tube of the correct size and length is employed (with spontaneous respiration).
2. Risk of trauma.
3. Subglottic œdema occasionally occurs post-operatively.

In neonates it is safer to pass the tube while the child is still conscious, since this is often easily achieved and it avoids the possibility of hypoxia due to spasm or obstruction. In the neonate the correct length of an endotracheal tube is 12 cm., with proximal end at the lips.† Children up to 1 year seldom tolerate a tube size larger than 4·5 mm. Children up to 5 years old will rarely take a tube larger than 5·5 mm. Size 2·5–3 mm. is usually satisfactory for the newborn. Cole‡ has designed a tube which is of much larger diameter in the pharynx than below the glottis. This minimizes obstruction to air flow and avoids inadvertent endobronchial intubation. It is modelled on an early version designed by Magill for the operation of repair of cleft palate. Tunstall and Hamer Hodges§ described a disposable modification of the Cole tube made of polyvinyl chloride. In small children and infants it is important to confirm that the endotracheal tube has not entered either main bronchus. Inspection and auscultation of the chest should be carried out.

* Sandiford, H. B. C., *Anæsthesia*, 1953, **8**, 122.
† Levin, J., *Ibid.*, 1958, **13**, 40.
‡ Cole, F., *Anesthesiology*, 1945, **6**, 627.
§ Tunstall, M. E., and Hamer Hodges, R. J., *Lancet*, 1961, **1**, 146.

Ayre's T-Piece.—This may be a T-tube or a Y-tube and has a minimal resistance to respiration. *See* pp. 119 and 264. Rees* has modified the system by fitting a 500-ml. bag with an open tail to the expiratory limb. This makes controlled ventilation possible.

Non-rebreathing Valves.—These are also popular. The simplest variety is a plastic or metallic cylinder containing two unidirectional valves attached to a small reservoir bag. *See also* p. 118.

Absorption Technique.—The to-and-fro system works well with children. The circle absorber has a higher resistance during spontaneous respiration and is not generally recommended for children, except in certain models which have been specially designed for pædiatric anæsthesia (Heidbrink infant circle filter or Foregger-Bloomquist† infant circle filter). Otherwise the Revell circulator‡ can be used for infants with the adult circle system ; the apparatus automatically circulates the gases round the adult circle at a rate which allows the infant to breathe gases without resistance.

Controlled Respiration.—Controlled respiration has the advantage that it relieves the respiratory muscles of work and prevents the gut from protruding. The rate of ventilation should be rapid. The Ayre T-piece is very useful for this, modified by Rees, and is better than a closed circle with absorption of carbon dioxide. A B.L.B. type bag, open at both ends, is fitted to the distal opening of a very short rebreathing tube, while a vulcanite tap or other form of leak at the other end of the bag is so manipulated that intermittent pressure applied to the bag expels the amount of gas required to maintain the equilibrium of the system. Anæsthesia can be maintained at light levels with nitrous-oxide–oxygen and a muscle relaxant, and recovery is rapid. Deep anæsthesia must be avoided, and occasional limb movements, a sign of light anæsthesia, can, with advantage, often be allowed.

Muscular Relaxation.—In babies, muscular relaxation requires neither deep anæsthesia nor relaxants. Protrusion of the intestines from the belly is due to diaphragmatic breathing and distension due to gas in the bowel, not to the muscular tone of the abdominal wall. Deep anæsthesia should only be produced for short periods at critical stages of the operation and the child deliberately allowed to become light at other times.

RELAXANTS IN CHILDREN.—The neonate§ is more sensitive to tubocurarine than the adult, though this sensitivity gradually decreases over the first month of life. Post-operative difficulties may be experienced if anticholinesterase drugs are not used, if hypothermia is allowed to occur, or when there is potentiation by ether or antibiotics. Initial dosage should be 0·2 mg. per lb. with supplementary doses of 0·125 mg. per lb. at about 40-min.

---

* Rees, G. J., *Brit. J. Anæsth.*, 1960, **32**, 132.

† Bloomquist, E. R., *Anesthesiology*, 1957, **18**, 787.

‡ Revell, D. G., *Canad. Anæsth. Soc. J.*, 1959, **6**, 98 and 104; and Roffey, P. J., Revell, D. G., and Morris, L. E., *Anesthesiology*, 1961, **22**, 583.

§ Stead, A. L., *Brit. J. Anæsth.*, 1955, **27**, 124; and Bush, G. H., and Stead, A. L., *Ibid.*, 1962, **34**, 721.

Muscular Relaxation, *continued.*

intervals. Atropine (0·008 mg. per lb.) followed by neostigmine (0·036 mg. per lb.) should be given at the end of operation.

Suxamethonium is probably the preferred relaxant in neonates for short operations and they require at least twice the dose (dose for weight) to produce comparable results as in adults, even though the pseudocholinesterase level is lower than in adults. A dose of 5 mg. can be given and repeated many times if necessary. It sometimes causes bradycardia in infants. Muscular fasciculation is not seen in infancy.

DOSES RECOMMENDED.—For neonates: tubocurarine 0·2 mg. per lb. initial dose, 0·125 mg. per lb. supplementary doses; gallamine 0·5 mg. per lb. initial dose and 0·125 mg. per lb. supplementary doses; suxamethonium, 0·5 mg. per lb. intravenously, 1 mg. per lb. with hyaluronidase intramuscularly, 2 mg. per lb. without hyaluronidase intramuscularly. For administering small doses to infants a 1-ml. tuberculin syringe has been found useful.

For older children: tubocurarine 1·5 mg. per 5 lb. (4–4·5 mg. per stone); gallamine 1 mg. per lb.

Dose of neostigmine : 0·03 mg. per lb. (0·5 mg. per stone) with atropine at least 0·3 mg. ($\frac{1}{200}$ gr.), 0·65 mg. ($\frac{1}{100}$ gr.) if over 1 year.

Dosage of intravenous agents.—Thiopentone 2–2·5 mg. per lb. (25 mg. per stone). Pethidine 0·1 to 0·5 mg. per lb.

A relaxant can be very useful in a child with tachycardia, tachypnœa, and fever, e.g., in a case of acute appendicitis or peritonitis when it is desirable to avoid deep anæsthesia. In neonates, a biphasic or dual block is apt to develop after suxamethonium and can be antagonized by neostigmine. To reduce the total amount of drug, intermittent injections are better than the continuous drip.

Causes of post-operative apnœa in the neonate are:—

1. Hypothermia, 85° F. (29·4° C.) or below.
2. Overdosage of relaxant.
3. Overdosage with inhalation agent.
4. Potentiation of non-depolarizing relaxant with ether.
5. Concurrent antibiotics.
6. A combination of the above.

Monitoring.—It may be difficult to obtain access to the radial pulse or to see the small infant's respirations under the towels, especially when a T-piece technique is used. It is valuable to strap a stethoscope over the precordium, which acts as a useful monitor of heart-sounds, rate, and rhythm. An œsophageal stethoscope can be used where a precordial stethoscope is impracticable.* A stethoscope attached to the side-arm of a T-piece provides audible monitoring of respiration. Otherwise pulse monitors can be attached to a digit, or the electrocardiogram used as a monitor.

Blood-loss and Replacement.†—The blood-volume of an infant is small (about 300 ml. in the newborn) and so blood replacement

---

* Cullingford, D. W. J., *Brit. J. Anæsth.,* 1964, **36,** 524.
† Carré, I. J., *Ibid.,* 1963, **35,** 488.

must be accurate. This can be done with the help of swab weighing to estimate blood-loss. Blood transfusion can be undertaken from small reservoirs, or a three-way tap and 20-ml. syringe can be used to transfuse an accurate volume in replacement. Other special apparatus is: (1) The Capon-Heaton pædiatric infusion unit which has a 30-ml. burette; (2) The Baxter Pedatrol controlled-volume unit, which has segments of 5 ml. controlled by a clamp.

Fluid infusion should not generally exceed 10 ml. per lb. in 24 hours. About 5 ml. per hour is enough for neonates for the first postoperative day.

The umbilical vein is not suitable for prolonged infusion in babies, only for short-term blood injections on the operating table. Thrombophlebitis as a sequel is common.

Temperature.—The newborn rapidly loses heat if placed in a cold environment. The heat-regulating mechanisms are unstable in the premature infant and in the mature newborn baby for some weeks. The newborn maintains its body heat through the metabolic activity of brown fat. This fat has a rich blood- and nerve-supply. It may be deficient in small or premature babies.* Care must be taken that undue heat loss does not occur on the operating table. Since the baby's head has a large surface area in relation to the rest of the body, it is useful to cover it with a stockinet cap to retain warmth.* Heat loss is increased when room temperature is low, when coverings are minimal, and when viscera are exposed. Transfusion of cold fluids intravenously may also produce hypothermia. For major operations on small babies it is wise to place the child on a mattress with circulating coils so that rewarming can be applied if necessary. Monitoring of temperature helps to give warning of accidental hypothermia.

Older children may develop hyperpyrexia on the operating table. This is likely to occur : (1) When the child is pyrexial ; (2) In hot climatic conditions ; (3) When there are too many coverings over the child, particularly if these include macintosh sheets ; (4) Inhibition of sweating following atropine premedication may interfere with heat loss. Hyperpyrexia is an aetiological factor in ether convulsions. A mattress with circulating coils placed under the patient may be useful for cooling.

Anæsthetic Agents.—

1. Ether is a useful agent, although explosive. It may be given with air on an open mask, or with nitrous-oxide–oxygen or oxygen from an anæsthetic machine. Respiration usually spontaneous.

2. Divinyl ether and ethyl chloride. Useful for induction of anæsthesia.

3. Halothane and oxygen. Particularly useful in children because it produces quiet respiration and muscular relaxation without explosive risk and without the need for intravenous injections. Respiration spontaneous or controlled.

---

* Tizard, J. P. M., *Proc. R. Soc. Med.*, 1967, **60**, 935.

Anaesthetic Agents, *continued.*

4. Intravenous techniques combined with nitrous-oxide–oxygen ar perhaps with controlled respiration. Rees* uses fine needl (26 S.W.G.) and recommends scalp veins in infants, employir special scalp-vein needles attached to a length of plastic tubin, the anterior aspect of the wrist between 6 months and 2 year and thereafter the dorsum of the hand or the antecubital foss.

5. Cyclopropane.† After atropine premedication, anæsthesia induced, using a Boyle's machine with Magill rebreathing attacl ment with the expiratory valve set at its slackest positior oxygen 1·25 l. per minute (which remains constant throughou the anæsthesia) and nitrous oxide 3 l. per minute are give from a face-mask and cyclopropane 750 ml. per minute a added, giving a cyclopropane percentage of 15. If deepe anæsthesia is required, the nitrous oxide is reduced to 2 l. pe minute and this increases the cyclopropane percentage to 2 The addition of a trace of ether vapour will increase relaxatior Respiration spontaneous or controlled.

6. Muscle relaxants. *See* p. 595.

Abdominal Surgery.—In neonates, muscular relaxation does nc require deep anæsthesia or relaxants, except in special cases suc as when a large volume of viscera has to be returned to the per toneal cavity. Older children may be satisfactorily anæsthetize with nitrous oxide and relaxants, cyclopropane, ether, or halc thane.

DIAPHRAGMATIC HERNIA.—Congenital herniation of ak dominal organs through the diaphragm prevents expansion c the lungs and displaces the mediastinum. The child exhibit bouts of cyanosis. Radiography shows loops of bowel in th left chest. Emergency operation should be carried out as soo: as the condition is diagnosed. Light general anæsthesia wit an orotracheal tube is indicated. Reduction of the hernia ma require profound muscular relaxation for a short time, and thi may be achieved with suxamethonium. Post-operativel, constant vigilance is required as fatalities have occurred due t atelectasis, pneumothorax, hyperpyrexia, etc.

OMPHALOCELE.—This requires emergency operation since ruptur of the thin sac covering the intestines will result in peritonitis Anæsthetic management is similar to that for diaphragmati hernia.

RAMSTEDT'S OPERATION.—The operation of pyloromyotom\ was first performed by Conrad Ramstedt (1868–1963) in 1911 Frequently performed under *local infiltration* of the abdomina wall, using up to 15 ml. of 0·5 per cent procaine and adrenalin or 0·25 per cent solution of lignocaine (3·5 mg. per lb.) witl adrenaline, 1–400,000.‡ During the 24 hours preceding opera tion, fluids must be pushed and the infant must come to th theatre with its stomach washings clean and a stomach tube i

---

* Rees, G. J., *Brit. J. Anæsth.*, 1960, **32**, 123.
† France, G. G., *Ibid.*, 1957, **29**, 76.
‡ Black, G. W., and Love, S. H. S., *Anæsthesia*, 1957, **12**, 430.

place. *Premedication* is nepenthe, 1 min., hypodermically, or chloral hydrate, 300 mg. (5 gr.), given 2 hours before operation, or rectal thiopentone, 15–20 mg. per lb. in 2 per cent solution given in the operating theatre with the buttocks held together—preceded by an enema.

Before *general anæsthesia*, atropine, 0·3 mg., may be used. The child is securely bandaged to a cross-splint and during the operation is fed a mixture of honey and syrup of chloral from a dummy. The patient must be kept warm.

Open ether, preceded by V.A.M. induction, also gives good results as does oxygen and halothane or oxygen and cyclopropane. Some workers prefer to use an endotracheal tube, while small doses of suxamethonium may be used to aid relaxation* (2·5 mg.). Infants weighing 7 lb. or less can be intubated in the conscious state. Heavier babies require 2·5 per cent thiopentone 1·5 mg. per lb. and suxamethonium 0·75 mg. per lb. for intubation. Subsequent doses of suxamethonium 2·5 mg. given as required intravenously. Denis Browne recommends that a ' bootlace ' stitch should be placed in the peritoneum before the pyloric tumour is delivered from the wound. During the operation this can be drawn aside. It avoids the need for increasing greatly the anæsthetic depth during closure.

Control of electrolytes must always precede operation, which is never an emergency. In the 2 hours following operation the infant may collapse and so needs careful watching. This may be due to deep anæsthesia or to hypercapnia.

Tracheo-œsophageal Fistula with Œsophageal Atresia.—Aspiration of food and secretions usually results in pneumonia within a few days of birth. Operation is a hazardous procedure and successful operations were not carried out before 1939 when Leven and Ladd (independently) in the U.S.A. performed multistage operations. Primary œsophageal anastomosis was introduced by Haight in 1941.

There are various anatomical variations. Much the commonest finding is the blind upper œsophageal pouch, with a fistula between the posterior trachea and lower œsophagus. The varieties of œsophageal atresia and the numbers of cases in a recent series is shown in *Fig.* 48.†

Anæsthetic management may be difficult. Endotracheal anæsthesia with controlled respiration is generally advocated. It is imperative that the anæsthetist be able to use effective suction in the airway at all times and a suitable fine catheter must be available. Intermittent positive-pressure respiration can result in gastric distension. Fortunately this is only a serious problem in a minority of cases, when gastrostomy may be necessary for its relief. Good relaxation enables ventilation to be carried out at minimal pressures. Accurate replacement of blood is essential.

---

* Booth, A. J., Nisbet, H. I. A., and Wilson, F., *Anæsthesia*, 1959, **14**, 355.
† Waterston, D. J., Bonham-Carter, R. E., and Aberdeen, E., *Lancet*, 1963, **2**, 55.

Tracheo-œsophageal Fistula with Œsophageal Atresia, *continued.*

RECOMMENDED TECHNIQUES. — Premedication : atrop
0·15 mg. ($\frac{1}{400}$ gr.). Set up intravenous infusion before induct
of anæsthesia. Intubate while the infant is awake. Anæsth

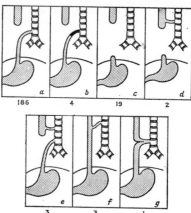

Fig. 48.—Varieties of œsophageal atresia, showing numbers of cases. (*By courtesy of 'Th
Lancet'.*)

agents : nitrous-oxide–oxygen, supplemented by minimal eth
or cyclopropane or muscle relaxants.

Cleft Palate and Hare-lip in Infants.*—The repair of cleft palate
usually done in two stages, while the hare-lip can be repair
during one of these operations or done independently. Ma
surgeons prefer to operate when the child is about 10–16 weeks o
for hare-lip and about one year old for the palate. The ch
should be fit and healthy.

Atropine, 0·3–0·4 mg., is suitable as premedication and i
children over the age of 2, pentobarbitone 40 mg. per ston
Endotracheal anæsthesia is indicated, using a Magill cleft-pala
tube (sizes 3, 4, 4·5, and 5). This consists of rubber dista.
and a coiled spring covered by thin rubber proximally, whe
there is also a small gas side-delivery tube. It can be used
an Ayre's T-piece by fixing to the proximal end 4–6 in. of rubb
tubing, to allow a little rebreathing. The Magill tube is ke
rigid during oral introduction by a metal stylet. The port
plastic tube is also useful for these cases. The oral route shou
be used when possible, as it allows the passage of a larger tub
Care is necessary to see that kinking of the tube does not occu
nor must it be occluded by the gag. The patient's hands shou

* *See also* articles by Davies, R. M., and Danks, Sylvia, *Anæsthesia*, 1953, **8**, 275 ; Nor
W., and Saunders, R. C. O., *Brit. J. Anæsth.*, 1955, **27**, 597.

be firmly secured. Anæsthesia can be induced on an open mask with vinyl ether or ethyl ether, or a nitrous-oxide–cyclopropane–ether–oxygen sequence can be used. Other workers give gas–oxygen and ether through an Ayre's T-piece, while there are those who use thiopentone (2 to 5 mg. per lb.), pethidine (2–7 mg. per stone), and tubocurarine (1 mg. per 5 lb.) or gallamine (1 mg. per lb.). If a rapidly acting relaxant is used for intubation the dose (of suxamethonium) should be 0·5 mg. per lb. intravenously or 1 mg. per lb. intramuscularly with hyaluronidase, or 2 mg. per lb. intramuscularly without hyaluronidase. Reflex resistance to intubation must be abolished. Intubation is facilitated if the glottis is first moistened with cocaine solution from the tip of a finger. Introduction of the endotracheal tube may be hindered by an anteriorly displaced premaxilla obstructing the field of vision. To prevent the blade of the laryngoscope from sinking deeply into the wide cleft, gauze packing or adhesive tape can be used or the gap can be bridged by a spatula. Dott's gag is useful as it allows the endotracheal tube to lie in the longitudinal slot in its blade. At least 30 per cent of oxygen should be given throughout, and volatile or non-volatile agents may be used to supplement the gas and oxygen. A total flow of 2–3 l. per min. is adequate once the patient has settled down, the gases flowing over the surface of the volatile anæsthetic. Only light anæsthesia is required.

Following removal of the tube and a careful oropharyngeal toilet, a patent airway can be ensured by a suture through the tongue. Post-operative œdema of glottis should be prevented by gentle technique and adequate depth of anæsthesia during intubation ; treatment is steam tent, oxygen tent, or tracheostomy. With gentleness, cleanliness, and care it should rarely be seen.

Tumours about the Face and Neck.—Cystic hygromas and other tumours may occur in these regions and may make endotracheal intubation difficult.*

Waters† has devised a method of guided blind endotracheal intubation for cases of cancrum oris. A Tuohy needle is introduced through the cricothyroid membrane and sterile vinyl plastic tubing threaded through the cords from below to coil up in the nasopharynx. A length of polythene tubing with a blunt hook is pushed through the nose to engage the vinyl catheter which is brought out through the nose. A Magill cuffed endotracheal tube is then passed round the catheter which is then withdrawn. He recommends the use of a small dose of thiopentone and tracheal injection of lignocaine to prevent undue distress in children.

Neurosurgical Operations.—These require light general anæsthesia via an oral endotracheal tube. Halothane is a useful agent in children, since respiration is usually quiet and there is no explosive risk. Tachypnœa is usually a drawback to trichloroethylene anæsthesia in small children.

Macdonald, D. J. F., *Anæsthesia*, 1966, **21**, 66.
Waters, D. J., *Ibid.*, 1963, **18**, 158.

Neurosurgical Operations, *continued.*

OPERATIONS FOR HYDROCEPHALUS.—Intubation may difficult due to the large forehead which makes visualizatio the larynx awkward.

OPERATIONS FOR CRANIOSTENOSIS.—Often done in the p position. Premature closure of the fissures restricts b development and must be relieved by removal of section skull. Hæmorrhage may be profuse and blood should be repla

MENINGOCELE.—Careful anæsthetic technique is required. operation is performed in the face-down position. Endotrac intubation is mandatory. Controlled ventilation is likely t required as spontaneous respirations, mainly diaphragmatic, embarrassed in this position.

Siamese Twins.*—These babies may require several anæsthe depending on how they are joined. *Radiological investigat* require quiet babies. Each twin must be anæsthetized se ately. Two anæsthetists should therefore be available. Induc of the first twin may be difficult. If there is a significant com circulation the anæsthetic agent will be drained away to the o twin so that the speed of induction is slowed. Conversely second twin is anæsthetized more readily since it has alre received some anæsthesia from the first. Depending on the of union, intubation may be technically difficult.

Operations for separation of Siamese twins are likely to be long to be associated with blood-loss. Separate anæsthetic te must therefore be assigned to each twin.

Post-operative Care.†—Intensive care is necessary in the neon Attention must be paid to: (1) Environmental temperature; Feeding: a weight-loss of 44 g. per day per kg. birth-weight r occur in the first two days of life. It is possible for the blood-su (normal level 50 mg. per cent at birth) to fall to undetectable le if early feeding is not commenced. Oral feeding is preferabl possible; (3) Acidæmia: if present must be corrected; (4) Oxy therapy: respiratory failure is a not uncommon complication assisted respiration may be necessary. Rates of 60–80 per mi may be required using air enriched with oxygen. Po_2 can necessary, be obtained using umbilical artery catheters; (5) Cr infection is a potential hazard; (6) Jaundice: this may occu any sick newborn baby due to low levels of glycuroniltransfe in the liver. After surgery, blood-clot provides an additic source of bile-pigments.

Respiratory Difficulties in Infants.—

1. ASPHYXIA OF THE NEWBORN. *See* Chapter XXV.
2. CONGENITAL LARYNGEAL STRIDOR.‡—Inspiratory stri from birth, usually gone by age 12–18 months. Commo ascribed to lax or superfluous aryteno-epiglottic folds. All ca must be investigated to exclude other causes.

---

* Ballantine, R. I. W., and Jackson, I., *Brit. med. J.*, 1964, **1**, 1339.
† *See* Tizard, J. P. M., *Proc. R. Soc. Med.*, 1967, **60**, 935.
‡ Editorial, *Brit. med. J.*, 1965, **1**, 1393.

3. CHOANAL ATRESIA.—Nearly always posterior. If bilateral the infant must breathe through the mouth. The airway must be kept patent by opening the mouth, keeping the child crying, or insertion of an oropharyngeal airway until surgical correction can be performed.

4. THE PIERRE-ROBIN SYNDROME.—Hypoplastic mandible with glossoptosis and a small epiglottis. This produces respiratory obstruction, which tends to disappear after the age of 2 years. It may be necessary to suture the tongue to the alveolar ridge of the mandible to relieve respiratory obstruction. Such cases may be very difficult to intubate. The child should be nursed in the prone position both before and after operation.

5. LARYNGOMALACIA.—This is caused by incomplete development of the laryngeal cartilages. Inspiratory obstruction to respiration occurs as the flaccid structures are drawn in. Usually improves after the age of 18 months.

6. TREACHER COLLINS SYNDROME.*—Rare. Receding chin and obtuse angle of mandible make it difficult to maintain an airway or pass an endotracheal tube. Other clinical features include abnormal ears, eyes, and maxillæ. Cleft palate may be present. There is a strong familial incidence.

(*See also* Symposium on Anæsthesia in Pædiatrics, *Brit. J. Anæsth.*, 1960, **32**, 97; Wilton, T. N. P., and Wilson, F., *Neonatal Anæsthesia*, 1965. Oxford: Blackwell; and Davenport, H. T., *Pædiatric Anæsthesia*, 1967. London: Heinemann.)

CHAPTER XXIV

DENTAL ANÆSTHESIA†

For the early use of nitrous oxide *see* p. 149. After the introduction of ether and chloroform, nitrous oxide fell into disfavour, until interest was revived in its use for dental extractions 100 years ago by G. Q. Colton and T. W. Evans. The latter demonstrated his method in London on 31 March, 1868.‡ Other pioneers of nitrous oxide anæsthesia include Edmund Andrews, who used it with oxygen, Sir F. Hewitt who designed an apparatus,§ and E. I. McKesson whose demand-flow machine is still in use.‖ In recent years there has been a re-appraisal of dental anæsthesia aimed at the prevention of hypoxia and the provision of better operating conditions for the surgeon. Improved anæsthetic technique allows the surgeon more time and increases the range of procedures which can be undertaken in the dental chair.

Recent advances include the use of halothane as a volatile supplement,¶ the use of intravenous techniques,** and the use of endotracheal

---

* Ross, E. D. T., *Anæsthesia*, 1963, **18**, 350.
† *See* Symposium on Dental Anæsthesia, *Brit. J. Anæsth.*, 1968, **40**, March.
‡ Evans, T. W., *Brit. J. Dent. Sci.*, 1868, **11**, 196; and *Ibid.*, 1868, **11**, 318.
§ Hewitt, F. W., *Anæsthetics and their Administration*, 1893. London: Griffin; and Hewitt, F. W., *The Administration of Nitrous Oxide and Oxygen for Dental Operations*, 1897. London: Ash.
‖ McKesson, E. I., *Brit. med. J.*, 1926, **2**, 1113.
¶ Walsh, R. S., *Brit. J. Anæsth.*, 1958, **30**, 578.
** Drummond-Jackson, S. L., *Dental Cosmos*, 1935, **77**, 130.

History, *continued.*

methods,* while the dangers of fainting when the patient is held in th
sitting position have been pointed out by Bourne.† The Society for th
Advancement of Anæsthesia in Dentistry has been active since 195
It is now possible to offer 'ultra-light' intravenous anæsthesia fo
conservative work in the dental chair employing, e.g., methohexiton
or propanidid.

NITROUS OXIDE AND OXYGEN

The addition of oxygen to nitrous oxide in dental anæsthesia wa
popularized by Frederick Hewitt.‡ If pure nitrous oxide is administere
the patient will pass through the stages of analgesia and excitemen
until the stage of surgical anæsthesia is reached. Oxygen must then b
added to prevent hypoxia, but the amount must be carefully regulate
as the margin between too light anæsthesia and dangerous hypoxia i
small. Skilled administration is necessary if smooth anæsthesia is t
be given consistently, and some degree of hypoxia has frequently to b
accepted. The signs are those of analgesia, excitement, and ligh
surgical anæsthesia. Deep planes of anæsthesia cannot be obtaine
using nitrous oxide alone, but the signs of hypoxia must be considerec
   The likelihood of hypoxia can be reduced: (1) By premedication
(2) By pre-oxygenation;§ (3) By using an intravenous or an inhalationa
supplement; (4) By skilled administration. Some groups of patient
are difficult to anæsthetize without gross hypoxia. These include
(1) The strong muscular man; (2) The frightened; (3) The alcoholic
(4) A combination of these factors.
   Most workers now think that at least 20 per cent of oxygen shoul
be given routinely.

The Signs of Anæsthesia.—
   1. ANALGESIA. STAGE I.—During induction of anæsthesia this i
      passed through quickly. Sustained analgesia can be produce
      by inhalation of 25–50 per cent nitrous oxide, and is useful i
      obstetrics, conservative dentistry, changing of painful dressings
      for post-operative physiotherapy, etc.
   2. EXCITEMENT, DELIRIUM. STAGE II.—Occurs most com
      monly in: (a) The frightened; (b) The tough and sturdy; (c) Th
      alcoholic. Due to removal of inhibition by the higher centres
      Can be lessened by: (1) Premedication; (2) A sympatheti
      approach. Many patients fear the unpleasant subjective feeling
      which may accompany induction. Others fear that surgery ma
      be started while they are still conscious. The anæsthetist shoul
      try to produce an atmosphere of quiet confidence and talk to th
      patient throughout induction.
   3. SURGICAL ANÆSTHESIA. STAGE III.—Onset of surgica
      anæsthesia is characterized by: (1) Automatic respiration,
      characteristic regular rhythm of respiration, inspiration, an
      expiration equal in duration, phonation absent. The change t

---

* Danziger, A. M., *Brit. dent. J.,* 1962, **113**, 426.
† Bourne, J. G., *Lancet,* 1957, **2**, 499.
‡ Hewitt, F., *Anæsthetics and their Administration,* 1893. London: Griffin.
§ Neff, W., and others, *Brit. med. J.,* 1950, **1**, 1400; and Mostert, J. W., *Ibid.,* 1958, **1**, 50

NITROUS-OXIDE–OXYGEN SIGN CHART OF THE THIRD STAGE OF ANÆSTHESIA
(McKesson)

	LIGHT ANÆSTHESIA	NORMAL ANÆSTHESIA	PROFOUND ANÆSTHESIA
	Due to too much oxygen in the mixture	Due to a properly balanced mixture of N_2O–O_2	Due to too little O_2 in the mixture, or to partial obstruction of respiratory passages
Respiration	a. Superficial slow breathing often irregular b. Prolonged inspiration c. Phonation due to reflexes of pain d. Holding breath, grunting	a. Full ' machine-like ' respirations. Regular and faster than normal b. Inspiration and expiration nearly equal c. No phonation d. Continuous uninterrupted respiration	a. Irregular rhythm (sobby) usually slower than normal. Spasmodic b. Prolonged expiration c. Phonation due to muscular spasm of vocal cords. Often crowing d. Temporary inefficient breathing. Cessation of respiration usually from spasm of muscles of exhalation
General muscles	a. Purposeful movements or rigid muscles b. Facial expression of pain, semi-consciousness c. Nausea, very rarely d. Reflex or purposeful resistance as result of trauma	a. Immobile and relaxed, but having normal muscular tonus b. Expression of normal sleep c. Quiet d. Quiet. Relaxed	a. Clonic movements, twitching or jerking in early minutes of induction, often start in upper eyelids b. Expression, wild looking c. Swallowing, retching, or vomiting common d. Tetanic spasm, marked rigidity—opisthotonos in some cases
The eye	a. Pupils large, contract to light actively b. Conjunctiva sensitive c. Eyeballs roll quite rapidly d. Eyelids resist opening, wink when touched	a. Pupils small or medium fixed b. Conjunctiva insensitive to touch c. Eyeballs fixed or slowly rolling d. Lids often slightly open, relaxed, no winking	a. Pupils fixed, enlarge progressively, and finally become irregular in outline* b. Conjunctiva insensitive c. Eyeballs fixed in some position, often downward, or jerk d. Eyelids stiff. Often wide open
Pulse-rate	Accelerated	Usually slightly above normal	Rapid or very slow, and sometimes irregular
Blood-pressure	Normal	Normal	Sometimes increased slightly, but usually decreased
Colour of skin and blood	a. Pink, or no change normally b. In anæmics, no colour change c. In plethorics, slight cyanosis	a. Varies from pink to decided cyanotic tint b. In anæmics, no colour change c. In plethorics, considerable cyanosis	a. Usually cyanotic b. In anæmics, slight flushing, rarely cyanotic c. In plethorics, very blue
Remedy	Decrease the percentage of oxygen in the mixture		Increase oxygen in the mixture, or inflate lungs with pure oxygen 1 to 3 times

* Jordanov, J., and Ruben, H., *Lancet*, 1967, **2**, 915, find that pupillary dilatation is not a feature of hypoxia until cardiac arrest becomes imminent.

23

The Signs of Anæsthesia, *continued.*

automatic respiration may occur quite suddenly in a single breath; (2) Loss of the eyelash reflex. Signs of established surgical anæsthesia include: (3) Loss of resistance to opening eye (4) Eyeballs roving and then becoming fixed. (5) The patient has minimal muscular movement and does not respond to surgical stimulation.

Clement* has separated this stage into:—

a. Light anæsthesia, reflex movements related to surgical stimuli
b. Normal anæsthesia, with relative muscular relaxation.
c. 'Deep anæsthesia', hypoxic rigidity, jactitation, purposeless and unrelated to surgical stimuli. Masseter spasm may prevent insertion of a gag.

4. THE SIGNS OF HYPOXIA.—(1) Hypoxic rigidity of muscles unrelated to surgical stimuli; twitching and jactitation; spasm of extra-ocular muscles pulling eyeballs downwards or in another direction; (2) Respirations become irregular and jerky; (3) Pupils enlarge; (4) Slow bounding pulse; (5) Finally, muscles become atonic and respirations cease, a grave prognostic state when death is imminent, though artificial respiration with oxygen will usually revive the patient.

Sweating, due to sympathetic stimulation, may occur in light anæsthesia. Retching and vomiting usually indicate oxygen lack.

Prolonged hypoxia may, in certain patients, cause permanent damage to the cells of the cerebral cortex. Results may take the form of Jacksonianism, athetoid movements, idiocy, or decorticate rigidity.

A full strong pulse indicates light or normal anæsthesia. An irregular pulse of poor volume or a rapid pulse is a sign of hypoxia.

During dental anæsthesia peak inspiratory flow rates may be between 50 and 200 l. per min., tidal volumes between 300 and 3000 ml., and inspiratory minute volume between 11 and 50 l. per min.†

CYANOSIS.—Cyanosis results when 3·3 g. to 5 g. or more of hæmoglobin in each 100 ml. of blood are circulating uncombined with oxygen. Some authors express it as a desaturation of venous blood exceeding 11·4 vol. per cent—the normal desaturation of venous blood being 6 vol. per cent. Cyanosis is not clinically recognizable until the saturation of oxygen is reduced to between 85 and 75 per cent, varying with different observers. The amount of oxyhæmoglobin in circulation does not influence cyanosis. As the blood of normal individuals contains 15 g. of hæmoglobin in each 100 ml., the onset of cyanosis leaves 10 g. available for carrying oxygen. In anæmia with a hæmoglobin estimation of 10 g. per 100 ml. the onset of cyanosis shows that only 5 g. are available for oxygen transport, which is thus reduced by half. In plethora with, say, 20 g. per cent cyanosis still leaves 15 g. for active duty.

Thus cyanosis must be correlated with the blood state of the patient. With severe anæmia there will be no cyanosis until

---

* Clement, F. W., *Nitrous Oxide–Oxygen Anæsthesia*, 3rd ed., 1951. London: Kimpton.
† Smith, W. D. A., *Brit. J. Anæsth.*, 1964, **36**, 696.

depression is grave, while the full-blooded patient is often cyanosed slightly, even when breathing fresh air. In normal patients under gas and oxygen anæsthesia a moderate cyanosis may not be harmful in the absence of muscular signs of hypoxia. In the plethoric patient, if anæsthesia with nitrous-oxide–oxygen is possible it will necessitate considerable cyanosis.

The chief guide from colour changes occurs once a patient is stabilized, when increasing cyanosis suggests increasing depth, and vice versa.

FACTORS MODIFYING CYANOSIS.—(1) Pigmentation of the skin either normal (e.g., race) or abnormal (e.g., in jaundice). (2) Thickness of epidermis. (3) Variation of density of capillary network in the observed skin area. (4) Temperature of skin—cold causes stagnation of circulation and consequent reduction of oxyhæmoglobin. (5) Increased venous pressure and high blood-volume, e.g., polycythæmia, favour cyanosis. Cyanosis may thus not be very obvious in shock.

PATHOLOGICAL CONDITIONS CAUSING CYANOSIS INDEPENDENT OF ANÆSTHESIA.—

1. Circulatory shunt from veins to arteries.—
   In Fallot's tetralogy; simple pulmonary stenosis with right to left interatrial shunt; pulmonary atresia; tricuspid atresia, etc.

2. In lung disease.—
   a. Lung consolidation, collapse, compression, or œdema.
   b. In diseases of the respiratory passages.
   c. Asthma.
   d. Emphysema.
   e. Ayerza's disease (cyanosis with right heart disease).
   f. When muscles of respiration are defective.

3. In heart disease.—
   a. Mitral disease.
   b. Congestive heart failure.
   c. Pulmonary atresia or stenosis.
   d. Tricuspid atresia.

4. In alterations in blood-pigment in sulphæmoglobinæmia and methæmoglobinæmia, following drugs (e.g., phenacetin and prilocaine).

5. In polycythæmia.

Apparatus.—For many years, intermittent-flow machines have been favoured for dental anæsthesia. Most popular have been the five Walton models* and the McKesson apparatus.† Since they operate on the demand system reservoir bags are not necessary (except in so far as a reservoir is an integral part of the machine itself, e.g., McKesson). Provision must be made, however, for accurate administration of known percentages of oxygen. Recent trends favour the use of continuous-flow machines. This is because of the greater use of non-hypoxic mixtures of nitrous oxide and oxygen together with volatile supplements. Accurate oxygen

---

* Smith, W. D. A., *Brit. J. Anæsth.*, 1961, **33**, 440.
† McKesson, E. I., *Brit. med. J.*, 1926, **2**, 1113.

Apparatus, *continued.*

percentages below 20 per cent are no longer required,* and doubt has been cast on the accuracy of many machines in general use.†

Recently, apparatus has been calibrated which allows the anæsthetist to give 20 per cent oxygen, 80 per cent nitrous oxide at various flow rates on a continuous-flow machine (the 'Salisbury').‡ Another development is the use of premixed gas cylinders‡ (50 per cent of each gas) together with a halothane vaporizer. Marrett has also described the Medrex apparatus for administration of halothane with nitrous oxide and oxygen.§

(*See also* good review of apparatus, Thompson, P. W., *Brit. J. Anæsth.*, 1968, **40**, 166.)

Classic Nitrous-Oxide–Oxygen Administration.—The stomach and bladder should be empty, the nose should be blown, and dentures should be removed. The anæsthetist must be sure that the patient is fit for the proposed operation and tight garments must be loosened in obese patients. Premedication is not given, but the patient should be treated sympathetically and the procedure explained to him. It is easy to suggest that pain and discomfort will ensue, and this is to be avoided. Dental forceps and other instruments should be prepared unobtrusively and an atmosphere of calm confidence engendered.

The patient should be seated comfortably in the chair, with the head rest adjusted to allow surgical access. The feet should be placed on the floor, not on the foot rest in case reactions in the excitement stage cause extension of the body or hypoxic spasm resulting in opisthotonos. The hands may be placed in the trouser pockets or arms comfortably folded. A lap belt may be valuable in the robust individual.

After insertion of a mouth prop, the patient is instructed to breathe through his nose, and pure nitrous oxide administered by nasal mask. This is continued until loss of consciousness is indicated by the onset of automatic respiration and loss of the eyelash reflex.

Difficulties during induction include: (1) Mouth breathing: This dilutes the nitrous oxide and delays induction. The patient should be exhorted to breathe through the nose, but if necessary an oral mask is used in addition; (2) Excitement: This is more likely in the frightened, the sturdy, and the alcoholic. The strange and sometimes unpleasant sensations which accompany induction induce panic states in susceptible individuals. Also some patients fear the commencement of surgery before the loss of consciousness. A quiet calm commentary by the anæsthetist helps to allay fears and allows the patient to know that the anæsthetist is aware that the patient is still awake.

When the patient is unconscious, oxygen must be added to the nitrous oxide being respired by the patient. A concentration of

* Vickers, M. D., and Pask, E. A., *Anæsthesia*, 1966, **21**, 261.
† Nainby-Luxmoore, R. C., *Ibid.*, 1967, **22**, 545.
‡ Latham, J., and Parbrook, G. D., *Ibid.*, 1966, **21**, 472; and *Ibid.*, 1967, **22**, 316.
§ Marrett, R., *Ibid.*, 1963, **18**, 290.

about 7 per cent is given initially, though this may be increased to 10 per cent or 15 per cent as time proceeds. The anæsthetist has several duties which he must perform simultaneously during the dental operation. These include: (1) Adjustment of the oxygen concentration according to the physical signs of light anæsthesia or hypoxia which may develop. (a) With too light anæsthesia purposeful movements occur in response to surgical stimuli. There may be phonation, withdrawal reflexes, and screwing up of the eyes. (b) With hypoxia, there are purposeless movements, hypoxic muscle spasms, and respirations may become jerky. The appropriate reduction or increase in oxygen percentage must be made. The experienced anæsthetist tries to anticipate events by changing the oxygen percentage before the situation gets out of hand. (2) Maintenance of a clear airway. This may be difficult during operations on the lower jaw when there is a tendency to flex the head and obstruct respiration. (3) Provide counter-pressure, if required by the dental surgeon. (4) See that a dental pack is used to prevent inhalation of blood and debris and to discourage mouth breathing. (5) Observe the vital signs, pulse and respiration, and take early action should untoward reactions (e.g., fainting) occur. (6) The anæsthetist must sometimes assist in the insertion of mouth gags, particularly when extractions on both sides of the mouth are necessary.

As soon as the operation is complete, nitrous oxide must be switched off and the patient allowed to recover consciousness. Pure oxygen may be given with advantage for a few minutes. The patient must be carefully observed at this stage, to ensure that blood-clot or debris is expelled from the mouth and not inhaled, and to control any signs of excitement during the recovery. Fainting can also occur after the operation is completed, and the anæsthetist must be prepared to flatten the chair and elevate the legs.

The tendency today is to give at least 20 per cent of oxygen with a volatile supplement if required from the beginning.

RESPIRATORY OBSTRUCTION.—Can be avoided by: (a) Careful holding of the lower jaw; (b) A pharyngeal airway; (c) A nasopharyngeal airway; (d) An endotracheal tube.

Airways and tubes should be smeared with lubricant containing a topical analgesic, e.g., amethocaine 1 per cent, cinchocaine 2–10 per cent, lignocaine 2 per cent. Their introduction may cause temporary gagging. A piece of Magill endotracheal tube, size 8–9·5, equal in length to the distance between the nostril and the external auditory meatus, can be used as a nasopharyngeal tube, its distal end lying just above the glottis, while its proximal end protrudes from the nostril prevented by a safety-pin from disappearing into the naris.

RESPIRATORY ARREST.—This may be due to:—

1. Respiratory obstruction—and is treated accordingly.
2. Breath-holding in light anæsthesia—treatment usually unnecessary.
3. Apnœa due to severe hypoxia. Treatment is by inflation of the lungs with oxygen. See that the airway is clear, close

Classic Nitrous-Oxide–Oxygen Administration, *continued.*

expiratory valve, hold mask firmly on to face, and see tha
oxygen under pressure makes the chest inflate, either by
touching the direct-pressure oxygen button, or by compressing
the reservoir bag, previously emptied and filled with pure
oxygen. Breathing pure oxygen, compared with breathing
air, raises the oxygen dissolved in blood by 11 per cent
Respiratory arrest usually precedes cardiac arrest, so resusci
tation by oxygen inflation is usually successful. Should it no
be so, other measures must be taken (*see* Chapter XXXIV).

4. Apnœa due to a sudden high oxygen tension following a perioc
of hypoxia. It results from a depression of the aortic anc
carotid body chemoreceptors by the high oxygen tensior
which removes their reflex-stimulating effect on the respiratory
centre.

Some Abnormal Types of Patient.—

1. Patients who are frightened and have a poor command of them
selves. These are difficult to control and may need premedi
cation.
2. Patients who resist all anæsthetics. Chronic alcoholics ; vigorous
young men. Supplements are often necessary to control such
patients.
3. Children under 4. These are not easily managed with nitrous-
oxide–oxygen, because of : (*a*) Emotional reaction ; (*b*) High
metabolic rate ; (*c*) Small volume of circulating blood which
causes rapid changes in level of anæsthesia and therefore a
small margin between too light and too deep anæsthesia.
Oxygen should be used from the beginning—about 15 per cent
later increasing. Premedication most useful. Minimal trichloroethylene or halothane very helpful as a supplement for
short operations.
4. Patients who are anæmic. They do not tolerate hypoxia. Induction should be slow with a high percentage of oxygen, 25–30
per cent, gradually increased or decreased according to the
patient's needs. Cyanosis may be a grave sign. With a
hæmoglobin of 5 g. per cent or less, death may occur before
the onset of cyanosis.
5. Patients with decompensated heart disease. These should be
treated like the anæmic group. It is often a good plan
to precede anæsthesia by the inhalation for ten minutes of
100 per cent oxygen. In the presence of valvular lesions, antibiotic cover should be given to prevent subsequent development
of subacute bacterial endocarditis.
6. Patients with hypertension. With good oxygenation these
patients do well. Struggling during induction should be
avoided.
7. Patients in shock. They are usually easily controlled, but
tolerate oxygen lack badly.
8. Diabetics. If receiving insulin, they can often be given a short
anæsthetic with safety just before a meal is due. They should be
kept under observation until they have received some nutriment
by mouth in case hypoglycæmia should develop.

9. Steroid therapy. For simple extractions steroid cover is not usually required. If there is doubt, the patient should take an extra tablet that day. Otherwise 100 mg. hydrocortisone may be given intravenously just prior to anæsthesia.

10. Mono-amine oxidase inhibitors. These drugs are contra-indications to the use of pethidine and related compounds. Nor should pressor drugs be used—e.g., adrenaline in local analgesic solutions.

11. It is seldom desirable to anæsthetize patients who are physically handicapped by nitrous-oxide–oxygen unsupplemented, except for short, minor operations.

Nitrous Oxide and Air.—Since nitrous oxide must often be given in concentrations approaching 90 per cent to sustain surgical anæsthesia, it is preferable to use pure oxygen as a diluent. Satisfactory anæsthesia of short duration has, however, been obtained with nitrous oxide and air. This can be done by removing the mask to allow a breath of air to every four or five breaths of nitrous oxide. Alternatively, some of the older pieces of apparatus are calibrated to allow use of air. A still older apparatus is the three-way stopcock which allows inspiration from gas supply or air. Nitrous-oxide–air anæsthesia is seldom justified in modern anæsthetic practice.

Modifications of the Technique.—There have been various attempts to minimize the hypoxia associated with nitrous oxide anæsthesia:

1. PRE-OXYGENATION.
2. AMNALGESIA.
3. PREMEDICATION.
4. USE OF VOLATILE SUPPLEMENTS.
5. USE OF INTRAVENOUS AGENTS.

PRE-OXYGENATION.—A technique of nitrous-oxide–oxygen anæsthesia for brief operations in healthy subjects has been described by Neff* and later by Mostert.† It depends on washing out nitrogen from the lungs by the administration of pure oxygen for 2 to 2½ min. prior to the administration of 100 per cent nitrous oxide. The administration of the pure gas continues for about 1 min. and the oxygen is added gradually until 20 per cent is being given. This makes hypoxia less likely and reduces the incidence of nausea and vomiting.

AMNALGESIA.‡—This is a plane between analgesia and anæsthesia and it allows 15–20 per cent of oxygen to be given (apart from a lower percentage for a few seconds during induction). In this plane operation can be performed without pain or the memory of it. When used for children pure gas is given for half a dozen breaths and this is followed by an 85 : 15 nitrous-oxide–oxygen mixture. Forty or fifty breaths are required before the dental surgeon should be allowed to make his extractions and at this time the breathing is free and regular and the eyelids are relaxed over expressionless eyes. In adults up to 20 per cent of

* Neff, W., and others, *Brit. med. J.*, 1950, **1**, 1400.
† Mostert, J. W., *Ibid.*, 1958, **1**, 502.
‡ Klock, J. H., *Curr. Res. Anesth.*, 1955, **34**, 379; Tom, A., *Brit. med. J.*, 1956, **1**, 1085; Klock, J. H., and Tom, A., *Nitrous Oxide Amnalgesia*, 1965. North Conway, New Hampshire: Reporter Press, Paul and Blanchardine; and Tom, H., *Brit. J. Anæsth.*, 1968, **40**, 177.

Modifications of the Technique, *continued.*

oxygen can be used. Cyanosis, stertor, and jactitation are o course unknown and the duration of analgesia can be considerable Reflex response to trauma may occur, but is not accompanied b the sensation of pain or the memory of it.

VOLATILE AGENTS.—These may be added to a nitrous-oxide-oxygen mixture, in which case the inspired oxygen concentratio should be at least 20 per cent, or they may be used independentl of nitrous oxide.

1. TRICHLOROETHYLENE.*—Minimal vaporization is begun at th first sign of light anæsthesia with nitrous-oxide–oxygen. Th oxygen concentration is gradually increased to at least 20 pe cent, and sufficient trichloroethylene added for the operativ need. Often used in a Rowbotham bottle attached to a intermittent-flow machine or A.E. Vaporizer.†

2. HALOTHANE.‡—Used in a similar manner to trichloroethylene but rather more potent. Used in a Goldman inhaler, a Penlor vaporizer, or in the Medrex apparatus.

4. METHOXYFLURANE.§—This agent has been used as a volatil supplement to nitrous oxide and oxygen. It should be intro-duced at the beginning of induction.

5. ETHYL CHLORIDE.—Useful in children, sprayed on a gauze mask as a single-dose anæsthetic for simple extractions. A poten agent to be used with care.

6. DIVINYL ETHER.—Used as a single-dose anæsthetic in children Ampoules of 3 ml. or 5 ml. are used in a Goldman or Oxford Inhaler.

Endotracheal anæsthesia has been advocated for the ambulant patient.‖ Tube may be inserted blindly or following suxameth-onium, but requires a high degree of skill.¶

INTRAVENOUS AGENTS.**—These may be given as an inductio agent prior to nitrous-oxide–oxygen anæsthesia, as a sole agent for simple extractions, or in intermittent doses for more pro-longed procedures.

1. THIOPENTONE.—A sleep dose can be used, continuing wit nitrous-oxide–oxygen. Larger doses may be used as a sol agent for extractions provided undue difficulty is not antici-pated, though it may be wise to lie the patient flat in cas hypotension should occur.

2. METHOHEXITONE.††—Thought to have a quicker recovery tha thiopentone and so preferred by many for the ambulant patient. Given as a 1 per cent solution, about 10 mg. pe

* Hewer, C. L., *Proc. R. Soc. Med.,* 1942, **35**, 463; and *Brit. med. J.,* 1944, **1**, 92.
† Hunter, J. D., and Fraser, A. L., *Brit. J. Anæsth.,* 1959, **31**, 367.
‡ Walsh, R. S., *Ibid.,* 1958, **30**, 578; and Goldman, V., *Curr. Res. Anesth.,* 1959, **38**, 192.
§ Unkles, R. D., and Murry Lawson, J. I., *Brit. J. Anæsth.,* 1965, **37**, 422.
‖ Danziger, A. M., *Brit. dent. J.,* 1962, **113**, 426.
¶ Bourne, J. G., *Studies in Anæsthetics,* 1967, p. 119. London: Lloyd-Luke.
** *See also Intravenous Anæsthesia,* 3rd ed., 1967, Society for the Advancement of Anæsthesia in Dentistry; Bourne, J. G., *Studies in Anæsthetics,* 1967. London: Lloyd-Luke; and Howells, T. H., *Brit. J. Anæsth.,* 1968, **40**, 182.
†† Green, R. A., and Jolly, C., *Ibid.,* 1960, **32**, 593; Coleman, J., and Green, R. A., *Anæsthesia,* 1960, **15**, 411; and Young, D. S., and Whitwam, J. G., *Brit. J. Anæsth.,* 1964, **36**, 31.

stone being an average dose. Can also be used in intermittent dosage for the 'ultra-light' anæsthesia required in conservative dentistry (0·75 mg. per kg.).

3. PROPANIDID.*—Used in a similar manner to methohexitone. The rather viscous 5 per cent solution being injected more easily if diluted to 2·5 per cent with saline or distilled water. It is thought to carry a higher incidence of nausea and vomiting if followed by nitrous oxide and oxygen, and so is often used as the sole agent, if necessary by intermittent injection. As relaxation of the jaw is often poor, it is best to insert a mouth prop prior to induction. The recovery of consciousness occurs about as rapidly as in the case of methohexitone, but the patient can leave the dental surgery earlier. The drug is rapidly destroyed and does not linger in the body as does methohexitone. More likely to cause venous thrombosis (5 mg. per kg.).

4. PETHIDINE can be given intravenously before nitrous oxide anæsthesia.

Fainting in the Dental Chair.†—Bourne has drawn attention to the possibility of fainting during the administration of nitrous oxide in the dental chair. The pulse should be frequently monitored, e.g., the carotid, superficial temporal or facial artery, in both the semi-recumbent and the sitting postures. Should the patient suddenly become pale, he must be immediately tilted into the horizontal position to prevent cerebral ischæmia. If this is neglected, delayed recovery from anæsthesia, permanent cerebral damage from hypoxia, or even death may result.‡ It is an arguable proposition that all dental operations should be performed with the patient in the horizontal position.§

Causes of Hypotension during Dental Anæsthesia may include :‖

1. Emotional factors, operative before or during early stages of anæsthesia.

2. Hypoxia. Some subjects faint when given hypoxic mixtures (10 per cent oxygen), in the absence of anæsthesia.

3. The effect of re-oxygenation following hypoxia. Collapse during oxygenation after a period of hypoxia has occurred in a variety of non-anæsthetic circumstances.

4. Pressure on the carotid sinus area when supporting the jaw.

5. Syncopal reactions associated with breathing against an increased pressure.

6. Bradycardia and hypotension due to surgical stimulation of vagal reflexes.

7. Cessation of anæsthesia. Anæsthesia may protect against syncopal reactions, which become manifest at the end of the procedure.

Conservative Dentistry.—Cavity fillings may be painful and require analgesia or even anæsthesia for their completion.

* Cadle, D. R., Boulton, T. B., and Spencer Swaine, M., *Anæsthesia*, 1968, **23**, 65.
† Bourne, J. G., *Lancet*, 1957, **2**, 499.
‡ Shanahan, J., *Ibid.*, 1966, **1**, 717; and Brierley, J. B., and Miller, A. A., *Ibid.*, 1966, **2**, 869.
§ Bourne, J. G., *Studies in Anæsthetics*, 1967, p. 131. London: Lloyd-Luke.
‖ Smith, W. D. A., *Brit. J. Anæsth.*, 1963, **35**, 28.

Conservative Dentistry, *continued.*

1. Local analgesic injection. Infiltration or inferior dental nerve-block. The most frequently employed method. Excellent results are usually obtained and it is the method of choice for most patients.

2. Inhalation of analgesic concentrations of nitrous oxide or trichloro-ethylene. Not frequently employed today.

3. 'Ultra-light' anæsthesia with methohexitone. A needle is inserted in a convenient arm vein and connected to a syringe by means of a length of disposable tubing. Anæsthesia is induced and intermittent supplementary injections given as required. Scrupulous attention must be paid to the airway and the insertion of a pack to prevent inhalation of water or tooth powder. The patient wakes within minutes of the final injection, but must rest a while before being accompanied home (0·75 mg. per kg.).

4. 'Ultra-light' anæsthesia with propanidid. A similar technique may be employed. It is better to dilute the drug to 2·5 per cent to allow easier injection through a length of tubing. The patient wakes within a few minutes of the final incremental injection, but is usually ready to leave the dental surgery or hospital earlier than when methohexitone has been given.*† The incidence of thrombosis of the vein is higher with propanidid than with methohexitone. Induction dose 5 mg. per kg.

5. The Jorgensen technique.‡ The aim is to provide good sedation while work is carried out under local analgesia. Intravenous pentobarbitone, pethidine, and hyoscine are given in incremental doses until the required degree of sedation is obtained.

6. Ataralgesia. Hayward-Butt§ has coined this neologism to describe a state of calmness and freedom from pain induced by the intramuscular injection of a mixture of pethidine, amiphenazole, and mepazine (Pacatal). One 'unit' consists of pethidine 100 mg., amiphenazole 25 mg., and mepazine 100 mg., and the average adult receives 3 units three-quarters of an hour before operation: minor surgery may then proceed. Occasionally thiopentone is necessary in addition.

7. The use of intravenous tranquillizers, e.g., diazepam, 10–20 mg. slowly over 2 min.†

ANÆSTHESIA FOR IN-PATIENTS

Dental patients are admitted to hospital and treated as in-patients when either the dental procedure exceeds the scope of the out-patient department, or when the general condition of the patient contra-indicates out-patient anæsthesia.

In-patients should receive a full general examination. Premedication can be prescribed. The anæsthetic technique usually involves endo-tracheal intubation with a throat pack to prevent aspiration of blood

---

* Cadle, D. R., Boulton, T. B., and Spencer Swaine, M., *Anæsthesia*, 1968, **23**, 65.

† Howell, T. H., *Brit. J. Anæsth.*, 1968, **40**, 182.

‡ Jorgensen, N. B., and Leffingwell, F., *Dental Clin. N. America*, 1961, July, p. 299; Jorgensen, W. B., and others, *J. Soc. Cal. Dent.*, 1963, **31**, 7; and *see also* Bourne, J. G., *Studies in Anæsthetics*, 1967, p. 116. London: Lloyd-Luke.

§ Hayward-Butt, J. T., *Lancet*, 1957, **2**, 972.

and debris. A nasotracheal tube is usually preferred, but an orotracheal tube is sometimes more acceptable to the surgeon, as when the site of operation is the upper incisor area (apicectomy, dental cysts, etc.). Complications and hazards include:—

1. Epistaxis and nasal trauma due to passage of a nasal tube. Can be minimized by prior spraying of the nasal mucosa with a vasoconstrictor (e.g., cocaine 4 per cent).

2. Sore throat. Due to the insertion of a throat pack, when bruising and abrasion of the mucus membrane of the palate and fauces can readily occur.

3. Suxamethonium. When this agent is used to facilitate intubation, post-operative muscle pains can be very distressing, since the patients are ambulant early. Can be abolished if other means are used to pass the tube; for example: (1) Use of gallamine; (2) Use of deep anæsthesia; (3) Blind intubation after use of carbon dioxide to produce hyperventilation; (4) Blind intubation during the hyperventilation produced by propanidid. All these methods have their disadvantages also, and many anæsthetists prefer suxamethonium because of the quick and smooth intubation which can be undertaken in light planes of anæsthesia.

4. Ventricular arrhythmias have been reported as a result of surgical stimuli during dental extractions.* These are, however, transient, and it would appear that their significance is not large provided the anæsthetic technique is impeccable. A pulse monitor may be useful to observe their occurrence.

The types of patient who present for in-patient operation because of their general physical condition include:—

1. Mental defectives, who are difficult to manage in the dental chair under local analgesia.

2. Cardiac patients, who require careful anæsthetic management, and may require antibiotic cover. At least 30 per cent oxygen should be administered.

3. Cases of chronic respiratory disease, particularly where there is gross derangement of ventilation–perfusion relationships.

4. Those with a hæmorrhagic disorder, e.g., hæmophilia, Christmas disease, thrombocytopenia, or where there is a history of severe post-extraction hæmorrhage. The blood should be examined for coagulation defects pre-operatively and, if necessary, appropriate treatment arranged.

The Hæmophiliac Patient.†—Operations are best performed on Thursdays or Fridays, since complications are likely to arise immediately, or on the fourth or fifth post-operative day. The day prior to operation the patient may be given epsilon aminocaproic acid (EACA), 6 g. 6-hourly. On the morning of operation an intravenous drip is started and the contents of 2 packets of freshly thawed cryoglobulin injected. Extreme gentleness is required during anæsthesia to avoid trauma. An oral tube is preferred to a nasal, and throat packs not used. Surgery should include meticulous hæmostasis. At the start of operation 1 unit of fresh

---

* Kaufman, L., *Proc. R. Soc. Med.*, 1966, **59**, 731.
† Davies, R. M., and Scott, J. G., *Brit. J. Anæsth.*, 1968, **40**, 202.

The Hæmophiliac Patient, *continued.*

frozen plasma is given and maintained for at least 1 hour post operatively. It is followed by an infusion of 12 g. EACA in normal saline. Infusions are maintained until the patient can take EACA by mouth. On the fifth post-operative day a second unit of fresh frozen plasma is administered.

FACIO-MAXILLARY OPERATIONS

Fractured Jaw.—This may be part of a grave emergency complicated by intra-oral hæmorrhage, obstructed airway, and associated injuries (including head injury and loss of consciousness). In these very severe cases the protective laryngeal reflexes may be obtunded with danger of aspiration of blood, teeth, and other debris. In other cases the jaw injury is less serious and operative treatment can be carried out subsequently as an elective operation.

The anæsthetist who is asked to deal with a fractured mandible and/or maxilla should look out for:—

1. Associated injuries, especially: (*a*) Head injuries—loss of consciousness, depressed fractures, raised intracranial tension; (*b*) Chest injuries—pneumothorax or hæmothorax; (*c*) Abdominal injuries —ruptured viscera; (*d*) Major bone fractures. The presence of associated injuries results in increased hæmorrhage and shock.

2. Presence of blood and debris in the pharynx, larynx, and trachea. There may be respiratory obstruction and the laryngeal reflexes may be obtunded. Occasionally it is necessary to bronchoscope the patient for tracheo-bronchial toilet.

3. Possibility of swallowed blood which may be regurgitated as anæsthesia is induced. It is seldom practical to ask the patient to swallow an œsophageal tube.

4. The possibility of food in the stomach if the operation is of an emergency nature.

First-aid treatment may include:—

1. In the unconscious patient, it may be wise to pass an endotracheal tube, usually via the nose. Rarely a tracheostomy may be required.

2. Temporary fixation with dental wire of large displaced fragments of bone.

3. Pharyngeal (or bronchial) toilet.

4. Treatment of shock, if present, by blood transfusion, etc.

ANÆSTHETIC TECHNIQUE.—

PREMEDICATION.—In the emergency case it is wise to restrict pre-medication to atropine or hyoscine. Respiratory depressants are to be avoided. An anti-emetic drug is sometimes used to prevent post-operative vomiting (when the jaws have been wired together).

INDUCTION.—This should only be commenced when the anæsthetist is satisfied that arrangements have been made to deal with any emergency that may arise and that he has adequate help. It is wise to place the patient on an operating table or trolley that can be instantly tipped. Suction should be available and switched on. Rarely bronchoscopy may be indicated. The anæsthetist should take the usual precautions regarding regurgitation of stomach contents.

Induction is usually carried out with thiopentone and short-acting relaxant. Visualization of the larynx may be rendered difficult if blood and debris are present—but the shattered tissues do not resist introduction of the laryngoscope and intubation can usually be performed without difficulty. It is wise to be as gentle as possible in order to avoid further mobilization of the fracture.

A nasotracheal tube is usually preferred. This may be cuffed.* A pharyngeal pack can also be inserted—but should be removed and pharyngeal toilet performed immediately before the jaws are wired together.

MAINTENANCE is usually by inhalation anæsthesia. Smooth anæsthetic technique is desirable, with rapid return of reflexes at the end of operation and absence of vomiting. Nitrous-oxide–oxygen–halothane or oxygen–halothane are suitable in most cases.

When the jaws have been wired together the patient should leave theatre with a nasopharyngeal airway in situ. A pair of wire cutters should remain near the patient, so that they can be used in an emergency to free the jaws and the mouth and pharynx can be sucked out. The nursing attendants should know how to use the instrument and which wires to cut. To cut the wires is not popular with the surgeon because the wires will then need to be replaced. In fact it is very seldom necessary, though on occasion it may be life-saving, in the presence of severe respiratory obstruction.

Post-operative sedatives and analgesics must be used sparingly, and only if the patient complains of pain.

(*See also* Davies, R. M., and Scott, J. G., *Brit. J. Anæsth.*, 1968, **40**, 202.)

CHAPTER XXV

ANÆSTHESIA AND ANALGESIA IN LABOUR

Pregnancy.†—The process of pregnancy and labour produces remarkable physiological and psychological changes in the mother.

1. CIRCULATORY SYSTEM.—The enlarged uterus pushes the diaphragm upwards. This results in a change in position of the heart which is lifted upwards, shifted to the left and anteriorly, and rotated towards a transverse position. The electrocardiogram may show a large Q-wave and inverted T-waves in Lead III. Heart-rate increases during pregnancy, reaching a peak between 28 and 36 weeks to about 10–12 beats above normal. There is a

---

* Davies, J. A. H., *Anæsthesia*, 1967, **22**, 153.
† *See also* Bonica, J. J., *Principles and Practice of Obstetric Analgesia and Anesthesia*, 1967, Vol. I, 'Fundamental Considerations'. Oxford: Blackwell.

Pregnancy, *continued.*

significant increase in cardiac output which reaches a peak 30–50 per cent above normal at about 28 weeks. Whereas the healthy heart compensates well for these changes, the diseased heart may be severely taxed. Peripheral resistance is reduced in pregnancy, and mean blood-pressure reaches lowest points at the time of maximal cardiac output. Venous pressure is normal, except where the gravid uterus may compress the inferior vena cava. Blood-volume is increased,* and uterine blood-flow is markedly increased.

2. RESPIRATORY SYSTEM.†—Upward displacement of the diaphragm results in decrease of vertical diameter of the thorax and increase in transverse diameter. X-rays show increased lung markings probably due to an increase of blood-volume in the pulmonary vessels. Minute ventilation rises to levels of 50 per cent above normal. Increased respiratory movements are due to an increase in thoracic breathing, the diaphragmatic component being neutralized. Oxygen consumption rises during the last trimester due to the metabolic needs of the uterus, placenta, and fœtus. Basal metabolic rate is increased by about 15 per cent.

3. FLUIDS AND ELECTROLYTES.‡—Water and salt retention occur. Probably related to the secretion of steroids by the placenta.

4. ENDOCRINE GLANDS.—There is hyperplasia of the anterior pituitary, thyroid, and adrenal cortex.

5. PSYCHOLOGY.—The emotional impact of pregnancy and parturition may have a considerable effect.

Supine Hypotensive Syndrome of Late Pregnancy.§—This is a condition of circulatory depression due to diminished venous return. It is caused by the gravid uterus pressing on the inferior vena cava. It is said to effect 3 per cent of pregnant women; most patients compensate by blood flowing through the azygos system via the paravertebral veins. It is relieved by a pillow under one side or the adoption of the lateral position.

Nerve-supply.—

1. SENSORY.—According to Cleland,‖ sensory fibres passed as follows: (a) Upper uterine segment via sympathetic nerves to T.11 and T.12; (b) Lower uterine segment via sacral parasympathetic, S.2, 3, 4; (c) Birth canal via the pudendal nerve. This has since been modified due to the increasing knowledge derived from various nerve-blocks. For example, uterine contractions are painless after extradural block between the segments T.10 to L.1,¶ and presacral sympathectomy results in

---

* Pritchard, J. A., *Anesthesiology*, 1965, **26**, 393.
† Prowse, C. M., and Gaensler, E. A., *Ibid.*, 1965, **26**, 381.
‡ Little, B., *Ibid.*, 1965, **26**, 400.
§ Kerr, M. G., Scott, D. B., and Samuel, E., *Brit. med. J.*, 1964, **1**, 532; and Holmes, F., *J. Obstet. Gynæc., Brit. Emp.*, 1958, **64**, 229.
‖ Cleland, J. G. P., *Surg. Gynec. Obstet.*, 1933, **57**, 51.
¶ Cleland, J. G. P., *Curr. Res. Anesth.*, 1952, **31**, 289; and Bromage, P. R., *Canad. Med. Ass. J.*, 1961, **85**, 1136.

relief from dysmenorrhœa (pain of cervical origin) as well as in pain relief during labour. It would therefore appear that sensory stimuli from the lower uterine segment also pass in sympathetic fibres, possibly from a sacral portion of the sympathetic chain.*

2. MOTOR.—The uterus receives both sympathetic and parasympathetic fibres, but the functions served by each are by no means clear-cut. (a) Sympathetic. Central connexions lie above level of T.6, so impulses are not cut off by spinal or extradural block unless they extend above this level. Fibres pass to the superior, middle, and inferior hypogastric plexuses and thence through the uterosacral ligaments and broad ligaments to the uterus. (b) Parasympathetic (S.2, 3, 4). Fibres join the sympathetic fibres in the pelvis or uterosacral ligaments. The accumulation of cells and fibres at the base of the broad ligament is called the great cervical plexus, or ganglion, of Frankenhauser.

Hormone Control.—An intact nerve-supply is not essential to the orderly initiation and progress of labour. Total spinal block does not inhibit uterine activity unless there is a marked fall of blood-pressure. Normal vaginal delivery can occur in the paraplegic patient.

The part played by hormones is complex and not well understood. We may consider: (1) Progesterone:† The pregnancy-stabilizing hormone. Labour commences when it is withdrawn. 2. Œstrogens: Promote the growth of the pregnant uterus. Production by the placenta increases in amount and effectiveness towards the end of pregnancy. (3) Oxytocin: From the posterior pituitary. Acts to increase the frequency and amplitude of spontaneous contractions. The synthetic analogue, syntocinon, is used therapeutically.

Uterine Contractions.—

1. Slight uteric contractions occur throughout pregnancy, but during the final 2 or 3 weeks before term they become rhythmical and co-ordinated. They increase progressively in frequency, intensity, and duration. (Painless contractions of Braxton Hicks.)
2. The first stage of labour. Not marked by a clear-cut change, though the contractions are more regular, more intense, and effect cervical dilatation.
3. The second stage. Frequent intense contractions are aided by reflex contraction of the abdominal muscles and diaphragm to force the descent and expulsion of the fœtus.
4. The third stage. Contractions continue, but with decreasing frequency. After expulsion of the fœtus they rapidly decrease in both frequency and intensity.

ANALGESIA IN NORMAL DELIVERY

The unprepared and untreated patient will feel pain during uterine contractions which occur in normal uncomplicated labour. The belief that primitive woman has no fear, no tension, and a painless labour is not founded in fact. The intensity of the pain is related to: (1) The

---

* Routledge, J. H., and Elliott, H., Amer. J. Obstet. Gynec., 1962, **83**, 701.
† See also Csapo, A., Clin. Obstet., Gynec., 1959, **2**, 275; and Ann. N.Y. Acad. Sci., 1959, **75**, 790.

Analgesia in Normal Delivery, *continued.*

intensity and duration of uterine contractions; (2) The degree of dilatation of the cervix, and how rapidly this is achieved with each contraction; (3) The distension of perineal tissue; (4) Other factors including age, parity, the size of the fœtus in relation to the birth canal, etc.

The ideal procedure should :—

1. Produce efficient relief from pain, with consciousness between pains and good co-operation from the patient.
2. Not depress the respirations of the fœtus.
3. Not depress the uterus, causing prolonged labour.
4. Be non-toxic.
5. Be safe for mother and child.

No agent at present in use fulfils all these conditions.

Analgesia is not necessary in every case of labour and sympathetic explanation may be all that is required.

The following have been found to be helpful : (1) Encouragement of muscular relaxation. (2) Congenial company in early stage, to maintain morale. (3) Rubbing of lumbar and sacral regions during early pains. (4) When pains become regular and distressing and os dilated to admit three fingers, pethidine 100–150 mg. injected intramuscularly. (5) If sleep is indicated, chloral hydrate 2 g. can be given with the pethidine. (6) Late first stage is very painful and intermittent gas–air may be necessary at this time. (7) With onset of second stage, patient is encouraged to push and this makes the pains easier to bear. (8) When the head distends the perineum, gas–air or trichloroethylene may be required, and towards the end may need to be given (not self-administered) almost continuously.

I. Non-pharmacological Methods

Since drugs administered may cross the placenta to depress the fœtus, any method which avoids or restricts their use deserves attention.

1. 'Natural Childbirth'—advocated by Dick-Read.* A naturalistic approach with emphasis on the positive attainment of relaxation of muscles. Patients are taught the art of relaxation and given exercises in a course of lectures and demonstrations.
2. Similar work in France involves a psychosomatic approach.†
3. Hypnosis.‡ This makes considerable demands on time for both patients and staff. Only about 25 per cent of patients can be successfully treated in this way. The method has, therefore, not proved popular for general use.
4. Decompression suit. Decompression of the abdomen and lower part of the thorax to 1–2 lb. per sq. in. below atmospheric pressure allows the uterus to become more spherical and to act at a greater mechanical advantage. It facilitates labour, shortens the first stage, and gives considerable pain relief.§

---

* Dick-Read, G., *Childbirth without Fear*, 4th ed., 1960. London: Heinemann.
† Vallay, P., *Childbirth without Pain*, 1st ed., 1960. London: Hutchinson and Allen & Unwin.
‡ Wahl, C. W., *Amer. J. Obstet. Gynec.*, 1962, **84**, 1869; and Moya, F., and James, L. S., *J. Amer. med. Ass.*, 1960, **174**, 2026.
§ Heyns, O. S., *J. Obstet. Gynæc., Brit. Emp.*, 1959, **66**, 220; Quinn, L. J., and others, *Amer. J. Obstet. Gynec.*, 1962, **83**, 458; and Quinn, L. J., and others, *J. Obstet. Gynæc., Brit. Cwlth*, 1964, **71**, 934.

II. Sedatives and Analgesics

1. Simple Sedatives.—*Chloral hydrate*, a soporific and mild analgesic, is only a cardiac depressant when given in large doses. It is excreted by the kidneys, with glycuronic acid. The syrup contains 20 g. in 100 ml. A safe dose is 2 g. Can be given as dichloral phenazonum (welldorm) or as trichlorethyl phosphate (triclofos) and if necessary with *tincture of opium* (1 ml.). These drugs can be given early in labour, well diluted to prevent vomiting, and can be repeated. They are useful in the early stages of labour, often allowing the patient to sleep between pains. Glutethimide (doriden) in 500-mg. doses is also a useful sedative in labour.*

2. Pethidine Hydrochoride, B.P. (*see also* p. 88).—Known also as dolantin, dolantal, isonipercain, meperidine hydrochloride U.S.P., and demerol, it is the hydrochloride of the ethyl ester of 1-methyl-4-phenyl-piperidine-4-carboxylic acid, and was synthesized in 1939 by Schaumann and Eisleb.

If certain rules propounded by the Central Midwives Board are observed, it can be used by midwives acting alone. Probably the most useful single drug employed in labour. First used in labour by Benthin in 1940. It does not result in lack of co-operation.

PHARMACOLOGY.—It relieves pain, having an action midway between morphine and codeine. A dose of 100 mg. of pethidine is roughly equivalent to 10 mg. of morphine. It does not produce amnesia, but causes sleepiness and drowsiness for about 2 hours. Side-effects are dizziness, faintness. Is somewhat uncertain in its action.

It reduces smooth-muscle spasm by :—
  a. A direct papaverine-like effect on the muscle-fibres.
  b. An atropine-like depressant effect on the parasympathetic nerve-endings.
Thus in labour it raises the pain threshold and reduces cervical spasm.

The blood-pressure may be depressed if given intravenously ; there is an increase in the incidence of vomiting, and the patient may experience vertigo and tingling of the extremities. It can produce addiction.

As it depresses fœtal respiration it should not be given within 3 hours of delivery : this depression is less marked than that due to morphine, but some infants require resuscitation. Analgesia is good in about 60 per cent of cases. There is no increase in the instrumental delivery rate. The patient usually sleeps during labour, which is shortened because of more rapid cervical dilatation. It is very useful in cases with a rigid, slowly dilating os. Sensitivity to the drug, with symptoms of circulatory and respiratory depression, has been described.

DOSAGE.—Initial dose 100 mg. when labour is well established. Should not be given too soon, as then it may abolish pains.

---

* Abbas, T. M., *Brit. med. J.*, 1957, **1**, 563.

Pethidine Hydrochloride, *continued.*

Usually given by intramuscular injection, when effect comes on in 15 minutes and is maximal 1–1½ hours after injection, in both mother and fœtus (respiratory depression). If given by mouth it may cause vomiting. Additional similar doses are given when required, e.g., every 2–3 hours. Maximum dosage allowed for a midwife working alone is 200 mg. in any one labour. (C.M.B. rule.)

It has been combined with pentobarbitone, and also with hyoscine to increase the amnesic effect. A well-recommended technique is to inject intramuscularly pethidine, 100 mg., and hyoscine, 0·4 mg., when contractions are occurring regularly and when the os shows definite dilatation. Repeat doses are given if required, but no pethidine should be injected within three hours of the expected delivery. The drug is of greatest use for first-stage labour pains. The same drugs and doses, well diluted in saline, can be injected very slowly intravenously on one or two occasions.

3. Morphine (*see also* p. 83).—Morphine was not much used in labour until Steinbuchel combined it with hyoscine in 1902: this was because of its depressant effect on fœtal breathing. An injection of morphine, 10 mg., or heroin, 5 mg., is often very useful in labour and is more efficient if given before severe pain comes on. The maximal effect on pain relief is shown ninety minutes after intramuscular injection. The drug must be given with care in shocked, exhausted, or exsanguinated patients. The maximal depression of fœtal respiration occurs about two hours after injection, so it should not be given within 2½–3 hours of the expected time of delivery. Oxymorphone (numorphan) 1·5 mg. has a similar effect to pethidine 100 mg. in labour.[*] *Heroin* effectively controls the pain of the first stage of labour.[†]

EFFECT ON MOTHER.—(1) Elevates pain threshold ; (2) Alters attitude of patient to her pain, producing relative indifference ; (3) Acts as a hypnotic.

EFFECT ON FŒTUS.—(1) Before labour—none which is harmful ; (2) During labour, it severely depresses the fœtal respiratory mechanism, soon crossing the so-called barrier of the placenta— worse in the premature than in the normal fœtus.

EFFECT ON PROGRESS OF LABOUR.—In small doses, morphine increases the intervals between pains ; in larger doses it may depress contractions.

Amiphenazole.—A respiratory stimulant can be given to the mother (30 mg. intramuscularly) shortly before the delivery of the child, or directly into the umbilical vein (3 mg.), in cases where morphine or pethidine has been injected into the mother at a rather late phase of labour. It reverses the respiratory depressant effects, but not the analgesic effects of the sedatives, morphine, levorphanol tartrate (dromoran), pethidine, etc.

Nalorphine.—Has a similar use. Dose : 10 mg. intravenously to the mother (*see* Chapter IV).

---

[*] Eames, G. M., and Pool, K. R. S., *Brit. med. J.*, 1964, **2**, 353.
[†] Beazley, J. M., and others, *Lancet*, 1967, **1**, 1038.

Levallorphan.—Dose: 0·5–2 mg. or 1 part to 80 of pethidine (*see* p. 95).

Tetrahydro-aminacrine (T.H.A.).—Dose : 15–20 mg. (*see* Chapter XVII).

4. **Hyoscine** (*see also* p. 102).—Introduced into obstetric practice in 1902. (1) Does not increase pain threshold. (2) Alters patient's reaction to pain by producing amnesia, excitement, and sometimes delirium resembling acute mania. Does not depress respiration of fœtus nor affect the course of the labour. Because it is an amnesic, it is sometimes combined with pethidine, barbiturates, etc. Has been known to cause œdema of uvula. It should not be given late in labour as then it may cause restlessness and lack of co-operation. It passes the placental barrier. One dose of morphine and hyoscine, or pethidine and hyoscine is often useful at the beginning of labour.

TWILIGHT SLEEP.—Morphine and hyoscine were used in 1902 by Gauss[*] and von Steinbuchel[†] of Freiburg. To-day it is not very popular because of:—

a. Its uncertain effects.

b. Its tendency to cause prolonged labour.

c. Its tendency to cause excitement and restlessness of the mother.

d. Its tendency to produce fœtal apnœa.

e. The requirement of skilled observers throughout the labour.

On the other hand, it is easy to give, has a rapid effect, is safe for the mother, and is not costly.

TECHNIQUE.—When labour has definitely started and is causing distress, the first injection is given of morphine, 10 to 16 mg. ($\frac{1}{6}$–$\frac{1}{4}$ gr.), with hyoscine, 0·4 to 0·6 mg. ($\frac{1}{150}$–$\frac{1}{100}$ gr.). Papaveretum can be substituted for the morphine. The patient, under careful observation throughout labour, is left to sleep in a darkened room, and in 1–1½ hours hyoscine, 0·15 mg., is injected, and repeated when amnesia is receding, as shown by the ability of the patient to recognize simple objects such as a safety-pin or powder-puff which have recently been shown to her. Injections average about once every 1–1½ hours. The dosage must be individualized to suit each patient. Moderate restraint may be required with the pains, but between them the patient should sleep. The method produces efficient amnesia in a reasonable percentage of cases.

Twilight sleep should not be commenced too early in labour, nor in cases of primary uterine inertia, because of the excessive doses which will be required. Thirst must be attended to, the bladder catheterized when necessary. During the second stage, other agents should be used to control pain, such as trichloroethylene or nitrous oxide.

5. **Barbiturates** (*see also* p. 96).—Pentobarbitone (nembutal) is most commonly employed, but butobarbitone sodium, quinalbarbitone, and sodium amytal have also been used. Barbiturates are less depressing to the fœtal respiration than morphine, but more so than rectal paraldehyde or ether-oil. The effects are uncertain,

---

[*] Gauss, C. J., *Zentral. f. Gynäk.*, Leipzig, 1905, 274.
[†] von Steinbuchel, N., *Ibid.*, 1902, 48.

Barbiturates, *continued.*

and restlessness, drowsiness, or delirium may result. The addition of alkali hastens the absorption of pentobarbitone. Reasonable doses of pentobarbitone sodium have no serious effect on the uterine contractions.

The initial dose of pentobarbitone or quinalbarbitone is 200 mg. (3 gr.) given when labour is well established with the cervix dilated to two fingers. Additional doses of 100 mg. (1·5 gr.) are given every 3–4 hours. It is unwise to exceed 600 mg. (9 gr.) in 12 hours. Chloral hydrate can be combined with pentobarbitone, 1·3 g. of the former being given ½ hour after initial dose of pentobarbitone. Small additional doses are given when required, with a safe maximum of chloral, 8 g., and pentobarbitone 500 mg., in 12 hours. Hyoscine, 0·4 mg., with 0·2 mg. later if required, has been added to pentobarbitone to increase its amnesic effect.

6. **Bromethol, B.P.** (Avertin) (*see also* p. 106).—The usual dose is 75 mg. per kilo, after deducting 6 kilos for the weight of the uterus and its contents. The effect lasts 1½–2 hours and may result in prolonged labour and fœtal apnœa. After bromethol, the patient takes light general anæsthesia, e.g., gas and oxygen, very well. This method is not recommended as an anæsthetic in labour but has its place in the treatment of eclampsia.

7. **The Phenothiazine Derivatives.—**

a. CHLORPROMAZINE HYDROCHLORIDE, B.P. (Largactil).—Opinions differ as to the utility of this drug in labour. It undoubtedly relieves nausea and vomiting, both before and during labour, and would appear to be relatively harmless to the child. It may, however, cause delay in labour and lower the maternal blood-pressure. The slow intravenous injection of pethidine 150 mg. with chlorpromazine 50 mg., 10 to 15 minutes before forceps delivery, has given good results in regard to both mother and infant.* It can be usefully combined with local infiltration of the perineum and internal pudendal nerve-block.

b. PROMETHAZINE HYDROCHLORIDE, B.P. (Phenergan).—Used with pethidine—25 mg. of promethazine and 50 mg. of pethidine, intramuscularly, repeated as required, the drugs form a useful sedative in labour and cause no harmful side-effects to mother or child if used in reasonable amounts. The mother becomes sleepy and contented, but can be roused and then becomes co-operative. Has been used to produce sedation before Cæsarean section. An antagonist to pethidine may be added.

c. PROMAZINE HYDROCHLORIDE (Sparine).—Has tranquillizing, analgesia-potentiating, and anti-emetic properties, making it a useful drug in labour.† May cause cholestatic jaundice.

III. Inhalation Methods

1. **Chloroform** (*see also* p. 180).—Chloroform is relatively safe in labour only because it is welcomed and not feared; hence ventricular fibrillation is seen less often than in other patients.

---

* Crawford, J. Selwyn, *Brit. med. Bull.*, 1958, **14**, 1, 34.
† Mathews, A. E. B., *Brit. med. J.*, 1963, **2**, 423.

John Snow employed Sir James Young Simpson's technique of light
chloroform analgesia during each pain when he administered
it to Queen Victoria in 1853 at the birth of Prince Leopold—
" anesthésie à la reine ".

Snow described his technique in his book *On Chloroform and Other
Anæsthetics* (1858) as follows : " It is desirable to give the
chloroform very gently at first, increasing the quantity a little
with each pain if the patient is not relieved. The practitioner
easily finds, with a little attention, the quantity of vapour it is
desirable to give at any stage of the labour and in each particular
case ; his object being to relieve the patient without diminishing
the strength of the uterine contractions and the auxiliary action
of the respiratory muscles, or with diminishing it as little as
possible. At first it is generally necessary to repeat the chloroform at the beginning of each pain ; but after a little time, it
commonly happens that sufficient effect has been produced to
get the patient over one or two uterine contractions without
suffering, before it is resumed. Complete anæsthesia is never
induced in midwifery, unless in some cases of operative delivery."
No better advice than this could be followed with chloroform or
with any other method of intermittent analgesia, e.g., trichloroethylene, gas and air, etc.

Chloroform can be given on a mask ; from ' brisettes '—small glass
capsules containing 20 min. of chloroform, which are broken on
to a mask and give relief for two or three pains ; from Simpson's
inhaler ; from Christie Brown's inhaler ; or from Junker's bottle*
or Mennell's modification of Junker's bottle. With the last
apparatus the patient compresses a bulb which blows air through
chloroform : she uses it when she needs it and cannot produce
true third-stage anæsthesia, as the vapour is too weak and
intermittent. Mennell's bottle cannot be connected up wrongly,
cannot spill, and cannot be overfilled. Chloroform can also
be given from an anæsthetic machine, using a Rowbotham or
Goldman bottle for its vaporization. Analgesia is brought about
by the inhalation of 0·1–0·3 per cent chloroform vapour in air.

Chloroform analgesia will retard labour, even given by Snow's technique ; it may predispose to post-partum hæmorrhage ; and
may cause toxic hepatitis. Chloroform will relax a labouring
uterus better than any other drug (except halothane).

Protection of the liver from the effects of chloroform include : (1) A
diet rich in carbohydrate, poor in fat ; (2) Addition of oxygen
to the inhaled gases. The drug is positively contra-indicated in
patients with depleted liver glycogen, e.g., in toxæmia or
starvation (persistent vomiting).

The sudden inhalation of a strong concentration may be dangerous
and may cause severe cardiac depression. Instant artificial
respiration with oxygen or air and perhaps external or internal
cardiac massage are then indicated.

2. Trichloroethylene (*see also* p. 188).—This is a useful drug in labour.
It gives better results in nervous, highly strung women than nitrous
oxide, and in patients whose labours are likely to be over within

---

* Junker, F. E., *Med. Times, London*, 1868, **1**, 171.

Trichloroethylene, *continued.*

six hours. If trichloroethylene is given intermittently for longer than six hours, the patient may show signs of drowsiness and lack of co-operation and anæsthesia if more is given. Such a state of affairs can be controlled by reducing the vapour strength of trichloroethylene to 0·35 per cent and by giving a dose of *pethidine*, 50 mg. Vapour of 0·5 per cent concentration and less does not

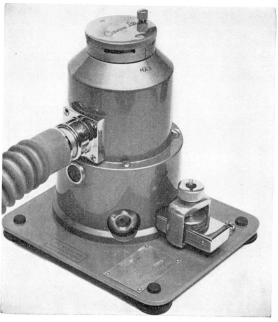

Fig. 49.—The Tecota Mark 6 trichloroethylene inhaler. (Cyprane Ltd.)

materially influence uterine contractions. Like other anæsthetic agents, it rapidly enters the fœtal circulation, but has not been proved definitely to harm the fœtus. In some animals, its concentration in fœtal blood soon exceeds that in maternal blood. It is possible that drugs used to augment action of trichloroethylene, such as pethidine or morphine, may be at least partly responsible for fœtal respiratory depression. Trichloroethylene–air, as compared with nitrous-oxide–air, causes a slight rise in systolic blood-pressure during second-stage pains. It has been given from: (1) The most accurate and elaborate apparatus designed for self-administration of trichloroethylene vapour, the Emotril Automatic

Inhaler* (*E*pstein, *M*acintosh, *O*xford, *Tri*lene) which delivers 0·5 per cent trichloroethylene in air and is compensated for changes in environmental temperature: it will also give a weaker vapour (0·35 per cent) should the patient become too drowsy with the higher concentration. (2) The Tecota Inhaler (*Fig.* 49) (*te*mperature *co*mpensated *t*richloroethylene *air*). (3) The Airlene Inhaler. (4) The Burns-Benson Inhaler.† (5) The Cyprane Inhaler which delivers a variable percentage vapour in air of 0·22 per cent to 0·54 per cent. (6) Freedman's Inhaler‡ (1943). This apparatus, which cannot be overfilled, is clamped to the bed and can be used by the patient unassisted. It consists of face-mask, corrugated tubing, and bottle, and, as a safety device, a hole is provided over which the patient places her finger. If this slips, due to too deep a level of analgesia, air is inhaled instead of trichloroethylene vapour. It delivers about 0·65 per cent trichloroethylene in air (by weight), but this vapour strength varies with environmental temperature, agitation of the bottle, etc., so that the authorities are not willing to place the apparatus in the hands of midwives working alone. (7) It has also been used in an Oxford vaporizer when 7·5 per cent on the ether scale gives a concentration of trichloroethylene in air of approximately 1·5 per cent with the normal hot water present. (8) Marrett's draw-over apparatus.§ (9) A Rowbotham's chloroform bottle attached to a gas–air or gas–oxygen machine.

The Central Midwives Board has approved the following apparatus for the administration of trichloroethylene by midwives: the Tecota Mark 6 (Cyprane Ltd.) and the Emotril Automatic Inhaler (Medical & Industrial Equipment Ltd.). They stipulate that such apparatus must be inspected periodically by the manufacturers to ensure accuracy and that midwives using them must be properly trained in their use.

3. Nitrous Oxide.—Nitrous oxide does not interfere with uterine contractions, nor has it any effect on the fœtus. The Russian, Klikowitsch,‖ introduced nitrous oxide into obstetrics in 1880. Guedel devised the first machine for self-administration of nitrous oxide in obstetrics in 1912.¶

ANALGESIA DURING FIRST STAGE OF LABOUR.—In the early first stage, if patient complains of pain, it is better to give a sedative such as tinct. opii, 1 ml., or chloral hydrate, 1·2 g. It is, nevertheless, better to start self-administration of gas too early rather than too late. Before gas is given, see that the machine is working well, that cylinders contain gas, and that dentures are removed. Inhalation must begin some seconds before the onset of the pain. If the patient holds her own mask, it will fall from her hand should unconsciousness supervene : this is a safety factor. Nitrous oxide 80 per cent and oxygen

* Epstein, H. G., and Macintosh, R. R., *Brit. med. J.*, 1949, **2**, 1092.
† Burns, T. H. S., *Ibid.*, 1954, **1**, 329.
‡ Freedman, A., *Lancet*, 1943, **2**, 696.
§ Marrett, H. R., *Brit. med. J.*, 1948, **1**, 643.
‖ Klikowitsch, H., *Arch. Gynaek.*, 1881, **18**, 81.
¶ Guedel, A. E., *N.Y. med. J.*, 1912, **95**, 387.

Nitrous Oxide, *continued.*

20 per cent is a suitable basis which may need altering to suit individual patients. Less than 20 per cent of oxygen will, if used for any length of time, cause fœtal hypoxia. Pethidine is a useful drug to combine with gas and oxygen, if delivery is not expected within 3–4 hours.

ANALGESIA DURING SECOND STAGE OF LABOUR.—Four or five breaths are taken, commencing just before the onset of the pain. After the last inspiration, the breath is held and patient bears down. If the pain is a long one, she may get out of breath before its cessation : in these cases three or four quick inspirations are taken, followed by bearing down during the remainder of the contraction. Late second stage pains are fairly regular, and it is often possible to commence inhalation a minute before the pain is expected and to continue until the pain is maximal, followed by bearing down. In this way, the blood is saturated with nitrous oxide during the most agonizing phase of the contraction. It must be remembered that when the baby is newly born, the oxygen content of the blood from its cord can be greater than that of the maternal venous blood. When the mother receives nitrous oxide and oxygen, the baby usually breathes spontaneously on delivery.

Self-administration is reasonable in early phase of labour, but when the second stage nears its end the anæsthetist should take over.

A little volatile supplement may be necessary for the crowning of the head, trichloroethylene being very suitable.

In self-administration, the patient must be sure to make a leak-proof junction between mask and face.

ANALGESIA DURING THIRD STAGE OF LABOUR.—Manual expulsion of the placenta can be made tolerable with analgesia, but perineal and vaginal repair requires analgesia or anæsthesia.

NITROUS-OXIDE–AIR.—The Minnitt Gas–Air machine* was introduced in 1933 and designed to deliver approximately 50 per cent nitrous oxide in air. The machine and its modifications are used for analgesia, the patient holding her own mask and using it as described above. The machines are intermittent-flow type and are arranged so that they deliver nitrous oxide 50 per cent in air approximately. In some varieties the percentages can be varied: in some others, a small air port is kept closed by the patient's finger so that if she becomes unconscious the finger slips, and air is breathed instead of the mixture. Care must be taken to instruct the patient in the technique before the onset of labour.

Bad results are usually due to lack of co-operation in hysterical patients ; leaks between face and mask ; a worn washer between the cylinder and the apparatus, leaking corrugated tubing, a sticking expiratory valve, and lack of care and interest on the part of the attendant ; starting the administration with each pain, too late.

---

* Minnitt, R. J., *Proc. R. Soc. Med.,* 1934, **27**, 1313.

THE ORIGINAL MINNITT APPARATUS (*Fig.* 50).—This was a modification of the McKesson oxygen therapy apparatus and was introduced in 1933. A reducing valve steps down the gas pressure to 60 lb. to the square inch, and gas is led from it

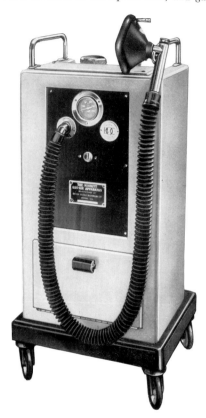

Fig. 50.—The Minnitt apparatus for gas–air analgesia in obstetrics.
(British Oxygen Gases Ltd.)

into a rubber bag enclosed in the familiar McKesson drum. After leaving the bag, gas is mixed with about 50 per cent of air. An expiratory valve is provided and the machine is of the usual intermittent-flow type, the patient's inspiration controlling the flow of gas. The weight, without cylinder, is 15 lb., while the weight of a 100-gallon cylinder is 8–9 lb. empty, $10\frac{1}{2}$ lb. full.

Nitrous Oxide, *continued.*

THE MINNITT-WALTON APPARATUS.—An Adams valve reduces gas
pressure to 4–5 lb. to the square inch. The rubber bag is
enclosed in a metal box. The working principles are the same
as in the original Minnitt machine.

THE LUCY BALDWIN APPARATUS (named after the first Countess
Baldwin of Bewdley who was interested in women's welfare

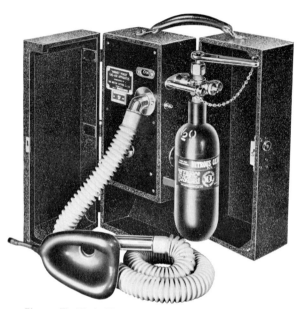

Fig. 51.—The Minnitt Minor apparatus.   (British Oxygen Gases Ltd.)

in the 1930's) is designed for the administration of nitrous
oxide and oxygen mixtures for analgesia in obstetrics. The
mixture delivered may be varied between 70 per cent nitrous
oxide/30 per cent oxygen, and 100 per cent oxygen, and does
not vary with different respiratory patterns. The gas mixture
flows only in response to the patient's inspirations and safety
cut-off valves eliminate any possibility of inhalation of pure
nitrous oxide in the event of undetected failure of the supply
of oxygen.

Considerable doubt has recently been cast on the accuracy of gas–
air machines to be found in hospitals.* On careful testing,

---

* Cole, P. V., and Nainby-Luxmore, R. L., *Anæsthesia*, 1962, **17**, 505.

many were shown to deliver more than 50 per cent of nitrous oxide and these could expose the fœtus to unnecessary danger, as the mother is inhaling less than 10 per cent of oxygen.

Fœtal distress should contra-indicate the continuance of gas–air analgesia. It is shown by:—

1. A fœtal heart-rate becoming progressively slower or faster between pains.
4. When fœtal heart does not increase after contractions, as previously it did.
3. When fœtal heart is irregular between pains.

PREMIXED NITROUS-OXIDE–OXYGEN.*—*See also* Chapter VI. Cylinders are now available containing a 50 per cent nitrous-oxide–oxygen mixture in a single gas phase at a pressure of 2000 lb. per sq. in. The use of premixed gases with the Entonox apparatus has now been approved by the Central Midwives Board for unsupervised use by midwives. At temperatures below −8° C., nitrous oxide separates as a liquid. When used, there is a danger that the initial gas will be oxygen-rich and the later issuing gas will be oxygen-deficient. This can be prevented by inverting the cylinder briskly three times prior to use to ensure reversion to a single-gas phase.

4. Methoxyflurane.—Although the uptake of this agent is slow, it possesses good analgesic properties, and it has been found to be more effective than trichloroethylene in a recent study.† It is suggested that a single fixed inhaled concentration of 0·35 per cent in air is satisfactory.‡

5. Other Agents.—Cyclopropane has been used in a concentration of 3–5 per cent. Halothane is not an analgesic in sub-anæsthetic concentrations.

IV. Regional Anæsthesia

1. Subarachnoid Block.—(*See also* Chapter XVI.) Can be used for mid or low forceps extraction or for normal delivery. For normal delivery or for outlet forceps with episiotomy, block should extend to S.1 (saddle block).§

This can be obtained if the patient is placed in the lateral position on a level delivery bed or table. In such a position, because the width of the hips is greater than that of the shoulders in most women, there is a slight head-down tilt of the vertebral canal. Other workers of experience‖ prefer to have a slight head-up tilt. Hyperbaric cinchocaine (1–200 with 6 per cent glucose), 0·8 ml., is injected between L.4 and L.5 and the patient immediately turned to the supine position with hips and knees flexed and the shoulders raised. The onset of analgesia takes about five minutes.

* Tunstall, M. E., *Lancet*, 1961, **2**, 964; *Brit. med. J.*, 1963, **2**, 915; and Gale, C. W., Tunstall, M. E., and Wilton-Davies, C. C., *Ibid.*, 1964, **1**, 732.
  † Major, V., Rosen, M., and Mushin, W. W., *Ibid.*, 1966, **2**, 1554.
  ‡ Major, V., Rosen, M., and Mushin, W. W., *Ibid.*, 1967, **4**, 767.
  § Parmley, R. T., and Adriani, J., *Amer. J. Obstet. Gynec.*, 1946, **52**, 636.
  ‖ Sears, R. T., *Brit. med. J.*, 1959, **1**, 755.

Subarachnoid Block, *continued.*

For high forceps or intra-uterine manipulation, block should reach T.11. This will require the injection of 1–1·2 ml. of hyperbaric cinchocaine and will abolish the traction pain associated with a high forceps delivery which will result if the sacral nerves alone are blocked. Spinal analgesia does not influence the course of established labour provided the level of block is not above T.10.*

Other techniques for performing sacral (saddle) block are :—

1. Injection into the sitting patient's subarachnoid space (L.3–4 or L.4–5) of :—

   a. Cinchocaine-hyperbaric 0·5 ml. with 0·5 ml. of cerebrospinal fluid.

   b. 30–50 mg. of procaine in 2 ml. of 5 per cent dextrose.

   c. 4 mg. of amethocaine in 2 ml. of 5 per cent dextrose.

   The patient remains sitting for thirty seconds and then lies flat on her back with a pillow under her shoulders.

2. In the U.S.A. a favourite technique for performing saddle block is to inject into the sitting patient, between L.4 and L.5, 0·2 ml. of 1 per cent pontocaine (amethocaine) solution, i.e., 2 mg., and 1 ml. of 10 per cent glucose. The addition of 0·25 to 0·5 ml. of 1–1000 adrenaline to these solutions will prolong the duration of block and slightly increase its extent, because of the extra volume of injected liquid. Perineal analgesia removes the bearing-down reflex but saddle block does not greatly delay normal labour if, when the cervix is fully dilated, the patient is encouraged to bear down during the pains and if fundal pressure is applied.

If used in congestive heart failure, to help spare the mother the exertion of pushing out the baby, subarachnoid injection should be made immediately the cervix is fully dilated.

In both subarachnoid and extradural block, a given dose of local analgesic solution will ascend higher in pregnant than in non-pregnant patients, so doses should be kept small.

Advantages of subarachnoid block : (1) No fœtal respiratory depression ; (2) Excellent relaxation of pelvic floor muscles ; (3) Absence of aspiration of stomach contents and risk of asphyxia, Mendelson's syndrome, pneumonia, etc. (4) Delivery of patient while she is conscious.

With all forms of regional block, blood-pressure fall must be avoided because of the risk of fœtal hypoxia, and to prevent this some workers give a pressor drug as a routine before the injection. Pressure should not be allowed to fall below 90 mm. Hg. Intravenous injection of ergometrine soon after a patient has received a vasopressor may cause dangerous hypertension or even apoplexy.

The method is not suitable if the head is high or if shock is present, e.g., in cases of failed forceps. The post-partum uterus contracts well. Post-operative headaches are rather frequent, but their incidence can be reduced if a very fine needle, preferably

* Friedman, E. A., *Anesthesiology*, 1965, **26**, 409.

with a conical point and lateral eye, is used.* Obstetric paralysis due to pressure of the fœtal head or the forceps on the lumbosacral trunk may occur even with intradural or extradural analgesia! Neuropathy due to the block itself is likely to be bilateral and to have a segmental (radicular) rather than a peripheral distribution.

Pressure drugs used to treat the hypotension associated with spinal analgesia do not necessarily improve the blood-flow to the uterus. It is best to avoid the α-stimulating pressor drugs. Recommended are ephedrine 12–25 mg. i.v. or metaraminol 0·002 per cent as an intravenous drip.†

Good results are reported by Steel,‡ Sadove,§ and Thorne.||

Extradural Lumbar Block.—This was first used in obstetrics by Graffagnino and Seyler in 1938,¶ and as a continuous technique by Flowers, Hellman, and Hingson in 1949.** Injection is between L.1 and L.2 or L.2 and L.3, with the patient on her side or sitting. The recommended dose of 1 per cent lignocaine is 5–20 ml., the smaller amount blocking the first-stage pains (T.11 and 12), the larger amount the second stage (S.2, 3, and 4). The continuous technique, using a plastic catheter, is satisfactory in labour. It has been suggested that a block up to T.10, paralysing the sympathetic efferent supply to the uterus, will dilate the cervix in cases of cervical dystocia.†† For the second stage, 15 ml. of solution injected at the L.4–5 interspace with the patient sitting up—one injection—is satisfactory. For forceps extraction in primiparæ the injection should be given at full dilatation and in multiparæ when the cervix is three-fifths dilated. Pain goes 5 min. after injection and the patient is ready for episiotomy and forceps extraction in 15 min.‡‡ Smaller than normal doses required in obstetrics.§§

Bupivacaine has recently been used with good results.|||| A dosage of 15–20 ml. 0·25 per cent solution with adrenaline 1–400,000 is satisfactory, and may be repeated if an indwelling catheter is used.

Extradural Sacral Block—Continuous Caudal Block.¶¶— (*See also* Chapter XVI.) Whatever the merits or demerits of continuous caudal block throughout labour, there is no doubt about the excellence of a single injection given for forceps delivery. In very obese patients, Alvarez recommends that the middle finger of the left hand should be inserted into the rectum, after the needle has pierced the skin, to facilitate location of the sacral hiatus and

* Cappe, B. E., and Deutsch, E. V., *Anesthesiology*, 1953, **14**, 398; also Harris, L. M., and Harmel, M. H., *Ibid.*, 1953, **14**, 390.
† Shnider, S. M., *Proc. 2nd Eur. Cong. Anæsth.*, 1966, **3**, 377.
‡ Steel, G. C., *Proc. R. Soc. Med.*, 1962, **55**, 933.
§ Sadove, M., and others, *Canad. Anæsth. Soc. J.*, 1961, **8**, 405.
|| Thorne, T. C., *Proc. R. Soc. Med.*, 1954, **47**, 301.
¶ Graffagnino, P., and Seyler, L. W., *Surg. Gynec. Obstet.*, 1938, **35**, 597.
** Flowers, C. E., Hellman, L. M., and Hingson, R. A., *Curr. Res. Anesth.*, 1949, **28**, 4.
†† Tunstall, M. E., *Brit. J. Anæsth.*, 1960, **32**, 292.
‡‡ Chaplin, R. A., and Renwick, W. A., *Canad. Anæsth. Soc. J.*, 1958, **5**, 414.
§§ Bromage, P. R., *Canad. med. Ass. J.*, 1961, **85**, 1136, and *Brit. J. Anæsth.*, 1962, **34**, 161.
|||| Duthie, A. M., Wyman, J. B., and Lewis, G. A., *Anæsthesia*, 1968, **40**, 20.
¶¶ Edwards, W. B., and Hingson, R. A., *Amer. J. Surg.*, 1942, **57**, 459; and *J. Amer. med. s.*, 1943, **121**, 225.

Extradural Sacral Block—Continuous Caudal Block, *continued.*

canal. Re-sterilization of the hands, of course, follows before injections are commenced. Continuous caudal block is relatively safe for mother and child, gives superlative relaxation of the lower birth canal, and gives good analgesia. Lignocaine 1 per cent solution or piperocaine, 1·5 per cent in Ringer's solution, 20–30 ml are the recommended agents and doses. Should continuation of the analgesia be decided upon, topping-up doses of 20 ml. can be given when necessary. The method should only be used when every means of resuscitation is to hand. It is not without its disadvantages and is accompanied by a high forceps rate and increased frequency of anomalies of rotation, e.g., persistent occipito-posterior position, and mid-transverse arrest of the head. The third stage is short and post-partum blood-loss minimal. The method is useful in uterine inertia and in cervical dystocia.

The dangers are: (1) Accidental subarachnoid block; (2) Infection; (3) Broken needle; (4) Intrafœtal injection.*

4. Paravertebral Block.—Paravertebral block of D.11 and D.12 on each side will abolish the pain of uterine contraction, but not that due to cervical or perineal stretching, and so has been used for giving relief from first-stage pains. The visceral afferent fibre must be blocked as they run in the white rami, mixed spinal nerve and posterior root. First used by Cleland, of Oregon, in 1933. Cinchocaine, 1–1500, or amethocaine, 0·2 per cent, is used, 10 ml being injected into each nerve. The effect lasts 2–3 hours.‡

For technique, *see* Chapter XV.

5. Pudendal Nerve-block and Local Infiltration.§—This may be used for :—

a. Normal delivery. It should be remembered that the sensory nerve-supply of the vulva comes from the ilio-inguinal nerve anteriorly and from the perineal branch of the posterior cutaneous nerve of the thigh posteriorly.

b. Episiotomy.

c. Outlet forceps.

d. Repair of laceration.

Indications may include fœtal distress, delayed second stage, assisted breech delivery, and multiple pregnancy. This should be used whenever possible for forceps delivery because it is associated with less danger, both for the mother and for the baby, than general anæsthesia.§

The hand cannot be inserted into the vagina without causing discomfort, and good relaxation for intra-uterine manipulation not provided by this technique. A recent study‖ suggested that many of the so-called nerve-blocks depended solely on local perineal and vulval infiltration for their effect. However, when the motor innervation of the levatores ani was successfully interrupted, the relaxation obtained made vaginal manipulation

* Sinclair, J. J., and others, *New Engl. J. Med.,* 1965, **273**, 1173.
† Cleland, J. G. P., *Surg. Gynec. Obstet.,* 1933, **57**, 51.
‡ Reikse, J. M., *Amer. J. Obstet. Gynec.,* 1959, **78**, 411.
§ Huntingford, P. J., *Brit. med. J.,* 1963, **1**, 1195.
‖ Scudamore, J. H., and Yates, M. J., *Lancet,* 1966, **1**, 23.

easier. The method can be used for well over half the cases of forceps delivery, including some mid-forceps extractions.* It can be combined with paracervical nerve-block (p. 636) or with pethidine or trichloroethylene.

ANATOMY OF PUDENDAL NERVE.—This comes from the anterior divisions of the second, third, and fourth sacral nerves, via the pudendal plexus. It passes through the greater sciatic foramen, crosses the spine of the ischium, medial to the internal pudendal vessels, and enters the pelvis through the lesser sciatic foramen. With the pudendal vessels it passes upwards and forwards in the pudendal canal, a tunnel in the fascia on the outer wall of the ischiorectal fossa, gives off an inferior rectal branch, and finally divides into the perineal nerve and the dorsal nerve of the clitoris.

TECHNIQUE.—Lignocaine 1 per cent, procaine 1 per cent, or amethocaine or cinchocaine, 1–2000, can be used. The addition of 150 turbidity reducing units of hyaluronidase to 30 ml. of analgesic solution aids efficiency of the infiltration.

a. NORMAL DELIVERY.—Injections are commenced when the head is appearing at the vulva but before it distends the perineum. A 12-cm. needle is required for the deep injections. The posterior part of the vulva must be infiltrated, including the levator ani muscles and the perineum. Injection is made down the posterior edge of each labium, across the fourchette, and between the vaginal wall and the rectum. Injection should also be made into each ischiorectal fossa to a depth of 5 cm. from weals midway between the anus and the tuberosity of each ischium so that the pudendal nerve can be blocked as it enters the pudendal canal at the level of the ischial spine, or its two branches, the perineal nerve and the dorsal nerve of the clitoris, as they leave the canal. The needle is guided by a finger of the left hand in the vagina. Some solution should be placed posteriorly to the tuberosity of the ischium to block the perineal branch of the posterior cutaneous nerve of the thigh. From the same weal the needle should be inserted subcutaneously in an anterior direction towards the symphysis pubis, to block the ilio-inguinal nerve, while, lastly, some more solution is injected from the weal towards the sphincter of the anus to reinforce the block of the inferior rectal nerve. Total volume of solution required is 20–35 ml. Adrenaline may inhibit labour pains and should not be used.

If the head is not yet distending the perineum, the transvaginal route for infiltrating the pudendal nerves may be preferable to the transperineal route.† To facilitate this, a needle director‡ and also a guide§ have been described.

b. FOR EPISIOTOMY.—Infiltration is made between the skin and the mucosa of the vagina, in the line of the proposed incision.

---

* Gate, J. M., and Dutton, W. A. W., *Brit. med. J.*, 1955, **2**, 99 ; Goldman, J. A., *Brit. J. Anœsth.*, 1959, **31**, 538 ; and Hawksworth, W., *Practitioner*, 1958, **180**, 679.
† Kobak, A. J., Evans, E. E., and Johnson, G. R., *Amer. J. Obstet. Gynec.*, 1956, **71**, 981 ; and Huntingford, P. J., *J. Obstet. Gynæc., Brit. Emp.*, 1959, **66**, 26.
‡ Cohen, H., *Brit. med. J.*, 1961, **2**, 1776.
§ Eaton, E. R., and Flanagan, M. B., *Lancet*, 1960, **1**, 1392.

Pudendal Nerve-block and Local Infiltration, *continued*.

    c. FOR REPAIR OF LACERATIONS.—A swab, soaked in 2 per cent lignocaine, 1–1000 amethocaine, or 5 per cent piperocaine, is placed in the raw area of the tear to effect surface analgesia. After a few minutes 0·5 per cent solution of lignocaine is infiltrated : (*a*) In a plane parallel to the perineal skin ; (*b*) In a plane parallel to the vaginal mucosa. In each case the needle is inserted from the raw area of the laceration.

Pudendal block may inhibit labour pains.

6. Paracervical Nerve-block.*—In this technique, pain sensation from the uterus is interrupted by the injection of local analgesic solution into the loose cellular tissue at the sides of the cervix. The nerve-fibres from the uterus and cervix form a plexus at the base of the broad ligament near the lateral vaginal fornix and pass to the presacral nerves.

    INDICATIONS.—Most useful towards the end of the first stage of labour. Very helpful : (1) to enable painless vaginal examinations to be carried out in nervous patients ; (2) to enable cervix to be dilated ; (3) to aid those patients who bear down at the end of the first stage. Not seen at its best when the head is low in the pelvis and the cervix is fully dilated. The technique does not appear to influence uterine activity.

    TECHNIQUE.—A 12- or 14-cm. hollow tube with bulbous end is employed, and through this a long needle is inserted and this can only project about 5–7 mm. beyond the end of the introducer. With the patient in the dorsal, lateral, or lithotomy position, the introducer is guided into the lateral fornix, at the three and nine o'clock positions, following the usual antiseptic safeguards ; 10 ml. of 1 per cent solution of lignocaine with adrenaline are now injected at the side of the cervix and the procedure repeated on the other side. Pain relief lasts for about an hour or two, and injections can be given more than once if necessary. Effects of 0·25 per cent bupivacaine last 3 hours.†

7. Presacral or Parasacral Block.—This involves block of the anterior primary divisions of the sacral nerves, of the sacrococcygeal plexus, and of the autonomic fibres in relation to the anterior surface of the sacrum. It is rarely done.

    INDICATION.—Forceps delivery ; manual rotation of occipitoposterior positions with forceps delivery : breech extractions Difficult cases of breech extractions requiring the hand to be inserted high into the uterus will require general anæsthesia in addition. A marked feature of the block is the good relaxation produced. Analgesia does not last as long as in extradural sacral (caudal) block. Relief of pain following hæmorrhoidectomy can be procured using this block.‡

---

* Cooper, K., and Moir, J. Chassar, *Brit. med. J.*, 1963, **1**, 1372 ; Cooper, K., *Proc. R. Soc. Med.*, 1963, **56**, 1096 ; Aldridge, C. W., and others, *Amer. J. Obstet. Gynec.*, 1961, **81**, 941; Page, E. P., and others, *Ibid.*, 1961, **81**, 1094 ; and Spanos, W. J., and Steele, J. C., *Obst. and Gynec.*, 1959, **13**, 129.
    † Gudgeon, D. H., *Brit. med. J.*, 1968, **2**, 403.
    ‡ Willis, J. H., *Ibid.*, 1965, **2**, 1002.

TECHNIQUE.—With the patient in the lithotomy position, the sacrococcygeal joint is identified by deep palpation. Two weals are raised, each 2 cm. from the midline at the level of the joint.

1. A long needle is inserted through a weal and makes contact with the edge of the last sacral vertebra. It is advanced, parallel to the sagittal plane of the body, along the anterior surface of the sacrum, for about 7 cm., when it will strike bone in the region of the second sacral foramen. As the needle is slowly withdrawn, 10–20 ml. of 1 per cent lignocaine with adrenaline are deposited between the second sacral vertebra and the sacrococcygeal joint.

2. The needle is again inserted at an angle of 15° to its former track, still keeping in the sagittal plane, this time for about 10 cm., when the sacrum should again be struck, in the region of the first sacral foramen, and 5–10 ml. of solution are injected in this area.

3. Finally, 10 ml. of solution are deposited between the rectum and the coccyx. The same procedure is repeated on the other side.

The empty rectum recedes before the needle point and is unlikely to be perforated. Some workers keep the index finger in the rectum throughout the injections.

Presacral block usually abolishes labour pains for 15–30 minutes, but they come on again.

In some cases local infiltration of the perineum is required in addition to ensure a painless delivery. The third stage of labour proceeds normally.

Administration of Analgesia by Midwives.—The Central Midwives Board lays down rules relating to analgesia in labour administered by midwives working alone. A practising midwife must not, on her own responsibility, administer an inhalation analgesic unless :

1. She has received special instruction in the essentials of obstetric analgesia at an institution approved by the Board, and has satisfied the institution or Board that she is thoroughly proficient in the use of the apparatus.

2. The patient has at some time during the pregnancy been examined by a registered medical practitioner who has signed a certificate that he finds no contra-indication to the administration of analgesia by a midwife. Should the patient subsequently contract an illness requiring medical attention, the onus is on the midwife to obtain confirmation that the certificate remains valid. In Scotland, the patient must be examined by a registered medical practitioner within one month of confinement and a certificate signed that the patient is fit for the administration of trichloroethylene.

3. One other person, acceptable to the patient, who in the opinion of the midwife is suitable for the purpose, is present at the time of the administration, in addition to the midwife.

The following apparatus are approved by the Board for the use of midwives :—

Minnitt gas–air machine (50 per cent nitrous oxide in air).

Jecta gas–air machine (50 per cent nitrous oxide in air).

Administration of Analgesia by Midwives, *continued.*

> The Entonox Apparatus for administration of premixed nitrous-oxide–oxygen (50 per cent of each).
>
> Emotril Trichloroethylene Automatic Inhaler (0·5 or 0·35 per cent in air).
>
> Tecota Mark 6 Trichloroethylene Inhaler (0·5 or 0·35 per cent in air).
>
> The trichloroethylene inhalers must be tested by the National Physical Laboratory before use and re-checked at 12-monthly intervals. The responsibility for checking devolves on the owner of the vaporizer.
>
> Pethidine can be administered by the midwife in doses of 100 mg. ; not more than 200 mg. may be given to any patient.
>
> The midwife can also administer the following drugs : chloral hydrate, syrup of chloral, potassium bromide, tincture of opium, Pil. opii, Dover's powder.

GENERAL ANÆSTHESIA

There is a definite maternal death-rate for which the anæsthetist must take some blame. This is associated with: (1) Aspiration of vomitus; (2) Hypotension and drug toxicity associated with regional analgesia; (3) Inadequate blood transfusion, too little, and too late.

Equipment.—Every labour ward should be equipped with: (1) A tipping table;* (2) An efficient suction apparatus; (3) Laryngoscope and endotracheal tubes; (4) Transparent face-mask. A bronchoscope may be occasionally necessary.

Prevention of Vomiting during Anæsthesia in Labour.†—Vomiting is always a real danger during labour as the patient may not be suitably prepared, while the gastric emptying time is delayed. There may, too, be associated hiatus hernia.‡ In addition, the rather light plane of anæsthesia required is often the cause of vomiting.

> DIET.—A satisfactory régime must be instituted to lessen the likelihood of acid stomach contents being present should general anæsthesia be required. Crawford§ suggests that patients be classified as 'normal' or 'high-risk' cases:—
>
> 1. 'NORMAL' CASES.—Unlikely to require general anæsthesia. The aim is to provide a light, easily digestible diet and to avoid large pieces of meat or vegetables with a high fibre content. Fried food should be avoided and the ingestion of milk curtailed. Sieved foods are allowed. Drinks should not contain more than 5 per cent glucose as stronger solutions delay gastric emptying. Small meals 3-hourly are preferable to large meals. Antacids,‡ such as aluminium hydroxide (aludrox) or magnesium trisilicate,‖ should be given 2-hourly to reduce gastric acidity.

---

* Wylie, W. D., *Lancet*, 1956, **1**, 840; Gibberd, G. F., *Ibid.*, 1955, **1**, 901; and Steel, G. C., *Brit. med. J.*, 1961, **1**, 963.

† *See also* McCormick, P. W., *Hosp. Med.*, 1967, **2**, 163.

‡ Dinnick, O. P., *Proc. R. Soc. Med.*, 1957, **50**, 547.

§ Crawford, J. S., *Principles and Practice of Obstetric Anæsthesia*, 2nd ed. 1965. Oxford: Blackwell.

‖ Taylor, G., and Pryse-Davies, J., *Lancet*, 1966, **1**, 288.

2. 'HIGH-RISK' CASES.—In these cases the obstetric history suggests that operative delivery may be required. Patients should be placed in the 'high-risk' category even if it is planned to use regional analgesia. Aspiration of vomitus can occur during spinal analgesia for Cæsarean section.* In these patients, once active labour is established, they should be given nothing by mouth except for antacids. They should receive intravenous fluids, 1 litre 5 per cent dextrose 4-hourly.

Before induction of anæsthesia, a No. 10 œsophageal tube may be passed if the anæsthetist cannot guarantee safety from aspiration of gastric contents without it. Trouble may arise from: (a) Gross obstruction by solid or liquid material. (b) An asthmatic and bronchospastic response due to the inhalation of irritating acid gastric contents (Mendelson's or the acid pulmonary aspiration syndrome).† Bronchopulmonary initiation is likely if the aspirated material has a pH of 2·5 or below.‡ (c) Bronchopneumonia and its later complications, e.g., lung abscess or bronchiectasis. Regional analgesia (pudendal, intra- or extradural block) avoids these dangers but may not always be convenient either to the patient or to her medical attendants.

Aspiration of stomach contents during general anæsthesia can be made less likely by :—

1. Giving only fluid and semi-solid material during labour.
2. The insertion of a No. 10 œsophageal (or No. 20 Wangensteen) tube before induction of anæsthesia.
3. Inducing anæsthesia with the head elevated. In a recent series of 2000 cases, deliberate gastric emptying was only employed in 1 per cent of cases and no aspirations of stomach contents occurred.§ (For Mendelson's syndrome see p. 220.)

The acid pulmonary aspiration syndrome can occur without definite vomiting or obvious regurgitation.||

A safe technique which gives good results is the following : Premedication, atropine 0·6 mg. The table is tilted steeply head-up and only returned to the horizontal after the airway is sealed off. Pure oxygen is given and ready access to a vein is assured. Unconsciousness results from thiopentone 200–250 mg. and this is followed by suxamethonium 50–100 mg. and the insertion of a cuffed endotracheal tube, the cuff of which is immediately inflated. Thereafter, gas and at least 30 per cent of oxygen are administered by I.P.P.V. and apnœa and muscular relaxation maintained by small additional doses of the relaxant. After the child is delivered, any form of light anæsthesia is employed.

Using this technique, many workers do not routinely employ an œsophageal tube to empty the stomach but rely on the

---

* Klein, M. D., and others, *N.Y. St. J. Med.*, 1953, **53**, 2861.
† Mendelson, C. L., *Amer. J. Obstet. Gynec.*, 1946, **52**, 191; and Hausmann, W., and Lunt, R. L., *Obstet. Gynæc.*, *Brit. Emp.*, 1955, **62**, 669.
‡ Taylor, G., and Pryse-Davies, J., *Lancet*, 1966, **1**, 288.
§ Hodges, R. J. H., and Tunstall, M. E., *Brit. J. Anæsth.*, 1961, **33**, 572.
|| McCormick, P. W., *Proc. R. Soc. Med.*, 1966, **59**, 66.

Prevention of Vomiting during Anæsthesia in Labour, *continued.*

head-up position to prevent regurgitation and the relaxant to prevent active vomiting. A tube should be used, however, if the anatomy of the patient is not conducive to smooth laryngoscopy and endotracheal intubation, or if there is gross alimentary distension.

A recent report on maternal deaths* showed that out of 3 deaths due to complications of anæsthesia, inhalation of stomach contents was a major cause in 17.

4. Using thiopentone (200–250 mg.) for induction and gas, oxygen, trichloroethylene, or ether for maintenance† on a bed which can be rapidly tilted head-down.‡

5. Inducing anæsthesia in the lateral position. Avoiding strapping face-piece on to face : using a face-piece made of transparent material.

6. Inducing anæsthesia with equal volumes of cyclopropane and oxygen with the head elevated to prevent regurgitation followed by the insertion of a cuffed endotracheal tube under suxamethonium (50 mg.).§

Methods 3 and 6 should only be used by anæsthetists of some experience. The tiro would perhaps do best with gas, oxygen, trichloroethylene, ether, with a little carbon dioxide in the early stages, and using the lateral position. The presence of a sucker would be an additional safety factor while Sellick's manœuvre of pressure on the cricoid cartilage to reduce the risk of regurgitation is helpful.‖

7. Intravenous injection of 1·5 mg. of apomorphine well diluted to induce vomiting. When the stomach has thus been emptied atropine 1·3 mg. is given slowly intravenously to combat the vagal effects sometimes seen after apomorphine. Anæsthesia is then induced. This treatment does not markedly disturb the patient.¶

TREATMENT OF ACID ASPIRATION SYNDROME.—

1. Milder cases may be treated by: (*a*) The Trendelenburg position (*b*) Lightening of anæsthesia to encourage coughing; (*c*) Pharyngeal suction.

2. Severe cases may require, in addition to careful tracheobronchial toilet, aspiration and lavage with solution of sodium bicarbonate, I.P.P.V. through an endotracheal tube with pure oxygen. Spontaneous respiration with pure oxygen may not be adequate to correct arterial desaturation in the presence of pulmonary œdema and profound acidosis.** Tracheostomy may be required: it reduces the respiratory dead space by

---

* Walker, A. L., and others, *Rep. publ. Health med. Subj.*, 1960, No. 103.
† Crawford, J. S., *Brit. J. Anæsth.*, 1956, **28**, 146 and 201.
‡ Wylie, W. D., *Lancet*, 1956, **1**, 840 ; Gibberd, G. F., *Ibid.*, 1955, **1**, 901 ; and Steel, G. C., *Brit. med. J.*, 1961, **1**, 963.
§ Wylie, W. D., *Proc. R. Soc. Med.*, 1955, **48**, 1089.
‖ Sellick, B. A., *Lancet*, 1961, **2**, 404.
¶ Holmes, J. M., *Proc. R. Soc. Med.*, 1957, **50**, 556.
** McCormack, P. W., Hay, R. G., and Griffin, R. W., *Lancet*, 1966, **1**, 1127.

50 per cent. Hydrocortisone in large doses reduces the inflammatory reaction and aids bronchodilatation.*

Thiopentone.—This should be used sparingly, because of its depressant effect on the fœtal respiratory centre. It would appear that the placenta forms no barrier to thiopentone and that the fœtal blood-level of the drug is at a maximum at the onset of anæsthesia and thereafter falls.† It is therefore suggested that fœtal respiratory depression may be less if delivery occurs 5–7 min. after induction of anæsthesia than if it is rapidly accomplished 2–3 min. after the thiopentone is injected. A dose of 200–250 mg. used for induction of anæsthesia is unlikely to have a serious depressant effect on the infant's breathing capacity, but further doses are probably undesirable.

For external version, thiopentone may not give adequate relaxation. It is often undesirable for forceps delivery, except as an inducing agent. If, however, a quick-working obstetrician can promise a rapid delivery, then 0·25 g. together with gas–oxygen, and perhaps *suxamethonium,* can be used for episiotomy and outlet forceps. It is unsuitable for complicated cases and premature labours.

Muscle Relaxants.—These agents are used in labour: (1) To relax the perineum and abdominal wall. (2) To aid endotracheal intubation. (3) To reduce reflex response to stimuli during light anæsthesia. There is evidence that gallamine enters the fœtal circulation more readily than tubocurarine or decamethonium, although clinical doses are without harmful effect on the fœtus. Ordinary doses of the remaining relaxants will probably do the infant no harm. Suxamethonium has been observed to cause an increase in uterine activity, so there is a possibility of intra-uterine hypoxia from interference with placental blood-flow.‡

The combination of thiopentone, nitrous oxide and oxygen anæsthesia with suxamethonium (30–60 mg.) or decamethonium (3–5 mg.) has given good results in cases of forceps delivery, delivery of the aftercoming head, episiotomy, and repair of the perineum. A cuffed endotracheal tube should be passed if there is any suspicion that the stomach is not empty. These drugs, used in appropriate dosage, do not appear to cross the placental barrier in significant amounts. They can also be used to prevent precipitate labour. (*See,* however, Older and Harris, 1968.§)

Halothane.—This drug must be used with care in obstetrics since it depresses the uterus. It offers some advantages if the anæsthetist is skilled in its use and avoids deep planes of anæsthesia. These are: (1) Induction is rapid; (2) Relaxation is quickly achieved; (3) Laryngospasm is absent; (4) Salivary and bronchial secretions are minimal; (5) Vomiting, both during induction and post-operatively, is reduced; (6) There is rapid recovery from anæsthesia.

* Nickold, R. M., and others, *Brit. med. J.,* 1967, **3**, 745.
† Crawford, J. S., *Brit. J. Anæsth.,* 1956, **28**, 146, 201.
‡ Felton, D. J. C., and Goddard, B. A., *Lancet,* 1966, **1**, 852.
§ Older, P. O., and Harris, J. M., *Brit. J. Anæsth.,* 1968, **40**, 459.

Halothane, *continued.*

While some anæsthetists of experience advocate its use,* other
believe it should be reserved for those occasions where uterin
relaxation is required.† In the authors' opinion, the main indicatio
for its use in obstetrics is for external versions. For forcep
delivery and Cæsarean section, other good methods are available
and halothane carries a risk of uterine relaxation and post-partur
hæmorrhage.

Cyclopropane.—A satisfactory agent for operative delivery provide
that deep anæsthesia is avoided, that delivery of the fœtus i
obtained without delay, and that anæsthesia is lightened as fa
as possible at the time of delivery. Not commonly used in Britai
to-day.

Nitrous Oxide.—This analgesic with thiopentone induction (200
250 mg.) and muscle relaxants is widely used in Britain to-day
The only complication, provided intubation can be speedil
achieved to prevent aspiration of stomach contents, is awarenes
during operation.

Trichloroethylene.—There is little place for this drug as a mai
anæsthetic agent for operative delivery, since it is slowly taken u
and eliminated, and a depth sufficient to permit tolerance of a
endotracheal tube will affect the fœtus.

Ether.—Although this agent has been used in obstetric anæsthesi
for many years, it is now less popular due to the use of muscl
relaxants with light planes of anæsthesia. If used, the depth o
anæsthesia should be as light as is consistent with the surgica
requirements as otherwise fœtal depression may occur.

Anæsthesia for External Version.—Halothane and oxygen is
satisfactory method. Uterine relaxation can be obtained wit
rapid recovery. Otherwise thiopentone and a muscle relaxant wil
relax the abdominal wall, though not the uterus. Where uterin
tone prevents version, deep anæsthesia with halothane or ethe
is required.

Anæsthesia for Internal Version.—If the obstetrician requires
well-relaxed uterus, high into which his hand and arm must b
introduced, deep anæsthesia is required, and this may be mos
readily obtained with ether or halothane.

Anæsthesia for Forceps Delivery.—An efficient anæsthetic fo
forceps delivery should produce together with complete safety
remembering the risk of the aspiration of stomach contents
(1) Adequate relaxation of the muscles of the pelvic floor an
perineum for the application of forceps. (2) Minimal depressio
of labour pains. (3) Minimal depression of post-partum uterin
contractions. (4) Minimal depression of the fœtal respiration
The method chosen will depend on the environment, the experi
ence of the anæsthetist, and the facilities available. In domiciliar

* Allard, E., and Guimond, C., *Canad. Anæsth. Soc. J.*, 1964, **11**, 83.
† Crawford, J. S., *Principles and Practice of Obstetric Anæsthesia*, 2nd ed., 1965. Oxford
Blackwell; and Bonica, J. J., *Principles and Practice of Obstetric Analgesia and Anesthesia*
1967, Vol. I. Oxford: Blackwell.

work, a pudendal block is the method of choice.* Otherwise light general anæsthesia must be employed using such agents and equipment as are available.

In hospital, low spinal analgesia has much to be said in its favour as it removes the risk of aspiration of gastric contents. Extradural sacral block is excellent, if time is available.

Thiopentone, suxamethonium, and nitrous-oxide–oxygen, given through a cuffed endotracheal tube, is rapidly gaining adherents as one of the safest techniques.†

Anæsthesia for Breech Delivery.‡—

1. In assisted breech delivery, good oxygenation and a smooth induction at the right time are necessary. In the first and early second stage, pethidine 100–150 mg. and gas–oxygen if necessary. When the presenting part appears, an episiotomy can be done under infiltration analgesia and pudendal block, and this gives adequate pain relief, for delivery of the aftercoming head by forceps and anæsthesia is not induced until the scapulæ are delivered. If it is then necessary it must be induced rapidly by one of the following methods : (1) Oxygen, thiopentone, suxamethonium, cuffed endotracheal tube, gas–oxygen ; (2) Thiopentone, gas–oxygen ; (3) Cyclopropane and oxygen.

2. For breech extraction there is no hurry to induce anæsthesia which can follow the usually accepted techniques. Good relaxation may be required.

Anæsthesia for Retained Placenta.—The patient may be shocked and a retraction ring may form an obstruction. Light thiopentone, light trichloroethylene and ether, gas–oxygen–ether—all are satisfactory. An endotracheal tube should be inserted and the cuff inflated if there are stomach contents present. Inhalation of one or two capsules of amyl nitrite may relax a retraction ring: if it does not, deeper anæsthesia will be necessary. This drug may also relax a contraction ring, earlier in labour. In the absence of facilities for general anæsthesia, trichloroethylene analgesia or intravenous opiates (e.g., morphine, 15 mg.) make the manœuvre of manual removal tolerable. Very rarely, in an emergency and to save life in severe post-partum hæmorrhage it may be justified to remove the placenta from a collapsed patient without any analgesia.

COMPLICATIONS

Eclampsia.§—May be controlled by heavy sedation, reduction of blood-pressure, or special techniques. These may include: (1) Infusion of trimetaphan; (2) Lumbar extradural blockade; (3) Intravenous barbiturate and muscle relaxant with I.P.P.V. Bromethol has frequently been used to produce a state of basal narcosis.

---

* Hawksworth, W., *Practitioner*, 1958, **180**, 679.
† Hodges, R. J. H., and Tunstall, M. E., *Brit. J. Anæsth.*, 1961, **33**, 572.
‡ Law, R. G., and Ransom, S., *Brit. med. J.*, 1953, **1**, 562.
§ *See also* Bonica, J. J., in *Clinical Anesthesia—Obstetric Complications* (Ed. Bonica, J. J.), 1965, Ch. 1. Oxford: Blackwell.

Amniotic Fluid Embolism.*—First described in 1941.† This is a dramatic catastrophe which can occur during labour and may be attributed to anæsthesia. A sudden infusion of amniotic fluid into the maternal circulation, after rupture of the membranes, gives rise to an acute shock-like state characterized by: (1) respiratory distress; (2) cyanosis; (3) chest pain; (4) peripheral vascular collapse; (5) coma; (6) hypofibrinogenæmia with excessive bleeding; this may occur without collapse and be the first sign of the condition. *Treatment* may include: (1) blood transfusion to combat defibrination; (2) administration of fibrinogen; (3) vasopressors (ephedrine or mephentermine are to be preferred as they do not cause pulmonary vasoconstriction); (4) artificial ventilation with oxygen; (5) bronchodilators; (6) steroids; (7) possibly digitalis.

Hypofibrinogenæmia.‡—May be due to: (1) Continued bleeding; (2) Destruction of fibrin and fibrinogen by plasma fibrinolysins; (3) Conversion of prothrombin to thrombin may be inactivated by release of heparin-like substance in amniotic fluid. Normal value at term is 450 mg. per cent. Less than 150 mg. per cent is dangerous. *Treatment*: (1) Give 4 g. fibrinogen rapidly and repeat in 1 hour if no significant improvement; (2) If there is a circulatory fibrinolysin give epsilon-aminocaproic acid, 4–5 g. initial dose intravenously over 1 hour, then 1 g. 8-hourly; (3) When heparin-like factor diagnosed, give 20–50 mg. protamine sulphate intravenously slowly. 500 ml. blood contains less than 1 g. of fibrinogen, 1000 ml. plasma provides 3 g. Purified concentrates are available.

Acute Inversion of the Uterus.—Shock is out of proportion to blood-loss. Immediate replacement is necessary with general anæsthesia (e.g., cyclopropane).

Shock.§—Causes of shock in the obstetric patient include:—
1. Hæmorrhage, e.g., ante-partum hæmorrhage, lacerations of birth canal, retained placenta, uterine atony.
2. Traumatic. Acute inversion of the uterus. Surgical trauma.
3. Septic shock.
4. Supine hypotensive syndrome. *See* p. 618.
5. Amniotic fluid embolism.
6. As a result of sodium loss.

ANÆSTHESIA FOR CÆSAREAN SECTION

The ideal anæsthetic or analgesic should provide:—
a. Good pain relief.
b. Absence of respiratory depression of the fœtus.
c. Good relaxation of the abdomen.
d. Absence of psychic trauma to mother.
e. Absence of toxicity of mother and infant.

* *See* Review article, Shnider, S. M., and Moya, F., *Anesthesiology*, 1961, **22**, 108.
† Steiner, P. E., and Lushbaugh, C. C., *J. Amer. med. Ass.*, 1941, **117**, 1245.
‡ Marx, G. F., *Anesthesiology*, 1965, **26**, 423; and Leader, *Brit. med. J.*, 1965, **2**, 955.
§ *See also* Little, D. M., in *Clinical Anesthesia—Obstetric Complications* (Ed. Bonica, J. J.), 1965, Ch. 2. Oxford: Blackwell; and Marx, G. F., *Anesthesiology*, 1965, **26**, 423.

f. Absolute safety, especially from aspiration of stomach contents. The fœtal mortality following elective section is greater than that following normal delivery.

Premedication.—Many workers prohibit all sedation and allow only atropine. Pentobarbitone and quinalbarbitone 100 mg. (1½ gr.) are probably free from serious effect on the child; similarly thiopentone, 0·25 g., is allowed by many if given immediately before delivery.

General Anæsthesia.—Proper measures to prevent aspiration of stomach contents must be taken (*see* p. 638). The oxygen, thiopentone, suxamethonium, cuffed tube, nitrous-oxide–oxygen, relaxant technique* is popular since it allows a very light plane of anæsthesia with minimal depression of the fœtus. The anæsthetic should not be started until the surgeon is scrubbed up and ready to operate. No hypoxia must be allowed. One of the disadvantages of the very light planes of anæsthesia allowed is that the mother may become aware of events during the operation.† Full doses of relaxant are seldom necessary in Cæsarean section. The abdominal muscles are stretched during pregnancy and muscle tone is seldom a problem. Relaxants are rather given to prevent undue reflex response during surgery with light anæsthesia. Hyperventilation has been used as an aid to the production of unconsciousness. Respiratory alkalosis in the mother may, however, produce hazard to the fœtus,‡ though this has been disputed.§ The critical level of maternal arterial Pco_2 may be as low as 17 mm. Hg.‖ Transmission of thiopentone through the placenta during anæsthesia for Caesarean section does not result in any close correlation between fœtal and maternal blood levels. The passage of time is no guarantee that fœtal blood level will be lowered.¶

Any general anæsthetic carefully given to lower Plane 1 or upper Plane 2 of surgical anæsthesia is suitable. After the delivery of the child, anæsthesia can be deepened if necessary. The more a general anæsthetic agent is pushed to produce relaxation, the more likely is the child to be born apnœic.

In all cases a high percentage of oxygen should be given to the mother immediately before the child is separated.

Muscular relaxation is seldom a problem as the abdominal wall has been stretched by the increasing size of the pregnant uterus. Provided coughing and straining are avoided the intestines are unlikely to obtrude. Relaxants are not often required to achieve relaxation but rather to ensure a tranquil operating field during the very light planes of anæsthesia employed. At the same time the anæsthetist should be aware of the possibility of the patient awakening paralysed during the operative procedure, and an adequate amount of nitrous oxide should be given by intermittent positive-pressure ventilation.

---

* Hodges, R. J. H., and Tunstall, M. E., *Brit. J. Anæsth.*, 1961, **33**, 572.
† Hutchinson, R., *Ibid.*, 1961, **33**, 463; and Waters, D. J., *Ibid.*, 1968, **40**, 259.
‡ Holmes, F., *Ibid.*, 1963, **35**, 433.
§ Coleman, A. J., *Lancet*, 1967, **1**, 813.
‖ Moya, F., *Amer. J. Obstet. Gynec.*, 1965, **91**, 76.
¶ Levy, C. J., and Owen, G., *Anæsthesia*, 1964, **19**, 511.

Cæsarean Section—General Anæsthesia, *continued.*

Dextran 40 (average M.W. 40,000) does not cross the placental barrier.*

Subarachnoid Block.—This is considered by many to be dangerous as an analgesic for Cæsarean section, though widely used in North America. A substantial number of maternal deaths have been reported. It is a method without bad effect on the child provided that the obstetrician extracts it as rapidly as possible after the onset of analgesia: should he dilly-dally at this time, fœtal hypoxia may result from the contracted uterus compressing the placenta. It ensures good retraction and absence of post-partum hæmorrhage. The enlarged uterus, by interfering with the movements of the diaphragm, tends to produce hypoxia of the mother. As Macintosh points out, this hypoxia may be the cause of some of the deaths that have been reported. Certainly 100 per cent of oxygen should be given to the mother from the outset. The blood-pressure should not be allowed to fall below 90 mm. Hg. Hypotension may be made worse by the supine position causing interference with venous return to the heart (the supine hypotensive syndrome of late pregnancy).†

Block should reach the costal margin and can be obtained with heavy cinchocaine, 1·4–1·6 ml. injected with the patient in the lateral position and afterwards turned on to her back on a level table. Hyperbaric amethocaine hydrochloride (8 mg. in 1 per cent solution with 1 ml. of 10 per cent dextrose) or procaine hydrochloride (100 mg. of crystals dissolved in 2 ml. of cerebrospinal fluid) can be used in the same way—all three solutions being hyperbaric. Supplementary anæsthesia should be withheld until the birth of the child, after which a little thiopentone or inhalation anæsthetic can be given, if necessary, and if it is certain that the stomach is empty.

Local analgesics are said to be specially toxic to the pregnant woman. Evidence has been produced to show that the circulation of the cerebrospinal fluid is altered during the later months of pregnancy, perhaps because of the pressure of the tumour on the large abdominal and thoracic veins. Nevertheless, in spite of objections from very experienced workers, subarachnoid block has gained some popularity as an analgesic method for Cæsarean section. It is the technique of choice in some clinics in the U.S.A. and is especially useful in patients suffering from diabetes. Great care is required, especially in control of the blood-pressure and in adequate oxygenation of the mother and hence of the child.

Extradural Lumbar Block.—Good results have been achieved with this method in non-urgent cases. Injection is between L.2 and L.3, 20 to 25 ml. of 1 per cent or 1·5 per cent lignocaine. Analgesia a little above the eighth thoracic dermatome appears in five to ten minutes, and may last 1½ to 2 hours. Early movement after operation is possible, as motor paralysis is not complete. The continuous technique, using a catheter, has its use here. It has been shown that patients in advanced pregnancy and labour

---

* Ricketts, C. R., and others, *Brit. med. J.*, 1966, **1**, 1050.
† Holmes, F., *J. Obstet. Gynæc., Brit. Emp.*, 1958, **64**, 229.

require smaller doses of local analgesic agents than normal women.* If necessary the patient can be kept asleep with nitrous oxide and oxygen. The blood-pressure should be maintained at 90 mm. Hg or above, while a continuous intravenous drip is useful.

Local Infiltration.—This is without serious effect on the mother or child, but is unsuitable for frightened or uncontrolled patients. The surgeon's co-operation is essential for success : he usually performs the injections himself.

Intradermal and subcutaneous infiltration is carried out in the line of the incision and solution should be deposited for about 1 in. on each side of the midline. Extra solution is injected into the pyramidales and into the retropubic space of Retzius. Solution injected into the rectus sheath will improve relaxation. The parietal peritoneum is infiltrated, likewise the tissue overlying the lower segment if the classic operation is not to be employed. Those interested in the technique should consult the paper by A. C. Beck (*Amer. J. Obstet. Gynec.*, 1947, **43**, 815). It is not very widely used to-day. Many obstetricians prefer the administration of 0·25 g. of thiopentone just before the uterus is incised, oxygen being given at the same time as the infiltration.

This whole difficult question was discussed at the Royal Society of Medicine,† to the reports of which readers are referred.

RESUSCITATION OF THE NEWBORN

The fœtal blood-hæmoglobin is 15 to 20 g. per 100 ml. and when fully saturated carries 22 vol. per cent of oxygen. But because of the low oxygen partial pressure at which maternal blood gives up its oxygen, fœtal hæmoglobin is only 50 per cent saturated. There is also a mild acidosis with Pco_2 of 55 mm. Hg and a pH fall to 7·25. To compensate for this hypoxia, fœtal hæmoglobin carries more oxygen at a lower tension, i.e., the dissociation curve of fœtal hæmoglobin is shifted to the left, while the dissociation curve of the maternal hæmoglobin is shifted to the right, making it give up oxygen more easily. The low metabolic rate of the fœtus allows this hypoxia to be tolerated.

At birth, the skin reflexes are ill developed except in the area supplied by the trigeminal nerve : mouth and pharyngeal stimulation may help to excite respiration.

In the newborn the amount of carbonic anhydrase is half that found in adult blood so that release of carbon dioxide in lungs is handicapped.

During the process of birth, anaerobic glycolysis may aid the survival of the infant, should respiratory embarrassment occur, oxygen being released from glycogen.

Intra-uterine respiration of the fœtus, the rhythmical amniotic tide into and out of the air-passages, was first demonstrated by Ahfelt in 1888 and then by the Italian, Ferroni, in 1899. Fluctuation in maternal carbon-dioxide tension may contribute to respiratory difficulties in the newborn, especially in premature infants. Maternal $Paco_2$ may fall

---

* Bromage, P. R., *Brit. J. Anæsth.*, 1962, **34**, 161.
† *Proc. R. Soc. Med.* (Sect. Anæsth.), 1947, **40**, 10, 557 ; *Ibid.*, 1957, **50**, 547; and *Ibid.*, 1962, **55**, 931.

Resuscitation of the Newborn, *continued.*

as a result of hyperventilation towards the end of the first stage of labour, but may rise during the second stage as a result of breath-holding.[*] The effect of hyperventilation during anæsthesia may be to depress the fœtus,[†] though blood-gas studies do not confirm this.[‡] The critical level of maternal arterial Pco_2 may be 17 mm. Hg.[§] Also, fœtal hypoxia fails to stimulate respiration, presumably because of the absence of the aortico-carotid body reflex in the fœtal and neonatal state. Hypoxia thus does not cause the initiation of respiration.

The signs of intra-uterine hypoxia are irregularity of the fœtal heart-rate going on to tachycardia and bradycardia. In a head presentation, the presence of meconium indicates hypoxic relaxation of the fœtal anal sphincter.

Causes of Hypoxia in Fœtus and Newborn.[||]—Hypoxia is of the hypoxic type; it may be either sudden, or continuous and prolonged, and is due to :—

1. Reduction of oxygen tension in maternal blood. For example, reduction of inspired oxygen concentration to 10 per cent results in fœtal heat-rate changes within 4 minutes.[¶]
2. The trauma of labour.
3. Interference of passage of oxygen from mother to fœtus through :—
   a. Hypotension due to spinal or extradural analgesia.
   b. Anæmia, e.g., hæmorrhage, cardiac failure, etc.
   c. Tetanic uterine contractions, sometimes caused by pituitary extract or spinal analgesia.
   d. Placental infarction or premature separation.
   e. Prolapse or knotting of cord.
4. Fœtal respiratory failure :—
   a. CENTRAL.—Due to : (i) Immaturity of respiratory centre, per-haps associated with gross fœtal abnormality. (ii) Damage to respiratory centre from trauma or from cerebral œdema due to diabetes or hydrops fœtalis. (iii) Oxygen lack perhaps associated with intrapartum fœtal asphyxia. (iv) Narcotics and sedatives given to mother. The threshold of maternal respiratory centre differs from that of the fœtal centre as a level of narcosis harmless to the mother may be depressing to fœtus. All general anæsthetics to mother are hazardous if the baby is premature.
   b. PERIPHERAL.—Due to : (i) Immaturity of lungs. (ii) Respira-tory obstruction. (iii) Muscular weakness. (iv) Fœtal lungs full of liquor amnii or meconium. (v) Intranatal pneumonia.
   The baby recovering from asphyxia first takes a series of gasps which give place to a series of single prolonged inspirations. Finally, rhythmic inspiration and expiration set in. Periodic breathing is not of bad prognostic significance in newborn babies and is usual in premature infants.

---

* Reid, D. H. S., *Lancet*, 1966, **1**, 784.
† Holmes, F., *Brit. J. Anæsth.*, 1963, **35**, 433; and Motoyama, E. K., and others, *Lancet*, 1966, **1**, 286.
‡ Coleman, A. J., *Ibid.*, 1967, **1**, 813.
§ Moya, F., and others, *Amer. J. Obstet. Gynec.*, 1965, **91**, 76.
|| Donald, I., *Brit. J. Anæsth.*, 1967, **29**, 553.
¶ John, A. H., *Ibid.*, 1965, **37**, 515.

Fœtal distress demands oxygen to the mother. There is evidence that asphyxia at birth may cause permanent cerebral or neurological damage. If placental function is suspect or labour shows the placental reserve to be low, e.g., if fœtal heart-rate falls ten beats per minute during the pains, then no form of analgesia lowering the maternal blood-oxygen tension should be used, such as gas–air. A maximal maternal blood-oxygen tension should be provided also in long labours, and in pregnancy toxæmia.

All anæsthetics, except nitrous oxide and oxygen, and all analgesic agents, other than bromide and chloral in reasonable dosage, depress the fœtal respiratory mechanism, an effect made worse by any hypoxia of the mother during labour. The placenta acts as no barrier to these agents. There is definite evidence that hypoxia of the fœtus during labour, and of the baby at birth or shortly afterwards, may be followed by impaired cerebral function in later life.* The danger is increased with premature infants.

Management of Asphyxia of the Newborn.—The fœtal circulation can withstand 10–15 min. of anoxia but deficient cerebral blood-flow may cause permanent damage. The fœtus in utero is cyanosed. The normally delivered child should breathe rhythmically from the beginning, air replacing liquor amnii as the fluid is respired. Alveoli are opened up by the negative pressure exerted by normal respiratory movements (−50 cm. water)—as in crying. In respiratory depression respiration begins differently, in gasps—the most primitive respiratory movement, involving many muscles.

Apgar† has described a system whereby the condition of a neonate can be assessed, one (or more) minutes after birth. A score of 0, 1, or 2 is given in each of five variables—heart-rate, respiratory effort, muscle tone, colour, and reflex irritability. The maximum score is 10. A single clinical assessment at one minute does not distinguish between primary apnœa (which will usually recover without treatment) and terminal apnœa (when active resuscitation is required).‡ Important factors are: (a) changes in heart-rate before resuscitation; (b) whether gasping precedes

APGAR SCORING SYSTEM

	HEART-RATE	RESPIRATORY EFFORT	MUSCLE TONE	COLOUR	REFLEX IRRITABILITY
0	Absent	Absent	Flaccid	Blue or white	No response
1	Slow, less than 100	Weak cry, hypoventilation	Some flexion of limbs	Blue hands or feet	Some movement
2	100 or over	Crying lustily	Well flexed	Healthy pink	Active movement

* Penfield, Wilder, *Curr. Res. Anesth.*, 1954, **33**, 145.
† Apgar, V., *Ibid.*, 1953, **32**, 260.
‡ Gupta, J. M., and Tizard, J. P. M., *Lancet*, 1967, **2**, 55.

Management of Asphyxia of the Newborn, *continued.*

an improvement in colour or vice versa; (c) whether or not apnœa supervenes in a baby who has initially gasped or cried.

Blue asphyxia seldom requires more than clearing the upper air-passages by suction, etc., using a rubber-ended rather than a metal-ended instrument, giving periods of negative pressure of 100–150 cm. water. A plastic suction catheter (No. 6 Fr.) is also useful for this purpose. Skin stimulation, passive limb movements, slapping, etc., are also very valuable, while oxygen given via a nasal catheter is beneficial. A useful method is to insufflate 2–3 l. per min. of oxygen, from a small rubber catheter into the infant's mouth, while its mouth and nares are occluded. This is sufficient to distend the lungs, and can be continued rhythmically for some time without causing trauma.* Better is the use of a neonatal inflating bag.† In feeble babies, a small stomach tube should be passed to evacuate the stomach of liquor amnii and prevent its aspiration into the lungs.

If no improvement takes place within 3–4 min. during which mouth, nose, and pharyngeal suction is carried out and oxygen is given from a plastic funnel (4 l. per min.) or from a nasal catheter (1 l. per min.), the trachea should be intubated, aspirated through a No. 6 Fr. plastic catheter, and the lungs inflated with oxygen. Incorrect insertion of an endotracheal tube may cause loss of the tube in the œsophagus requiring removal under general anæsthesia.‡ Any baby born apnœic, flaccid, or with a slow heart-beat should be intubated. To obtain proficiency in intubating neonates, a model 'resusci-baby' (Oxygenaire, Ltd.) is most useful.

Suitable tubes include the Magill 3 mm.; the Portsmouth Riplex tube§ with a shoulder separating the tracheal from the pharyngeal part, which is a modification of Cole's tube;|| the St. Thomas's Hospital tube,¶ a 3-mm., 6-in. plastic tube. The last two are supplied ready sterilized. Blind oral intubation in neonates has been advocated.**

Oxygen is carried to the lungs by: (1) a Jackson Rees modification of Ayre's T-piece,†† with manual compression of the reservoir bag; or (2) pressure from an oxygen cylinder giving 2–3 l. per min. where the gas is led from a water manometer which can deliver pressures of 40 cm. water for inflation of an atelectatic lung, or 10–15 cm. water for use when the lungs have been inflated. A small hole in the tubing is occluded by the finger to build up controlled pressure so that frequent half-second puffs of oxygen can be given. The pressure needed to expand the

---

* Knowles, G. S. A., *Brit. med. J.*, 1952, **2**, 1151.
† Mushin, W. W., and Hillard, E. K., *Ibid.*, 1967, **1**, 416.
‡ Dickson, J. A. S., and others, *Ibid.*, 1967, **2**, 811.
§ Tunstall, M. E., and Hodges, J. J. H., *Lancet*, 1961, **1**, 146.
|| Cole, F., *Anesthesiology*, 1945, **6**, 87 and 627.
¶ Barrie, H., *Lancet*, 1963, **1**, 650.
** Doss, A. F., *Brit. med. J.*, 1964, **2**, 1331.
†† Rees, G. Jackson, in *General Anæsthesia*, Vol. 2, p. 191 (Ed. Evans, F. T., and Gray, T. C.), 1959. London : Butterworths.

newborn lung is less than 50 cm. water. Pressures greater than this may cause rupture of the lung.*

To intubate a neonate the patient should be on a flat table with no pillow. Intubation should not be attempted in a cot. The head should not be extended over the end of the table. The blade of the infant laryngoscope should be inserted as far as the glottis and then lifted vertically. Rhythmic inflation of oxygen often has beneficial results (probably because of changes in intrabronchial pressure rather than because of expansion of collapsed alveoli). There is evidence that a positive pressure of 30–50 cm. of water applied through an endotracheal tube for repeated short periods will cause a collapsed lung to expand.†

Closed chest massage, if required, can be carried out by pressure of two fingers over the mid-sternum.‡

Premature babies must not be given pure oxygen for any length of time. If they are cyanosed they may receive 40 per cent oxygen for short periods only, thus reducing the danger of retrolental fibroplasia.

DRUGS.—Injection into the umbilical vein of *alpha-lobeline* 3 mg. may help, while 0·1 to 0·5 mg. of *N-allyl nor-morphine* (nalorphine, lethidrone), similarly injected, will counteract any respiratory depression following injection of pethidine or morphine into the mother. It may have to be repeated as its stimulant effect may be shorter than the depressant effect of the sedative. Another method is to give an intravenous dose of 10 mg. to the mother just before delivery, if she has recently received morphine or one of its congeners. The drug *amiphenazole* (daptazole) gives promise as a respiratory stimulant. Like nalorphine it can be given either to the mother who has recently received morphine or pethidine (20 mg. intramuscularly), or into the infant's umbilical vein (3 mg.). It is said to be relatively harmless and does not abolish the analgesic effects of opiates, etc., in the mother. Its effects are less prolonged than those of morphine in labour. It reduces but does not abolish neonatal apnœa caused by morphine.§ *Nikethamide* (0·5 ml. of 5 per cent solution) and *vanillic acid diethylamide* (vandid) (0·5 ml. of 25 per cent solution) placed on the tongue both have an appreciable stimulant effect on respiration.‖

Severe asphyxia has been successfully treated by *hypothermia* with a colonic temperature of 73° F. (23° C.) to 87° F. (30° C.) together with a small transfusion of oxygenated blood.¶

An entirely new approach to the treatment of hypoventilation or apnœa in the newborn baby has been described by Cooke and Bryce-Smith.** The child is placed within a *transparent airtight cabinet* and its trachea connected up to the exterior by a tube. Into this tube oxygen can be drawn and exhaled

* Rosen, M., and Laurence, K. M., *Lancet*, 1965, **2**, 721.
† Goddard, R. F., *Curr. Res. Anesth.*, 1955, **34**, 1.
‡ Moya, F., and others, *Anesthesiology*, 1961, **22**, 644.
§ Holmes, J. M., *Lancet*, 1956, **2**, 765.
‖ Barrie, H., and others, *Ibid.*, 1962, **2**, 742.
¶ Weston, B., and others, *Surgery*, 1959, **45**, 868.
** Cooke, M., and Bryce-Smith, R., *Anæsthesia*, 1962, **17**, 133.

Management of Asphyxia of the Newborn, *continued.*

gas can be extruded by subatmospheric pressure, intermittently produced by a hand bellows connected to the airtight cabinet.

Hyperbaric Oxygen.—A special pressure oxygen cabinet with a maximal working pressure of 4 atmospheres absolute (45 lb. per sq. in.) has been constructed. The infant is placed inside and is supplied with an oxygen flow of 7 l. per min. to wash out CO_2.* In a recent study, hyperbaric oxygenation and tracheal intubation with I.P.P.V. were equally effective methods of resuscitation.†

Electrical stimulation of the phrenic nerves through an intact skin was first applied by Hufeland in 1783 and again by Ziemssen in 1857. Sarnoff (1948) and Cross (1950) have recently reported good results following its use. Stimulation of the phrenic by a suitable electric current will cause contraction of the diaphragm and inspiration.‡ It cannot cause emphysema. The phrenic motor point lies anterior to the scalenus anterior muscle and is most readily palpated if the supine patient faces directly upwards. The airway must of course be patent. The method has also been used successfully in adults.

Focal epilepsy in later life can often be ascribed to neonatal hypoxia or to improper head compression during labour.§
(*See also* review by Barrie, H., *Lancet*, 1963, **1**, 650.)

Hyaline Membrane Disease.‖—The idiopathic respiratory distress syndrome of the newborn is the commonest cause of death in liveborn premature infants. The incidence is related to the degree of prematurity and is rare in infants born at term. One baby out of every 200 born alive dies of respiratory failure in the first few days of life. An equal number have respiratory distress but recover normal function. The distress may show itself from birth or may come on several hours later, and is characterized by severe retraction of the chest wall during inspiration, cyanosis, an increased respiratory rate, and an expiratory grunt. Recovery is usual in those babies who survive beyond the third day. The lungs are grossly atelectatic, and the radiographic appearances are those of 'ground glass'. The alveoli and terminal bronchioles are lined by a hyaline membrane, first described in 1925.¶ The material interfering with ventilation is probably formed from the lung itself and not inhaled. It is believed that lack of a surface tension-lowering substance—surfactant—in the alveolar spaces, is causal.** Surfactant is a lipoprotein containing dipalmitryl

---

* Sutnick, A. I., and Soloff, L. A., *Amer. J. Med.*, 1962, **35**, 31; and Patkin, M., *Anæsthesia*, 1965, **20**, 351.
† Hutchison, J. H., Kerr, M. M., Inall, J. A., and Shanks, R. A., *Lancet*, 1966, **1**, 935.
‡ *See also* Cross, K. W., and Roberts, P. W., *Brit. med. J.*, 1951, **1**, 1043; and Sarnoff, S. J., *Ibid.*, 1951, **1**, 1515.
§ Penfield, Wilder, *Curr. Res. Anesth.*, 1954, **33**, 145.
‖ *See* Leading Article, *Brit. med. J.*, 1967, **1**, 1.
¶ Johnson, W. C., and Meyer, J. R., *Amer. J. Obstet. Gynec.*, 1925, **9**, 151; *see also* Strang, L. B., *Brit. med. Bull.*, 1963, **19**, 1, 45.
** Avery, M. E., and Mead, J., *Amer. J. Dis. Child.*, 1959, **97**, 515; and Hutchison, J. H., and others, *Lancet*, 1963, **2**, 1019.

lecithin. Its function is to confer stability on the terminal air spaces, or to act as an anti-atelectasis factor.* The condition is most frequently seen in premature babies, which include babies born to mothers suffering from diabetes, toxæmia, or placenta prævia. Cæsarean section is probably not a cause.

A biochemical explanation has been suggested† and it has been shown that in neonates a metabolic acidosis is usual. If inadequate respiration allows acid-base imbalance, hyperkalæmia may occur. It has also been suggested that routine placental transfusion of blood may reduce the incidence of the condition. The infant should be nursed in an incubator in a humid atmosphere and at a temperature (95° F., 35° C.) to minimize oxygen consumption.‡ Careful monitoring of blood gases and pH is mandatory, and metabolic acidosis corrected by sodium bicarbonate which may be given orally or intravenously. The atmosphere should be oxygen enriched to maintain an arterial oxygen tension as near normal as possible. I.P.P.V. may be required, though survival is then unusual, infants dying with severe lung damage.§

This whole question is well discussed in *Proc. R. Soc. Med.*, 1962, **12**, 1095.

CHAPTER XXVI

CHOICE OF ANÆSTHETIC AGENTS AND METHODS AS INFLUENCED BY GENERAL CONDITION OF PATIENT

Anæsthesia is now a very safe procedure in the fit healthy patient. The risk is increased when systemic disease is present. In a study where patients were classified according to physical status (p. 75), 16,000 cases of physical status I were operated on without any death attributable to anæsthesia. In patients of physical status V, there was a 10 per cent mortality rate.‖

Old Age.—The following may occur : dehydration, tissue wasting, cardiac enlargement and perhaps dilatation ; arteriosclerosis of renal, cerebral, and cardiac vessels ; stiffening of thoracic cage with ossification of cartilages, emphysema, narrowing of bronchioles, and dilatation of alveoli ; atrophy of brain and increase in cerebrospinal fluid volume with dilatation of cerebral ventricles ; atrophy of mandibles and increased brittleness of bones ; atrophy of tissue cells and proliferation of connective tissue ; diminution of blood-volume and hæmoglobin and decreased cardiac reserve with slowing of circulation time ; decreased thoracic and increased

---

* *See also* Avery, M. E., and Normand, C., *Anesthesiology*, 1965, **26**, 510.
† Reardon, H., and others, *J. Pediat.*, 1960, **57**, 151 ; *see also* Annotation in *Lancet*, 1960, **2**, 1071.
‡ Scopes, J. W., *Brit. med. Bull.*, 1966, **22**, 88.
§ Hawker, J. W., and others, *Lancet*, 1967, **2**, 75.
‖ Dripps, R. D., Lamont, A., and Eckenhoff, J. E., *J. Amer. med. Ass.*, 1961 ,**178**, 261.

Old Age, *continued.*

abdominal respiration ; decreased tidal volume and vital capacity, with consequent tachypnœa. In the post-operative state there may be diminished activity of the cough reflex which may predispose to atelectasis.

In old age, the most incurable of all diseases, the emotions are often well under control, so that the patient is easy to manage. Muscular relaxation is also often easy to produce. As metabolism is low, sedatives should be ordered with care and atropine substituted for hyoscine as the latter may produce stimulation of the central nervous system with restlessness and delirium. It has been suggested that adverse cerebral effects of anæsthesia in old people are more common than is realized.* But a recent very careful survey† investigating the pre- and post-operative condition of a large group of elderly patients showed that anæsthesia had no effect on the physiological or mental activity or on the personality. Toothless gums and flabby cheeks may cause difficulty with the airway. Too much premedication may cause the patient to appear pale and collapsed. Hypoxia is not well tolerated as the blood oxygen tension is reduced in old people.

PRE- AND POST-OPERATIVE SEDATION.—Old people may become confused ; a common cause for this being cerebral hypoxia due to cardiovascular or respiratory abnormality. Barbiturates will make this disorientation worse. To produce sleep, alcohol is useful for those accustomed to it, while a chloral hydrate derivative, e.g., dichloral phenazone 0·5–2 g., trichlorethyl phosphate 250–500 mg., may be suitable. Paraldehyde by mouth or intramuscularly in 5-ml. doses, or chlorpromazine 100 mg. intramuscularly, is also useful. Confusion caused by sedatives should not be treated by further sedation. For post-operative depression, imipramine hydrochloride (tofranil) 30–100 mg. is useful.

For severe pain, methadone (physeptone) 10 mg. is less depressing to the respiratory centre, and is as good an analgesic as morphine or pethidine, while for the pain of incurable cancer, chlorpromazine can be combined with it.

Extra- and intradural analgesia is often very suitable for operations below the umbilicus. Blood-pressure-raising drugs should not be injected, if indeed they are used at all, until it is known that the block is working well, lest a blood-pressure too high for the inelastic vascular system should be produced, with a resulting vascular accident.

Thiopentone is well tolerated as a rule, if dosage is kept down.

Early post-operation ambulation is usually desirable, to prevent the development of phlebothrombosis, while rapid recovery of the cough reflex is important in the prevention of post-operative atelectasis.

In old people with emphysema, general anæsthesia with halothane, maintaining spontaneous respiration, has given good results and

---

* Bedford, P. D., *Lancet*, 1955, **2**, 259.
† Simpson, B. R., Williams, M., Scott, J. F., and Crampton-Smith, A., *Ibid.*, 1961, **2**, 887.

for upper abdominal surgery may well be combined with small doses of relaxants or bilateral intercostal nerve-block to aid relaxation.* Good speedy operating is valuable at all times and is especially to be desired in elderly people.

Pregnancy.—Physiological changes associated with pregnancy of interest to anæsthetists include water and salt retention ; increased total blood-volume ; a tendency to secondary anæmia ; an increased pulse-rate unaccompanied by changes in blood-pressure ; increased pulmonary ventilation, sometimes accompanied by dyspnœa ; movement to the right of the oxygen dissociation curve of hæmoglobin ; a lowered renal threshold sometimes causing glycosuria.

Anæsthetics are well tolerated, but should, if possible, be avoided during the menstrual epochs in the early months, lest anæsthesia gets the blame for possible abortion. Curare does not increase uterine tone in pregnancy, nor do intradural and extradural blocks. Hypoxia and hypotension must be avoided.

The hypotensive supine syndrome of late pregnancy must be borne in mind and many such patients are better anæsthetized in the lateral position.†

Hiatus Hernia.‡—The presence of this abnormality, often unknown or unsuspected, may result in regurgitation during induction or maintenance of anæsthesia. It is most likely to occur in middle-aged obese patients or those in advanced pregnancy and is fostered by a pressure differential between the stomach and the œsophagus. This can be caused by: (1) Increased intragastric pressure, as in obesity, abdominal tumour, distension, ascites, late pregnancy or posture (lithotomy or head-down positions) ; (2) Relative decrease in intra-œsophageal pressure in cases of inspiratory obstruction with hyperpnœa, part of a reduced intrathoracic pressure.

If there is a history suggestive of hiatus hernia with complaints of pyrosis with retrosternal pain and reflux into the œsophagus induced by gravity, then such patients should be treated by the anæsthetist as if they are suffering from acute intestinal obstruction in order to reduce the likelihood of regurgitation and subsequent aspiration of gastric contents into the lungs.

Asthma.—

PRE-OPERATIVE TREATMENT OF PATIENTS WITH SEVERE BRONCHIAL ASTHMA.—(1) Bronchodilators : (a) Aerosol containing 2 per cent phenylephrine with 0·4 per cent isoprotorenol ; (b) Oral ephedrine, 25 mg., 4-hourly, and aminophylline, 200–300 mg., 4-hourly—this can also be given intravenously in dextrose (500 mg.) or per rectum, 500 mg. dissolved in 30 ml. water; or (c) Orciprenaline (alupent) 20 mg. by mouth. (2) Steroids. To reduce œdema and relieve spasm. Oral prednisone, 10–25 mg., 4-hourly, for 4 days before operation, and 50–100 mg. intravenously during operation ; orally in decreasing

---

* Scott, D. L., *Brit. J. Anæsth.*, 1961, **33**, 354.
† Holmes, F., *J. Obstet. Gynæc., Brit. Emp.*, 1958, **44**, 229.
‡ Dinnick, O. P., *Lancet*, 1961, **1**, 470.

Asthma, *continued.*

doses after operation. Antacids to prevent hyperchlorhydria in addition.

Anæsthetics well tolerated. Ether and halothane, being bronchodilators, are especially suitable, while it is of great importance that upper respiratory tract reflexes should be completely suppressed from the outset. Thiopentone not contra-indicated but must be used with care, as both it and cyclopropane may cause bronchospasm and wheezing. Hexobarbitone or propanidid is often preferable to thiopentone in asthmatic patients.

In cases of grave bronchospasm when the lungs will not deflate, benefit may follow the insertion of a tube into the pleural cavity and deflation by oxygen pressure, or open chest lung massage.*

Status asthmaticus has been successfully treated by I.P.P.V. and also by continuous high extradural block.†

Anæmia.—This should, when possible, be treated medically before operation. Hypoxia must be avoided. Barbiturates reduce the number of circulating red cells by causing their absorption by the spleen. Cyclopropane is most satisfactory in these cases. If hæmoglobin percentage is less than 50, a transfusion should be given. Extradural analgesia not suitable for patients with anæmia or who are likely to undergo severe blood-loss. Anæmia causes atony of muscles, including myocardium. It also causes impairment of conduction of nerve impulses. In anæmia, grave hypoxia may not be accompanied by cyanosis. There is an oxygen lack in the circulating blood—a reduction in oxygen content, not in oxygen tension.

Sickle-cell Anæmia and Sickle-cell Trait‡ (Drepanocytosis).—This is a recessive disease not infrequently seen in patients of tropical African descent and commonest in children. It is due to the replacement of normal hæmoglobin A by abnormal hæmoglobin S. The clinical condition was first described by Herrick in 1910 while hæmoglobin S was first described by Pauling in 1949.§ In *sickle-cell anæmia* all the hæmoglobin is of the S variety, in the *trait* hæmoglobin S represents 30–40 per cent of the total hæmoglobin, the remainder being of the normal type. Hæmoglobin S is vulnerable to various changes in the physical and chemical environment of the patient, especially to reduction in the oxygen tension of the blood. Should this be less than 45 mm. Hg the reduced hæmoglobin forms liquid crystals called 'tactoids' which distort and finally rupture the red cells. These altered cells cause capillary and venous thromboses and later infarction and their destruction results in anæmia. In the trait the Po_2 must fall to 25 or below before changes in the hæmoglobin occur. Increasing the Po_2 does not reverse these changes. Acute crises may interrupt the chronic state.

In addition to the anæmia which may be either hæmolytic or aplastic (due to bone changes and infarction) there may be:

---

* Smolnikoff, V. P., *Anæsthesia*, 1960, **15**, 40.

† Bromage, P. R., 1967, personal communication.

‡ *See also* Lehmann, H., and Huntsman, R. G., *Man's Hæmoglobins*, 1966, Ch. 8. Amsterdam: North Holland Publishing Co.

§ Pauling, L., and others, *Science, N.Y.*, 1949, **110**, 543.

(1) Thrombotic lesions in the lungs, kidneys, bones, or brain; (2) Hæmorrhages in various organs including the ocular vitreous and abdominal viscera; (3) Shift of the oxygen-hæmoglobin dissociation curve to the right; (4) Enlarged heart; (5) Enlarged liver.

Patients may present for surgery because of: (1) Abdominal pain due to vascular lesions; (2) Osteomyelitis; (3) Priapism; (4) Leg ulcers; (5) Gall-stones.

MANAGEMENT.—All Negroes should be tested for sickling before operation. In those affected the following must be avoided: (1) Hypoxia; (2) Hypothermia; (3) The use of tourniquets.

Blood transfusion must be reserved for patients with a hæmoglobin of less than 4 g./100 ml., while a level of 8 g./100 ml. is required before operation is undertaken. Anticoagulants are useless before operation but low molecular weight dextran may be helpful. Before operation sodium bicarbonate should be given 0·5–1 g./kg. daily or in emergency 3·3 mEq./kg. intravenously. The higher the alkali reserve the greater the degree of hypoxia necessary to cause sickling.

Regional analgesia should be preferred to general anæsthesia where suitable, while the latter should always be accompanied by the administration of an excess of oxygen. The halothane–oxygen technique may be very satisfactory. Sickling can occur in what seems to be a faultless anæsthetic procedure. Postoperative hypoxæmia must be prevented and anticoagulants may be required after surgery to prevent pulmonary embolism, especially if thrombosis or pain in the bones is present.

(*See also* Walters, J., and others, *Proc. R. Soc. Med.*, 1964, **57**, 1147; Gilbertson, A. A., *Brit. J. Anæsth.*, 1965, **37**, 614; Brown, R. A., *Ibid.*, 1965, **37**, 181; and Gilbertson, A. A., and Boulton, T. B., *Anæsthesia*, 1967, **22**, 607.)

Idiopathic Myoglobinuria (Idiopathic Recurrent Rhabdomyolysis).—A syndrome with muscle pain and red urine with a normal urinary sediment in the absence of intravascular hæmolysis. It is possible that the fasciculations caused by suxamethonium and decamethonium may exacerbate the condition (like muscular exercise) and even lead to renal failure from tubular blockage with pigment.*

Methæmoglobinæmia.†—If a patient appears cyanosed in the absence of heart or lung disease, the blood should be spectroscopically examined for abnormal pigments. The condition may be idiopathic or secondary to exogenous toxins, e.g., nitrites, sulphonamides, phenacetin, prilocaine, etc. Methæmoglobinæmia can be dangerous during anæsthesia as the oxygen-carrying capacity of the blood is reduced, the oxygen dissociation curve being shifted to the left. The condition is treatable by the intravenous injection of methylene blue (1 to 2 mg. per kg. given over 5 minutes) which specifically converts methæmoglobin to normal hæmoglobin.

---

* Bennike, K., and Jarum, S., *Brit. J. Anæsth.*, 1964, **36**, 730; and Jensen, K., Bennike, K., Hanel, H. K., and Olesen, H., *Ibid.*, 1968, **40**, 329.
†Joseph, D., *Ibid.*, 1962, **34**, 309.

Sulphæmoglobinæmia.—This is produced by an oxidizing agent (often in the presence of a bowel upset) or a sulphur-containing drug. In some patients methæmoglobin and sulphæmoglobin are both present. Sulphæmoglobin cannot be reversed. It stays in the red cell for the remainder of its life span.

Hæmophilia.*—There are between 1500 and 2000 male hæmophiliacs in Britain. Diagnosis may be difficult but the thromboplastin-generation test will detect almost every case. There is no such thing, surgically, as a mild hæmophiliac. If a female carries the hæmophilia gene she is herself unaffected but has a 1 : 2 chance of passing the disorder on to her sons, or a carrier state to her daughters. With good pathological backing, most patients with this disorder can withstand necessary operations. About 88 per cent of coagulation defects are due to hæmophilia A, 8 per cent being due to hæmophilia B or Christmas disease. In the former there is a deficiency of Factor VIII, in the latter of Factor IX. The missing factor must be replaced before operation, in the case of hæmophilia, by antihæmophilic globulin (A.H.G.). In this disease the Factor VIII may vary from 0 to 20 per cent (normal is 100 per cent). For safe surgery 25 per cent is required. The half-life of A.H.G. is about 14 hours, so repeated high dosage is required to keep the level greater than 25 per cent. A small number of hæmophiliacs have in addition, a circulating anticoagulant which destroys all A.H.G. injected and so makes them unsuitable for surgery.

REPLACEMENT OF A.H.G.—(1) *Plasma*: Reasonable amounts will not raise the A.H.G. much above 20 per cent, so it and also fresh blood are only useful for trivial operations. (2) *Human A.H.G.*: This is in short supply and should be used mainly for children. (3) *Animal A.H.G.*: This is obtained from the cow and the pig and, though potent and effective, is antigenic. Its use cannot be continued for more than 10–14 days nor given on more than two or three occasions. It is very expensive. Dosage is controlled by estimations of the A.H.G.†

Local analgesia is not contra-indicated, e.g., for dental extractions, but in general anæsthesia gentleness is necessary to prevent minor trauma which might cause bleeding.

DENTAL EXTRACTIONS.—(1) For extraction of deciduous teeth in children and single teeth in adults, fresh frozen plasma is adequate. (2) For extraction of 2–9 teeth in adults human A.H.G. is given for the first 2 days and then plasma. (3) For extraction of a larger number of teeth or of impacted lower third molars, human A.H.G. 13–15 units per kg. is an average dose.‡ Epsilon-aminocaproic acid can be used.§ *See also* p. 615.

For management, during dental surgery, of patients on anticoagulants, *see* McIntyre, H., *Lancet*, 1966, **2**, 99.

---

* McIntyre, H., Nour-Eldin, F., Isreals, M. C. G., and Wilkinson, J. F., *Lancet*, 1959, **2**, 642.

† Livingstone, G., *Proc. R. Soc. Med.*, 1965, **58**, 65.

‡ Biggs, R., and others, *Lancet*, 1965, **1**, 969.

§ Cooksey, M. W., and others, *Brit. med. J.*, 1966, **2**, 1633; and Davies, R. M., and Scott, J. G., *Brit. J. Anæsth.*, 1968, **40**, 202.

Christmas Disease has the same mode of inheritance and clinical features as hæmophilia, but the Christmas factor is more stable than antihæmophilic globulin and is present in stored normal blood.

Myasthenia Gravis.*—The *myasthenic state* may be present as follows :
1. Myasthenia gravis: (a) Classic; (b) Undiagnosed; (c) During remission. First described by Friedrich Jolly (1844–1904).†
2. Associated with other diseases : (a) Thyrotoxicosis ; (b) Collagen diseases ; (c) Carcinoma, especially of the bronchus.
3. Caused by drugs : (a) Neomycin ; (b) Streptomycin.

The treatment of myasthenia by the anticholinesterase drug physostigmine was first described by M. Walker in 1934 in Greenwich. It appears to be a condition in which the response of the motor end-plate to acetylcholine no longer gives a short depolarizing block, but results in a more prolonged dual block and consequent muscular weakness.

The first thymectomy for myasthenia gravis was performed by F. Sauerbruch in 1911 and the operation was further developed by Blalock‡ in 1936. Geoffrey Keynes did the first such operation in Britain in 1942.§

The injection of blood fractions contained in globulin from patients with myasthenia into normal rats causes neuromuscular block which has features of both depolarizing and non-depolarizing block.‖

Myasthenia gravis is a chronic disease of disputed aetiology, characterized by exacerbations and remissions. It may occur at any period of life including childhood and old age, and while severe cases are easily diagnosed, mild ones can be overlooked and may cause anæsthetic difficulties. Some of the muscles of the head and neck are usually involved and may give rise to ptosis, dysphagia, and easy fatigue of the jaw muscles. Muscle weakness comes on after exercise and improves following rest. The myoneural block which is present may be non-depolarizing in some end-plates (and so reversible), but depolarizing in others. The myoneural junction may react to choline with the production of a non-depolarizing block.¶

A *cholinergic crisis* consists of a state of muscle weakness and fasciculation, lacrimation, sweating, and abdominal colic due to relative overdosage with anticholinesterase drugs. It is distinguished from myasthenic weakness by the response to edrophonium which temporarily exacerbates the cholinergic crisis but improves myasthenic weakness.

TESTS FOR MYASTHENIA GRAVIS.—
1. Edrophonium, 2 mg., is injected intravenously and if in half a minute there is no response a further 8 mg. are given. In myasthenics there is a full but temporary return of muscular

---

* Matthews, W. A., and Derrick, W. S., *Anesthesiology*, 1957, **18**, 443 ; and McClelland, R. M. A., *Brit. J. Anæsth.*, 1960, **32**, 81 ; *see also* review article, Foldes, F. F., and McNall, P. G., *Anesthesiology*, 1962, **23**, 837.

† Jolly, F., *Neurol. Zbl.*, 1895, **14**, 34.

‡ Blalock, A., and others, *Ann. Surg.*, 1939, **110**, 544.

§ Keynes, G., *Brit. J. Surg.*, 1946, **33**, 201.

‖ Parkes, J. D., and McKinna, J. A., *Lancet*, 1966, **1**, 388.

¶ Grob, D., and others, *Bull. Johns Hopk. Hosp.*, 1956, **99**, 115.

Myasthenia Gravis, *continued.*

power. In normal patients and myasthenics who are adequately treated there may be muscular fasciculations, colic, salivation, and diarrhœa, but muscular weakness is unaffected.

2. Decamethonium. In the stage of the disease before clinical signs develop (the stage of resistance), myasthenic muscle can withstand an abnormally large dose of decamethonium without showing weakness. In the later stage (the stage of dual block) the drug produces not a depolarizing block but a dual or biphasic block reversible by edrophonium and neostigmine. The last stage is the stage of myopathy with muscle wasting or atrophy.* The combination of decamethonium and electromyography can be used in the diagnosis of myasthenia.†

PRE-OPERATIVE PREPARATION.—The serum potassium should be estimated (normal value 4–5 mEq. per l.) as hypokalæmia aggravates myasthenia. A chest radiograph is desirable. Respiratory infection should contra-indicate all but the most urgent operations. Neostigmine should be given by mouth until the optimum dosage is reached but should be slightly reduced just before operation to avoid anticholinesterase excess.

Sedative premedication should be minimal. Opiates and barbiturates should be avoided.

USE OF RELAXANTS IN MYASTHENIA GRAVIS.—

1. Non-depolarizing relaxants cause hypersensitivity of affected muscles only. Other muscles behave normally.

2. Decamethonium is abnormally well tolerated in mild cases but causes hypersensitivity in severe cases, but the block is a non-depolarizing one, preceded by a brief depolarizing block, i.e., it is a dual block. Suxamethonium should be given very carefully as it causes a muscular paralysis of dual or biphasic type and recovery is neither as rapid nor as complete as in normal patients.

ANÆSTHETIC MANAGEMENT.—The chief concern is to ensure adequate respiration both during and after the operation, while the special difficulties to be borne in mind are muscular weakness and bronchial secretion from neostigmine. Regional analgesia which does not depress respiration, e.g., intra- or extradural block to T.10, may be suitable. Ether and thiopentone should be used most sparingly if at all, but cyclopropane and halothane are satisfactory agents. Relaxants are better avoided. The non-depolarizers are contra-indicated and it must be remembered that decamethonium may act as a non-depolarizer in this disease. Suxamethonium is the preferred relaxant but this too must be given as sparingly as possible. The dual or biphasic response it causes is of shorter duration than that caused by decamethonium because of hydrolysis; it can be reversed by neostigmine or edrophonium if its effects are unduly prolonged. Some myasthenic patients are very resistant to suxamethonium and decamethonium. Endotracheal intubation may well be advisable,

---

* *See also* Jenkins, L. C., and others, *Canad. Anæsth. Soc. J.*, 1964, **11**, 633.
† Wylie, W. D., and Churchill-Davidson, H. C., *A Practice of Anæsthesia*, 1960, p. 624. London : Lloyd-Luke.

both to ensure a perfect airway and to facilitate tracheobronchial aspiration. Neostigmine or edrophonium may be given intravenously with care either during or after operation if respiration is peripherally depressed (but overdosage after operation can give rise to a cholinergic crisis), while aspiration of secretions from the upper respiratory tract must be performed with frequency, enthusiasm, and efficiency. The possible need for artificial respiration after operation, perhaps from a machine, and for tracheostomy must be provided for.* Many workers now agree that elective tracheostomy, with I.P.P.V. if indicated by blood-gas analysis, is indicated in patients who have even mild involvement of the respiratory or pharyngeal muscles.† Anticholinesterase drugs may then be avoided in the immediate post-operative period, with the result that a cholinergic crisis does not occur, and a better effect may be expected if and when they are resumed. Only when the eye and limb muscles are involved and the pharyngeal and respiratory muscles spared, is spontaneous respiration allowed.

Neonatal myasthenia has been described. It develops within a few hours or days after birth in some infants born of myasthenic mothers. If the diagnosis is suspected edrophonium, 0·5–1·0 mg., may be given intramuscularly. The effect of pregnancy on the mother is variable. In about one-quarter of patients there is improvement, and in about one-third there is an exacerbation during or after pregnancy. In most cases the pregnant mother has no change in the myasthenic state.

MYASTHENIC SYNDROME COMPLICATING BRONCHIAL CARCINOMA.—A condition of muscular weakness developing at the periphery in a patient with bronchial carcinoma, usually in older males. Was formerly called 'carcinomatous neuropathy'.‡ A small minority of patients with bronchial carcinoma, less than 1 per cent, may develop prolonged apnœa after anæsthesia. The condition was first described as a distinct entity by Eaton and Lambert in 1957.§ It differs from myasthenia gravis as follows: (1) It involves the proximal muscles of the limbs rather than the bulbar and extra-ocular muscles; (2) The presence of aching muscular pains in the limbs; (3) Diminished tendon reflexes; (4) A poor response of the myoneural block to neostigmine; (5) A very marked sensitivity to tubocurarine, even 5 mg. sometimes causing prolonged apnœa; (6) An increased sensitivity to depolarizing relaxants; (7) Electromyographic characteristics: (a) Low-voltage action potentials at twitch rates of supramaximal stimulation; (b) Growth of potentials with tetanic rates of stimulation.‖

MANAGEMENT OF MYASTHENIC EMERGENCIES (UNDER-VENTILATION).—These may be related to, or unassociated

* Harland, J. H., and Stephen, C. R., Canad. Anæsth. Soc. J., 1958, 5, 325.
† Schwab, R. S., and others, J. Amer. med. Ass., 1964, 187, 850; and Baird, W. L. M., and Norris, W., Brit. J. Anæsth., 1965, 37, 174.
‡ Croft, P. B., Brit. med. J., 1958, 1, 181.
§ Eaton, M. L., and Lambert, E. H., J. Amer. med. Ass., 1957, 163, 1117.
‖ Wise, R. P., Brit. J. Anæsth., 1963, 35, 558; and Anæsthesia, 1962, 17, 448.

Myasthenia Gravis, *continued.*

with, anæsthesia and surgery. The first and most important factor is to ensure a clear airway and adequate respiratory exchange, using an endotracheal or tracheostomy tube and intermittent positive pressure. The emergency may be due to (1) Myasthenia in exacerbation ; (2) Cholinergic crisis ; (3) A less clear-cut entity associated with insensitivity of the neuromuscular junction to acetylcholine. It is advisable to withhold all drugs until the nature of the emergency has been diagnosed

1. Exacerbation of myasthenia. When this is the cause of the emergency neostigmine may be given intravenously over several minutes, the first dose not more than 0·3 mg., and preceded by atropine 0·4–0·6 mg. intravenously.

2. Cholinergic crisis. Atropine 0·4–1·0 mg. may be given intravenously to control muscarinic reactions. All anticholinesterase medication must be withdrawn, if necessary for several days, until tests with edrophonium indicate that the end-plates have regained their sensitivity to acetylcholine.

3. Insensitivity of end-plates to acetylcholine. All cholinesterase medication should be withdrawn and respiration maintained artificially. Churchill-Davidson and Richardson have gone further than this and administered tubocurarine to ' rest the end-plate, maintaining artificial ventilation for several days.*

4. Intravenous potassium should be administered if there is hypokalæmia (0·3 per cent KCl).

5. Other measures should include suction of the tracheobronchial tree, antibiotics, general nursing care, etc.

Rheumatoid Arthritis.—Potential difficulties may arise from (1) Flexion deformity of cervical vertebræ and involvement of temporomandibular joints making laryngoscopy difficult ; (2) Involvement of small joints of larynx and neuropathy of laryngeal muscles causing stridor ; (3) Amyloidosis of kidneys ; (4) Tendency to respiratory depression and interstitial pneumonia after operation; (5) Steroid therapy. Thus there may be difficulty in intubation together with the need for great care after operation.†

Ankylosis of Jaw.—This may be part of a generalized arthritis and may render laryngoscopy difficult. It must be diagnosed before induction, and sometimes blind intubation is of service.

Ankylosing Spondylitis.—The lungs in this condition perform efficiently, and sufferers from it may undergo operation on the lungs, heart, or abdomen without pulmonary complications as the diaphragm provides good compensation for the reduced chest movement.‡

Stiffness of the cervical spine and of the atlanto-occipital joint may cause difficulty during endotracheal intubation, so that occasionally the blind technique must be employed.

* Churchill-Davidson, H. C., and Richardson, A. T., *Lancet*, 1957, **1**, 1221.
† Gardner, D. C., and Holmes, F., *Brit. J. Anæsth.*, 1961, **33**, 258.
‡ Zorab, P. A., *Quart. J. Med.*, 1962, **31**, 267.

Kyphoscoliosis.—These patients are likely to have reduced vital capacity so their tidal volume is limited and cannot increase, e.g., in response to premedication which may slow the breathing-rate. Airway obstruction is seldom a feature. Fluoroscopic assessment of diaphragmatic movement is helpful in estimating operative risk.[*] Underventilation in these patients is a danger even before anæsthesia is induced and may be present also after operation. They show respiratory handicap and may have a lowered blood oxygen saturation and an abnormal ventilation perfusion ratio. The resulting hypoxia and hypercapnia eventually leads to fluid retention and to pulmonary hypertension as the result of pulmonary vasoconstriction. Right heart failure may follow as in chronic obstructive lung disease.[†] Cardiac failure secondary to severe scoliosis does not occur in children.

Achondroplasia.—There may be difficulties with endotracheal intubation, due to abnormalities at the base of the skull.[‡]

Paraplegia.[§]—Patients with transection of the cord at or above T.5 may get severe hypertension after certain visceral stimuli, e.g., distension of the bladder or rectum. Hexamethonium may be required to relieve this. About 40 per cent of such patients about to undergo operation will require anæsthesia as it is difficult to be sure that the lesion of the cord is complete.

The following factors must be borne in mind : (1) Excitability of autonomic reflexes ; (2) Psychiatric difficulties ; (3) Chronic infection ; (4) Nutritional difficulties ; (5) Disturbed temperature regulation ; (6) Problems of pain ; (7) Problems of respiration ; (8) Problems of position on the operating table.

Dystrophia Myotonica.[||]—This is a hereditary disease. Patients may show one or more of the following characteristics: (1) Expressionless face; (2) Sternomastoid wasting; (3) Limb weakness with inability to let go after a handshake; (4) Cataract; (5) Frontal baldness; (6) Atrophy of gonads; (7) Thyroid adenomata; (8) Percussion myotonia; (9) Familial incidence.

It is a primary disorder of muscular fibres and not of the myoneural junction. The sufferer may have respiratory muscle weakness giving rise to reduced pulmonary ventilation and an increased P_{CO_2}. There may be cardiovascular impairment and adrenal cortical dysfunction.

ANÆSTHETIC MANAGEMENT.[¶]—Lung function should be investigated by : (1) Measurement of vital capacity ; (2) Forced expiratory volume (1 second); (3) Fluoroscopy of chest to see if there is myotonia of the diaphragm.

Respiratory depressants should be avoided before, during, and after operation. Thiopentone has no specific peripheral

---

* Zorab, P. A., *Brit. med. J.*, 1966, **1**, 1155.
† Hanley, T., and others, *Quart. J. Med.*, 1958, **27**, 155.
‡ Mather, J. S., *Anæsthesia*, 1966, **21**, 244.
§ Guttmann, L., and Whitteridge, D., *Brain*, 1947, **70**, 36 ; and Rollo, A. G., and Vandam, L. D., *Anesthesiology*, 1959, **20**, 348.
|| Kaufman, L., *Proc. R. Soc. Med.*, 1960, **53**, 183 ; Bourke, T. D., and Zuck, D., *Brit. J. Anæsth.*, 1957, **29**, 135 ; Lodge, A. B., *Brit. med. J.*, 1958, **1**, 1043 ; and Dundee, J. W., *Curr. Res. Anesth.*, 1952, **31**, 257.
¶ Kaufman, L., *Proc. R. Soc. Med.*, 1960, **53**, 183.

Dystrophia Myotonica, *continued.*

depressant effect as it has in porphyria but if it is used it should be given in 50-mg. doses while its effects are watched. Assisted respiration may be required during operation, while I.P.P.V. perhaps through a tracheostomy may be necessary in the immediate post-operative period. Intubation is usually possible without the use of relaxants.

Spinal analgesia does not relax myotonia but injection of local analgesic solution into the muscle may do so. Non-depolarizing relaxants do not abolish myotonia but may be given very sparingly. Depolarizing relaxants usually have their normal effect, but a case of generalized myotonia following suxamethonium has been reported.* Decamethonium too has caused a generalized myotonic response. The increased muscle tone may represent an exaggerated fasciculation which gives place to ordinary depolarizing relaxation with injection of additional doses of the drug.† Thus the safety of these drugs in this condition is doubtful. The possibility of this disease, along with diabetes, should be borne in mind in anæsthetizing young patients with cataracts.

Progressive Muscular Dystrophy.‡—This disease causes changes not only in striated muscle but also in cardiac muscle and in the smooth muscle of the alimentary tract.

PREMEDICATION.—These patients have a tendency to tachycardia, so excitement must be avoided and atropine may be less suitable than hyoscine.

ANÆSTHESIA.—Thiopentone should only be given in small doses, its effects being carefully watched. The disease does not involve the myoneural junctions but both types of relaxant should only be given in small doses and their effects watched before additional amounts are injected. Inhalation agents may be suitable but the concentration of halothane should be increased with care.

COMPLICATIONS.—As the myocardium may be involved in the disease process, tachycardia is frequent and should not be made worse by the anæsthetic ; pre-operative digitalis may be desirable. Acute dilatation of the stomach may be seen after operation and may be due to a disorder of the smooth muscle of the wall of the viscus. It should be preventable by parenteral fluid therapy during the first day or two after operation and by assumption of the prone position for periods during the first 24 or 48 hours. If these measures fail, then a Ryle's tube must be passed.

Porphyria§ (from the Greek *porphyros* = purple).—First described by Stokvis, a Dutch physician, in 1889.|| Rare in England, prevalent

* Paterson, I. S., *Brit. J. Anæsth.*, 1962, **34**, 340.
† Thiel, R. E., *Ibid.*, 1967, **39**, 815.
‡ Wislicki, L., *Anæsthesia*, 1962, **17**, 482 ; and McClelland, R. M. A., *Brit. J. Anæsth.*, 1960, **32**, 81; and Cobham, I. G., and others, *Curr. Res. Anesth.*, 1964, **43**, 22.
§ Norris, W., and Macnab, G. W., *Brit. J. Anæsth.*, 1960, **32**, 505; Rimington, C., *Proc. R. Soc. Med.*, 1964, **57**, 511; Murphy, P. C., *Brit. J. Anæsth.*, 1964, **36**, 801; Bush, G. H., *Proc. R. Soc. Med.*, 1968, **61**, 171; and Symposium, *Ibid.*, 1968, **61**, 191.
|| Stokvis, B. J. E., *Ned. Tijdschr. Geneesk.*, 1889, **25**, 409.

in South Africa and Scandinavia. Classified by Waldenström* (1937) into: (1) Acute intermittent porphyria; (2) Congenital form with skin lesions and sensitivity to light; (3) Porphyria cutanea tarda with some features of both types. Cutaneous porphyrias are little if at all sensitive to barbiturates. Porphyria is a congenital metabolic defect and is characterized in its active phase by the passage of red or brown urine. If the condition is suspected the urine should be tested for the characteristic pigment by spectroscopy. The defect is inherited as an irregular Mendelian dominant, affected persons being heterozygous. The condition in South Africa is thought to have been carried by two early settlers from Holland. Acute attacks may arise *de novo* or may be associated with infection, pregnancy, or the ingestion of such drugs as barbiturates, alcohol, or sulphonamides. Clinical features are: (1) Gastro-intestinal: Abdominal pain; (2) Neurological: Lower motor neuron lesion, sensory disturbance, epilepsy, mental symptoms, rarely coma; (3) Cardiovascular: Tachycardia and raised blood-pressure when disease active. Pathologically it is characterized by widespread demyelinization of the central and peripheral nervous systems together with such biochemical abnormalities as a raised blood-urea and low values for serum potassium, sodium, and chloride. Clinically, the disease may present as an acute abdominal emergency of doubtful causation, or in obstetric patients undergoing Cæsarean section or forceps delivery.

Barbiturates as premedication and thiopentone and its congeners are absolutely contra-indicated as their administration may be followed by lower motor neuron paralysis, mental disturbances, or even death. In the acute phase, artificial ventilation may be required.

Medicolegal rather than scientific reasons make some workers avoid regional analgesia in these patients.

Liver Disease.—Even light planes of general anæsthesia reduce by about 25 per cent the blood perfusing the liver.† This may be due to vasoconstriction or to reduction in the blood-pressure. Chloroform and bromethol contra-indicated. Thiopentone fairly well tolerated in small doses, but as detoxication is largely in the liver, large doses may easily cause prolonged narcosis: moreover, large doses can actually cause additional damage to the liver cells. Excretion of pethidine delayed. Patients with a low value for pseudocholinesterase, as is commonly seen in liver disease, may require larger amounts of non-depolarizing and smaller amounts of depolarizing drugs than normal patients. Liver function is often slightly depressed as a result of operation and anæsthesia. A progressive fall in the serum pseudocholinesterase which reaches its maximum about the fifth post-operative day occurs, and this suggests a mild dysfunction of the liver parenchyma.

Patients with liver disease, including those with obstructive jaundice, need several days of careful preparation before operation. Carbohydrates and protein should be given in large quantities.

---

* Waldenström, J., *Acta med. scand.*, 1937, Suppl. 2.
† Shackman, R., and others, *Clin. Science*, 1953, **12**, 307.

Liver Disease, *continued.*

These patients should undergo a prothrombin time test, to avoid overlooking a dangerous hypoprothrombinæmia. Prothrombin, a necessary link in the clotting mechanism, is synthesized by the liver under the influence of vitamin K, which is absorbed from the gut. As it is fat-soluble, absence from the intestine of bile-salts will give rise to poor absorption, deficiency of the vitamin, and so reduced prothrombin formation. If the prothrombin time is greater than 25 seconds, or below 40 per cent of normal, the patient is a potential bleeder. Prothrombin deficiency is treated by the administration of synthetic vitamin K, either by mouth or by injection : a water-soluble variety of the drug is used. For the most rapid effect vitamin K_1 should be given intravenously, 100–350 mg. in cases of severe hæmorrhage, 10–50 mg. in less serious cases. Hypoprothrombinæmia due to vitamin-K deficiency is the only type of this condition which responds to vitamin-K therapy. If the state is due to decreased liver function or to liver disease, fresh blood transfusion is the correct treatment.

Severe prothrombin deficiency may exist in the absence of jaundice as synthesis of prothrombin by the liver depends on at least four factors : (1) Adequate amount of vitamin K in the intestine ; (2) Presence of bile-salts in intestine ; (3) Normal intestinal absorption ; (4) A healthy liver. Thus patients inadequately nourished, those with biliary fistula, and those with pyloric obstruction may be potential bleeders.

Prothrombin concentration should be as high as possible before operation is performed, and some vitamin K must be continued post-operatively as long as prothrombin deficiency persists.

After a severe attack of infective hepatitis it is probably wise to defer elective surgery for at least 6 months.

Polyarteritis Nodosa.*—In this disease there may be an abnormal response to suxamethonium because of associated liver dysfunction. Before depolarizing relaxants are used in this condition, investigation of liver function should be undertaken. The same response may occur in the presence of polymyositis, dermatomyositis, and systemic lupus erythematosus.

Thyrotoxicosis.—The anæsthetist, noticing an enlarged thyroid, should inquire about the existence of thyrotoxicosis. Minor degrees of this do not matter but if it is severe, right heart failure, atrial fibrillation, and liver damage may be present. The patient should be euthyroid before operation.

In the pre-operative control of restlessness or tachycardia, reserpine, 5 mg. thrice daily, or potassium iodide, five drops of the saturated solution thrice daily, will inhibit the release of thyroxine but may require 1–3 weeks' treatment. More serious states of thyrotoxicosis should be controlled by: (1) Methyl- or propyl-thiouricil—100 mg. four times daily gradually reducing the dosage. (2) Carbimazole (neomercazole)—10–15 mg. thrice daily.

---

* Potts, M. W., and Thornton, J. A., *Brit. J. Anæsth.,* 1961, **33**, 405.

Both these groups prevent thyroxine synthesis. (3) Potassium perchlorate—250 mg. thrice daily. Prevents iodine uptake by thyroid. Contra-indicated in pregnancy. (4) Radioactive iodine (^{131}I) by mouth. Contra-indicated in pregnancy. A post-operative thyroid crisis should be treated by hypothermia, chlorpromazine, potassium iodide, or intravenous hydrocortisone. *See also* Chapter XX.

ypothyroidism.—In this condition, metabolism of drugs, especially sedatives used in pre-medication and narcotics, is likely to be delayed, and respiratory depression is easily produced. There may be secondary changes in the pituitary gland and the adrenal cortex which may impair the normal response to stress. Post-operative hypotension should be treated by intravenous hydrocortisone.

Oral thyroxine takes 10 days to exert its effect. To correct hypothyroidism before operation 25 μg. of tri-iodothyroxine can be given intravenously in a drip or a solution of 0·1 mg. per l. in 5 per cent dextrose at 20 drops per minute with E.C.G. control (look for flattened T-waves or ST depression), using special caution in those patients over 50 and those suffering from angina. Intravenous hydrocortisone is also beneficial.

The nitrous oxide, oxygen, relaxant sequence, with I.P.P.V. is perhaps the most suitable anæsthetic technique.*

idney Disease.—Bromethol and thiopentone detoxicated more slowly in severe renal failure. Moderate doses of thiopentone may cause prolonged narcosis in such patients, and in those with a high blood-urea. Gallamine excretion is delayed in patients with renal disease of very severe degree. Ether may cause albuminuria. Uræmia may be associated with pericardial effusion, thus adding a cardiac hazard to the conduct of the anæsthesia. Methylamphetamine raises the blood-pressure without causing renal vasoconstriction, so in the presence of oliguria is probably the pressor drug of choice.

ardiovascular Disease.—Anæsthesia may affect the heart :—

1. To cause arrhythmias, including ventricular fibrillation.
2. By direct depressant effect on the myocardium, including asystole.
3. As a result of hypotension, especially when the heart cannot compensate by increasing the cardiac output (tight valvular stenosis, constrictive pericarditis).
4. As a result of hypoxia and hypercapnia.

In general, patients with compensated heart disease tolerate anæsthesia well, provided it is carefully administered and overdosage, hypoxia, and hypotension avoided.

1. HYPERTENSION AND ARTERIOSCLEROSIS.—Patients usually tolerate anæsthesia well, though it should be given carefully. Marked falls of blood-pressure are likely when ganglion-blocking drugs, halothane, large doses of thiopentone, and high spinal block are given. If the patient is under treatment with drugs for hypertension, problems may arise as the depressant effects of anæsthetic agents on the heart can only be corrected by a

---

* Abbott, T. R., *Brit. J. Anæsth.*, 1967, **39**, 510.

Cardiovascular Disease, *continued.*

functioning sympathetic nervous system. The effects of methy
dopa and of guanethidine may persist for up to 10 days followir
withdrawal of the drug. Patients under treatment may rea
badly to rapid changes in position, to a reversed Trendelenbur
position, and to I.P.P.V.*

2. HYPOTENSION.—Seldom causes anæsthetic difficulties, unle
secondary to other pathology (Addison's disease, shock).

3. DECOMPENSATION.—These cases are serious risks. The ons
of acute pulmonary œdema is to be guarded against and, if
shows itself, properly treated, e.g., a small dose of thiopenton
with oxygen given under pressure. Spinal analgesia has als
been used to treat the acute œdema. Intravenous fluid mus
not be allowed to overload the circulation. Intra- and extr
dural analgesia may suit some of these patients. Hypoxi
must be definitely avoided. Thiopentone, apart from sma
doses for induction, must be used very carefully and combine
with oxygen. Endotracheal intubation is often indicate
Cyclopropane is not contra-indicated in these cases, provide
satisfactory respiratory exchange is maintained. Pulmonar
congestion predisposes to post-operative pulmonary morbidit
Before induction these patients are often benefited by an intr
venous dose of digoxin (1 mg.) or double that amount by mout
if they are not already taking it or one of its allies. A suitab
diuretic, e.g., frusimide (lasex) 20–40 mg. intravenously,
helpful. Induction of anæsthesia in the semi-sitting positio
may be desirable.

4. ACUTE RHEUMATISM.—This should contra-indicate all bu
emergency operations. Tonsils and adenoids should be remove
if necessary, during a period of quiescence.

5. CARDIAC INFARCTION.—A period of 2–3 months, at leas
should, if possible, elapse between an attack and a surgic
operation. In one series† 18 per cent of patients died who we
operated on during the acute stage. An interval of 3 yea
between infarction and operation does not greatly increase th
operative risk over the normal patient.‡

6. CORONARY DISEASE.—Anoxia of the heart muscle must b
avoided by maintaining an adequate diastolic blood-pressur
as coronary flow depends on the diastolic pressure. A turbulen
second stage should be avoided. The mechanics of respiratio
must be safeguarded to ensure adequate filling of the right hear
The mortality rate of 517 patients with chronic coronary diseas
was 2·9 per cent compared with a rate of 2 per cent in 415
patients with no clinical evidence of coronary disease.† On th
other hand, in a large series of operations, the post-operativ
mortality was 6·6 per cent in patients with atherosclerotic hear
disease and 2·9 per cent in those without.§ In a total of ove

* Dingle, H. R., *Anæsthesia*, 1966, **21**, 151; and Annotation, *Lancet*, 1966, **2**, 269.
† Etsten, B., and Proger, S., *J. Amer. med. Ass.*, 1955, **159**, 845.
‡ Topkins, M. J., and Artusio, J. F., *Curr. Res. Anesth.*, 1964, **43**, 716.
§ Mattingley, T. W., *Amer. J. Cardiol.*, 1963, **12**, 279.

12,000 male surgical patients over the age of 50 the incidence of post-operative coronary occlusion in patients without previous coronary heart disease was 0·66 per cent as compared with an incidence of 6·5 per cent in patients with a known pre-operative occlusion. The mortality-rates from the heart attacks were 26 and 70 per cent in the two groups.*

7. COMPLETE HEART-BLOCK.†—In complete atrioventricular dissociation the idioventricular rate is about 35 beats per minute. The vagus produces no direct influence on the ventricle, while the sympathetic nervous system still exerts considerable control. Stokes-Adams attacks may occur during anæsthesia. Pre-operative treatment : (a) Digitalis may be useful if cardiac failure is present, but may itself cause heart-block ; (b) Atropine 1 mg. intravenously will detect and treat those cases where vagal action has produced the block ; (c) Oral ephedrine or sublingual isoprenaline can be administered to stimulate the idioventricular centre and abolish the Stokes-Adams attacks. The anæsthetic technique should be impeccable. The actual technique chosen is probably not so important as the skill with which it is used, though agents such as cyclopropane, halothane, chloroform, and trichloroethylene may cause ventricular arrhythmias when the sympathetic nerves alone influence the ventricle. In complete heart-block there is a decreased cardiac output and the heart is unable to compensate by increasing the rate. Thiopentone should therefore be administered carefully (cf. constrictive pericarditis). Gallamine is probably the relaxant of choice. Drugs such as quinidine and procaine amide should never be given to treat a ventricular arrhythmia. It may in fact be preferable to give an intravenous sympathomimetic amine in an attempt to speed the idioventricular rhythm and thereby abolish multifocal foci. The use of artificial pacemakers is discussed on p. 589.

8. ATRIAL FIBRILLATION.—Should be controlled pre-operatively by digitalization until the ventricular rate is reasonably slow.

9. CONGENITAL HEART DISEASE.—Patients require careful supervision and smooth anæsthesia. It is wise to administer antibiotic cover if there is danger of subacute bacterial endocarditis.

10. CONSTRICTIVE PERICARDITIS.—Thiopentone has a bad reputation in this disease.‡ The heart is unable to compensate for sudden changes in hæmodynamics such as may occur when peripheral resistance is altered.

In dealing with patients who have heart disease and who are about to have an operation and anæsthetic, the following six questions must be answered§ :—

1. Will the operation and anæsthetic overtax the heart beyond its limits, precipitating congestive failure?
2. Does the heart require treatment before operation?

---

* Topkins, M. J., and Artusio, J. F., Curr. Res. Anesth. 1964, **43**, 716.
† Ross, E. D. T., Brit. J. Anæsth., 1962, **34**, 102.
‡ Parry Brown, A. I., and Sellick, B. A., Anæsthesia, 1953, **8**, 4; and Brit. med. Bull., 1955, **11**, 174.
§ Ernestene A. C., Cleveland Clin. Quart., 1946, **13**, 189.

Cardiovascular Disease, *continued.*

3. Is the cardiac prognosis so grave that the operation needs to be postponed or limited to a palliative procedure?
4. Is the cardiac condition likely to lead to sudden death under anæsthesia?
5. What bearing does the state of the heart have on the choice of anæsthetic?
6. What, if any, cardiovascular complications are likely to follow operation, or occur in the immediate post-operative period?

Patients with organic heart disease who can carry on their daily jobs usually tolerate anæsthesia and operation well.

The following conditions should be detected before anæsthesia as they may lead to sudden death, especially if hypoxia or sudden alteration in the blood-pressure should occur :—

1. Recent cardiac infarction.
2. Angina pectoris.
3. Aortic stenosis.
4. Syphilitic aortic reflux, and aortitis with narrowing of the orifices of the coronary arteries.
5. Complete heart-block with Stokes-Adams attacks.

Suxamethonium, in patients with valvular incompetence, takes longer to act—up to 2 minutes—and may have to be given in larger doses (e.g., 100 mg.), than in normal patients, before intubation, due to a slow time of onset consequent on a reduced cardiac output.* In the digitalized patient arrhythmias may occur.†

Gallamine may so increase the cardiac rate as to initiate decompensation, so it must be used most carefully in heart conditions associated with tachycardia. A pulse-rate above 130 per minute, if prolonged, may cause trouble.

Congestive heart failure occurring as a post-operative complication may be difficult to diagnose. The appearance of triple rhythm or auricular fibrillation may give a clue, while orthopnœa may precede signs of pulmonary congestion in early left heart failure. Increase in venous filling in the neck heralds right heart failure. Measurement of central venous pressure may be useful (*see* Chapter XXXIII).

Diabetes.‡—Diabetes is a disease affecting the metabolism of fat and sugar and causes symptoms due to§ :—

1. A rising blood-sugar—polyuria, thirst, pruritus, etc.
2. Ketosis, i.e., metabolic acidosis causing hyperventilation, loss of extracellular sodium and water, dehydration leading to circulatory collapse and coma.
3. Peripheral vascular disease and neuritis. A severe diabetic is one who easily becomes acidotic if deprived of insulin, usually the younger age-groups—not necessarily the patient requiring large doses of insulin. During stress more insulin than normal may be needed.

---

* Harrison, G. C., *Anæsthesia*, 1966, **21**, 28.
† Dowdy, E. G., and Fabian, L. W., *Curr. Res. Anesth.*, 1963, **4**, 501.
‡ Foster, P. A., and Francis, B. G., *Brit. J. Anæsth.*, 1955, **27**, 291; Keen, H., *Hospital Medicine*, 1968, **2**, 760; and Bloom, A., *Ibid.*, 1968, **2**, 766.
§ Cates, J. E., *Brit. J. Anæsth.*, 1956, **28**, 222.

When properly controlled the risk to diabetics is little more than to ordinary patients, when they undergo surgical operations.

Regional analgesia, gas and oxygen, halothane, trichloroethylene, cyclopropane, thiopentone, ether—are the choice of anæsthetics in approximately that order. Chloroform, ether, and bromethol must be avoided when possible, as they cause a pronounced rise in blood-sugar. Relaxants are well tolerated.

The diabetic may also have pulmonary tuberculosis.

SCHEMES OF CONTROL FOR OPERATION PERIOD.—There is no single scheme to cover all cases. Generally speaking, it is wiser to have a slightly increased blood-sugar than to risk hypoglycæmia. The patient should be admitted several days before operation, so that he can be assessed for a reasonable period. He should be seen by the anæsthetist at the earliest possible moment. Important factors are :—

1. Are hypoglycæmic drugs being used? Mild diabetics treated by diet alone seldom give cause for concern.

2. How much insulin is being given? Except for minor operations it is wise to restabilize the patient on soluble insulin for 2 or 3 days.

3. Is the diabetes stable? History of diabetic coma or hypoglycæmic coma may indicate an unstable diabetic state. Particular care should therefore be used over the operative and post-operative period.

4. What is the nature of the surgical operation? Factors to be considered include the likelihood of a quick recovery, the duration of intravenous feeding, and the inability to obtain urine specimens (e.g., after prostatectomy or implantations of the ureters).

5. Are there associated lesions? Peripheral vascular disease or neuritis.

Any scheme must be worked out with common sense, taking these factors into account. Some general schemes :—

1. Give an amount of glucose equal to the patient's carbohydrate requirements by intravenous drip, and give soluble insulin 4- or 6-hourly, calculating the dose according to his previous requirements, checked by urine-sugar estimations or blood-sugar estimations.*

2. Give a fixed amount of glucose in place of each meal by intravenous drip, e.g., 50 g. (500 ml. 10 per cent glucose), and give enough insulin to cover this either by subcutaneous injection or in the drip. Calculate the dosage of insulin in the light of the patient's usual requirements. Some authorities recommend 25 units of soluble insulin per 50 g. glucose, but this should be varied according to the patient's usual insulin requirements.

3. If in doubt, it is a good general rule to add 10 to 12 units of soluble insulin to every pint of 5 per cent glucose solution used for intravenous infusion.

4. In mild cases, for minor operations, it is sometimes justifiable to omit both food and insulin pre-operatively.

---

* King, R. C., *Anæsthesia*, 1957, **12**, 30.

Diabetes, *continued.*

5. In emergency operations, consider each case on its merits. In the absence of urinary ketones by the ferric chloride test, 50–100 g. glucose may be given intravenously with 25 units soluble insulin. When ketonuria is present 100 g. glucose may be given with 100 units of insulin as an intravenous drip until the urine no longer shows a positive ferric chloride test for ketones. One pint of 5 per cent dextrose contains 28 g. Emergency operations for acute infections should be undertaken with the minimum delay, since drainage of pus and improvement in the surgical condition often results in an improvement in the diabetic condition.

6. The patient who takes no insulin or who is on oral hypoglycæmic drugs needs no special régime. It is sufficient to omit food and drugs pre-operatively. Afterwards urine specimens should be tested frequently in case insulin should then be required.

In cases of doubt a physician's advice should be sought.

Glucose should never be given by mouth as a pre-operative measure because of the risk of vomiting or regurgitation.

There is a real danger of vomiting during induction in the diabetic with ketosis. Hexamethonium may enhance the action of insulin and cause severe hypoglycæmia. Diabetic patients sometimes develop a syndrome simulating an acute abdomen. The effects of soluble insulin last for four to six hours. Hyperglycæmic coma takes time to develop whereas hypoglycæmia can come on during an operation and may be characterized by sweating, pallor, tachycardia, dilated pupils, normal eyeball tension, etc. It should be treated by intravenous glucose 25 per cent followed by 5 per cent solution and 25–50 units of insulin. It may be the cause of a delayed return to consciousness. Normal diet must be restored as soon as possible in the diabetic after operation.

Should the diabetes become unstable in the post-operative period, it is a good plan to prescribe soluble insulin according to 4-hourly urine testing; i.e., 2 per cent sugar—give 20 units; 1 per cent sugar—15 units; ½ per cent sugar—10 units.

For discussion of anæsthesia for the *surgical treatment of hyperinsulinism see* Bourke, A. M., *Anæsthesia*, 1966, **21**, 239.

Obesity.—This condition, usually the result of superalimentation, is perhaps the most common abnormality present in patients who require surgical operations. It is a serious handicap to surgeon and anæsthetist alike.

RESULTS.—Decrease in the expiratory reserve volume. Restriction of both diaphragmatic and chest movements, made worse in the head-down and lithotomy positions. Work of breathing increased. Hypoxic constriction of the pulmonary vessels causes pulmonary hypertension and enlargement of the right ventricle.

The following difficulties may occur: With venepuncture; with regional blocks; with airway patency; with low chest compliance; with increased chance of atherosclerosis including coronary artery disease; with increased likelihood of bronchitis; with monitoring; with hiatus hernia, especially during induction;

with handling if anything goes wrong; with nursing; with increased likelihood of post-operative pulmonary complications; with post-operative movement; with surgical access. This condition is usually preventable but seldom prevented. Pre-operative dietetic guidance should be more common. *See also* p. 76.

Pulmonary Disease.—

1. ACUTE.—Inhalation anæsthesia is better avoided: if it must be given halothane or gas and oxygen are the most suitable, while trichloroethylene is well tolerated. Antibiotics should be given to prevent post-operative lung complications.

2. CHRONIC.—Sputum should be coughed up before anæsthesia, by postural drainage for two hours, if necessary. Both halothane and small intravenous doses of pethidine—bronchial dilators—are fairly well tolerated. Post-operative respiratory depression must be avoided. Thiopentone is not well borne if there is bronchospasm, and soluble hexobarbitone is preferable.

There are anæsthetists of skill and experience who do not regard acute and chronic lung disease as contra-indications to the use of ether, and when much bronchospasm is a feature, ether maintenance, following cyclopropane induction, may go far to relieve the spasm and its resulting hypoxia.

Chronic Pulmonary Emphysema.*—These patients hyperventilate because of defective chest mechanics; the stretch receptors are overstimulated and ventilation is thereby limited. There may be a horizontal flattened diaphragm which pulls the lower ribs inwards during inspiration, and early use of the sternomastoids and scalene muscles. The arterial P_{CO_2} rises and the respiratory centre becomes less sensitive although some chemoreceptors still respond to oxygen lack. When a chest infection is superadded, hypoventilation is made worse. They are a problem to anæsthetists and the following points merit attention: (1) Hypersensitivity of respiratory reflexes (bucking, bronchospasm, etc.), to irritant vapours, thiopentone, secretions, and intubation. (2) Piston-type respiration where diaphragm moves up and down like a piston in a cylinder, while the thoracic cage fails to expand. This can seriously impede the abdominal surgeon in his work. (3) Dependence on chronic hypoxia for the respiratory drive, via the aortic and carotid bodies. This is impaired if the patient breathes an oxygen-rich atmosphere during or after anæsthesia. The pink colour due to this hyperoxæmia may mask hypoventilation so that carbon dioxide narcosis goes unnoticed. (4) Undue sensitivity to such respiratory depressants as opiates and barbiturates. (5) During controlled breathing there may be difficulty in inflation, necessitating the use of high pressure, with adverse effects on the circulation, and reduced elastic recoil leading to inefficient expiration. (6) Patient may be accustomed to a relatively high P_{CO_2}. (7) Tendency for neostigmine, owing to its muscarinic effect, to cause bronchospasm after operation.

---

* Dornhorst, A. C., *Brit. J. Anæsth.*, 1958, **30**, 130; and Nunn, J. F., *Ibid.*, 1958, **30**, 134.

Pulmonary Disease, *continued.*

VENTILATION.—The alveolar CO_2 tension can be inferred from the rebreathing method of estimating the mixed venous P_{CO_2}. Underventilation may have many causes but in the non-anæsthetized patient the commonest is airway obstruction due to chronic bronchitis, emphysema, or asthma ; it can be estimated by the use of the Wright Peak Flow Meter† or from a fast respiratory spirogram. The forced expiratory volume (F.E.V) is the volume of air which can be expired in a given time after a full inspiration. If the 1-sec. F.E.V. is less than 70 per cent of the vital capacity (taken at the same time) there is likely to be airway obstruction. In the absence of metabolic imbalance a change in the serum bicarbonate level will indicate whether carbon dioxide is being retained.

VENTILATION-PERFUSION RELATIONSHIPS.—These are disturbed. In some areas of the lung pulmonary capillary blood does not come into contact with alveolar gases.

ANÆSTHETIC MANAGEMENT.—

PRE-OPERATIVE CARE.—This should include amelioration of bronchospasm and infection ; reduction in body-weight and correction of anæmia.

PREMEDICATION.—Promethazine, pethidine, and atropine are well tolerated. Opiates and barbiturates may cause undue respiratory depression. Ephedrine and aminophylline may be helpful.

ANÆSTHESIA.—Regional block, e.g., extradural or brachial plexus when suitable. Good reasons can be advanced for preferring either spontaneous‡ or controlled respiration.§ If no relaxation is required, spontaneous respiration with a smooth induction and perhaps a little ether or halothane, avoiding too much oxygen so as to keep the respiratory drive active. When relaxation is required or when piston respiration makes conditions difficult, controlled respiration may be necessary following the use of a relaxant. This need not be followed by difficulty in restarting respiration if curarization is properly reversed, even if the P_{CO_2} is lower than the patient's normal level.‖ Hypoxæmia must be avoided and care taken with the P_{CO_2}: hypercapnia may paralyse the respiratory centre while hypocapnia may fail to stimulate it if the tension is much less than that to which the patient has become accustomed. Alternately raising and lowering the amount of CO_2 in the blood, a trial and error method, may be required until the correct P_{CO_2} is found. For bronchoscopy, topical analgesia is often better than general anæsthesia in emphysematous patients.

POST-OPERATIVE CARE.—Oxygen may be needed and ventilation may have to be stimulated : (1) Chemically, by nikethamide

* Campbell, E. J. M., and Howell, J. B. L., *Brit. med. J.*, 1962, **2**, 630 ; and *Ibid.*, 1962, **1**, 458.
† Wright, B. M., and McKerrow, C. B., *Ibid.*, 1959, **2**, 1041.
‡ Johnstone, M., *Anæsthesia*, 1956, **11**, 165.
§ Nunn, J. F., *Brit. J. Anæsth.*, 1958, **30**, 134.
‖ Utting, J. E., and Gray, T. C., *Ibid.*, 1962, **34**, 785.

10 ml. well diluted, $\frac{1}{2}$-hourly or as a continuous intravenous drip, or amiphenazole 150 mg. in 2 per cent solution, repeated if necessary,* or dichlorphenamide (daranide) 50 mg. 4-hourly. It is also a carbonic anhydrase inhibitor. (2) Mechanically, by ventilation, perhaps through a tracheostomy.

Diffusion of nitrous oxide into gas-filled body cavities, e.g., pneumothorax, may be quicker than diffusion of nitrogen outwards if nitrous oxide is inhaled. This increase in total gas pressure may be transmitted to the great veins causing cardiorespiratory difficulty.†

Disease of the Nervous System.—Spinal analgesia and extradural block are usually inadvisable because future symptoms and signs may be blamed on these methods of analgesia. A history of frequent headaches may also make spinal analgesia undesirable.

Alcoholism.—Alcohol addicts may require large doses of thiobarbiturates and volatile anæsthetics. Alcohol may well play a useful part in their premedication.

Narcotic Addiction.‡—These patients may manufacture symptoms to earn an operation in order to obtain morphine afterwards. Withdrawal symptoms may include cramp, vomiting, and diarrhœa, while intestinal obstruction is often simulated. There may be multiple abscesses from unhygienic injections, with thrombophlebitis, so that the external jugular veins remain the only usable channels for intravenous therapy. Frequent history of viral hepatitis and asthma. Sedative premedication may involve large doses of drugs to be effective. Hypotension is common in the operating theatre. The patient may interfere with the wound to prolong stay in hospital, so that great care and discipline are required after operation.

Diseases of the Adrenal Glands

Primary Adrenal Failure.—May be seen following :—
1. Removal, i.e., adrenalectomy.
2. Destruction, e.g., Addison's disease ; adrenal apoplexy.
3. Exhaustion, e.g., starvation and toxæmia.
4. Dysfunction, virilizing hyperplasia.

Secondary Adrenal Failure.—This may occur as a result of :—
1. Removal of the pituitary gland (hypophysectomy).
2. Destruction of the pituitary gland, e.g., tumours ; Simmonds's disease.
3. Inhibition of the pituitary gland due to steroid therapy. Death due to circulatory failure may occur in patients who, having been on doses of cortisone for long periods, are suddenly deprived of it before the stress of anæsthesia and operation.

Addison's Disease.—Patients with this complaint are susceptible to infection, to loss of sodium chloride, and to narcotics. These patients are likely to be debilitated, hypotensive, and perhaps

---

* Little, G. M., *Brit. med. J.*, 1962, **1**, 223.
† Hunter, A. R., *Proc. R. Soc. Med.*, 1955, **48**, 765.
‡ Eisman, B., and others, *J. Amer. med. Ass.*, 1964, **159**, 748.

Addison's Disease, *continued.*

tuberculous. They are bad anæsthetic risks as Addisonian crises are easily precipitated. These start with loss of sodium chloride in the urine and so of large amounts of water. The circulating fluid is reduced, while diarrhœa and vomiting make the plasma volume smaller. Dehydration and circulatory collapse follow, and, in addition, there is often autonomic imbalance. If such a patient is operated on and Addison's disease not diagnosed, severe post-operative collapse may occur. If the disease is, however, recognized, adequate pre-operative treatment greatly lessens the risk, although post-operative hypotension is likely. If it occurs it should be treated by transfusion and the intravenous injection of cortisone. Pre-operative management consists in giving sodium chloride and fluid, dextrose, and cortisone to maintain the circulating blood-volume as near normal as possible. Neither hypotension nor anoxia must be produced by the anæsthetic technique. Thiopentone may cause a serious fall in blood-pressure.

Adrenal Apoplexy.—This is usually fatal, and is often associated with meningococcal septicæmia (Waterhouse-Friderichsen syndrome). Hyperpyrexia and circulatory collapse are the usual modes of death. Rarely the condition comes to operation because of associated arterial embolism or peritonitis. Cortisone is indicated.

Cushing's Syndrome.—This is often associated with or perhaps caused by cortical hypertrophy or tumour. Surgical removal may cause Addisonian crises, and similar measures must be taken to combat them (*see above*). Pre-operative sodium chloride, etc., should be given for two days pre-operatively and also post-operatively. Intravenous noradrenaline and cortisone may be required.

Hypopituitarism.—Chronic hypopituitarism is most commonly due to ischæmic necrosis of the anterior lobe of the pituitary following hæmorrhage or shock in labour. It may be suspected if there is absence of a palpable thyroid, absence of pubic hair, and genital hypoplasia. General anæsthesia is liable to precipitate coma in these patients. Cortisone may be helpful. Barbiturates and opiates too may have a very prolonged action.*

Steroid Therapy.—Steroid therapy suppresses the formation of ACTH by the anterior pituitary with resultant adrenocortical atrophy. The cortex is then unable to secrete extra hormones in response to the stress of anæsthesia, operation, or trauma. Collapse, with fall of blood-pressure, may ensue even though the operation is of a trivial character.†

Adrenocortical reserve is *diminished* :—

1. In Addison's disease, whether treated or untreated.
2. After bilateral adrenalectomy.
3. During steroid therapy.
4. When a patient has received steroids in the past. It may be that adrenocortical reserve is sufficient to meet the ordinary needs of life, but that the reserve is inadequate to meet the extra burden

---

* Sheehan, H. L., *Brit. med. J.*, 1955, **2**, 1022.
† Dundee, J. W., *Brit. J. Anæsth.*, 1957, **29**, 166.

of anæsthesia and operation. As short a course as 1 week may produce depression of the cortex. Depression may last as long as 1–2 yr., and in some cases of prolonged therapy the cortex may never regain its full functional reserve.

There are no satisfactory simple tests for adrenocortical reserve. The response of the cortex to ACTH given intravenously over 8 hours is reflected as a fall of eosinophils in peripheral blood and a rise in corticoids and 17-ketosteroids in the 24-hour urine. Such tests are cumbersome and unsuited to routine use. Where facilities for blood-cortisol estimation are available, a pre-operative stress test can be carried out. A small dose of insulin is given, and frequent estimations of blood-sugar and blood cortisol carried out. A fall in blood-sugar indicates a successful test, a rise of blood cortisol a satisfactory response indicating the presence of adrenocortical reserve, and steroid cover is not required. A rough test* has been suggested, requiring only 5 ml. of blood and urine. Adrenocortical insufficiency may be suspected when the serum sodium is less than 130 mEq. per l. and the urinary sodium more than 100 mEq. per l.

In the light of present knowledge it is best to assume that there is some diminution of reserve whenever a course of steroids has been given during the past two years. It is generally safer to give cortisone cover than to omit it in cases of doubt. The normal adult secretes 20–30 mg. of hydrocortisone daily and this may reach 400 mg. daily in response to surgery and anæs-thesia. A chronic excess causes Cushing's syndrome but dangerous effects are unlikely if the daily dose does not exceed 75 mg. (prednisone 15 mg. daily).

CORTISONE COVER should commence 24–48 hr. pre-operatively. Intramuscular injections of cortisone acetate are absorbed slowly and must be given at least 12 hours before operation, or the drug may be given by mouth. In an emergency hydrocortisone hemisuccinate should be given intravenously. Some workers, however, believe that there is no need to commence cover earlier than 1–2 hours before surgery. They believe that a rapidly acting steroid such as hydrocortisone should be given intramuscularly at the time of pre-operative medication. The intramuscular route is preferred, except in an emergency situation, since the plasma steroid levels are maintained for several hours, whereas after intravenous injection they fall more rapidly.

DOSAGE of cortisone acetate or hydrocortisone, in an adult, should be 100–200 mg. daily, starting 1–2 days before operation, and continued until the stress of the operative and the post-operative period is over. Dosage should then be reduced gradually over several days either to the normal maintenance dose or to zero.

Should unexplained hypotension occur, or when the emergency nature of an operation does not allow time for full preparation, hydrocortisone hemisuccinate can be given intravenously in doses of 100 mg.

---

* Perlmutter, M., *J. Amer. med. Ass.*, 1956, **160**, 117.

Steroid Therapy, *continued.*

OTHER STEROID DERIVATIVES include prednisone and prednisolone (3 to 5 times as potent as cortisone), triamcinolone (15 times as potent), betamethasone and dexamethasone (35 times as potent). *See also* the drugs listed in the Appendix.

Carcinoid Tumours.—Arise from Kultschitzky cells of the crypts of Lieberkuhn of the gastro-intestinal tract. 50–90 per cent originate in the area of the appendix. About 25 per cent of malignant carcinoids produce and secrete 5-hydroxytryptamine (serotonin).

MALIGNANT CARCINOID SYNDROME.—There are big variations in the clinical manifestations. The syndrome does not occur unless there are hepatic secondaries with secretion of 5-hydroxytryptamine into the hepatic veins. It may be characterized by :—

1. A growing intra-abdominal malignancy.
2. Cutaneous flushes, involving mainly the upper part of the body. The flush changes in colour from fiery red to dusky cyanosis. It may last minutes, hours, or days and normal colour is restored from the centre outwards, so that the fingers lose their cyanosis last.
3. Other symptoms may include : profuse perspiration, nausea and vomiting, abdominal distension and cramps, diarrhœa.
4. Dyspnœa, respiratory stridor, asthmatic attacks.
5. Tachycardia and fall in blood-pressure.
6. Long-term manifestations : valvular fibrosis of the right side of the heart (pulmonary stenosis, tricuspid insufficiency), arthritis, sclerodermic changes, telangiectasia of the face, dependent œdema.

Attacks may be precipitated by : (1) Palpation of the tumour ; (2) hypotension ; (3) fear ; (4) eating, drinking, defæcation.

Diagnosis is confirmed by measuring urinary secretion of 5-hydroxy indole acetic acid. Normal 2–9 mg. per 24 hours, greater than 25 mg. per 24 hours is diagnostic. Up to 1000 mg. per 24 hours have been obtained.

5-Hydroxytryptamine causes contraction of the smooth muscles of blood-vessels, bronchi, uterus, and pulmonary blood-vessels. It releases histamine and is antidiuretic.

Anæsthesia may be uneventful, but may provoke an attack of the syndrome with an acute flushing and severe bronchospasm. This is particularly likely if hypotension is allowed to occur and so spinal techniques are not recommended. Treatment of an attack during anæsthesia is to avoid stimuli and maintain ventilation of the lungs, using high inflation pressures if necessary.

The 5-hydroxytryptamine blood level is also increased in argent-affinoma of the lung, non-tropical sprue, and intestinal lipodystrophy.*

(*See* Review article, Stone, H. H., and Donnelly, C. C., *Anesthesiology,* 1960, **21**, 203.)

Leprosy.†—Leprosy patients are often on steroids and so need appropriate preparation for operation. Cosmetic surgery for the

---

* Wulfsohn, W. L., and Politzer, W. M., *Anæsthesia,* 1962, **17**, 64.
† Davidson, J. T., and Aladjemoff, L., *Brit. J. Anæsth.,* 1963, **35**, 484.

amelioration of deformities is often undertaken in these patients. Because of the analgesia sometimes caused by the disease, small operations may be possible without any other agent than a mild sedative.

Anæsthetic apparatus must be sterilized after use to prevent transfer of the disease but its infectivity is not high.

Epidermolysis Bullosa.*—A rare skin disease, characterized by the formation of vesicles and bullæ in response to trauma. The simplex type affects the skin only, does not result in scarring, and is of no great concern to the anæsthetist. The dystrophic type affects skin and mucous membranes. Healing occurs with formation of scar tissue, and secondary infection is common. The condition may be associated with porphyria and patients have often been treated with steroids.

The anæsthetist should avoid trauma of any kind. Endotracheal intubation should thus be avoided unless absolutely necessary. Muslin soaked in 0·5 per cent hydrocortisone may be placed over the face to afford protection against face-masks. Beware of barbiturates (in case of porphyria).

Pharmacogenetics and Anæsthesia.—
1. Pseudocholinesterase variants.
2. Group of patients who become hyperthermic.†
3. Acute intermittent porphyria.
4. Myotonic syndromes.
5. Familial dysautonomia (the Riley-Day syndrome).‡
6. Sickle-cell anæmia.
7. Diabetes.
8. Congenital heart disease.
9. Telangiectasia.
10. Hæmophilia.

(*See also* Kalow, W., *Anesthesiology*, 1964, **25**, 377; and discussion, *Proc. R. Soc. Med.*, 1968, **61**, 167 et seq.)

CHAPTER XXVII

SHOCK§

Shock may be described as any hæmodynamic disturbance causing such a degree of reduced capillary flow that tissue hypoxia leading to functional and/or morphological changes is produced. In the past the main emphasis has been on indirect blood-pressure and pulse-rate measurement. It is now becoming realized that we must also take

---

* Wilson, F., *Brit. J. Anæsth.*, 1959, **31**, 26; and Marshall, B. E., *Ibid.*, 1963, **35**, 724.
† Denborough, M., and Lovell, R. R. H., *Lancet*, 1960, **2**, 45.
‡ Riley, C. M., and others, *Pediatrics*, 1949, **3**, 468.
§ See *The Treatment of Wound Shock*, The Wound Shock Working Party, 1957. London: The Medical Research Council, H.M.S.O.; Symposium on Trauma, *Brit. J. Anæsth.*, 1966, **38**, April; and Weil, M. H., and Shubin, H., *Diagnosis and Treatment of Shock*, 1967. Baltimore: Williams and Wilkins.

Introduction, *continued.*

account of venous return and venous pressure, cardiac competence, peripheral resistance, velocity of blood-flow, and tissue perfusion.

The term 'shock' was first used in the sense in which it is now employed by James Latta in 1832.*

Theories of causation have included the following:†—

1. Vasomotor collapse or vasodilatation (Crile, 1899).
2. Vasoconstriction (Malcolm, 1905).
3. Carbon-dioxide depletion—acapniac theory of shock (Yandell Henderson, 1909).‡
4. Increased capillary permeability leading to hypovolæmia, the cause being toxic substances liberated in the injured area (Cannon and Bayliss, 1919).
5. Fluid loss at site of injury (Blalock, 1930).
6. Vasoconstriction due to hypovolæmia (Freeman, 1933).
7. Left ventricular failure as a contributing factor (Wiggers, 1947).

The chief factor in shock is depletion of blood-volume, and replacement of that volume is the major therapeutic weapon. Irreversible shock has now come to mean shock which cannot be controlled by blood or similar fluid transfusion. Other factors may be the inability of the liver to inactivate the vasodepressor material circulating in the blood or exhaustion of the adrenocortical reserve.

In irreversible shock congestion and hæmorrhagic necrosis of mucosa of the small intestine may occur. Bacterial endotoxins may play a part in the production of the syndrome.

What was formerly known as primary shock is now termed ' vaso-vagal collapse ', which is characterized by a slow pulse, unlike the tachycardia associated with true (secondary) shock.

Signs.—Pallor, best seen in the face ; cold moist skin, best seen in the extremities ; rapid weak pulse ; declining pulse-pressure ; blood-pressure drop is not an early sign ; collapse of superficial veins due to compensatory peripheral vasoconstriction and fall in venous pressure; a production of urine less than 10–30 ml. per hour; cyanosis of lips and nail beds; thirst; rapid shallow breathing; vomiting; restlessness; diminished sensibility; subnormal temperature; anxiety; drowsiness; and coma. The peripheral circulation time increases with fall in blood-pressure, whereas the increase in the pulmonary circulation time is relatively less.

Causes.§—

1. **HÆMORRHAGE.**—A loss up to two pints is usually well compensated by splanchnic and cutaneous vasoconstriction. If bleeding continues, true oligæmic shock is seen. Heart-rate 100–120, which will probably be made faster by anæsthesia. In early stages, hæmoglobin percentage is no index of blood lost. The decreased blood-volume and the blood dilution cause a decreased venous pressure, a decreased venous return, and so a decreased cardiac output. Blood-pressure is well maintained at first, but falls later.

* Latta, J. A., *Lancet*, 1832, **1**, 274.
† Bloch, J. H., and others, *Brit. J. Anæsth.*, 1966, **38**, 234.
‡ Henderson, Y., *Amer. J. Physiol.*, 1908, **21**, 126 et seq.
§ *See* Hershey, S. G., *Anesthesiology*, 1960, **21**, 303.

Should the patient with hæmorrhagic or wound shock not receive intravenous fluid he may :—

a. Become rehydrated from his own tissue fluids, his cardiac output returning to normal : but he remains anæmic. This is the hyperkinetic phase and in it rapid blood or fluid transfusion may overload the circulation and cause heart failure. A slow drip of packed red-cell suspension is required, or—

b. He fails to rehydrate himself and passes into peripheral circulatory failure. A normal man has a blood-volume of 5 litres.

2. REDUCTION IN THE VOLUME OF FLUID IN THE VASCULAR BED.—e.g., (a) plasma, electrolyte fluid, due to burns or trauma; and (b) dehydration.

3. INADEQUATE MYOCARDIAL PUMPING MECHANISM.—e.g., cardiac infarction.

4. VASCULAR OBSTRUCTION, SYSTEMIC OR PULMONARY.—e.g., embolus.

5. VASOMOTOR IMPAIRMENT.—After neurological injury or deep anæsthesia.

6. HORMONAL DEFICIENCIES.—e.g., adrenals.

7. ACUTE HYPERSENSITIVITY REACTION; ANAPHYLAXIS.—Classically, a reaction to foreign protein. Can occur with penicillin. Onset usually occurs within a few minutes of exposure and is characterized by pruritis, urticaria, dyspnœa, wheezing, syncope, nausea and vomiting, rhonchi and râles in the chest, hypotension, cyanosis, and flushing or pallor. Treatment may include: adrenaline intramuscularly or subcutaneously, up to 0·5 ml. 1–1000 solution, attention to pulmonary ventilation and removal of secretions, an intravenous drip with vasopressors, corticosteroids.*

8. TISSUE TRAUMA.—Circulating poisons, the results of tissue autolysis or infection, are absorbed into the circulation from damaged tissue. They injure the endothelial lining of the capillaries, causing leakage of fluid into tissue spaces and producing a reduced blood-volume. Sympathetic-adrenal activity helps to compensate for this by causing vasoconstriction, contraction of the spleen, and cardiac stimulation. The peripheral circulation is reduced and extremities become cold and pale, so that vital organs can be better supplied with blood. If condition is progressive, venous return to heart and cardiac output are reduced and blood-pressure falls. But this fall is not a sign of incipient shock; rather it is a sign that the circulatory system is not able to cope with the emergency.
Renal failure may be due to the effect of these same toxins on the renal epithelium.

9. NERVE TRAUMA.—Operative trauma may cause shock of sudden onset, e.g., disarticulation of the hip-joint ; rapid dilatation of a pregnant cervix uteri ; traction on the spermatic cord ;

---

* Abernathy, R. S., in *Diagnosis and Treatment of Shock* (Ed. Weil, M. H., and Shubin, H.), 1967, Ch. 11. Baltimore: Williams and Wilkins.

Causes, *continued.*

traction on the gall-bladder or cardiac end of the stomach. Signs often disappear with the cessation of the stimulus. The anoci-association theory of G. W. Crile is not now regarded as of major importance.*

10. SEPTIC SHOCK.†—Septic infection, usually with Gram-negative organisms, can cause a state of acute hypotension, oliguria, and reduced peripheral blood-flow. The condition may come on acutely over a period of a few hours. Treatment includes intravenous fluids, antibiotics, pressor agents, corticosteroids,‡ and adjustment of acid-base balance.

Shock may be made worse by :—

1. Bad Anæsthetic Technique.—Overdose of anæsthetic or hypoxia can cause depression of the circulation.
2. Prolonged operating time.
3. Rough movement of the patient while under anæsthesia.

Metabolic Effects of Shock.§—

1. Decreased oxygen consumption.
2. Fall in body temperature.
3. Hyperglycæmia in the initial period, followed by hypoglycæmia in late shock as glycogen stores are depleted.
4. Rise of blood lactate and pyruvate. In severe and prolonged shock a greater rise in blood lactate is observed.‖ The lactate/pyruvate or L/P ratio may be valuable if an early estimation is available for comparison.
5. Metabolic acidosis, and perhaps respiratory acidosis.
6. Depletion of body protein, with increase of urinary nitrogen.
7. Fall in serum sodium and chloride and rise in potassium. Reduced excretion of sodium, chloride, and water.
8. Fall in serum levels of ascorbic acid and decreased excretion of ascorbic acid, riboflavin, thiamine, and nicotinamide.¶
9. Increase of hypothalamic–pituitary–adrenal activity. Increase of ACTH secretion.**
10. Impairment of liver function—tests may be abnormal.
11. The kidneys.†† During shock the rate of urine flow indicates parallel changes in glomerular filtration rate. The urine may contain protein casts. The relationship of shock to the development of acute renal insufficiency is not clear. Patients particularly at risk include those who have shock in association with septic abortion, Gram-negative septicæmia, hæmoglobinæmia,

---

* Crile, G. W., *Lancet*, 1913, **2**, 7.

† *See also* Weil, M. H., and Shubin, H., *Diagnosis and Treatment of Shock*, 1967, Ch. 10. Baltimore: Williams and Wilkins.

‡ Lansing, A. M., *Canad. Anæsth. Soc. J.*, 1963, **89**, 583 ; and Annotation in *Lancet*, 1963, **2**, 1265.

§ *See* Levenson, S. M., in *Diagnosis and Treatment of Shock* (Ed. Weil, M. H., and Shubin, H.), 1967, Ch. 4. Baltimore: Williams and Wilkins.

‖ Broder, G., and Weil, M. H., *Science, N.Y.*, 1964, **143**, 1457.

¶ Levenson, S. M., and others, *Ann. Surg.*, 1946, **124**, 840; and Lund, C. C., and others, *Arch. Surg.*, 1947, **55**, 557.

** Melby, J. C., in *Diagnosis and Treatment of Shock* (Ed. Weil, M. H., and Shubin, H.), 1967, Ch. 5. Baltimore: Williams and Wilkins.

†† Berman, L. B., *Ibid.*, 1967, Ch. 5. Baltimore: Williams and Wilkins.

myoglobinuria, intra-abdominal trauma, aortic surgery, acute liver failure, and burns.

The following conditions may be confused with shock :—

FAT EMBOLISM.*—This was first described in man by Zenker in 1862, was first diagnosed clinically by von Bergmann in 1873,† and may be wrongly diagnosed as shock. Due to escape of droplets of fat into the circulation, and their deposition in the lungs, brain, or skin. Often associated with fractures of lower-limb bones. Onset of symptoms may rapidly follow the injury or may be delayed for two or three days.

Pulmonary symptoms include dyspnœa, pallor, cyanosis, pyrexia, frothy sputum.

Cerebral symptoms usually seen in the first twenty-four hours after operation or injury, with pyrexia and there may be restless-ness, leading to coma, convulsions, and paralysis; deep coma carries a bad prognosis; fat emboli may be seen in the retinal vessels with an ophthalmoscope.

Skin signs are likely to be a purpuric eruption with petechiæ over the upper chest, neck, and conjunctivæ and are seen on the second or third day.

The lung manifestations are the most common but cause few symptoms.

TREATMENT.—Because of the similarity of the clinical picture of fat embolism to that of acute head injury (coma, decerebration, tonic convulsions, and fever) it has been treated by hypo-thermia with surface cooling and the 'lytic cocktail' and dehydration.‡ This reduces the oxygen requirements of the brain, lowers intracranial pressure, and depresses both the autonomic and the somatic nervous systems. The temperature aimed at is 30–35° C. and as improvement in the patient's condition develops the amount of the chlorpromazine–promethazine–pethidine mixture needed to maintain vaso-dilatation can be reduced.§ Hypothermia with I.P.P.V. has been recommended.‖

An early sign of fat embolism may be urinary incontinence. It has been said that collapse in the second hour after operation is likely to be due to shock ; in the second day, to fat embo-lism ; in the second week, to pulmonary embolism.

AIR EMBOLISM.—This may cause collapse or cardiac standstill. The patient should be turned on to his left side to relieve the ' air trap ' in the right ventricle. Cardiac massage may be required, preceded by aspiration of air from the ventricles. The condition can often be diagnosed in its early stages by ausculta-tion (*see also* p. 546).

Differential Diagnosis of Oligæmic Shock.—The following con-ditions may give rise to a shock-like state: (1) Coronary

* Sevitt, S., *Lancet*, 1960, **2**, 825; Peltier, L. F., *Surg. Gynec. Obstet.*, 1965, **121**, 371; and Corn, D., *Med. Clin. N. Amer.*, 1964, **48**, 1459.
† Von Bergmann, E., *Berl. med. Wschr.*, 1873, **10**, 385.
‡ Hamilton, W. H., *Lancet*, 1964, **2**, 994.
§ Aladjemoff, L., and others, *Ibid.*, 1963, **1**, 13.
‖ Galloon, S., and Chakravarty, K., *Brit. J. Anæsth.*, 1967, **39**, 71.

Differential Diagnosis of Oligæmic Shock, *continued*.

thrombosis. (2) Perforation of viscera. (3) Acute high intestinal obstruction. (4) Adrenal cortical insufficiency. (5) Severe fluid loss, e.g., vomiting or diarrhœa. (6) Severe burns. (7) Certain obstetrical manœuvres. (8) Introduction of certain foreign proteins into tissues. (9) Toxæmia, e.g., *B. welchii* or diphtheria. (10) Certain drugs used in anæsthesia, e.g., opiates, phenothiazines, pethidine, halothane. (11) Adrenal hæmorrhage due to infection or trauma. (12) Interference with venous return to heart due to position, or to pressure on the vena cava from abdominal tumours, e.g., the pregnant uterus near term. (13) Following intradural or extradural analgesia.

Methods of Estimating Blood-loss.—*See* Chapter XXXIII.

The Treatment of Shock before Operation.—Moderate warmth and rest. Elevate foot of bed. For restlessness and anxiety not due to pain, give barbiturates, e.g., pentobarbitone, intravenously. Thirst may be more distressing than pain, but is better relieved by mouth-washes and intravenous fluid than by drinks, if operation is pending.

Morphine should be injected intravenously and given only if the patient complains of pain. If given subcutaneously or intramuscularly, absorption will be much delayed. This will render the drug useless as an anodyne, and may result in sudden absorption on improvement of the peripheral circulation. Abdominal wounds are much more painful than thoracic. Only about one-quarter of seriously injured and shocked patients require morphine for pain relief and rarely should 10 mg. (⅙ gr.) be exceeded. It should not be given if there is severe brain injury or respiratory depression.

Transfusion of whole blood is of paramount importance, especially if hæmorrhage has been marked, and it should be given at a rapid rate. If the patient does not respond to intravenous blood transfusion, an intra-arterial transfusion should be set up, as even 100–200 ml. given by this route may be helpful.

Oxygen inhalation helpful. Very useful in cases where oxygenation is deficient, e.g., wounds of chest, patients who are cyanosed. May be given if there is severe hæmorrhage, tachycardia, or respiratory depression and may need to be combined with I.P.P.V.‡

If there is hæmoconcentration, dextran, plasma, or serum is indicated, but two pints are usually sufficient except in cases of burn shock. Serum contains no fibrinogen and when reconstituted contains 14 per cent of protein ; plasma contains 8–9 per cent of protein. These two are very useful in shock unassociated with much hæmorrhage, e.g., after crush injury.

The amount of fluid given will depend on the patient's reaction to it. The aim is to restore the blood-pressure to normal as quickly as

* Hercus, V. M., and others, *Brit. med. J.*, 1961, **2**, 1467.
† Alsop, W., and others, *Ibid.*, 1963, **1**, 125 ; *see also* Gardiner, A. J. S., and Dudley, H. A. F., *Brit. J. Anæsth.*, 1962, **34**, 653 ; and Thornton, J. A., and others, *Ibid.*, 1963, **35**, 91.
‡ Weale, F. E., *Lancet*, 1963, **1**, 673.

possible. Each pint of blood should raise the systolic blood-pressure 10–20 mm. Hg, and the hæmoglobin percentage 6–8 per cent.

INTRAVENOUS INFUSION.—The drip bulb was described in 1909.* Suitable veins are the veins in the forearm or at the bend of the elbow; the saphenous vein anterior to the medial malleolus; veins on the dorsum of the hand; veins above the wrist. The saphenous vein should very seldom be used as flow rates are unpredictable and complications not infrequent. The femoral vein just below the inguinal ligament is attached to the surrounding structures and so does not collapse at this point when other veins are in venospasm. Subclavian vein puncture, first described by Aubaniac in 1952, has been used when other veins are inaccessible. The patient lies supine looking upwards and an 18-gauge needle is inserted on the right side (to avoid the thoracic duct) just below the clavicle at the junction of its inner and middle thirds. It is thrust backwards, inwards, and slightly upwards, with a 5-ml. syringe attached, keeping very near the clavicle. The method should not be used routinely as a hæmatoma may result.† Another technique of subcutaneous subclavian venepuncture has recently been described‡ (see also Wilson, J. H., and others, Ann. Surg., 1962, **85**, 563). In infants the internal or external jugular or scalp veins can be used or the umbilical vein during laparotomy.§ For puncture of the internal jugular vein the child should be wrapped in a blanket enclosing the arms with its head overhanging the end of the table and rotated. A needle is inserted near the posterior border of the sternomastoid near its midpoint and advanced beneath the muscle, perhaps as much as $1\frac{1}{2}$–2 inches. The femoral vein is approached below the inguinal ligament where it lies medially to the artery. A sandbag should be under the infant's buttocks.

To speed up the rate of flow, often slowed down by the venous spasm associated with shock, 10 ml. of 1 per cent procaine solution injected into the tubing through an intradermal needle is useful. Nikethamide, 2 ml., can also be used for this purpose. Raising the bottle well above the patient's limb may be helpful, while air pressure can be raised in the bottle, above the level of the fluid, by means of a hand pump attached to the air vent tube. This last method must never be used if there is any air in either the filter chamber or the drip chamber,‖ for fear of air embolism. A Martin rotary pump or an oxygen-driven blood infusion pump can be employed.¶ A three-way syringe can be used in infants.

There is a real danger in giving blood too fast to patients with myocardial weakness (which may be due to anæmia, the reason for the transfusion).

---

* Laurie, R. D., Lancet, 1909, **1**, 248.
† Aubaniac, R., Pr. méd., 1952, **60**, 1456 ; and Davidson, J. T., and others, Lancet, 1963, **2**, 1139.
‡ Yoffa, D., Ibid., 1965, **2**, 614.
§ Wilkinson, A. W., Ibid., 1963, **1**, 86.
‖ Bewes, P. C., Ibid., 1961, **1**, 429.
¶ Salt, R. H., Hall, M. R. P., and Taylor, W. H., Ibid., 1961, **1**, 642.

The Treatment of Shock before Operation, *continued.*

To make veins more prominent moist heat should be applied to the whole limb for half an hour before venepuncture.

For prolonged infusion, a plastic catheter or cannula can be inserted through a needle percutaneously into a vein or a cannula can be tied into the saphenous vein at the ankle. Alternatively, a polythene cannula can be inserted into the cephalic vein at the anterior axillary fold, and passed up to a point just short of the angle in the vein where it passes through the clavi-pectoral fascia.* A similar tube can also be inserted into the superior vena cava from a small incision in the basilic vein, 2 in. (5 cm.) above and anterior to the medial epicondyle. Femoral vein transfusion may also be useful. Cava infusion† also has a place but should not be used in the presence of local or general infection.‡

A 540-ml. bottle of fluid at 40 drops a minute takes 4 hours ; at 60 drops a minute, 2½ hours ; at 200 drops a minute, 45 minutes.

To prevent thrombophlebitis from intravenous drips :—

1. Use plastic rather than rubber tubing.
2. Remove drip each eight hours and insert into a different vein.
3. Use a plastic cannula rather than a needle.
4. Add hydrocortisone 10 mg. per litre to the infused fluid.
5. If glucose is infused it should be sterilized by filtration rather than by autoclaving.
6. Avoid leg veins.

The *p*H of intravenous fluids may be a factor in causing thrombo-phlebitis.§ *See also* Chapter XXXI.

BLOOD TRANSFUSION.—First described in animals in 1666 by Richard Lower and in man by Denis of France in 1667, using lamb's blood. First successful man-to-man transfusion reported by J. Blundell in 1818, an obstetrician.‖ Transfusions were first given to alter the patient's temperament. Hustin (1882–1967) of Belgium in 1914¶ demonstrated the usefulness of sodium citrate as an anticoagulant. In 1900, Landsteiner (1868–1943)** first observed agglutination of human red cells by serum belonging to other individuals, and described the ABO groups. The Rh system was discovered in 1939–40 (Landsteiner and Weiner).†† One bottle of blood will raise the hæmoglobin about 1 g. per cent (7 per cent Haldane). If the hæmoglobin is less than 6 g. per cent (40 per cent), a transfusion is necessary. If a major operation is to be performed and the hæmoglobin is less than 10 g. per cent (70 per cent), a blood transfusion is required. A low value for hæmoglobin delays healing. Blood banks were established in the 1930's in Moscow and in Cook County Hospital, Chicago,‡‡

* Jones, P. F., *Postgrad. med. J.*, 1957, **33**, 446.
† Verel, D., *Lancet*, 1958, **1**, 716.
‡ Chambers, V. W., and Smith, G., *Brit. J. Surg.*, 1957, **45**, 160.
§ Elving, G., and Saikku, K., *Lancet*, 1966, **1**, 953.
‖ Blundell, J., *Med. Chir. Trans.*, 1818, **9**, 56.
¶ Hustin, A., *Bull. Soc. Roy. Sci. méd. Brux.*, 1914, **72**, 104.
** Landsteiner, K., *Zbl. Bakt.*, 1900, **27**, 357.
†† Landsteiner, K., and Wiener, A. S., *Proc. Soc. exp. Biol., N.Y.*, 1940, **43**, 233.
‡‡ Fantus, B., *J. Amer. med. Ass.*, 1939, **109**, 128.

and in 1939 in Barcelona, during the Spanish Civil War. (For history of blood transfusion *see* Diamond, L. K., *J. Amer. med. Ass.*, 1965, **193**, 40.)

Hæmoglobin can be estimated by:—

1. The oxyhæmoglobin method.
2. The cyanmethæmoglobin method—currently fashionable.
3. The alkaline hæmatin method, where there may be sulphæmoglobin in the blood.

Stored, refrigerated blood (at a temperature of 2–6° C.) is good for increasing hæmoglobin, and for raising blood-volume, up to about three weeks from the time of its collection, but the clotting factor together with immune bodies deteriorate in stored blood. Thus if the transfusion is planned in the treatment of sepsis, hæmorrhagic disease, or lack of clotting power, blood less than twenty-four hours old should be used.

Rh-negative blood should whenever possible be given to Rh-negative patients, who form about 15 per cent of the population in Britain. It is specially desirable in :—

1. Rh-negative patients of either sex who have either had a previous transfusion or may require a subsequent one.
2. Rh-negative girls and women of child-bearing age.
3. Mothers of infants who have hæmolytic disease.
4. Infants with hæmolytic disease. With no preliminary testing at all, incompatibility (ABO) will only occur once in three times.*

Packed red-cell transfusion is carried out by siphoning off the supernatant fluid from two bottles of blood, and adding the red-cell deposits together. It is useful in the treatment of anæmia before operation, anæmia associated with myocardial disease, and anæmia associated with nephritis. By giving sedimented red cells, three-quarters of the sodium content of whole blood is removed. Such blood should be given within a few hours of processing to prevent the harmful results of possible bacterial contamination.

DIRECT CROSS-MATCHING TEST.—When the services of a pathologist are not available, one drop of the recipient's serum is placed on a white tile and one drop of 5 per cent suspension of donor's blood in saline (2 or 3 drops of blood in 1 or 2 ml. of normal saline) is added to it. The two sera are mixed with a loop, the tile tilted and left for 10 to 15 minutes and again agitated, and examined with a hand lens for agglutination.

In a grave emergency, uncross-matched group ORh negative is the least dangerous to use.

COMPLICATIONS.—Each blood transfusion carries a certain risk and single bottle transfusions are seldom necessary.† The possible hazards are the following:—

1. HÆMOLYTIC REACTION.—
   a. Intravascular.—Due to incompatible transfusion and the destruction of the donor's red cells by the action of specific antibodies in the recipient's circulation—chiefly anti-A,

---

* Mollison, P. L., *Brit. med. J.*, 1959, **2**, 1035.
† Graham-Stewart, C. W., *Lancet*, 1960, **2**, 421.

The Treatment of Shock before Operation, *continued.*

anti-B, and anti-D of the Rhesus system. Usually ABO incompatibility causes a more violent reaction than one due to the Rhesus factor. General anæsthesia masks the effects. The blood-pressure and pulse-rate should be taken every five minutes for the first quarter-hour with each new bottle of blood. If there is a fall of the blood-pressure or a rise in pulse-rate or cyanosis for which no other cause can be found, the transfusion should be stopped.

b. Extravascular.—Due to transfusion of lysed blood which is : (i) Old (i.e., more than 3–4 weeks after collection) ; (ii) Heated above 38° C. ; or (iii) Frozen (i.e., less than 2° C.).

Treatment of anuria due to incompatible transfusion, *see* p. 703.

Signs of incompatible transfusion : All patients receiving blood should be carefully watched during the first 15 minutes to detect possible trouble : (A) *In the conscious* : (1) Fullness of the head ; (2) Tingling of limbs ; (3) Precordial pain ; (4) Lumbar pain ; (5) Dyspnœa ; (6) Restlessness ; (7) Suffused face ; (8) Nausea and vomiting ; (9) Pyrexia ; (10) Circulatory collapse ; (11) Later, hæmoglobinæmia, hæmoglobinuria, and oliguria. (B) *Under anæsthesia* : (1) Hypotension ; (2) General oozing from wound ; (3) Later, jaundice and oliguria in 5–10 per cent of these patients. These changes start to occur early on in the transfusion.

Investigation of transfusion reactions : The following specimens are needed :—

1. The blood samples used for the compatibility test before the transfusion.

2. The remains of the blood in the bottle or bottles used for the transfusion.

3. A sample of the patient's blood taken 3 hours after the transfusion reaction, collected into a dry sterile bottle with a dry sterile needle and syringe ; 10 ml. will suffice. In addition 2 ml. should be put into an oxalated bottle.

4. A sample of clear urine.

(*See also Notes on Transfusion,* issued by the Ministry of Health for the National Blood Transfusion Service, 1958.)

2. USE OF INFECTED BLOOD.—Most frequent following packed red-cell transfusion. Blood left out of the refrigerator for more than 30 minutes should not be used.

3. CIRCULATORY OVERLOADING.—During rapid transfusion, a low arterial and a raised venous pressure are evidence of cardiac overloading. To prevent acute pulmonary œdema, especially in patients with severe anæmia, frusimide, 40 mg., can be given into a vein at the outset of the transfusion; if renal function is good a diuresis of 2 litres will occur over a period of 2 hours if it is not good. Thus 1 litre of blood can be given in 2 hours without increase of blood-volume. The rate of drip should be 0·5–1 ml. per lb. per hour. The signs are: (*a*) Tightness in the chest. (*b*) Cough. (*c*) Dyspnœa. (*d*) Cyanosis. (*e*) Engorgement of neck veins. (*f*) Tachycardia.

(g) Basal crepitations. (h) Pulmonary œdema. (i) Increase in central venous pressure.

The condition may be relieved by inhalation of oxygen, venesection, digitalis, aminophylline, and tourniquets to the limbs.

Treatment.—Stop transfusion. Give digitalis and atropine. Prop patient up. Apply heat to dilate the skin vessels and enlarge the vascular bed.

4. AIR EMBOLISM.—The intravenous injection of 10 ml. of air may prove fatal.

5. TRANSMISSION OF DISEASE.—(a) Virus hepatitis, 6–16 weeks afterwards. (b) Malaria. (c) Syphilis. (d) Yaws. (e) Relapsing fever. (f) Kala-azar.

The incidence of virus hepatitis in patients receiving an average of two bottles of blood is 0·8 per cent; in those receiving large-pool plasma it is 11·9 per cent; in those receiving small-pool plasma (less than 10 bottles) it is 1·3 per cent.* During the Korean War, it was estimated that 3·6 per cent of patients given blood and 31·9 per cent of patients given blood and plasma developed viral hepatitis.† Work in Japan indicates that a higher proportion of cases receiving transfusions during major surgery develop subclinical viral hepatitis.‡ One in 200 healthy donors may be a carrier of hepatitis virus. Transference of malaria can be prevented by giving 600 mg. of chloroquine diphosphate before transfusion to the recipient. Elevation of serum levels of S.G.O.T. (aspartate transaminase) and S.G.P.T. (alanine transaminase) without jaundice has been found in one-fifth of those patients receiving two bottles of blood.§

6. FEBRILE AND ALLERGIC REACTIONS.—Are said to occur in about 1–2 per cent of transfusions, usually only mild urticaria resulting. Rarely asthma, angioneurotic œdema, and laryngeal œdema are seen and must be treated by stopping the transfusion and giving adrenaline. The addition of 10 mg. of chlorprophenpyridamine (piriton) to each pint of blood reduces the incidence of reactions in allergic patients.‖

7. POTASSIUM INTOXICATION.—Cardiac arrest due to this condition may occur during or shortly after transfusion of stored whole blood or overconcentrated plasma. Hyperkalæmia is more likely if there is accompanying metabolic acidosis.

The potassium/calcium ratio may be upset by the following factors :—

a. Old stored blood may contain 25 mEq. per l. of potassium, over five times the normal amount, due to the diffusion of the ion out of the red cells. In shock the fatal dose of potassium may be reduced by one-third.

* Annotation, *Brit. med. J.*, 1966, **1**, 997; and *Ibid.*, 1967, **1**, 256.
† Johnstone, M., *Brit. J. Anæsth.*, 1964, **36**, 718.
‡ Shimizu, Y., and Kitamota, O., *Gastroenterology*, 1963, **44**, 740.
§ Hampers, C. L., and others, *New Engl. J. Med.*, 1964, **271**, 747.
‖ Hobsley, M., *Lancet*, 1958, **1**, 459.

The Treatment of Shock before Operation, *continued.*

 b. The liver releases potassium due to many different stimuli
e.g., anoxia, hypercapnia, adrenaline liberated from the
adrenals in response to hæmorrhage.

 Signs of potassium intoxication may include a failing myocardium
a raised venous pressure, and peaking and elevation of the
T-wave on the E.C.G. Pre- and post-operative digitalization
will counteract the toxic effects of potassium.

8. The Low Temperature of Transfused Blood is also harmful
to the myocardium and may result in arrhythmia or even
ventricular fibrillation. If voluminous transfusion is necessary
the drip tubing can be warmed and fresh blood should be
employed.

9. Citrate Intoxication.—Storage with acid citrate dextrose was
a great advance and allowed blood to be kept for 21 days with
70 per cent viability of red cells.*

Whole blood is citrated :—

 a. By adding to 420 ml. of blood 100 ml. of 3 per cent tri
sodium citrate in distilled water, plus 20 ml. of 15 per
cent glucose in distilled water. Such blood must be
used within fourteen days.

 b. By adding to 420 ml. of blood 2 g. of disodium citrate
plus 3 g. of glucose in 120 ml. of distilled water. Such
blood lasts twenty-one days if stored at 2-6° C. About
70 per cent of red cells are supposed to survive for 2
days in this solution. The oxygen dissociation curve of
the hæmoglobin is shifted to the left, and potassium may
be liberated so that its concentration may rise from 5 to
25 mEq. per l.

The citrate in citrated blood is altered fairly rapidly into
water and carbon dioxide, and partly excreted as calcium
citrate. *Tetany* can result from the removal of calcium ions
in this way if a large amount of citrated blood (e.g., 4 litres
in one hour) is transfused over a short period. A high plasma
citrate level is unlikely unless the transfusion rate is greater
than 540 ml. per 5 minutes, except in the following states
(1) Liver disease ; (2) Anuria ; (3) Impairment of liver circu
lation ; (4) Hypothermia, which retards citrate clearance. A
suitable ionizable calcium salt should be given after every
1000 ml. of citrated blood. It should be injected rapidly
into another vein (to avoid clotting in the drip tubing) (e.g.
1 g. of calcium gluconate or calcium chloride). *Cardiac
depression* may be caused by citrated blood due to : (1) Citrate
toxicity. (2) Acidity of citrated blood. The pH is 7·1 when
fresh. (3) Removal of ionizable calcium by citrate. (4) Hyper
kalæmia—in intra-arterial transfusions. (5) Paralysis of the
cardiac vagus.† Injection of calcium gluconate, 10 per
cent, 5–10 ml. for each bottle of blood which is rapidly
transfused, will benefit cardiac depression,‡ and preserve the

* Loutit, J. F., and Mollison, P. L., *Brit. med. J.*, 1943, **2**, 744.
†'Argent, D. E., *Brit. J. Anæsth.*, 1957, **29**, 136.
‡ Burton, G. W., *Proc. R. Soc. Med.*, 1965, **58**, 777

calcium : potassium ratio. The oxygen released from blood stored in an acid citrate dextrose medium, after transfusion, may be decreased, so the blood of an anæmic patient may, for a few hours after transfusion, be unable to release as much oxygen as it did before (*see* p. 58). There is progressive loss of viability of stored red cells so that after 21 days about one-quarter of them are removed from the recipient's circulation within 24 hours of transfusion. *Increased oozing* may also occur.

In open heart surgery and in renal dialysis, heparinized blood may be preferred, 30 mg. of heparin being added to 540 ml. of blood. Any hæmorrhagic tendency thereafter can be controlled by protamine sulphate, 1 mg. for each mg. of heparin. Heparinization does not interfere with calcium stores in the body and citrate intoxication does not arise.

10. HYPOTHERMIA.—Massive transfusion of cold blood may cause body cooling, and this has been incriminated in a recent analysis of transfusion arrests.*

11. METABOLIC ACIDOSIS.—The pH of stored blood varies between 6·58 and 6·72, acidæmia being due to an accumulation of lactic acid, pyruvic acid, and citric acid, and raised Pco_2. This may be important in massive transfusion.

12. HÆMORRHAGIC TENDENCY.—This may be seen after massive transfusion and requires fresh blood.

GLUCOSE, 50–100 ml. of 50 per cent solution, raises the blood-pressure quickly and keeps it elevated for 20–30 minutes.

Ordinarily 5 per cent glucose solution is used, but if a combination of saline and glucose is to be employed, the proportion should be ⅕ normal saline with 4·3 per cent glucose : this mixture is isotonic and will not irritate the veins. Thrombophlebitis can be minimized by neutralization to a pH of 6·8 with a phosphate buffer.† When stored blood is followed by glucose, the filter should be renewed to prevent hæmolysis. Glucose of 10 per cent or over may produce thrombosis : 5 per cent solution is isotonic and should be the routine solution for intravenous drips designed for fluid replacement and to keep open an intravenous route for medication. Solution should be filtered rather than autoclaved.

NORMAL SALINE.—The rapid infusion of this solution will raise the blood-pressure significantly for 15–20 minutes, without change in the pulse-rate.‡

The pH of 5 per cent dextrose in water is 4·55, an acid load of 0·28 mEq./l.

The pH of 5 per cent dextrose in normal saline is 4·03, an acid load of 0·70 mEq./l.

The pH of normal saline is 4·00, an acid load of 0·80 mEq./l.

PLASMA or serum is used in the liquid state or after adding distilled water to the dried powder. Plasma is prepared from citrated

---

* Bryan, C. P., and Howland, W. S., *J. Amer. med. Ass.*, 1963, **183**, 58; and Leader, *Lancet*, 1966, **1**, 1193.
† Elfving, G., and others, *Ibid.*, 1966, **2**, 226.
‡ Askrog, V., *Brit. J. Anæsth.*, 1966, **38**, 455.

The Treatment of Shock before Operation, *continued.*

blood which does not clot and therefore contains fibrinogen. Serum is separated from blood which has been allowed to clot and so does not contain fibrinogen. Reconstituted plasma or serum should be used within three hours and not stored for future use. These substances are retained in the circulation ; they do not leak through the capillary walls, nor do they leave via the kidneys. Plasma is preferred to dextran as a blood-volume restorer in conditions where hypofibrinogenæmia is apt to develop, e.g., in cases of accidental hæmorrhage, amniotic fluid embolism, dead fœtus in utero, or hydatidiform mole. It may be necessary to use it in triple strength. Dried serum or plasma should be stored at a temperature below 20° C. (68° F.) in the dark. It need not be stored in a refrigerator. Rapid infusion of triple-strength plasma may cause death from hyperkalæmia; when this is given routine calcium should accompany it.*

POVIDONE (P.V.P.; Plasmosan; Periston N.; Subtosan).†—This is a 3·5 per cent solution of polyvinyl pyrrolidone in normal saline. It also contains ions of potassium, calcium, and magnesium. It was suggested first by Hecht and Weese in Germany in 1943.‡ It is a stable plasma substitute, having a viscosity and colloid osmotic pressure similar to plasma, with a molecular size of 30,000–60,000. Is not antigenic and contains no protein. It is a substance foreign to the body. Does not interfere with blood-clotting or antibacterial activity. Can be given through same apparatus as plasma, but a saline wash-through should be interposed between it and blood. Detectable in body up to two weeks after infusion, although 75 per cent of it is excreted by the kidneys during the first ten days and more is broken down in the body. It may interfere with interpretation of results of: (1) Blood-sugar, (2) Urinary albumin, and (3) Erythrocyte sedimentation estimations. It does not interfere with blood grouping or cross-matching. It diminishes platelet adhesiveness.§ It is now seldom used in Britain. It is taken up by cells of the reticulo-endothelial system and is said to be carcinogenic.

DEXTRAN (Intradex ; Dextraven ; Macrodex ; Expandex ; Plavolex ; Gentran).—A plasma substitute originally prepared in Sweden and suggested as a plasma expander in 1944 by Gronwall and Ingleman. It is a 6 per cent solution in normal saline or dextrose solution of polydispersoid glycose polymer. It is formed by bacterial action (*Leuconostoc mesenterioides*) on sucrose. Its viscosity is between that of blood and plasma, while its specific gravity is slightly greater than that of plasma, with a molecular size of between 70,000 and 150,000; the average being near the latter figure. The molecules have a high colloid-osmotic (oncotic) pressure. Dextran contains antigens which occasionally give rise to skin sensitivity and other mild allergic

* Zorab, J. S. M., *Brit. med. J.*, 1965, **1**, 105.
† De Freitas, F. M., and others, *J. clin. Invest.*, 1965, **44**, 3.
‡ Hecht, G., and Weese, H., *Münch. med. Wschr.*, 1943, **90**, 11.
§ Sanbar, S. S., and others, *Lancet*, 1967, **2**, 917.

lesions which can be ameliorated by the injection of antihistamine drugs. Such reactions do not detract from its usefulness. It is non-toxic, electrically neutral, and chemically inert. Although it is eventually eliminated completely from the body, it remains in the circulation, in gradually decreasing amount, up to a week, and some of its larger molecules are stored for some time in the cells of the reticulo-endothelial system. Only 50 per cent can be recovered from the urine. Has proved useful as a plasma substitute in cases of burns and surgical shock; prophylaxis of shock during operations and in the treatment of circulatory depression in toxæmic states, e.g., poisoning with barbiturates, salicylates, etc., peritonitis. It increases the venous return to the heart. During manufacture, the size of its molecules must be made to approach that of plasma-protein molecules: if too small, dextran molecules pass through the glomerular filter; if too large, kidney damage may follow. Reactions occur in rather less than 2 per cent of patients, the chief being mild pyrexia. Very occasionally circulatory collapse, cyanosis, and vomiting have been reported. Some samples may interfere with blood grouping and cross-matching results, owing to rouleaux formation, so specimens should be taken for this purpose before dextan is infused. If this is not done, recipient cells must be washed before testing. It may interfere with plasma protein determinations. Dextran molecules greater in size than 50,000 increase the E.S.R., those smaller decrease it. Blood sugar values not increased and diabetics tolerate it well. Can also be obtained in a salt-free solution with 5 per cent dextrose and as a 10 per cent solution for use in cases of nephrotic and pregnancy œdema. Contra-indicated in severe congestive heart failure and in anuria.

The sulphuric ester of dextran has similar antithrombin activity to heparin, which it structurally resembles. Ordinary dextran is not an anticoagulant.

LOW MOLECULAR WEIGHT DEXTRAN (about 40,000).—This is a 10 per cent solution in either normal saline or 5 per cent dextrose. It has been used to aid the circulation as a blood-flow improver in: (1) Severe burns; (2) Severe hæmorrhage; (3) Crushing injuries; (4) Toxæmias; (5) Fat embolism; (6) Oliguria; (7) Incipient gangrene; (8) Impairment of arterial or venous circulation, etc. The rate of infusion should average 500 ml. in half to 1 hour. It is removed from the body in about 2 hours, more rapidly than high molecular weight dextran. Has been used with blood (1 part to 3–4 parts of blood) to prime pump-oxygenators. It is said to prevent intravascular aggregation of red cells[*] or so-called 'sludging';[†] and to reverse peripheral ischæmia.[‡] It does not interfere with cross-matching, blood grouping, or with coagulation.

Dextran of low molecular weight has been combined with neomycin to make the antibiotic non-absorbable from the peritoneal cavity.[§]

* Gelin, L. E., and Ingelman, B., *Acta chir. scand.*, 1961, **122**, 294.
† Bigelow, W. G., Heimbecker, R. O., and Harrison, R. I., *A.M.A. Arch. Surg.*, 1949, **59**, 667.
‡ Ratliff, A. H. C., *Lancet*, 1963, **1**, 1188.
§ Markalous, P., *Anæsthesia*, 1962, **17**, 427.

The Treatment of Shock before Operation, *continued.*

ACACIA, 6 per cent (Bayliss, 1917), in saline; PECTIN, 5 per cent; GELATIN, 6 per cent; have also been used.

Plasma substitutes cause no homologous serum jaundice (which occurs in 1·3 per cent of cases receiving small pool plasma) and this is a good reason for preferring them to plasma. Up to 1 litre can be infused, but larger amounts are not desirable. A pint of substitute to two pints of blood or plasma is a convenient and beneficial proportion. Their great advantage is their availability and stability in emergency, especially in cases of : (1) Acute hæmorrhage, while waiting for blood ; (2) Traumatic shock ; (3) Burns ; (4) Crush injuries ; (5) Dehydration. They must be used carefully in cases of intestinal obstruction, as they may be excreted into the bowel lumen, when their osmotic properties are likely to withdraw fluid from the blood. They contain no nutriment, are not oxygen carriers, and are not buffering agents.

Whole blood is indicated :—

    1. In acute hæmolytic crises.

    2. In acute hæmorrhage.

    3. In subacute hæmorrhage which has led to secondary anæmia.

Fresh blood is needed :—

    1. In prothrombin deficiency.

    2. In hæmophilia and Christmas disease.

Packed red cells are needed :—

    1. In anæmia of infection, before operation.

    2. After acute hæmorrhage not treated by transfusion (the hyper-kinetic phase of shock). Should be given within 24 hours of preparation to prevent infection.

    3. In congestive cardiac failure or recent myocardial disease.

Small pool plasma or dextran is indicated:—

    1. In acute hæmorrhage when blood is not available.

    2. In trauma and operation.

    3. In burns.

Fresh plasma may be indicated in :—

    1. Prothrombin deficiency.

    2. Hæmophilia.

Concentrated platelet transfusion may be required before splenectomy for thrombocytopenic purpura. If whole blood is centrifuged at a suitable speed the plasma will contain a high platelet fraction.

INTRA-ARTERIAL TRANSFUSION.—Intra-arterial transfusion was advocated in 1906 by Crile and Dolley and it was again advocated by Kemp in 1933. The left radial artery is cannulated 2 in. proximal to the styloid process under local analgesia or brachial plexus or stellate ganglion block to relieve spasm. Application of 1–40 papaverine solution also helps to release arterial spasm. The vessel is tied in continuity when the cannula is withdrawn. Apparatus may consist of two giving bottles connected in series with a Macintosh-Pask drip chamber to prevent injection of air, together with a bellows and manometer. In emergency, a syringe and a three-way tap may be used. Indications : (1) When in severe shock the response to intravenous transfusion is poor. (2) During surgery when there is rapid and severe hæmorrhage. The aorta may have to be used to receive blood. (3) When blood is in short supply.

The risk of gangrene is slight, while it is usually no more difficult to cannulate an artery than a collapsed vein. Because of the high plasma potassium level in stored blood, fresh blood should be used. Intra-arterial transfusion is less popular than it was.

THE RISKS OF OVER-TRANSFUSION.—Harm is unlikely if the rate is slowed up when the blood-pressure is back to normal or, if this is not known, to 100 mm. Hg. The heart pumps out 5 l. of blood each minute. Seldom should more than 500 ml. of fluid be run in at speed under pressure. Care should be taken if the venous pressure in the superior vena cava is greater than 12 cm. of water with I.P.P.V. or 5 cm. with spontaneous respiration.

In severe anæmia, the pulse may be full and bounding, the pulse-pressure high, and the cardiac output increased in spite of a handicapped myocardium. In these cases large rapid transfusions may cause acute pulmonary œdema. Raising the head of the bed to encourage venous pooling in the legs, together with intravenous digoxin 1 mg., are useful, should the heart begin to fail. One or two bottles should be given slowly, or, better still, a transfusion of concentrated corpuscles should be given, i.e., the corpuscles of two or more bottles are mixed, after siphoning off part of the plasma.

Overload is dangerous, too, in patients with severe arterio-sclerosis or coronary disease in whom a rise in pulse-rate and fall in blood-pressure during transfusion may signify developing heart failure, rather than further hæmorrhage.

Excessive amounts of plasma or serum dilute the blood and so produce anæmia.

Glucose and saline are not retained in the circulation ; so excessive amounts may cause acute pulmonary œdema, owing to overfilling of vascular bed. For prolonged infusion in cases of dehydration, forty drops a minute is a suitable rate, giving one pint of fluid every four hours.

INTRAMEDULLARY INFUSION.—See p. 300.

HYPODERMOCLYSIS.—This can be : (1) Subpectoral ; (2) Into the outer side of the thigh ; (3) Into axilla ; (4) Into sub-scapular region ; (5) Into anterior abdominal wall, especially in infants.

To prevent pain, 1 g. of procaine may be added to each litre of fluid.

Normal saline or 5 per cent glucose should be used.

HYALURONIDASE.*—This is a ' spreading factor ' which aids absorption of fluid injected into the subcutaneous and intra-muscular tissues. It is a mucolytic enzyme which hydrolyses

---

* See article by Gaisford, W., and Evans, D. G., Lancet, 1949, **2**, 505.

The Treatment of Shock before Operation, *continued*.

hyaluronic acid, a viscous polysaccharide found in interstitial spaces which normally obstructs diffusion of invasive substances. It takes the line of least resistance and will not diffuse through an infected area because of the fibrin acting as a barrier. It is an enzyme first isolated by Mayer and Palmer in 1934, and described by Duran Reynals in 1929. It is a testicular extract. Prepared under the names of hyalase, rondase, wydase, diffusin, as a white powder, sterile and soluble in water. The contents of one ampoule, 1 mg., should be added to 500–1000 ml. of fluid for hypodermoclysis; the substance must be used as soon as possible after it is dissolved. It is non-toxic and has no side-actions. An international standard of assay has now been defined by the W.H.O. at Geneva. It must not be contaminated with antiseptic, which might inhibit its action.

USES.—(*a*) In pædiatrics, where veins are difficult to find; (*b*) In infiltration anæsthesia. where it increases the area of effective analgesia. It does not increase the efficiency of nerve-block and may make the infiltrated area painful in the hours following injection. No hyaluronic acid has been demonstrated in the extradural space and the enzyme is useless as an aid to extradural block. It is no substitute for precise anatomical knowledge but may be helpful in skin and subcutaneous analgesia, hernia block, splanchnic and pudendal block, and in the reduction of fractures (e.g., Colles's) under local analgesia. It has been reported to increase the toxic effects of local analgesia. (*c*) To maintain the fluid balance pre- and post-operatively, instead of intravenous infusions.

PROCTOCLYSIS.—If a slow sustaining effect is required, 5 per cent glucose in water is beneficial, or tap water alone, using a drip.

PRESSOR DRUGS.—The intravenous injection—usually via a continuous drip—of sympathomimetic drugs has a part in the treatment of shock, but conflicting opinions exist as to its proper place. They should be given early, as anoxia, if allowed to develop, diminishes their effect. Noradrenaline may redistribute available blood and may be useful in the periods when blood is not available. It has, too, a positive inotropic effect (unlike, e.g., phenylephrine, methoxamine, and metaraminol. As the drug, after a time, comes to lose its pressor effect so the drip must be gradually withdrawn.

The reasons given for this are :—

1. It eventually depresses the vasomotor centre.
2. It eventually causes ganglionic blockade.
3. It may, after a time, unite with a metabolite to form a vaso-dilator substance.

ISOPRENALINE.—When given by intravenous infusion (1–450,000) this causes peripheral vasodilatation and has achieved success, especially in cases of endotoxic shock.*

STROPHANTHIN G† (Ouabaine).—The injection, intravenously, of 0·5 mg. with or without replacement of blood volume improves

---

* Du Toit, H. J., and others, *Lancet*, 1966, **2**, 143.
† *See* articles by Horton, J. A. G., and others, *Brit. med. J.*, 1953, **2**, 1249; Brown, A. S., *Lancet*, 1953, **2**, 745.

the circulation in many patients, and is useful if the response to fluid therapy is disappointing, during, before, or after operation, and as a preventative of circulatory depression during induction and maintenance of anæsthesia. The drug appears to do no harm, acts quickly and for a short time, and is rapidly excreted. It should not, however, be used in a patient who has received a digitalis glycoside within the past two weeks. Indications include:*—

1. In shock, as an aid to blood-volume replacement.
2. To restore blood-pressure when transfusion is undesirable, e.g., in congestive failure.
3. When there is peripheral vasoconstriction or tachycardia which might contra-indicate pressor drugs.
4. In sudden hypotension associated with induction of anæsthesia or movement of the patient.
5. In congestive heart failure and when the central venous pressure is raised and the blood-volume is low or normal.

The following agents may have a part to play in the management of shock:—

SODIUM BICARBONATE.—For the correction of any metabolic acidosis which may be present. A reasonable first dose would be 40–80 mEq. (40–80 ml. of 8·4 per cent solution). Further doses would depend on laboratory findings.

TROMETAMOL (Tromethamine, THAM, Tris, Trihydroxymethyl aminomethane).—This alkaline buffer may also be used to combat metabolic acidosis and to buffer lactic and pyruvic acids formed by anaerobic metabolism.

HYDROCORTISONE.—This has, as well as anti-inflammatory, positive inotropic and α-blocking effects.† Dose: 25–50 mg. per kg., i.e., up to 2 g. intravenously in a short period. The plasma volume must be maintained as vasodilatation results.

CHLORPROMAZINE.—This antagonizes the constrictor response of small vessels to the increased levels of catecholamines and promotes tissue perfusion. Dose: 5 mg., carefully repeated as necessary.

PHENOXYBENZAMINE (Dibenzyline).—This is a blocker of α-adrenergic receptors, the effects of which come on rapidly after intravenous injection and last for about 24 hours. The dose is 1 mg. per kg. repeated as required, keeping a close watch on the blood-pressure. Plasma volume must be maintained.‡

Evidence is accumulating to show that as much good or more can be achieved in the treatment of shock by promoting tissue perfusion than by raising the blood-pressure. Pressure is not perfusion. The administration of vasodilator agents must always be accompanied by infusion of adequate amounts of plasma volume expanders.

Anæsthesia for the Patient in Shock.—Operation should not be undertaken, except in cases of grave emergency, until the patient

---

* Horton, J. A. G., and Davison, M. H. Armstrong, *Brit. J. Anæsth.*, 1955, **27**, 139.
† Lillehei, R. C., and others, *Ann. Surg.*, 1964, **160**, 682.
‡ Lillehei, R. C., and others, *Int. Anæsth. Clin.*, 1964, **2**, 297.

Anæsthesia for the Patient in Shock, *continued.*

is resuscitated. Here again, the aim is still uncertain: Is it restoration of blood-pressure or of tissue perfusion? Are vasopressors to be preferred to vasodilators with adequate fluid replacement? Pressure rise is not necessarily accompanied by increased perfusion. Full fluid replacement before use of vasodilator drugs is imperative. Once improvement has occurred, the longer operation is delayed the worse it is for the patient. The blood-pressure should, if possible, be restored to at least 100 mm. Hg and the clinical condition should show signs of improvement. A systolic blood-pressure above 100 mm. Hg indicates that blood-volume is probably not less than 70 per cent of normal.

Shocked and recently resuscitated patients require much smaller amounts of anæsthetic agents than do normal patients, and only light anæsthesia is usually necessary. Vomiting may occur at this light plane as shock is an important cause, along with fear and anxiety, of delayed gastric emptying.

Hypoxia must be avoided most carefully. There is evidence that in the treatment of hæmorrhagic shock the patient should be hyperventilated to prevent hypoxia ; the osmolarity of the extracellular fluid should be raised ; and the metabolic acidosis corrected by infusion of 2·74 per cent sodium bicarbonate solution. Hypertonic solutions should be infused during or prior to blood transfusion.*

Premedication should be given intravenously, just before induction of anæsthesia, so that suitable dosage can be arrived at. On account of respiratory depression, morphine may be contraindicated, atropine alone being usually sufficient.

Induction.—A full stomach may complicate induction.

Maintenance.—Ether may cause, theoretically, increase in vasodilatation and capillary leakage. Actually, light ether is a suitable anæsthetic.

Cyclopropane is well tolerated and does not cause a further fall in blood-pressure. It may be useful in the actively bleeding patient until blood-volume is restored, but prolonged administration in shock may be harmful as among other effects it reduces renal blood-flow. Halothane and oxygen must be used carefully as hypotension may be potentiated. Renal blood-flow tends to be enhanced. Should relaxation prove difficult, small doses of a muscle relaxant can be satisfactorily combined with either agent.

Thiopentone is satisfactory if used in minimal doses but it must be remembered that, in shock, the distribution of thiopentone to non-nervous tissues is interfered with, so that removal of the drug from the blood-stream has to be by the slow process of detoxication rather than by the more normal process of redistribution to other tissues. It should be combined with inhalation of either pure oxygen or mixtures of oxygen and nitrous oxide in equal proportion.

A cuffed endotracheal tube is often desirable both to minimize the chances of underventilation and to guard against aspiration of gastric contents.

---

* Brooks, D. K., and others, *Anæsthesia*, 1963, **18**, 363.

Regional analgesia may be very satisfactory. (*See* Brindenbaugh, L. D., and Moore, D. C., *Management of the Patient in Shock* (Ed. Orkin, L.), 1965, Ch. 5. Oxford: Blackwell.)

The blood-pressure and pulse-rate should be charted regularly. Some patients seem to benefit from the injection of 0·25–0·5 mg. of ouabaine during operation (*see* p. 696).

The Treatment of Shock during Operation.—

1. Lower head of table.
2. Lighten anæsthesia if necessary and see that oxygen is reaching the alveoli. I.P.P.V. may be beneficial.
3. Arrange for blood, dextran, plasma, or saline intravenous infusion.
4. Consider the use of hydrocortisone.

SALT AND WATER BALANCE

Fluid Requirements.—Water balance is the ratio between the water taken in by all routes over the water leaving the body by all routes. Loss of fluid may occur independently of, but more usually together with, loss of electrolytes, chiefly sodium chloride. The fluid balance is worked out as follows :—

Intake		Output	
As food	1100 ml.	As urine	1500 ml.
As drink	1500 ml.	As fæces	100 ml.
		Vapour from lungs	400 ml.
		Vapour from skin	600 ml.
Total	2600 ml.	Total	2600 ml.

In hot climates, insensible loss may be 2 l. in 24 hours.

The healthy kidney can concentrate the day's waste products (average 35 g.) into 500 ml. of urine, the specific gravity of which may be as high as 1032. Twice or thrice this volume of urine may have to be secreted to remove the waste solids, if the kidneys are handicapped.

If water depletion is suspected, a fluid balance chart should be kept. The following three types of water and salt depletion are described :

1. No liquid intake, e.g., œsophageal obstruction : treatment is plenty of water ; only a little salt.
2. No intake, plus loss of secretion, e.g., pyloric obstruction: treatment is little water ; plenty of salt.
3. Normal intake with loss of secretion, e.g., diarrhœa : treatment is little water ; plenty of salt.

Fluid Loss.—When the patient appears clinically to be dehydrated, about 6 per cent of his body-weight in water has already been lost, and this amount must be replaced to restore hydration.

a. CAUSES.—

i. Inability to ingest adequate fluid after operation and anæsthesia ; coma ; severe prostrating illness ; dysphagia.

ii. Loss of fluid from alimentary canal. Seven and a half to ten litres of fluid are daily excreted into the gut and reabsorbed into its more distal segments. This gastro-intestinal fluid

Fluid Loss, *continued.*

circulation is two or three times the volume of the averag
amount of fluid taken by mouth in twenty-four hours. It
thus seen that vomiting, suction drainage, diarrhœa, intestina
fistulæ, etc., may have a powerful effect on the fluid economy
Disturbances in this circulation have been given by Nadler a
follows :—

1. Removal of fluid from proximal gut ; e.g., vomiting, gastri
   and duodenal fistulæ, high intestinal obstruction, intestina
   suction drainage.
2. Failure of secretions to reach absorptive area, as in ileus
   acute dilatation of stomach, intestinal obstruction.
3. Escape of secretions and wastage ; e.g., biliary drainage
   pancreatic and intestinal fistulæ.
4. Increased peristalsis, leaving insufficient time for reabsorp
   tion, as in diarrhœa.

These fluids are isotonic with serum, so salt is lost too.

iii. Excessive sweating, which may cause great fluid loss. Swea
contains 0·2 per cent sodium chloride, so loss of one litre o
it produces a loss of one litre of water, the excess salt (0·8
per cent minus 0·2 per cent) remaining in the body until it i
excreted by the kidney because there is not sufficient wate
to support it as normal saline in the body. The salt is never
theless excreted, so the one litre of sweat results in loss o
one litre of normal saline. Treatment is normal saline.

b. DIAGNOSIS.—On clinical and laboratory evidence.

CLINICAL.—Thirst, dryness of mouth, because of scantiness o
saliva and oliguria. Thirst is more characteristic of fluid tha
of salt depletion.

LABORATORY.—Raised blood-urea, because urinary volume is no
sufficient adequately to carry away the non-protein nitrogen
High specific gravity of urine. If one pint of urine is passe
each eight hours, and is of low specific gravity, all is probabl
well as far as fluid balance is concerned. If, in addition, th
urinary chlorides are normal (3–5 g. per litre) salt depletio
is not serious.

c. TREATMENT.—Abnormal loss of fluid should be replaced by a
equal volume of fluid to that lost, in addition to the normal flui
requirements of the body. In exceptional cases, as much a
eight pints a day may be necessary, e.g., ileus, persistent diar
rhœa.

i. PROPHYLACTIC.—Tap water, one and a half pints, can usefull
be given per rectum while patient is on the table, as thi
volume of fluid is often lost during a major operation ; i
cannot cause overloading with either salt or water an
is specially useful in children (in proportionately smalle
amounts).

ii. CURATIVE.—Water by mouth, rectum, vein, or hypodermo
clysis. Glucose, 5 per cent in distilled water, is an isotonic
fluid useful for this purpose, providing in addition 200 calories
per litre. As salt loss frequently accompanies fluid loss, one
fifth normal saline with 4·3 per cent glucose can often be

substituted. Normal saline, containing 9 g. of salt per litre, should not be used in the absence of abnormal salt loss so that the kidneys are not presented with excess of salt to excrete ; renal impairment may result in œdema from salt retention should this occur.

The average requirements after operation are as follows : First day, 3·5 l. ; second and third days, 3 l.—by any available route. Too much fluid is harmful, as pulmonary œdema and cardiac embarrassment may result.

3. Salt Requirements.—Basic need of body for salt is 1–2 g. per day, but as much as 15 g. may be taken with food, the excess being excreted in the urine (normal, 5 g. per litre). In cases of salt lack as soon as the plasma-salt level falls below normal (560–630 mg. per 100 ml.), the kidneys cease to excrete salt.

4. Salt Depletion.—

a. CAUSES.—Usually occurs when salt is lost but fluid intake is normal as in vomiting, diarrhœa, intestinal fistulæ or drainage, intestinal obstruction, etc.

b. SYMPTOMS.—Lassitude, apathy, weakness, anorexia, vomiting, peripheral circulatory failure. Urine normal in amount.

c. RESULTS.—

i. A loss of total osmotic pressure of extracellular fluid leading to excretion of water by the kidney and thus to decreased extracellular fluid volume with secondary or extracellular dehydration. Later follows a fall in plasma chlorides with a low value for urinary chlorides as shown by Fantus's test. There may be a rise in blood-urea.

ii. There is a disturbance of acid-base balance if the loss of chloride and sodium ions is disproportionate. With continued loss of gastric juice there is hypochloræmia with the production of alkalosis which may be accompanied by a rise in the plasma-bicarbonate level, as the freed sodium combines with carbonic acid. On the other hand, with continued loss of fluid from the gut distal to the pylorus, there is a greater loss of sodium ions, with resulting acidosis, and decrease of the plasma-bicarbonate. The alkali reserve, normally 55–75 ml. of carbon dioxide per 100 ml. of plasma, may be over 100 ml. or less than 20 ml. after vomiting or diarrhœa respectively.

Sweat contains 80 mEq./l. of sodium but in acclimatized patients in hot countries it may be only 10 mEq./l.

d. DIAGNOSIS.—On the clinical signs and symptoms. On the urinary chloride estimation or test of Fantus.

FANTUS'S TEST.—Ten drops of urine are accurately measured into a test-tube with a pipette. After washing out the pipette, one drop of 20 per cent potassium chromate solution is added, and the pipette rinsed again. Next, 2·9 per cent solution of silver nitrate is added drop by drop, the test-tube being shaken after each drop. The end-point is a sharp colour change from yellow to brown and the number of drops needed to produce it gives the concentration of sodium chloride in the urine expressed as grammes per litre ; 5 drops, i.e., 5 g. per litre, is normal.

Salt Depletion, *continued.*

If the end-point change occurs with the first drop, chloride is absent. If the urinary specific gravity is 1020, anything less than 3 g. per litre suggests salt depletion. If it is 5 g. per litre and the patient is not suffering from Addison's disease and is not receiving intravenous saline, he is probably not short of salt.

This test assumes the presence of relatively normal kidneys. If this is not so, plasma chloride estimations are required. Its accuracy and usefulness have recently been called in question.

The combination of a high urinary chloride with a low plasma chloride should suggest the possibility of potassium deficiency which can be corrected by giving Darrow's solution intravenously or potassium chloride by mouth. If supplemented intravenously, electrocardiographic control may be desirable.

e. TREATMENT.—Normal saline by any suitable route. When the symptoms are relieved and the urinary chlorides return to normal, one-fifth normal saline with 4·3 per cent glucose can be substituted. Coller, Bartlett, and Maddock advise the administration of 3·2 g. of salt per stone of body-weight for every 100 mg. that the plasma-chloride level needs to be raised to normal (560 mg. per cent).

5. Potassium.—Most of the body potassium is found within the cells, and only about 2 per cent is in the extracellular compartment. The average dietary intake of a normal healthy adult is 75–100 mEq. (3–4 g.) per 24 hours, out of which about 10 per cent is lost in the stools. Normal plasma levels are 3·5–5·0 mEq. per l. Daily urine loss is about 50–75 mEq.

POTASSIUM DEPLETION.—

CAUSES.—(i) Excessive loss from the gastro-intestinal tract, vomiting, diarrhœa, biliary fistula, etc. (ii) Excessive loss in the urine if diuresis is marked. (iii) Absence of normal potassium intake. This may aggravate depletion in the presence of excessive loss. (iv) In cirrhosis of the liver. (v) In congestive heart failure. (vi) May occur when patients are receiving intravenous glucose and saline drips for long periods.

RESULTS.—A clinical picture of lethargy, apathy, anorexia, and nausea related to disordered function of the three types of muscle: (*a*) Smooth muscle—causing constipation, distension, and ileus; (*b*) Skeletal muscle—causing hypotonia, weakness, and paralysis; (*c*) Cardiac muscle—causing hypotension, arrhythmia, and arrest. There may be accompanying sodium retention and metabolic alkalosis.

DIAGNOSIS.—Suspicion should arise when there is excessive fluid loss from urinary or gastro-intestinal tracts, particularly when potassium intake is low or absent. It may be a factor in prolonged paralytic ileus or metabolic alkalosis not responding to normal treatment. Diagnosis is confirmed by : (i) Plasma potassium estimation, though this can sometimes be normal in the presence of intracellular depletion—less than 5 per cent of the body's potassium is contained in the extracellular fluid, so a normal serum concentration may not give a true picture of the body's potassium content. (ii) E.C.G. changes: depression of ST-segment, lowering, widening, or inversion of T-waves, prolongation of QT-interval, appearance of U-waves—these are a reflection of intracellular potassium deficiency. (iii) Response to treatment.

TREATMENT.—A good mixed diet contains 60–80 mEq. potassium daily. The oral route is used, when possible, to eliminate the danger of an untoward rise in serum potassium. It may be given as potassium chloride, 2 g. (30 gr.) 6-hourly, or potassium citrate 2·6 g. (40 gr.) 6-hourly. Intravenous replacement must be cautious because of the dangers of hyperkalæmia (*see below*). It is recommended that it should be given only when there is good urinary output, that the concentration of infused fluid should not exceed 40 mEq./l. (i.e., KCl, 3 g. per l. or 0·3 per cent), the rate should not exceed 20 mEq. per hour, and the total dose should not exceed 100 mEq. in 24 hours* (2500 ml. 0·3 per cent KCl).

Effervescent potassium tablets (B.P.C.) each contain 6·5 mEq. of potassium. Dissolved in a glass of water they are not too unpleasant.

POTASSIUM INTOXICATION.—A dangerous rise in serum potassium may occur with over-zealous intravenous replacement therapy, or when urine output is depressed or absent. Toxic manifestations may occur at concentrations above 7 mEq./l., when the E.C.G. shows a tall peaked T-wave with a narrow base. Ventricular fibrillation may supervene at levels of 12 mEq./l. or above. Note that stored blood may contain 25 mEq./l. (*see* p. 689).

ANURIA.—Acute tubular necrosis leading to oliguria and anuria is a serious condition. May result from severe hypotension associated with shock as well as from mismatched transfusion. Spontaneous recovery may take place in 1 to 4 weeks if the patient can be protected from the disturbances of water and electrolyte balance which occur. Death is often due to potassium poisoning, on about the tenth to twelfth day, when serum levels as high as 14–16 mEq./l. may be reached.

TREATMENT is to carefully supervise the intake of water and electrolytes to prevent overloading. *See* Chapter XXXV. Once urine flow returns, intake should be increased by an equivalent amount of water and salt. A period of diuresis is accompanied by considerable loss of potassium in the urine and it may be necessary to add potassium to the intake to prevent hypokalæmia at this stage.

If recovery is greatly delayed, the use of an artificial kidney may be indicated.

6. The Metabolic Response to Injury.—This occurs after operation and is characterized by :—

---

* LeQuesne, L. P., *Fluid Balance in Surgical Practice*, 1955, 87. London : Lloyd-Luke.

The Metabolic Response to Injury, *continued.*

    a. Impairment of water excretion. Lasts 24–36 hours. Independent of salt and water intake.

    b. Impairment of sodium excretion. Lasts 4–6 days. Independent of sodium intake.

    c. Increased potassium excretion. Maximal in 24 hours. Usually lasts only 48 hours.

    This response is associated with an increased secretion of adrenocortical hormones, an impairment of their breakdown, and an increased production of antidiuretic hormone. The essential stimulus is probably via a nervous reflex, relaying in the hypothalamus.

COMPOSITION OF SOME FLUIDS USED FOR INTRAVENOUS INFUSION

	CONSTITUENTS	g. per cent	mEq./l.			
			Na	K	Cl	Lactate
Isotonic saline	NaCl	0·9	153	—	153	—
¼ normal saline	NaCl	0·18	30·25	—	30·25	—
Sodium lactate (⅙ molar)	Na lactate	1·86	167	—	—	167
Potassium chloride	KCl	0·3	—	40	40	—
Potassium chloride Sodium chloride in 2·5 per cent glucose (isotonic)	KCl NaCl	0·3 0·225	— 40 ‾ 40	40 — ‾ 40	40 40 ‾ 80	— — ‾ —
Saline lactate (Hartmann or Darrow)	NaCl Na lactate	0·6 0·62	102 56 ‾ 158	— — ‾	102 — ‾ 102	— 56 ‾ 56
Ringer lactate	NaCl Na lactate KCl CaCl₂	0·6 0·31 0·03 0·02	102 28 — — ‾ 130	— — 4 — ‾ 4	102 — 4 4 ‾ 110	— 28 — — ‾ 28
Darrow's solution (K lactate)	NaCl Na lactate KCl	0·4 0·62 0·27	68 56 — ‾ 124	— — 36 ‾ 36	68 — 36 ‾ 104	— 56 — ‾ 56
Extracellular fluid (for comparison)			140	5·0	103	—

$$\text{mEq./l.} = \frac{\text{mg. per cent} \times 10 \times \text{valency}}{\text{atomic weight}}.$$

It is wise, before undertaking fluid therapy, to assess thoroughly the following three points :—

1. Is fluid really necessary?
2. What fluid should be given?
3. What quantity of the correct fluid should be given?

AVERAGE FIGURES FOR ELECTROLYTE LOSSES
IN SECRETIONS FROM VARIOUS SITES*

	mEq./l.		
	Na	K	Cl
Stomach	60·4	9·2	84·0
Small intestine	111·3	4·6	104·2
Bile	148·9	4·98	100·6
Pancreatic juice	141·1	4·6	76·6
Recent ileostomy	129·4	11·2	116·2
Established ileostomy	46	3·0	21·4
Cæcostomy	52·5	7·9	42·5

Parenteral Feeding.—This can be safe, reliable, and efficient in patients who develop major complications of surgery. Prolonged recovery from severe trauma or operation may result in severe weight-loss and malnutrition. A constant nitrogen balance and constant body-weight can be maintained by intravenous feeding, but it is better to prevent than to treat bad nutritional states, e.g., in severe ulcerative colitis, chronic renal failure, and severe burns. The acidity of solutions and their hypertonicity may cause thrombophlebitis, so a large central venous catheter is required after 2 days' treatment. Care of electrolyte balance is imperative. Materials injected may include: (1) Amino-acid solutions: (a) Enzymatic hydrolysates of casein which contain up to 66 per cent of free amino-acids; (b) Mixtures of pure amino-acids, in which the total nitrogen and amino-acid concentration is higher than in (a) and the *p*H also higher. There is no evidence that either is superior to the other. (2) Fat emulsions. Large amounts of caloric fuel can be contained in a small volume; soya-bean oil emulsion is very satisfactory. Prolonged fat infusion increases the coagulability of the blood so heparin is required, but it does not increase the incidence of thrombophlebitis.* *See also* Chapter XXXV.

---

* Johnston, I. D. A., *Proc. R. Soc. Med.*, 1966, **59**, 575.

CHAPTER XXVIII

PRODUCTION OF ISCHÆMIA DURING OPERATIONS

Increased Bleeding during Anæsthesia.*—

ANÆSTHETIC CAUSES.—The production of unconsciousness causes release of vasomotor tone at the periphery and while those vessels supplying the skin and muscles dilate, those going to the kidney and splanchnic area constrict.

Bleeding may be made worse by :—

1. Respiratory obstruction.
2. Hypercapnia due to : (a) Inefficient carbon dioxide elimination ; (b) Hypoventilation.
3. Coughing during induction and maintenance, especially in surgery involving the head and neck.
4. Resistance in the anæsthetic circuit, including a tight expiratory valve causing a rise in intrathoracic pressure during expiration.

NON-ANÆSTHETIC CAUSES.—

1. Venous congestion secondary to: (a) Posture; (b) Heart disease; (c) Lung disease; (d) Overtransfusion.
2. Conditions causing a rise in the basal metabolic rate.
3. Operations involving vascular tissues, e.g., muscle or gland.
4. A rise in blood-pressure. This does not always increase bleeding, however.
5. Bleeding associated with systemic disease.
   a. Platelet deficiency. This may occur in idiopathic thrombocytopenic purpura ; purpura associated with leukæmia or with aplastic anæmia. Bleeding may occur if the platelet count is less than 50,000 per c.mm. The remedy is fresh blood.
   b. Liver disease.
   c. Uræmia.
   d. Polycythæmia.
   Acidosis, low serum calcium, low vitamin C level, low serum protein may all result in increased oozing.
6. Hæmorrhagic tendency due to treatment.
   a. Massive blood transfusion.
   b. Citrate intoxication.
   c. Incompatible blood transfusion.
   d. Previous administration of anticoagulants, requiring either vitamin K, protamine sulphate, or polybrene.
   e. Trauma to the blood in extracorporeal circulation.

---

* Feldman, S. A., and Marks, V., *Anæsthesia*, 1961, **16**, 410 ; and Biggs, R., and Macfarlane, R. G., *Blood Coagulation and its Disorders*, 1957. Oxford : Blackwell Scientific Publications Ltd.

7. Congenital hæmorrhagic disorders.
   a. Hypofibrinogenæmia, requiring estimation of clotting time ; remedy : fresh whole blood or human fibrinogen.
   b. Hypoprothrombinæmia, requiring estimation of prothrombin time ; remedy : fresh frozen plasma.
   c. Hæmophilia, almost always in males, requiring thromboplastin generation test and prothrombin consumption test ; remedy : fresh blood or plasma, fresh frozen plasma, or antihæmophilia globulin preparation, the human type of which is non-antigenic.

A pathologist investigating a case with a history of bleeding may want to perform the following tests :—

1. The examination of a stained blood-film, with white cell and platelet count ; this should exclude leukæmia and thrombocytopenia.
2. A one-stage prothrombin time estimation.
3. A thromboplastin generation test to help to exclude hæmophilia and Christmas disease.
4. An estimation of bleeding time.
5. Whole-blood clotting time, useful in detection of hæmophilia.

Sometimes no exact cause can be found for excessive bleeding.

ISCHÆMIA DURING OPERATION HAS BEEN PRODUCED BY :—

1. Total spinal analgesia (Griffiths, H. W. I., and Gillies, J., *Anæsthesia*, 1948, 3, 134; Koster, H., *Amer. J. Surg.*, 1928, **5**, 554; and Vehrs, G. R., *Northw. Med.*, Seattle, 1931, **30**, 256, 322). *See* p. 403.
2. High extradural block (Bromage, P. R., *Ibid.*, 1951, **6**, 26). *See* p. 403.
3. Ganglionic blocking agents (Enderby, G. E. H., and Davison, M. H. Armstrong, *Proc. R. Soc. Med.*, 1951, **44**, 829 ; Aserman, D., *Brit. med. J.*, 1953, **1**, 961 ; Payne, J. P., *Brit. J. Anæsth.*, 1953, **25**, 134 ; Hampton, L. J., and Little, D. M., *Lancet*, 1953, **1**, 1299 ; Wyman, J. B., *Proc. R. Soc. Med.*, 1953, **46**, 605 ; Enderby, G. E. H., *Proc. World Congress of Anesthesiologists*, 1956, 143, Minneapolis : Burgess Publishing Co.; and Postgraduate Courses, 71, *First European Congress of Anæsthesiology*, 1962, Wiener medizinischen Akademie, Vienna). *See below.*
4. Controlled arteriotomy (Gardner, W. J., *J. Amer. med. Ass.*, 1946, **132**, 572; and Bilsland, W. L., *Anæsthesia*, 1951, **6**, 20). Used chiefly in neurosurgery, but is now seldom employed.
5. Application of negative pressure to the lower limbs after moderate hypotension has been induced by a ganglionic blocking agent (Saunders, J. W., *Lancet*, 1952, **1**, 1286).
6. Infiltration with adrenaline-saline 1–250,000 to 1–500,000. Very useful to prevent oozing from the skin-flaps in thyroid surgery, craniotomy, and in vagino-perineal surgery.
7. Tourniquets during operations on limbs.

In the above groups (1) to (3) hypotension is normovolæmic with no reduction of circulating blood-volume. In groups (4) and (5) hypotension is hypovolæmic as there is a reduction in the volume

Increased Bleeding during Anæsthesia, *continued.*

of circulating blood. The hypotension reduces the pressure in the great veins and reduces venous return and consequently cardiac output. A fall in blood-pressure results, which in its turn by its effect on the carotid and aortic sinuses leads to tachycardia (Marey's law).

Hypovolæmic hypotension is accompanied by intense vasoconstriction. On the other hand, high intra- and extradural block result in the interruption of sympathetic vasoconstrictor impulses which travel through the anterior spinal roots, mixed spinal nerves, and white rami communicantes. Hypotension does not depend solely, however, on the number of white rami or anterior roots blocked. Interruption of vasomotor impulses causes dilatation of the arterioles and pre-arteriolar capillaries so that the blood-pressure falls. The effect is helped by reduction of the venous return and by paralysis of the sympathetic cardio-accelerator fibres, resulting in further reduction of cardiac output. Hypotension here is accompanied by vasodilatation.

Ganglionic blocking agents and sympathetic vasoconstrictor blockade produce their hypotension by increasing the capacity of the vascular bed relative to the volume of circulating fluid.

The 'normal' blood-pressure during sleep is often little above 80 mm. Hg.*

GANGLIONIC BLOCKING AGENTS
Hexamethonium (and Pentamethonium)

Pentamethonium was first used as an antidote to the myoneural blocking effects of decamethonium by Organe, Paton, and Zaimis in 1949,[†] while in the same year, M. H. Armstrong Davison warned against its severe hypotensive action.[‡] Scurr in 1949[§] was the first deliberately to use the drug to lessen bleeding during surgery.

The formula of pentamethonium halide (C_5) is :

$$(CH_3)_3 \overset{+}{N} (CH_2)_5 \overset{+}{N} (CH_3)_3$$

Hexamethonium has the following formula :

$$(CH_3)_3 \overset{+}{N} (CH_2)_6 \overset{+}{N} (CH_3)_3$$

The bromide of *pentamethonium* (lytensium) comes in 1-ml. ampoules of 10 per cent solution, and its iodide (antilusin) is put in ampoules of 2·5 ml. containing 50 mg. It is to-day seldom used. Hexamethonium bromide (vegolysen), B.P.C., is sold in 10-ml. ampoules of 1 per cent and 2·5 per cent and in 1-ml. ampoules of 10 per cent solution, and hexamethonium iodide (hexathide) in 2·5-ml. ampoules containing 2 per cent solution. Hexamethonium tartrate, B.P., is sold as vegolysen-T,

---

* Richardson, D. W., and others, *Clin. Science*, 1964, **26**, 445.
† Organe, G. S. W., Paton, W. D. M., and Zaimis, E. J., *Lancet*, 1949, **1**, 21.
‡ Davison, M. H. A., *Ibid.*, 1950, **1**, 252.
§ Scurr, C. F., *Anesthesiology*, 1951, **12**, 253; and Enderby, G. E. H., *Lancet*, 1950, **1**, 1145.

and hexamethonium chloride as methium chloride, hexameton, esormid, and bistrium; 50 mg. of the bromide is roughly equivalent to 70 mg. of the tartrate.

The *hexamethonium* salts are rather more constant in action than pentamethonium salts, but even they fail to produce a dry operating field in 20 to 40 per cent of cases. Duration of effect is half to three-quarters of an hour. The addition of procaine amide hydrochloride, guanethidine, or halothane will frequently convert these failures into successes.

Penta- and hexamethonium act by blocking the transmission of pre-ganglionic stimuli to post-ganglionic neurons, and act at all autonomic ganglia : all pre-ganglionic nerves are cholinergic. Three types of blocking mechanism have been described :* (1) By depolarization of the ganglion cells, an acetylcholine-like action, preceded by excitation, e.g., by nicotine, tetramethyl ammonium salts. (2) By increasing the threshold for acetylcholine at the receptor cells—competitive inhibition : the inhibition is not preceded by an excitatory stage—e.g., hexamethonium, pendiomid, pentolinium, tetraethyl ammonium salts, trimetaphan camsylate. This block can be reversed by sympathomimetic (or parasympathomimetic) drugs. (3) By decrease in the amount of acetylcholine liberated by the post-ganglionic endings, e.g., procaine and procaine amide : thus procaine amide increases the ganglionic block produced by hexamethonium.

Hexamethonium then acts by competitive inhibition of acetylcholine, but is better not called an anticholinergic drug. Its action on the ganglia is analogous to that of tubocurarine at the motor end-plate.

Pharmacology.—When given to the conscious patient hexamethonium and pentamethonium cause postural hypotension, fall in intra-ocular pressure, dilated pupils (ciliary ganglion), and dryness of the eyes (sphenopalatine ganglion) ; dilatation of retinal and conjunctival vessels, dry mouth and nose (otic and sphenopalatine ganglia and chorda tympani) ; dryness of the larynx (vagal ganglia) and skin, reduction in gastric secretion and tone, reduction in intestinal tone with constipation, anorexia (enteric ganglia), and difficulty in micturition and impotence (pelvic ganglia). Fall in temperature, relief of causalgia due to increase in blood-supply. In diabetics there is a hypersensitivity to insulin through an effect on the adrenal medulla, so that a patient may go into hypoglycæmia without warning, if otherwise normal doses of insulin are given. This may be shown during anæsthesia by progressive tachycardia.

During anæsthesia they cause : (1) Low blood-pressure or postural sensitivity of blood-pressure. (2) Release of autonomic tone by paralysis of ganglia at the pre-ganglionic synapses of both sympathetic and parasympathetic systems, the former predominating. (3) Diminution of muscle tone and non-depolarizing myoneural block. (4) Disturbance of cardiac function. (5) Respiratory depression. (6) Dilated pupils. (7) Reduction of operative shock.

Different ganglia are sensitive to these drugs in the following order :
  1. Parasympathetic ganglia to salivary gland.

Hexamethonium and Pentamethonium—Pharmacology, *continued.*

    2. Superior cervical ganglion.
    3. Vasomotor ganglia.
    4. Visceral ganglia.
    5. Vagal ganglia in heart.

On the other hand, except in very large doses, they cause no stimulation of nerve terminations or of muscle ; have no atropine-like action; do not liberate histamine; and have no anticholinesterase activity. During hypotension, vessels retain their sensitivity to adrenaline and the pressor amines. A neuromuscular blocking effect has been demonstrated in animals.[*]

Hypotension and decreased hæmorrhage may be due to : (1) The effects of gravity on blood distribution when the blood-pressure is low ; (2) The effects of gravity on venous blood, causing it to pool in the distended veins of the lower and dependent parts of the body ; (3) The reduced cardiac output consequent on the reduced venous return to the heart. As both sympathetic and parasympathetic ganglia are blocked, hypotension depends on the original balance of these two. Where there is great parasympathetic tone, its release will cause tachycardia, so that hypotension will not be maximal. Myocardial ischæmia may occur.

Hypercapnia antagonizes the hypotension caused by ganglionic blocking drugs but potentiates that due to extra- or intradural sympathetic block.[†]

The drugs pass the placental barrier but do not cause ill effects in the fœtus. Their action on the bronchi is not yet settled. Hypotension may stimulate pressor receptors in the walls of the aortic and carotid sinuses, resulting in reflex bronchodilatation. On the other hand, the release of sympathetic tone may favour bronchoconstriction, and atelectasis has been described after its use. Hexamethonium and pentamethonium do not interfere with the anticurare effects of neostigmine.

Renal Blood-flow.—During general anæsthesia, ganglionic blockade has no significant effect on renal blood-flow because the glomerular filtration rate, the renal plasma flow, and the flow of urine are already greatly diminished by the state of anæsthesia and are reduced in proportion to the depth of anæsthesia. A pressure below 50 or 60 mm. Hg, however, may depress renal function.

The Liver.—A blood-pressure below about 60 mm. Hg has been seen to cause a turgidity and cyanosis of the liver, and death has been reported owing to liver necrosis. In practice, little harm appears to result.

Cerebral Blood-flow.—Opinions vary about this, some investigators finding a reduced cerebral blood-flow, others finding it well maintained due to decreased cerebrovascular resistance.[‡] In cerebral atheroma, the vessels cannot relax to decrease vascular resistance

---

   * Deacock, A. R. deC., and Davies, T. D. W., *Brit. J. Anæsth.*, 1958, **30**, 217.
   † Payne, J. P., *Anæsthesia*, 1958, **13**, 185.
   ‡ Slack, W. K., and others, *Lancet*, 1963, **1**, 1082; Eckenhoff, J. E., and others, *J. Appl. Physiol.*, 1963, **18**, 1130; and Eckenhoff, J. E., *Lancet*, 1964, **2**, 711.

and ischæmia may therefore occur in such patients. The brain is said to be more sensitive than the heart to acute hypotension.* Hypotension may cause alteration of cerebral function as shown by the flicker fusion test of Berg,† while psychiatric disorders have been noticed after its use.‡

Coronary Blood-flow.—The state of the coronary vessels probably plays a large part in the development of cardiac ischæmia when hypotension occurs, but low blood-pressure reduces cardiac work and the demand of the myocardium for oxygen. There is no evidence that hypotensive anæsthesia causes any permanent damage to the myocardium§ seen on electrocardiogram evidence, although marked T or S–T wave alterations may indicate acute ischæmia.

Lung Changes.—Organized fibrinous pulmonary œdema with dyspnœa has followed the use of hexamethonium, but only when it has been given over a long period. The physiological dead space is increased by hypotension under I.P.P.V. as it also is by the head-up position, by hæmorrhage, and by the rise in the mean intrathoracic pressure associated with I.P.P.V. Thus an excess of oxygen (40–50 per cent) should always be provided.‖

Excretion.—The drugs are not metabolized in the body, but are excreted via the renal glomeruli, 50 per cent of it in two hours and 90 per cent within twenty-four hours after intravenous injection. If the blood-pressure drops below about 50 mm. Hg glomerular filtration ceases and excretion will no longer take place.

Pentolinium Tartrate (B.P.)
(Pentapyrrolidinium, Ansolysen)

This was synthesized in 1952 by Libman and used in anæsthesia by Enderby.¶ Chemical composition is pentamethylene 1-5-*bis* (1-methyl-pyrrolidinium). Its action is similar to that of hexamethonium, but it is said to be five times more potent, has an action slower in onset but longer in duration, causes less tachycardia, does not antagonize the neuromuscular blocking action of decamethonium, and produces less parasympathetic ganglionic block than does hexamethonium (i.e., less tendency to ileus). Excreted in the urine. Average intravenous dose is 10–20 mg. in 0·5 per cent solution, which takes about three minutes to produce a maximum fall in blood-pressure.

Trimetaphan Camsylate, B.P. (Camphorsulphonate)
(Arfonad)

This compound, a thiophanium derivative, was described by Randall and others** in 1949 and is *d*-3, 4-(1′, 3′-dibenzyl-2′-ketoimidazolido)-1,

---

* Robson, J. M., and Keele, C. A., *Recent Advances in Pharmacology*, 2nd ed., 1956. London : Churchill.
† Nilsson, E., *Brit. J. Anæsth.*. 1953, **25**, 24.
‡ Brierley, J. B., and Cooper, J. E., *J. Neurol. Psychiat.*, 1962, **25**, 24.
§ Rollason, W. N., and Cumming, A. R. R., *Anæsthesia*, 1956, **11**, 319 ; and Rollason, W. H., and Hough, C. M., *Brit. J. Anæsth.*, 1960, **30**, 276 and 286.
‖ Eckenhoff, J. E., and others, *Ibid.*, 1963, **35**, 750.
¶ Enderby, G. E. H., *Lancet*, 1954, **2**, 1097.
** Randall, L. O., and others, *J. Pharmacol.*, 1949, **97**, 48.

Trimetaphan Camsylate, *continued.*

2-trimethylene thiophanium *d*-camphorsulphonate. It is supplied as the dry substance in 250-mg. ampoules. It was used to reduce the blood-pressure by Sarnoff in 1952[*] and reported on by Magill, Scurr, and Wyman in 1953.[†] It is a ganglion-blocking agent and has a direct dilator effect on peripheral vessels. It liberates histamine. During anæsthesia it can be given as an intravenous drip in a strength varying from 0·05 per cent to 0·2 per cent—0·1 per cent being the most commonly used (1 mg. per ml.). With this concentration the drip starts at 60 drops per minute (3–4 mg. per min.). The drug can be given as 5 per cent solution (the dose being 2·5 to 5 mg.) by repeated single injections.[‡] It inhibits pseudocholinesterase. Hypotension depends on the speed of the drip, and after the drip is stopped recovery is usually moderately rapid.

It is incompatible with thiopentone and other strongly alkaline solutions, gallamine triethiodide, iodides, and bromides ; its hypotensive effect is antagonized by methylamphetamine and similar pressor drugs. It causes less tachycardia than does hexamethonium, and causes more hypotension in arteriosclerotic patients than in those with normal blood-pressure, interferes with the heat-regulating mechanism, causing hypothermia after long operations, and reduces the need for anæsthesia once a low pressure has been established. It may, however, result in tachyphylaxis, tachycardia, and rather prolonged hypotension. Partially excreted by the kidneys after destruction by cholinesterase. After large doses excretion may be slow and hypotension prolonged. The maximum dose should not exceed 1 g.

It would seem that this drug with its rapid onset and short duration of action is a great improvement on the longer-acting ganglionic blocking agents.

Reserpine, 1 to 2·5 mg. intravenously, half to two hours before operation, potentiates the hypotensive action of trimetaphan.

Phenacyl-homatropinium
(Trophenium)

This drug was investigated by Johnston and Spencer in 1956 and described clinically as a hypotensive agent in anæsthesia by Robertson, Gillies, and Spencer (Robertson, J. D., Gillies, J., and Spencer, K. E. V., *Brit. J. Anæsth.*, 1957, **29**, 342).

It causes hypotension by virtue of its ganglionic blocking action, and has no effect either as a liberator of histamine or as a vascular dilator. It causes a non-depolarizing neuromuscular block,[§] and with large doses, tachyphylaxis and respiratory depression may result.[‖] It is ten times as potent and lasts half as long as hexamethonium, and is slightly more effective and lasts a similar time to trimetaphan. The hypotension which it causes is readily reversed by such vasopressors as methoxamine, methylamphetamine, and noradrenaline. Its solution is

---

[*] Sarnoff, S. J., and others, *Circulation*, 1952, **6**, 63.
[†] Magill, I. W., Scurr, C. F., and Wyman, J. B., *Lancet*, 1953, **1**, 219.
[‡] Kilduff, C. J., *Ibid.*, 1954, **1**, 337.
[§] Deacock, A. R. deC., and Hargrove, R. L., *Brit. J. Anæsth.*, 1962, **34**, 357.
[‖] Eyre-Walker, D. W., *Anæsthesia*, 1961, **16**, 74.

compatible with thiopentone and it has been given as a 0·2 per cent intravenous drip in saline or dextrose (2 mg. per ml.). The rate at the beginning should be 100–200 drops a minute, and when the pressure has reached almost to the desired low level, this may be reduced to 40–60 drops each minute. Pressure should be stabilized at the required level before the operation commences. The clinicians responsible for the introduction of this hypotensive agent recommend that the head should be kept level or tilted downwards throughout the operation.

In spite of its chemical constitution, trophenium does not inhibit structures innervated by post-ganglionic cholinergic nerves, i.e., it has no atropine-like action.

Potentiation of Hypotension.—

1. BY PROCAINE AMIDE.—Mason and Pelmore* have reported on their use of procaine amide in association with hexamethonium in those patients who develop a tachycardia with indifferent hypotension after hexamethonium alone. Procaine and its amide antagonize the stimulating action of acetylcholine on the ganglion cells and at the same time decrease the amount of acetylcholine liberated by the post-ganglionic endings so the ganglionic inhibition is further increased. Procaine amide does not achieve its effect by a direct cardiac action. Intravenous injection of 0·5–1 g. is given when hexamethonium causes a tachycardia greater than 110 beats per minute. By this means, ischæmia is greatly increased.

2. BY GUANETHIDINE SULPHATE (Ismelin).†—When vasomotor nerve impulses reach post-ganglionic nerve-endings, this drug prevents the production and release of adrenaline and noradrenaline and causes hypotension with bradycardia. It has no effect on the parasympathetic nerves and so may cause a parasympathetic predominance. Its effects are maintained for several days after its oral administration ceases. It increases the pressor response to adrenaline and noradrenaline but antagonizes that to ephedrine and methylamphetamine. In hypotensive anæsthesia the intravenous injection of 20 mg. before ganglionic blockade slows the pulse and increases ischæmia. Its effects may be prolonged.

3. BY HALOTHANE.—This agent can be used alone to produce hypotension. It can also be employed with ganglionic blocking agents : (1) Before these agents are used, or (2) It can be added to the inhaled gases in those patients in whom the blood-pressure cannot be completely controlled by the classic hypotensive technique.‡

   The anæsthetist should, however, be warned against overdosage with halothane in an effort to lower systolic blood-pressure.

---

* Mason. A. A., and Pelmore, J. F., *Brit. med. J.*, 1953, **1**, 250.
† Holloway, K. B., Holmes, F., and Hider, C. F., *Brit. J. Anæsth.*, 1061, **33**, 648 ; Enderby, G. E. H., Postgraduate Courses, 71, *First European Congress of Anæsthesiology*, 1962, Wiener medizinischen Akademie, Vienna; and Eckenhoff, J. E., and others, *Brit. J. Anæsth.*, 1963, **35**, 750.
‡ Enderby, G. E. H., *Anæsthesia*, 1960, **15**, 25.

Potentiation of Hypotension, *continued.*

4. BY PROPRANOLOL.—This β-adrenergic blocking agent can be
used to prevent tachycardia and its associated oozing, which
may accompany ganglionic blockade, with or without halothane
and I.P.P.V. The dose should be 0·5 mg. repeated carefully until
the pulse is at the required rate.*

Because tachycardia may increase oozing, both atropine and
gallamine should be withheld if hypotension is thought to be
desirable. Tubocurarine lowers the blood-pressure.

Uses of Hypotensive Agents during Anæsthesia.—It must be
remembered that in the absence of hypotensive drugs there are
great blood-pressure fluctuations during anæsthesia. The technique under consideration is said to have two great advantages :
it reduces bleeding and prevents shock but is only justified if it
enables a better operation to be performed.

When a normal patient stands up after lying down, his cardiac
output is lessened and a reflex is initiated which causes vasoconstriction to maintain blood-pressure. After general anæsthesia and still more after the use of ganglion-blocking drugs,
this reflex vasoconstriction does not occur, and so, cardiac output being reduced because of the position, profound hypotension results. The technique of controlled hypotension aims
to block the sympathetic ganglia, so causing hypotension.

TECHNIQUE.—Agents may be classified as : (*a*) Longer-acting,
e.g., hexamethonium and pentolinium ; (*b*) Shorter-acting, e.g.,
trimetaphan and phenactropinium. Both of these can be made
more effective and more controllable by the use of halothane
and/or guanethidine. Many workers now use the shorter-acting
agents in repeated small doses of 10 mg. rather than as a continuous intravenous drip.

POSTURE.—Gravity acting on the tilted patient results in blood
pooling in the dilated (capacity) veins, and this leads to
decreased venous return and hypotension. Posture is also
used to make the operation site ischæmic. The blood-
pressure is said to be reduced 2 mm. Hg for each inch of
vertical height above heart level, so that when the head is
tilted 25° upwards, the cerebral blood-pressure is likely to
be about 16 mm. Hg less than the blood-pressure at heart
level. Many, but not all, experienced workers consider it
reasonably safe in normal patients to allow a 25° head-up tilt
with a brachial arterial blood-pressure of 60–70 mm. Hg.†

INTERMITTENT POSITIVE-PRESSURE VENTILATION.—Increased airway pressure is transmitted to the great veins and so venous
return to the heart is decreased; this lowers the blood-pressure.
If the Pco_2 is allowed to rise, the resulting liberation of
catecholamines may cause both a rise in blood-pressure and
cardiac arrhythmias, also when the Pco_2 returns to normal.

---

* Helliwell, P. J., and Potts, M. W., *Brit. J. Anæsth.*, 1966, **38**, 794; Rollason, W. N., *Ibid.*,
1967, **39**, 183; and Hewitt, P. B., and others, *Anæsthesia*, 1967, **22**, 82.
† Annotation, *Brit. med. J.*, 1962, **2**, 1523.

On the other hand, hyperventilation, by causing a low P_{CO_2}, may result in an increased venous tone and consequent interference with venous pooling in the capacity vessels and so may reduce ischæmia in the operative field.*

The technique is simple, but must be meticulous. Both the airway and the patient's ventilation must be faultless, and afferent impulses must be properly blocked. Any of the ordinary anæsthetic combinations may be used, such as thiopentone, gas and oxygen, pethidine, relaxant, or volatile agents. It is often convenient to insert a Mitchell needle into a vein for intravenous injections. As full oxygenation is essential, endotracheal intubation is usually employed. Before induction, the blood-pressure is taken and it is again taken after the anæsthesia has become stabilized. The patient is then placed in the optimal position for operation and a third blood-pressure reading is made. A labile blood-pressure is an indication that small dosage will probably be adequate ; other such indications for small dosage are increasing age and low metabolic rate. Arteriosclerotics require a small dose and little posture to get a profound effect, while young, fit patients, besides often developing tachycardia, require a steep head-up tilt and high initial dosage to show a good ischæmia. In upper abdominal operations, the elevation of the gall-bladder bridge lowers blood-pressure perhaps by interfering with the passage of blood up the inferior vena cava, as also does the actual opening of the peritoneal cavity. In lower abdominal operations ischæmia is not easy to produce, nor is it when the patient is in the lithotomy position.

The blood-pressure is taken at regular and frequent intervals and for this an oscillometer is most useful as it gives a clear reading at low levels of blood-pressure; facilities for blood transfusion must be to hand as bleeding is a dangerous complication because the normal response to it, vasoconstriction, is impossible. Great care and constant attention must be given throughout the operation and afterwards to the patient, who is taken near to the point of death.

A carefully evolved and well-tried technique is used by Bodman† in patients over the age of 50 for prostatectomy and similar operations in the pelvis. After oral premedication with trimeprazine tartrate, 60 mg., and intubation under thiopentone and suxamethonium, the patient is given a gas–oxygen mixture containing 40–50 per cent of oxygen together with 2 per cent halothane for 3 minutes by spontaneous respiration. The halothane is then reduced to about 0·5 per cent and the table tilted 10° head down for pelvic operations and the same angle head up for head and neck procedures. Hexamethonium and tubocurarine, 20 mg. of each to patients of 75 years and under, and 15 mg. of each to those over 75, are now injected and the endotracheal tube connected to a mechanical ventilator. The

* Enderby, G. E. H., Postgraduate Courses, 71, *First European Congress of Anæsthesiology*, 1962, Wiener medizinischen Akademie, Vienna.

† Bodman, R .I., in *Recent Advances in Anæsthesia and Analgesia* (Ed. Hewer, C. Langton), 10th ed., 1967, Ch. 4. London: Churchill.

Uses of Hypotensive Agents during Anæsthesia, *continued*.

halothane is now switched off. Ventilation is at a rate of about 10 litres a minute with a slow rate and large volume. Further relaxation and hypotension are provided by addition of a little more halothane. The blood-pressure runs at about 60 mm. Hg. At the end of the operation the patient is allowed to get lighter and usually the blood-pressure rises to 80 mm. Hg before he leaves the table which he does on a head-down tilted trolley. Blood-loss must be measured and replaced and a most careful watch must be kept on the blood-pressure throughout. Pressor drugs are very seldom needed and are usually undesirable. Hypotension should not be prolonged. Patients under 50 years of age usually require larger doses of the drugs.

In other techniques, suggested initial doses which may be given with the patient horizontal are:* (1) For normotensives, 100–200 mg. of hexamethonium or 10–20 mg. of pentolinium, or 30–50 mg. of trimetaphan. (2) For hypertensives and patients over 55 years of age, 50–80 mg. of hexamethonium, 5–10 mg. of pentolinium, or 20–30 mg. of trimetaphan. The initial dose is the most important. Other workers employ a dosage scheme such as the following—using hexamethonium : (i) To young adults, 50 mg. (ii) To patients between 40 and 60, 30 to 40 mg. (iii) To hypertensives, arteriosclerotics, and those over 60, 20 mg. Three minutes after injection the effects are assessed, and more drug is given if required then or later, usually in doses of 10 to 25 mg. The first dose is, however, the important one. A large initial dose causes maximal hypotension, but may be dangerous in inexperienced hands. The last injection of hexamethonium should be given not less than twenty minutes before the end of the operation.

Armstrong Davison† recommends the following technique : premedication with papaveretum and promazine (30–50 mg.) 1½ hours pre-operatively ; inhalation induction and intubation (ether) ; muscular paralysis with tubocurarine and hyperventilation with a ventilator ; 10° head-up or foot-up tilt, depending on site of operation ; 40 mg. hexamethonium bromide after positioning completed ; control of blood-pressure by adjustment of respiratory rate and volume. A systolic level of 80–85 mm. Hg is aimed at. Strophanthin G (0·25–0·5 mg.) is used to treat a more severe fall of blood-pressure.

Failure to produce good ischæmia with ganglionic blocking agents may be due to : (a) Incomplete block of sympathetic ganglia. (b) Increased cardiac output due to tachycardia. (c) Presence of pressor agents, e.g., noradrenaline or adrenaline, in the circulation. (d) The presence of a phæochromocytoma.

Signs of excessive hypotension include : (1) A completely dry wound. (2) Irregular respiration, if breathing is spontaneous. (3) The onset of cardiac irregularity.

---

* Enderby, G. E. H., *Proc. World Congress of Anesthesiologists*, 1956, 227. Minneapolis : Burgess Publishing Co. ; *Brit. J. Anæsth.*, 1961, **33**, 109 ; and Postgraduate Courses, 71, *First European Congress of Anæsthesiology*, 1962, Wiener medizinischen Akademie, Vienna.
†Davison, M. H. Armstrong, *Anæsthesia*, 1962, **17**, 322.

To raise the blood-pressure at the end of the operation, or before that if necessary, a return to the horizontal position is usually sufficient. Hypertensive drugs and also infusions may be used. Methylamphetamine, 4–8 mg. intravenously, is satisfactory, but may cause cerebral stimulation and restlessness. Phenylephrine, methoxamine, and noradrenaline are also used. Pressor drugs do not, however, restore vasomotor control and may restore blood-pressure at the expense of tissue perfusion. Towards the end of the operation the blood-pressure is allowed to rise slowly, and no patient should leave the table unless his blood-pressure is 80 mm. Hg. The journey back to the ward is made on a tilting trolley, and if necessary the head-down position is employed for the first few hours. Blood-pressure readings must be taken frequently in the post-operative period.

The results in successful cases are: (1) A bloodless field of operation. (2) Easier surgical dissection. (3) Reduction of amount of ligatured or cauterized tissue and consequent reduction in infection. (4) Decreased oozing beneath skin-flaps and hence better healing. (5) Reduction of operative shock. (6) Reduction of vomiting after operation. (7) Delayed recovery from anæsthesia.

The Dangers.—Many workers think that the technique should be confined to those cases where it makes the impossible possible. It should not be used to make the possible easy. Other workers employ it more liberally. Its advantages to the patient must be weighed against the increased risks. Hypothermia decreases the dangers of hypotension.*

Trouble has been reported from cerebral and coronary thrombosis, renal and hepatic ischæmia, reactionary hæmorrhage, ileus, cerebral damage, arterial thrombosis (e.g., the carotid, central retinal artery, and limb arteries), and massive atelectasis. Primary heart failure is an ever-present anxiety. *See also* Discussion *below*.

Indications.—These are not yet established, but may include the following :—

1. Neurosurgery, especially in operations for vascular tumours and aneurysms. Hypotension causes shrinkage of the brain.
2. Peripheral vascular surgery, e.g., coarctation of the aorta to reduce bleeding from enlarged vessels in the chest wall.
3. Removal of vascular tumours, e.g., carcinoma of the breast.
4. Operations associated with voluminous hæmorrhage, e.g., total cystectomy, abdomino-perineal resection of the rectum, panhysterectomy, and pelvic exenteration.
5. Plastic surgery.
6. Operations on the inner ear when the operating microscope is in use.
7. When a patient's abnormal blood group makes transfusion difficult.
8. The possible prevention of shock by autonomic paralysis.

---

* Gray, T. C., *Lancet*, 1957, **1**, 383.

Ganglionic Blocking Agents—Indications, *continued*.

9. Pelvic floor repair operations.*
10. Prostatectomy.†

Contra-indications.—These of course vary in the practice of different workers. The following conditions may increase the danger: (1) Respiratory inadequacy from any cause, especially obstructive airways disease; (2) Bronchospasm and asthma; (3) Diabetes, because ganglionic blocking agents increase the patient's response to insulin, and hypoglycæmia may result; (4) Cerebral and coronary vascular disease requires careful consideration; (5) Previous steroid therapy; (6) Where there is poor renal or hepatic function; (7) In Addison's disease; (8) In pregnancy; (9) *When the technical skill and experience of the anæsthetist are not of a high order.*

Discussion.—Eckenhoff‡ reports the results of his investigations in 350 patients whose blood-pressure was lowered during operations for plastic surgery, using Enderby's technique, and no detectable mental changes resulted (apart from 1 patient who was disorientated for 2 days, probably due to sedative drugs, and who made a complete recovery). In another study,§ two groups of elderly patients were compared, and those in whom hypotension was induced did as well as those receiving normal anæsthetics. Linacre* reported on 1000 patients undergoing gynæcological operations under hypotensive anæsthesia in the horizontal or head-down position, with no cerebral complications.

On the other hand, a report has recently appeared‖ in which a patient aged 45 had her blood-pressure deliberately reduced during an operation and whose return to consciousness was delayed and who subsequently developed organic dementia; she died two years later from another cause and had well-marked histopathological changes in the brain. The anæsthetic details in this case are not stated.

Thus it would seem that in expert and experienced hands, induced hypotension in normal patients with the blood-pressure reduced to 70–80 and with 25° head-up tilt is reasonably safe. What is certain is that the technique can be lethal if its details are not fully understood and if it is not conducted impeccably.

The subject is excellently reviewed by Bodman, R. I., in *Recent Advances in Anæsthesia* (Ed. Hewer, C. Langton), 10th ed., 1967, p. 90. London: Churchill.

Hypotension before Operation.—

1. THE NORMOVOLÆMIC PATIENT.—No special treatment is usually required to raise the blood-pressure before anæsthesia, but techniques which increase hypotension unduly, e.g., rapid

---

* Linacre, J. L., *Brit. J. Anæsth.*, 1961, **33**, 45.
† Shepperd, N. L., and Grace, A. H., *Proc. R. Soc. Med.*, 1961, **54**, 127; Bodman, R. I., *Ibid.*, 1964, **57**, 1184; and Bodman, R. I., *Brit. J. Surg.*, 1965, **52**, 757.
‡ Eckenhoff, J. E., *Proc. R. Soc. Med.*, 1962, **55**, 942; and Eckenhoff, J. E., and Rich, J. C., *Curr. Res. Anesth.*, 1966, **45**, 21.
§ Rollason, W. N., and Hough, J. M., *Brit. J. Anæsth.*, 1960, **30**, 276 and 286.
‖ Brierley, J. B., and Cooper, J. E., *J. Neurol., Psychiat.*, 1962, **25**, 24.

intravenous injection of barbiturates and spinal blockade should be used, if at all, most cautiously.

2. THE HYPOVOLÆMIC PATIENT.—The volume of circulating fluid should be corrected before anæsthesia, whenever possible.

CONTROLLED HYPOTENSION BY ARTERIOTOMY

This technique is seldom used to-day as it depends for its success on vasoconstriction and tissue underperfusion. Blood withdrawn from the radial artery into bottles containing sodium citrate in amounts of 500 ml. or less, until the blood-pressure is reduced to about 80 mm. Hg, and afterwards retransfused, was first advocated by Gardner in 1946.* The amount required to reach such a blood-pressure varies between 300 and 3000 ml. and it can be returned to the circulation when needed either before the end or at the end of the operation. Intra-arterial retransfusion, by raising the coronary blood-pressure and myocardial circulation, soon raises the systemic blood-pressure. Hæmorrhage probably liberates a hormone causing vasoconstriction.

The technique is to induce anæsthesia and maintain it with any of the usual agents. A brachial plexus block is performed to cause maximal dilatation of the radial vessels and to prevent their reflex spasm as part of a generalized compensatory vasoconstriction. A cannula is tied into the artery, which is afterwards carefully sutured, and, through it, blood is taken and given back as required.

During bleeding from any cause, a time comes when vasopressor compensation reaches its limit, and thereafter further bleeding causes a progressive hypotension.

It has been stated that in cranial surgery, controlled arteriotomy has four advantages : (1) It makes bleeding more easily controllable because of hypotension and consequent vasoconstriction. (2) It causes shrinkage of the cerebral cortex. (3) It gives a relatively bloodless field in the vicinity of vascular tumours such as aneurysms of the circle of Willis. (4) It reduces the need for blood donors.† *See also* Jackson, I., *Anæsthesia*, 1954, **9**, 13.

CHAPTER XXIX

INDUCED HYPOTHERMIA

Induced hypothermia is a method used to lower the metabolism of the body as a whole, and to reduce the dangers from hypoxia and the cellular damage resulting from regional occlusion of the circulation of the brain, the heart, the liver, the kidneys, and the legs. Cooling enables certain specialized tissues of the body to withstand periods of hypoxia which in its absence would cause harm. It has also been used to treat hyperpyrexia during and after operation and to treat shock.

The name first used in 1941.‡

* Gardner, W. J., *J. Amer. med. Ass.*, 1946, **132**, 572.
† Mortimer, P. L. F., *Anæsthesia*, 1951, **6**, 128.
‡ Talbott, J. H., *New Engl. J. Med.*, 1941, **224**, 305.

History.—

1798. Dr. James Currie, of Liverpool, published observations on the effect on man of immersion in cold water.

1905. Simpson and Herring coined the term 'artificial hibernation' and showed that cold—below about 28° C.—could act as a general anæsthetic.*

1938. Temple Fay treated carcinoma by lowering the body temperature—cryotherapy.†

1947. Delorme of Edinburgh showed that hæmorrhagic shock was better tolerated by cooled dogs than by dogs at normal temperatures.

1950. Bigelow and his colleagues from Toronto‡ showed that with progressive cooling the rectal temperature and the oxygen consumption of the body showed an almost linear relationship, that even slight shivering doubled oxygen consumption, and that no oxygen debt was incurred by the tissues. Surface cooling was the method used.

1951. Blood-stream or pervascular cooling employed by Delorme of Edinburgh§ and by Boerema of Holland.||

1953. Pioneer work was done by Swan, Virtue, and their colleagues in Denver.¶

1959. Deep hypothermia with cardiopulmonary by-pass and blood-stream cooling described by Drew.**

The so-called artificial hibernation of Laborit and Huguenard in France (1951) using chlorpromazine, etc.,†† should not be confused with induced hypothermia.

TECHNIQUES OF HYPOTHERMIA‡‡

Surface Cooling.—The original method of Bigelow§§ and the simplest. The patient is anæsthetized, intubated, and placed in a cold environment. The anæsthetic technique must provide : (1) Peripheral vasodilatation to promote heat exchange ; (2) Absence of shivering (which prevents cooling and increases oxygen utilization). METHODS.—

1. IMMERSION IN COLD WATER.||||—The quickest surface method. The patient is immersed in a bath of water and ice added to bring the water temperature to 6–10° C., stirring continuously. Lower temperatures may cause skin necrosis.

2. ICE-BAGS.¶¶—The patient is laid on a mattress filled with crushed ice, and ice-bags are packed around the body, particularly

* Simpson, S., and Herring, P. T., *J. Physiol.*, 1905, **32**, 305.
† Fay, T., and Henry, G. C., *Surg. Gynec. and Obstet.*, 1938, **66**, 512.
‡ Bigelow, W. G., and others, *Amer. J. Physiol.*, 1950, **160**, 125 ; and *Canad. J. Med. Sci.*, 1952, **30**, 185.
§ Delorme, E. J., *Lancet*, 1952, **1**, 1108; and *Ibid.*, 1952, **2**, 914.
|| Boerema, I. A., and others, *Arch. chir. neerl.*, 1951, **3**, 25.
¶ Swan, H., and others, *J. Amer. med. Ass.*, 1953, **153**, 1081.
** Drew, C. E., and others, *Lancet*, 1959, **1**, 745.
†† Laborit, H., and Huguenard, P., *Pr. Méd.*, 1951, **59**, 1329.
‡‡ McMillan, I. K. R., and Machell, E. S., *Brit. med. Bull.*, 1961, **17**, 32.
§§ Bigelow, W. G., and others, *Ann. Surg.*, 1950, **132**, 531.
|||| Sellick, B. A., *Lancet*, 1957, **1**, 443.
¶¶ Burrows, M. M., and others, *Anæsthesia*, 1956, **11**, 4.

near the major arteries (groins, axillæ, etc.). Position of the bags should be changed at frequent intervals.

3. REFRIGERATED BLANKETS.—The patient lies between two blankets which incorporate coils of tubing. The tubing is filled with a solution containing anti-freeze and connected to a cabinet which incorporates a refrigeration/warming unit and a pump to circulate the fluid. The method is cleaner than the above, but more expensive. The underneath mattress can remain in situ during operation and be used for rewarming.

4. AIR COOLING.—Use of fans and damp sheets. Particularly useful in the ward to produce moderate hypothermia or to prevent hyperpyrexia (e.g., head injuries, or post-operative). A cabinet has been designed for air cooling in the operating theatre.*

5. COLD WATER SPRAY.—This method keeps a constant supply of cold water in contact with the patient's skin, and prevents water acting as an insulator.

Time taken to reduce the temperature to 30°–28° C. is between ¾ hr. and 3 hr., largely depending on the size and build of the patient. It takes longer in large and obese patients, not so long in children who present a large surface area per unit mass of body-weight.

Surface cooling produces extreme vasoconstriction of the peripheral vessels, even when vasodilators are administered. This delays cooling of the main body mass and hastens the development of metabolic acidosis. Recent suggestions to increase the peripheral blood-flow during surface cooling include the administration of carbon dioxide† and the use of 'warm' water at 25° C.‡ instead of 6°–10° C.

After-drop.—The temperature continues to fall after active cooling has been discontinued. This is due to loss of heat from the core or main body mass of the patient to the skin or superficial regions. It may be of the order of 2°–6° C. Active cooling should, therefore, cease a few degrees above the desired temperature and care taken that undue fall with its increased risk of ventricular fibrillation does not occur.

Internal or Body Cavity Cooling.—

a. Pleural, when chilled saline is poured into the pleural cavity after thoracotomy.

b. Gastric, when a balloon is inserted into the stomach and ice-cold water is made to circulate through it,§ in the anæsthetized patient. By this means the blood in the large abdominal vessels and in the neighbouring viscera is cooled. This method has also been used to inhibit the acid-producing cells in the gastric mucosa in the treatment of peptic ulcer.‖

---

* Forrester, A. C., *Anæsthesia*, 1958, **13**, 289.
† Broom, B., and Sellick, B. A., *Lancet*, 1965, **2**, 452.
‡ Keen, R. I., *Proc. 2nd Eur. Cong. Anæsth.*, 1966, **1**, 684.
§ Khalil, H. H., *Lancet*, 1957, **1**, 185.
‖ Wangensteen, O. H., and others, *Ann. Surg.*, 1962, **156**, 579 ; and Nicoloff, D. M., and others, *Surg. Gynec. Obstet.*, 1962, **114**, 495.

Extracorporeal Methods.—Blood is taken from the circulation, cooled by means of a heat exchanger in an extracorporeal circulation, and then returned to the body. This method of cooling is faster than surface cooling. It has its main application in cardiac surgery, when the heart can be examined under direct vision and when the surgeon can immediately start cardiac massage should ventricular fibrillation supervene.

1. VENO-VENOUS.*—A catheter is inserted through the right auricular appendage into the superior vena cava : blood is withdrawn from it, passed by a rotary pump through a plastic cooling coil immersed in a jar containing a mixture of alcohol, saline, and solid carbon dioxide at a temperature of −2° C.† The blood, after cooling, is returned to the inferior vena cava via a catheter in the same incision in the right auricular appendage. Clotting does not occur in the tubing at low temperatures. Circulatory arrest can fairly safely last 5–10 minutes at 28° C., and ventricular fibrillation is not common above this temperature. Below 25° C. the ventricles tend to fibrillate spontaneously.

2. CARDIOPULMONARY BY-PASS.‡—*See* Chapter XXII. A heat exchanger is incorporated to provide direct blood cooling. Since the circulation is maintained by an extracorporeal pump, ventricular fibrillation is unimportant and hypothermia may be carried to low levels (15° C.).

Rewarming.—This must be undertaken with care as there is a danger of burning the patient if rewarming is overzealous. After surface cooling the patient can usually be allowed to regain heat normally. Rewarming can be expedited by use of a mattress with circulatory fluid, by the use of warm blankets, warm water, or warm air if care is taken. A temperature higher than 40° C. should not be used. In the case of direct blood cooling the heat exchanger can be used to warm up the blood passing through it.

It is usual to rewarm to 35° C. or until consciousness has returned before taking the patient out of the operating theatre to the recovery room.

Measurement of Body Temperature.—Body temperature varies slightly in different regions of the body. When hypothermia is induced different organs and tissues are cooled at varying rates according to their blood-supply, the method of hypothermia, etc. Thus when the blood is cooled directly the temperature of the heart falls before that of the brain.

It is wise to place thermometers in several different situations during hypothermia. Œsophageal temperature approximates to the heart, nasopharyngeal to the brain. Rectal temperature may differ from both.

To convert Fahrenheit to Centigrade, take away 32 and multiply by ⅝. Centigrade to Fahrenheit, multiply by ⅝, then add 32.

---

* Ross, D. N., *Lancet*, 1954, **1**, 1108 ; *Brit. med. Bull.*, 1955, **11**, 225 ; and Brock, R. C., *Proc. R. Soc. Med.*, 1956, **49**, 347.
† Lucas, B. G. B., *Ibid.*, 1956, **49**, 345.
‡ Drew, C. E., and others, *Lancet*, 1959, **1**, 745 and 748.

TEMPERATURES

Fahrenheit (deg.)	Centigrade (deg.)
59	15·0
60	15·5
62	16·6
65	18·3
68	20·0
70	21·1
72	22·2
74	23·3
76	24·4
78	25·5
80	26·6
82	27·7
84	28·8
86	30·0
88	31·1
90	32·2
92	33·3
94	34·4
96	35·5
98	36·6
100	37·7
102	38·8
104	40·0
106	41·1
108	42·2
110	43·3
120	48·8
130	54·4
140	60·0
150	65·5
200	93·3
212	100·0

Temperature can be measured in the following ways :—
1. The clinical thermometer (mercury-in-glass).
2. Thermocouple.
3. Resistance (metal).   Platinum resistance thermometry.
4. Thermistor (resistance of semi-conductor).
5. Dial thermometers (mercury-in-steel, vapour pressure, or bimetallic elements).

For further information *see* Chapter XXXIII.

Effects of Hypothermia.—
1. THE CARDIOVASCULAR SYSTEM.—Arrhythmias occur at temperatures below 30° C. ; spontaneous ventricular fibrillation may be seen, but is not likely above 28° C.   Factors in its causation may include : (a) hypothermia, (b) hyperkalæmia, (c) sudden pH and Pco₂ changes, (d) citrate intoxication.   Bradycardia not due to vagal overaction is progressive.   The blood-pressure, pulse-rate, and cardiac output fall progressively as the temperature gets lower.   E.C.G. changes include lengthening of the

Effects of Hypothermia, *continued.*

QRS complex and prolongation of the P–R interval.* Vaso-constriction of skin vessels. Sympathetic block is said to afford some protection against ventricular arrhythmias, e.g., trimetaphan (arfonad) drip.†

2. RESPIRATION.—Measurements of human cerebral oxygen consumption indicate that at 30° C. it is 39 per cent and at 28° C. 35 per cent of normal.‡ The oxygen dissociation curve is shifted to the left so that liberation of oxygen to the tissues is hindered; although more oxygen is dissolved in plasma there is reduced availability of oxygen to the tissues due to: (*a*) depressed respiration; (*b*) decreased cardiac output; (*c*) vasoconstriction; (*d*) increased blood viscosity; (*e*) arteriovenous shunts. Tissue oxygenation may be improved by: (*a*) Controlled ventilation; (*b*) Hyperbaric oxygenation (not practical during surgery); (*c*) Controlled cooling; not more than 1° C. fall per 5 min.; (*d*) Controlled hypercapnia; deliberate addition of carbon dioxide to inhaled gases;§ (*e*) Intravenous alcohol;‖ (*f*) Hæmodilution to reduce viscosity; use of Ringer or dextrose solutions in disposable bubble oxygenators during cardiopulmonary by-pass. The solubility of carbon dioxide in blood is increased. The respiration-rate falls and breathing ceases at a temperature of 26° C.

3. ACID-BASE BALANCE.—Acidosis tends to be a feature of hypo-thermia. Factors which may produce acidosis include :—

   a. Increased solubility of carbon dioxide.

   b. Respiratory insufficiency.

   c. Increase in formation of lactic acid as a result of a metabolic deficit during circulatory arrest, hypoxia, shivering, surgical trauma, or anæsthesia.

   d. Decreased breakdown of lactic acid due to impaired liver func-tion.

   e. Depression of renal function prevents correction of acidosis.

   Rapid changes of pH may be a cause of cardiac irregularities.

4. CENTRAL NERVOUS SYSTEM.—The cerebral cortex can tolerate the acute hypoxia due to complete circulatory arrest for 5–10 minutes at a temperature of 28° C. and for 50 minutes at 15° C. There is a reduction in brain volume and cerebro-spinal fluid pressure, changes appreciated by the neurosurgeon. Consciousness is usually lost between 28° and 30° C. Cerebral blood-flow is reduced due to increased viscosity.

5. METABOLISM.—With each fall of 1° C. the metabolism is reduced 6–7 per cent. The functions of the liver and kidneys are depressed during hypothermia so that intravenous agents, e.g., thiopentone, gallamine, etc., which are excreted via the kidneys must be given in small amounts. Utilization of glucose is depressed, and continued intravenous infusion of glucose solu-tion may result in a high blood-glucose level, not affected by

* Emslie-Smith, D., and others, *Brit. Heart J.*, 1959, **21**, 343.
† Albert, S. N., and others, *J. Amer. med. Ass.*, 1957, **163**, 1435.
‡ Stone, H. H., and others, *Surg. Gynec. Obstet.*, 1956, **103**, 313.
§ Broom, B., and Sellick, B. A., *Lancet*, 1965, **2**, 452.
‖ Hewer, A. J. H., *Int. Anæsth. Clin.*, 1964, **2/4**, 919.

insulin. Metabolism of substances like heparin, lactic acid, and citrate is inhibited. Large blood transfusions of citrated blood may cause citrate intoxication; the typical E.C.G. change of QT prolongation is an indication for the administration of calcium gluconate or chloride. Renal blood-flow and glomerular filtration are diminished. Below 30° C. there is a secretion of dilute urine. Following profound hypothermia (below 20° C.) this water diuresis may persist into the post-operative period. Cellular damage in the liver, kidneys, and adrenals has been reported.

6. ELECTROLYTES.—There may be a rise in serum potassium associated with acidosis, prolonged circulatory arrest, anoxia, or large transfusions of stored blood. Calcium gluconate is given to cover each unit of donor blood to prevent lowering of ionized calcium. The cold heart is more sensitive to potassium, so small changes are of significance.

7. THE NEUROMUSCULAR JUNCTION.—The duration and magnitude of block by depolarizing drugs are increased. The effect of non-depolarizing drugs is reduced. These effects are reversed on rewarming.*

8. THE BLOOD.—Clotting mechanisms are depressed, platelet count falls rapidly, and 'sludging' may occur in capillaries at very low temperatures. Viscosity is increased. As the metabolic demand for oxygen decreases, the saturation in venous blood rises. Oxygen is more soluble in plasma at low temperatures.

Methods of Anæsthesia.—The anæsthetic requirements are : (1) light general anæsthesia ; (2) prevention of shivering ; (3) peripheral vasodilatation (with surface methods). During hypothermia minimal amounts of anæsthetic drugs are required, and their de-toxication and excretion may be delayed. The actual choice of anæsthetic agents is not critical provided they are used with care. Chlorpromazine has been used in premedication or during anæs-thesia to prevent shivering, and promote vasodilatation and heat loss. Muscle relaxants, in conjunction with light anæsthesia, prevent shivering. Halothane has been employed to promote peripheral vasodilatation.

Monitoring of temperature, blood-pressure, pulse-rate, electro-cardiogram, and perhaps of electro-encephalogram is advisable.

Important points to note are :—

1. VENTRICULAR FIBRILLATION.—This is the principal acute danger during hypothermia. (a) Facilities should be available for immediate cardiac massage. (b) Prevent respiratory acidosis from hypoventilation. (c) Continuous electrocardiography gives early warning.

2. SKIN DAMAGE.—Make sure that ice does not come into contact with skin. Change position of ice-packs frequently. Cold skin is particularly susceptible to damage from pressure or heat. Be careful of : (a) pressure points ; (b) warming devices (which should not exceed 40° C.).

---

* Zaimis, E., Cannard, T. H., and Price, H. L., *Science*, 1958, **128**, 34.

Techniques.—

1. With spontaneous respiration. Premedication with chlorproma-zine and pethidine is useful. Thiopentone, suxamethonium, topical analgesia to the larynx and trachea, intubation, nitrous-oxide–oxygen supplemented with thiopentone, pethidine, trichloroethylene, ether, or halothane as required. Or halothane may be used with oxygen as the main anæsthetic agent.

2. With controlled respiration. A muscle relaxant is used to facili-tate controlled respiration and to prevent shivering. A thio-pentone–relaxant–nitrous-oxide–oxygen sequence is satisfactory. If peripheral vasoconstriction occurs blood-pressure may be hard to obtain by the Riva-Rocci method and intra-arterial recording may be useful.

3. In the patient who is not having an operation, cooling may be combined with intramuscular chlorpromazine and pethidine to prevent shivering. These drugs may be given intravenously if occasion demands. Inhalation of nitrous-oxide–oxygen mix-tures is also useful to prevent shivering but this requires close supervision.

Complications of Hypothermia.—

1. VENTRICULAR FIBRILLATION.—Causes : (1) Deep anæs-thesia. (2) Respiratory acidosis. (3) Physical irritation of heart. (4) Defective coronary circulation.* Treatment in-volves : (1) Restoration of cerebral circulation by cardiac compression. (2) Restoration of heart beat. If this occurs during an operation on the heart and if the temperature is low enough to abolish circulation temporarily, the cardiotomy is performed and defibrillation left until the operative intervention is complete. In other cases, cooling is terminated, the heart massaged to make it tonic and then it is electrically depolarized or defibrillated. A noradrenaline drip may be required to sustain the blood-pressure. Intracoronary injection of neo-stigmine, vigorous hyperventilation, and avoidance of tempera-ture below 28° C. reduce the likelihood of this complication.

2. TENDENCY TO HÆMORRHAGE.—Uncontrolled oozing is sometimes seen after hypothermia, especially if it has been pro-longed. It is due to a reduced coagulability of the blood, perhaps due to a high heparin level. It is also present when an artificial pump oxygenator is used. Damage to platelets may also be a factor in causation.

3. BRAIN DAMAGE.—This may follow a too prolonged interrup-tion of the cerebral circulation.

4. ATELECTASIS.—May occur.

5. HISTOPATHOLOGICAL CHANGES.—These have been re-ported to occur in vital organs.†

6. LOCAL EFFECTS.—Frostbite due to local injury. Burns due to overzealous rewarming.

---

* Lucus, B. G. B., *Brit. med. Bull.*, 1958, **14**, 1, 47.
† Knocker, P., *Lancet*, 1955, **2**, 837.

Uses of Hypothermia.—

1. Cardiac surgery.—
   a. Repair of atrial septal defects (ostium secundum). These can usually be undertaken within the 10-minute period of circulatory arrest which is allowable at 30° C. Hypothermia may be produced by surface or veno-venous cooling. Simple hypothermia is also suitable for operations for atrial tumours, simple pulmonary valvular stenosis, and aneurysm of the thoracic aorta.
   b. May be continued with extracorporeal circulation to produce profound hypothermia.
2. Neurosurgery.—
   a. Resection of aneurysms.
   b. Reduces brain tension.
   c. Makes hypotension safer.
3. Operations on the great vessels. Enables circulation to be interrupted during resection of aneurysms, arterial grafting, endarterectomy, or organ transplant.
4. Therapeutic uses.—
   a. Cerebral ischæmia due to œdema following head injuries, anoxic episodes.
   b. Chronic anoxia in association with shock states.
   c. Malignant disease.
   d. Treatment of hyperpyrexia such as may occur in febrile children undergoing operation, thyrotoxic crisis, etc.

Profound Hypothermia.*—At temperatures much below 28° C. the risk of ventricular fibrillation becomes prohibitive. Lower temperatures can, however, be safely achieved during cardiac or cardiopulmonary by-pass. A heat exchanger is incorporated in the arterial lead of the pump and can be used for cooling or warming. After by-pass has started, body temperature can be rapidly lowered to 15° C. This affords a high degree of protection to the brain. During rewarming the heart is started by defibrillation and massage. *See also* p. 794.

The reader is referred to further articles on hypothermia.†

REFRIGERATION ANALGESIA

Refrigeration analgesia is the application of cold to a localized part of the body to block local nerve conduction of painful impulses. It is not to be confused with induced hypothermia which is the application of cold in order to reduce the oxygen needs of the tissues during temporary interruption of the circulation.

---

* Drew, C. E., *Brit. med. Bull.*, 1961, **17**, 37.

† *See* the following articles : Scurr, C. F., *Proc. R. Soc. Med.*, 1955, **48**, 1077 ; Lucus, B. G. B., *Ibid.*, 1956, **49**, 345 ; Ross, D. N., *Ibid.*, 1956, **49**, 365 ; Brock, R., *Ibid.*, 1956, **49**, 347 ; Gray, T. C., *Lancet*, 1957, **1**, 384 ; Gray, T. C., *Med. Ann.*, 1957, Special Article, 175 ; Annotation, *Lancet*, 1959, **1**, 675; Malphee, I. W., Gray, T. C., and Davies, S., *Ibid.*, 1958, **2**, 1196; Cooper, K., and Ross, D., *Hypothermia in Surgical Practice*, 1960. London: Cassell; Sellick, B. A., in *Recent Advances in Anæsthesia and Analgesia* (Ed. Hewer, C. Langton), 10th ed., 1967. London: Churchill; *Brit. med. Bull.*, 1961, **17**, No. 1; and Forrester, A. C., in *Thoracic Anæsthesia* (Ed. Mushin, W. W.), 1963, Ch. 16. Oxford: Blackwell.

Refrigeration Analgesia, *continued.*

A method of analgesia revived by Fredk. M. Allen, of New York City.* Very seldom used to-day. It involves chilling and not freezing of the tissues. It acts on all the cells of the part, not just on the nerve-cells as do other anæsthetics and analgesics. It was used by Baron Dominique Jean Larrey (1766–1862) at the battle of Preuss Eylan in 1807 and also during Napoleon's retreat from Moscow in 1812; and by James Arnott (1797–1883), of Brighton, in 1847.† Benjamin Ward Richardson, the biographer of John Snow, used an ether spray to produce refrigeration analgesia in 1866,‡ and this gave rise to the term 'freezing' for local analgesia. The ether spray was replaced in 1890 by ethyl chloride by Redard,§ while in 1938 Fay and Smith described cryotherapy for the relief of pain and for the treatment of cancer.

The effects of chilling:—

1. Interference with conduction of nerve impulses.
2. Reduction of metabolic rate and oxygen requirements.
3. Inhibition of bacterial growth and infection.
4. Retardation of healing.

Technique.—Before a tourniquet can be applied, the tissue underlying it must be chilled for an hour by the close application of thin rubber ice-bags. Any convenient site proximal to the operation site is chosen for the tourniquet, which is then most carefully put on. A ½-in. rubber tube is very suitable. If the limb below the tourniquet becomes congested, the tourniquet is inefficient and must be reinforced. A pale blanched limb shows that the tourniquet is efficient.

A rubber sheet is placed beneath the limb and firmly fastened by a safety-pin 2–3 in. above the tourniquet. Cracked ice is now piled around the limb and kept in place by a few turns of a bandage around the rubber sheet. If the head of the bed is elevated the melted ice will drain into a bucket. The rubber sheet is undone occasionally to see that the limb is kept surrounded by ice. Patients do not complain of discomfort due to cold and seldom to the tourniquet : a small intravenous dose of morphine will control discomfort if it is present.

A loose tourniquet has the following disadvantages :—

1. Complete refrigeration and analgesia are hindered.
2. Chilling of the remainder of the patient is favoured.
3. Venous congestion in the limb increases amount of blood lost.

A tourniquet can be dispensed with :—

1. When the limb is rendered ischæmic by arteriosclerosis, trauma, or embolism.
2. When operation site is superficial ; e.g., skin-grafts can be cut after the tight application of ice-bags for two hours.

Other methods of cooling involve bandaging around the limb thin rubber ice-bags, and immersing the limb in a bucket of ice and

---

* *See* Allen, F. M., and Crossman, L. W., "Refrigeration Anæsthesia and Treatments", *Curr. Res. Anesth.*, 1943, **22**, 5; and *Anesthesiology*, 1943, **4**, 12. *See also* Furnas, D. W., *Ibid.*, 1965, **26**, 344.

† Arnott, J., *Lancet*, 1848, **2**, 98 (*see* Bird, H. M., *Anæsthesia*, 1949, **4**, 10).

‡ Richardson, B. W., *Med. Times Gaz.*, 1866, **115**, 3 Feb.; and *Dublin J. Med. Sci.*, 1867, **42**, 463.

§ Redard, C., *Cong. Franç. Chir.*, Paris, 1891, p. 431. Paris: Germer, Baillière, et Cie.

water if the operation is on the distal part of a limb. Electrical apparatus can also be used. With any of these methods, the skin temperature should be about 5° C. (40° F.). If necessary, a thermometer can be used to verify this.

Duration of refrigeration depends on the bulk of tissue. For a thigh, 2–3 hours ; for a leg or arm, 1½–2 hours ; for a hand or foot, 1 hour ; for fingers and toes, 20–30 minutes. If the surgeon is prepared to inject local analgesic solution into major nerves as he comes to them, refrigeration time can be reduced by about 50 per cent. About three buckets of chipped ice are required for an amputation through the thigh.

The patient in his bed is brought to the operating theatre, and, when the surgical team is ready, is placed on the table, the limb dried and painted, and the operation proceeded with. Cold lotions are used and warm objects kept away from the wound. Analgesia will last about an hour if the tourniquet is kept efficiently in place.

When main vessels have been tied, the tourniquet is released, spurting vessels are dealt with, and the wound closed. No evidence of thrombosis is seen in the stump.

Analgesia lasts long enough after removal of the tourniquet for the wound to be sutured.

After dressing, the stump can be surrounded by ice-bags for two or three days if infection is present. In clean cases no further chilling is necessary as it delays healing.

Ulceration of tissue does not occur if undue pressure of ice-bags and actual freezing are avoided.

The method can be used for the treatment of badly traumatized limbs requiring amputation.

Preliminary chilling reduces pain and infection and, by limiting absorption of toxins, lessens shock. The patient's general condition can be treated with blood, plasma, etc., and later, amputation performed under refrigeration analgesia, without producing further shock. In these cases, the tourniquet is only applied an hour or two before operation.

Advantages.—Specially indicated in amputation of leg in arteriosclerotic or diabetic gangrene. Mortality strikingly reduced in these operations by this method of analgesia. A useful, if rather messy technique even in the 1960's.

There is absence of post-operative pain ; absence of shock ; less chance of stump infection ; less upset of the patient's general condition.

Disadvantages.—Fussy technique. Delayed healing in arteriosclerotic tissues.

Refrigeration analgesia can be used for operations on the fingers and toes, hands and wrists, etc. Duration of chilling is 20–30 minutes and a tourniquet can be applied either at the base of a digit or above the wrist. Healing in healthy wounds is not delayed. Application of an ice-bag for 20–30 minutes over a superficial abscess or boil will enable incision to be performed painlessly.

The pain from post-operative wounds can be eased if an ice-bag is placed over the wound, which is protected by a double layer of cellophane, kept in place by adhesive strapping.

CHAPTER XXX

ANÆSTHESIA IN ABNORMAL ENVIRONMENTS

ABNORMAL AMBIENT PRESSURE

Altitude.—The sum of the partial pressures of oxygen, nitrogen, carbon dioxide, water vapour, and anæsthetic agents in alveolar gases equals the atmospheric pressure. At high altitudes the barometric pressure is low, and the pressure of alveolar oxygen falls disproportionately as compared with carbon dioxide and water vapour.

BAROMETRIC PRESSURE RELATED TO ALTITUDE AND
ALVEOLAR TENSIONS

Altitude (feet)	Barometric Pressure (mm. Hg)	Alveolar Oxygen Tension (mm. Hg)	Alveolar Carbon-dioxide Tension (mm. Hg)	Alveolar Water-vapour Tension (mm. Hg)
0	760	103	40·0	47
5,000	632	81	37·5	47
10,000	523	61	35·5	47
15,000	429	45	32·5	47
18,000	380	38	31·0	47
20,000	349	35	30·0	47

The anæsthetist working at high altitudes should consider:—

1. The low alveolar and arterial oxygen tension which is normally present. Since this may be further lowered should respiratory depression or altered ventilation–perfusion relationships occur, high concentrations of oxygen should always be given in anæsthetic mixtures for inhalation.

2. Nitrous oxide is a weak agent. The partial pressure needed in the alveolar gases to produce its effect may approach and even exceed the barometric pressure. It is the absolute tension and not the percentage in a mixture with oxygen which must be considered. Nitrous oxide is therefore less useful at altitude, particularly as increased concentrations of oxygen are needed to prevent hypoxia.

3. Vaporizers and flow-meters are not pressure compensated and so do not read true when barometric pressure is low. This applies to any apparatus which has not been recalibrated for altered pressure, including instruments such as the Fluotec. Actual flows and actual concentrations will be higher than the scale reading.

4. Altitude is often associated with low temperatures (*see below*).

5. The pathophysiology of both the unacclimatized and acclimatized resident at high altitude. Changes include pulmonary hyperventilation, polycythæmia, hypervolæmia, rise in pulmonary blood-volume, pulmonary hypertension, and increase in diffusion

capacity. Acute pulmonary œdema indicates I.P.P.V. with 100 per cent oxygen and descent to lower levels. (*See also* Safar, P., *Ann. Surg.*, 1956, **144**, 835; Ramo Rao, K. R., *Indian J. Anæsth.*, 1964, **12**, 4; and Safar, P., and Tenicela, R., *Anesthesiology*, 1964, **25**, 515.)

Hyperbaric Chambers.—For patients undergoing radiotherapy in a single-person hyperbaric chamber, intravenous anæsthesia, endotracheal intubation, and spontaneous respiration are satisfactory.* For major surgery more sophisticated techniques may be required.

1. EXPLOSIVE RISK.—Flammable agents such as ether and cyclopropane are contra-indicated. Halothane is non-flammable below 4 atmospheres' pressure,† but it should not be used with a nitrous-oxide–oxygen mixture since this widens the flammability range. Methoxyflurane is also non-flammable at pressures used in surgical hyperbaric chambers. Oil or grease must be excluded absolutely from ventilators, etc., because of the fire hazard. Electrically operated ventilators should not be used owing to the hazard from sparking.

2. THE EFECTS ON STAFF.—Decompression must be carried out with due care when staff are required to work in hyperbaric chambers.

3. NITROUS OXIDE.—The partial pressure required to produce its effect can be achieved using a relatively smaller percentage in a mixture. However, the solubility of the gas in body tissues is such that there is a danger of nitrous-oxide bubbles forming at the time of decompression. Nitrous oxide also extends the flammability range of halothane. Most authorities believe that it has little place in anæsthesia under hyperbaric conditions. Halothane and oxygen are usually preferred.

4. APPARATUS.—(*a*) Reducing valves are not affected by changes in ambient pressure unless the supply pressure falls to levels near the delivery pressure from the valve. Pipeline pressure of 60 lb. per sq. in. will need to be increased in order to operate valves within a hyperbaric chamber.‡ (*b*) Rotameters are not accurate under hyperbaric conditions. They read high unless they have been recalibrated for the increased ambient pressure.§ (*c*) Vaporizers. The Fluotec and other vaporizers are not pressure compensated and will deliver lesser percentages than the scale readings under hyperbaric conditions. Vaporizers when not in use should be removed from the anæsthetic machine or have the filler plug open during changes in ambient pressure. Otherwise explosion or implosion can occur. There is also a danger that liquid anæsthetic agent can be forced back up the inlet pipe.

5. CHANGES IN GAS VOLUME during compression and decompression. Cuffs on endotracheal tubes or Foley catheters should

* Sanger, C., Churchill-Davidson, I., and Thompson, R. N., *Brit. J. Anæsth.*, 1955, **27**, 436; and Churchill-Davidson, I., Sanger, C., and Thomlinson, R. H., *Brit. J. Radiol.*, 1957, **30**, 406.
† McDowall, D. G., *Anæsthesia*, 1964, **19**, 321; and Gottlieb, S. F., Fegan, F. J., and Tieslink, J., *Anesthesiology*, 1966, **27**, 195.
‡ Slack, W. K., in *Recent Advances in Anæsthesia and Analgesia* (Ed. Hewer, C. Langton), 10th ed., 1967, Ch. 9. London: J. & A. Churchill.
§ McDowall, D. G., *Anæsthesia*, 1964, **19**, 321.

Hyperbaric Chambers, *continued.*

be filled with water or left open. Similar considerations apply to thoracotomy drainage tubes, intragastric tubes, etc. [Intravenous transfusions require careful handling during decompression to prevent possible explosion, rapid transfusion, or air embolism. Plastic bags without air inlets are preferable to glass bottles. Multi-dose containers for drugs are not recommended. Aerosol sprays may behave inconsistently. Drugs subject to oxidation should not be exposed to hyperbaric conditions.

6. MONITORING.—Samples for blood-gas analysis taken within a hyperbaric chamber cannot be passed to the outside because the gases in solution pass out of solution as soon as ambient pressure falls. If blood-gas analysis is required, it must be carried out within the chamber, and then only if the equipment can be guaranteed by the manufacturers as safe for use under hyperbaric conditions. Expired gases can be led through a fine tube to an infra-red analyser outside the chamber, though it must be appropriately calibrated. Alveolar carbon dioxide and oxygen tensions may not equate with arterial tensions under hyperbaric conditions.

(*See also* Slack, W. K., in *Recent Advances in Anæsthesia and Analgesia* (Ed. Hewer, C. Langton), 10th ed., 1967, Ch. 9. London: Churchill. McDowall, D. G., *Anæsthesia*, 1964, **19**, 321; and Severinghaus, J. W., in *Fundamentals of Hyperbaric Medicine*, Ch. 9. Pub. No. 1298, Nat. Acad. Sci. Nat. Res. Council, Washington, D.C.)

ABNORMAL AMBIENT TEMPERATURE

Low Temperatures.—These may be encountered at altitude or in polar regions, particularly when surgery has to be carried out under field conditions. The patient must be kept warm, and techniques of local analgesia are often unsatisfactory.

Tropical Conditions.—Care must be taken to keep certain drugs cool to prevent deterioration (e.g., suxamethonium). Gas cylinders are filled to specified standards (filling ratio) to prevent the danger of increased pressure within cylinders should the temperature rise. Tropical conditions do not prevent the use of open ether.* Rubber articles are liable to perish.

FIELD SITUATIONS

Anæsthesia may have to be administered without the facilities of the modern general hospital: (1) In industrial accidents (e.g., mine-workings); (2) Following major disasters (earthquake, nuclear explosions); (3) On board ships at sea; (4) During exploration of remote regions; (5) In underdeveloped countries.

Apparatus.—Medical gases are likely to be in short supply. Volatile agents may be vaporized in air, or perhaps oxygen-enriched air. Draw-over apparatus is useful, and should be light and portable. A Venturi system for oxygen enrichment is economical.

* Boulton, T. B., *Anæsthesia*, 1966, **21**, 513.

Apparatus for intravenous anæsthesia is easily carried, and the use of disposable syringes and needles obviates the need for sterilization immediately prior to use. Endotracheal tubes, laryngoscopes, and connexions make anæsthesia safe. Where laryngoscopes are not available, simple equipment can be improvised,* or intubation achieved during transillumination† or a tube passed blindly through mouth‡ or nose.

Inhalation Methods.—

1. OPEN MASKS.—The Schimmelbusch mask may be used for ether, chloroform, or halothane. It is rather wasteful since vapour is lost to the atmosphere without being inhaled. Also there is no provision for artificial ventilation of the patient.

2. THE EPSTEIN MACINTOSH OXFORD VAPORIZER FOR ETHER.§—The apparatus has a water jacket and an automatic thermocompensator and delivers known concentrations of ether in air. Special versions for halothane, azeotropic ether–halothane mixture, and trichloroethylene are available. Halothane should not be placed in the ether vaporizer since the metal is attacked. Capacity 450 ml.

3. THE OXFORD MINIATURE VAPORIZER.‖—Delivers 0–3·5 per cent halothane and was designed to smooth induction with ether using the Oxford vaporizer for ether (above). Has a sealed water jacket but is not thermocompensated. Interchangeable scales for trichloroethylene and chloroform are available, approximate conversion factors being × 3 and × ⅔ respectively. Capacity 20 ml.

4. THE BRYCE-SMITH INDUCTION UNIT.¶—The wick is charged by soaking in a limited quantity of halothane. The unit is then used to smooth the introduction of ether from the Oxford vaporizer. It delivers up to 5 per cent halothane initially, falling to zero over 5 or 6 minutes.

5. THE PENLON DRAW-OVER VAPORIZER.**—Designed for halothane (up to 6 per cent) though other volatile agents can be used. A special vaporizer is made for methoxyflurane (up to 2 per cent). The conversion factor when ether is used in the methoxyflurane apparatus is × 10.

6. THE BLEASE UNIVERSAL VAPORIZER (Gardner; Fraser Sweetman).—Thermocompensated. Interchangeable control units for ether, halothane, azeotrope, trichloroethylene, and methoxyflurane. Capacity 180 ml. Incorporated in a range of Portablease models together with bellows, oxygen enrichment, or a complete apparatus.

7. THE FLUOXAIR.††—Designed for Service use. Halothane is vaporized in air with oxygen enrichment and a bellows is provided for I.P.P.V. The Oxford ether vaporizer can be connected to the air-inlet if desired.

---

* Gillett, G. B., and Patkin, M., *Anæsthesia*, 1964, **19**, 595.
† Tate, N., *Lancet*, 1955, **2**, 980.
‡ Siddall, W. J. W., *Anæsthesia*, 1966, **21**, 221.
§ Macintosh, R. R., *Brit. med. J.*, 1955, **2**, 1054.
‖ Parkhouse, J., *Anæsthesia*, 1966, **21**, 498.
¶ Bryce-Smith, R., *Ibid.*, 1964, **19**, 393.
** Merrifield, A. J., and others, *Brit. J. Anæsth.*, 1967, **39**, 50.
†† Stephens, K. F., *Ibid.*, 1965, **37**, 67.

Inhalation Methods, *continued.*

8. HEWER'S EMERGENCY APPARATUS.*—Consists of an Ambu bag, a Goldman vaporizer, and a Ruben valve. Provides halothane and air with I.P.P.V.

9. THE FLAGG CAN.†—Devised during World War I. The patient breathes to and fro through a can containing ether. Recent modifications facilitate some variation of vapour strength by admitting air as a diluent via a suction union.‡

10. IMPROVISED VAPORIZERS can be made out of materials which are readily available.‡ Flagg cans can be easily constructed using empty coffee jars. Inhalers can also be made from two suitable food tins with a layer of gauze between if the Schimmelbusch mask is not available.

11. SIMPLE APPARATUS for administration of a non-explosive mixture of cyclopropane have been described: (*a*) Cyclopropane, 50 per cent; nitrogen, 25 per cent; oxygen, 25 per cent.§ (*b*) Cyclopropane, 40 per cent; oxygen, 30 per cent; helium, 30 per cent.‖ (*c*) The CON apparatus (cyclopropane, 40 per cent; oxygen, 30 per cent; nitrogen, 30 per cent).¶

Suction Apparatus.—Portable foot-operated suction pumps are now available (e.g., Ambu or Smith-Clarke).

Artificial Ventilation.—Portable hand-operated bellows include the Ambu bag, the Oxford inflating bellows, the Cardiff bellows, the Penlon bellows, etc. *See also* Chapter VIII.

Field Techniques.—Intravenous apparatus, induction agents, and muscle relaxants are easily carried and may be used in conjunction with endotracheal methods and a portable apparatus as described above. Ether and halothane are the two most promising agents for inhalation. There may, however, be some restrictions preventing the carriage of inflammable agents in aircraft. Examples:—

1. Thiopentone and muscle relaxant, combined with ether in air from the Oxford vaporizer with I.P.P.V. using the Oxford inflating bellows.

2. Halothane and air, using the Fluoxair, with I.P.P.V., thiopentone, and muscle relaxants, if indicated.

   It should thus be possible to provide good operating conditions to allow the performance of major surgery, even where medical gas cylinders are not available.

(*See also* Boulton, T. B., and Cole, P. V., *Anæsthesia*, 1966, **21**, 268; *Ibid.*, 1966, **21**, 379; *Ibid.*, 1966, **21**, 513; *Ibid.*, 1967, **22**, 101; *Ibid.*, 1967, **22**, 435; Davenport, H. T., *Canad. med. Ass. J.*, 1964, **90**, 687; and Farman, J. V., *Brit. J. Anæsth.*, 1962, **34**, 877.)

---

* Hewer, C. L., *Lancet*, 1961, **2**, 1290.
† Flagg, P. J., *The Art of Anesthesia*, 7th ed., 1954. Philadelphia: Lippincott.
‡ Boulton, T. B., *Anæsthesia*, 1966, **21**, 513.
§ Bourne, J. G., *Nitrous Oxide in Dentistry*, 1960. London: Lloyd-Luke.
‖ Hingson, R. A., *J. Amer. med. Ass.*, 1958, **167**, 1077.
¶ Stephens, K. F., and Bourne, J. G., *Lancet*, 1960, **2**, 481.

ANÆSTHESIA IN THE DARK

Diminution of room lighting, or near-total darkness, may be requested during some endoscopy and radiological procedures. The patient, not under the direct observation of the anæsthetist, is exposed to the hazards of unrecognized cyanosis, respiratory obstruction, exhaustion of gas cylinders, etc. Adequate lighting should always be provided when possible. When lights have to be extinguished, the anæsthetist should pay particular attention to the following points:—

1. That gas cylinders, particularly oxygen, contain adequate reserves of gas.
2. Endotracheal anæsthesia obviates the danger of airway obstruction.
3. Monitoring of vital signs by auditory and tactile signs, e.g., finger on pulse, hand on reservoir bag or chest, precordial or œsophageal stethoscope, auditory bleep such as is provided on some commercial pulse monitors and electrocardiograms.
4. A torch should be available for occasional inspection of the fingers, etc., for cyanosis and for emergency use.
5. In some anæsthetic machines, vital parts may be fluorescent, e.g., the plastic sheet behind the rotameters.

CHAPTER XXXI

THE COMPLICATIONS AND SEQUELÆ OF ANÆSTHESIA

PULMONARY COMPLICATIONS*

These are usually due to the inability of the patient to remove secretions by coughing, because of post-operative pain.

Abdominal operations adversely affect mechanical lung function by reducing total lung capacity and maximal inspiratory and expiratory flow-rates, due to mechanical obstruction, bronchospasm, and spasm of the muscles of the anterior abdominal wall secondary to pain.

These may be expected to occur in 5 per cent of all operations ; in at least 10 per cent of abdominal operations. In a recent large series, 13 per cent of post-operative deaths were due to pulmonary complications.†

Post-operative atelectasis was described by Wm. Gairdner, of Glasgow, in 1850.‡ It was later described by Barr and by Pasteur in the first decade of the present century.§ A later erroneous theory of causation still held by some is that the post-operative chest is due to the irritating properties of anæsthetic gases and vapours.

As early as 1900 J. von Mikulicz-Radecki (1850–1905) showed that, over a 4-year period, chest complications followed general and local

---

* *See also* Anscombe, A. R., *Pulmonary Complications of Abdominal Surgery*, 1957. London : Lloyd-Luke.
† Vosschulte, K., *Arch. Klin. Chir.*, 1958, **288**, 328.
‡ Gairdner, W. T., *Month. J. Med. Sci.*, 1850, **11**, 122, 230.
§ Barr, J., *Brit. med. J.*, 1907, **2**, 289; Pasteur. W., *Lancet*, 1908, **2**, 1351; and *Ibid.*, 1910, **2**, 1080.

Pulmonary Complications, continued.

anæsthesia with equal frequency. Even now, nearly 70 years later, there are those who regard the anæsthetic gas or vapour as the main cause.

Pathology.—The conditions arise in association with :—

1. Primary blocking of bronchi. The most common.
2. Primary interference with pulmonary blood-supply.
3. Primary bacterial invasion of lungs.
4. Spread from disease in abdomen.
5. Pneumothorax—rarely.

The commonest complication is segmental atelectasis (Coryllos, J., *J. Amer. med. Ass.*, 1929, **93**, 98) due to retention of sputum and absorption of air distal to the block.

1. PRIMARY BLOCKING OF BRONCHI AND RETENTION OF SPUTUM while blood-supply remains intact.

   a. Poor expulsive mechanism after operation due to : (i) Pain. (ii) Reduced movement of diaphragm. (iii) Sedatives. (iv) A tight binder or dressing. (v) Spasm of muscles of abdominal wall. The smaller bronchi are cleared by cilia and these may be inhibited by the anæsthetic used, increased stickiness of sputum, hypoxia, hypercapnia, etc.

   b. Constriction of the bronchi. This, together with engorgement of the mucosa, may : (i) Follow reflexly from stimuli inflicted at too light a plane of anæsthesia (intubation, traction on mesentery, etc.). (ii) Result from post-operative pain. (iii) Be due to cholinergic drugs, e.g., cyclopropane, thiopentone, neostigmine. (iv) Be due to irritant anæsthetics. (v) Be due to aspiration of stomach contents, blood, etc.

   c. Excessive production of sputum due to : (i) Smoking. (ii) Infection, etc.

   Mendelson* describes a post-operative, exudative pneumonitis in women in labour following the aspiration of acid, irritating gastric contents characterized by asthma, cyanosis, dyspnœa, and, in severe cases, acute pulmonary œdema. It can be relieved by aspiration, bronchial lavage with normal sodium bicarbonate solution, oxygen, and hydrocortisone. The pH to be seriously irritating must be 2·5 or below. Magnesium trisilicate, half an hour before anæsthesia, has prophylactic value.

2. PRIMARY INTERFERENCE WITH PULMONARY BLOOD-SUPPLY.—

   a. Emboli—blood-clot, fat, liquor amnii, or tumour (e.g., hypernephroma).

   b. Acute pulmonary œdema and cardiac asthma. Most common in hypertensive patients and in coronary disease. May be brought on by too much intravenous fluid.

3. PRIMARY BACTERIAL INVASION OF LUNGS.—

   a. From aspirated material.

   b. From contaminated anæsthetic equipment, e.g., tubes, face-masks, etc. (For prevention *see* Chapter XXXVIII.)

   Secondary bacterial invasion soon follows in patches of atelectasis.

---

* Mendelson ,C. L. ,*Amer. J. Obstet. Gynec.*, 1946, **52**, 191.

4. SPREAD FROM DISEASE IN ABDOMEN.—The lymphatics can readily transmit infection through the diaphragm from the abdomen to the thorax, e.g., in cases of subphrenic abscess or peritonitis. Empyema or suppurative pneumonitis may result, perhaps with bronchial fistula. Multiple small lung abscesses may be part of a general pyæmia following peritonitis or acute abdominal infection.

5. PNEUMOTHORAX.—May occur spontaneously. May follow trauma to pleura in operation on kidney, gall-bladder, structures deep in the neck, thyroid, etc. May follow intercostal block.

Factors influencing Chest Complications.—
TYPE OF OPERATION.—Most common after upper abdominal operations, especially long ones. Fairly common following operations for hernia. Of non-abdominal operations, thyroidectomy is most often followed by chest complications. Pulmonary embolism commonest after pelvic operations.

After laparotomy there is reflex fixation of the diaphragm and of the muscles of the anterior abdominal wall, while reflex bronchospasm may also occur.

The situation of the incision is important and if this can avoid the anterior abdominal wall so much the better (e.g., Mayo's incision for renal surgery ; a transthoracic incision for high gastrectomy, etc.).

Relationship to Pneumoperitoneum.[*]—There is a close correlation between pneumoperitoneum and post-operative pulmonary collapse. Pneumoperitoneum can be prevented by :—

1. Closing the incision round a catheter after laparotomy and aspirating air before completing the suture. Simpler methods include :—
2. Expelling air from under the diaphragm by replacing the liver and obliterating dead space.
3. Blowing the intestines gently into the wound as the peritoneum is being sewn up, just as the lung is blown up at the end of a thoracotomy.
4. Avoidance of tenting of the peritoneum during its closure.
5. Application of light pressure to the abdominal wall just before the peritoneum is closed.

Other Relationships.—
ORAL SEPSIS.—Pulmonary suppuration may occur in patients with dental sepsis : (1) Independently of operation ; (2) Following operation under general anæsthesia ; (3) Following dental extraction. Resulting pathology may be : (a) suppurative bronchitis, (b) suppurative pneumonitis, (c) lung abscess, (d) empyema. Pulmonary abscess is very rare in edentulous patients. The onset may be delayed for three weeks after operation. As a routine, dental sepsis should be removed three weeks before operation. In patients undergoing major dental operations, a careful pre-operative oral toilet, adequate packing

---

[*] Bevan, P. G., *Brit. med. J.*, 1961, **2**, 609.

Pulmonary Complications—Other Relationships, *continued.*

of the pharynx, head-down position, avoidance of drugs depressing the laryngeal reflexes, and antibiotics are all useful preventive measures. If inhalation of a foreign body is suspected, early radiography and bronchoscopy are necessary.

SEX.—Males affected three times as frequently as females.

AGE.—More frequent in older age-groups.

SEASON.—More frequent in cold weather.

SMOKING.—By causing bronchial exudation, smoking greatly increases incidence of chest complications.

ANÆSTHETIC.—Very little to choose between different agents and techniques, if administration is skilful. The longer the duration of deep anæsthesia, the greater will be the incidence of chest complications. Contamination of airways, tubes, lubricants may be a factor and *Pseudomonas aeruginosa* has caused infection from unsterile analgesic lubricant.*

Possible Causes.—

1. Operation and anæsthesia reduce and inhibit ciliary action, and lower resistance to endogenous and exogenous infection, the latter either travelling via the air-passages or through the lymphatics of the diaphragm from infected areas in the abdomen.

2. Hypoventilation during and immediately after operation, due to :—

   a. Injudicious use of muscle relaxants.

   b. Prolonged, deep general anæsthesia.

   c. High intradural or extradural analgesia with intercostal paralysis.

   d. Pre-operative and post-operative sedative drugs which depress respiration, e.g., opiates.

   e. Pain from operation site, preventing adequate breathing and coughing. This was recognized as long ago as 1900 by J. von Mikulicz-Radecki, and in 1902 by Campiche, of Lausanne.

   f. Reflex inhibition of diaphragmatic or thoracic movement, associated with abdominal operation.

   g. Awkward position on operation table, as in gall-bladder and kidney operations when the bridge is used, lithotomy, and Trendelenburg positions.

   h. Tight bandages.

   Pulmonary mechanical function may be decreased by 50–70 per cent after upper abdominal operation and by 25–35 per cent after lower abdominal operation.† When the patient is in the lateral position, bronchospirometry has shown that the ventilation of the lower lung is greater than that of the upper lung.‡

---

* Phillips, I., *Lancet*, 1966, **1**, 903.

† Anscombe, A. R., *Pulmonary Complications of Abdominal Surgery*, 1957, p. 56. London: Lloyd-Luke.

‡ Wade, D. L., and Gilson, J. C., *Thorax*, 1951, **6**, 103 ; and Rothstein, E., and others, *J. thorac. Surg.*, 1950, **19**, 821.

3. Rapid absorption of gases from alveoli and the absence there of sustaining gases, e.g., nitrogen (a mechanism first described in 1878*).
4. Intrabronchial aspiration of foreign material.
5. Prolonged shock.
6. Septic emboli from site of operation in infected cases.
7. Atelectasis may be part of a reflex respiratory spasm, the result of stimuli applied at too light a plane of anæsthesia.

Clinical Types.—May vary from mild bronchitis to massive collapse, but lobular atelectasis is the commonest finding. It is likely to be basal and unilateral with onset some time during the first 48 hours. Progressing insidiously it may develop until there are malaise, pyrexia, slight cyanosis together with the signs of consolidation. The differential diagnosis is from : (a) Lobar or bronchopneumonia. (b) Pulmonary embolism. (c) Cardiac infarction. (d) Pulmonary tuberculosis. (e) A surgical complication. (f) Temporary paralysis of the diaphragm, sometimes seen after operation.

1. Bronchitis. This may be difficult to differentiate from lobular atelectasis.
2. Atelectasis.
   a. Lobular.
   b. Lobar.
3. Bronchopneumonia.
4. Aspiration pneumonitis.
5. Pulmonary embolism.

Diagnosis.—Atelectasis need cause no symptoms, but it is likely to lead to trouble if it is associated with bronchial obstruction, infection, or a persistent interference with circulation associated with an arteriovenous shunt through the area of collapse. Onset of symptoms in first 48 hours probably points to bronchitis or atelectasis; occasionally to massive pulmonary embolism. Atelectasis should be suspected if in the immediate post-operative period the temperature rises to 101° F. (38° C.); if the pulse-rate is greater than 100 per minute, and the respiration-rate more than 20 per minute —always providing that there is no surgical reason to account for these signs. Involved area may be anything between a whole lung and a few alveoli. Extensive collapse can occur on the operating table and then may give rise to difficulty in breathing, cyanosis, right heart failure, and death. Blood flowing through a non-ventilated lung undergoes a right-to-left shunt, causing a lowered Po_2 and a raised Pco_2.

Onset several days after operation is probably due to secondary bronchopneumonia from aspiration, etc., especially if signs of a fulminating pneumonitis develop in a patient suffering from such conditions as intestinal obstruction, persistent vomiting, etc.

Primary bronchopneumonia can occur without previous atelectasis. Primary lobar pneumonia can also occur. It is important not to overlook the possible coexistence of abdominal abnormality, e.g., peritonitis, which may cause chest symptoms.

Sudden onset in second week is probably due to pulmonary embolism.

---

* Lichtheim, L., *Arch. exp. Path. Pharmakol.*, 1878, **10**, 54.

Pulmonary Complications—Diagnosis, *continued.*

SIGNS AND SYMPTOMS OF ATELECTASIS.—

1. Rapid breathing—30–60 per minute.
2. Rapid heart-rate.
3. Absence of pain on inspiration, unless pleural surface of lung is involved.
4. Dilatation of alæ nasi and slight cyanosis.
5. Restricted movements of affected side of chest.
6. Diminution of breath-sounds and perhaps decreased resonance are almost normal after abdominal operations. When the condition is established, signs of consolidation are present. Rhonchi may be present. Râles rare.
7. Lower lobes usually involved.
8. Mediastinal displacement towards affected side, in gross cases.
9. Radiographic appearance may resemble that of broncho-pneumonia.

   Elevation of one or other side of diaphragm very common after upper abdominal operations, in absence of clinical atelectasis. In atelectasis there is contraction of lung tissue ; in bronchopneumonia, swelling. Occasionally, an unresolving chest condition after operation is tuberculous. Massive collapse causes pain in the chest of sudden onset, dyspnœa, cyanosis, fever, tachycardia, and mediastinal shift.

The complications of atelectasis are bronchopneumonia, pleural effusion, and bronchiectasis.

SIGNS AND SYMPTOMS OF ASPIRATION PNEUMONITIS.—

1. Cyanosis, unrelieved by oxygen therapy.
2. Tachypnœa.
3. Tachycardia.
4. Prostration.
5. Coarse asthmatic rhonchi on auscultation—may not occur for some hours.
6. Chest radiograph shows areas of density.
7. Cardiovascular failure may supervene. Hypotension, pulmonary œdema ; usually lasts 2–4 hours if the patient survives.

Management.—

1. Repeated tracheal aspiration, perhaps associated with periodic intratracheal injections of up to 10 ml. normal saline.
2. Oxygen administration.
3. Treatment of cardiovascular failure. Digitalization. Pressor drugs or intravenous fluids may produce pulmonary œdema.
4. Bronchodilator drugs, e.g., aminophylline, aerosol isoprenaline.
5. Hydrocortisone may be useful : (*a*) to treat hypotensive state ; (*b*) to reduce lung reaction.
6. Antibiotics to prevent infection.
7. Intermittent positive-pressure ventilation may be required.[*]

SIGNS AND SYMPTOMS OF PULMONARY EMBOLISM.[†]—

This is more common in medical than in surgical wards, especially in patients with heart disease and carcinoma. Massive thrombosis

[*] McCormick, P. W., Hay, R. G., and Griffin, R. W., *Lancet*, 1966, **1**, 1127; and McCormick, P. W., *Proc. R. Soc. Med.*, 1966, **59**, 66.
[†] Barritt, D. W., and Jordan, S. C., *Lancet*, 1961, **1**, 729.

and embolism more frequent in old than in young patients and in septic cases and those having undergone long and difficult operations. Prolonged bed-rest, e.g., in patients with hip fractures, causes special risk.* The operative and peri-operative period are critical times for the development of hypercoagulable states and the prophylactic administration of heparin may reduce the incidence of this grave catastrophe.† Condition usually associated with venous thrombosis in legs or pelvis. Onset may coincide with getting up or straining at stool. Sudden onset of pain in chest from second to fourteenth day after operation. Usually during second week.

Signs.—Tachycardia, a rise in the venous pulse—distended neck veins; hypotension; cyanosis; sometimes gallop rhythm; râles and friction sounds and later, dullness and bronchial breathing. *Radiographs of chest* may show right-sided cardiac enlargement; elevation of dome of diaphragm; shadow in the lower zone and, later, clouding in costophrenic angle due to pleural effusion. *Electrocardiograph* is abnormal in about one-half the cases and may show an S wave in limb Lead I and a Q wave in Lead III, T wave inversion in Lead III; these represent right heart strain.

Symptoms.—Faintness, dyspnœa, substernal discomfort, pleural pain, and hæmoptysis. Pain is usually less severe than that in myocardial infarction.

Jaundice, due to hæmolysis of the blood in the infarct, may be seen. If the embolus is massive, there is profound shock, sweating, pallor, air hunger, raised venous pressure, and anxiety. Death usually follows quickly, but recoveries have been reported. Trendelenburg's operation of embolectomy has been done occasionally. Small emboli are often overlooked, the patient complaining only of faintness, tightness in chest : duration short, no physical signs. Non-fatal attacks are three or four times as common as fatal attacks. The classic causes of pulmonary embolism during operation are : (1) Hypernephroma; (2) Liquor amnii (in obstetric patients).

Diagnosis.—In typical cases after operation, there is a short period of fever suggesting thrombosis, followed by apyrexia and then the onset of embolism. Should be thought of when there is tachycardia, hæmoptysis, jaundice, or unilateral effusion after operation. It is often misdiagnosed as atelectasis or pneumonia. Sudden pain in the chest within three weeks of operation is due to embolism unless it can be proved otherwise. The condition accounts for about 6 per cent of deaths associated with surgical operation. Ventilation of the non-perfused lung reduces the alveolar CO_2 below that of the blood.

Treatment.—Sedation, anticoagulants to prevent chronic pulmonary hypertension, and oxygen. If further emboli appear after the prothrombin time is prolonged, ligation of a femoral vein or even of the inferior vena cava must be considered. Benefit is said to have resulted from stellate ganglion block, i.e., assuming

---

* Fagan, D. G., *Lancet*, 1964, **1**, 846; and Sharnoff, J. G., and others, *Ibid.*, 1964, **1**, 845
† Sharnoff, J. G., *Ibid.*, 1966, **2**, 876.

Pulmonary Complications—Diagnosis, *continued*.

the existence (which is doubtful) of neurogenic reflex vaso-constriction in the pulmonary vessels.

SIGNS AND SYMPTOMS OF LUNG ABSCESS.—When foreign material is introduced into the trachea, it gravitates into the dependent apex of the lower lobe with the patient lying supine, and into the dependent upper lobe with the patient on his side : these are the commonest sites of abscess. Onset may be mild, after a latent period of two to ten days, simulating bronchitis or early bronchopneumonia. Cough, dry and hacking, appears, together with wasting, chills, anorexia, etc. A leucocytosis develops, and the temperature starts to swing. Radiology in the early stages usually shows an area of consolidation. When the abscess erodes into a bronchus, foul mucopurulent sputum is coughed up and a minority of patients achieve spontaneous cure. Those who do not require postural drainage, suitable antibiotic treatment, and, perhaps, operation. Occasionally, a lung abscess ruptures into the pleura, forming an empyema and, of course, a bronchopleural fistula. Such an empyema should be drained with the patient sitting, not lying down ; local analgesia should be used : these measures prevent the patient from being drowned in his own pus.

The earliest sign is a patch of consolidation ; later a fluid level may be seen.

Prevention of Chest Complications.—All patients before under-going an abdominal operation should have a chest radiograph. Causal factors should be avoided as much as possible.

1. PRE-OPERATIVE.—Pre-operative investigation of pulmonary mechanical efficiency deserves more attention than it now receives.

Simple tests of ventilatory function include: (1) Maximal breathing capacity. (2) Forced expiratory volume. (3) Peak expiratory flow-rate (Wright portable meter). If the results of these are abnormally low they should be repeated after the use of bronchodilators. Reversible airway obstruction should be reversed immediately before and after operation. (*See also* pp. 75 and 673.)

Avoid operations during acute infections of upper respiratory tract. See that chronic infections are treated. Avoid smoking for three weeks before operation. Have a physiotherapist go over with a patient the breathing exercises necessary after operation so that maximal thoracic breathing is possible. Arrange for postural drainage in patients with much secretion. Have teeth attended to, and sinus infection cleared up. Penicillin should be given before operation to patients in whom the risk of pulmonary complications is likely to be high : 1,000,000 units should be injected, and, if a cough develops, 250,000 units may be given six-hourly. There is, however, evidence that this is useless.* Inhalations of penicillin are also helpful (60,000 units of calcium penicillin in

---

* Griffiths, E., *Brit. med. J.*, 1957, **1**, 803.

2 ml. of water). Encourage loss of weight before operation when necessary. Obese patients are more liable to post-operative complications because of : (1) Associated respiratory and circulatory disease. (2) The reduced vital capacity in obesity. (3) The poor tone of the fat-laden respiratory muscles. (4) The increased technical difficulty of the operation.

Palmer and Sellick* advise a routine which, in their hands, definitely reduces the incidence of atelectasis. It consists of the inhalation of isoprenaline (neoepinine, aleudrine, isupren, neodrenal) and postural drainage with vibratory and clapping percussion to the chest wall, before and after operation. 1 ml. of 1 per cent isoprenaline solution is inhaled by mouth from a hand inhaler, three times daily, followed by fifteen to twenty minutes' postural drainage during which time the basal regions of the chest wall are submitted to clapping and vibratory percussion during expiration. It is done with the patient in the prone and in each lateral position. This thrice-daily drill is continued until tipping produces no sputum, during the immediate pre-operative period. The patients are tipped and given the inhalation, just before the premedication is injected, and on return to the ward are similarly dealt with as soon as conditions allow, starting off with inhalation alone. Treatment is maintained for about five days or until no more sputum can be coughed up. Lævo-isoprenaline—isolevin—is less toxic than ordinary isoprenaline. It is said to have ten times the bronchodilator action of adrenaline. Each ml. contains 4·2 mg. of active base.

Another method of easing cough and liquefying sputum is the inhalation after nebulization of alevaire, a detergent in sterile alkaline solution. It lowers the surface tension of the sputum and facilitates its removal by coughing. Each treatment should last about half an hour and can be repeated three or four times daily.†

2. AT OPERATION.—Avoid over-sedation, but use adequate atropine or hyoscine. Employ careful anæsthetic technique. See that the patient is as little depressed at the end of the operation as possible. It is, however, an interesting fact that chest complications do not appear to increase in patients who have prolonged post-operative sedation, the result of the phenothiazine derivatives. Endeavour to remove the respiratory depressant action of muscle relaxants before the patient leaves the theatre. To prevent bronchoconstriction during and after operation, the administration, during the operation, of 1 per cent isoprenaline sulphate aerosol has been recommended.‡ Suck upper air-passages clear of secretions, blood, vomitus, etc., after operation, using a bronchoscope if contamination has been gross. Post-operative bronchoscopy is not, however, without its dangers. It may cause hypoxia and consequent circulatory

* Palmer, K. N. V., and Sellick, B. A., *Lancet*, 1953, **1**, 164.
† Ruben, E. J., and others, *Anesthesiology*, 1955, **16**, 801.
‡ Linton, S., and Odell, J. R., *Anæsthesia*, 1959, **14**, 68.

Prevention of Chest Complications, *continued.*

depression and should be preceded and accompanied by oxygen insufflation and an intravenous injection of atropine to damp down vagal reflexes. If the pleura has been opened during operation the lungs must be reinflated as the chest is closed, and the pleural cavity kept free of air and exudation in the post-operative period.

If the patient has been in the lateral position, the lower lung cannot be adequately ventilated during controlled respiration and absorption atelectasis may develop. At the end of the operation, the patient should be maintained in controlled respiration in the supine position to re-expand this lower collapsed zone.[*]

3. POST-OPERATIVE.—Avoid excessive sedation and prohibit use of atropine. Get the patient moving about in bed as early as possible. Encourage deep breathing and coughing at least once each hour.[†] Periodic overinflation of the lungs during the operation, and at its end, with nitrogen-containing gas may reduce the incidence of miliary atelectasis. Alveolar collapse can be produced by denitrogenation and requires renitrogenation for its prevention.[‡] The nurse should be constantly rallying the patient, to avoid hypoventilation and hypostasis. Diaphragmatic excursion is not improved by getting patient from the supine to the sitting position. Cough should be especially encouraged soon after a dose of morphine; the abdomen can be held firm while the patient is coughing. Premixed nitrous oxide in oxygen (25 : 75) inhaled for 15 minutes diminishes post-operative pain as proved by an increase in vital capacity measurements.[§] Trichloroethylene can be used in a similar way.[||] Pot. iod. in adequate dosage, i.e., 1–3 g. t.d.s., definitely liquefies viscous secretions and increases their amount, and so permits their expectoration. It should not be given for more than three or four days consecutively, as a tolerance develops. Steam, too, decreases the viscosity of bronchial secretions, but does not increase their amount. Sputum viscosity can be efficiently reduced by the inhalation of an aerosol of water, for one hour.[¶] Urea as an aerosol has a powerful mucolytic effect and facilitates expectoration.[**]

I.P.P.V. during inspiration with aerosol isoprenaline during the first few days after operation has been suggested recently and gives good results.

Control of pain by extradural analgesia allows free movement of the chest and good expectoration. A catheter is inserted in

[*] Potgeiter, S. V., *Brit. J. Anæsth.*, 1959, **31**, 472.
[†] Brock, R. C., *Guy's Hospital Reports*, 1936, **86**, 191; and Dripps, R. D., and Waters, R. M., *Amer. J. Nurs.*, 1941, **41**, 530.
[‡] Dery, R., and others, *Canad. Anæsth. Soc. J.*, 1965, **12**, 531.
[§] Parbrook, G. D., and Kennedy, B. R., *Brit. med. J.*, 1964, **2**, 1303; and Petrovsky, B. V., and Yefuni, S. N., *Brit. J. Anæsth.*, 1965, **37**, 42.
[||] Ellis, M. W., and Bryce-Smith, R., *Brit. med. J.*, 1965, **2**, 1412; and Hovell, B. L., and others, *Anæsthesia*, 1967, **22**, 284.
[¶] Palmer, K. N. V., *Lancet*, 1960, **1**, 91.
[**] Waldron-Edwards, D., and Skoryna, S. C., *Canad. med. Ass. J.*, 1966, **94**, 1249.

the high or mid-thoracic region. Small volumes of analgesic solution achieve pain relief without fall of blood-pressure.*

PREVENTION OF PULMONARY EMBOLISM.—This involves frequent post-operative movement of the legs, feet, and toes with active and frequent calf-muscle exercises and deep breathing. Post-operative thrombophlebitis is most frequent in old, fat patients who have suffered from shock or hæmorrhage. Pre-existing varicose veins are a predisposing factor. There is an abrupt rise in platelet count and shortening of clotting time within a few hours of the start of an operation.† The mutual adhesiveness of the blood-platelets increases from the fourth to the twelfth post-operative day. Prolonged bed-rest favours the condition. The possible sites of thrombosis should be examined frequently, e.g., the calf, groins, and feet. Homan's sign—pain in the calf on passive dorsiflexion of the foot—indicates phlebothrombosis of calf and may demand ligation of the vein proximal to the clot. A low fever after a pelvic operation, unless otherwise explained, is probably due to thrombophlebitis, which may be improved by lumbar paravertebral sympathetic block (L.2, L.3 ganglia). Should thrombophlebitis be suspected, the blood-prothrombin level should be lowered. The intravenous injection of alphatocopherol 300–600 mg. daily has been recommended for the prevention of the condition.‡

ANTICOAGULANTS.—
1. Direct anticoagulant : heparin.
2. Indirect anticoagulants : the coumarins and the indanediones. These are both hypothrombinæmic agents.

HEPARIN.—First discovered in 1916 and probably produced in the mast cells of Ehrlich. Commercially prepared from the lungs and liver of beef cattle by enzymatic digestion. It is a sulphonated mucopolysaccharide with a strong electronegative charge. Must be given intravenously, 100–130 units being equal to 1 mg.

Action.—Inhibits conversion of prothrombin to thrombin and interferes with action of thrombin on fibrinogen, thus delaying or preventing blood coagulation. Effects come on a few minutes after injection and if dose is small, pass off in an hour.

Prophylactic Uses.—Following operation if there is a history of thrombosis or embolism or if the chances of abnormal clotting are greater than usual, e.g., with severe varices, in vascular surgery, and heart disease.

Therapeutic Uses.—In pulmonary embolism, thrombophlebitis, coronary thrombosis, peripheral vascular disease, or injury.

Laboratory Uses.—As an anticoagulant before taking blood samples for E.S.R. and Wassermann tests, and in blood transfusion for erythroblastosis fœtalis.

* Simpson, B. R., Parkhouse, J., Marshall, R., and Lambrechts, W., Brit. J. Anæsth., 1961, 33, 628; and Bromage, P. R., Ibid., 1967, 39, 721.
† Sharnoff, J. G., J. Amer. med. Ass., 1959, 108, 688.
‡ Shute, W. E., and Shute, E. V., Lancet, 1954, 1, 625.

Prevention of Chest Complications, *continued.*

Dosage.—Intravenously, 6000–10,000 units. Intramuscularly 25,000 units with 0·5 per cent procaine. Estimation of clotting time should be 15–20 minutes after injection.

Reversal.—Protamine sulphate 1 per cent solution given slowly (to prevent hypotension). It is a protein with a strong electropositive charge—5000 units reverse 5 ml. of heparin; 100 units contained in 1 mg. Dosage should be controlled by coagulation-time estimations, as excess protamine itself prolongs coagulation time.

COUMARINS AND INDANEDIONES.—They act, probably, on the liver but only after being absorbed into the body and there is a delay of about 12 hours before their effect takes place. Usually taken orally. The coumarins include nicoumalone, dicoumarol, ethyl biscoumacetate (tromexan), and warfarin sodium (marevan). This last agent can also be given by intravenous or intramuscular injection. The indanediones include diphenadione and phenindione (dindevan).

CONTROL OF ANTICOAGULANT EFFECT.—Heparin effect is measured by estimating the clotting time of whole blood. The oral anticoagulant drugs are assessed by the prothrombin time of Quick and by the thrombotest on capillary blood. The coagulating mechanism should be depressed so that it is 2–2½ times control value by the Quick test or 10–20 per cent with the thrombotest.

THERAPEUTIC USES.—For an immediate effect, intravenous heparin 10,000–15,000 units repeated 6- or 8-hourly for 48 hours. For the prevention of pulmonary embolism or venous thrombosis oral drugs are usually adequate. Suggested initial doses are: dicoumarol 200–300 mg.; ethyl biscoumacetate (tromexan) 1000–1500 mg.; warfarin sodium (marevan) 25–50 mg.; phenindione (dindevan) 200–400 mg. The effects are assessed in 36 hours.

CONTRA-INDICATIONS.—History of bleeding; pregnancy; liver or kidney failure; malignant hypertension; subacute endocarditis.

ANTIDOTES.—For heparin, protamine sulphate or hexadimethrine bromide (polybrene) 1 mg. for every 100 units given in the last dose of heparin, e.g., 5 ml. of 1 per cent, slowly. For oral anticoagulants, phytomenadione (vitamin K_1) 5–10 mg. repeated as necessary by mouth, intramuscularly, or intravenously. (*See* " Current Practice ", *Brit. med. J.*, 1963, **1**, 801.)

There is evidence that phenindione effectively prevents thrombosis in veins and eliminates the risk of pulmonary embolism in patients under its influence, provided that the drug is given early, for sufficient time, and under laboratory control. With a plasma prothrombin time between two and three times normal, hæmorrhage at operation is not a problem (e.g., in the surgery of fracture of the neck of femur).*

---

* Sevitt, S., and Gallagher, N. G., *Lancet*, 1959, **2**, 981.

Treatment of the Post-operative Chest.—

1. BRONCHITIS.—Sulphonamides, expectorants, or sedatives as may be required. Inhalations of steam with menthol or tinct. benzoini co. are soothing in cases of tracheitis. Penicillin.

2. ATELECTASIS.—The hourly " shake-up treatment " :—

   a. Turn patient in the bed.

   b. See that he takes at least a dozen really deep breaths.

   c. See that he coughs effectively, if possible bringing up sputum.

If the chest is forcibly knocked with the fist over the site of the collapse, a plug of mucus may be dislodged from a bronchus during coughing. Postural drainage, to prevent the patient coughing uphill, may also be employed. It involves putting the patient in such a position that an area of collapse is above the bronchus supplying it. Diaphragmatic excursion is not improved by moving patient from supine position to sitting position. Fowler's position does not make coughing any easier and may cause cerebral ischæmia and hypotension. Inhalation of alevaire is useful in treatment as well as in prevention.

Good results have followed the intravenous injection of 5 ml. of nikethamide (preceded if necessary by 0·1 to 0·2 g. of intravenous thiopentone). The explosive cough produced may clear the air-passages. Intravenous injection of 2 ml. of paraldehyde has a similar effect.

A few ml. of penicillin solution can be injected into the trachea from the front of the neck, through a fine needle. The irritation of the carina so produced may result in a useful cough. This irritation can be repeated as often as necessary if an extradural nylon catheter is introduced into the trachea from a Tuohy needle inserted into the cricothyroid ligament : through the catheter, saline or other liquid can be dropped on to the carina.*

Carbon dioxide and oxygen inhalations can be given, and when hyperpnœa is maximal, strong ether vapour can be added to produce coughing.

Intravenous procaine drips (0·1 per cent) have been advocated both to relieve pain and to dilate the bronchial tree. The analgesia unaccompanied by respiratory depression which they produce enables coughing and deep breathing to take place and lessens the need for sedatives of a depressant type.

The application of cocaine solution to the pyriform fossæ, to paralyse the internal laryngeal nerves and aid bronchial dilatation, has been recommended.

Should these treatments not be successful, a Magill's tube should be inserted into the trachea, blindly if possible after topical analgesia of the larynx, and a suction catheter introduced into the lower air-passages. The coughing so produced is usually beneficial. In grave cases, bronchoscopic suction should be carried out, on one or more occasions using topical analgesia or internal laryngeal nerve-block, and intravenous atropine. Tracheostomy may sometimes be necessary, with frequent bronchial suction, and in gross cases I.P.P.V. may be required.

---

* Keown, K. K., *Curr. Res. Anesth.*, 1960, **39**, 570 ; and Buchwald, H., *Surgery*, 1962, **51**, 760.

Treatment of the Post-operative Chest, *continued.*

If the secretions seem to be imprisoned by bronchospasm, the slow intravenous injection of 0·25 g. of aminophylline is helpful in relieving the bronchospasm.

The great danger of atelectasis is that it may be followed by bronchopneumonia and this is likely if re-expansion does not take place. Pneumonia can be treated by penicillin, 2 million units daily by injection together with either full doses of a suitable sulphonamide or with 0·5 g. of tetracycline daily by mouth, for a week, or until radiograph appearances return to normal. Unsuccessful treatment may result in bronchiectasis.

POST-OPERATIVE RESPIRATORY INSUFFICIENCY.—This may be due to: (1) Inadequate ventilation from mechanical causes following abdominal or thoracic surgery; (2) Central respiratory depression due to: (*a*) drugs; (*b*) hypocapnia; (3) Suxamethonium, when this has been used with a low pseudocholinesterase level; (4) Non-depolarizing relaxants when these have been used, due to: (*a*) too little neostigmine; (*b*) myasthenia; (*c*) hyperthermia (the warm bed potentiating the relaxant);* (5) Carbon dioxide narcosis.

Hypoxæmia after General Anæsthesia.—Measurement of oxygen tension is a more sensitive index of hypoxæmia than measurement of arterial oxygen saturation, due to the shape of the oxygen hæmoglobin dissociation curve (*see* p. 57). The Po_2 may fall as low as 40 mm. Hg without evidence of cyanosis. There is an inverse correlation between age and Po_2 before surgery in patients awaiting operation† and also in the post-operative period.‡ Some recent investigations have shown that the arterial oxygen tension falls at the end of even minor operations.§ It remains low for up to 24 hours although the Pco_2 becomes normal at the end of 1 hour. The cause of this hypoxæmia is probably a shunt resulting from spontaneous alveolar collapse, perhaps due to progressive inactivation of pulmonary surfactant through failure to take periodic deep breaths post-operatively. Disturbance of the ventilation/perfusion relationships within the lungs; a form of regional relative underventilation is probably a less important cause. Underventilation and reduction of diffusion are unlikely to account for the condition and radiological evidence of atelectasis is not seen. In the light of these findings it is advised that oxygen should be given after operation to all ill patients, to those with hypoventilation from any cause, and to those having a metabolic acidosis or a fixed low cardiac output. Periodic deep breathing is of the greatest importance. Other work fails to agree with this concept of hypoxæmia.‖

The effect of atropine on hypoxæmia after operation is greater if it is given subcutaneously than if injected intravenously. It is

* Bigland, B., and others, *J. Physiol.*, 1958, **141**, 475.
† Conway, C. M., Payne, J. P., and Tomlin, P. J., *Brit. J. Anæsth.*, 1965, **37**, 405.
‡ Nunn, J. F., *Lancet*, 1965, **2**, 466.
§ Nunn, J. F., and Payne, J. P., *Ibid.*, 1962, **2**, 631.
‖ Stephen, C. R., and Talton, I., *J. Amer. med. Ass.*, 1965, **191**, 743.

said to increase the dead space, both physiological and anatomical. There is a local pulmonary alveolar vascular reflex which regulates perfusion in response to ventilation: atropine blocks this and leads to the removal of blood from the lungs into the systemic circulation. This may well be of more theoretical than practical importance.[*]

For the administration of an oxygen-enriched mixture, Conway and Payne[†] have shown that the disposable Oxygenaire mask supplied with oxygen at a flow-rate of 2 l. per min. relieves desaturation and does not cause significant hypercapnia; 30–40 per cent oxygen is beneficial.

Delayed Post-anoxic Encephalopathy.[‡]—The neuropathological changes following death due to acute anoxia are degeneration of nerve-cells in the deeper layers of the cerebral cortex, in the Ammon's horn area of the hippocampus, and in the globus pallidus. A form of encephalopathy which may often be fatal has been described which may follow some days or weeks after apparent clinical recovery from the anoxic episode due to either cardiac standstill or carbon monoxide poisoning.[§] It is recommended that all patients who have recovered from severe anoxia should be treated by complete bed-rest for at least 10 days, where they can be kept under close observation.

GASTRO-INTESTINAL COMPLICATIONS

Nausea and Vomiting.—May be influenced by one or more of the following factors :—

1. ANÆSTHETIC AGENT AND TECHNIQUE.—Most likely to be produced by chloroform, ether, cyclopropane, trichloro-ethylene, pethidine, and halothane in this order. Thiopentone, regional analgesia, and myoneural blocking agents are not so frequently followed by vomiting. Nitrous oxide and oxygen resulted in vomiting in 14·7 per cent of 3000 consecutive patients in an out-patient department. Children were more prone to vomit than adults, while some types of operation carried a higher vomiting rate than others.[||] Intradural and extradural block usually cause less vomiting than inhalation of a volatile anæsthetic. Hypoxia predisposes to vomiting. Duration of operation and depth of anæsthesia are unfavourable factors.

2. TYPE OF PATIENT.—Some patients are ready vomiters, e.g., in travelling ; after simple dietary indiscretions ; sufferers from 'bilious' attacks. Suggestion, and the example of surrounding patients, are important factors. Suitable pre-operative reassurance and 'sales talk' are important.

3. CONDITION OF STOMACH.—Vomiting is likely unless the stomach is empty. Reflex pylorospasm due to anxiety may delay gastric emptying. Swallowing of ether-impregnated

[*] Tomlin, P. J., Conway, C. M., and Payne, J. P., *Lancet*, 1964, **1**, 14.
[†] Conway, C. M., and Payne, J. P., *Brit. med. J.*, 1963, **1**, 844.
[‡] Annotation, *Lancet*, 1962, **2**, 546.
[§] Plum, F., and others, *Arch. intern. Med.*, 1962, **110**, 18.
[||] Bodman, R. I., Morton, H. J. V., and Thomas, E. T., *Brit. med. J.*, 1960, **1**, 1327.

Nausea and Vomiting, *continued.*

mucus or blood is a cause which can be lessened by suction from the mouth and pharynx after operation. Sipping of water, soon after recovery of consciousness, may cause vomiting. Post-operative thirst should be treated by mouth-washes and rectal tap water.

4. OPIATES AND PETHIDINE.—Given before and after operation, make some 30 per cent of patients vomit. Heroin is said to cause less vomiting, although more respiratory depression, than morphine. Papaveretum is not superior to morphine in preventing nausea and vomiting. A barbiturate or phenothiazine derivative before operation may be substituted.*

5. TYPE OF OPERATION.—Vomiting is most frequent after laparotomy and especially after operation on the biliary tract. Dilatation of the cervix uteri often produces vomiting after operation. Length of operation predisposes to vomiting.†

6. SEX.—More frequent in women than in men, and in the young than in the old.

TREATMENT.—This consists largely in preventing the causal factors, whenever possible.

a. Cyclizine hydrochloride (marzine) 50 mg. by deep subcutaneous injection, half an hour before and several times after operation, is said to be free from unpleasant side-effects and to reduce vomiting.‡ It can be given by suppository.§ Its solution is pharmaceutically incompatible with the tetracyclines and penicillin. It is an anticholinergic and antihistaminic. It has been added to morphine in an effort to prevent nausea and vomiting—15 mg. to morphine 10 and 15 mg.—cyclimorph.

b. Promethazine 50 mg. intramuscularly during operation, and 25 mg. post-operatively for four doses, four-hourly, is said to reduce vomiting after operation most definitely.‖

c. Chlorpromazine will also reduce the incidence of vomiting and can be given before and after operation by mouth (25 mg. the night before operation, repeated before and immediately after operation) ; by injection ; and per rectum as a 300-mg. suppository.¶

d. Sod. phenobarbitone 150 mg. hypodermically may also be useful.

e. Pyridoxine, 100 mg. before, and once after, operation, is said to lessen the incidence of vomiting.

f. The antihistamine drug dimenhydrinate (dramamine) given 50 mg. before operation, 50 mg. immediately afterwards, and then four-hourly for four doses, is said to reduce the rate of vomiting after operation by 50 per cent.

---

* Riding, J. L., *Proc. R. Soc. Med.*, 1960, **53**, 671 ; and Bellville, J. W., *Anesthesiology*, 1961, **22**, 773.
† Smith, J. M., *Brit. med. J.*, 1945, **2**, 217.
‡ Marcus, P. S., and Sheehan, J. C., *Anesthesiology*, 1955, **16**, 423 ; and Moore, D. C., and others, *Ibid.*, 1956, **17**, 690.
§ Bonica, J. J., *Ibid.*, 1958, **19**, 582.
‖ Gordon, R. A., and others, *Canad. Anæsth. Soc. J.*, 1955, **1**, 95.
¶ Boulton, T. B., *Anæsthesia*, 1955, **10**, 233.

    g. Perphenazine* (trilafon ; fentazin) 5 mg. given intramuscularly at the end of the operation reduces vomiting significantly. It is occasionally followed by acute dystonic reactions.†

    h. Prochlorperazine (stemetil) 12·5 mg. intramuscularly.‡

    i. Thiethylperazine dihydrogen maleate (torecan) is said to have a sedative action on both the chemoreceptor trigger zone and on the vomiting centre. Each ml. contains 5 mg., the dose being 0·08 ml. per kg. body-weight intramuscularly on return from the operating room. Effects are said to last six hours and hypotension, narcosis, and extrapyramidal signs are seldom seen.

    j. The non-phenothiazine trimethoxybenzamide (tigan) in 400 mg. doses.§

    k. Droperidol 5–10 mg. It has a specific effect on the chemoreceptor trigger zone.

Glucose given for a day or two before operation may be helpful, especially in children. A glucose (10 per cent) enema can be given immediately after the operation and can be combined with 10 units of insulin. A little solid carbohydrate food, given soon after recovery of consciousness, is sometimes helpful.

Vomiting persisting for more than twenty-four hours may be helped by :—

    a. The rapid swallowing of a pint of warm water containing a teaspoonful of sodium bicarbonate. This will probably be returned and will wash out the stomach, with benefit.

    b. The intramuscular injection of dilute solution of chlorpromazine (12·5–25 mg.).

    c. The insertion of a Ryle's stomach tube through the nose, with frequent gastric lavage and aspiration.

    (*See* Discussion on Post-operative Vomiting, *Proc. R. Soc. Med.*, 1960, **53**, 671.)

INTESTINAL DISTENSION.—Frequently follows laparotomy when it can be a very troublesome complication ; due to handling of intestine, traction on mesentery, and stimulation of autonomic ganglia. Other causes are air swallowing and partial inflation of the stomach from assisted or controlled respiration. *Treatment*: (1) Heat to abdomen. (2) Use of a rectal tube. (3) Pitressin, 10 units hypodermically ; it relaxes the small bowel while stimulating the colon (morphine has the opposite effect). (4) Neostigmine (0·5 mg.) stimulates the small gut and inhibits the colon. (5) Hypertonic sodium chloride, 20 ml. of 10 per cent solution, intravenously. (6) Enemata. (7) Pantothenic acid, part of the vitamin B complex, given as the calcium salt, 50 mg. in 1 ml., injected intramuscularly. This dose can be repeated.

Hiccup.—Persistent hiccup may follow anæsthesia, either general or regional. It is a state of intermittent spasm of the diaphragm,

---

* Scurr, C. F., and Robbie, D. S., *Brit. med. J.*, 1958, **1**, 922 ; and Moore, D. C., and others, *Anesthesiology*, 1958, **19**, 72.
† Montgomery, R. D., and Sutherland, V. L., *Brit. med. J.*, 1959, **1**, 215.
‡ Howat, D. D. C., *Anæsthesia*, 1960, **15**, 289 ; and Robbie, D. S., *Ibid.*, 1959, **14**, 349.
§ Simonsen, L. E., and Vandewater, S. L., *Canad. Anæsth. Soc. J.*, 1962, **9**, 51.

Hiccup, *continued.*

accompanied by sudden closure of the glottis. The central part of the diaphragm is supplied by the phrenic nerves, the peripheral parts by the lower six or seven intercostal nerves. The phrenic nerves contain motor, sensory, and sympathetic fibres ; the intercostals, mostly sensory fibres.

CAUSES.—Stimulation of sensory nerve-endings of phrenic, which are connected with the cœliac and other intra-abdominal autonomic plexuses. The vagus may also act as part of the afferent arc of the reflex. Thus, through these pathways, hiccup may arise from impulses in any abdominal or thoracic viscus.

Central stimulation of the medulla may be causal in, e.g., alcoholic intoxication, uræmia, encephalitis.

TREATMENT.—

1. Periodic inhalation of carbon dioxide to produce hyperpnœa. This may be carried out for as long as it is beneficial.
2. Intravenous injection of 4–8 mg. of methylamphetamine.*
3. Inhalation of amyl nitrite.
4. Deflation of the gut by neostigmine, pitressin, etc.
5. Sedatives.
6. Intravenous fluid.
7. Injection of atropine.
8. Benzyl benzoate 2 ml. of 20 per cent solution by mouth, two-hourly.
9. Quinidine, 9 gr. by mouth or intramuscularly, repeated two or three times at hourly intervals.
10. Muscle relaxants.
11. Hexamethonium salts.
12. Block of phrenic nerves—either unilateral or bilateral. 20 ml. of 1 per cent procaine or 1–1000 cinchocaine or amethocaine, with adrenaline, is used. Injection is made at a depth of $\frac{1}{4}-\frac{1}{2}$ in. along a line extending 2 in. laterally from a point $\frac{1}{2}$ in. above the sternoclavicular joint.
13. Division of phrenic nerves—either unilateral or bilateral.

Radiology may determine which side of the diaphragm is at fault, before division of the phrenic nerve, in extreme cases. Unfortunately, even bilateral division of the phrenic nerves may fail to cure hiccup, because of the associated spasm of the intercostal and accessory respiratory muscles.

Liver Failure.—

1. There is delayed recovery from the anæsthetic, merging into semicoma and death within forty-eight hours, preceded by hyperpyrexia. Post-mortem findings—necrosis of liver cells.
2. After four or five days' normal post-operative progress, patient becomes drowsy and comatose and dies, death being preceded by oliguria. Post-mortem—liver necrosis and kidney tubule necrosis.

Treatment is by intravenous amino-acids and glucose.

Halothane has now been shown to differ little from other anæsthetic agents in the occurrence of jaundice after its use. It is possible,

---

* Burke, C. B., *Brit. med. J.*, 1963, **1**, 944.

however, that very rarely a hypersensitivity type of reaction may occur with repeated administration. *See also* p. 198. Fever of unknown origin developing within a few days of the operation is a warning sign and may be followed by jaundice or even by liver failure. Jaundice occurring after halothane administration must be differentiated from jaundice due to blood transfusion, shock, septic cholangitis, and coincidental virus hepatitis. Only with the last of these does it share the same histology (by liver needle biopsy).*

MECHANISMS OF INJURY.—

1. TOXIC HEPATITIS.—A direct toxic effect. Few drugs satisfy the rigid criteria:† (*a*) Liver injury should occur in all patients if administered in sufficient dosage; (*b*) Severity of lesion should be directly related to dose; (*c*) Identical lesions should be obtained in experimental animals; (*d*) The histological pattern should be characteristic and distinctive; (*e*) The latent period between exposure and injury should be constant and brief (e.g., carbon tetrachloride).

2. SENSITIVITY REACTIONS.—Most drugs that produce hepatic damage behave as sensitizing agents rather than as true hepatotoxins. The characteristics of these reactions are: (*a*) The lesion occurs in only a small proportion of individuals exposed; (*b*) The occurrence and extent of the lesion are not dose related; (*c*) Morphological changes are variable and less distinctive than in toxic hepatitis; (*d*) The latent period is highly variable; (*e*) Other manifestations of hypersensitivity such as fever, skin rashes, arthralgia, and eosinophilia may accompany the hepatic lesion.

3. CHOLESTATIC HEPATITIS.—Clinical and laboratory findings mimic those found in extrahepatic biliary obstruction, and there is stasis of bile within the canaliculi. Parenchymal damage is less than in (2) above. There may be an underlying hypersensitivity reaction.

EFFECT OF ANÆSTHETIC AGENTS.—

1. CHLOROFORM.—The most dangerous of anæsthetic drugs. Considered by many to be a true hepatotoxin. Others believe that the dangers have been magnified and that many older studies are invalid because of inadequate control of conditions surrounding the administration.‡ However, instances of fatal delayed chloroform poisoning have been reported in recent years.§

2. ETHER.—Changes in liver function and histology have been reported. Bile secretion is said to be stimulated in light anæsthesia, but depressed in deep planes. Liver glycogen is mobilized and there is a rise in blood-sugar.

3. DIVINYL ETHER.—Central zonal necrosis can be produced routinely in dogs, after relatively short exposures. Liver necrosis has been reported in man.

---

* Sheila Sherlock, *Proc. R. Soc. Med.*, 1964, **57**, 305.
† Klatskin, G., *Gastroenterology*, 1960, **38**, 789.
‡ Davidson, M. H. A., *Anæsthesia*, 1959, **14**, 127; and Poe, M. F., and Mayfield, J. R., *Anesthesiology*, 1960, **21**, 508.
§ Marx, G. F., Kikkawa, Y., and Orkin, L. R., *Curr. Res. Anesth.*, 1962, **41**, 575.

Liver Failure, *continued.*

4. TRICHLOROETHYLENE.—Although cases of massive hepatic necrosis have occurred following trichloroethylene anæsthesia, a cause-and-effect relationship has not been established. Studies of liver function in man have shown only slight and transient dysfunction.

5. CYCLOPROPANE.—Abnormal liver-function tests do not occur more frequently than with other potent anæsthetic agents.

6. NITROUS OXIDE.—No evidence of toxic effects.

7. HALOTHANE.—Extensive investigations have failed to show that halothane causes liver damage. *See* p. 198.

8. METHOXYFLURANE.—Transient changes in liver-function tests have been reported, as with other anæsthetic agents.

9. THIOPENTONE.—Little evidence that the drug itself produces liver damage.

10. LOCAL ANALGESICS.—These have little toxic effect. Liver damage has been reported following spinal analgesia, but this may be due to hypotension.

Cases of massive hepatic necrosis have been reported after anæsthesia with all of the commonly used anæsthetic agents. Transient changes in liver-function tests are commonly reported. Only in the case of chloroform and divinyl ether does there seem to be definite evidence of hepatotoxicity. In other cases it seems likely that other factors associated with the period of anæsthesia and surgery are more important than the drug itself in the production of post-operative liver damage.

OTHER FACTORS.—

1. Hypoxia.* The oxygen consumption of the liver is normally one-third that of the entire body, or 40 ml. per minute per sq. metre body surface.

2. Hypercapnia† is a factor in producing liver damage.

3. Hypotension. The normal value for hepatic blood-flow in man is 1·5–1·8 l. per minute, of which 20–40 per cent is from the hepatic artery, the remainder from the portal vein. The portal vein is loaded with absorbed materials, has an oxygen saturation of 60–75 per cent, and a pressure of 8–10 mm. Hg.

4. Nutritional status.

5. Blood transfusion. *See* p. 689.

6. Non-anæsthetic drugs.

7. Viral hepatitis. It is estimated that about 100 patients per million may develop coincidental viral hepatitis in the weeks following anæsthesia.

8. Other infectious processes.

9. The nature and site of surgical trauma.

10. Repeated exposure producing hypersensitivity.

[*See also* Little, D. M., and Wetstone, H. J., *Anesthesiology*, 1964, **25**, 815; and Johnstone, M., *Brit. J. Anæsth.*, 1964, **36**, 718.]

* Marx, G. F., Kippawa, Y., and Orpin, L. R., *Curr. Res. Anæsth.*, 1962, **41**, 575.
† Sims, J. L., Morris, L. E., Orth, O. S., and Waters, R. M., *J. Lab. Clin. Med.*, 1951, **38**, 388.

MISCELLANEOUS COMPLICATIONS

Air Embolism.*—
  CAUSES.—
    1. SURGICAL.—
        a. Operations involving injury to veins in the neck, thorax, breast, and pelvis : operations on the brain and cord in the sitting position.
        b. Operations on the heart.
        c. Uterine curettage and insufflation, including criminal abortion and vaginal insufflation of powder.
    2. DIAGNOSTIC AND THERAPEUTIC INJECTION OF AIR INTO—
        a. Peritoneum.
        b. Pleural cavity.
        c. Large joints.
        d. Urinary bladder.
        e. Tissue spaces, e.g., the perinephric area.
        f. Nasal antra.
        Carbon dioxide is safer than air for diagnostic tests as it dissolves in the blood more readily.
    3. SURGICAL EMPHYSEMA.
    4. ACCIDENTAL ENTRANCE OF AIR.—
        a. During intravenous infusions.
        b. During intra-arterial transfusion under positive pressure.
        The air may enter either an artery or a vein, but it can reach the left side of the heart from entry via a vein, by passage through arteriovenous communications in the lungs.
        Factors of Importance.—(1) The volume of air. (2) The speed of injection. (3) The pressure in the veins. (4) Posture. (5) General condition of patient.
            For air to enter a vein there must be a subatmospheric pressure in the vein or positive pressure from outside it.
  SIGNS AND SYMPTOMS.—If air enters the veins in any quantity it will cause a hissing sound in the wound and it will go to the right heart and lung, causing an air-lock obstruction in the pulmonary artery. This may result in a loud precordial murmur, the so-called ' mill-wheel murmur '. There will also be sudden cyanosis, hypotension, engorged neck veins, tachycardia, irregular gasping respiration, progressing through tachypnœa and hypopnœa and followed by cardiac arrest. Early diagnosis can be made if an œsophageal stethoscope is in place.
  TREATMENT.—(1) Prevent further entrance of air into the circulation. (2) Lower the head end of the table to keep air out of the cerebral vessels. (3) Place patient on his left side so that bubbles are carried away from the mouth of the pulmonary artery. (4) Give pure oxygen. (5) Infuse large volumes of intravenous fluid to wash out froth. (6) Papaverine (30–60 mg.) to dilate pulmonary vessels. (7) Vasopressors. (8) If rapid improvement is not noticed, the right thorax should be opened, air aspirated from the heart, and manual cardiac compression carried out : this will clear air out of the heart and

---

* Emery, E. R. J., *Anæsthesia*, 1962, **17**, 455.

Air Embolism, *continued.*

great vessels. If air has been injected into an artery causing convulsions and rapid collapse, or if it has passed through a congenital defect into the left heart, manual systole will milk it away from the orifices of the coronary vessels. Defibrillation may be necessary, as also may the aspiration of froth from the ventricles, via a large-bore needle.

Post-mortem radiographs of cases dying suddenly on the operating table might reveal this as a cause of death, not infrequently.

In neurological operations in the sitting position it has been suggested that pressure on the internal jugular vein should be applied at 5-minute intervals so that bleeding will occur at the point of entry of air, and this can be dealt with by the surgeon.*

Encephalopathy.—A. R. Hunter† has described a type of encephalopathy following general anæsthesia, characterized by light coma, without definite localizing symptoms in the central nervous system, some hours after apparent recovery from general anæsthesia. All the cases ended fatally, and at post-mortem there is found cerebral congestion, subarachnoid hæmorrhage, and areas of cerebral softening. It is not due to fat embolism, cerebral thrombosis, or hypoxia, and is not associated exclusively with any particular anæsthetic or operation, although several of the cases followed gas–oxygen and trichloroethylene anæsthesia for radical mastectomy.

Seldon and his colleagues have reported similar cases from the Mayo Clinic,‡ one of them a radical mastectomy. They suggest that the cause is cerebral œdema and advise the intravenous injection of 100-ml. doses of 25 per cent human serum albumin. Their cases completely recovered.

Generalized Muscular Hypertonicity.—This may follow the use of suxamethonium and may result in grave hyperpyrexia.§ It may be due to the injection of contaminated solutions, e.g., by *Alcaligenes fæcalis.* May be preceded by muscular rigidity associated with either suxamethonium or halothane or methoxyflurane. Disturbance of oxidative phosphorylation may be a cause.‖ May be familial or due to inborn error of metabolism. Abnormal rigidity should be a warning of possible trouble to follow and hypothermia, with correction of any metabolic acidosis, should be considered. (*See* Saidman, L. J., and others, *J. Amer. med. Ass.*, 1964, **190**, 1029; Bieler, J. A., and others, *Ibid.*, 1951, **146**, 551; and Thut, W. H., and Davenport, H. T., *Canad. Anæsth. Soc. J.*, 1966, **13**, 425.)

Hyperpyrexia.—This may be seen after anæsthesia, and may progress to convulsions and death.¶

Post-operative Paralysis of Upper Extremity.—First reported by Büdinger in 1894. The most dangerous position is the Trendelenburg tilt, with arm abducted to a right angle, fully supinated, and

---

* Hunter, A. R., *Anæsthesia*, 1962, **17**, 467.
† Hunter, A. R., *Lancet*, 1949, **1**, 1045.
‡ Seldon, T. H., and others, *Proc. Mayo Clin.*, 1949, **24**, 14.
§ Relton, J. E. S., and others, *Canad. Anæsth. Soc. J.*, 1967, **14**, 22.
‖ Wilson, R. D., and others, *Anesthesiology*, 1966, **27**, 231.
¶ Brown, R. L., *Brit. med. J.*, 1954, **1**, 1526.

externally rotated. The condition, formerly thought to be due to pressure on nerves, e.g., by shoulder braces, is now thought to be secondary to stretching of nerves over the head of the humerus which the abducted position makes prominent. Additional factors are tying the arm or arms to an armboard behind the coronal plane of the body, and full rotation of the head and neck towards the opposite side. Cases have occurred following the use of the gall-bladder bridge. The upper part of the brachial plexus is more commonly involved than the lower part : effects usually on motor nerves, not sensory. To avoid stretching the plexus, the following measures should be taken : (1) Shoulder braces must be padded and must make contact with acromion as far laterally as possible, but they are better done away with, the patient being supported on a non-slip mattress (Langton Hewer*) ; (2) Armboard must be built up with pads to prevent backward displacement of arm ; (3) Hyperextension and external rotation of elbow must be avoided ; (4) Intravenous injections should be given with the arm at the patient's side, using an apparatus such as that described by Lee,† or folded across the chest.‡ Prognosis is good, but recovery may take months. The deltoid, biceps, and brachialis are the muscles usually affected.

Post-operative Paralysis of Lower Extremity.—Femoral nerve injury from pressure due to abdominal retractors can easily be ascribed to intra- or extradural block. In 3 cases reported, 2 had intradural block and sustained unilateral palsy while 1 patient received general anæsthesia and sustained bilateral palsy.§

Neurological Complications following General Anæsthesia.— Neurological complications can follow general as well as spinal analgesia. A case of diplopia following thiopentone, curare, and cyclopropane ;‖ a case of ascending spinal paralysis under gas-oxygen, ether, and gallamine,¶ peroneal nerve palsy, and meningitis** have all been reported. (*See also* Britt, B. A., and Gordon, R. A., *Canad. Anæsth. Soc. J.*, 1964, **11**, 514.)

Ophthalmological Complications.—
1. CORNEAL ABRASION.—This should be prevented by tulle gras or a drop of oil into the conjunctival sac before anæsthesia. It can be diagnosed if a drop of 0·5 per cent amethocaine is put into the eye, followed by fluorescine, when the abraded cornea will take up the stain. Treatment consists of a firm pad and bandage.
2. ACUTE GLAUCOMA in susceptible patients who will complain of pain in and around the eye of a different nature to that due to foreign bodies or abrasions. On examination the eye is red, the cornea cloudy, and the pupil dilated. There may be nausea and

* Hewer, C. L., *Anæsthesia*, 1953, **8**, 198.
† Lee, J. A., *Ibid.*, 1952, **7**, 256.
‡ Macintosh, R. R., *Brit. med. J.*, 1955, **2**, 1054.
§ Ruston, F. G., and Politi, V. L., *Canad. Anæsth. Soc. J.*, 1958, **5**, 428.
‖ Norman, J. E., *Anæsthesia*, 1955, **10**, 88.
¶ Sinclair, R. N., *Ibid.*, 1954, **9**, 286.
** Lett, Z., *Brit. J. Anæsth.*, 1964, **36**, 266.

Ophthalmological Complications, *continued.*

vomiting. Treatment in emergency: Acetazolamide, 500 mg. intravenously; eserine or pilocarpine drop, 1 per cent, into the conjunctival sac.

3. VITREOUS HÆMORRHAGE.—This has followed hypotensive techniques.*

4. RETINAL INFARCTION from pressure of an anæsthetic mask on the eyeball.

5. RETINAL EMBOLI.

Local Complications of Intravenous Therapy.†—When infusions are taken down within 12 hours, thrombophlebitis is rare, but the incidence rises steeply thereafter. The internal saphenous vein should be used only if no other vein exists. Dextrose in any concentration is more likely to cause thrombophlebitis than other solutions, but the addition of 1 mg. of hydrocortisone to each 100 ml. of solution is helpful. Caval catheters can be dangerous, especially if there is sepsis in the body.

Post-operative Pressure Alopecia.‡—A sudden loss of hair over a circumscribed area on the posterior scalp following a period of unconsciousness, e.g., a prolonged operation. The hair loss is temporary and growth occurs within 120 days. Prevention: Quicker surgery!

Rubber Dermatitis.§—This is usually due to the accelerator mercapto-benzo-thiazole (M.B.T.) used to speed up vulcanization.

Perforation of Ear Drums.‖—This is due, in the absence of an endotracheal tube, to intermittent positive-pressure ventilation compressing the air in the mouth and pharynx, so that with widely dilated Eustachian tubes and a thin and atrophic tympanic membrane, perforation may occur. Cleanliness and, if necessary, antibiotics form the correct treatment.

Failure to pass Urine.—There is a normal oliguria for the first 24 hours after operation. Due to:—

1. PRERENAL.—Fall in blood-pressure.

2. RENAL.—Damage to renal tubules by: (*a*) Anoxia. (*b*) Toxins—(i) Bacterial, (ii) Products of tissue autolysis. Clinically, acute glomerulonephritis, bilateral cortical nephrosis, and acute tubular necrosis are described. The last may be an acute toxic nephrosis due to chemicals such as mercury or may be a lower nephron nephrosis due to hæmolysis, sulphonamide sensitivity, or shock. (*c*) Mismatched blood. (*d*) Reflex anuria. (*e*) Hypoxia. (*f*) Hypotension. (*g*) Low fluid intake.

3. POSTRENAL.—Ureteral obstruction, bladder-neck obstruction, etc., neurological conditions, following the injection of ephedrine.

If there is oliguria or anuria, fluid should not be pushed and a continuous intragastric drip set up consisting of glucose 400 g.,

* White, D. C., *Anæsthesia*, 1964, **19**, 573.
† McNair, T. J., and Dudley, H. A. F., *Lancet*, 1959, **2**, 365.
‡ Abel, R. R., *Anesthesiology*, 1964, **25**, 869.
§ Gilston, A., *Brit. J. Anæsth.*, 1961, **33**, 274.
‖ Whittingham, J. K. R., *Brit. med. J.*, 1954, **2**, 970.

peanut oil 100 g., and water 1 litre, emulsified with acacia. This gives limited fluid and calories, but neither protein nor salts. Spontaneous cure may come about during the second week of such treatment. *See* p. 813.

Blockage of the sympathetic nerves supplying the kidney may be useful and may be accomplished by one of the following routes : (1) Sacral extradural ; (2) Lumbar extradural ; (3) Subarachnoid ; (4) Paravertebral. The block must ascend to the eighth thoracic nerve-root.

Difficulty in Micturition.—Occurs more frequently after spinal than after other methods of anæsthesia. Occurs in about 10 per cent of cases following general anæsthesia. It is influenced by:—

1. TYPE OF PATIENT.—Most common in anxious, apprehensive type. Patients with an enlarged prostate, although managing well before operation, may develop retention after operation.

2. TYPE OF OPERATION.—Most common after abdominal and pelvic operations, including hæmorrhoidectomy. A rectal tube predisposes to difficulty with micturition.

3. ATTITUDE OF SISTERS AND NURSES.—Incidence of condition differs from hospital to hospital. In some wards it is expected and so is frequently encountered.

4. DEEP SEDATION.—By removing desire for micturition, deep sedation may allow the bladder walls to become stretched, with subsequent difficulty in voiding.

TREATMENT.—

1. Encouragement and suggestion.

2. Sit patient up in bed, if possible with legs over side of bed. Hot bath.

3. Drugs : potassium acetate, 4 g. two-hourly for three doses ; potassium acetate is both a diuretic and a parasympathetic stimulant. Carbachol, pituitrin, neostigmine, etc.

4. Catheterization should not be left too long, otherwise stretching of bladder wall will occur, making natural voiding more difficult.

Minor Sequelæ.—

Reasonable care and common sense will prevent most of them :— Cutting of lips ; bruising of face and tongue ; excoriation of pharynx and larynx ; chipping or knocking out of teeth ; damage to eyes ; strain of muscles of back and limbs.

Cardiovascular Accidents.—May occur during or soon after anæsthesia, while mental changes may be noticed afterwards, especially in elderly patients. Abnormalities which are present before operation should be written in the clinical notes, so that operation and anæsthesia are not blamed for them.

Awareness during Surgery.—Some patients, anæsthetized with nitrous-oxide, oxygen, and muscle relaxants, have reported awareness during anæsthesia.* It is possible if hypnosis is used

---

* Parkhouse, J., *Postgrad. med. J.*, 1960, **36**, 674; and Hutchinson, R., *Brit. J. Anæsth.*, 1961, **33**, 463.

Awareness during Surgery, *continued.*

that memory may be recalled for incidents occurring during operation.*

Acute Adrenocortical Deficiency.—This usually shows itself during the first day or two after operation as acute circulatory collapse with hypotension, tachycardia, pallor, and sometimes pyrexia and unconsciousness. The state of adrenocortical deficiency may arise in those patients who have been treated for some time with cortisone and from whom the drug has been suddenly withheld before operation. The treatment is intravenous hydrocortisone in full doses.† Sometimes noradrenaline is required in addition.

(*See also* good article, " The Pre- and Post-operative Care of Patients receiving Cortisone or Other Steroid Therapy ", by de Mowbray, R. R., *Postgrad. med. J.*, 1957, **33**, 632.)

Surgical Convalescence.—This can be subdivided into four phases : (1) The period of injury. Associated with catabolism, loss of protein from tissue, mostly muscle, with increase in urinary nitrogen secretion and negative nitrogen balance. There is also fat loss and an accumulation of fluids and electrolytes. (2) The period of convalescence, or the turning point. Protein loss and urinary nitrogen excretion diminished. Peristalsis returns and salt and water diuresis begins. (3) The phase of anabolism. Protein is built up by skeletal muscle and a high protein diet becomes important. Vitamins C and the B complex are also required. (4) The phase of weight gain with increase in both protein and fat which were depleted in the immediate post-operative phase.

The Body's Response to Injury.—During the first few days after injury or operation, the following changes occur, but normally require no treatment : (1) Rise in temperature and pulse. (2) Reduced urinary secretion due to antidiuretic hormone. (3) Loss of nitrogen for the first three to seven days followed by a positive nitrogen balance. (4) Potassium loss for two to five days, then potassium retention. (5) Sodium retention. (6) Water retention. (7) Loss of weight due to oxidation of fat. (8) Reduction in eosinophils, which is delayed by general anæsthesia. (9) Increased excretion of steroid hormones. (10) A temporary period of starvation and relative calorie deficiency. (*See also* Chapter XXVII.) (*See* Moore, F. D., and Ball, M. R., *The Metabolic Response to Surgery*, 1952. Oxford: Blackwell.)

The Neurohumoral Response to Injury.—Pituitary adrenocorticotrophic hormone secretion stimulates the secretion of corticosteroids, aldosterone, adrenaline, noradrenaline, and antidiuretic substance. This results in maintenance of blood-pressure. Aldosterone increases the depleted blood-volume by mobilizing intracellular water and causes an exchange of extracellular hydrogen and sodium for intracellular potassium. The antidiuretic effects of anæsthesia, which sometimes lead to oliguria, differ from those

---

* Cheek, D. B., *Amer. J. clin. Hypnosis*, 1959, **1**, 101; *Ibid.*, 1960, **3**, 101; and Levinson, B. W., *Brit. J. Anæsth.*, 1965, **37**, 544.
† Lundy, J. S. *Anesthesiology*, 1953, **14**, 376.

due to surgical trauma by decreasing both glomerular filtration and renal plasma flow. (Clinical Anæsthesia Conference, *N.Y. St. J. Med.*, 1960, **60**, 890.)

Post-operative Hypotension.*—Causes may be : (1) Cardiovascular. (2) Respiratory. (3) Pharmacological. (4) Neurogenic. (5) Hæmatological. (6) Endocrine. (7) Postural.

It may result in minor or major brain damage, sudden heart failure, renal damage, vascular thrombosis or embolism, and may be specially serious in elderly patients. The facilities of a post-operative observation room should be more widely provided.

Delayed Recovery from Anæsthesia.—This may be due to : (1) *Drugs used during operation* in relative overdosage, e.g., phenothiazine derivatives, pethidine, opiates, thiopentone, volatile agents, especially methoxyflurane. Unconsciousness associated with prolonged apnœa. (2) *Disturbances of physiology resulting from anæsthesia*, e.g., hypercapnia ; a hypoxic episode during anæsthesia ; acid-base disturbances ; fainting, especially in the dental chair ; induced hypotension. (3) *Disturbances resulting from surgery*, e.g., shock, metabolic acidosis, fat embolism, air embolism, operative trauma in brain surgery. (4) *Incidental diseases*, e.g., cerebral embolism, thrombosis or hæmorrhage occurring during operation ; myxœdema ; hypopituitarism ; hypoglycæmia with its picture of the sweaty flushed patient with raised blood-pressure ; hyperglycæmic coma with ketosis, air-hunger, low intra-ocular pressure, hypotension, and glycosuria ; adrenal deficiency ; uræmia ; liver failure. The patient may have been unconscious before operation, or may be moribund. (5) *Drugs given before operation*, e.g., monoamine oxidase inhibitors (with pethidine during operation) ; sedatives.

Unfavourable Effects of Prolonged Anæsthesia.†—May include: (1) Accumulation of anæsthetic agents in depots with slow subsequent elimination; (2) Development of shock; (3) Blood-volume may be diminished; (4) Post-operative respiratory difficulties; (5) Effect on fluid and electrolyte balance; (6) Metabolic disturbances; e.g., reduced B.M.R., hyperglycæmia, use of blood-lactate; (7) Subsequent mental changes; (8) Higher infection rate; (9) Nitrous oxide may enter air-spaces within the body. Effect on bone-marrow after prolonged use.

---

* Barbour, C. M., and Little, D. M., *J. Amer. med. Ass.*, 1957, **165**, 1529; and Smith, L. L., and Moore, F. D., *New Engl. J. Med.*, 1962, **267**, 733.
† Vandam, L. D., *Canad. Anæsth. Soc. J.*, 1965, **12**, 107.

CHAPTER XXXII

EXPLOSION RISKS IN ANÆSTHESIA*

The vapours of certain volatile anæsthetic agents, and some gases, form flammable mixtures with air or oxygen. Nitrous oxide also supports combustion. Mixtures which correspond exactly with the chemical equation, so that combustion is complete, are said to be *stoichiometric*. The most powerful deflagrations occur when the concentration of reactants approach stoichiometric values. There are limits of flammability, when the mixture becomes too weak, or the oxygen content too low.

Detonations or explosions are usually associated with a high oxygen content in the mixture.

Under average conditions, explosive anæsthetic mixtures become diluted with the air of the theatre to a non-flammable range before reaching a distance of 2 ft. from a point of leak of anæsthetic vapours involving the quantities of these vapours used in ordinary surgical procedures.

The following table, published by the U.S. Bureau of Mines, shows the limits of flammability of anæsthetics :—

	In Air Per cent	In Oxygen Per cent	In Nitrous Oxide Per cent	Density (Air = 1)
Ethylene	3·05 to 28·6	2·9 to 79·9	1·9 to 40·7	0·97
Cyclopropane	2·4 to 10·3	2·48 to 60·0	1·6 to 30·3	1·45
Ethyl chloride	4·0 to 14·8	4·05 to 67·2	2·1 to 32·8	2·23
Divinyl ether	1·7 to 27·0	1·85 to 85·5	1·4 to 24·8	2·42
Diethyl ether	1·85 to 36·5	2·1 to 82·0	1·5 to 24·2	2·56

The halothane-ether azeotrope is non-flammable up to 7·25 per cent (by volume) in oxygen.

Fluroxene (fluomar) is non-flammable up to 4 per cent in oxygen.

Before an explosion can occur, a source of heat sufficient to raise a liquid to its flash point, or a vapour to its ignition temperature, is required.

Ether.—Mixtures of nitrous oxide, oxygen, and ether are always explosive and more dangerous than ether and oxygen alone. Pure ether vapour will not explode. The addition of reasonable percentages of carbon dioxide will not prevent explosion. Ether vapour is made more dangerous when mixed with oxygen or nitrous oxide than when mixed with air. Ether in air burns slowly, the flame being unlikely to travel to the patient's air-passages. Explosions only occur in ether–air mixtures in large containers, or with wide long pipes, and with powerful ignition sources. In the relatively narrow, short tubes of anæsthetic systems, detonation in

* See *Report of a Working Party on Anæsthetic Explosions, including Safety Code for Equipment and Installations* (Anæsthetic members : Drs. Marston, Low, Morton, and Galley). London : H.M.S.O. 1956. 2s. 6d. Also *Physics for the Anæsthetist*, 3rd ed., 1963, Macintosh, M. M., Mushin, W. W., and Epstein, H. G. Oxford : Blackwell. Also Hill, D. W., *Physics Applied to Anæsthesia*, 1967, Ch. 8. London: Butterworths.

ether–air mixtures does not occur.* Ether–air mixtures are not easily ignited by a spark. The most easily ignited ether–air mixture requires a spark energy comparable to that of the least ignitable ether–oxygen mixture. Ether vapour is heavier than air and so sinks to the floor. A source of ignition may be safe if it is held above the ether–air mixture (open mask), providing no draughts spread the ether vapour. The presence of peroxides will enable it to ignite at still lower temperatures. Ether peroxides are less volatile than ether and so may accumulate in ether bottles or anæsthetic machines if residual ether is not frequently discarded. Ether will not ignite spontaneously. Hot wires and surfaces— below the temperature of visible, dull-red heat (i.e., 300° C.)— may set going an invisible cool flame in ether vapour. This may travel.

If the administration of ether is discontinued five minutes before a possible source of ignition is exhibited, the patient's exhalations are unlikely to burn or explode provided an open circuit is used after the ether is discontinued.† Further anæsthesia can be maintained with a non-explosive agent. Open ether (without added oxygen) has never been known to cause injury to a patient from ignition or explosion.

Ethyl Chloride.—This burns actively if ignited and will then explode if its vapour is in an oxygen mixture.

Divinyl Ether.—Behaves in a similar manner to diethyl ether.

Cyclopropane.—This is very explosive when mixed with oxygen, and can be ignited by a spark of less energy than that required to explode an ether–oxygen mixture. As cyclopropane is present in the tissues after 20–30 minutes, diathermy should not be used in body cavities when this anæsthetic is being given. Nor must diathermy be applied to the lungs. The possibility of broncho-pleural fistula must be borne in mind. When cyclopropane is used, both the trichloroethylene and the halothane vaporizers should be removed from the apparatus to prevent possible solution of the gas in the liquids, with its possible discharge into the anæsthetic circuit subsequently.

Trichloroethylene.—This is not flammable in air under operating-theatre conditions. A vapour strength of or over 10 per cent in air enriched with oxygen is flammable, but such a strength should never be used when it is considered that a vaporizing bottle of a Boyle machine with the plunger up is unlikely to deliver a concentration greater than 1·5 per cent.

Halothane.—Is non-flammable and non-explosive. The halothane–ether azeotrope is non-flammable up to a concentration of 7·25 per cent in oxygen. While such concentrations may arise in anæsthetic systems during induction, lower concentrations are generally required during maintenance.

---

* Macintosh, R. R., Mushin, W. W., and Epstein, H. G., *Physics for the Anæsthetist, including a Section on Explosions*, 3rd ed., 1963, p. 340. Oxford: Blackwell.
† Vickers, M. D., *Anæsthesia*, 1965, **20**, 315.

Methoxyflurane.—Methoxyflurane is non-flammable and non-explosive at room temperature in either air or oxygen.

Oxygen.—If oxygen under pressure comes into contact with oil or grease, ignition may occur. Thus no oil must be used on valves, etc. The same applies to nitrous oxide and oil or grease.

Sources of Ignition.—

1. HEAT.—From open flames or fires; from hot surfaces or wires; from overheating electric bulbs, e.g., on endoscopes; from thermocautery. Pipes, lighters, cigarettes. The minimal temperature which will ignite an explosive anæsthetic mixture is stated to be 180° C. (355° F.).

2. ELECTRIC CURRENT.—(a) Normal; (b) Faulty.

   a. NORMAL.—Diathermy which comes next in order of importance after static electricity as a cause of explosions; electric cautery; sparks from motors; sparks from X-ray machines; sparks from switches, etc.

   b. FAULTY.—Short-circuits in electrical apparatus; faulty wires and cables; breaking of bulbs.

   All portable electrical apparatus should be fitted with explosion-proof switches and three-wire flex, the third wire being connected to the outer casing of the apparatus and to the third point in a wall plug. The plug should incorporate a locking device making it impossible to remove the plug while the current is switched on.

3. STATIC ELECTRICITY.—The most frequent cause of explosions in operating theatres. To reduce the hazard of such explosions to a minimum meticulous precautions must be taken. Static electricity is produced when two dissimilar surfaces are brought into intimate contact and then separated. It also occurs just before the point of contact of a highly charged non-conductor with a conductor.

   The way to banish the danger from static sparks is to arrange for static charges to be carried away to earth, and the conducting floor should be the common connexion through which all objects in a theatre are intercoupled. A good conducting floor should have an electrical resistance between 25,000 and 500,000 ohms when measured between two electrodes placed 3 ft. apart, at any point on the floor. Floor conductivity having been attained, it becomes necessary for all equipment and personnel to be brought into electrical continuity with it.

   One obvious way of preventing the development of static electricity would be to eliminate non-conductors and, wherever possible, conducting materials should be used.

   The following items are all charge producers and non-conductors: rubber mattresses, plastic sheet material, plastic caps, plastic pillow covers, woollen blankets, cotton sheets, woollen suits, rayon, terylene, and nylon garments and hosiery, cotton overalls and gowns, rubber stool tops, painted stool tops, rubber gloves. The next group comprises commonly used insulators: non-conductive castors on tables and trolleys, non-conductive rubber stool tips, interior non-conducting parts of anæsthetic machines. The following are both charge producers and insulators : non-conductive floors, non-conductive shoes, non-conductive rubber tyres, non-conductive rubber tubes of anæsthetic machines, and anæsthetic masks. Undergarments are not included in the list as they do not add to a person's electrostatic charge when covered with a cotton gown.

To ensure the neutralization of all charges—with consequent avoidance of sparks, the non-conductive material should be bridged by suitable conductors to a conducting floor. One easy way of lessening danger in the absence of conducting rubber is to connect the metal parts of the table, anæsthetic machine, and anæsthetist's stool with the floor, by means of a wet towel, which itself makes contact with the anæsthetist's leather-soled shoes. This forms a makeshift electrical inter-coupler. It is virtually impossible to design conditions in which a dangerous static discharge will never occur.

The Vapotester* is essentially a Wheatstone bridge in which the electric current is balanced. It enables the anæsthetist to measure accurately the concentration of the anæsthetic agent and the explosibility of the mixture.

The Statometer* detects the presence of static electricity, its source and intensity.

SPONTANEOUS IGNITION.—This may occur if oil or grease is allowed to react with nitrous oxide or oxygen under pressure, e.g., when escaping from a cylinder. This absolutely contra-indicates the use of lubricants on reducing valves and gas cylinders.

Explosions can arise from ignition of such gases as hydrogen, methane, and sulphuretted hydrogen arising from the stomach or bowel from fermentation.†

Recommendations for Prevention.‡—

1. Explosive anæsthetics should not be used when the following potentially dangerous pieces of apparatus are employed : diathermy, cautery, X-rays, electric motors, electric and gas heating equipment—unless suitable precautions are taken. It is probably safe to give open ether in an anæsthetic room and then to bring in the anæsthetized patient for examination.

2. Administration of ignitable anæsthetics should be stopped 5 minutes before diathermy or cautery is used. Ether bottles should be removed—not merely turned off—and air should be blown through apparatus. Maintenance of anæsthesia can be by a non-flammable agent.

3. Oxygen and nitrous oxide, although not flammable, increase the danger of other agents.

4. Small electric bulbs should not be overrun : voltage should not be greater than the 2·5 to 6 volts for which they are designed.

---

* *Anesthesiology*, 1949, **10**, 479 ; and *Ibid.*, 1960, **21**, 83.
† Galley, A. H., *Brit. J. Anæsth.*, 1954, **26**, 189; *Proc. R. Soc. Med.*, 1955, **48**, 502; and Carroll, K. J., *Brit. med. J.*, 1964, **2**, 1178.
‡ *See also* article in *Hospitals*, the journal of the American Hospitals Association, 1949, Dec.

Recommendations for Prevention, *continued.*

The use of batteries, instead of electric mains, prevents accidental overrunning.

5. Electric wiring and apparatus should be inspected frequently by an electrician, even though their function is not impaired. All electrical apparatus should have a third wire for positive grounding.

6. Foot switches must be flame-proof, as ether vapour falls towards the floor. Wall plugs should be 5 ft. above the floor if they are not flame-proof. Electric connexions, ideally, should all be flame-proof.

7. In all rooms where explosive anæsthetics may be used, a conducting floor should be provided. This includes X-ray rooms, where the risk of electric shock from the high potentials used is remote. Swabbing theatre floor with 4 per cent calcium chloride solution is said to increase its electrical conductivity while damp sheets have the same effect. Wax polish must not be allowed on conducting floors.

8. Conducting rubber or vinyl thermoplastic products having antistatic properties should be used for tyres of trolleys, tables, stool tips, etc. The resistance of antistatic material should be between 10 megohms and 50,000 ohms. It should be used for breathing tubes, face-masks, reservoir bags. The conductivity of antistatic rubber is attributed to microscopic chains of carbon particles. Resistance does increase gradually with time, and periodical checks are necessary. Where antistatic rubber is not available the risk can be reduced if the rubber is wetted internally and externally before use. Non-conducting mattresses, rubber sheeting, aprons, etc., can be made reasonably safe if they are completely enclosed in a close-fitting cover of such antistatic material as cotton, linen, or viscose rayon. All personnel should wear either conducting rubber or leather footwear, each shoe having a resistance between 0·1 and 1 megohm (if less than 0·1 megohm there is a danger of accidental electrocution should contact with electrical mains occur); cotton blankets and sheets should replace woollen articles in the theatre suite, and should not be allowed to become too dry. When a patient comes to the theatre covered by woollen blankets, they should never be removed quickly and should be taken out of the theatre suite before the patient is anæsthetized. Woollen stockings should not be rapidly pulled off. It is possible that if all theatre suites were equipped with antistatic rubber exclusively and if all woollen blankets were prohibited, explosions from static electricity, the commonest cause of anæsthetic explosions, would almost disappear.

9. The relative humidity of the atmosphere should not be allowed to fall below 50 per cent. It may be most difficult to raise the humidity. Static sparks are more frequent when the air is dry and the barometric pressure high. Humidity of the atmosphere will not prevent explosions taking place in the anæsthetic apparatus.

10. Ignitable gas-flow should be turned off if metallic unions have to be made or unmade during anæsthesia.

11. Avoid spilling ether, etc., about the theatre.

12. Avoid cigarettes, matches, etc., in the anæsthetic room.

13. Remember that spirit lotions may ignite.

14. When diathermy is applied to the bladder, hydrogen is given off and may ignite inside the bladder. Prolonged use of diathermy may cause a strong positive charge on the patient, which may lead to spark formation unless he is adequately earthed. If the diathermy electrode is actually touching the tissues or the hæmostat before the current is switched on, arcing is minimized.

15. When there is risk of explosion, use an intravenous barbiturate, trichloroethylene, gas–oxygen, regional, halothane, or chloroform anæsthesia.

16. See that fire-fighting equipment is available and in good order.

17. The use of a tube containing radon, to neutralize static electricity.* The use of a hair-dryer containing a radioactive salt has been recommended.

18. When cautery or diathermy is applied to the mouth or bowel, nitrogen or carbon dioxide should be run in to wash out ignitable gases, e.g., hydrogen and methane, because they do not support combustion.

    Nitrogen or carbon dioxide can also be used to flush out deep wounds (e.g., thoracotomy) should diathermy become necessary when an explosive agent has been given.

19. Dilution of cyclopropane–oxygen mixtures with nitrogen or helium to prevent the chance of explosion† (see p. 162).

20. The stomach may be a reservoir of flammable gases (as distinct from gases due to fermentation). Gases may be flammable up to 45 minutes after administration is stopped.‡

    This vast question is excellently discussed in a brochure published by the U.S. Bureau of Mines (Report of Investigations 4833) entitled " Static Electricity in Hospital Operating Suites : Direct and Related Hazards and Pertinent Remedies ", by P. G. Guest, V. W. Sikora, and B. Lewis, 1952. Pittsburgh, Pa., U.S.A.

---

* Gordh, T., and Egmark, A., *Curr. Res. Anesth.*, 1952, **31**, 400.

† Bourne, J. G., *Nitrous Oxide in Dentistry*, 1960, Ch. X. London: Lloyd-Luke; and Corcoran, J. W., and Hingson, R. A., *Dent. Dig.*, 1955, **61**, 303.

‡ de Nava, B. L., and McDermott, T. F. J., *J. Amer. med. Ass.*, 1960, **174**, 2023.

CHAPTER XXXIII

MONITORING*

BLOOD-PRESSURE†

Stephen Hales (1677–1761) in 1733 was the first to attempt measurement of the blood-pressure of animals by direct cannulation of an artery.‡ Herrison, 1834, devised a crude instrument to be placed directly over an artery for clinical measurement of blood-pressure. Vierordt, 1855, was the first to estimate the amount of counter-pressure necessary just to obliterate the arterial pulse. Etienne Jules Marey (1830–1904) in 1875, Mosso in 1895, and Gärtner in 1899 designed apparatus in the nature of a finger plethysmograph.

Riva-Rocci (1863–1937) introduced the blood-pressure cuff in 1896,§ though the cuff he used was only 5 cm. in width. In 1901, von Recklinghausen drew attention to the importance of the width of the pneumatic cuff and E. A. Codman in 1894 and Harvey Cushing¶ advocated the use of blood-pressure readings regularly during anæsthesia. Korotkoff in 1905 described the sounds heard over an artery at a point just below the compression cuff.

The Compression Cuff.—This should be of the correct width. If the cuff is too narrow, readings will be high ; if too wide, readings will be low. In general it is recommended that the cuff should cover approximately two-thirds of the length of the upper arm or 20 per cent greater than the diameter of the arm. The length of the cuff should be such as to encircle at least half of the limb and the centre should lie over the artery. The cloth cover should be made of non-extensible material so that pressure is exerted uniformly.

Recommended sizes of cuff at different ages :—

	Width
Newborn infant	2·5 cm.
1–4 years	6·0 cm.
4–8 years	9·0 cm.
Adult (arm)	12 cm.
Adult (leg)	15 cm.

Palpation Method.—The cuff is inflated until the peripheral pulse is obliterated. It is then decompressed at a rate of 2–3 mm. Hg per

---

* *See also Clinical Anesthesia—Instrumentation and Anesthesia* (Ed. Dornette, W. H. L.), 1964. Oxford: Blackwell; Collins, V., *Principles of Anæsthesiology*, 1966, Ch. 3. London: Kimpton; and Atkinson, R. S., in *Recent Advances in Anæsthesia and Analgesia* (Ed. Hewer, C. Langton), 10th ed., 1967, Ch. X. London: Churchill.

† *See* Graham, G. R., *Brit. J. Anæsth.*, 1962, **34**, 646 ; and Burch, G. E., and DePasquale, N. P., *Primer of Clinical Measurement of Blood Pressure*, 1962. St. Louis: Mosby.

‡ Willius, F. A., and Keyes, T. E., *Cardiac Classics*, 1941, Vol. I, p. 131. St. Louis: Mosby.

§ Riva-Rocci, S., *Gaz. med. di Torino*, 1896, **47**, 981, reprinted in English translation in *Foundations of Anesthesiology* (Ed. Faulconel, A., and Keys, T. E.), 1965, p. 1043. Springfield, Ill.: Thomas.

¶ Cushing H. W., *Ann. Surg.*, 1902, **36**, 321; and *Boston Med. Surg. J.*, 1903, **148**, 291.

heart-beat. The level of pressure at which the radial pulse returns is recorded as the systolic blood-pressure.

The Korotkoff Sounds.*—The cuff is inflated until the pulse is obliterated, and then decompressed at a rate of 2–3 mm. Hg per heart-beat. As blood begins to flow through the compressed artery, turbulence is produced and this is transmitted as vibrations or sounds which can be detected by a stethoscope placed over the brachial artery. The point of first sound is taken as the systolic pressure; the point at which there is an abrupt decrease in intensity (muffling) is taken as the diastolic pressure. During surgical operations it may be preferable to fix the stethoscope over the brachial artery on the medial side of the arm above the elbow where it is covered by the cuff.†

Venous congestion must be avoided as it may give rise to an abnormally high diastolic and an abnormally low systolic reading (i.e., the cuff should not remain inflated longer than necessary).

Sometimes the Korotkoff sounds fade completely between systolic and diastolic pressures. This is known as the auscultatory gap. A false systolic reading may be obtained unless pressure has first been checked by the palpation method.

The pressure can also be obtained by watching the oscillations of the needle of the anaeroid manometer.

Flush Method.—Useful in newborn babies and infants. The limb is elevated and milked of blood. The cuff is then inflated and slowly deflated. The pressure at which a flush appears is taken as the systolic pressure. It may in fact be nearer to a mean arterial pressure.

Pressure may be measured by a mercury column or by an anaeroid manometer. The former is accurate, but is relatively bulky and must be held upright. The latter is small and compact but requires frequent calibration against a mercury column.

Continuous Recording by Indirect Method.—The systolic blood-pressure can be continuously recorded by the "Blood-pressure Follower" (Winston Electronic Ltd.). A small piezo-crystal is placed over the digital artery and a small cuff put over the finger. The cuff is blown up automatically until the crystal no longer picks up arterial pulsations and then deflates. The process is at once repeated to give a continuous recording. The position of the arm may be important, since the reading obtained varies according to the height of the blood column between heart and the digital cuff.

Oscillometer.—The armlet contains two rubber cuffs, the first proximal and overlapping the second distal bag. The cuffs are connected to an anaeroid which can be switched to either cuff by means of a lever. The two cuffs are inflated above the systolic pressure. A discharge valve is opened to create a slight leakage while the distal cuff remains in communication with the anaeroid pressure chamber. The needle deflexions which occur show a definite increase at the level of systolic blood-pressure and a

---

* Korotkoff, N. S., *Izvest. imp. Voyenno-Med. Acad. St. Petersburg*, 1905, **11**, 365.
† Collins, V. J., and Magora, F., *Curr. Res. Anesth.*, 1963, **42**, 443.

Oscillometer, *continued*.

definite decrease at the level of diastolic pressure. At each of these
points the lever must be switched to connect the anaeroid with the
proximal cuff to determine the actual pressure.

Direct Intra-arterial Methods.—A needle or catheter is inserted
into an artery and connected via a column of fluid to a manometer.*
The most suitable type is the electronic pressure transducer in
which the pressure change transmitted along the column of fluid
causes displacement or distortion of a membrane or similar device
to produce an electrical current. The current is then amplified
to form a visual record upon a cathode-ray oscilloscope or direct
writer. The transducer may be one of four main types : (1) resis-
tance-wire strain gauge ; (2) capacitance manometer ; (3) variable
inductance pressure gauge ; (4) semi-conductor gauge. Accurate
reproduction of a pressure wave requires a frequency response of
the entire system which is the tenth harmonic of the fundamental
wave frequency. The frequency response is limited to that of the
slowest link in the chain. Thus it is important that the connexion
between artery and transducer should be as short and rigid as
possible. Too narrow tubing increases frictional resistance to
the movement of fluid ; too wide tubing increases the inertia as
the mass of fluid is larger. With these methods, an immediate
trace of pressure and waveform is obtained. Each heart-beat is
recorded and a permanent record can be made. Direct measurement
is the only practical method during cardiopulmonary by-pass
when the circulation is not pulsatile, and when intense vasoconstriction renders the peripheral pulse impalpable. Direct methods
are subject to technical difficulties, cause discomfort to the patient,
and may carry a risk to the artery used. Indirect methods are, in
general, preferable.

A *pneumatic pressure transducer*† has been described—simple to
calibrate and requires no knowledge of electronic technique.

PULSE MONITORS

The most popular type of monitor consists of a photo-electric cell or
carbon microphone fixed over a digit. The output is fed into a simple
electrical circuit which signals each systole by the flick of a needle,‡ the
flash of a light, or a sound from a loudspeaker. The apparatus may be
combined with a sphygmomanometer for rapid blood-pressure estimations,§ and a device may be added to count the pulse-rate and record
it on a dial.‖

Pulse monitors of this type function best under conditions of vasodilatation and may be less reliable in the presence of vasoconstriction.

---

* Mallard, T. R., Payne, T. P., and Peachey, C. J., *J. Physiol.*, 1963, **167**, 10; Sivapragasam,
S., and Sandison, J. W., *Brit. J. Anæsth.*, 1967, **39**, 986; Severinghaus, J., *Anesthesiology*,
1957, **81**, 906; Blackburn, J. P., *Anæsthesia*, 1966, **21**, 108; and Fink, B. R., *Anesthesiology*,
1963, **24**, 872.
   † Thompson, C. W., and others, *Lancet*, 1967, **1**, 1364.
   ‡ Keating, V. J., *Brit. med. J.*, 1952, **1**, 1188.
   § Bishop, C., *Anæsthesia*, 1958, **13**, 329.
   ‖ Molyneux, L., and Pask, E. A., *Brit. J. Anæsth.*, 1955, **27**, 261 ; and Lawton, W., and
Wulfsohn, N. L., *Anæsthesia*, 1958, **13**, 352.

During halothane anæsthesia, the amplitude of deflexion of the needle increases until maximal vasodilatation occurs. This may be called the 'peak amplitude'. Reduction of amplitude is then indicative of either vasoconstriction (due to lightening of anæsthesia or pressor drugs) or a fall in systolic pressure. With deepening halothane anæsthesia the amplitude of deflexion (measured in geometric degrees) is proportional to systolic blood-pressure. The apparatus can, therefore, be used, within limits, as a monitor of blood-pressure from heart-beat to heart-beat, and is particularly useful during controlled respiration with halothane and oxygen (V.I.C.).[*]

Pulse monitors are particularly valuable :—

1. In small children and infants when access to a palpable pulse may be difficult.
2. During controlled respiration, when changes in respiration would not give warning of circulatory arrest.
3. To observe ectopic or coupled beats during anæsthesia with agents such as cyclopropane or halothane.
4. As an index of failing blood-pressure during halothane anæsthesia.
5. In situations where air embolism may occur.

A number of efficient and reliable pulse monitors are now commercially available. Some models can be attached to ear-lobe or lips. The photo-electric cell is now more popular than the carbon microphone. Examples of useful monitors include the Cotel-Keating monitor,[†] the Videograph (M.I.E.), etc.

The pulse can also be monitored by the use of a precordial stetho-scope, a method particularly suited to use in infants.[‡] In neonates and adults undergoing major surgery an œsophageal stethoscope may be useful.[§]

A continuous electrocardiogram acts as an excellent pulse monitor.

CARDIAC OUTPUT

1. The Fick Principle.—This is used to measure pulmonary blood-flow which is equal to cardiac output. Specimens of central venous blood are obtained from a catheter passed via an antecubital vein to the right ventricle or pulmonary artery. Arterial blood is obtained from the radial or femoral artery. Oxygen consumption is measured by use of a spirometer. Calculations are made according to the formula:

$$\text{Cardiac output (ml./min.)} = \frac{\text{Total body oxygen consumption (ml./min.)}}{\text{Arteriovenous oxygen difference (ml. per cent)}} \times 100.$$

Inaccuracies occur if there are changes in the lung reserve volumes which affect the spirometer reading.

[*] Beddard, J. R. J., *Brit. J. Anæsth.*, 1965, **37**, 354.
[†] Keating, V. J., *Brit. med. J.*, 1952, **1**, 1188.
[‡] Roberts, B., and Thompson, P. W., *Brit. J. Anæsth.*, 1963, **35**, 746 ; and Mushin, W. W., *Brit. med. J.*, 1958, **1**, 455.
[§] Cullingford, D. W. J., *Brit. J. Anæsth.*, 1964, **36**, 524.

2. Dye Dilution Methods.—Dye is injected via a catheter threaded up to the pulmonary artery, and blood samples taken from a peripheral artery and analysed by a photo-electric method. Successive measurements are plotted on a graph, and the area under the curve must then be determined. This can be accomplished using: (a) A planometer, (b) mathematical methods,* (c) computers.† Recirculation of the dye must not be included in the measurement, and this can be avoided if the graph is plotted on semi-logarithmic paper. Since the decay of the dye dilution curve is exponential it will then appear as a straight line which can be extended to exclude the secondary recirculation peak.

$$\text{Cardiac output (ml./min.)} = \frac{\text{Mass of dye injected}}{\text{Area under curve}} \times 60.$$

3. Measurement of temperature changes as blood flows through the lungs and heart. Not yet a clinical method.

THE ELECTROCARDIOGRAM

Ludwig and Waller (1887) first recorded the electric current which is associated with activity of the heart. Development of the string galvanometer (Einthoven, the Leyden physiologist (1860–1927), in 1903)‡ led to clinical and experimental studies of the electrocardiogram. To-day the best fidelity is obtained with vacuum tube amplifiers and the cathode-ray oscilloscope.

The Standard Leads.—

LEAD I.—Between right and left arms.

LEAD II.—Between right arm and left leg.

LEAD III.—Between left arm and left leg.

The series of waves obtained are arbitrarily designated as the **P** wave, the **QRS** complex, the **T** wave, and the **U** wave. The electromotive forces that are responsible for the **P** wave and the **QRS** complex actually occur before the auricular and ventricular muscle-fibres respectively contract and not as a result of their contraction.

P WAVE.—Does not normally exceed 0·11 sec. Represents the depolarization wave of the auricle.

P–R SEGMENT.—Represents the delay in transmission at the A.V. node.

P–R INTERVAL.—From beginning of **P** wave to beginning of **QRS** complex. Normal upper limit of duration 0·20 sec.

QRS COMPLEX.—The depolarization complex of the ventricular muscle. Does not normally exceed 0·10 sec.

S–T SEGMENT.—Represents the depolarized state, or the duration of the excited state of the ventricles.

T WAVE.—Ventricular repolarization.

U WAVE.—An " after-potential " wave, usually of low amplitude.

---

* Hill, D. W., *Physics Applied to Anæsthesia*, 1967, Ch. 1. London: Butterworths.

† Sinclair, S., and others, *Surgery*, 1965, **57**, 414; and Hamer, J., and others, *Brit. Heart J.*, 1966, **28**, 147.

‡ Einthoven, Willem, *Pflügers Arch. f. d. ges. Physiol.*, 1903, **99**, 472 (translated in *Cardiac Classics* (Ed. Willius, F. A., and Keyes, T. E.), 1941, Vol. 2, p. 722. St. Louis: Mosby.

Precordial Leads are obtained by placing the exploring electrode over the chest wall. These leads are popular in coronary care and intensive therapy units since they can be attached to the patient with little disturbance.* Readers are referred to standard texts of electrocardiography for further information.

The Electrocardiogram during Anæsthesia.†—The electrocardiogram acts as an excellent pulse monitor. At the same time it gives further information about the nature of irregularities. Under no circumstances does it afford a measure of the efficiency of myocardial contraction or of cardiac output ; in fact a normal electrical activity may occur when there is no measurable blood-pressure.

ARTEFACTS.—Tracings during anæsthesia and surgery are particularly liable to artefacts which must be differentiated from changes originating in the heart. They may be caused by disconnexion of an electrode, superimposition of potential from another person in contact with the patient, diathermy, improper earthing of apparatus, etc. It is possible for interference to take the form of a sine wave giving rise to the appearance of ventricular tachycardia.

EXTRASYSTOLES.—This is the disorder of rhythm most frequently observed in the operating room ; may be atrial, nodal, or ventricular.

TACHYCARDIA.—This is usually a sinus tachycardia. It is, however, important to distinguish between a supraventricular (atrial) and a ventricular paroxysmal tachycardia, since the treatment and prognosis of each are different. In the electrocardiogram P waves may be hard to distinguish and other criteria may be helpful. Thus, supraventricular paroxysmal tachycardia will often respond to vagal stimulation (carotid sinus or eyeball pressure) and to methoxamine, phenylephrine, and neostigmine. Ventricular tachycardia seldom exceeds 180 beats per minute ; supraventricular tachycardia may range from 140 to 300 beats per minute. The most rapid rates are seen in atrial flutter with a 1 : 1 ventricular response.

Tachycardia is generally well tolerated in the absence of myocardial disease. Treatment is indicated when it results in fall in blood-pressure or cardiac failure. Ventricular arrhythmias are more dangerous since they may deteriorate into ventricular fibrillation. A pulse-rate not exceeding 140 is seldom likely in itself to cause serious cardiac embarrassment.

THE DYING HEART.—The dying heart pattern may occur when the patient is near death from any cause and after cardiac standstill or ventricular fibrillation when resuscitative measures have had partial success. As myocardial function deteriorates the QRS complex becomes widened, heart-rate slows, and various disorders of rhythm may be seen. The last recognizable activity

---

* Fluck, D. C., and Burgess, P. A., *Lancet*, 1966, **1**, 1405.

† *See* Cannard, T. H., Dripps, R. D., Helwig, J., and Zinsser, H. F., *Anesthesiology*, 1960, **21**, 194; Rollason, W. N., *Electrocardiography for the Anæsthetist*, 1964. Oxford: Blackwell; and Price, J. H., in *Clinical Anesthesia—Instrumentation and Anesthesia* (Ed. Dornette, W. H. L.), 1964, Ch. 4. Oxford: Blackwell.

The Electrocardiogram during Anæsthesia, *continued.*

is usually a broad sine wave which may continue for some minutes after death is apparent. The ventricles may fibrillate at any stage in this course of events.

This pattern reflects a grave disorder which is likely to end in death. It may, however, be reversed if resuscitative measures can be applied. These must be directed to oxygenation of the myocardium and cardiac compression correction of metabolic acidosis, etc.

CENTRAL VENOUS PRESSURE

Venous Tone.—About half the total blood-volume is accommodated in the systemic venous system. Alterations in venous tone play a large part in the regulation of the hæmodynamics of the circulatory system.

Factors which increase venous tone:—
1. Skin stimulation.
2. Hypocapnia.
3. I.P.P.V.
4. Low arterial pressure.
5. Catecholamines.
6. Heart failure.
7. Cold.

Factors which diminish venous tone:—
1. Sleep.
2. Hypercapnia.
3. Ganglion-blocking drugs.
4. Thiopentone.
5. Histamine.
6. Nitrites.
7. Warmth.

Central Venous Pressure Measurement.*—A catheter is inserted in a peripheral vein and threaded up to the vena cava. The cutaneous veins of the arm or the external jugular are popular. Puncture of the skin below the middle of the clavicle to enter the subclavian vein directly† carries a risk of accidental pneumothorax. The catheter is connected to a simple saline manometer. Occurrence of respiratory fluctuations confirm that the tip lies within the thoracic cage. Sudden increase in pressure with fluctuations in time with the heart-beat indicates that the tip has entered the ventricle of the heart and it should be withdrawn.

READINGS.—The zero must be alined to a chosen reference point, i.e., the midaxillary line or the manubriosternal angle. This may be facilitated by the use of a spirit level on a long piece of wood, or by a horizontal 'gunsight'.‡ More elaborate methods using a transducer and automatic recording equipment can also be used. Normal central venous pressure may be taken as 30–100 mm. H_2O (2–8 mm. Hg). Values over 200 mm. H_2O may indicate heart failure.

---

* Sykes, M. K., *Ann. R. Coll. Surg. Engl.*, 1963, **33**, 185.
† Wilson, J. N., and others, *Arch. Surg.*, 1962, **85**, 563.
‡ Bethune, D. W., Gillett, G. B., Watson, A. C., and Crichton, T. C., *Lancet*, 1966, **2**, 684.

INDICATIONS.—

1. Open-heart surgery.* The amount of blood in the circulation can be adjusted to maintain a venous pressure around 50–100 mm. H_2O during the immediate post by-pass period.
2. Whenever massive infusions or transfusions are required. Central venous pressure gives a measure of the adequacy of replacement and early warning of overloading.
3. When circulatory hæmodynamics are unstable, e.g., during and following removal of a phæochromocytoma.†
4. In acute circulatory failure of obscure origin. Useful in the critically ill patient treated in an intensive therapy unit.
5. In severe shock.
6. In pædiatric surgery where accurate replacement is essential.‡

URINE OUTPUT

Renal function is a useful index of cardiovascular function in the patient with healthy kidneys. Collection and measurement of urine flow by indwelling catheter is a simple and useful procedure during cardiac operations. About 30 ml. urine should be secreted per hour if the renal perfusion is adequate.§

MEASUREMENT OF BLOOD-LOSS

Gravimetric Method.—The simplest and most commonly employed method. Blood-loss is estimated by measurement of the gain in weight of swabs and towels, together with measurement of suction bottles ; 1 ml. of blood weighs 1 g.

Colorimetric Method.‖—Swabs and towels are mixed thoroughly with a large known volume of fluid, which is then estimated colorimetrically. Errors may occur due to incomplete extraction or contamination with bile. The patient's pre-operative hæmoglobin must be known.

$$\text{Blood-loss (ml.)} = \frac{\text{Colorimeter reading} \times \text{Volume of solution (ml.)}}{200 \times \text{Patient's Hb (g. per cent)}}$$

In operations involving complex exchanges of blood (e.g., extracorporeal circulation), it may be useful to weigh the whole patient before and after operation.

Estimation of Blood-volume.¶—It is sometimes useful to measure blood-volume before operation and also as a check on the adequacy

---

* Ross, D., *Proc. R. Soc. Med.*, 1966, **60**, 359; and Feldman, S., in *Recent Advances in Anæsthesia and Analgesia* (Ed. Hewer, C. Langton), 10th ed., 1967, Ch. 6. London: Churchill.

† Schnelle, N., and others, *Surg. Clin. N. Amer.*, 1965, **45**, 991; de Blasi, S., *Brit. J. Anæsth.*, 1966, **38**, 740; and Engelbrecht, E. R., Hugill, J. T., and Graves, H. B., *Canad. Anæsth. Soc. J.*, 1966, **13**, 598.

‡ Dawson, B., and Lynn, H. B., *Surg. Clin. N. Amer.*, 1965, **45**, 949.

§ Ross, D., *Proc. R. Soc. Med.*, 1966, **60**, 359.

‖ *See also* Thornton, J. A., and others, *Brit. J. Anæsth.*, 1963, **35**, 91; Thornton, J. A., *Ann. R. Coll. Surg., Engl.*, 1963, **33**, 164; Rustad, M., *Lancet*, 1963, **1**, 1304; and Mainland, J. F., *Brit. J. Anæsth.*, 1966, **38**, 76.

¶ Albert, S. N., *Blood Volume*, 1963. Springfield, Ill.: Thomas; Underwood, P. S., and Howland, W. S., in *Clinical Anesthesia—Instrumentation and Anesthesia* (Ed. Dornette, W. H. L.), 1964, Ch. 7. Oxford: Blackwell; and Davies, J. W. L., *Brit. J. Anæsth.*, 1966, **38**, 250.

Estimation of Blood-volume, *continued*.

of transfusion. Normal blood-volumes can be obtained from nomograms according to height and weight. Where body-weight and height are in reasonable proportion, a rough guide is to take blood-volume as 7·7 per cent of body-weight.*

Plasma volume can be obtained by dye-dilution or radioactive-iodine-dilution methods. Semi-automatic instruments are now available for the radioactive-iodine method. Dilution is measured after a 15-minute mixing time, calculations being made automatically. Labelling of red cells with radioactive chromium can also be carried out and a dilution test made, but the method is more elaborate as cells have to be first separated for labelling.

ANALYSIS OF GAS MIXTURES

1. **Oxygen.**—Paramagnetic analysers are useful.† Gases are classed as paramagnetic or diamagnetic according to their behaviour in a magnetic field. The former seek the area of strongest, the latter of weakest flux. Of the gases of interest to the anæsthetist only oxygen, nitric oxide, and nitrogen dioxide are paramagnetic, others are weakly diamagnetic. This principle is used in commercial apparatus for analysis of oxygen concentrations in a gas mixture.

2. **Carbon Dioxide.**—The infra-red analyser is used. Gases whose molecules contain two dissimilar atoms or more than two atoms absorb radiation in the infra-red region of the spectrum.

3. **Halothane.**—The analyser depends upon the principle of ultra-violet absorption.‡ Useful in checking the calibration of vaporizers and for monitoring the concentration in closed-circuit anæsthesia.

4. **Simultaneous analysis** of various gases can be carried out using: (*a*) The Mass Spectrometer—molecules are ionized, accelerated by an electric field, and deflected by a magnetic field. The angle of deflexion is related to molecular weight. Does not differentiate between carbon dioxide and nitrous oxide which have the same molecular weight. Not satisfactory for large organic molecules, e.g., halothane. A bulky and expensive apparatus, suitable only for research purposes. (*b*) Gas Chromatography.§ Separation of components by means of a partition column. The estimation takes several minutes, so does not follow the changes in a single breath.

RESPIRATION

Tidal Volume and Minute Volume.—

1. THE DISPLACEMENT METER.—This is the type of gas meter used for domestic purposes. It is most conveniently used to measure expired gases—that is, by connecting it to the outlet port of a non-rebreathing valve.

2. INFERENTIAL METERS.—Volume is inferred from the number of revolutions of a vane rotated by the gas stream. Now commercially available as small and light apparatus, which may be

---

* Scholar, H., *Amer. Heart J.*, 1965, **69**, 701.
† Nunn, J. F., and others, *Brit. J. Anæsth.*, 1964, **36**, 666.
‡ Robinson, A., and Denson, J. S., *Anesthesiology*, 1962, **23**, 391.
§ Youngman, P. M. E., *Biomed. Eng.*, 1966, **1**, 157.

connected directly to a facepiece or catheter mount : (1) **Wright Anemometer** ;* gas passes through ten tangential slots in a cylindrical stator ring to turn a flat two-bladed rotor ; (2) Dräger Volumeter ; two lightweight lozenge-shaped meshing rotors ; (3) Bennett Ventilation Meter ; two interlocking rotors of light alloy which run in jewelled bearings.

3. SPIROMETRY.—This is a complex method since allowances must be made for fresh gases entering the system.† A simplified method has, however, proved useful as a monitor during neurosurgery.‡ Certain characteristic patterns give early warning of untoward reactions, e.g., ischæmia of the brain-stem due to retraction, etc.

Arterial Oxygen Tension.—

THE OXYGEN ELECTRODE.—This consists of a platinum cathode and a silver anode in an electrolyte solution. Platinum gives up electrons to oxygen and the resulting voltage change can be measured and expressed in terms of oxygen tension. Platinum receives a deposition of protein when used in biological fluids, so the electrode system must be isolated from the blood sample by a thin gas-permeable membrane. The Clark electrode§ is the basis of the modern oxygen electrode though modifications have been produced.||

BLOOD SAMPLES.¶—Must be drawn from an artery into a syringe whose dead space has been filled with heparin. The oxygen consumption of whole blood at 38° C. is sufficient to cause a fall in Po_2 of about 3 mm. Hg per minute. Samples should therefore be analysed at once, or kept cool to reduce oxygen consumption.

HYPOXÆMIA.—'Normal' values may be as low as 70 mm. Hg in the over 70 age-group.** Arterial oxygen tension is a more sensitive index of oxygen lack than oxygen saturation—*see* the dissociation curve (*Fig.* 2). Hypoxæmia may occur postoperatively, as a result of respiratory depression, and as a result of chest injury or disease. Changes in ventilation–perfusion relationships in the lungs occur in a variety of clinical states. (*See also* Adams, A. P., Morgan-Hughes, J. A., and Sykes, M. K., *Anæsthesia*, 1967, **22**, 575.)

Venous Oxygen Content is an index of adequate cardiac output and tissue perfusion.††

Oximetry (the measurement of oxygen saturation of the blood).—The oximeter is attached to the lobe of the ear. Suitably filtered light passes through the ear and is measured by a photocell. The instruments are delicate and have not found a regular use during anæsthesia.

* Wright, B. M., *J. Physiol.*, 1955, **127**, 25.
† Nunn, J. F., *Brit. J. Anæsth.*, 1956, **28**, 440.
‡ Hewer, A. J. H., *Proc. R. Soc. Med.*, 1966, **60**, 362.
§ Clark, L. C., *Trans. Amer. Soc. artif. Int. Org.*, 1956, **2**, 41.
|| Laver, M. B., and Seifen, A., *Anesthesiology*, 1965, **26**, 73.
¶ Nunn, J. F., *Brit. J. Anæsth.*, 1962, **34**, 621.
** Nunn, J. F., *Lancet*, 1965, **2**, 466; and Dobkin, A. B., and others, *Proc. 2nd Eur. Cong. Anæsth.*, 1966, **1**, 542.
†† Ross, D., *Proc. R. Soc. Med.*, 1966, **60**, 359; and Valentine, P. A., and others, *Lancet*, 1966, **2**, 837.

Arterial Carbon Dioxide Measurement.—

DIRECT METHODS.—A sample of blood may be taken by direct arterial puncture. 'Arterialized' capillary blood from the back of the hand is an acceptable alternative provided there is no stasis and the skin temperature is at least 35° C. (vasodilatation from general anæsthesia will usually produce these conditions).

The hydrogen electrode is the prototype of electrodes for pH measurement, though it has been superseded by the glass electrode for practical use. In clinical practice pH must be measured with much greater accuracy than is the case in industry. Every part of the measuring system must be maintained at a high standard of accuracy.

If water or bicarbonate solution is separated from a solution of a gas mixture containing carbon dioxide by a membrane permeable to this gas, the pH of the water or bicarbonate solution will be related to the Pco_2 of the phase on the other side of the membrane. It is, therefore, a measure of it. This is the principle of the Severinghaus carbon dioxide electrode.*

INTERPOLATION.—The Micro-Astrup Apparatus (p. 779) can be used to measure the acid-base state of a microspecimen of blood, the arterial Pco_2 being read off the Siggaard-Andersen nomogram.

INDIRECT MEASUREMENTS.—Samples of expired gases are analysed.

1. END-TIDAL SAMPLES.—Carbon dioxide content can be measured using the Haldane or Dräger apparatus or by a colorimetric method.

2. CONTINUOUS ANALYSIS.—This requires an analyser capable of responding to changes within a single breath. Infra-red analysers are of this type. Physical methods of gas analysis are reviewed by Mapleson, W. W., *Brit. J. Anæsth.*, 1962, **34**, 631.

3. REBREATHING METHODS.—These methods of determining Pco_2 avoid the necessity for arterial puncture. The principle of the method is that gases rebreathed in a closed system come rapidly into equilibrium with those in mixed venous blood. This equilibrium will occur within 20 sec. (less than the circulation time) provided that the difference in concentration is not too great.

   a. *Method of Campbell and Howell.*†—1·5 litres of oxygen are rebreathed for 90 sec. The patient is rested for 2 min., and the bag contents rebreathed for a further 20 sec. or 5 breaths. Carbon dioxide is then estimated by the modified Haldane apparatus.

   b. *Method of Cooper and Smith.*‡—Five per cent carbon dioxide in oxygen is rebreathed either spontaneously or artificially

---

* Severinghaus, J. W., and Bradley, A. F., *Applied Physiol.*, 1958, **13**, 513 ; Severinghaus, J. W., *Anesthesiology* 1960, **21**, 717 ; and Lunn, J. N., and Mapleson, W. W., *Brit. J. Anæsth.*, 1963, **35**, 666.

† Campbell, E. J. M., and Howell, J. B. L., *Brit. med. J.*, 1960, **1**, 458 ; and *Ibid.*, 1962, **2**, 630.

‡ Cooper, E. A., and Smith, H., *Anæsthesia*, 1961, **16**, 445.

for 5 breaths. After 60-sec. rest, the contents are re-breathed for 3 periods of 15 sec., with a rest period of 60 sec. between each. Carbon dioxide is then analysed.

c. *Modification by Godfrey* to overcome the discomfort felt by some patients.*

d. *Modification for use in infants and children.*†

The carbon dioxide figure is correlated with 713 mm. Hg (the sum of the tensions of gases less water vapour in expired air) to obtain Pco_2. The arterial Pco_2 is 6 mm. Hg lower than the figure obtained which is for mixed venous blood. Other simple CO_2 analysers have recently been described.‡

(*See also* Woolmer, R. F., in *Modern Trends in Anæsthesia* (Ed. Evans, F. T., and Gray, T. C.), 1962, Vol. 2, Ch. 2. London : Butterworths ; Nunn, J. F., *Brit. J. Anæsth.*, 1958, **30**, 254 ; *Symposium on pH and Blood Gas Measurement* (Ed. Woolmer, R. F.), 1959. London : Churchill ; Robinson, J. S., *Brit. J. Anæsth.*, 1962, **34**, 611; and Adams, A. P., Morgan-Hughes, J. O., and Sykes, M. K., *Anæsthesia*, 1968, **23**, 47.)

ACID-BASE BALANCE

Laboratory techniques are now available to measure the degree of acidosis or alkalosis in a blood sample and to separate them into respiratory and metabolic components. Blood samples may be taken by direct arterial puncture, but where the patient is vasodilated 'arterialized' blood from the dorsum of the hand or capillary blood is satisfactory.§ Venous blood is not of value unless a specimen of mixed venous blood from the vena cava can be obtained. Blood specimens should be kept sealed where blood gases are to be measured.

Measurement of pH.‖—It may be necessary to measure to 0·005 of a pH unit and the glass electrode has now been perfected for this purpose. It consists of a lattice of oxygen and silica atoms with metal cations in the interstices. Hydrogen ions enter the lattice and displace cations to produce a potential difference. Electrodes are temperature-sensitive, and measurements must be made at a standard temperature of 38° C.

The Siggaard-Andersen Nomogram.‡—When pH is plotted against log Pco_2, buffer lines can be constructed for particular blood samples. The position and slope of the buffer line depend on the acid-base composition of the sample. Nomograms are provided so that base excess can be read off. *See also* Chapter II.

The Micro-Astrup Method.¶—This is an interpolation technique based on measurement of pH and the use of the Siggaard-Andersen nomogram. Three estimations of pH are required. In order to

---

* Godfrey, S., *Brit. med. J.*, 1966, **1**, 1163.
† Hodson, W. A., Chernick, V., and Avery, M. A., *Lancet*, 1966, **1**, 515.
‡ Austin, W. T. S., Harris, E. A., and Slawson, K. B., *Ibid.*, 1963, **2**, 984 ; Essex, L., and Pask, E. A., *Ibid.*, 1964, **1**, 311.
§ Harrison, E. M., and Galloon, S., *Brit. J. Anæsth.*, 1965, **37**, 13.
‖ *See* Robinson, J. S., *Ibid.*, 1962, **34**, 31.
¶ Andersen, O. S., and Engel, K., *Scand. J. Clin. Lab. Invest.*, 1960, **12**, 177; and Astrup, P., Jorgensen, O. S., Andersen, O. S., and Engel, K., *Lancet*, 1960, **1**, 1935.

The Micro-Astrup Method, *continued.*

construct the buffer line it is necessary to equilibrate the blood sample with a known high and a known low tension of carbon dioxide, and *p*H measured. These two points (A and B) are entered on the graph and joined by a straight line. Where this

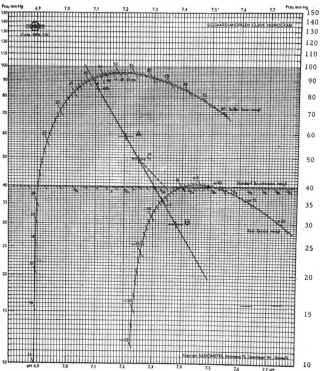

Fig. 52.—The full Siggaard-Andersen nomogram. (*By permission of Dr. Siggaard-Andersen and 'Radiometer', Copenhagen.*)

line crosses the base excess nomogram, the value for base excess is read off. Note that metabolic acidosis is evidenced by a base deficit, but this is conventionally expressed as a negative base excess. The third estimation of *p*H is carried out on the blood sample without equilibration. Its point is then entered on the buffer line (C) and the Pco_2 read off. (*Fig.* 52.)

The information required is now available: (1) The base deficit (negative base excess) as an expression of metabolic acidosis; (2) The arterial Pco_2 which expresses respiratory acidosis or alkalosis.

Correction of Metabolic Acidosis.*—The figure for base deficit obtained by the Micro-Astrup method is expressed in mEq. per litre blood. To find the deficit in mEq. total for the extracellular fluid compartment of the whole body, a simple formula can be used:—

Base deficit × 0·3 × body-weight in kg. = Dose of bicarbonate
required in mEq.

(*See also* Adams, A. P., Morgan-Hughes, J. O., and Sykes, M. K., *Anæsthesia*, 1968, **23**, 47.)

THE ELECTRO-ENCEPHALOGRAM†

Electrical activity of the brain in animals noted by Richard Caton in 1875. Hans Berger‡ (1931) described alpha rhythms in man. Adrian and Matthews (1934) developed the technique of the electro-encephalogram.

Types of Wave.—
1. DELTA WAVES.—0·5–3·5 cycles per sec. ; amplitude 100 microvolts. Occur in infants and sleeping adults.
2. THETA WAVES.—4–7 cycles per sec. 10 microvolts.
3. ALPHA WAVES.—8–13 cycles per sec. 20 microvolts in infants, 75 in children, 50 in adults. Augmented by closing eyes or mental repose. Reduced by visual and mental activity.
4. BETA WAVES.—14–25 cycles per sec. 20 microvolts.
5. GAMMA WAVES.—26 cycles per sec. or more. 10 microvolts. Rare in normal subjects.

Multiple electrodes may be inserted to obtain patterns from different axes of the scalp. In anæsthetic practice simple monitoring is satisfactory by means of a single lead between frontal and occipital regions. Artefacts may occur due to movement of the patient or to superimposition of an electrocardiogram if an electrode is placed directly over an artery.

Changes during Anæsthesia.—
1. RELATION TO DEPTH OF ANÆSTHESIA.—Changes in electrical activity follow a characteristic pattern when most general anæsthetics are given. Seven electrocardiographic levels have been described.§ The first level is relatively flat, the second shows high-amplitude rhythmical discharges, the third is complex and irregular, and succeeding levels show an increasing suppression until the seventh level which is characterized by a complete absence of measurable waves (*Fig.* 53). The electro-encephalograph is not a reliable indicator of consciousness or unconsciousness during nitrous-oxide–oxygen–relaxant anæsthesia.‖

* Mellemgaard, K., and Astrup, P., *Scand. J. Clin. Lab. Invest.*, 1960, **12**, 187.
† *See also* Faulconer, A., and Bickford, R. G., *Electro-encephalography in Anesthesiology*, 1960. Springfield, Ill.: Thomas; Clutton-Brock, J., in *Thoracic Anæsthesia* (Ed. Mushin, W. W.), 1963, Ch. 19. Oxford: Blackwell; and Marshall, M., and others, *Brit. J. Anæsth.*, 1965, **37**, 845.
‡ Berger, H., *Arch. f. Psychiat.*, 1931, **94**, 16.
§ Faulconer, A., *Anesthesiology*, 1952, **13**, 361.
‖ Clutton-Brock, J., in *Thoracic Anæsthesia* (Ed. Mushin, W. W.), 1963, Ch. 19. Oxford: Blackwell.

Changes during Anæsthesia, *continued.*

　　2. EFFECT OF HYPOXIA.—Causes slowing of the frequency of
　　　the waves. After about 20 sec. of complete anoxia the recording
　　　becomes a straight line. Lesser degrees of hypoxia may not
　　　affect the tracing until a level of 40 per cent arterial oxygen
　　　saturation is reached.

LEVEL OF ANESTHESIA

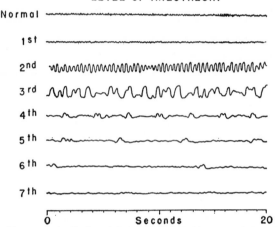

Fig. 53.—A classification of electro-encephalographic pattern changes during
increasing depth of ether–oxygen or nitrous-oxide–oxygen–ether anæsthesia of
human beings. The first and second patterns occur during induction. Patterns
3, 4, and 5 occur during light, moderate, and deep surgical anæsthesia. Patterns
6 and 7 are seen during excessively deep anæsthesia. (*By courtesy of Albert Faulconer,
jun., and the Publishers of 'Anesthesiology.'*)

　　3. EFFECT OF RAISED CARBON DIOXIDE TENSION.—
　　　Potentiates the effect of other anæsthetic drugs.
　　4. HYPOTENSION.—A rapid fall of blood-pressure is associated
　　　with slow high-amplitude waves or temporary cessation.
　　5. HYPOTHERMIA.—Below 35–31° C. some decrease in amplitude
　　　and frequency occurs. At 20° C. there may be little activity.
　　6. CIRCULATORY ARREST.—Activity ceases. The recording can
　　　be used as a measure of cerebral circulation during cardiac
　　　massage.

Servo Device.—The electro-encephalograph has been used as a servo
　　device to maintain a steady state of anæsthesia.*

Index of Cerebral Circulation.—The main application of the electro-
　　encephalograph in the operating theatre is as a measure of the
　　circulation to the brain. In this respect it is a more sensitive

---

　　* Kiersey, D. K., Bickford, R. G., and Faulconer, A., *Brit. J. Anæsth.*, 1951, **23**, 141 ;
and Soltero, D. E., Faulconer, A., and Bickford, R. G., *Anesthesiology*, 1951, **12**, 574.

index of the failing heart than the electrocardiogram, and it is a valuable monitor during operations involving extracorporeal circulation.

ELECTROMYOGRAPHY

The electromyogram is a record of action potential from the contracting muscle. It gives a rough guide to the degree of activity of the particular muscle. Monitoring of the abdominal wall muscles has been used to regulate the administration of suxamethonium during laparotomy.[*] It can also be used to distinguish depolarizing from non-depolarizing myoneural block and to diagnose myasthenia from the myasthenic state associated with bronchial carcinoma (see Chapter XXVI).

TEMPERATURE

The founder of clinical thermometry was C. A. Wunderlich (1815–1877), Professor of Medicine at Leipzig, whose classic work appeared in 1868.[†]

Thermometers are required for a number of purposes:—

1. THE STANDARD MERCURY-IN-GLASS CLINICAL THERMOMETER.—Fragile, unsuitable for insertion in body cavities, slow response time. Not suitable for use during hypothermia.

2. DIAL THERMOMETERS.—Simple instruments: (a) A flat bimetallic spiral spring which winds or unwinds as temperature changes; (b) The pressure gauge (Bourdon gauge)—a hollow ribbon of metal which winds or unwinds as temperature changes produce pressure changes within the coil.

3. THERMOCOUPLE.—A circuit of two dissimilar metals produces an e.m.f. when the two junctions are at different temperatures. The e.m.f. is measured and calibrated according to temperature. The apparatus can be made small, and it has a rapid response.

4. PLATINUM RESISTANCE THERMOMETRY.—The resistance of a metal varies according to temperature, and the former is measured by means of a Wheatstone bridge. A platinum coil can be mounted within the lumen of a hypodermic needle for insertion in body tissues.

5. THERMISTOR (thermally sensitive resistor).—A small bead of semiconductor material can be sealed into hypodermic needles. Semiconductors have negative coefficients of resistance, which can be measured using a Wheatstone bridge.

6. SKIN THERMOMETERS.—Difficulties arise due to poor contact with the skin and because skin temperature itself falls as heat passes to the thermometer: (a) The magnetic thermometer—temperature affects its field strength. (b) The radiometer—infrared rays, which are emitted by all substances at temperatures above absolute zero, are focused on a thermistor device.

(See also Cliffe, P., Anæsthesia, 1962, **17**, 215; Levine, S. D., in Clinical Anesthesia—Instrumentation and Anesthesia (Ed. Dornette, W. H. L.), 1964, Ch. 6. Oxford: Blackwell; and Hill, D. W., Principles of Electronics in Medical Research, p. 965. London: Butterworths.)

* Fink, B. R., Anesthesiology, 1960, **21**, 178.
† Wunderlich, C. A., Medical Thermometry, 2nd ed., 1871, translated by Woodman, W. B. London: New Sydenham Society. See also Brit. med. J., 1965, **1**, 1449.

ANÆSTHETIC RECORDS*

Record cards should be used in all major operations. They are doubly useful : they enable the anæsthetist to assess accurately the condition of the patient during the operation ; they are invaluable for reference.

Nosworthy's cards are most useful and convenient and the fourth type is now published by the Copeland Chatterson Co. They enable the sex, age, physical state, pre-operative complications, anæsthetic techniques, complications during anæsthesia, plane of anæsthesia, site of operation, duration of operation, pre-medication, anæsthetics used, post-operative complications, etc., to be accurately charted, while they allow for a 5-minute record of the pulse and blood-pressure readings. By converting a series of circles into notches, rapid sorting is possible with the aid of a knitting needle.

Some types of record combine pre-operative assessment with a record of vital signs during operation. Other record systems incorporate carbon copies which may be retained as departmental records when the originals are filed in the case notes.

In every case, the agents, doses, and methods of administration should be written in the operation book, followed by the anæsthetist's signature.

A record of all intravenous fluids given during operation should be entered on the case-sheet, including the identification numbers of any bottles of blood.

A clean sheet of paper and a pencil are still the best tools for collecting worth-while data which will be useful in the future.

Automatic recording may be useful in the intensive therapy unit. Various systems such as the 'Monitron' can be used to print out serial estimations of several parameters simultaneously in a way which allows easy visual interpolation.†

COMPUTERS IN ANÆSTHESIA

The computer is a machine capable of performing any specified data-procedure at great speed. Its use is not restricted to calculation. There are as many data-procedures as thought processes. The setting down of data-procedures in a suitable form for the computer is called *programming*.

The first electronic digital computer was made in 1946. Since then there have been rapid advances in design, including miniaturization.

Computers work on the principle that any calculation whatsoever can be expressed as a sequence of a few elementary operations. These include addition, subtraction, and discrimination between positive and negative, zero and non-zero. The design of every practical digital computer is dominated by the need to store alphabetical and numerical data reliably and cheaply and to operate on the data at very high speeds. For practical reasons it is convenient to use a binary system.

---

* See also Collins, V., *Principles of Anesthesiology*, 1966, Ch. 2. London: Kimpton.
† Cliffe, P., *Postgrad. Med. J.*, 1967, **43**, 195; Atkinson, R. S., in *Recent Advances in Anæsthesia and Analgesia* (Ed. Hewer, C. Langton), 10th ed., 1967, Ch. 10. London: Churchill.

For further information the reader is referred to Payne, L. C., *An Introduction to Medical Automation*, 1966. London: Pitman.

Computers have so far been used in anæsthesia in a limited, exploratory, and specialized manner. The fields which would appear most promising at the present time include:—

1. MEDICAL RECORDS.—Use for data acquisition and retrieval.
2. SIGNAL ANALYSIS.—
    a. DIAGNOSIS.—For example, the computer can give a more rapid and certain analysis of infarction in the E.C.G. than the conventional twelve-lead interpretation by the human eye.[*]
    b. MONITORING.—Work is in progress regarding the analysis of measurements and trends to give early warning of impending complications.[†] This would be particularly valuable in coronary care units, intensive therapy units, and after cardiac surgery,[‡] as well as during anæsthesia itself.[§] Useful in cardiac output estimations.[||]
3. SIMULATION STUDIES.—Computer analysis may be valuable in the study of phenomena such as the uptake and elimination of anæsthetic drugs.[¶]
4. Computers have been used in the preparation of physiological nomograms.[**]
5. In the education of the anæsthetist.

---

[*] Stack, I., Dickson, J. F., Whipple, G. H., and Horibe, H., *Ann. N.Y. Acad. Sci.*, 1965, **126**, 851.
[†] Sayers, B. McA., *Proc. R. Soc. Med.*, 1967, **60**, 756; and Cliffe, P., *Postgrad. med. J.*, 1967, **43**, 195.
[‡] Osborne, J. J., Badia, W., and Gerbode, F., *J. thorac. cardiovasc. Surg.*, 1963, **45**, 500.
[§] Wilber, S. A., and Derrick, W. S., *J. Amer. med. Ass.*, 1965, **191**, 893.
[||] Sinclair, S., and others, *Surgery*, 1965, **57**, 414; and Hamer, J., and others, *Brit. Heart J.*, 1966, **28**, 147.
[¶] Mapleson, W. W., *Brit. J. Anæsth.*, 1964, **36**, 129.
[**] Kelman, G. R., and Nunn, J. F., *J. appl. Physiol.*, 1966, **21**, 1484.

CHAPTER XXXIV

RESUSCITATION

Historical.—Expired air ventilation has been used throughout history in an effort to revive the apparently dead.* Tracheostomy was performed in the twelfth and thirteenth centuries in the treatment of drowned persons. Paracelsus (1493–1541) is usually credited with the introduction of the bellows to ventilate the lungs.

Modern history begins in the middle of the eighteenth century. This was a period when a wave of humanitarianism spread through Europe. A Society for the Recovery of Drowned Persons was founded in Amsterdam in 1767. In Britain the Humane Society, later the Royal Humane Society, was established by William Hawes in 1771. Classic early contributions to the literature include those of John Hunter† in 1776 and Kite‡ in 1788.

Artificial ventilation of the lungs was advocated by Marshall Hall§ in 1856, who described a method of rotating the patient's body combined with pressure on the back to aid expiration. Silvester described his method in 1857, and Holger Nielsen‖ published details of a new technique in 1932. In the same year Eve introduced the tilting board method.¶ These methods were popular for many years. Only in the past decade has positive-pressure ventilation to the mouth displaced these methods.**

Reports of deaths during anæsthesia, in the years following 1846, led to interest in the study of cardiac arrest. The first successful internal cardiac massage was probably performed in Norway in 1901.†† The first in Britain was reported by Starling‡‡ in 1902. Beck§§ successfully defibrillated the human heart in 1937. External cardiac compression became popular following the work of Kouwenhoven and others in 1960.‖‖

CARDIAC ARREST

The term is difficult to define. Milstein¶¶ suggests that it is used to mean failure of the heart action to maintain an adequate cerebral circulation, in the absence of a causative or irreversible disease. Cardiac arrest may be reversible or irreversible. Examples of reversible cardiac arrest include asystole due to vagal stimulation and asystole or fibrillation due to anæsthetic drugs, hypercarbia, etc. In these cases, as long

---

* 2 Kings iv, 34–35.
† Hunter, J., *Phil. Trans.*, 1776, **66**, 412.
‡ Kite, C., *An Essay on the Recovery of the Apparently Dead*, 1788. London: Dilly.
§ Ellis, R., *Lancet*, 1868, **2**, 538.
‖ Nielsen, H., *Ugeskr. Laeger*, 1932, **94**, 1201.
¶ Eve, F. C., *Lancet*, 1932, **2**, 995.
** Safar, P., *J. Amer. med. Ass.*, 1958, **167**, 335.
†† Keen, W. W., *Ther. Gaz.*, 1904, **28**, 217.
‡‡ Starling, E. A., *Lancet*, 1902, **2**, 1397.
§§ Beck, C. S., and Mautz, F. R., *Ann. Surg.*, 1937, **106**, 525.
‖‖ Kouwenhoven, W. B., and others, *J. Amer. med. Ass.*, 1960, **173**, 1064.
¶¶ Milstein, B. B., *Cardiac Arrest and Resuscitation*, 1963. London: Lloyd-Luke.

as oxygenation is maintained, the heart may be expected to respond to cardiac compression. Irreversible cardiac arrest may be due to myocarditis, myocardial failure from gross hypertrophy or infarction, coronary artery embolism (except air), hyperkalæmia from fresh-water drowning, uræmia, etc. In such cases treatment is not likely to be successful.

Cessation of the heart-beat occurs in two entirely different forms: (a) cardiac asystole, (b) ventricular fibrillation. The two cannot be differentiated by clinical observation, but only by electrocardiography or direct inspection of the heart.

Asystole and ventricular fibrillation can change one to the other, either spontaneously or as a result of treatment.

ASYSTOLE.—The heart is relaxed, soft, blue, and motionless. The coronary veins are black, tense, and prominent.

VENTRICULAR FIBRILLATION.—There is a fine or coarse irregular uncoordinated twitching. The heart is pale and cyanotic. Metabolism continues at about the normal rate. Fine fibrillation may be confused with asystole, coarse fibrillation with ventricular tachycardia if the observer is inexperienced, particularly if the pericardium is not opened. During fibrillation blood-pressures of 20–30 mm. Hg have been observed, but this is due to residual vascular tone and there is no flow of blood.

CAUSES OF CARDIAC ARREST.—

1. *Effect of Anæsthetic Drugs.*—Has occurred during administration of all the anæsthetic agents in common use, including local and spinal techniques. In retrospect, the arrest can often be shown to be due to errors in technique, overdosage, or hypoxia. Anæsthetic drugs may exert an effect on the heart in a variety of ways : (a) Direct myocardial depression (specific impairment of contraction of the muscle-fibres) ; (b) Vagotonic effect ; (c) Sympathetic stimulation ; (d) Increased excitability of ventricular muscle ; (e) Hypotension, especially in patients with inability to increase cardiac output (severe valvular stenosis, constrictive pericarditis) ; (f) Hypoxia as a result of respiratory depression ; (g) Hypercapnia associated with respiratory depression.

2. *Vagal Reflex Mechanisms.*—Sources of stimuli which may provoke bradycardia or asystole include the rectum, uterus, and cervix, the throat, glottis, and bronchial tree, bladder and urethra, mesentery, the carotid sheath, and traction on extra-ocular muscles (especially the internal rectus).

3. *Electrolyte Changes.*—Administration of *potassium* ions leads to loss of conductivity, contractility, and a decreased threshold to vagal stimulation. Eventually, if potassium is given slowly, the heart action ceases in diastole. If given quickly, potassium causes ventricular fibrillation. *Calcium* administration leads to increased contractility, prolongation of systole, shortening of diastole, and eventual cardiac arrest in systole. The ratio of potassium to calcium in the blood is important. Rise of serum potassium occurs in

Cardiac Arrest, *continued*.

anuria, dehydration, diabetic ketosis, drowning in fresh water, extensive tissue breakdown, in transfusion of stored blood, and in hypoxia. When large volumes of stored blood are transfused calcium gluconate may be given, 5–10 ml. of 10 per cent solution per pint of blood transfused (after first 2 pints). The deleterious effect of potassium on the myocardium can also be offset by administration of digitalis.

4. *Hypoxia and Anoxia.*—In clinical practice hypoxia is one of the commonest factors to be incriminated in the causation of cardiac arrest. It is, however, difficult to reproduce sudden cardiac arrest in the laboratory by subjecting animals to acute anoxia—changes take place over several minutes.

Hypoxia may be due to : (*a*) Respiratory obstruction ; (*b*) Inadequate oxygen supply in inspired gas (unobserved empty oxygen cylinder) ; (*c*) Respiratory depression or apnœa ; (*d*) Impaired organ perfusion (anæmia, hæmorrhage, right-to-left circulatory shunts).

Hypoxia results in : (*a*) Tachycardia and rise of blood-pressure (sympathetic stimulation) leading to bradycardia, nodal rhythms, partial or complete heart-block, and eventual asystole ; (*b*) Release of potassium from all tissues of the body, especially the liver. The serum potassium may rise by 50 per cent in 5 min. ;[*] (*c*) Potentiation of the depressant effects of drugs. The end-result is usually cardiac asystole, but there is a stage when the conducting mechanism has been affected before the ventricular muscle and when a mechanical stimulus (e.g., pin-prick) may precipitate ventricular fibrillation.

5. *Hypercapnia.*—Results in: (*a*) Increase of circulating catecholamines ; (*b*) Increase of serum potassium level ; (*c*) Prolongation of the period of asystole induced by vagal stimulation ; (*d*) Depression of conductivity and contractility of the heart muscle (at pH 7·0 or below). There is an arrhythmic $Paco_2$ threshold with some volatile anæsthetics. This is of the order of 96 mm. Hg with halothane and 72 mm. Hg with cyclopropane.[†]

In a healthy patient, moderate hypercapnia is well tolerated in the absence of hypoxia.

Sudden hypocapnia after a period of hypercapnia is associated with severe arrhythmias and even ventricular fibrillation in dogs, the Brown and Miller effect.[‡]

In asphyxia there is both anoxia and hypercapnia.

6. *Circulating Catecholamines.*—Adrenaline increases the conductivity, contractility, and excitability of the ventricular muscle. The latter effect leads to ventricular arrhythmias

[*] Gordon, A. S., and Jones, T. C., *J. thorac. Surg.*, 1959, **38**, 618.

[†] Price, H. L., and others, *Anesthesiology*, 1959, **20**, 563; and Price, H. L., *Ann. Surg.*, 1960, **152**, 1071.

[‡] Brown, F. B., and Miller, F., *Amer. J. Physiol.*, 1952, **169**, 56.

which are associated with an uptake of potassium by the myocardium. Rapid rise of serum adrenaline also leads to a rise of serum potassium due to release from the liver. The heart is more sensitive to adrenaline in the presence of anæsthetic drugs, especially chloroform, cyclopropane, halothane, trichloroethylene, and in the presence of myocardial hypoxia. Other causes of a rise in the blood catecholamine level include anxiety, adrenal tumours, and after haemorrhage.

7. *Effect of Non-anæsthetic Drugs.*—Large doses of digitalis, quinidine, procaine amide. Contrast media used in X-ray studies.

8. *Air Embolism.*—Air can gain access to the venous circulation through any vein if the physical factors are right. Thus a neck vein with the head raised, or a pelvic vein in the steep Trendelenburg position may, if injured, enable air-bubbles to be sucked in. This prevents proper emptying of the right heart and occlusion of the pulmonary artery. The initial signs may be cardiac irregularity or standstill and fall of blood-pressure. On auscultation, a loud pathognomonic murmur is heard with the stethoscope over the heart. Death occurs from acute circulatory obstruction. Air must be aspirated from the right ventricle before cardiac massage is instituted; otherwise it passes into the pulmonary bed where it cannot be relieved. The head-down, left lateral position results in displacement of the bolus of air to the apex of the right ventricle and thus allows blood to occupy the outflow tract of the ventricle.* Coronary artery air embolism gives rise to ventricular fibrillation which is amenable to cardiac massage which displaces the air-bubbles.

9. *Hæmorrhage.*—Massive hæmorrhage may cause cardiac arrest due to a fall in coronary perfusion pressure, especially hæmorrhage from the left atrium which interferes with filling of the left ventricle. Note also the danger of hyperkalæmia in massive transfusions of stored blood.

10. *Fainting.*—This may be fatal if the patient is prevented from assuming the horizontal position. There is a danger of this during anæsthesia (e.g., in the dental chair) and in the post-operative period if the patient is sat up in bed.†

11. *Cardiac Disease.*—Certain forms of cardiac disease are particularly prone to sudden arrest : (*a*) where there is a danger of acute circulatory obstruction (atrial myxoma or ball-valve thrombus with change of posture) ; (*b*) where the cardiac output is low and the heart cannot compensate for fall in peripheral resistance due to exercise or anæsthesia (tight valvular stenosis, constrictive pericarditis, severe pulmonary hypertension, cardiac tamponade) ; (*c*) cardiac myopathies.

* Oppenheimer, M. J., Durant, T. M., and Lynch, P., *Amer. J. med. Sci.*, 1953, **225**, 362.
† *Lancet*, 1957, **2**, 499; and Bourne, J. G., *Nitrous Oxide in Dentistry: Its Dangers and Alternatives*, 1960, p. 140. London: Lloyd-Luke.

Cardiac Arrest, *continued.*

The grossly hypertrophied or hypoxic heart is also liable to develop ventricular fibrillation if stimulated mechanically. Cardiac arrest may occur in rheumatic and diphtheritic myocarditis, toxæmia from severe infections, familial cardiomegaly, heredo-familial muscular dystrophies, and Friedrich's ataxia.

12. *Cardiac Catheterization and Angio-cardiography.*—Ventricular fibrillation may occur, most likely when the tip of the catheter is in the right ventricle. Catheterization is particularly dangerous in the presence of Ebstein's malformation of the tricuspid valve (characterized clinically by gallop rhythm, cyanosis, diastolic scratch, globular heart, clear lung fields, and right bundle-branch block), ischæmic heart disease, severe pulmonary hypertension, and left bundle-branch block. The incidence is 0·2 per cent or less, overall.

13. *Coronary Occlusion.*—Arrest is usually associated with ventricular fibrillation, but sometimes with asystole. It is thought to be due to an imbalance in electrical activity and is not necessarily related to the size of the infarct. Recovery is likely in a significant proportion of these cases of sudden arrest if treatment can be instituted at once.*

14. *Electrocution.*—This is an increasing hazard to the surgical patient with the greater use of electrical monitoring equipment, pacemakers, etc. Alternating currents are likely to be fatal at lower voltages than direct currents. Other factors include the state of the skin (i.e., wet or dry). The effect on the heart is determined by that part of the current which flows through it. Low currents cause ventricular fibrillation, high voltages cause a violent systolic contraction followed by slow relaxation after which a slow regular beat may resume. A current of i milliamps should be interrupted within t seconds for fibrillation to be prevented, in the formula:—

$$i = \frac{165}{\sqrt{t}},$$

which is valid between 8 milliseconds and 5 seconds.†

15. *Drowning.*—In fresh-water drowning there is a sudden massive ionic imbalance which gives rise to ventricular fibrillation. Asystole may be the immediate cause of death associated with hypoxia.

16. *Hypothermia.*—*See* Chapter XXIX.

PREVENTION OF CARDIAC ARREST.—Since cardiac arrest during anæsthesia is frequently associated with errors in technique, overdosage, or hypoxia, the anæsthetist must pay careful attention to the condition of his patient at all times. The experienced anæsthetist is more likely to prevent a sequence of events which may lead to cardiac arrest than a more junior colleague. Some points of particular importance may be noted :—

---

* Annotation, *Lancet*, 1960, **2**, 1333.
† Lee, W. R., *Brit. med. J.*, 1965, **2**, 616.

1. Pre-operative assessment and choice of methods.

2. Premedication with atropine to lessen the dangers of vagal inhibition. Note that atropine, 0·6 mg., does not cause complete vagal block.

3. Apparatus must be carefully maintained and safety devices incorporated where available. It should be impossible to connect cylinders to the wrong yoke. Drugs must be carefully labelled after they have been drawn up in a syringe or added to an intravenous infusion.

4. Monitoring equipment may give early warning of a dangerous situation or that cardiac arrest has in fact occurred. Thus the occurrence of extrasystoles during cyclopropane or halothane anæsthesia may be a warning to assist ventilation or reduce the inhaled concentration of the agent. Pulse monitors may also be valuable during controlled respiration when cessation of respiration would not warn the anæsthetist that cardiac arrest had occurred.

5. The anæsthetist should note the general condition of the patient and correct any undesirable departure from the norm, i.e., assist respiration, replace blood-loss, etc.

6. The anæsthetist should be particularly alert at the times when cardiac arrest most commonly occurs, viz., during induction, at the end of operation, and in the first 30–60 min. post-operatively. The post-operative recovery room is useful in maintaining careful observation at this time. The anæsthetist should not commence induction of anæsthesia for the next case until he is quite satisfied with the condition of the patient who is leaving the theatre.

DIAGNOSIS OF CARDIAC ARREST.—

1. *The Pulse.*—Inability to palpate any arterial pulsation. Note that it is sometimes impossible to feel a peripheral pulse in the obese, vasoconstricted, or shocked patient, even though a circulation to the brain is obviously maintained, since other vital functions are present. Continuous monitoring of the pulse is valuable in rapid diagnosis. The electrocardiogram is useful if it has been giving a continuous record and in the differential diagnosis between asystole and ventricular fibrillation. But normal tracings do not necessarily imply that the circulation is effective.

2. *The Pupils.*—The pupils dilate, but they may be dilated due to hypoxia, drugs, etc. The intensely constricted pupil (e.g., after morphine) may not dilate at once under arrest.

3. *Absence of Bleeding.*—Venous bleeding may occur (e.g., in the thoracotomy incision), and should not be confused with arterial bleeding which is absent.

4. *Respiration.*—Blood-flow to the respiratory centres ceases and respiratory arrest occurs, which may be preceded by some irregular gasps.

5. *On ophthalmoscopy* the veins of the fundus show segmentation of the blood column.

6. *General Appearance of the Patient.*—Cyanosis occurs and there are no signs of a circulation.

The Effects of Cardiac Arrest on the Brain.—

1. Unconsciousness supervenes in 7–8 seconds.
2. E.E.G. changes occur in 4 seconds, and the tracing is flat within 20–30 seconds.
3. The Po_2 of cerebral blood falls to 20 mm. Hg at the time consciousness is lost. Tissue Po_2 falls to zero within 1 minute.*
4. Histological changes.† Diffuse neuronal damage is not restricted to any particular vascular territory of the brain. Petechial hæmorrhages also occur. The sequence of changes in the nerve cells is: (a) Swelling of the cell, pale staining, occasional vacuoles in cytoplasm, Nissl substance fragmented; (b) Cell shrunken, darkly staining nucleus, angular outline, Nissl substance aggregated; (c) Cell disintegrates and is surrounded by small round neuroglial cells.

Treatment of Cardiac Arrest

The person who should treat cardiac arrest is the person immediately available. The anæsthetist must therefore be prepared to initiate treatment while assistance is summoned. There are two vital factors which must be accomplished quickly if adequate cerebral circulation is to be restored: *Pulmonary ventilation* and *cardiac compression or massage.* Avoid wasting time giving intracardiac injections, intravenous infusions, or waiting for asepsis.

Expired Air Ventilation.—This is the method described by Safar‡ and others. They showed that it was possible to obtain a reasonable blood oxygen level and carbon dioxide output by this method in the curarized volunteer. The patient lies in the supine position and the airway must be maintained by extending the neck and holding the jaw forwards. The nares are occluded, and the operator expires directly into the mouth of the patient. Alternatively, the mouth-to-nose method may be used. In either case, movements of the chest should be observed to check that adequate expansion of the lungs has occurred. A simple pharyngeal airway is a valuable aid, and two airways may be cemented by their flanged ends to provide a mouthpiece for the donor. The Brook airway§ is a more elaborate apparatus, which has a valve permitting exhaled gases from the patient to escape directly to the atmosphere. When available, apparatus such as the Globe resuscitator,‖ Cardiff inflating bellows,¶ Porton bellows,** self-inflating bags,†† or the anæsthetic bag and mask with an oxygen supply may be used.

I.P.P.V. with oxygen is of course always to be preferred, if available.

---

* Meyer, J. S., Gotoh, F., and Tazaki, Y., *J. Neuropath.*, 1962, **21**, 4.
† Lindenberg, R., *Amer. J. Path.*, 1956, **32**, 1147; and Lucas, B. G. B., *Proc. R. Soc. Med.*, 1950, **43**, 606.
‡ Safar, P., *J. Amer. med. Ass.*, 1958, **167**, 335.
§ Brook, M. H., and others, *Brit. med. J.*, 1962, **2**, 1564.
‖ Sykes, M. K., in *Recent Advances in Anæsthesia and Analgesia* (Ed. Hewer, C. Langton), 10th ed., 1967, Ch. 11. London: Churchill.
¶ Hilliard, E. K., and Mushin, W. W., *Brit. med. J.*, 1960, **2**, 729.
** Lucas, B. G. B., and Whitcher, H. W., *Ibid.*, 1958, **2**, 887.
†† Ruben, H., and Ruben, A., *Lancet*, 1957, **2**, 373.

Cardiac Compression.—

1. EXTERNAL CARDIAC COMPRESSION.—Developed by Kouwenhoven and others.* The heart is compressed against the vertebral bodies. The patient should be on a rigid surface such as the operating table or the floor. Pressure is applied to the lower sternum about sixty times a minute. The legs should be elevated 30° to 40° to facilitate venous return to the heart. This does not provide adequate ventilation of the lungs which must be inflated independently. Advantages lie in the simplicity of the technique and its ready applicability both inside and outside the operating theatre. It has also been applied to the newborn infant. Criticisms of the method include: (a) doubts about its effectiveness,† which is not supported by other observers,‡ (b) possibility of damage to ribs, liver, and lungs,§ (c) ventricular fibrillation cannot be treated unless an external defibrillator is available, and requires electrocardiographic diagnosis. External defibrillators utilize a high voltage and must be used with great care. (d) Should not be used for treatment of arrest due to air embolism—since massage is dangerous unless air has been aspirated from the right ventricle. This can only be done satisfactorily through the open chest. Cardiac tamponade is a contra-indication to external compression, since it is necessary to open the pericardium for drainage.

Apparatus is now available to perform cardic compression automatically, thus freeing the operator for other duties.‖

External cardiac compression should be abandoned and the chest opened: (a) when such massage is ineffective, shown by absent carotid pulse; (b) when ventricular fibrillation occurs in the absence of an external defibrillator. For a discussion on the relative efficiency of external and direct cardiac compression *see also* Sykes.¶

2. DIRECT CARDIAC COMPRESSION.—This was first done in animals by Schiff of Florence in 1874 and in man by Igelsrud in 1901. Electrical defibrillation came later, the first successful case in man being by Beck,** of Cleveland, in 1947. The first successful cardiac massage in England was by Arbuthnot Lane (1856–1943) of Guy's Hospital in 1902, at the suggestion of Ernest Starling.††

a. TRANSTHORACIC ROUTE.—This is the method of choice as it is more efficient than the abdominal approach, and also allows electrical defibrillation to take place should it be necessary.

---

* Kouwenhoven, W. B., and others, *J. Amer. med. Ass.*, 1960, **173**, 1064; and *Brit. med. J.*, 1960, **2**, 1582.
† Weale, F. E., and Rothwell-Jackson, R. L., *Lancet*, 1962, **1**, 990.
‡ Jude, J. R., Kouwenhoven, W. B., and others, *J. Amer. med. Ass.*, 1961, **178**, 1063.
§ *Brit. med. J.*, 1961, **2**, 440.
‖ Bailey, R. A., Browse, N. L., and Keating, V. J., *Brit. Heart J.*, 1964, **26**, 481; Knight, I. C. S., *Brit. med. J.*, 1964, **1**, 894; and Nachlas, M. M., and Siedband, M. P., *Amer. J. Cardiol.*, 1965, **15**, 310.
¶ Sykes, M. K., in *Recent Advances in Anæsthesia and Analgesia* (Ed. Hewer, C. Langton), 10th ed., 1967, Ch. 11. London: Churchill.
** Beck, C. S., and Mautz, F. R., *Ann. Surg.*, 1937, **106**, 525.
†† Starling, E. A., and Lane, W. A., *Lancet*, 1902, **2**, 1397.

Cardiac Compression, *continued.*

An incision, large enough to admit the hands, is made in the fourth or fifth left intercostal space, stopping 1 in. from the sternum to avoid dividing the internal mammary artery and extending to the mid-axillary line. Avoid injuring the lung by making a small hole in the pleura before incising it. The left arm of the patient should be abducted. To start with, the heart and the pericardium should be lifted up against the sternum and compressed against it 50–60 times per minute; later, if necessary, the pericardium should be incised so that the heart can be drawn out and compressed between both palms (not finger-tips—for fear of cardiac rupture). A rib retractor may be necessary after a minute or two, to ease the pressure on the surgeon's wrists. Time must be allowed for the refilling of the heart after each compression; elevation of the legs and intravenous infusion will encourage filling. When oxygenated blood has been squeezed from the heart into the aorta for a minute or two, the situation is reviewed, and the diagnosis made of asystole or ventricular fibrillation, the former being more common.

Further Treatment of Asystole.—This is not standardized, but the following measures have been suggested: (i) Continue cardiac compression until a normal beat returns. (ii) If the returning beat is weak, stimulate the myocardium by injection into the left auricle—or the thoracic aorta proximal to a clamp applied to divert all the circulating blood towards the brain—of 3–5 ml. of a mixture of noradrenaline in saline (1 ml. of 1–1000 solution to 10 ml.).* (iii) If the response is still unsatisfactory, 10 ml. of 1 per cent calcium chloride or 5–10 ml. of 10 per cent calcium gluconate† should be similarly injected to restore the cardiac tone. These injections may initiate ventricular fibrillation, which must be appropriately treated. Pumping may be necessary for a long period.

Further Treatment of Fibrillation.—After the tone of the heart muscle has been improved by compression for several minutes and the fine almost invisible fibrillation gives way to coarse fibrillation, electrical defibrillation must be attempted. Adrenaline 0·5–2·0 ml. of 1 in 10,000 solution may be injected into the right ventricle to convert a slow fibrillation to a rapid fibrillation prior to administering the shock. Correction of metabolic acidosis is also an aid to successful defibrillation. The average adult can safely be given 200 ml. of 2·74 per cent $NaHCO_3$ (67 mEq.) in 10–15 minutes, and 500 ml. (166 mEq.) should be given over 20–30 minutes if necessary. Calcium salts can also be used to convert slow to rapid fibrillation. In the adult 5 ml. of 10 per cent calcium gluconate can be injected into the right ventricle and repeated. Calcium chloride, which is more

* McMillan, I. K. R., Cockett, F. B., and Styles, P., *Thorax,* 1952, **7**, 205; and Redding, J. S., and Pearson, J. W., *Anesthesiology,* 1963, **24**, 203.
† Milstein, B. B., *Proc. R. Soc. Med.,* 1960, **53**, 845.

highly ionized, may be preferable. The passage of an electrical current through the heart causes all its muscular fibres to have their refractory period simultaneously: a normal beat is then stimulated by manual compression.

i. *A.C. defibrillation*: (α) 50–300 V. internally; (β) 300–750 V. externally. The current is passed for 0·1–0·2 second with increments of 50–100 V. if necessary. Sometimes a series of shocks at 0·5-second intervals succeed after failure with a single shock.

ii. *D.C. defibrillation*: (α) 15–100 watt-seconds internally; (β) 100–400 watt-seconds externally. The D.C. shock is produced by the discharge from a condenser, is of brief duration, and is measured in watt-seconds or joules. D.C. defibrillation is now displacing A.C. defibrillation as it is thought to be more effective and to cause less myocardial damage.* D.C. defibrillators can also be used for synchronous discharge in the treatment of atrial fibrillation or ventricular tachycardia.

The operating team should wear rubber gloves to protect themselves from electric shock. If electrical methods are unavailable or unsuccessful, 5 ml. of 4 per cent potassium chloride, 10 ml. of 1 per cent procaine in doses of 100–200 mg., or lignocaine 25 mg. (2·5 ml. of 1 per cent solution), may be tried. The chest should not be closed until the heart has been beating healthily for some minutes. The pericardium is partly closed by interrupted sutures, leaving plenty of room for drainage of fluid which may otherwise collect, and the costal cartilages sutured if they have been divided, and the chest closed using an underwater seal.

For simple units for testing defibrillators, *see* Hesse, G. E., *Anæsthesia*, 1965, **20**, 215.

b. TRANSABDOMINAL ROUTE.—This should be tried only if the abdomen is already open, and while the surgeon is opening the thorax, by one hand under the diaphragm and the other over the sternum. Very rarely, it may be the only practicable method because of fixation of the chest wall.† Pumping is carried out as above. If after half a minute the heart-beat has not been restored, the transthoracic approach should be proceeded with.

To raise the blood-pressure and stimulate the coronary circulation once the beat has been restored, noradrenaline is useful, as it is, in addition to being a coronary dilator, a general vasoconstrictor. It has little direct effect on the myocardium. It should be injected into the ventricle or into the great veins. Ampoules of noradrenaline each containing 200 micrograms in 2 ml. should be readily available for resuscitation: up to 100 micrograms may be used. Isoprenaline sulphate may be useful when myocardial contraction is weak and the rate slow. Acting almost exclusively on the β-receptors it is a potent

---

* Cox, A. R., Dodds, W. A., and Trapp, W. G., *Canad. med. Ass. J.*, 1963, **89**, 1193.
† Feldman, S. and Ellis, H., *Principles of Resuscitation*, 1967. Oxford: Blackwell.

Cardiac Compression, *continued.*

cardiac stimulant; 2 mg. may be added to 540 ml. isotonic saline and infused at a rate just sufficient to maintain adequate blood-pressure. β-adrenergic blocking agents, propranolol 10–20 mg. i.v., may sometimes be of value in preventing a recurrence of ventricular fibrillation.* The blood-pressure may need support for some hours from intravenous infusions. Hydrocortisone, 100–300 mg. i.v., may also have a pressor effect. To aid the circulation further, Woodward† recommends the application of Esmarch bandages to the elevated limbs, especially when collapse follows shock or spinal analgesia.

Biochemical Changes during Cardiac Arrest.—These occur as a result of tissue hypoxia, and inadequate removal of the products of metabolism. Even with external or internal cardiac compression, the flow of blood is not sufficient to perfuse tissues normally. There is thus a maximum arteriovenous-oxygen and carbon-dioxide difference. As a result of tissue hypoxia, there is a movement of water and sodium into the cells and a movement of potassium ions out of cells into extracellular fluid. This results in a rise in packed-cell volume, and in plasma proteins, while plasma-potassium concentration can reach levels as high as 7 mEq./l. in a few minutes. There is a rise in lactic acid in the blood, together with a fall of bicarbonate. pH may fall to levels as low as 6·8 or 6·9. Blood-sugar also rises as a result of hypoxia and levels of 300–400 mg. per cent are commonly observed.

CORRECTION.—*Bicarbonate infusion* is given to correct the metabolic acidosis. About 500–1000 ml. of 2·75 per cent solution may be required in an adult, with further doses on subsequent days as indicated by biochemical measurement of the deficit. It has been suggested that the initial dose may be related to the estimated duration of arrest‡:—

Dose of bicarbonate in mEq. =

$$\frac{\text{Wt. of patient in kg.}}{5} \times \frac{\text{Duration of arrest in minutes}}{2}.$$

Calcium ions act upon the myocardium as an antagonist to potassium ions. Calcium chloride may be preferable to the gluconate since it is more highly ionized. Calcium can itself cause ventricular fibrillation, especially in the presence of digitalis intoxication, though this may be neutralized by the use of potassium. Calcium is less effective in the presence of metabolic acidosis.

THAM (Tri-hydroxymethyl-amino-methane; tromethamine) is also effective in assisting defibrillation of the heart. It can enter cells to neutralize intracellular acidosis. It lowers blood-sugar and plasma potassium, and corrects acidosis.§

AFTER TREATMENT.—The main cause of hypoxic brain damage is cerebral œdema from damage to the cerebral capillaries.

* Sloman, G., Robinson, J. S., and McLean, K., *Brit. med. J.*, 1965, **1**, 895.
† Woodward, W. W., *Lancet*, 1960, **2**, 1120.
‡ Gilston, A., *Ibid.*, 1965, **2**, 1039.
§ Nahas, G. G., *Clin. Pharmac. Therap.*, 1963, **4**, 784.

CLINICAL SIGNS OF CEREBRAL HYPOXIA.—These may follow either an acute hypoxic episode after cardiac standstill or a prolonged period of suboxygenation. Recovery may occur after the episode and the patient may regain consciousness after the anæsthetic, but may relapse into coma later. Respiration is gasping and stertorous and may be accompanied by a tracheal tug. There may be sweating, hyperpyrexia, dilated pupils, and a coarse nystagmus. There may be restlessness, rigidity, choreo-athetosis, or fits and twitching. These may progress to deepening coma, periodic breathing, tachycardia, and death.

TREATMENT.—Dehydration. This must be started early and the following solutions may be used: (1) Urea, 30 per cent in invert sugar which is longer lasting and three times more powerful as an osmotic agent than glucose. Dose 1 g. per kilo infused over 1-hour period, then half this amount over the next 4 hours if necessary. (2) Mannitol 20 per cent, 1 litre per 24 hours. (3) Sucrose in 50 per cent solution, intravenously, 50 ml., then a further similar dose in half an hour, if necessary. It is excreted by the kidneys and does not pass into the theca. (4) Dextran 10 per cent. (5) Quadruple strength plasma. (6) Massive doses of hydrocortisone.

The following measures may be required. Reduction of body temperature by surface cooling. Elevation of the head. Support of the circulation ; physiotherapy ; antibiotics ; tracheostomy and respiratory assistance or control. (*See* Cope, D. H. P., *Proc. R. Soc. Med.*, 1960, **53**, 678, and subsequent discussion.)

The use of induced hypothermia to combat the sequelæ of cerebral hypoxia has been questioned since there is little evidence that induced hypothermia is of therapeutic value. It has been suggested that the use of hypothermia be limited to the prevention of hyperpyrexia following brain injury from any cause.*

RESPONSIBILITY FOR DEATH ASSOCIATED WITH OPERATION.—In the case of a death on the operating table, legal responsibility will exist only if either the surgeon or the anæsthetist has failed in the proper execution of his functions as a person of professional skill. The anæsthetist, no more than the surgeon, is legally responsible if death has resulted from a genuine error of judgement, but he is expected to exercise care, skill, and judgement in all that has to do with the anæsthetic procedure, including the assessment of the patient's fitness to withstand the strain of anæsthesia successfully. The actual decision to operate together with the choice of operation is the responsibility of the surgeon.

DROWNING

About 2000 fatalities from drowning occur in the U.K. every year, about a quarter in the sea.

---

* Strong, M. J., and Keats, A. S., *Anesthesiology*, 1967, **28**, 920.

Fresh Water.—Due to the difference in osmotic pressure, water passes rapidly from the lungs to the general circulation. There may be a 50 per cent increase in circulatory volume within 3 min. This results in hæmolysis, and ventricular fibrillation, resistant to treatment, occurs at an early stage. The heart is submitted to hypoxia, over-filling, potassium excess, and sodium deficit. The clinical features can be demonstrated readily in animals, but there is evidence that the hæmodilution is much less in man, and it is possible that some other factor may be operative.* The prognosis is poor.

Salt Water.—The osmotic effect is exerted in the opposite direction. Fluid passes out from the circulation into the alveoli to produce pulmonary œdema.

Vagal Inhibition.—Death from vagal inhibition can occur without entrance of fluid into the lungs. Or vagal inhibition may prevent fluid entering the lungs for several minutes. Prompt resuscitation is likely to be successful in this type of case.

Treatment.—Speed is vital. Experiments in Denmark on cadavers suggest that the lungs cannot be emptied by posture, and that regurgitation from the stomach does not occur except with inflation pressures greater than 25 cm. H_2O. Treatment should consist of: (i) very quick efforts to clear the mouth and pharynx of debris; (ii) artificial ventilation, mouth-to-mouth, mouth-to-nose, or by means of an apparatus, if possible while the subject is still in the water; (iii) external cardiac compression; (iv) exchange transfusion.

Prognosis.—Better after immersion in salt water than in fresh water. Recovery unlikely if the lungs have been flooded with fresh water for a period of over 2 min., owing to the rapid circulatory changes with irreversible ventricular fibrillation. However, a case has recently been reported when a 5-year-old boy survived a period of 22 min. immersion in fresh water in conditions of hypothermia.†

RESPIRATORY INSUFFICIENCY

The anæsthetist has a most useful part to play (with his colleagues) in the management of patients suffering from respiratory insufficiency.

Causes of Respiratory Failure.—

1. ORGANIC DISEASE OF THE CENTRAL NERVOUS SYSTEM.—
   a. Bulbospinal poliomyelitis.
   b. Encephalitis lethargica.
   c. Polyneuritis.
   d. Spinal cord injury.
   e. Acute cerebral compression.
   f. Brain-stem hæmorrhage.
   g. Motor neuron disease.

2. DISEASES INVOLVING MUSCLES.—
   a. Myasthenia gravis.
   b. Dystrophia myotonica.

---

* Fuller, R. H., *Milit. Med.*, 1963, **128**, 22.
† Kvittingen, T. D., and Naess, A., *Brit. med. J.*, 1963, **1**, 1315.

3. POISONING BY.—
   a. Narcotics.
   b. Coal gas.
   c. Strychnine.
   d. Anticholinesterases.
   e. Carbon dioxide narcosis.
4. CHEST DISEASE AND CHEST SURGERY.—
   a. Emphysema.*
   b. Kyphoscoliosis.
   c. Cor pulmonale.
   d. Stove-in chest.
   e. Status asthmaticus.
5. TETANUS.
6. STATUS EPILEPTICUS.†
7. IATROGENIC.—
   a. Prolonged effect of neuromuscular relaxants.
   b. Neuromuscular block due to antibiotics.
   c. High subarachnoid or extradural block.
   d. Hyperventilation.
   e. Depression of respiratory centre by drugs.
8. RESPIRATORY DISTRESS OF THE NEWBORN.

The Airway.—Respiratory obstruction must be relieved at once, by supporting the jaw. A pharyngeal airway may be useful, but endotracheal intubation is preferable when respiratory insufficiency is other than short term. Direct laryngoscopy may not be easy unless the patient is in deep coma, but the experienced anæsthetist can pass a blind nasal tube in a high proportion of cases, with little disturbance to the patient. Tracheostomy may be considered later.

Prolonged Nasotracheal Intubation.‡—This has recently been advocated as an alternative to tracheostomy in infants and young children where the incidence of complications is unduly high.§ Tubes have been left in situ for up to 4 weeks. The Jackson Rees tube has been devised to facilitate management.‖

TRACHEOSTOMY

History.—Performed by Pedro Virgili (1699–1776) of Cadiz for the relief of quinsy. George Martine (1702–41) was the first to employ it in a case of diphtheria in Britain. Heister introduced the term "tracheotomy" in place of "bronchotomy" in 1718 and this gave place to "tracheostomy" at the suggestion of Negus in 1938 (*see* Wath, J. M., *Brit. J. Surg.*, 1963, **50**, 954).

Tracheostomy reduces the anatomical dead-space by 30–50 per cent.

---

* Bradley, R. D., and others, *Lancet*, 1964, **1**, 854.
† Robinson, J. S., and others, *Ibid.*, 1964, **1**, 770.
‡ McDonald, I. H., and Stocks, J. J., *Brit. J. Anæsth.*, 1965, **37**, 161; Allen, T. H., and Stevens, I. M., *Ibid.*, 1965, **37**, 566; and Coul, J. F., and Wolffensperger, W. A. G., *Anæsthesia*, 1965, **20**, 227.
§ Glas, W. W., King, O. J., and Lui, A., *Arch. Surg., Chicago*, 1962, **85**, 56.
‖ Jackson Rees, G., and Owen-Thomas, J. B., *Brit. J. Anæsth.*, 1966, **38**, 901.

Indications in Resuscitation.—
1. In obstruction of the upper airway.
2. To permit artificial ventilation.
3. For aspiration of the bronchial tree.
4. To prevent inhalation of foreign material, usually in the unconscious patient.
5. To reduce dead space when respiration is handicapped.

Except in the rare case of sudden complete obstruction to the upper airway, tracheostomy is not an operation of extreme urgency. It is best performed after transfer to an operating theatre where adequate lighting and skilled help are available. It is usually possible to maintain artificial ventilation and to keep a clear airway by means of an endotracheal tube, intermittent suction, and intermittent positive-pressure ventilation.

Apparatus Required.—Although emergency tracheostomy has on occasion been carried out with simple instruments, such as scissors or penknife, it is desirable to have a proper range of instruments available. An emergency tracheostomy set should include scalpel, dissecting forceps, artery forceps, small retractors, scissors, a selection of tracheostomy tubes and tapes, tracheal dilators, cricoid hook, ligatures and needles, swabs and towels, syringes and needles for local analgesia (if necessary). Suction apparatus should be available.

Technique.*—General anæsthesia is preferable to local analgesia unless it is contra-indicated. Prior intubation of the trachea is useful to maintain a clear airway, when the operation is performed under general anæsthesia or on the unconscious patient. In children the presence of an endotracheal tube aids identification of the soft trachea. The endotracheal tube should be withdrawn as the tracheostomy tube is inserted.

The position of the patient is important. The neck should be extended by placing a sandbag between the shoulders. This may, however, sometimes render a partially obstructed airway completely obstructed, and the patient should be carefully observed at this time.

The incision may be vertical from the lower thyroid border to the suprasternal notch, or transverse midway along this line. While the latter may be better from the cosmetic point of view, the former is recommended for the tiro.

Dissection should be continued in the midline, to keep away from the major vessels in the neck. The pre-tracheal muscles may be held apart by retractors. If necessary the isthmus of the thyroid gland is divided between clamps.

The trachea is opened, after injection of 4 per cent lignocaine into the lumen, by a small transverse incision between the second and third rings. A window is cut by removing portions of the front of the second and third or third and fourth rings. Experienced

---

* *See also* Wilson, K., *Proc. R. Soc. Med.*, 1966, **59**, 32.

surgeons may fashion a flap from the trachea to the lower skin incision (Björk) to aid changing of tubes.

After insertion of the tracheostomy tube, which should be of the largest size which will fit comfortably, the wound is loosely closed with a few skin stitches and dressed with petroleum-jelly gauze.

Mediastinal emphysema and pneumothorax are frequent complications of tracheostomy and can be prevented more easily when the operation is planned than when it is done in an emergency. Their cause is the increased negative intrathoracic pressure resulting from the obstruction and this results in air being sucked into the wound before the trachea is opened.

Types of Tube.—

1. The King's College Hospital pattern silver tube. Size 32 or 34 for men. Size 28 for women. The lumen is relatively large in proportion to the diameter, and the inner tube can easily be removed for cleaning. Later a valved tube can be inserted which enables the patient to speak.

2. Cuffed plastic tracheostomy tube. The cuff can be inflated to prevent pharyngeal secretions passing into the tracheobronchial tree and to prevent escape of gas during intermittent positive-pressure ventilation.

3. Radcliffe tracheostomy tube. Made of rubber. Provided with inflatable cuff. A magnetic insert can be used to discourage separation from airway connexions during intermittent positive-pressure ventilation.[*]

Laryngostomy.

—Easier to perform than tracheostomy, but may be followed by permanent narrowing of larynx. A transverse incision of the skin is made between the thyroid and cricoid cartilages, with the patient's neck extended. With an introducer or artery forceps the cricothyroid membrane is pierced and the short, flat laryngostomy tube or any available tube introduced and secured.[†] As soon as possible it should be converted to a formal tracheostomy, certainly within 24 hours, to lessen the danger of subsequent stenosis. Should not be done in children.

As a desperate measure if the patient is *in extremis*, a large-bore needle may be inserted through the cricothyroid membrane into the larynx and through it either air is rapidly injected with a syringe, or oxygen is delivered to the needle under slight pressure: allowance must of course be made for emptying the lungs.

Complications of Tracheostomy.—

1. EARLY COMPLICATIONS INCLUDE.—Hæmorrhage; displacement or obstruction of the tube; injury to the trachea, tracheitis, crust formation; respiratory complications; surgical emphysema and pneumothorax.

2. INFECTION.—May arise from: (a) Contamination during tracheal suction. Aseptic 'no-touch' methods,[‡] with the use of disposable

* Agerholm, M., and Salt, R. H., *Lancet*, 1965, **1**, 468.
† Cawthorne, T., *Ibid.*, 1964, **1**, 1081.
‡ Plum, F., and Dunning, M. F., *New Engl. J. Med.*, 1956, **254**, 193.

Complications of Tracheostomy, *continued.*

gloves, helps to minimize this; (*b*) The wound itself is liable to become infected. Hourly spraying with polybactrin aerosol is helpful, and so is application of nystatin; (*c*) The humidifier.* This can be prevented by raising the temperature of the water to 140° F. (60° C.) so that pasteurization occurs.† Despite all measures, tracheostomy wounds may become infected. Most serious is the antibiotic-resistant Staphylococcus. Cross-infection with *Pseudomonas pyocyaneus* and *Bacillus proteus* may occur also.

3. TRACHEAL ULCERATION.—Erosions of the tracheal mucous membrane are not uncommon.‡ In some cases, ulceration has produced exposure of the tracheal rings, secondary hæmorrhage from erosion of a major vessel, and even ulceration into the œsophagus.

4. TRACHEAL DILATATION.§ Mechanism not fully understood.

5. TRACHEAL STENOSIS.‖—A fibrous, granulomatous, polypoid mass may form, probably due to irritation from the tracheostomy tube. Such cases will require dilatation.

The operation of tracheostomy is not without risk. McClelland¶ found an overall mortality of 3·4 per cent over a 10-year period. The incidence of complications is higher in children.

Humidification.—When the normal humidifying mechanisms of the upper respiratory tract are by-passed by an endotracheal tube or tracheostomy, there is a tendency for fibrinous exudation with crusting to occur in the trachea and larger bronchi. In 1 hour, 20 ml. water are lost from the lungs. This represents 480 ml. water vapour per minute.

During artificial ventilation a humidifier should be incorporated between the ventilator and the patient. During spontaneous respiration through a tracheostomy, crusting can be discouraged by blowing humidified air into a plastic mask fitting loosely over the tracheostomy.**

METHODS OF HUMIDIFICATION.††—

1. The classic humidifier is a can of warm water over which the gases are blown. Tubing between humidifier and patient should be lagged to prevent condensation. A water trap placed between expired gases and a volume meter helps to prevent false readings caused by condensation. Colonization by bacteria has proved to be a major disadvantage, but it can be prevented if a temperature of the water is maintained at 140° F. (60° C.) so that a process of pasteurization occurs.‡‡

2. Nebulizers are used to produce a supersaturated mist.

---

* Bradley, R. D., Spencer, G. T., and Semples, S. J. G., *Lancet*, 1964, **1**, 854.
† Phillips, I., and Spencer, G. T., *Ibid.*, 1965, **2**, 1325.
‡ Stiles, P. J., *Thorax*, 1965, **20**, 517.
§ Robbie, D. S., and Feldman, S. A., *Brit. J. Anæsth.*, 1963, **35**, 771.
‖ Hunter, A. R., *Recent Advances in Anæsthesia and Analgesia* (Ed. Hewer, C. Langton), 10th ed., 1967, Ch. 8. London: Churchill.
¶ McClelland, R. M. A., *Brit. med. J.*, 1965, **2**, 567.
** Spalding, J. M. K., *Lancet*, 1956, **2**, 1140.
†† *See also* Morgan, J. G., in *Modern Trends in Anæsthesia*, No. 3 (Ed. Evans, F. T., and Gray, T. C.), 1967. London: Butterworths.
‡‡ Phillips, I. and Spencer, G. T., *Lancet*, 1965, **2**, 1325.

3. **Ultrasonic humidifiers.*** Water drops on to a vibrating plate and is broken up into particles of 1–2 micron size.

4. **Condenser humidifiers** ('artificial nose').† Layers of wire gauze may be interposed between the tracheostomy tube and the external air. May offer some resistance to respiration.‡ Can also act as reservoirs of infection.§

5. **A simple method,** requiring no sophisticated apparatus, is to insufflate oxygen via a catheter placed in the mouth of the tracheostomy tube, at 2 l. per min. A fine needle is inserted through the wall of the catheter and water allowed to pass through at a rate of 4 drops per min., using a standard transfusion set.

6. **Acetylcysteine** (Airbron). Useful for the liquefaction of sputum. It is dropped down the airway in 5–10 per cent solution or nebulized in 20 per cent solution. Not more than 2 ml. should be used at one time.

Whatever method of humidification is used it is important to make sure that the patient is well hydrated.

Nursing Care of Patient with Tracheostomy.‖—The following points are important :—

1. All conscious patients should have a bell, pencil and paper, and mirror at hand.

2. Clean the inner tube of a silver tracheostomy tube at regular (4-hourly) intervals.

3. Deflate the cuff of a cuffed tube at regular intervals (4-hourly) and re-inflate the cuff with just enough air to make an air-tight seal. Suck out the pharynx before, and the trachea after, carrying out such a manœuvre.

4. Use a humidifier to prevent crusting. Maintain hydration.

5. Suck out trachea as indicated. All catheters should be sterile and used only once.

6. Sterile dressing to tracheostomy wound daily.

Artificial Ventilation of the Lungs.—*See* Chapter VIII.

Oxygen Therapy.—*See* Chapter X.

(*See also* Feldman, S., and Ellis, H., *Principles of Resuscitation*, 1967. Oxford: Blackwell; Brooks, D. K., *Resuscitation*, 1967. London: Arnold; and Sykes, M. K., *Recent Advances in Anæsthesia and Analgesia* (Ed. Hewer, C. Langton), 10th ed., 1967, Ch. 11. London: Churchill.)

---

* Herzog, P., Norlander, O., and Engström, G.-G., *Acta anæsth. scand.*, 1964, **8**, 79.

† Walley, R. V., *Lancet*, 1956, **1**, 781; and Mapleson, W. W., Morgan, J. G., and Hillard, E. K., *Brit. med. J.*, 1963, **1**, 300.

‡ Hingorani, B. K., *Brit. J. Anæsth.*, 1965, **37**, 454.

§ Pennington, J. H., Lumley, J., and O'Grady, F., *Anæsthesia*, 1966, **21**, 211.

‖ Robbie, D. S., and Feldman, S. A., *Brit. J. Anæsth.*, 1963, **35**, 771 ; and Matheson, M. A., and others, *Lancet*, 1963, **2**, 31.

CHAPTER XXXV

THE INTENSIVE THERAPY UNIT

These units provide for the management of the critically ill patient who requires facilities greater than those available in the traditional ward. They provide additional space, staff, and equipment. The vital functions of the body can be continuously observed and when necessary supported promptly and efficiently.

The criteria for admission to the unit have yet to be fully established and will vary from hospital to hospital. Certain broad groups may be defined:—

1. Patients requiring the use of an artificial machine to support a vital system (e.g., ventilator, renal dialysis, pacemaker).
2. Patients requiring continuous monitoring (e.g., certain cases of cardiac infarction).
3. Patients with complex metabolic disturbances.
4. Head injuries and multiple injuries, including stove-in chests.
5. Those who require heavy or specialized nursing (e.g., difficult tracheostomy, the comatose patient).

Patients should not be admitted to an intensive therapy unit when the disease process is irreversible. The number of beds set aside for this purpose has been stated to be 1 per cent of the acute bed complement of a hospital.*

The anæsthetist, because of his special knowledge and experience of ventilatory and resuscitation problems, has a major role to play in the management of patients in the unit.

Design of the Unit.†—A unit of 6–8 beds is an economic size. The plan should be as flexible as possible to allow for future changes. Mobile partitions are useful. About 200–300 sq. ft. floor space should be allowed for each bed. The danger of cross-infection is a particular hazard. Division into cubicles and the wearing of gowns and masks by staff help to reduce this. Equipment must be sterilized between use. Adequate storage space for equipment must be provided, and a small laboratory is advantageous.

ACUTE MYOCARDIAL INFARCTION‡

Patients with recent infarction are liable to develop cardiac asystole or ventricular fibrillation. This is thought to be due to an electrical imbalance in the myocardium and is not necessarily related to the size of the infarct. If resuscitation can be carried out promptly, and cerebral hypoxia is prevented, there is a good chance of restoration of cardiac function and the prognosis is hopeful.

Such patients require intensive monitoring. The electrocardiogram is usually recorded continuously, and alarm systems are activated if the

---

* B.M.A. Planning Unit Report No. 1, *Intensive Care*, November, 1967.
† Robinson, J. S., *Brit. J. Anæsth.*, 1966, **38**, 132; Sherwood Jones, E., *Postgrad. med. J.*, 1967, **43**, 339; and B.M.A. Planning Unit Report No. 1, *Intensive Care*, November, 1967.
‡ *See also* Annotation, *Lancet*, 1967, **2**, 665; Brooks, D. K., *Resuscitation*, 1967, p. 206 *et seq.* London: Arnold; and Lawrie, D. M., and others, *Lancet*, 1967, **2**, 109.

heart-rate rises above or falls below preset limits. Apparatus for cardiac resuscitation is kept immediately at hand so that defibrillation or cardiac pacing can be carried out at once if required. The electrocardiogram reflects the electrical activity of the heart and provides information about the nature of arrhythmias which may develop. It is not, however, a measure of the hæmodynamic action of the heart muscle, and it is possible to have a normal electrocardiogram in the presence of grave hypotension and inadequate tissue perfusion. Bloodpressure must therefore be recorded frequently and some workers prefer a direct arterial line for continuous recording. In certain specialized units a multiplicity of parameters are monitored. They may include electrocardiogram, arterial blood-pressure, central venous pressure, and blood-gas analysis.*

Treatment.—

1. RELIEF OF PAIN.—Morphine is given for relief of severe pain in doses of 10–15 mg. In the shocked patient it may be given intravenously slowly. Some workers prefer diamorphine (heroin), as it is thought to have fewer side-effects (e.g., vomiting).

2. OXYGEN.—May be given by mask or tent. Hyperbaric oxygen has been used.†

3. ARRHYTHMIAS.‡—About 80 per cent of patients show some form of arrhythmia in the first few days following infarction. Occasional atrial or ventricular ectopic beats may be ignored. Treatment is recommended if they occur early in the cardiac cycle, in salvos of two or more, or at a frequency greater than 5 per minute. Slow intravenous injection of lignocaine 25–75 mg. (or 1–2 mg. per kg.) is now commonly advocated.§ Otherwise procainamide at a rate not exceeding 100 mg. per min. may be tried. Oral quinidine 100–200 mg. 4-hourly or oral procainamide 200–600 mg. 4-hourly are also used. Supraventricular bradycardia may be treated by atropine in doses of 0·3 mg. up to a total of 2 mg. Heart block, when complete and associated with a failing circulation, must be treated by electrical pacing. The use of β-adrenergic blocking agents is controversial because of their negative inotropic effect.

4. CARDIAC SHOCK.—Some authorities recommend the use of pressor agents, since profound hypertension is frequently fatal in outcome. Failure to raise blood-pressure results in further impairment of coronary perfusion. L-Noradrenaline can be used if other pressor drugs are ineffective, though it will not be effective if gross metabolic acidosis is present. Infusion of dextrose solution has also been recommended.‖

5. DIGITALIS.—This may be indicated in the presence of cardiac shock. It may be given intravenously if there has been no digitalis administered during the previous 5–6 weeks. The

---

* Shillingford, J. P., *Proc. R. Soc. Med.*, 1965, **58**, 101.

† Moon, A. J., Williams, K. G., and Hopkinson, W. I., *Lancet*, 1964, **1**, 18; and Cameron, A. J. V., Hutton, I., Kenmuir, A. C. F., and Murdoch, W. R., *Ibid.*,, 1966, **2**, 833.

‡ *See also* McNicol, M. W., *Postgrad. med. J.*, 1967, **43**, 207.

§ Spracklen, F. H. N., and others, *Brit. med. J.*, 1968, **1**, 89.

‖ Nixon, P. G. F., and others, *Postgrad. med. J.*, 1967, **43**, 212; and Annotation, *Brit. med. J.*, 1966, **2**, 481.

Acute Myocardial Infarction—Treatment, *continued.*

most rapidly acting digitalis preparation is oubain, digitalizing dose 0·25–0·75 mg. Otherwise, digoxin, 0·75–1·0 mg., may be given.

6. CORTICOSTEROIDS.—Intravenous hydrocortisone may have a profound effect on cardiac shock. Large doses may be required, 100 mg. i.v. every 10 minutes up to 300 mg., then 100 mg. every 2 hours for a further four or five doses. Steroids should always be given when there is a history of steroid therapy in the previous 2 years.

7. ANTICOAGULANTS.—Heparin may be given if anticoagulant therapy is decided upon.

8. CARDIAC FAILURE.—If failure occurs, it must be treated along conventional medical lines.

9. MEASUREMENT OF ACID-BASE STATE.—This may show the presence of metabolic acidosis. Non-acidotic patients probably have a better prognosis, and when acidosis is present, correction with intravenous sodium bicarbonate may result in a rise in systolic blood-pressure.[*]

10. POTASSIUM AND GLUCOSE BY MOUTH, TOGETHER WITH SUBCUTANEOUS INSULIN.—May favour potassium entry into damaged cardiac cells with resulting diminution of the effects of ischæmia and reduction of incidence of arrhythmias.[†]

11. SLEEP RÉGIME.—Maintaining the patient in a light sleep by means of pethidine and promethazine for 1–7 days, waking him thrice daily for feeding, washing, and physiotherapy.[‡]

ACUTE EXACERBATIONS OF CHRONIC BRONCHITIS AND EMPHYSEMA

An acute infection may precipitate acute respiratory failure. Arterial oxygen tension falls and arterial carbon dioxide tension rises. Respiration is maintained by the hypoxic drive via the carotid body reflexes. There is a danger that oxygen administration may remove this so that further depression of respiration occurs and a state of carbon dioxide narcosis results. Oxygen must, however, be administered to relieve hypoxia and respiration maintained. This may be achieved by :—

1. The use of controlled concentrations of oxygen.[§] Hypoxic hypoxia is always very sensitive to the PO_2 of the inspired air. Raising this from normal 150 mm. to 200 mm. Hg (28 per cent O_2) has a very significant effect. Intermittent oxygen therapy may be dangerous because on cessation hypoxia may become intense while retained carbon dioxide is excreted. In patients with carbon dioxide retention the inspired oxygen concentration should be increased gradually.

2. Respiratory stimulants (nikethamide, amiphenazole, vanillic acid diethylamide). May be useful in marginal cases.

3. Trometamol (THAM tri-hydroxymethyl-amino-methane; tromethamine). A buffering agent, at present experimental.

4. Intermittent positive-pressure ventilation via tracheostome.

[*] Neaverson, M. A., *Brit. med. J.*, 1966, **2**, 383.
[†] Mittra, B., *Lancet*, 1965, **2**, 607.
[‡] Nixon, P. G. F., and others, *Ibid.*, 1968, **1**, 726.
[§] Campbell, E. J. M., *Ibid.*, 1960, **2**, 10.

STATUS ASTHMATICUS

Status asthmaticus can be defined as a severe episode of broncho-spasm, causing distress to the patient, and not relieved by conventional therapy. Reports of deaths show an incidence of between 1·6 and 7·07 per 100,000 population per annum in various series.*

Treatment.†—

1. OXYGEN.—Arterial oxygen tensions as low as 30 mm. Hg are common in severe cases. The aim should be to maintain it above 50 mm. Hg. As hypercapnia may be present and the chemo-receptor drive lost, oxygen must be given with care, in controlled concentrations.

2. BRONCHODILATORS.—Adrenaline subcutaneously 0·5–1·0 ml. of 1 in 1000 solution over 10 minutes is a time-honoured therapy. Subjective relief does not correlate with P_aO_2 and its use is now questioned. Aminophylline may be given intravenously or per rectum. Oral treatment is not satisfactory in the acute case. Isoprenaline is useful as an aerosol inhalation.

3. CORTICOSTEROIDS.—These should be given, especially when the patient is already on long-term steroid therapy.

4. ANTIBIOTICS.—Unless the precipitatory factor is obviously allergic or psychological, it is wise to give a bactericidal anti-biotic such as penicillin and streptomycin or ampicillin.

5. FLUID REPLACEMENT to correct dehydration.

6. SEDATION.—Drugs which cause respiratory depression should be avoided unless I.P.P.V. is being undertaken. Promazine, 50–100 mg. intramuscularly, or amylobarbitone sodium, 100–200 mg. orally, are recommended.

7. RESUSCITATION of the moribund asthmatic who has failed to respond to the above measures may require I.P.P.V.* and bronchial lavage.‡ Relatively large inflation pressures may be required.

POLIOMYELITIS

This may be : (a) Spinal, (b) Bulbar, (c) Bulbospinal.

a. Spinal poliomyelitis may cause respiratory paralysis but gives rise to no trouble with upper respiratory tract secretions and can be treated in a cabinet respirator (iron-lung), or in mild or recovering cases in a cuirass respirator. When the vital capacity is less than 50 per cent of normal, such an appliance should be used.

b. Bulbar poliomyelitis patients can breathe but cannot maintain the integrity of their upper air-passages. The semi-prone, head-down position, together with suction, will keep such patients from harm. Intubation is not necessary.

c. Bulbospinal poliomyelitis is the dangerous type, especially if the bulbar component is not noticed at the beginning of treatment in the cabinet respirator. A patient lying supine in such a respirator will, if he vomits (a likely event in this

---

* Rees, H. A., *Postgrad. med. J.*, 1967, **43**, 225.
† Riding, W. D., and Ambiavagar, M., *Ibid.*, 1967, **43**, 234; and Ambiavagar, M., and Sherwood Jones, E., *Anæsthesia*, 1967, **22**, 375.
‡ Thompson, H. T., and others, *Thorax*, 1966, **21**, 557.

Poliomyelitis, *continued.*

illness), have the vomitus drawn into his lungs by the pressure changes induced by the machine. Saliva collects in the pharynx where it may obstruct respiration or be inhaled into the tracheobronchial tree.

Signs of bulbar involvement are : (i) A rattle in the throat ; (ii) Dysphagia ; (iii) Dysphonia ; (iv) Regurgitation of fluids through the nose ; (v) Facial weakness ; (vi) Weakness of neck muscles. These signs call for head-down position, suction and prone position, followed by tracheostomy, the insertion of a cuffed endotracheal tube, and intermittent positive-pressure ventilation.*†

The high tracheostomy and cuffed tube technique‡ provide for suction of the airways, protection of the airway from soiling, and an easy route for intermittent positive-pressure ventilation. For transport to hospital, a cuffed endotracheal tube is passed under local or general anæsthesia, while portable suction apparatus, breathing machine (or manual reservoir bag and gas supply), and personnel trained in their use travel with the patient. Later a planned high tracheostomy is performed under local or general anæsthesia and a cuffed rubber or metal tube is inserted through the wound. The problems associated with assisted or artificial ventilation are discussed in Chapter VIII. *See also Essentials of Artificial Ventilation of the Lungs*, Hunter, A. R., 1962. London: Churchill; and *Clinical Practice and Physiology of Artificial Respiration*, Spalding, J. M. K., and Crampton-Smith, A., 1963. Oxford : Blackwell Scientific Publications.

TETANUS

Tetanus presents some problems very similar to those seen in poliomyelitis. There may be pharyngeal and laryngeal paralysis and respiratory insufficiency due to spastic not flaccid muscles. It has been treated by intermittent positive-pressure ventilation via a cuffed endotracheal tube through a high tracheostome with tubocurarine,§ or suxamethonium to relax the muscles.‖ Chloral hydrate or other sedatives or nitrous-oxide–oxygen can be used to produce sedation. Good reports have also followed a continuous mephanesin drip with spontaneous respiration.¶

Yet another method of treating tetanus is by the injection of the phenothiazine derivatives sometimes combined with gas and oxygen anæsthesia.** This is said to control the convulsions and virtually to eliminate the problem of secretions in the chest. The patient breathes spontaneously and no relaxants are required. A dose of 25 mg. each of chlorpromazine, promethazine, and pethidine is given when required.

* Crampton-Smith, A., Spalding, J. M. K., and Russell, W. Ritchie, *Lancet*, 1954, **1**, 939.
† Russell, W. Ritchie, *Brit. med. J.*, 1955, **1**, 98.
‡ Lassen, H. C. A., *Lancet*, 1953, **1**, 37.
§ Crampton-Smith, A., and others, *Ibid.*, 1956, **2**, 550.
‖ Shackleton, P., *Ibid.*, 1954, **2**, 155.
¶ Docherty, D. F., *Ibid.*, 1955, **1**, 437.
** Bodman, R. I., Morton, H. J. V., and Thomas, E. T., *Ibid.*, 1955, **2**, 230.

Prolonged administration of nitrous oxide may depress the bone-marrow, causing aplastic anæmia.

Successful treatment of tetanus by chlordiazepoxide has been reported.*

MYASTHENIA GRAVIS

Cases may require I.P.P.V. and careful supervision over a long period. For details of management, *see* p. 659.

LONG-TERM VENTILATION

Nursing Care of Patient on Artificial Ventilation.—In addition to care of the tracheostomy (*see* p. 803):—

1. Never leave the patient unattended.
2. Make sure that, in case of mechanical failure, alternative means of ventilation are available and understood by the nursing attendant.

The Control of Long-term Ventilation.—

1. CLINICAL.—The underventilated patient may show discomfort, restlessness, rise in pulse-rate, rise in blood-pressure, sweating, cyanosis (if air is used). The overventilated patient may show increased muscular irritability leading to tetany.
2. ANALYSIS OF BLOOD GASES.—*See* Chapter XXXIII.

General Care of the Patient.—

1. FLUID BALANCE AND CALORIE INTAKE.—Generally speaking, the intake (via gastric tube) should be above 5 l. of fluid and 2000 calories per day. For information about parenteral and tube feeding, *see* p. 814.
2. INFECTION.—Chest infections may occur unless prophylactic measures are taken. Suction catheters should be sterile and used on one occasion only before resterilization. Antibiotic cover is advisable. Patients should be turned at regular intervals (2-hourly) and physiotherapy three or four times daily helps to prevent atelectasis. Visitors may be required to wear gowns and masks.
3. PRESSURE AREAS.—These require careful nursing attention.
4. SEDATION.—This may be required: (1) to help the patient to become accommodated to the artificial ventilation, particularly in the early stages when intravenous pethidine may be useful; (2) to ensure adequate rest at night.
5. COMMUNICATION.—Make sure that the conscious patient has bell, pencil, and paper.
6. EYES.—If the external muscles of the eye are paralysed corneal abrasions may occur. Spalding and Crampton Smith† recommend the following régime: (i) bathe the eyes with sterile saline swabs, (ii) insert a drop of 1 per cent atropine and 0·5 per cent chloramphenicol, (iii) hold the lids open and insert 5 drops of plasma, followed by 2 drops of nor-thrombin (200 N.I.H. units in 10 ml. isotonic saline) from a separate pipette and hold

* Phillips, L. A., *Lancet*, 1965, **1**, 1097.
† Spalding, J. M. K., and Crampton Smith, A., *Clinical Practice and Physiology of Artificial Respiration*, 1963. Oxford: Blackwell.

Long-term Ventilation—General Care of the Patient, *continued.*

lids apart until fibrin clots are formed, (iv) strap the eyelids together lightly. The régime is repeated 8-hourly.

7. BLADDER AND BOWELS.—Function may become automatic in the unconscious or immobilized patient. Manual removal of fæces and manual compression or catheterization of the bladder may be necessary.

8. MONITORING.—Frequent notes must be made of blood-pressure, pulse, tidal volume, respiratory rate, etc. Special record charts are useful. Daily blood-gas estimation, chest radiographs, and examination of sputum for organisms and sensitivity are helpful.

9. PSYCHOLOGICAL ASPECTS.—These are important in long-term cases on ventilator treatment. Special arrangements must be made to enable patients to read newspapers and books, watch television, etc.

See also Chapter VIII.

POISONING

Barbiturates.—Produce coma, which may be associated with airway obstruction and respiratory depression. Some barbiturates are more readily dialysable by the artificial kidney than others, so it is of help to know which particular barbiturate has been ingested. Phenobarbitone is easy to eliminate in this way ; amylobarbitone and butobarbitone less easy ; pentobarbitone is difficult to remove, and secobarbitone almost undialysable. Elimination of barbiturates in the urine is hastened by diuresis and at any rate in the case of phenobarbitone, by alkalinity of the urine.* (*See also* Chapter IV.)

A rapid method of screening for barbiturates is reported.† Only 0·2– 2 ml. of blood are required and while the test takes five minutes to perform, it needs no costly reagents or equipment.

Salicylates.—Metabolic acidosis results and prompt treatment with intravenous sodium bicarbonate is necessary, despite a coincident respiratory alkalosis. Hyperventilation, due to central respiratory centre stimulation, exhausts the patient. A serum level of 50 mg. per cent requires urgent treatment, while a figure above 70 mg. per cent may indicate the preparation of equipment for hæmo-dialysis. Forced alkaline diuresis is the method of treatment advised, the aim being to achieve a urinary output of 500 ml. hourly. If this therapy does not rapidly lower the serum level, hæmodialysis should be begun.

Treatment of Overdosage.—It is often not known what particular poison has been ingested by the patient. Treatment is, however, similar in principle :—

1. Precedence must be given to correction of respiratory difficulty ; intubation of the trachea, artificial or assisted respiration.

2. Aspiration of stomach contents prevents further absorption of the drug and aids identification.

---

* Annotation, *Lancet*, 1963, **2**, 1367.
† Curry, A. S., *Brit. med. J.*, 1963, **2**, 1040.

3. There is little evidence that antidotes, respiratory stimulants, etc., have any significant effect on the ultimate prognosis. They may be useful in first-aid treatment to overcome undue depression before the patient reaches hospital.

4. Dialysis. Use of the artificial kidney to reduce the blood concentration of the drug. Elimination can also be aided by osmotic diuresis.* Urea, sodium bicarbonate, sodium lactate, and mannitol have been used for this purpose.

5. General nursing care is very important, especially as the patient may remain unconscious for several days. Antibiotics should be administered in these cases.

It is an interesting fact that poisoning seldom has a fatal outcome in children.

MULTIPLE INJURIES

First-aid treatment of multiple injuries is very important: 25 per cent of those severely injured in accidents die in respiratory obstruction,[†] and it is important that a clear airway be established as a first priority in the unconscious subject. Ambulance crews should be trained in the positioning of patients, in the maintenance of a clear airway, and in techniques of artificial ventilation. The services of an experienced anæsthetist may be invaluable, as urgent endotracheal intubation may be required. Tracheostomy can nearly always be deferred for at least 24 hours.

Chest Injuries.[‡]—Respiration is embarrassed should bleeding occur into the airway or into the pleural cavity. Blood-clot, saliva, stomach contents, and other debris may be inhaled to produce suffocation. The flail chest renders physiological ventilatory exchange impossible as some degree of paradoxical respiration occurs. Pain may also prevent proper excursion of the diaphragm and thoracic cage. In some cases, intermittent positive-pressure ventilation will be required.[§]

Head Injuries.[||]—It is vital that proper oxygenation of the brain is maintained. Primary efforts should therefore be directed to maintenance of the airway and adequate pulmonary ventilation, arrest of any serious hæmorrhage, and maintenance of an adequate blood circulation. Uncomplicated head injury should not prevent the treatment of abdominal injuries, compound limb fractures, or hæmothorax, though faciomaxillary fractures can usually be left to a later date.

MIDDLE MENINGEAL HÆMORRHAGE.—This is the most important remediable head injury and requires urgent operation. The most important physical signs are:—

1. Progressive deterioration of consciousness.

---

* Linton, A. L., Luke, R. G., Speirs, I., and Kennedy, A. C., *Lancet*, 1964, **1**, 1008.

† *See also* Ambiavagar, M., *Postgrad. med. J.*, 1967, **43**, 256.

‡ Wilson, D., *Proc. R. Soc. Med.*, 1967, **60**, 946.

§ Jackson, J. W., *Ibid.*, 1967, **60**, 947; and Collie, J. A., and Lloyd, J. W., *Anæsthesia*, 1967, **22**, 392.

|| Potter, J. M., *Proc. R. Soc. Med.*, 1967, **60**, 949.

Head Injuries, *continued.*

2. Progressive dilatation of a previously normal pupil.
3. Progressive bradycardia, perhaps with a rising systolic blood-pressure.
4. Swelling on the side of the larger pupil.
5. Radiological evidence of a fracture crossing a branch of the middle meningeal artery; sometimes of a calcified pineal body shifted to the side away from the injury.
6. Progressive weakness of the face, arm, and even leg on the side opposite to the injury.

Continued observation is necessary, and not all the signs may be present.

Other injuries which require surgical treatment include the depressed fracture, though this does not carry the same degree of urgency as the middle meningeal hæmorrhage.

Epileptic fits may occur within hours of a head injury. These are usually best treated by intramuscular paraldehyde, 5–8 ml. Epanutin may also be given, 250 mg. parenterally, followed by 50–100 mg. 8-hourly by mouth, gastric tube, or parenterally. This is better than phenobarbitone which may depress the level of responsiveness in early head injuries.

Abdominal Injuries.—All penetrating wounds of the abdomen require laparotomy. The signs of intra-abdominal trauma may be misleading in the presence of other injuries, but an accurate diagnosis should not be necessary in making the decision to perform laparotomy.

Blood Transfusion.—This will often be required where there are multiple injuries. An estimate of blood-loss from fractures can be made as follows: Humerus, 500–1000 ml.; radius and ulna, 500 ml.; pelvis, over 3000 ml.; femur, 500–2000 ml.; tibia and fibula, 500–1000 ml.* Monitoring of central venous pressure may be very helpful in these cases, and a blood-volume estimation carried out later as a check on the adequacy of replacement.

See a symposium on 'Early Treatment of Multiple Injuries', *Proc. R. Soc. Med.*, 1967, **60**, 945 *et seq.*

INTENSIVE CARE OF THE NEONATE†

1. TEMPERATURE.—The neonate is liable to heat loss on the operating table, and care should be taken not to expose the baby unnecessarily. A mattress with coils for circulation of warm water is useful. Note that a stockinet cap is valuable since the head has a larger proportion of body-surface area than in the case of the adult. The normal neonate makes use of the metabolic activity of the brown fat to maintain body temperature. Small or premature babies or babies who have suffered from intra-uterine malnutrition may have a lack of brown fat and so are at a disadvantage in a heat-losing environment.

2. FEEDING.—This must be considered under the headings of water,

---

* Wilson, J. N., *Proc. R. Soc. Med.*, 1967, **60**, 951.
† Tizard, J. P. M., *Ibid.*, 1967, **60**, 935.

electrolytes, and calories. Dehydration can lead to fever, acidæmia, shock, and brain damage. The normal weight-loss in the first two days of life may be taken as 44 g. per day per kg. birth-weight— about half as urine and fæces, and about half as insensible fluid loss. Though healthy neonates starve for 48 hours, the small or premature baby is liable to severe hypoglycæmia if unfed, and this may be severe enough to produce brain damage or death.

3. ACIDÆMIA.—If present this should be corrected before surgery.

4. OXYGEN.—This is important in that while hypoxæmia may be dangerous, administration of high concentrations of oxygen may result in retrolental fibroplasia. Arterial oxygen tension can be measured, sampling being undertaken from umbilical artery catheters. Hypoxæmia results in inhibition of the brown-fat mechanism (*see above*). Assisted respiration may be necessary.

5. CROSS-INFECTION.—One hazard particular to the neonate is that the cord stump can act as a culture medium for pathogenic organisms. This can be reduced by the use of a polybactrin spray to the cord stump daily. *Pseudomonas pyocyanea* is a hazard and polymixin methane sulphonate may be given as a protection. In babies on respirators it can be instilled into the trachea.

ACUTE RENAL FAILURE

Acute reversible intrinsic renal failure (acute tubular necrosis) must be differentiated from pre-renal failure due to inadequate perfusion of the kidney, and occult post-renal obstruction.

Treatment.*—

1. Careful control of fluid intake. The present view is that daily intake should be restricted to 400 ml. plus the volume of any sensible fluid loss. Daily weight-loss should average 200–500 g. Overhydration may be revealed as failure to lose weight and hyponatræmia.

2. Routine sodium administration should not be given unless there is obvious loss. Where it cannot be avoided (e.g., as sodium bicarbonate to treat acidosis) care must be taken to avoid overloading.

3. Control of hyperkalæmia. Potassium is released from depleted glycogen stores, destruction of tissue protein, etc. If serum potassium is more than 7 mEq./l. urgent therapy with hypertonic sodium bicarbonate is required. These effects (antagonism of cardiac effects of potassium and movement of the ion into cells as a result of treatment of acidosis) are short-lived and must be reinforced by use of exchange resins or dialysis. Other treatment includes use of hypertonic glucose with insulin, hypertonic sodium chloride, and calcium gluconate.

4. Control of calorie intake. High carbohydrate diet is indicated with restriction of protein. The oral route should be used when possible. 'Hycal' is a useful preparation, since 4 bottles daily will provide 1700 calories with only 400 ml. water. For intravenous feeding, 20 per cent fructose is preferable to glucose in the uræmic patient.†

---

* Blagg, C. R., *Postgrad. med. J.*, 1967, **43**, 290.
† Luke, R. G., and others, *J. Lab. clin. Med.*, 1964, **64**, 731.

Acute Renal Failure—Treatment, *continued*.

　　5. Anabolic steroids. If these drugs are used, it may be wise to give a more liberal food intake, including some milk and eggs, provided facilities for dialysis are available.

　　6. Prevention and early treatment of infection.

　　7. Dialysis. For details of techniques *see* Blagg.*

ARTIFICIAL FEEDING

Minimal Nutritional Requirements.—The daily basal requirements of main food constituents may be stated as follows:†

	REQUIREMENT PER KG. BODY-WEIGHT	REQUIREMENT FOR 70-KG. MAN	CALORIES SUPPLIED PER G.
Water	25–35 ml.	1500–2500 ml.	—
Protein	1 g.	70 g.	4·0
Carbohydrate	2 g.	140 g.	4·0
Fat	2 g.	140 g.	9·0
Calories	30 cal.	2100 cal.	—

Minerals and vitamins are also necessary.

Tube Feeding.—When the patient cannot swallow, a liquid diet must be given by intragastric tube. This is preferable to intravenous feeding, which carries a definite complication rate, whenever the function of the gastro-intestinal tract allows.

　　Eggs and powdered milk have the highest biologic degree of utilization and surpass other natural nutrients for tube feeding.† Various artificial foods are available. 'Complan' is widely used. Each 100 g. of 'Complan' contains 44 g. of carbohydrate, 31 g. of protein, 16 g. of fat as well as minerals and vitamins, and provides 450 calories.‡ One recommended régime is: 'Complan' 100 g. and glucose 100 g. dissolved in 1 litre water; methylcellulose 3 g. is added to provide roughage which reduces the incidence of diarrhœa; 125 ml. of the mixture are given hourly via the gastric tube.§

Parenteral Feeding.‖—

　　CARBOHYDRATES.—

　　　　1. GLUCOSE.—One litre of isotonic (5 per cent) solution provides only 200 calories. Concentrated solutions are therefore necessary to produce a high-calorie intake without over-hydration. After fasting the glucose tolerance is low and consequently sugar may be lost in the urine. Insulin may be given to increase glucose retention.

　　　　2. LÆVULOSE (FRUCTOSE).—Enters into metabolism without the action of insulin and builds up carbohydrate stores rapidly.

　* Blagg, C. R., *Postgrad. med. J.*, 1967, **43**, 290.
　† Steinbereithner, K., in *Modern Trends in Anæsthesia* (Ed. Evans, F. T., and Gray, T. C.), 1967, No. 3, Ch. 11. London: Butterworths.
　‡ Peaston, M. J. T., *Postgrad. med. J.*, 1967, **43**, 317.
　§ Sherwood Jones, E., and Peaston, M. J. T., *Practitioner*, 1966, **196**, 271.
　‖ *See also* Steinbereithner, K., in *Modern Trends in Anæsthesia* (Ed. Evans, F. T., and Gray, T. C.), 1967, No. 3, Ch. 11. London: Butterworths.

It does not, however, enter into metabolism directly, and so is not of value in the treatment of hypoglycæmia caused by insulin. Blood-sugar estimations may give a false picture, as a high concentration may be found when blood-glucose is low.

3. LACTOSE.—This has been used for parenteral feeding, but is less popular since the finding that it is not well tolerated by over half the adult population.

4. INVERT SUGAR.—Can be given at a rate of 1 g. per kg. per hour without serious glycosuria.

5. SORBITOL.—Useful only as an additive to amino-acid solutions. Administration rates over 0·33 g. per kg. per hour result in osmotic diuresis.

6. GLYCEROL.—Used only as an additive to fat emulsions. High doses cause serious side-reactions—hæmolysis and muscle cramps.

7. DEXTRAN.—Not a practical substitute for other carbohydrates.

PROTEINS.—

1. BLOOD, ALBUMIN, AND PLASMA.—The 'half-life' is several weeks. Should be reserved for those patients with reduced blood-volume or hypoproteinæmia.

2. PROTEIN HYDROLYSATES.—Produced by enzymatic fission. Side reactions occur due to incomplete fission, though high molecular polypeptides can be reduced by dialysis.

3. CRYSTALLINE AMINO-ACID MIXTURES.—These may be pure lævo-rotatory acids, or equimolecular mixtures of lævo- with the unphysiological dextro-rotatory forms. Some D-amino acids can be catabolized, but the major part is lost by renal excretion. Amino-acid mixtures should fulfil the following criteria:—

   a. Low incidence of side-reactions.
   b. Adequate content of essential and semi-essential amino-acids, in the correct proportions.
   c. Must be biologically adequate.
   Contra-indications to their use include:—
   a. Coronary insufficiency.
   b. Potassium deficiency.
   c. Liver disease.
   d. Renal insufficiency.
   e. Acidosis.

Commercial amino-acid preparations which are now available include 'Aminosol' and 'Trophysan'.

FAT.—Fat administration is necessary for complete parenteral nutrition. Advantages include lack of osmotic effects and tolerance by vessels. No losses occur in fæces or urine. A fat emulsion should fulfil the following criteria:—

1. Particles must be less than 4 μ in diameter to avoid embolism.
2. The stability of the solution on storage must be beyond reproach.
3. It must be pure.
4. The emulsion must be made isotonic by addition of glucose or glycerol.

The use of fat emulsions is contra-indicated in all conditions

Parenteral Feeding, *continued.*

associated with hyperlipæmia, diabetes, nephrotic syndrome, coagulation disorders, and liver disease.

Suitable commercial preparations which are now available include 'Intralipid' and 'Lipiphysan'.

Technique.—Intravenous feeding may be used to supplement oral or tube feeding or as complete parenteral nutrition.

The following régime has been recommended:*—

Bottle 1: 500 ml. 'Aminosol-fructose-ethanol' with 25 mEq. KCl added.

Bottle 2: 500 ml. 20 per cent w/v 'Intralipid'.

Bottle 3: As No. 1.

Bottle 4: 500 ml. 10 per cent 'Aminosol'.

Bottle 5: As No. 1.

Bottle 6: As No. 2.

Bottles are given in this order. The incidence of thrombophlebitis has been found to be reduced if the infusions are given in pairs through a Y-shaped connector.† Thus bottles 1 and 2, 3 and 4, 5 and 6 are given, each pair over an 8-hour period.

CHAPTER XXXVI

INTRACTABLE PAIN

THE PAIN CLINIC‡

The patient with intractable pain requires careful evaluation and sympathetic understanding. Active treatment can often be offered to those with terminal malignant disease. The main avenues of treatment are:—

1. Use of analgesics. These may be required in high dosage. Problems of tolerance and addiction may arise.

2. Surgical rhisotomy and cordotomy. Useful in selected cases, but they involve surgical procedures in patients who are not good operative risks.

3. Specific nerve-blocks. It is here that the skill of the anæsthetist may be required. Disappointments may arise since pain is often not strictly anatomical.

Somatic Nerve Pain.—Can be relieved by injection of local analgesic solution into suitable nerves if they are approached from the skin surface. The following are examples:—

The trigeminal nerve and its branches in patients not suitable for retro-Gasserian ganglionectomy who are suffering from tic douloureux ;§ inferior dental block in some cases of fractured lower jaw ; infra-orbital, supra-orbital, supratrochlear, and mental nerve-block for herpes zoster ; facial nerve-block for

---

* Sherwood Jones, E., and Peaston, M. J. T., *Practitioner*, 1966, **196**, 271.
† Peaston, M. J. T., *Postgrad. med. J.*, 1967, **43**, 317.
‡ Swerdlow, M., *Anæsthesia*, 1967, **22**, 568.
§ Rollason, W. N., *Brit. J. Anæsth.*, 1955, **27**, 354.

intractable spasm ; superior laryngeal nerve-block for carcinoma of larynx (*see* p. 329) ; accessory nerve-block for traumatic
torticollis (together with superficial cervical plexus block). Injection into the temporomandibular joint in severe cases of painful
clicking jaw. Suprascapular nerve-block for subacromial bursitis
and pain on abduction of the arm.* (*See* p. 334.) Phrenic
nerve-block in intractable hiccup (*see* p. 752). Intercostal
nerve-block for herpes zoster, post-operative abdominal pain,
post-operative or post-traumatic atelectasis, fractured ribs,† or
pain following the insertion of a drainage-tube. Block of
lumbar nerves for intractable neuritis (*see* pp. 346, 347), herpes
zoster, lightning pains of tabes.‡ Periarticular injections for
severe sprain, and injections into painful amputation stump
and scars, flat-feet ;§ and anterior and posterior femoral
cutaneous nerve-block for hip-joint pain.|| When long-acting
relief is required, it may be necessary to employ phenol 5 per
cent or chlorocresol 2 per cent in glycerin, or alcohol in some
of these patients.

INTRATHECAL BLOCK.—Both phenol¶ and alcohol** may be
injected intrathecally to relieve the intractable pain of malignant
disease. Both will destroy nervous tissue. Histological studies††
on patients who have received intrathecal phenol for terminal
malignant disease show degeneration of nerve-fibres in the
posterior roots and in the posterior columns of the cord. It is
suggested that the injected solution tends to run along nerve-
roots with which it makes contact, spreading both centrally and
peripherally. There is little evidence of local action on the ganglia.
  In the selection of patients the risks must be weighed against
the anticipated benefits. Regardless of care and technique the
following can be produced: (i) patchy degeneration in the spinal
cord, (ii) degeneration of motor fibres, (iii) arachnoiditis. Note
also that destruction of the sensory component of the sacral roots
leads to loss of control of bladder and bowel.
  Phenol, 5 per cent in glycerin, may be injected in the region
of the segments involved. If more than three segments are
involved, more than one injection is required. Only one side
is treated by a single injection (gravity).

TECHNIQUE.—Lateral position, painful side down. Break the
    table so that the area to be treated is at the lowest point.
    Insert the needle and ensure a free flow of cerebrospinal fluid.
    Then rotate the patient towards the operator to an angle of
    30° with the vertical. Inject solution slowly in increments
    of 0·3 ml., waiting 3–5 min. between injections. Maximum

---

* Wertheim, H. M., and Rovenstine, E. A., *Anesthesiology*, 1941, **2**, 541.
† Powell, H. D. W., *Brit. med. J.*, 1955, **2**, 829.
‡ Fowler, W., *Brit. J. vener. Dis.*, 1947, **23**, 90.
§ Hipps, H. E., and Neely, H., *Nav. med. Bull.*, 1945, **44**, 262.
|| Lundy, J. S., and others, *Proc. Mayo Clin.*, 1951, **26**, 281.
¶ Maher, R. M., *Lancet*, 1955, **1**, 18 ; and Nathan, P. W., and Scott, T. G., *Ibid.*, 1958, **1**, 76.
** Dogliotti, A. M., *Pr. méd.*, 1931, **39**, 1249.
†† Smith, M. C., *Brit. J. Anæsth.*, 1964, **36**, 387.

Somatic Nerve Pain, *continued.*

dose in any one site is 1 ml. Maintain the position for 30 min. and return patient to bed in the supine position.*

For alcohol injection, the patient should lie with the affected side uppermost and 30° head-down tilt. The patient should be rolled as far as possible into a prone position. Sterilized absolute alcohol in a glass ampoule is used. Initial dose should be 0·4–0·5 ml. and may be repeated after 5 days in dosage up to 1 ml. There is a greater danger of side-effects with the larger dose.†

Sympathetic Block.—Sympathetic dysfunction can cause symptoms due to vasospasm, the production of pain, and alteration of function, so that therapy is directed to vasodilatation, relief of pain, and restoration of function.

Vasomotor block may be performed at any of four levels :—

a. Peripheral nerve-block, e.g., the ulnar nerve, causing vasodilatation of the skin of the little finger.

b. The sympathetic ganglia, e.g., the stellate or the second and third lumbar ganglia, causing release of vasomotor tone in the upper and lower limbs.

c. Extradural block.

d. Subarachnoid block.

The last two are examples of pre-ganglionic block and must extend in the case of the lower limb to the tenth thoracic segment so as to paralyse all the pre-ganglionic fibres going to the limb.

INDICATIONS FOR SYMPATHETIC BLOCK.—

PAINFUL LIMBS DUE TO VASCULAR DISEASE.—Raynaud's phenomena ; vasospasm associated with lesions of the spinal cord, e.g., poliomyelitis and some cases of pyramidal disease ; arteriosclerosis and thrombophlebitis obliterans ; chronic ulceration of the extremities ; embolism of major vessels ; thrombophlebitis ; erythromelalgia.

CONDITIONS DUE TO IDIOPATHIC AND POST-TRAUMATIC PAIN OF LIMBS.—Causalgia ; amputation stump neuralgias ; Sudeck's atrophy.

UNCLASSIFIED CONDITIONS OF THE LIMBS.—Hyperhidrosis ; after embolectomy ; in the post-hyperæmic stage of the immersion foot syndrome.

THORACIC AND ABDOMINAL DISEASE.—Angina pectoris ; painful aortic aneurysm ; bronchial asthma ; megacolon and cardiospasm ; biliary and renal colic ; pancreatitis (bilateral block of T.7, 8, and 9) ; post-partum hæmorrhage ; eclampsia ; to arrest bleeding after prostatectomy ; to differentiate organic from functional disease of the bowel.

STELLATE GANGLION BLOCK (*see* p. 329).—Although nervous control of intracranial vascular tone is now discounted it has been successfully used in the treatment of recent cerebral embolism and thrombosis‡ (not in cases of apoplexy, e.g., if there is

---

* Gordon, R. A., and Goel, S. B., *Canad. Anæsth. Soc. J.*, 1963, **10**, 357.
† Russell, W. R., *Lancet*, 1936, **1**, 595 ; and Greenhill, J. P., *Brit. med. J.*, 1947, **2**, 859.
‡ Leriche, R., *Ibid.*, 1952, **1**, 231.

cervical rigidity); block should be bilateral; in neonates born with hemiplegia due to birth injury; in central arterial or venous occlusion of the retina, e.g., in quinine amblyopia ;* in cases of vascular spasm of the arm ; for painful shoulder ; for treatment of Bell's palsy;† as an aid to orbital phlebography during injection of contrast medium into angular vein in diagnosis of orbital tumours.‡

TECHNIQUE.—

1. *Upper Extremity.*—The second and third thoracic sympathetic ganglia. Brachial plexus block. Stellate ganglion block.

2. *Heart and Aorta.*—Paravertebral sympathetic block of the second to the fifth thoracic ganglia on the left side.

3. *Abdomen.*—Subarachnoid injection of absolute alcohol is suitable for the relief of pain below the groin and iliac crests, i.e., in the lumbosacral distribution. The intraspinal segmental technique can be employed in which a plastic catheter is passed into the theca, its exact position being checked by radiography. Relief of visceral pain due to malignant disease can be obtained by block of the cœliac plexus; 40–50 ml. of 50 per cent alcohol may be injected after a test injection of 25 ml. 0·1 per cent amethocaine.§ Hirschsprung's disease in children has yielded to high subarchnoid block (to T.5).‖ Anuria, if due to cortical ischæmia, has been improved by block to T.8. Paravertebral block of T.7 and T.8, and sometimes of T.6 and T.9 in addition, will ease the pain of biliary colic, while block of T.12 and L.1 will relieve renal colic. If the eighth, ninth, and tenth thoracic ganglia are blocked, the pain of acute pancreatitis will be relieved.

Retroperitoneal hæmatoma has followed paravertebral blocks. No blocks should be undertaken in a patient who is being treated with anticoagulants unless their action is first reversed by protamine sulphate or vitamin K_1. *See also* Bonica, J. J., *The Management of Pain*, 1953. London, Kimpton; Bonica, J. J., *Clinical Applications of Diagnostic and Therapeutic Nerve Blocks*, 1958. Oxford, Blackwell; and Ball, H. J. C., Pearce, D. J., and Davies, J. A. H., *Anæsthesia*, 1964, **19**, 250.

INTRAVENOUS PROCAINE
(*See also* p. 296)

Good reports of its use, which is generally in 0·2 per cent solution, are reported in a large variety of conditions, including :—

1. Lower nephron nephrosis.
2. Painful vasomotor and trophic conditions, such as frost-bite and intermittent claudication.
3. Amblyopia following retinal vascular occlusion or massive hæmorrhage.

---

* Glick, L., and Mumford, J., *Brit. med. J.*, 1955, **2**, 194; and Bricknell, P. P., *Ibid.*, 1967, **4**, 400.
† Korkis, F. B., *Arch. Otolaryng.*, 1959, **70**, 562.
‡ James, P., *Anæsthesia*, 1965, **20**, 285.
§ Bridenbaugh, L. D., and Moore, D. S., *J. Amer. med. Ass.*, 1964, **190**, 877.
‖ Telford, E. D., and Haxton, H. A., *Brit. med. J.*, 1948, **1**, 827.

Intravenous Procaine, *continued.*

4. Orchitis and epididymitis.
5. To speed up intravenous drips by relaxing the vein walls.
6. Pruritus.
7. Serum sickness and other states of sensitivity ; urticarias associated with blood transfusions.
8. To control post-operative pain.
9. To relieve the pain of chest injury.
10. To relieve the pain and reduce the intra-ocular tension in acute glaucoma.

Intravenous procaine is seldom employed to-day.

Lignocaine has also been given with success intravenously. It has proved beneficial in the pain of general carcinomatosis, in severe cardiac arrhythmia, and as an analgesic during labour and also during surgery.*

CHAPTER XXXVII

POST-OPERATIVE OBSERVATION ROOM†

These rooms, which should be close to the operating theatre, and supervised by members of the departments of anæsthesia and surgery, serve a most useful purpose. Respiratory and circulatory depression are detected early and efficiently treated by the skilled nursing sister in charge of the room, which is suitably equipped with oxygen therapy appliances, intravenous drip apparatus, beds which can be easily tipped, proper lighting, and suction apparatus.

The advantages of such a room are obvious : It prevents duplication of equipment, economizes skilled nursing staff, and saves lives. It must be remembered in this connexion that almost half the deaths occurring in the immediate post-operative period are due to inadequate nursing care including respiratory obstruction.

Such a room should be staffed for twenty-four hours each day, three beds being sufficient for one operating theatre. Sex differentiation is unnecessary as by the time the patient is sufficiently conscious of his or her sex the time has come for transference to the ordinary ward.

In some modern hospitals, each patient is connected to a central observation post where the nurse in charge can monitor such parameters as temperature, pulse-rate, E.C.G., blood-pressure, respiration, blood gases, and even the comfort of the patient.

---

* de Clive Lowe, G. C., Desmond, J., and North, J., *Anæsthesia*, 1958, **13**, 138.
† Jolly, Clive, and Lee, J. A., *Ibid.*, 1957, **12**, 49. *See also* discussion, *Proc. R. Soc. Med.*, 1958, **51**, 151.

CHAPTER XXXVIII

CARE AND STERILIZATION OF EQUIPMENT

METHODS OF STERILIZATION

1. Heat Sterilization.—

  a. MOIST HEAT.—Moisture increases cellular permeability and heat coagulates protein. Boiling (100° C.) for 15 min. kills bacteria, but spores may escape destruction. Increased pressure makes it possible to produce higher temperature ; 10 to 15 min. at 15 lb. pressure at 250° F. in an autoclave will kill all living organisms provided the material treated is properly wrapped to allow penetration. Deterioration of rubber and plastics is hastened by this method. Sharp instruments become dulled.

  b. DRY HEAT.—160° C. for 1 hr. Useful for powders, greases, oils, and glass syringes.

2. Chemical Sterilization.—Useful for objects which will not withstand heat. Chemicals kill by coagulation or alkylation of proteins. Non-sporing bacteria, viruses, the tubercle bacillus, and spores are resistant to destruction in that order. Chemicals only act on exposed surfaces, some react with metals, some impregnate materials (e.g., rubber) and remain as a source of irritation. Rubber and plastics are particularly subject to destruction by strong chemicals.

  a. FORMALDEHYDE.—Can be used for endoscopic equipment, catheters, etc. Residual formaldehyde persists after prolonged airing and may harm the skin.

  b. ETHYLENE OXIDE (C_2H_4O).—A colourless gas which is a good bactericidal agent, although very toxic to inhale. It has good penetrability and few materials are harmed. It is effective against all organisms, but is slow (8–12 hours). The gas is explosive and it is necessary to use a mixture of 15 per cent ethylene oxide and 85 per cent carbon dioxide to eliminate the explosive risk. A relative humidity of 30 per cent is essential. A good method of sterilizing complicated and delicate apparatus (e.g., pump oxygenators, Ruben's valves, plastic tubing, catheters, etc.), though the method is expensive and takes time. It has also been used for sterilization of artificial ventilators after prolonged use in dirty cases.* *See also Lancet*, 1962, **1**, 732.

  The cylinders containing the mixture are identified by aluminium paint; the shoulder is red and below it is a circular band of yellow paint.

  c. LIQUIDS.—

  i. PHENOL (1–5 per cent).—Used to clean surfaces of apparatus. Should not be used on equipment which comes into contact with the patient. Does not kill spores.

---

* Bishop, C., Potts, M. W., and Molloy, P. J., *Brit. J. Anæsth.*, 1962, **34**, 121; Bishop, C., and others, *Ibid.*, 1964, **36**, 53; and Boultree, P. J., and others, *Ibid.*, 1964, **36**, 531.

Chemical Sterilization, *continued*.

    ii. IODINE (0·5–2 per cent in alcohol).—May irritate or burn the skin.

    iii. ETHYL ALCOHOL (70–80 per cent).—Is more efficient than absolute alcohol. Isopropyl alcohol, 50–70 per cent.

    iv. HEXACHLOROPHENE (pHisoHex).—One of the few antiseptics that does not lose its properties in the presence of soap.

    v. CHLORHEXIDINE (Hibitane).—0·1 per cent aqueous solution for 20 min. for sterilization of endotracheal tubes and other anæsthetic equipment.* 0·5 per cent in 50 per cent ethyl alcohol for skin sterilization (30 sec.).†

    vi. RESIGUARD.—A commercial preparation containing picloxydine digluconate 1 per cent, octylphenoxy polyethoxyethanol, 11 per cent, and benzalkonium 12 per cent, and active against a wide range of organisms including *Pseudomonas pyocyanea*. Can be used in 1–160 concentration for storage of endotracheal tubes, etc. (though metallic instruments may rust), and in association with a fogging apparatus for sterilization of theatres or rooms. A concentration of 1–80 has been recommended for sterilization of the East-Radcliffe ventilator.‡

3. Gamma Rays.—Lethal dose for bacteria is 2·5 megarads. Usually obtained from a cobalt 60 source. Tubes, catheters, etc., can be sterilized in a transparent plastic envelope.

4. Ultra-violet Light.—Has been used to kill organisms by submitting the whole operation area to the light. Patients and staff must be protected from sunburn. All skin must be covered and plain spectacles worn with an eyeshade.

5. Filtration.§—Filters are used to prevent the entry of organisms (e.g., ventilators). They will remove all particles down to a diameter of 0·5 micron with a 99·99 per cent efficiency. The filters themselves can be autoclaved.

Endotracheal Tubes, Suction Catheters, Airways.—These may be washed with soap and water and well rinsed. A suitable brush should be used to clear the inside of tubes and airways. They may then be sterilized by boiling, although this tends to soften the rubber endotracheal tubes. Portex tubes should be boiled with a stylet in situ so that they retain their curvature. Armoured latex tubes should be handled with care since they may be compressed by Chealte's forceps when hot. Alternatively, tubes may be soaked in a solution of 0·1 per cent chlorhexidine (hibitane) and 0·02 per cent Tween 80 in distilled water for 30–60 min.‡ or in Resiguard (1–160). They should be stored in dust-free containers. It has been suggested that sterile endotracheal tubes, airways, and suction catheters should be provided from a Central Sterile Supply, even though repeated autoclaving might mean replacing the tubes after six uses.||

  * Stratford, B. L., Clark, R. R., and Dixson, S., *Brit. J. Anæsth.*, 1964, **36**, 471.
  † Beeuwkes, H., and v. d. Vijver, A. E. D., *Ibid.*, 1959, **31**, 363.
  ‡ Meadows, G. A., Richardson, J. C., Fish, E., and Williams, A., *Ibid.*, 1968, **40**, 71.
  § Bishop, C., and others, *Ibid.*, 1963, **35**, 32.
  || Stark, D. C. C., and Pask, E. A., *Anæsthesia*, 1962, **17**, 195.

Expensive apparatus, such as endobronchial tubes, must be handled carefully and subjected to minimum periods of boiling to prevent deterioration.

Another recommended method is to place all suitable equipment in a domestic dish-washer in which temperatures of 70° C. are reached. A commercially supplied detergent, providing 33 p.p.m. of available chlorine, is used. Although this does not guarantee absolute sterility, the method kills those pathogenic organisms with which anæsthetic equipment is likely to be contaminated, except spores and some viruses.*

Face-masks.—These may deteriorate with repeated boiling. It has been found that placing in a bowl of water between 60° and 70° C. for 2 min., followed by rinsing under running tap-water at the same temperature for 2 min., will reduce the number of pathogens present to a very small number.†

Laryngoscope Blades.—(1) May be boiled or autoclaved, provided they are detachable. (2) Stand in 1–20 carbolic for 30 min. (3) Formalin oven. (4) Simple treatment between cases is to wipe with 70 per cent alcohol or 0·1 per cent chlohexidine in 70 per cent alcohol.

Do not boil the Macintosh spray as the rubber of the internal tube swells slightly. A jet is then delivered instead of a fine spray.

Rebreathing Tubes. Reservoir Bags.—Repeated boiling destroys the antistatic properties of rubber. It is common practice, therefore, to wash, rinse, and allow the tubing to dry between cases. It may be boiled once a week for 10 min., or after particularly contaminated cases. Corrugated tubing, face-masks, and reservoir bags can be pasteurized (75° C. for 10 min.). Only vegetative organisms need be killed as spores are relatively unimportant. Common organisms present may be the *Streptococcus pyogenes*, *Staphylococcus aureus*, and *Pseudomonas pyocyanea*.‡

Water's Canisters.—These should be sterilized daily, or after each anæsthetic where the patient is suffering from tuberculosis or upper respiratory tract infection.

Circle Absorbers.—These can be sterilized by gamma radiation, formaldehyde vapour, or ethylene oxide. Alternatively, they should be frequently dismantled, cleaned, and disinfected with spirit. Another approach is to prevent entry of organisms by using a filter on the expiratory limb of the circuit.§

Ventilators.—Proper sterilization is essential when they are used in intensive therapy units. The methods available include: (1) Use of an absolute filter to prevent entrance of organisms; (2) Ethylene oxide; (3) Internal irrigation with antiseptics (e.g., Resiguard), provided the circuit is watertight.||

* Barrow, M. E. H., and Meynell, M. J., *Brit. J. Anæsth.*, 1966, **38**, 907.
† MacCallum, F. O., and Noble, W. C., *Ibid.*, 1960, **32**, 192.
‡ Jenkins. J. R. E., and Edgar, W. M., *Anæsthesia*, 1964, **19**, 177.
§ Helliwell, P. J., and others, *Ibid.*, 1965, **20**, 334.
|| Meadows, G. A., Richardson, J. C., Fish, E., and Williams, A., *Brit. J. Anæsth.*, 1968, **40**, 71.

Contamination with Tubercle Bacilli.—This may be expected after anæsthesia in the presence of open pulmonary tuberculosis. The endotracheal tubes, suction catheters, rebreathing tubing, etc., may be placed immediately in an antiseptic solution (e.g., 0·1 per cent chlorhexidine for 1 hr.). They can then be cleaned and scrubbed with soap and water with less danger to personnel. After this they can be sterilized by boiling or autoclaving. Boiling for 3 min. will kill tubercle bacilli.

The to-and-fro system is preferable to the circle absorber in the presence of tuberculosis since it is more easily cleaned and sterilized.

Syringes and Needles.—The most satisfactory methods are autoclaving or dry heat. Cleaning, packing, and sterilization can be most conveniently carried out in a special department providing a Syringe Service.

Syringes must be dismantled and thoroughly cleaned. They may be immersed in detergent solution. An ultra-sonic washer is useful for loosening fragments of blood-clot or foreign material. Needles must be similarly treated, blown through with water, and sharpened. The parts must be dried and the syringe barrels lubricated lightly with silicone diluted in industrial alcohol. They are then reassembled, packed in individual containers, and sterilized (e.g., 1 hr. dry heat at 160° C.). All-glass syringes are essential for dry heat sterilization, as the cement of glass-metal syringes may be softened.

Boiling is an acceptable alternative method of sterilization only in the absence of autoclave or dry heat facilities. Syringes should be dismantled, glass pieces wrapped in gauze and placed in warm water which is brought slowly to 100° C. Syringes should be reserved for anæsthetic purposes only.

Syringes should be neither sterilized nor stored in disinfectant solution, since all organisms are not killed and sometimes pathogens may be harboured.

Syringes and needles to be used for extradural or intradural block should not be contaminated with either detergents or alcohol.

Plastic, disposable, presterilized needles are now generally used.

Instruments for Local Blocks.—Special packs should be made up for each type of procedure and should contain all the needles, syringes, towels, swabs, and other apparatus required. Local analgesic solutions, such as lignocaine, amethocaine hydrochloride, and cinchocaine, will withstand autoclaving at 160° C. for 20 min. at 20 lb. pressure, but not dry heat. They should not be subjected to repeated sterilization. Adrenaline ampoules may also be sterilized in this way on one occasion.

Tests for Sterility.—The inclusion of a Browne's tube in the set is a safeguard. If the appropriate temperature has been reached, there is a change in colour from red to green.

(*See also* Helliwell, P. J., in *Recent Advances in Anæsthesia and Analgesia* (Ed. Hewer, C. Langton), 10th ed., 1967, Ch. 12. London: Churchill.)

APPENDIX

Conversion Table for the More Generally Used Sizes of Needles

Size	Diameter		Length	
	mm.	s.w.g.	mm.	in.
19	·45	26	17·5	$\frac{11}{16}$
18	·45	26	19	$\frac{3}{4}$
17	·50	25	23·5	$\frac{15}{16}$
16	·55	24	25	1
15	·60	23	25	1
14	·60	23	30	$1\frac{3}{16}$
12	·65	23	30	$1\frac{3}{16}$
2	·70	22	33	$1\frac{5}{16}$
1	·80	21	38	$1\frac{1}{2}$
0	·90	20	41·5	$1\frac{8}{8}$

Conversion Tables

Length.—

1 inch	..	..	..	..	..	2·54 cm.
1 cm.	..	..	..	..	..	0·394 in.

Volume.—

1 gallon (Imperial) ..		..	..	..	..	4·55 litres
1 gallon (U.S.)	..	..	..	..	..	0·833 gallon (Imp.)
1 litre	..	..	..	..	..	0·22 gallon (Imp.)
1 pint	..	..	..	..	..	568 ml. (c.c.)
1 litre	..	..	..	..	..	35·3 fl. oz.
1 litre	..	..	..	..	..	1·76 pints
Pints × 0·5682	..	..	..	..	=	litres
Gallons (Imp.) × 4·5459	..	..	..	=	litres
1 fl. oz.	..	..	..	..	..	28·4 ml. (c.c.)
1 ml.	..	..	..	..	..	16·95 minims
1 minim	..	..	..	..	..	0·06 ml.
1 ml.	..	..	..	..	..	0·061 c. in.
Cubic centimetres × 0·0352	..	..	=	fl. oz.
5 fl. oz.	..	..	..	..	..	142 ml.
15 minims	..	..	..	..	..	0·89 ml.
5 minims	..	..	..	..	..	0·3 ml.
1 per cent solution	..	..	..	4·4 grains per oz.

1 ml. of a 1 per cent solution contains 10 mg.
1 ml. of a 1 in 1000 solution contains 1 mg.
1 ml. of a 1 in 1500 solution contains 0·67 mg.

Weight.—

1 kilogram (kg.)	..	..	..	..	..	2·2 lb.
1 pound	..	..	..	..	..	0·454 kg.
1 stone	..	..	..	..	..	6·4 kg.
1 ounce	..	..	..	..	..	28·4 grammes
Grains × 0·9648	..	..	..	..	=	grammes
Grammes × 15·432	..	..	..	=	grains
1 grain	..	..	..	..	..	60 mg.
1 gramme (g.)	..	..	..	..	..	15·4 grains
1½ grains	..	..	..	..	..	100 mg. (approx.)
¼ grain	..	..	..	..	..	15 mg.
⅛ grain	..	..	..	..	..	10 mg.
1/64 grain	..	..	..	..	..	1 mg.
1/100 grain	..	..	..	..	..	0·6 mg.
1/150 grain	..	..	..	..	..	0·4 mg.

Pressure.—

1 atmosphere	..	..	..	..	.. 760 mm. mercury
1 atmosphere	..	..	..	..	.. 14·7 pounds per sq. in.
1 mm. mercury	..	..	..	..	.. 1·36 cm. water
1 cm. water	..	..	..	..	.. 0·73 mm. mercury

SOME NORMAL PHYSIOLOGICAL VALUES

Air.—

Oxygen content	..	..	..	.. 20·93 per cent (160 mm. Hg)
Carbon dioxide content	..	..	..	0·04 per cent

Alveolar Air.—

P_AO_2	..	..	..	..	.. 104 mm. Hg
P_ACO_2	..	..	..	..	.. 40 mm. Hg

Arterial Blood.—

Oxygen saturation	..	..	..	..	.. 95 per cent
P_aO_2	..	..	..	..	.. 97 mm. Hg
P_aCO_2	..	..	..	..	.. 40 mm. Hg

Mixed Venous Blood.—

Oxygen saturation	..	..	..	..	.. 75 per cent
P_VO_2	..	..	..	..	.. 40 mm. Hg
P_VCO_2	..	..	..	..	.. 46 mm. Hg

SOME NORMAL BIOCHEMICAL VALUES

1. *Blood.—*

Hæmoglobin (men) ..	..	..	..	.. 13·5–18 g. per 100 ml.
				14·6 g. equals 100 per cent.
Hæmoglobin (women)	..	..	..	12–16·4 g. per 100 ml.
*p*H ..	..	..	..	.. 7·36–7·44
Plasma-protein	..	..	..	.. 6–8 g. per 100 ml.
Red cells (men)	..	..	..	.. 4·75–6 million per c.mm.
Red cells (women)	..	..	..	.. 4·3–5·3 million per c.mm.
White cells ..	..	..	..	.. 4000–9000 per c.mm.
Fasting blood-sugar	..	..	..	60–120 mg. per 100 ml.
Urea ..	..	..	..	.. 20–40 mg. per 100 ml.
Volume ..	..	..	..	.. 4–8 litres
Alkali reserve	..	..	..	.. 53–77 ml. CO_2 per 100 ml. plasma
Chlorides (NaCl)	..	..	..	560–620 mg. per 100 ml. plasma

2. *Urine.—*

Reaction ..	..	..	..	.. *p*H 4·8–7·4
Specific gravity	..	..	..	.. 1010–1025
Daily output	..	..	..	.. 1000–1800 ml.

CONCENTRATIONS OF ELECTROLYTES IN PLASMA

Sodium	142	milliequivalents per litre		
Potassium	5	,,	,,	,,
Calcium	5	,,	,,	,,
Magnesium	3	,,	,,	,,
Bicarbonates	27	,,	,,	,,
Chlorides	102	,,	,,	,,
Phosphates	2	,,	,,	,,
Sulphates	1	,,	,,	,,
Protein	16		,,	,,

Sodium   100–250 milliequivalents in 24 hours
Potassium   35– 90   ,,   ,, ,, ,,
Chloride   170–250   ,,   ,, ,, ,,
Phosphates   30– 90   ,,   ,, ,, ,,

1 milliequivalent of chloride = 35·5 mg.
1 milliequivalent of sodium = 23 mg.

SOLUTIONS

A *molar solution* contains the molecular weight of a substance expressed in grammes dissolved in 1 litre.

A milliequivalent per litre (mEq./l.) is the equivalent weight in grammes per litre, divided by 1000. To convert milligrammes per cent into milliequivalents per litre (mEq./l.) divide the concentration in milligrammes per litre by the atomic weight of the substance and multiply by its valency.

Strength of Solution :—
    1–4000 = 0·025 per cent; 1–2000 = 0·05 per cent; 1–1333 = 0·075 per cent; 1–1000 = 0·1 per cent; 1–666 = 0·15 per cent; 1–500 = 0·2 per cent; 1–400 = 0·25 per cent.

UNITS OF METRIC SYSTEM

milli (m) .. 10^{-3}
micro (μ) .. 10^{-6}
nano (n) .. 10^{-9}

A 1 per cent solution contains 10 mg. per ml.

DRUGS USED IN THE MEDICAL TREATMENT OF PATIENTS WHICH MAY INFLUENCE ANÆSTHESIA

1. *Mono-amine Oxidase Inhibitors.*—
    Iproniazid (Marsilid).
    Nialamide (Niamid).
    Phenelzine (Nardil).
    Pheniprazine (Cavodil).
    Pivhydrazine (Tersavid).
    Isocarboxazid (Marplan).
    Phenoxypropazine (Drazine).
    Mebanazine (Actomol).
    Pargyline (Eutonyl).
    Tranylcypromine (Parnate).
    Tranylcypromine with trifluoperazine (Parstelin).

These drugs are concerned in the inactivation of noradrenaline and 5-hydroxytryptamine. Sympathomimetic agents (especially methyl-amphetamine by intravenous injection), rauwolfia alkaloids, guan-ethidine, imipramine, pethidine, morphine, barbiturates (and certain foods, e.g., cheese, broad-beans, meat extracts and yeast extracts) may all be influenced by the prior administration of mono-amine oxidase inhibitors.

2. *Antihypertensives.*—
    a. Ganglion-blocking agents :—
        Hexamethonium (Vegolysen).
        Pentolinium (Ansolysen).

Chlorisondamine (Ecolid).
Mecamylamine (Inversine) 2·5- and 10-mg. tablets.
Pempidine (Perolysen, Tenormal).

b. Adrenergic blocking agents :—
  Bretylium (Darenthin).
  Guanethidine (Ismelin) 10- and 25-mg. tablets.
  Propranolol (Inderal).
  Bethanidine (Estabal).

c. Drugs which interfere with normal synthesis of noradrenaline:—
  Methyldopa (Aldomet).

d. Less potent drugs :—
  Reserpine (Serpasil).
  Rauwolfia (Rauwiloid).
  Hydrallazine (Apresoline).
  Methoserpidine (Decaserpyl).

e. Chlorothiazides :—
  Chlorothiazide (Saluric).
  Hydrochlorothiazide (Direma ; Esidrex ; Hydrosaluric).
  Cyclopenthiazide (Navidrex ; Navidrex K).
  Bendrofluazide (Aprinox ; Centyl ; Neo-nallex).
  Polythiazide (Nephril).
  Hydroflumethiazide (Di-adenil).
  Methyclothiazide (Enduron).
  Benzthiazide (Fovane).

f. Chlorothiazides in combination with antihypertensives :—
  Ismelin Navidrex K. (Guanethidine + cyclopenthiazide + KCl).
  Salupres (Hydrochlorothiazide ; Reserpine KCl).
  Serpasil-Esidrex K. (Reserpine hydrochlorothiazide KCl).
  Decaserpyl Plus (Methoserpidine benzthiazide).
  Adelphane (Di-hydrallazine reserpine nepresol).

3. *Corticosteroids.*—
  Cortisone (5- and 25-mg. tablets).
  Prednisone (De-cortisyl ultra corten). 1- and 5-mg. tablets. One-fifth dosage of cortisone.
  Prednisolone (Precortisyl; Delta-Cortril). 1- and 5-mg. tablets. One-fifth dosage of cortisone.
  Triamcinalone (Adcortyl; Ledercort). 1- and 4-mg. tablets. Dosage one-third less than prednisolone.
  Methyl prednisolone (Medrone). 4-mg. tablets. Ten times the activity of cortisone.
  Dexamethasone (Decadron). 0·5- and 1·0-mg. tablets. Daily dosage one-tenth to one-fifth of prednisolone.
  Betamethasone (Betnelan). 0·5-mg. tablets. Six to ten times as potent as prednisolone.
  Fluorocortisone (Florinef). 0·1-mg. tablets. 1·0-mg. tablets.

4. *Disulpharim* (Antabuse). Synergistic depressant effect with thiopentone.

5. *Premidone* (Mysoline) an anticonvulsant used in the treatment of epilepsy may make the patient susceptible to barbiturates.

6. *Digitalis.* Patients on digitalis, if given atropine, may become decompensated because of the tachycardia produced. A rise in

the serum potassium (e.g., following massive blood transfusion) may inactivate digitalis, unless calcium is given too. Hypothalæmia (e.g., in intestinal obstruction) may dangerously potentiate digitalis.

7. *Ergometrine.* May potentiate the effects of pressor amines.
8. *Pitocin.* May result in coronary spasm when cyclopropane is administered, perhaps going on to ventricular fibrillation.

RADIATION

The anæsthetist's exposure to radiation during radium application is of the same order of magnitude as that received during diagnostic X-ray procedures.*

---

* Trachtenberg, H. A., *J. Amer. med. Ass.*, 1965, **191**, 763.

INDEX